ESSENTIAL
OTOLARYNGOLOGY

Eighth Edition

ESSENTIAL OTOLARYNGOLOGY

Head & Neck Surgery

Edited by

K. J. Lee, MD, FACS
Associate Clinical Professor
Section of Otolaryngology
Yale University School of Medicine

Managing Partner
Southern New England Ear, Nose, Throat,
   and Facial Plastic Surgery Group

Chairman and CEO
MedWin of Connecticut, LLC

Chief of Otolaryngology
Hospital of Saint Raphael

Attending Otolaryngologist
Yale–New Haven Hospital

New Haven, Connecticut

McGraw-Hill
MEDICAL PUBLISHING DIVISION

New York   Chicago   San Francisco   Lisbon   London   Madrid   Mexico City
Milan   New Delhi   San Juan   Seoul   Singapore   Sydney   Toronto

McGraw-Hill

A Division of The McGraw·Hill Companies

ESSENTIAL OTOLARYNGOLOGY
Eighth Edition

1234567890 DOCDOC 098765432

ISBN 0-07-137322-5

This book was set in Times Roman by Circle Graphics.
The editors were Marc Strauss and Muza Navrozov.
The production supervisor was Catherine H. Saggese.
The cover was designed by Mary McKeon.
The index was prepared by Alexandra Nickerson.

R. R. Donnelley and Sons Company was printer and binder.

This book is printed on acid-free paper.

Library of Congress Cataloging-in-Publication Data

Essential otolaryngology : head and neck surgery / [edited by] K. J. Lee—8th ed.
    p. ; cm.
   Includes bibliographical references and index.
   ISBN 0-07-137322-5
   1. Otolaryngology—Outlines, syllabi, etc. 2. Head—Surgery—Outlines, syllabi, etc. 3.
Neck—Surgery—Outlines, syllabi, etc. I. Lee, K. J. (Keat Jin), date—
   [DNLM: 1. Otorhinolaryngologic Diseases—surgery—Outlines. 2.
Otorhinolaryngologic Surgical Procedures—Outlines. WV 18.2 E78 2003]
   RF58 .E88 2003
   617.5'1—dc21
                                                                                    2002016662

INTERNATIONAL EDITION ISBN 0-07-121249-3

Copyright © 2003. Exclusive rights by *The McGraw-Hill Companies, Inc.*, for manufacture and export.
This book cannot be re-exported from the country to which it is consigned by McGraw-Hill.
The International Edition is not available in North America.

Contents

Contributors*

Thomas J. Balkany, MD [23]
Hotchkiss Professor and Chairman
Department of Otolaryngology
University of Miami Ear Institute
Miami, Florida

Nigel J. P. Beasley, MB, FRCS [27]
Clinical Fellow, Head and Neck Surgery
Wharton Head and Neck Center
Princess Margaret Hospital
Toronto, Ontario, Canada

William E. Bolger, MD [19]
Associate Professor
Chief of Rhinology and Sinus Surgery
Department of Otorhinolaryngology—
    Head and Neck Surgery
University of Pennsylvania Health System
Philadelphia, Pennsylvania

Derald E. Brackmann, MD, FACS [3]
Clinical Professor of Otolaryngology—
Head and Neck Surgery
Clinical Professor of Neurosurgery
University of Southern California School of Medicine
President, House Ear Clinic
Board of Directors, House Ear Institute
Los Angeles, California

Hilary A. Brodie, MD, PhD [7]
Professor and Chairman
Department of Otolaryngology—
    Head and Neck Surgery
University of California, Davis
Sacramento, California

Craig A. Buchman, MD, FACS [23]
Assistant Professor
Department of Otolaryngology—
    Head and Neck Surgery
University of North Carolina at Chapel Hill
Chapel Hill, North Carolina

Nicolas Y. Busaba, MD [32]
Assistant Professor
Department of Otology and Laryngology
Harvard Medical School
Associate Chief
Division of Otolaryngology
Boston VA HealthCare System
Assistant Surgeon
Department of Otolaryngology
Massachusetts Eye and Ear Infirmary
Boston, Massachusetts

Maria N. Byrne, MD, FACS [21]
Attending
Hospital of St. Raphael
Yale–New Haven Hospital
New Haven, Connecticut

Vincent N. Carrasco, MD [8]
Private Practice
Hurdle Mills, North Carolina

Mack L. Cheney, MD [34]
Director, Division of Facial Plastic
    and Reconstructive Surgery
Massachusetts Eye and Ear Infirmary
Boston, Massachusetts

*Numbers in brackets following the author's name refer to chapter(s) written or co-written by the contributor.

ix

Mark A. D'Agostino, MD   [38]
Staff Otolaryngologist
Yale–New Haven Hospital
Hospital of St. Raphael
Middlesex Hospital
Milford Hospital
MidState Medical Center
Griffin Hospital
Assistant Professor of Surgery
Uniformed Services University
    of Health Sciences
Bethesda, Maryland
Clinical Instructor
Yale University School of Medicine
Section of Otolaryngology
New Haven, Connecticut

Anthony C. De la Cruz, MD   [4]
Department of Otolaryngology
Massachusetts Eye and Ear Infirmary
Harvard Medical School
Boston, Massachusetts

Antonio De la Cruz, MD   [4]
Director of Education
House Ear Institute
Vice President, House Ear Clinic, Inc.
Professor of Clinical Otolaryngology
University of Southern California School
    of Medicine
Los Angeles, California

Mark D. DeLacure, MD, FACS   [29, 35]
Chief, Division of Head and Neck Surgery
    and Oncology
Associate Professor of Otolaryngology
    and Reconstructive Plastic Surgery
New York University Medical Center
New York, New York

Manuel Don, MD, PhD   [3]
Head, Department of Electrophysiology
House Ear Institute
Los Angeles, California

Paul J. Donald, MD   [7]
Professor, Department of Otolaryngology—
    Head and Neck Surgery
Director, Center for Skull Base Surgery
University of California, Davis
Sacramento, California

David E. Eibling, MD   [22]
Professor of Otolaryngology
University of Pittsburgh
Eye and Ear Institute
Pittsburgh, Pennsylvania

David N. F. Fairbanks, MD   [20]
Clinical Professor, Otolaryngology—
    Head and Neck Surgery
George Washington School of Medicine
Washington, DC

Jay B. Farrior, MD   [10, 24]
Clinical Associate Professor
University of South Florida
Department of Otolaryngology—
    Head and Neck Surgery
Farrior Ear Clinic
Tampa, Florida

Thomas M. Fynan, MD   [17]
Assistant Clinical Professor of Medicine
Yale University School of Medicine
Attending Physician
Hospital of St. Raphael
Yale–New Haven Hospital
New Haven, Connecticut

Helmuth W. Gahbauer, MD   [37]
Director of Neuroradiology and MRI
Hospital of St. Raphael
Assistant Clinical Professor
Yale University
New Haven, Connecticut

Isaac Goodrich, MD   [15]
Associate Clinical Professor of Neurosurgery
Yale University School of Medicine
Chief of Neurosurgery
Hospital of St. Raphael
Yale–New Haven Hospital
New Haven, Connecticut

Patrick J. Gullane, MD   [27]
Director, Head and Neck Program
Wharton Chair, Head and Neck Surgery
Professor of Surgery and Otolaryngology
Toronto, Ontario, Canada

Tessa Hadlock, MD   [34]
Division of Facial Plastic
    and Reconstructive Surgery
Massachusetts Eye and Ear Infirmary
Boston, Massachusetts

F. Christopher Holsinger, MD   [26]
Fellow, Head and Neck Surgical Oncology
Department of Head and Neck Surgery
University of Texas
M. D. Anderson Cancer Center
Houston, Texas

Jean Edwards Holt, MD [14]
Clinical Professor of Ophthalmology
University of Texas Health Science Center
San Antonio, Texas

John R. Houck, MD [12]
Associate Professor of Otorhinolaryngology
University of Oklahoma Health Sciences Center
Oklahoma City, Oklahoma

John W. House, MD [6]
President, House Ear Institute
Clinical Professor
Department of ORL-HNS
University of Southern California Medical School
Los Angeles, California

David W. Kennedy, MD [19]
Professor and Chairman
Department of Otorhinolaryngology—
    Head and Neck Surgery
University of Pennsylvania Health System
Philadelphia, Pennsylvania

Randall C. Latorre, MD [39]
Private Practice
Latorre Cosmetic Facial Surgery/ENT
Tampa, Florida

K. J. Lee, MD, FACS [1, 2, 4, 5, 8, 9,
    10, 13, 14, 15, 21, 24, 29, 36, 38, 39]
Associate Clinical Professor
Section of Otolaryngology
Yale University School of Medicine
Managing Partner
Southern New England Ear, Nose, Throat, and Facial
    Plastic Surgery Group
Chairman and CEO
MedWin of Connecticut, LLC
Chief of Otolaryngology
Hospital of St. Raphael
Attending Otolaryngologist
Yale–New Haven Hospital
New Haven, Connecticut

Mark E. Lee [9]
Quincy House
Harvard University
Cambridge, Massachusetts

Joshua D. Levine, MD [23]
Chief Resident
Department of Otolaryngology
University of Miami School of Medicine
Miami, Florida

Thomas C. Logan, MD [8]
Ear, Nose and Throat Surgery
Evansville, Indiana
Henderson, Kentucky
Owensboro, Kentucky

W. Bruce Lundberg, MD [18]
Associate Clinical Professor of Medicine
Yale University School of Medicine
Section Chief
Medical Oncology and Hematology
Department of Medicine
Hospital of St. Raphael
Attending Physician, Medicine
Yale–New Haven Hospital
New Haven, Connecticut

James C. McVeety, MD [15]
Assistant Clinical Professor of Neurology
Yale University School of Medicine
Attending Physician
Hospital of St. Raphael
New Haven, Connecticut

Frank R. Miller, MD [16]
Assistant Professor of Otolaryngology—
    Head and Neck Surgery
Director, Head and Neck Surgery
University of Texas Health Science Center
San Antonio, Texas

Eric J. Moore, MD [11]
Assistant Professor, Department of Otolaryngology—
    Head and Neck Surgery
Mayo Clinic
Rochester, Minnesota

Jeffrey N. Myers, PhD, MD [26]
Assistant Professor of Surgery
Department of Head and Neck Surgery
University of Texas
M. D. Anderson Cancer Center
Houston, Texas

James E. Peck, PhD, CCC-A [2]
Associate Professor, Department of Otolaryngology
    and Communicative Sciences
Audiologist, Communicative Disorders
University of Mississippi Medical Center
Jackson, Mississippi

David A. Randall, MD [30]
Private Practice
Springfield, Missouri
Associate Adjunct Professor of Surgery
Uniformed Services University of the Health Sciences

Gregory W. Randolph, MD   [28]
Director, General Otolaryngology Service
  and Thyroid Division
Massachusetts Eye and Ear Infirmary
Assistant Professor of Otology and Laryngology
Harvard Medical School
Boston, Massachusetts

Rollie E. Rhodes, MD   [12]
Clinical Professor of Otorhinolaryngology
University of Oklahoma Health Sciences
Tulsa, Oklahoma

Weldon Selters, PhD   [3]
Audiologist
House Ear Clinic
Los Angeles, California

Craig W. Senders, MD, FACS   [11]
Professor, Department of Otolaryngology
Director, Cleft and Craniofacial Surgery Program
University of California, Davis
Sacramento, California

Larry J. Shemen, MD   [25]
Assistant Clinical Professor
  of Otorhinolaryngology
Weill Medical College, Cornell University
Chief of Head and Neck Services—
  New York Hospital, Queens
Co-Chief of Head and Neck Services—
  Manhattan Eye, Ear and Throat Hospital
Attending Surgeon, St. Vincent's Hospital
Attending Surgeon, Lenox Hospital
Attending Surgeon, New York Eye and Ear Infirmary
New York, New York

Kathleen C. Y. Sie, MD   [33]
Associate Professor
University of Washington School of Medicine
Children's Hospital Regional Medical Center
Seattle, Washington

Peak Woo, MD   [31]
Associate Professor
Mount Sinai School of Medicine
Clinical Director
Grabscheid Voice Center
New York, New York

Eiji Yanagisawa, MD, FACS   [31, 37]
Clinical Professor of Otolaryngology
Yale University School of Medicine
New Haven, Connecticut

Ken Yanagisawa, MD, FACS   [37]
Clinical Instructor
Section of Otolaryngology
Yale University School of Medicine
New Haven, Connecticut

Carlton Jude Zdanski, MD   [8]
Assistant Professor
University of North Carolina Hospital
Department of Otolaryngology—
  Head and Neck Surgery
Chapel Hill, North Carolina

Preface

The first edition of *Essential Otolaryngology,* published in 1973, was based predominantly on my own notes that had helped me through my Board examination. Since that time, seven editions have been published. Because of the enthusiastic reception among practicing clinicians and the universal acceptance of this book among residents in the United States and abroad, I have found keeping this book current a most satisfying endeavor. Dr. Anthony Maniglia arranged for the sixth edition to be translated into Spanish by Drs. Blanco, Cabezas, Cobo, Duque, Reyes, and Santamaria. The seventh edition was also translated into Spanish by Drs. Rendón, Araiza, Pastrana, Enriquez, González. It was translated into Turkish and other languages. We have received even more requests to translate the eighth edition.

Since the medical world has grown far more complex, this eighth edition of *Essential Otolaryngology* contains new material in addition to the original compilation of one doctor's notes. Although the original material still forms the core of the book, a broad panel of authorities in several subspecialties present additional information which is considered the most current in their areas of expertise.

Neither a complete review of otolaryngology nor a comprehensive textbook on the subject, *Essential Otolaryngology, Eighth Edition,* remains true to its original intent—to serve as a guide for Board preparation as well as a practical and concise reference text reflecting contemporary concepts in clinical otolaryngology. Senior medical students, residents and fellows, Board-eligible otolaryngologists, primary care physicians, and specialists in other fields will all find this edition to be an even more useful and indispensable resource.

K. J. Lee

Acknowledgments

First of all, I would like to thank the one person who has been by my side, even before the appearance of the very first edition of this book—my lovely and devoted wife, Linda. And now that our three sons, Ken, Lloyd, and Mark are all old enough to have helped with editorial assistance on the subsequent editions, I would like to thank them as well. Jeannie Grenier, my nurse and editorial associate, has worked hard to see that the eighth edition is published on time. I thank the McGraw-Hill staff for their diligence, hard work, and congeniality.

Concerning the material within this book, I remain forever grateful to those men at the forefront of otolaryngology who have taught me so much—the late Dr. Harold F. Schuknecht, the late Dr. Daniel Miller, and Dr. William W. Montgomery, to name but three.

And to those newcomers to the frontiers of medical science who have contributed to this edition, I also extend my thanks for taking the time to share their own expertise and, in doing so, helping to keep this book up to date.

K. J. Lee

Anatomy of the Ear

1

1. The temporal bone forms part of the side and base of the skull. It constitutes two-thirds of the floor of the middle cranial fossa and one-third of the floor of the posterior fossa. There are four parts to the temporal bone:
    a. Squamosa
    b. Mastoid
    c. Petrous
    d. Tympanic
2. The following muscles are attached to the mastoid process:
    a. Sternocleidomastoid
    b. Splenius capitis
    c. Longissimus capitis
    d. Digastric
    e. Anterior, superior, posterior, auricular (The temporalis muscle attaches to the squamosa portion of the temporal bone and not to the mastoid process.)
3. The auricle (Figure 1-1) is made of elastic cartilage, the cartilaginous canal of fibrocartilage. The cartilaginous canal constitutes one-third of the external auditory canal (whereas the eustachian tube is two-thirds cartilaginous); the remaining two-thirds is osseous.
4. The skin over the cartilaginous canal has sebaceous glands, ceruminous glands, and hair follicles. The skin over the bony canal is tight and has no subcutaneous tissue except periosteum.
5. Boundaries of the *external auditory canal* are:

Anterior:	mandibular fossa
	parotid
Posterior:	mastoid
Superior:	epitympanic recess (medially)
	cranial cavity (laterally)
Inferior:	parotid

    The anterior portion, floor, and part of the posterior portion of the bony canal are formed by the tympanic part of the temporal bone. The rest of the posterior canal and the roof are formed by the squamosa.
6. Boundaries of the *epitympanum* are:

Medial:	lateral semicircular canal and VII nerve
Superior:	tegmen
Anterior:	zygomatic arch
Lateral:	squamosa (scutum)
Inferior:	fossa incudis
Posterior:	aditus

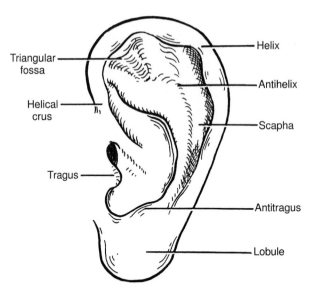

Figure 1-1. Auricle.

7. Boundaries of the *tympanic cavity* are:

Roof:	tegmen
Floor:	jugular wall and styloid prominence
Posterior:	mastoid, stapedius, pyramidal prominence
Anterior:	carotid wall, eustachian tube, tensor tympani
Medial:	labyrinthine wall
Lateral:	tympanic membrane, scutum (laterosuperior)

8. The *auricle* is attached to the head by:
   a. Skin
   b. An extension of cartilage to the external auditory canal cartilage
   c. Ligaments
      (1) Anterior ligament (zygoma to helix and tragus)
      (2) Superior ligament (external auditory canal to the spine of the helix)
      (3) Posterior ligament (mastoid to concha)
   d. Muscles
      (1) Anterior auricular muscle
      (2) Superior auricular muscle
      (3) Posterior auricular muscle

9. *Notch of Rivinus* is the notch on the squamosa, medial to which lies Shrapnell's membrane. The tympanic ring is not a complete ring, with the dehiscence superiorly.

10. *Meckel's cave* is the concavity on the superior portion of the temporal bone in which the gasserian ganglion (V) is located.

11. *Dorello's canal* is between the petrous tip and the sphenoid bone. It is the groove for the VI nerve. *Gradenigo syndrome,* which is secondary to petrositis with involvement of the VI nerve, is characterized by:
   a. Pain behind the eye

b.   Diplopia
c.   Aural discharge
12.   The suprameatal triangle of *Macewen's triangle* is posterior and superior to the external auditory canal. It is bound at the meatus by the spine of Henle, otherwise called
the *suprameatal spine*. This triangle approximates the position of the antrum medially. *Tegmen mastoideum* is the thin plate over the antrum.
13.   *Trautmann's triangle* is demarcated by the bony labyrinth, the sigmoid sinus, and the
superior petrosal sinus or dura.
   Citelli's angle is the *sinodural* angle. It is located between the sigmoid sinus and
the middle fossa dura plate. Others consider the superior side of Trautmann's triangle
to be Citelli's angle.
   Solid angle is the angle formed by the three semicircular canals.
   Scutum is the thin plate of bone that constitutes the lateral wall of the epitympanum. It is part of the squamosa.
   Mandibular fossa is bound by the zygomatic, squamosa, and tympanic bones.
   Huguier's canal transmits the chorda tympani out of the temporal bone anteriorly. It is situated lateral to the roof of the protympanum.
   Huschke's foramen is located on the anterior tympanic plate along a nonossified
portion of the plate. It is near the fissures of Santorini.
   Porus acusticus is the "mouth" of the internal auditory canal. The canal is divided
horizontally by the *crista falciformis.*
14.   There are three parts to the inner ear (Figure 1-2).
a.   Pars superior: vestibular labyrinth (utricle and semicircular canals)

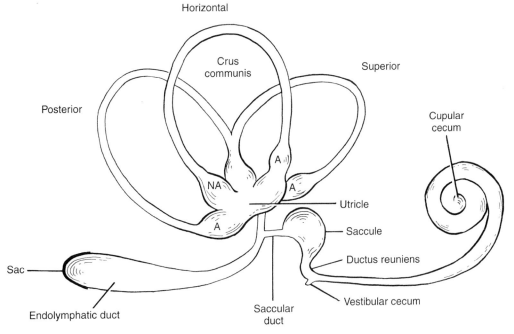

Figure 1-2.   Membranous labyrinth. A, ampulated end; NA, nonampulated end.

        b.   Pars inferior: cochlea and saccule

        c.   Endolymphatic sac and duct

15. There are four small outpocketings from the perilymph space:
    a.   Along the endolymphatic duct
    b.   Fissula ante fenestram
    c.   Fossula post fenestram
    d.   Periotic duct

16. There are four openings into the temporal bone:
    a.   Internal auditory canal
    b.   Vestibular aqueduct
    c.   Cochlear aqueduct
    d.   Subarcuate fossa

17. The *ponticulum* is the ridge of bone between the oval window niche and the sinus tympani.

18. The *subiculum* is a ridge of bone between the round window niche and the sinus tympani.

19. *Korner's septum* separates the squamosa from the petrous air cells.

20. Only one-third of the population has a pneumatized petrous portion of the temporal bone.

21. *Scala communis* is where the scala tympani joins the scala vestibuli. The helicotrema is at the apex of the cochlea where the two join (Figure 1-3).

22. The *petrous pyramid* is the strongest bone in the body.

23. The upper limit of the internal auditory canal diameter is 8 mm.

24. The *cochlear aqueduct* is a bony channel connecting the scala tympani of the basal turn with the subarachnoid space of the posterior cranial cavity. The average adult cochlear aqueduct is 6.2 mm long.

MIDDLE EAR

Tympanic plexus = V_3, IX, and X.

V_3 ⟶   auriculotemporal nerve

IX   ⟶   Jacobson's nerve

X   ⟶   auricular nerve

INNER EAR

Superior and horizontal semicircular canals

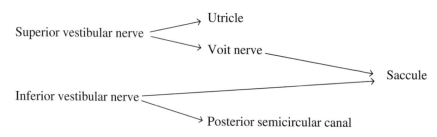

BLOOD SUPPLY

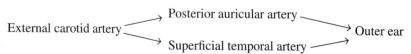

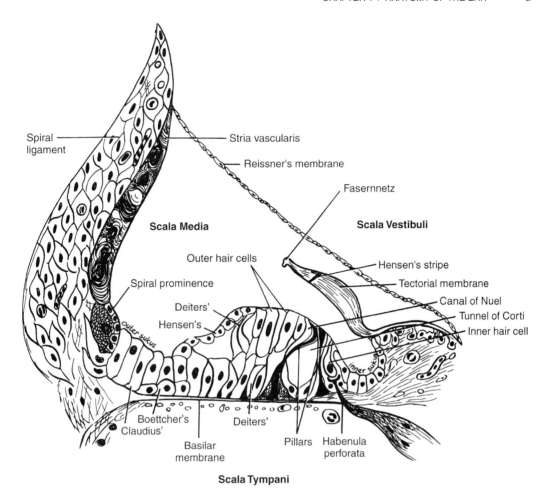

Spiral ligament

Stria vascularis

Reissner's membrane

Fasernnetz

Scala Media

Scala Vestibuli

Outer hair cells

Hensen's stripe

Spiral prominence

Tectorial membrane

Deiters'

Canal of Nuel

Hensen's

Tunnel of Corti

Outer sukus

Inner hair cell

inner sukus

Boettcher's
Claudius'

Deiters'

Basilar
membrane

Pillars

Habenula
perforata

Scala Tympani

Figure 1-3. Organ of Corti.

Anterior tympanic branch

↑

External carotid artery → Interior maxillary artery

Superior tympanic branch

↓   ↗

Middle meningeal artery   Middle ear

↙

Superficial petrosal branch

Internal carotid artery → Caroticotympanic artery → Anastomoses with
branches from
stylomastoid, internal
maxillary, and ascending
pharyngeal arteries

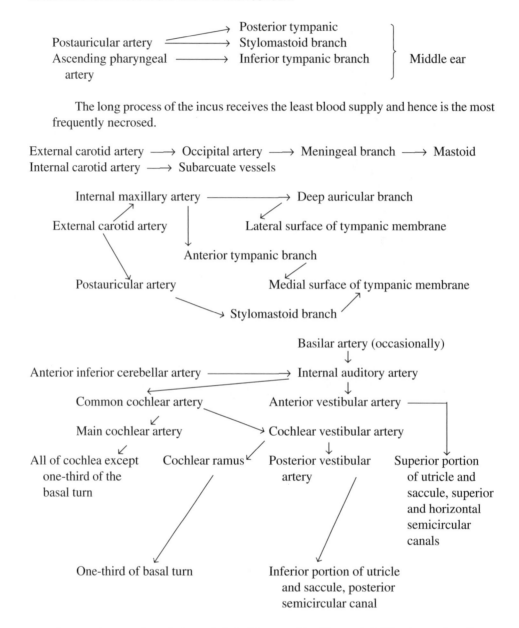

Postauricular artery ⟶ Posterior tympanic
                    ⟶ Stylomastoid branch   } Middle ear
Ascending pharyngeal ⟶ Inferior tympanic branch
artery

The long process of the incus receives the least blood supply and hence is the most frequently necrosed.

External carotid artery ⟶ Occipital artery ⟶ Meningeal branch ⟶ Mastoid
Internal carotid artery ⟶ Subarcuate vessels

Internal maxillary artery ⟶ Deep auricular branch

External carotid artery   Lateral surface of tympanic membrane

                          Anterior tympanic branch

Postauricular artery   Medial surface of tympanic membrane

                          Stylomastoid branch

                                    Basilar artery (occasionally)
                                            ↓
Anterior inferior cerebellar artery ⟶ Internal auditory artery
                                            ↓
        Common cochlear artery   Anterior vestibular artery

    Main cochlear artery   Cochlear vestibular artery

All of cochlea except   Cochlear ramus   Posterior vestibular   Superior portion
  one-third of the   artery   of utricle and
  basal turn   saccule, superior
                                                                    and horizontal
                                                                    semicircular
                                                                    canals

    One-third of basal turn   Inferior portion of utricle
                                       and saccule, posterior
                                       semicircular canal

Sensory innervation of the auricle is illustrated in Figure 1-4. The internal auditory canal is shown in Figure 1-5 and the dimensions of the tympanic membrane in Figure 1-6.

TYMPANIC MEMBRANE

The tympanic membrane has four layers:

1. Squamous epithelium
2. Radiating fibrous layer

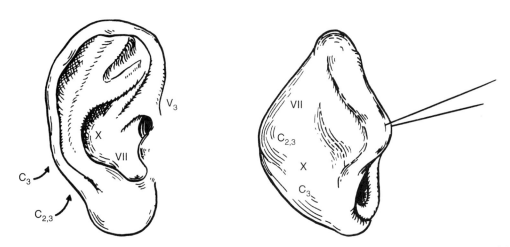

Figure 1-4. Sensory innervation of the auricle. C_3 via greater auricular nerve; $C_{2,3}$ via lesser occipital nerve; X, auricular branch; V_3, auriculotemporal nerve; VII, sensory twigs.

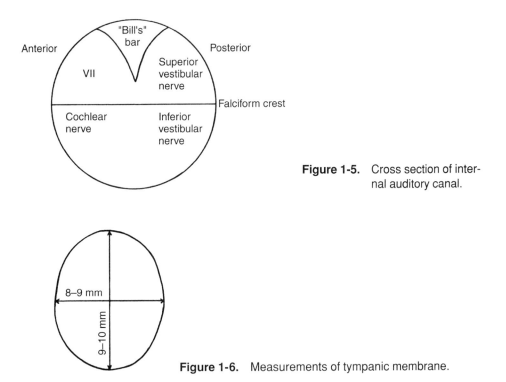

Figure 1-5. Cross section of internal auditory canal.

Figure 1-6. Measurements of tympanic membrane.

3. Circular fibrous layer
4. Mucosa layer

Average total area of tympanic membrane: 70 to 80 mm^2
Average vibrating surface of tympanic membrane: 55 mm^2

VENOUS DRAINAGE

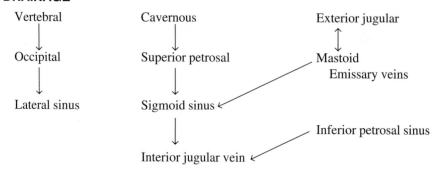

OSSICLES
Malleus
1. Head
2. Neck
3. Manubrium
4. Anterior process
5. Lateral or short process

Incus
1. Body
2. Short process
3. Long process (lenticular process)

Stapes
1. Posterior crus
2. Anterior crus
3. Footplate (average 1.41×2.99 mm)

LIGAMENTS
Malleus
1. Superior malleal ligament (head to roof of epitympanum)
2. Anterior malleal ligament (neck near anterior process to sphenoid bone through the petrotympanic fissure)
3. Tensor tympani (medial surface of upper end of manubrium to cochleariform process)
4. Lateral malleal ligament (neck to tympanic notch)

Incus
1. Superior incudal ligament (body to tegmen)
2. Posterior incudal ligament (short process to floor of incudal fossa)

Stapes

1. Stapedial tendon (apex of the pyramidal process to the posterior surface of the neck of the stapes)
2. Annular ligament (footplate to margin of vestibular fenestrum)
   Malleal: Incudal joint is a diarthrodial joint.
   Incudo: Stapedial joint is a diarthrodial joint.
   Stapedial: Labyrinth joint is a syndesmotic joint.

MIDDLE EAR FOLDS OF SIGNIFICANCE

There are five malleal folds and four incudal folds.

1. Anterior malleal fold: Neck of the malleus to anterosuperior margin of the tympanic sulcus
2. Posterior malleal fold: Neck to posterosuperior margin of the tympanic sulcus
3. Lateral malleal fold: Neck to neck in an arch form and to Shrapnell's membrane
4. Anterior pouch of von Troltsch: Lies between the anterior malleal fold and the portion of the tympanic membrane anterior to the handle of the malleus
5. Posterior pouch of von Troltsch: Lies between the posterior malleal fold and the portion of the tympanic membrane posterior to the handle of the malleus

Prussak's space (Figure 1-7) has the following boundaries:

1. Anterior: Lateral malleal fold
2. Posterior: Lateral malleal fold
3. Superior: Lateral malleal fold
4. Inferior: Lateral process of the malleus
5. Medial: Neck of the malleus
6. Lateral: Shrapnell's membrane

The *oval window* sits in the sagittal plane.

The *round window* sits in the transverse plane and is protected by an anterior lip from the promontory. It faces posteroinferiorly as well as laterally.

The *tensor tympani* inserts from the cochleariform process onto the medial surface of the upper end of the manubrium. It supposedly pulls the tympanic membrane medially, thereby tensing it. It also draws the malleus medially and forward. It raises the resonance frequency and attenuates low frequencies.

The stapedius muscle most frequently attaches to the posterior neck of the stapes. Occasionally, it is attached to the posterior crus or head and rarely to the lenticular process. It is attached posteriorly at the pyramidal process. It pulls the stapes posteriorly, supposedly increases the resonant frequency of the ossicular chain, and attenuates sound.

EUSTACHIAN TUBE

1. It is 17 to 18 mm at birth and grows to about 35 mm in adulthood.
2. At birth the tube is horizontal and grows to be at an incline of 45° in adulthood. Thus, the pharyngeal orifice is about 15 mm lower than the tympanic orifice.
3. It can be divided into an anteromedial cartilaginous portion (24 mm) and a posterolateral bony (11 mm) portion. The narrowest part of the tube is at the junction of the

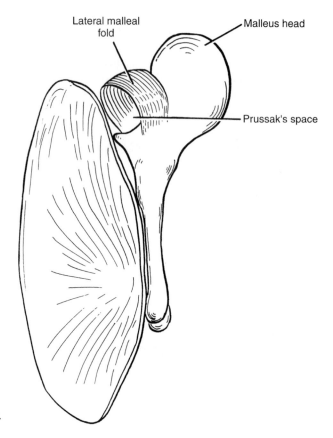

Figure 1-7.   Prussak's space.

bony and the cartilaginous portions. (Reminder: The external auditory canal is one-third cartilaginous and two-thirds bony.)

4. The cartilaginous part of the tube is lined by pseudostratified columnar ciliated epithelium, but toward the tympanic orifice it is lined by ciliated cuboidal epithelium.

5. It opens by the action of the tensor palati (innervated by the third division of the V nerve) acting synergistically with the levator veli palatini (innervated by the vagus). In children the only muscle that works is the tensor palati because the levator palati is separated from the eustachian tube cartilage by a considerable distance. Therefore, a cleft palate child with poor tensor palati function is expected to have eustachian tube problems until the levator palati starts to function.

6. In a normal individual a pressure difference of 200 to 300 mm H_2O is needed to produce airflow.

7. It is easier to expel air from the middle ear than to get it into the middle ear (reason for more tubal problems when descending in an airplane).

8. A pressure of minus 30 mm Hg or lower for 15 minutes can produce a transudate in the middle ear. A pressure differential of 90 mm Hg or greater may "lock" the eustachian tube, preventing opening of the tube by the tensor palati muscle. It is called the critical pressure difference.

9. If the pressure differential exceeds 100 mm Hg, the tympanic membrane may rupture.
10. A Valsalva maneuver generates about 20 to 40 mm Hg of pressure.
11. The lymphoid tissues within the tube have been referred to as the tonsil of Gerlach.
12. The tympanis ostium of the tube is at the anterior wall of the tympanic cavity about 4 mm above the most inferior part of the floor of the cavity. The diameter of the ostium is 3 to 5 mm. The size of the pharyngeal ostium varies from 3 to 10 mm in its vertical diameter and 2 to 5 mm in its horizontal diameter.

Figures 1-8 to 1-22 are temporal bone horizontal sections from HF Schuknecht's Research Laboratory at the Massachusetts Eye and Ear Infirmary.

EMBRYOLOGY OF THE EAR

Auricle

During the 6th week of gestation condensation of the mesoderm of the first and second arches occurs, giving rise to six hillocks called the hillocks of His. The first three hillocks are derived from the first arch, and the second arch contributes to the last three (Figure 1-23).

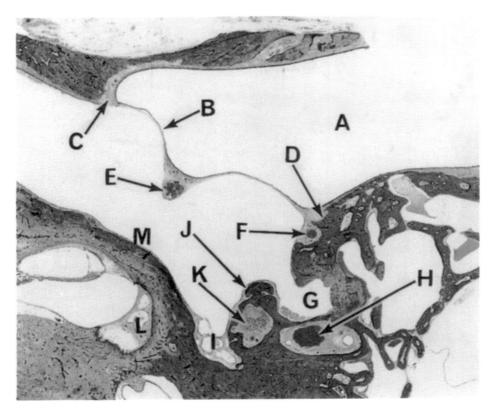

Figure 1-8. A, external auditory canal; B, tympanic membrane; C, fibrous annulus; D, tympanic sulcus; E, malleus handle; F, chorda tympani; G, facial recess; H, facial nerve; I, sinus tympani; J, pyramidal process; K, stapedius muscle; L, round window; M, promontory.

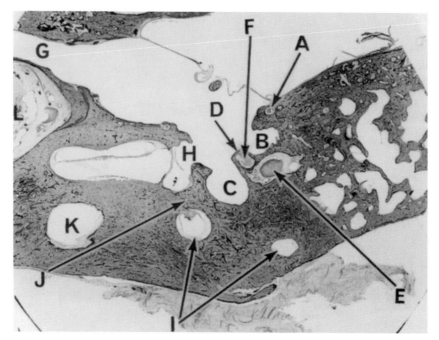

Figure 1-9. A, chorda tympani; B, facial recess; C, sinus tympani; D, pyramidal process; E, facial nerve; F, stapedius muscle; G, eustachian tube; H, round window niche; I, posterior semicircular canal; J, microfissure with no known significance; K, internal auditory meatus; L, carotid canal.

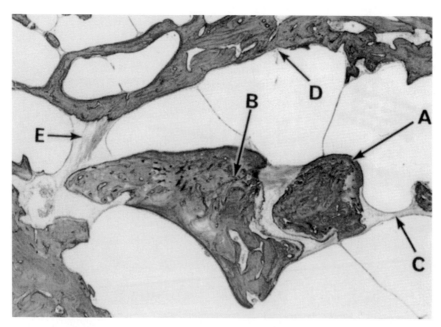

Figure 1-10. A, malleus head; B, incus body; C, anterior malleal ligament; D, lateral wall of the attic; E, posterior incudal ligament.

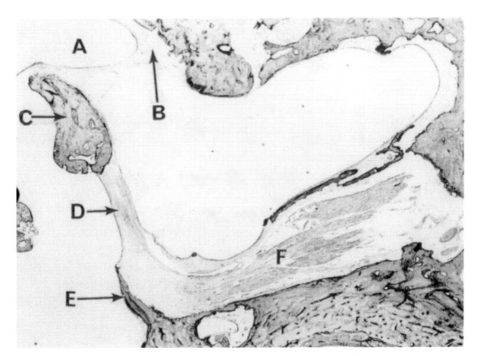

Figure 1-11. A, external auditory canal; B, fibrous annulus; C, malleus; D, tendon of tensor tympani; E, cochleariform process; F, tensor tympani muscle.

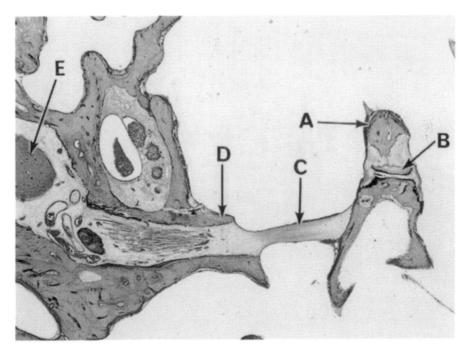

Figure 1-12. A, incus; B, lenticular process; C, stapedius tendon; D. pyramidal process; E, facial nerve.

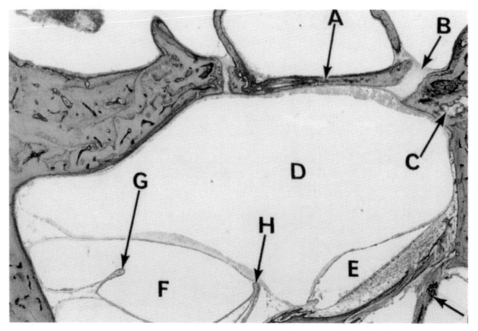

Figure 1-13. A, stapes footplate; B, annular ligament; C, fissula ante fenestram; D, vestibule; E, saccule; F, utricule; G, inferior utricular crest; H, utriculoendolymphatic valve; I, saccular nerve.

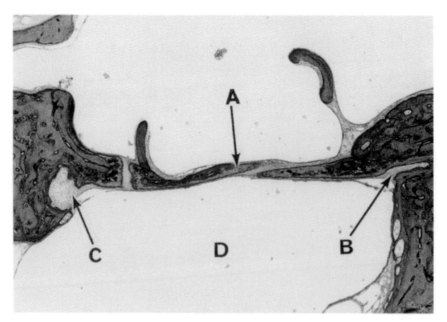

Figure 1-14. A, stapes footplate; B, fissula ante fenestram; C, fossula post fenestram; D, vestibule.

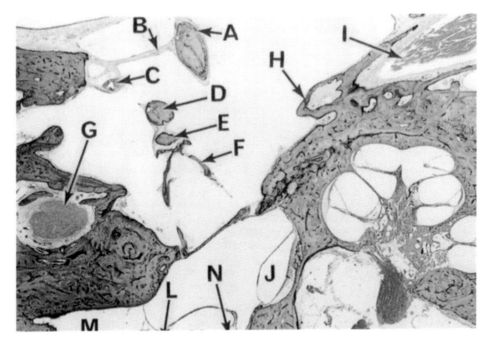

Figure 1-15. A, malleus; B, tympanic membrane; C, chorda tympani; D, incus; E, lenticular process; F, stapes; G, facial nerve; H, cochleariform process; I, tensor tympani; J, saccule; L, inferior utricular crest; M, lateral semicircular canal; N, sinus of endolymphatic duct; O, internal auditory canal.

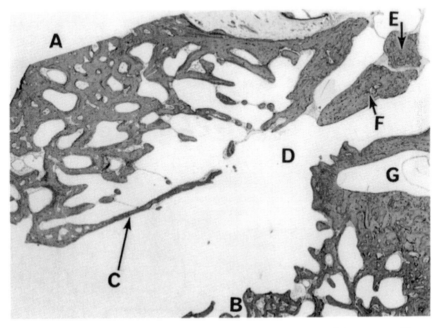

Figure 1-16. A, squamosa part of the temporal bone; B, petrous part of the temporal bone; C, Korner's septum; D, aditus; E, malleus; F, incus; G, lateral semicircular canal.

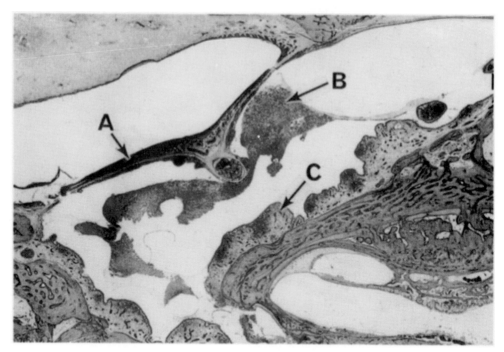

Figure 1-17. Acute otitis media. A, tympanic membrane; B, purulent material; C, thickened middle ear mucosa; D, carotid; E, eustachian tube.

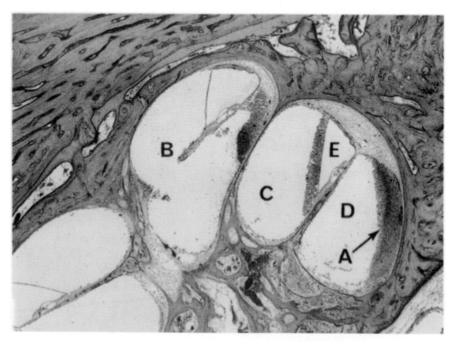

Figure 1-18. Acute labyrinthitis. A, leukocytes; B, helicotrema; C, scala vestibuli; D, scala tympani; E, scala media.

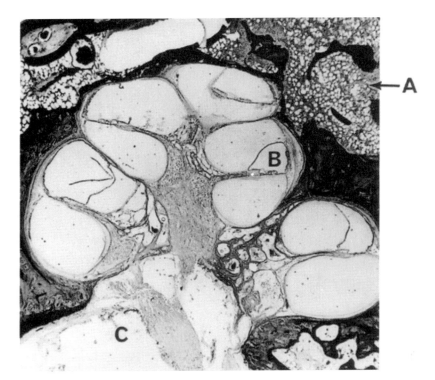

Figure 1-19. Congenital syphilis. A, leutic changes in the otic capsule; B, endolymphatic hydrops; C, internal auditory canal.

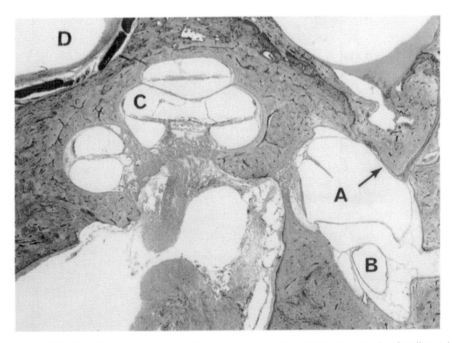

Figure 1-20. Ménière disease. A, enlarged saccule against footplate; B, utricule; C, "distended" cochlear duct; D, carotid artery.

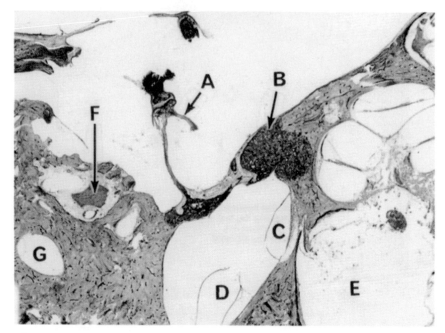

Figure 1-21.   Otosclerosis. A, stapes; B, otosclerotic bone; C, saccule; D, utricle; E, internal auditory canal; F, facial nerve; G, lateral semicircular canal.

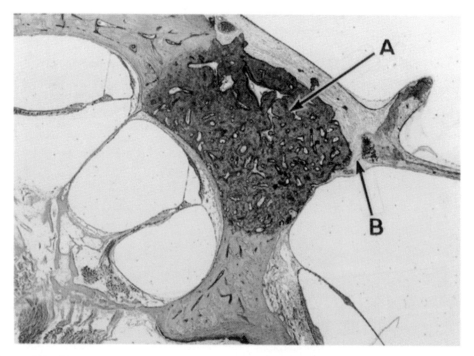

Figure 1-22.   Otosclerosis. A, histologic otosclerosis without involving the footplate; B, annular ligament.

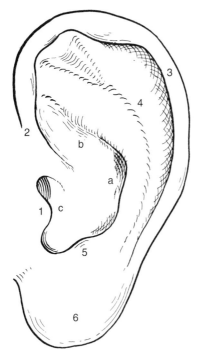

Figure 1-23. Embryology of the auricle.

First arch: First hillock   ⟶ tragus (1)
                 Second hillock   ⟶ helical crus (2)
                 Third hillock   ⟶ helix (3)
Second arch: Fourth hillock   ⟶ antihelix (4)
                 Fifth hillock   ⟶ antitragus (5)
                 Sixth hillock   ⟶ lobule and lower helix (6)

Seventh week: Formation of cartilage is in progress.

Twelfth week: The auricle is formed by fusion of the hillocks.

Twentieth week: It has reached adult shape, although it does not reach adult size until age 9.

The concha is formed by three separate areas from the first groove (ectoderm) (see Figure 1-23).

1. Middle part of the first groove: Concha cavum
2. Upper part of the first groove: Concha cymba
3. Lowest part of the first groove: Intertragus incisor

External Auditory Canal

During the 8th week of gestation, the surface ectoderm in the region of the upper end of the first pharyngeal groove (dorsal) thickens. This solid core of epithelium continues to grow toward the middle ear. Simultaneously, the concha cavum deepens to form the outer one-third of the external auditory canal. By the 21st week this core begins to resorb and "hollow out" to form a channel. The innermost layer of ectoderm remains to become the superficial layer of the tympanic membrane. Formation of the channel is completed by the 28th week. At birth the external auditory canal is neither ossified nor of adult size. Completion of ossification occurs around age 3, and adult size is reached at age 9.

Eustachian Tube and Middle Ear

During the 3rd week of gestation, the first and second pharyngeal pouches lie laterally on either side of what is to become the oral and pharyngeal tongue. As the third arch enlarges, the space between the second arch and the pharynx (first pouch) is compressed and becomes the eustachian tube. The "outpocketing" at the lateral end becomes the middle ear space. Because of the proximity to the first, second, and third arches, the V, VII, and IX nerves are found in the middle ear. By the 10th week, pneumatization begins. The antrum appears on the 23rd week. It is of interest that the middle ear is filled with mucoid connective tissue until the time of birth. The 28th week marks the appearance of the tympanic membrane, which is derived from all three tissues.

Ectoderm $\longrightarrow$ squamous layer
Mesoderm $\longrightarrow$ fibrous layer
Entoderm $\longrightarrow$ mucosal layer

Between the 12th and the 28th weeks, four primary mucosal sacs emerge, each becoming a specific anatomic region of the middle ear.

Saccus anticus $\longrightarrow$ anterior pouch of von Troltsch
Saccus medius $\longrightarrow$ epitympanum and petrous area
Saccus superior $\longrightarrow$ posterior pouch of von Troltsch, part of the mastoid, inferior incudal space
Saccus posterior $\longrightarrow$ round window and oval window niches, sinus tympani

At birth the embryonic subepithelium is resorbed, and pneumatization continues in the middle ear, antrum, and mastoid. Pneumatization of the petrous portion of the temporal bone, being the last to arise, continues until puberty.

The middle ear is well formed at birth and enlarges only slightly postnatally. At age 1 the mastoid process appears. At age 3 the tympanic ring and osseous canal are calcified.

The eustachian tube measures approximately 17 mm at birth and grows to 35 mm in adulthood.

Malleus and Incus

During the 6th week of embryonic development, the malleus and incus appear as a single mass. By the 8th week they are separated, and the malleoincudal joint is formed. The head and neck of the malleus are derived from Meckel's cartilage (first arch mesoderm), the anterior process from the process of Folius (mesenchyme bone), and the manubrium from Reichert's cartilage (second arch mesoderm). The body and short process of the incus originate from Meckel's cartilage (first arch mesoderm) and the long process from Reichert's cartilage (second arch mesoderm). By the 16th week, the ossicles reach adult size. On the 16th week, ossification begins and appears first at the long process of the incus. During the 17th week, the ossification center becomes visible on the medial surface of the neck of the malleus and spreads to the manubrium and the head. At birth the malleus and incus are of adult size and shape. The ossification of the malleus is never complete, so that part of the manubrium remains cartilaginous. (The lenticular process is also known as "sylvian apophysis" or "os orbiculare.")

STAPES

At 4.5 weeks the mesenchymal cells of the second arch condense to form the blastema. The VII nerve divides the blastema into stapes, interhyale, and laterohyale. During the 7th week the stapes ring emerges around the stapedial artery. The lamina stapedialis, which is of the otic mesenchyme, appears to become the footplate and annular ligament. At 8.5 weeks the incudostapedial joint develops. The interhyale becomes the stapedial muscle and tendon; the laterohyale becomes the posterior wall of the middle ear. Together with the otic capsule, the laterohyale also becomes the pyramidal process and facial canal. The lower part of the facial canal is said to be derived from Reichert's cartilage.

During the 10th week, the stapes changes its ring shape to "stirrup" shape. During the 19th week, ossification begins, starting at the obturator surface of the stapedial base. The ossification is completed by the 28th week except for the vestibular surface of the footplate, which remains cartilaginous throughout life. At birth the stapes is of adult size and form.

Inner Ear

During the 3rd week, neuroectoderm and ectoderm lateral to the first branchial groove condense to form the otic placode. The latter invaginates until it is completely submerged and surrounded by mesoderm, becoming the otocyst or otic vesicle by the 4th week. The 5th week marks the appearance of a wide dorsal and a slender ventral part of the otic vesicle. Between these two parts, the endolymphatic duct and sac develop. During the 6th week the semicircular canals take shape, and by the 8th week, together with the utricle, they are fully formed. Formation of the basal turn of the cochlea takes place during the 7th week, and by the 12th week the complete 2.5 turns are developed. Development of the saccule follows that of the utricle. Evidently, the pars superior (semicircular canals and utricle) is developed before the pars inferior (sacculus and cochlea). Formation of the membranous labyrinth without the end-organ is said to be complete by the 15th week of gestation.

Concurrent with formation of the membranous labyrinth, the precursor of the otic capsule emerges during the 8th week as a condensation of mesenchyme precartilage. The 14 centers of ossification can be identified by the 15th week, and ossification is completed during the 23rd week of gestation. The last area to ossify is the fissula ante fenestram, which may remain cartilaginous throughout life. Other than the endolymphatic sac, which continues to grow until adulthood, the membranous and bony labyrinth are of adult size at the 23rd week of embryonic development. The endolymphatic sac is the first to appear and the last to stop growing.

At the 3rd week the common macula first appears. Its upper part differentiates into the utricular macula and the cristae of the superior and lateral semicircular canals, whereas its lower part becomes the macula of the saccule and the crista of the posterior semicircular canal. During the 8th week, two ridges of cells as well as the stria vascularis are identifiable. During the 11th week, the vestibular end-organs, complete with sensory and supporting cells, are formed. During the 20th week, development of the stria vascularis and the tectorial membrane is complete. During the 23rd week, the two ridges of cells divide into inner ridge cells and outer ridge cells. The inner ridge cells become the spiral limbus; the outer ones become the hair cells, pillar cells, Hensen's cells, and Deiters' cells. During the 26th week, the tunnel of Corti and canal of Nuel are formed.

The neural crest cells lateral to the rhombencephalon condense to form the acoustic-facial ganglion, which differentiates into the facial geniculate ganglion, superior vestibular ganglion (utricle, superior, and horizontal semicircular canals), and inferior ganglion (saccule, posterior semicircular canal, and cochlea).

At birth, four elements of the temporal bone are distinguishable: petrous bone, squamous bone, tympanic ring, and styloid process. The mastoid antrum is present, but the mastoid process is not formed until the end of the second year of life; pneumatization of the mastoid soon follows. The tympanic ring extends laterally after birth, forming the osseous canal.

CLINICAL INFORMATION

1. Congenital microtia occurs in about 1:20,000 births.
2. The auricle is formed early. Therefore, malformation of the auricle implies a malformation of the middle ear, mastoid, and VII nerve. On the other hand, a normal auricle with canal atresia indicates abnormal development during the 28th week, by which time the ossicles and the middle ear are already formed.
3. Improper fusion of the first and second branchial arches results in a preauricular sinus tract (epithelium lined).
4. Malformation of first branchial arch and groove results in:
    a. Auricle abnormality (first and second arches)
    b. Bony meatus atresia (first groove)
    c. Abnormal incus and malleus (first and second arches)
    d. Abnormal mandible (first arch)
    When the maxilla is also malformed, this constellation of findings is called Treacher–Collins syndrome (mandibular facial dysostosis).
    a. Outward-downward slanted eyes (antimongoloid)
    b. Notched lower lid
    c. Short mandible
    d. Bony meatal atresia
    e. Malformed incus and malleus
    f. Fishmouth
5. Abnormalities of the otic capsule and labyrinth are rare because they are phylogenetically ancient.
6. An incidence of 20 to 30% dehiscent tympanic portion of the VII nerve has been reported.
7. The incidence of absent stapedius tendon, muscle, and pyramidal eminence is estimated at 1%.
8. Twenty percent of preauricular cysts are bilateral.
9. In very young infants, Hyrtl's fissure affords a route of direct extension of infection from the middle ear to the subarachnoid spaces. The fissure closes as the infant grows. Hyrtl's fissure extends from the subarachnoid space near the glossopharyngeal ganglion to the hypotympanum just inferior and anterior to the round window.[1]

Reference

1. Eggston AA, Wolff D. *Histopathology of the Ear, Nose and Throat.* Baltimore: Williams & Wilkins, 1947.

Bibliography

Allam A. Pneumatization of the temporal bone. *Ann Otol Rhinol Laryngol* 1969;78:49.

Anson B, Donaldson JA. *Surgical Anatomy of the Temporal Bone,* 3rd ed. Philadelphia: WB Saunders, 1980.

Bailey B. *Head and Neck Surgery—Otolaryngology.* Vols 1 & 2. Philadelphia: JB Lippincott, 1993.

Ballenger JJ. *Diseases of the Nose, Throat, Ear, Head and Neck,* 13th ed. Philadelphia: Lea & Febiger, 1985.

Hough J. Malformations and anatomical variations seen in the middle ear during the operation for mobilization of the stapes. *Laryngoscope* 1958; 68:1337.

Hough JVD. *Malformations and Anatomical Variations Seen in the Middle Ear During Operations on the Stapes.* American Academy of Ophthalmology and Otolaryngology Manual, 1961.

May M. Anatomy of the facial nerve (spacial orientation of fibres in the temporal bone). *Laryngoscope* 1973;83:1311.

Moore GF, Ogren FP, et al. Anatomy and embryology of the ear. In: Lee KJ, ed. *Textbook of Otolaryngology and Head and Neck Surgery.* New York: Elsevier Science Publishing Co., Inc., 1989.

Pearson AA, et al. *The Development of the Ear.* American Academy of Ophthalmology and Otolaryngology Manual, 1967.

Proctor B. The development of the middle ear spaces and their surgical significance. *J Laryngol* 1964; 78:631.

Proctor B. Embryology and anatomy of the eustachian tube. *Arch Otolaryngol* 1967;86:503.

Proctor B. Surgical anatomy of the posterior tympanum. *Ann Otol Rhinol Laryngol.* 1969;78:1026.

Schuknecht HF. *Pathology of the Ear,* 2nd ed. Philadelphia: Lea & Febiger, 1993.

Audiology 2

ACOUSTICS

1. *Sound:* energy waves of particle displacement, both *compression* (more dense) and *rarefaction* (less dense) within an elastic medium; causes sensation of hearing.
2. *Amplitude* of sound: extent of vibratory movement from rest to furthest point from rest in compression and rarefaction phases of energy waves.
3. *Intensity* of sound: amount of sound energy through an area per time; refers to sound strength or magnitude; psychoacoustic correlate is loudness.
4. *Sound pressure:* sound force (related to acceleration) over a surface per unit time.
5. *decibel (dB):* unit to express intensity of sound; more specifically the logarithm of the ratio of two sound intensities. One-tenth of a bel (named for Alexander Graham Bell).
6. *Frequency:* number of cycles (complete oscillations) of a vibrating medium per unit of time; psychoacoustic correlate is pitch. Time of one cycle is period.
7. *Hertz (Hz):* in acoustics, unit to express frequency (formerly cycles per second, or cps). Human ear capable of hearing from approximately 20 to 20,000 Hz.
8. *Pure tone:* single-frequency sound; rarely occur in nature.
9. *Complex sound:* sound with more than one frequency.
10. *Noise:* aperiodic complex sound. Types of noise in audiology are white noise (containing all frequencies in the audible spectrum at average equal amplitudes), narrowband noise (white noise with frequencies above and below a center frequency filtered out), and speech noise (white noise with frequencies above 3000 and below 300 Hz reduced by a filter).
11. *Resonant frequency:* frequency at which a mass vibrates with the least amount of external force. Determined by elasticity, mass, and frictional characteristics of the medium. Natural resonance of external auditory canal is 3000 Hz; of middle ear, 800–5000 Hz, mostly 1000 to 2000 Hz; of tympanic membrane, between 800 and 1600 Hz; of ossicular chain, between 500 and 2000 Hz.

The Decibel

The decibel scale is:

1. A logarithmic expression of the ratio of two intensities.
2. Nonlinear (eg, the energy increase in going from 5 to 7 dB is far greater than the increase in going from 1 to 3 dB).
3. A relative measure (ie, 0 dB does not indicate the absence of sound).
4. Expressed with different reference levels, such as sound pressure, hearing, and sensation levels.

Sound Pressure Level

The referent of sound pressure level (SPL) is the most common measure of sound strength.

1. Decibels SPL are referenced to micropascals (but can be referenced to dynes per centimeter squared or microbars).

24

2. Sound pressure is related to sound intensity.
3. The formula for determining the number of decibels is

$$\text{dB intensity} = 10 \log I_o/I_r$$

where

$$I_o = \text{intensity of output sound being measured}$$
$$I_r = \text{intensity of reference}$$

However, intensity is proportional to pressure squared, as

$$I \propto p^2$$
$$\therefore \text{dB SPL} = 10 \log (p_o^2/p_r^2) \text{ or}$$
$$\text{dB SPL} = 10 \log (p_o/p_r)^2$$
$$= 10 \times 2 \log (p_o/p_r)$$
$$= 20 \log (p_o/p_r)$$

where

$$p_o = \text{pressure of the output of sound being measured}$$
$$p_r = \text{pressure of the reference, usually 20 } \mu\text{Pa}$$

Hearing Level

When the reference is hearing level (HL):

1. 0 dB HL at any frequency is the least intensity needed for a normal ear to perceive a sound 50% of the time.
2. This scale (dB HL) was developed because the ear is not equally sensitive to all frequencies. The human ear, for example, cannot perceive 0 dB SPL at 250 Hz; rather, a 250-Hz sound must be raised to 26.5 dB SPL before it is heard. This level is assigned the value 0 dB HL. The referent is to a normal ear (Table 2-1).

TABLE 2-1. NUMBER OF dB SPL NEEDED TO EQUAL 0 dB HL AT DIFFERENT FREQUENCIES FOR TDH–49 AND TDH–50 EARPHONES

Frequency (Hz)	dB SPL
125	47.5
250	26.5
500	13.5
1000	7.5
1500	7.5
2000	11.0
3000	9.5
4000	10.5
6000	13.5
8000	13.0

From American National Standard Specifications for Audiometers. ANSI S3.6–1996. New York: American National Standards Institute, Inc., 1996.

3. This scale takes into account differences in sensitivity for the various frequencies: normal hearing is 0 dB HL across the frequency range rather than 47.5 dB SPL at 125 Hz, 26.5 dB SPL at 250 Hz, 13.5 dB SPL at 500 Hz, 7.5 dB SPL at 1000 Hz, and so on.[1]
4. HL is the reference used on audiometers.

Sensation Level
When the reference is sensation level (SL):

1. The referent is an individual's threshold.
2. 0 dB SL is the level of intensity at which an individual can just perceive a sound in 50% of the presentations.
3. For example, if a person has a threshold of 20 dB HL at 1000 Hz, 50 dB SL for that individual would equal 70 dB HL.

It is important to state a reference level when speaking of decibels. Table 2-2 lists typical sound pressure levels for various situations.

THE AUDITORY MECHANISM
Outer Ear

1. The outer ear is composed of the auricle or pinna (the most prominent and least useful part), the external auditory canal or ear canal (it is approximately 1 inch or 2.5 cm in length and 1/4 inch in diameter, and it has a volume of 2 cm^3), and the outer surface of the tympanic membrane or eardrum.
2. The pinna is funnel-shaped and collects sound waves. The ear canal directs the sound waves, which vibrate the eardrum.
3. The pinna also aids in the localization of sound and is more efficient at delivering high-frequency than low-frequency sounds.

TABLE 2-2.   DECIBEL LEVELS (dB SPL) OF SOME ENVIRONMENTAL SOUNDS

Sound	Decibels (dB SPL)	
Rocket launching pad	180	Noises greater than 140 dB SPL may cause pain
Jet plane	140	
Gunshot blast	140	
Riveting steel tank	130	
Automobile horn	120	
Sandblasting	112	
Woodworking shop	100	Long exposure to noises over 90 dB SPL may eventually harm hearing
Punch press	100	
Boiler shop	100	
Hydraulic press	100	
Can manufacturing plant	100	
Subway	90	
Average factory	80–90	
Computer printer	85	
Noisy restaurant	80	
Adding machine	80	
Busy traffic	75	
Conversational speech	66	
Average home	50	
Quiet office	40	
Soft whisper	30	

4. The external auditory canal is a resonance chamber for the frequency region of 2000 to 5500 Hz. Its resonant frequency is approximately 2700 Hz and varies according to ear canals.

Middle Ear

1. The middle ear is an air-filled space approximately $\frac{5}{8}$ inch high (15 mm), $\frac{1}{8}$ to $\frac{3}{16}$ inch wide (2–4 mm), $\frac{1}{4}$ inch deep, and 1 to 2 cm³ in volume.
2. Sound waves from the tympanic membrane travel along the ossicular chain, which consists of three bones (the malleus, incus, and stapes), to the oval window. The displacement of the ossicular chain varies as a function of the frequency and intensity of the sound.
3. The malleus and incus weigh about the same, but the stapes is about one-fourth the mass of the other ossicles. It is this difference that facilitates the transmission of high frequencies.
4. The tympanic membrane and ossicular chain most efficiently transmit sound between 500 and 3000 Hz. Thus, the ear has greatest sensitivity at those frequencies most important to understanding speech.
5. The middle ear transforms acoustic energy from the medium of air to the medium of liquid. It is an impedance-matching system that ensures energy is not lost. This impedance matching is accomplished by:
   a. *The area effect of the tympanic membrane.* Although the area of the adult tympanic membrane is between 85 and 90 mm², only about 55 mm² effectively vibrates (the lower two-thirds of the drum); the stapes footplate is 3.2 mm². Thus, the ratio of the vibrating portion of the tympanic membrane to that of the stapes footplate results in a 17:1 increase in sound energy.
   b. *Lever action of the ossicular chain.* As the eardrum vibrates, the ossicular chain is set into motion about an axis of rotation from the anterior process of the malleus through the short process of the incus. Because the handle of the malleus is approximately 1.3 times longer than the incus long process, the force (pressure) received at the stapes footplate, through the use of leverage, is greater than that at the malleus by about 1.3:1. Thus, the transformer ratio of the middle ear is about 22:1 (the result of the area effect of the tympanic membrane and the lever action of the ossicles: $17 \times 1.3 = 22$). This translates to approximately 25 dB.
   c. *The natural resonance and efficiency of the outer and middle ears* (500–3000 Hz).
   d. *The phase difference between the oval window and the round window.* When sound energy impinges on the oval window, a wave is created within the cochlea that travels from the oval window, along the scala vestibuli and the scala tympani, to the round window. The phase difference between the two windows results in a small change (approximately 4 dB) in the normal ear.

Inner Ear

Once the sound signal impinges on the oval window, the cochlea transforms the signal from mechanical energy into hydraulic energy and then, ultimately at the hair cells, into bioelectrical energy. As the footplate of the stapes moves in and out of the oval window, a traveling wave is created in the cochlea (Békésy's traveling wave theory). As the wave travels through the cochlea, it causes movement of the basilar membrane and the tectorial membrane. Because these two membranes have different hinge points, this movement results in a "shearing" motion that bends the hair cell stereocilia. This bending depolarizes the hair cells, which in turn, sets off afferent electrical nerve impulses.

The energy wave travels from base to apex along the basilar membrane until the wave reaches a maximum. The basilar membrane varies in stiffness and mass throughout its length.

The point of maximum displacement of the traveling wave is determined by the interaction of the frequency of the sound and the basilar membrane's physical properties. The outer hair cells (OHCs) are motile, reacting mechanically to the incoming signal by shortening and lengthening according to their characteristic (best) frequency. Under strong efferent influence, the OHCs are part of an active feedback mechanism, adjusting the physical properties of the basilar membrane so that a given frequency maximally stimulates a narrow group of inner hair cells (IHCs). This is the "cochlear amplifier." It is the IHCs that trigger the preponderance of the afferent nerve responses; 95% of all afferent fibers innervate the IHCs.

The cochlea is organized spatially according to frequency, ie, tonotopic arrangement. For every frequency there is a highly specific place on the basilar membrane where hair cells are maximally sensitive to that frequency: the basal end for high frequencies and the apical end for low frequencies. Frequency-selective neurons transmit the neural code from the hair cells through the auditory system. For multiple frequencies (complex sound), there are several points of traveling wave maxima, and the cochlear apparatus constantly tunes itself for best reception and encoding of each component frequency. The auditory mechanism's superb frequency resolution rests mostly on this resonation of the highly tuned hair cell response rather than on processing at higher auditory centers.

The cochlea is nonlinear, acting like a compression circuit by reducing a large range of acoustic inputs into a much smaller range. The compression mainly occurs around the OHCs' characteristic frequency. This nonlinearity allows the auditory system to manage a very wide range of intensities, which is represented by the nonlinear, logarithmic decibel scale.[2] Perception of pitch and loudness is based on complex processes from the outer ear up through the higher auditory centers. However, the major factor is in the periphery, where the cochlea acts as both a transducer and an analyzer of input frequency and intensity. Table 2-3 lists the enzymes found in the organ of Corti and stria vascularis. Table 2-4 lists normal labyrinthine fluid levels.

Central Pathway

Once the nerve impulses are initiated, the signals continue along the auditory pathway from the spiral ganglion cells within the cochlea to the modiolus, where the fibers form the cochlear branch of nerve VIII. The fibers pass to the cochlear nucleus at the pontomedullary junction of the brain stem, the first truly central connection. The fibers and nucleus are tonotopically organized. All fibers synapse at the ipsilateral cochlear nucleus. The majority of fibers cross through the acoustic striae and trapezoid body to the contralateral superior olivary complex in the lower pons of the brainstem. This is the first point of decussation, where signals from both ears first interact to allow binaural function. Fibers ascend to the nuclei of the lateral lemniscus in the pons and to the inferior colliculus in the midbrain. The medial geniculate body in the thalamus is the last nucleus before the cortex. From there, the nerve fibers radiate to the auditory cortex. Tonotopic organization is largely maintained throughout.

TABLE 2-3. ENZYMES IN THE ORGAN OF CORTI AND STRIA VASCULARIS

Succinate dehydrogenase
Cytochrome oxidases
Diaphorases (DPN, TPN)
Lactic dehydrogenase
Malic dehydrogenase
α-Glycerophosphate dehydrogenase
Glutamate dehydrogenase

TABLE 2-4. NORMAL LABYRINTHINE FLUID VALUES

	Perilymph				Endolymph		
	Serum	CSF	Scala Tympani	Scala Vestibuli	Cochlea	Vestibule	Endolymph Sac
Na (mEq/L)	141	141	157	147	6	14.9	153
K (mEq/L)	5	3	3.8	10.5	171	155	8
Cl (mEq/L)	101	126	—	—	120	120	—
Protein (mg/dL)	7000	10–25	215	160	125	—	5200
Glucose (mg/dL)	100	70	85	92	9.5	39.4	—
pH	7.35	7.35	7.2	7.2	7.5	7.5	—

The central pathway is a complex system with several crossovers and nuclei. Not all neuronal tracts synapse with each auditory nucleus sequentially in "domino" fashion; rather, they may encounter from two to five synapses. There is a proliferation of fibers from about 25,000 in nerve VIII to millions from the thalamus. Along with the various nuclei, there are afferent and efferent fibers, all exerting a mutual influence on one another. It would be an enormous task to examine all of the possible pathways, nuclei, and the processing involved in this neural transmission. A mnemonic for the auditory structures leading up to the medial geniculate body is ECOLI: *E*ighth nerve, *C*ochlear nucleus, *O*livary complex, *L*ateral lemniscus, and *I*nferior colliculus.

TUNING-FORK TESTS

Tuning-fork tests serve as a basic hearing screening. Every otologic patient is tested with a tuning fork before an audiogram is performed. If the responses to the tuning fork do not agree with the audiogram, the difference is resolved with repeated testing and audiometric studies. Clinically, the most useful fork is the 512-Hz fork. A negative Rinne response to the 512-Hz fork indicates a 25- to 30-dB or greater conductive hearing loss. A 256-Hz fork may be felt rather than heard. In addition, ambient noises are also stronger in the low frequencies, around 250 Hz. A negative Rinne response to a 256-Hz fork implies an air–bone gap of 15 dB or more. A negative Rinne response to a 1024-Hz fork implies an air–bone gap of 35 dB or more. It is essential to strike the fork gently to avoid creating overtones. The maximum output of a tuning fork is about 60 dB. See Table 2-5 for a summary of these tests.

Weber Test

1. The Weber test is a test of lateralization.
2. The tuning fork is set into motion and its stem is placed on the midline of the patient's skull. The patient must state where the tone is louder: in the left ear, right ear, both ears, or the midline.
3. Patients with normal hearing or equal amounts of hearing loss in both ears (conductive, sensorineural, or mixed loss) will experience a midline sensation.
4. Patients with a unilateral sensorineural loss will hear the tone in their better ear.
5. Patients with a unilateral conductive loss will hear the tone in their poorer ear.

Rinne Test

1. The Rinne test compares a patient's air and bone conduction hearing.
2. The tuning fork is struck and its stem is placed first on the mastoid process (as closely as possible to the posterosuperior edge of the canal without touching it), then approxi-

TABLE 2-5. SUMMARY OF TUNING-FORK TESTS

Test	Purpose	Fork Placement	Normal Hearing	Conductive Loss	Sensorineural Loss
Weber	To determine conductive versus sensorineural loss in unilateral loss	Midline	Midline sensation; tone heard equally in both ears	Tone louder in poorer ear	Tone louder in better ear
Rinne	To compare patient's air and bone conduction hearing	Alternately between patient's mastoid and entrance to ear canal	Positive Rinne: tone louder at ear	Negative Rinne: tone louder on mastoid	Positive Rinne: tone louder at ear
Gellé	To determine if tympanic membrane and ossicular chain are mobile and intact	Mastoid	Decrease in loudness when pressure is increased	No decrease in loudness when pressure is increased if tympanic membrane and/or ossicular chain are not mobile or intact	Decrease in loudness when pressure is increased
Bing	To determine if the occlusion effect is present	Mastoid	Positive Bing: tone is louder with ear canal occluded	Negative Bing: tone is not louder with ear canal occluded	Positive Bing: tone is louder with ear canal occluded
Schwabach	To compare patient's bone conduction to that of a person with normal hearing	Mastoid	Normal Schwabach: patient hears tone for about as long as the tester	Prolonged Schwabach: patient hears tone for longer time than the tester or normal Schwabach	Diminished Schwabach: patient stops hearing the tone before the tester

mately 2 inches lateral to the opening of the external ear canal. The patient reports whether the tone sounds louder with the fork behind or in front of the ear.

3. Patients with normal hearing or sensorineural hearing loss will perceive the tone as louder in front of the ear (positive Rinne).

4. Patients with conductive hearing loss will perceive the sound as louder behind the ear (negative Rinne).

Bing Test

1. The Bing test examines the occlusion effect.

2. The tuning fork is set into motion and its stem is placed on the mastoid process behind the ear while the tester alternately opens and closes the patient's ear canal with a finger.

3. Patients with normal hearing and sensorineural hearing loss will report a pulsating tone (it becomes louder and softer) (positive Bing).

4. Patients with conductive hearing loss will notice no change in the tone (negative Bing).

Schwabach Test

1. The Schwabach test compares the patient's bone conduction hearing to that of a normal listener (usually the examiner).

2. The tuning fork is set into motion and its stem is placed alternately on the mastoid process of the patient and that of the examiner. When the patient no longer hears the sound, the examiner listens to the fork to see whether he or she can still perceive the sound.

3. Patients with normal hearing will stop hearing the sound at about the same time as the tester (normal Schwabach).
4. Patients with sensorineural hearing loss will stop hearing the sound before the examiner (diminished Schwabach).
5. Patients with conductive hearing loss will hear the sound longer than the examiner (prolonged Schwabach).

Gellé Test

1. The tuning fork is struck and placed on the patient's mastoid.
2. The loudness of the sound heard by the patient is assessed while varying amounts of pressure are applied to the tympanic membrane.
3. Patients with a mobile and intact tympanic membrane and ossicular chain will report a decrease in loudness of bone-conducted sound as the pressure against the tympanic membrane is increased.
4. Patients with ossicular discontinuity or fixation will report no decrease in loudness of bone-conducted sound as the pressure against the tympanic membrane is increased.

Lewis Test

1. The tuning fork is set into motion and placed against the patient's mastoid.
2. When the tone is no longer heard, the fork is placed against the tragus while the examiner gently occludes the meatus.
3. The patient is asked whether the sound is heard.
4. Interpretation of the test is neither simple nor consistent.

STANDARD AUDIOMETRIC TESTING

Typical Equipment

1. Audiometer to test hearing for pure tones and speech
2. Immittance analyzer to assess middle ear function
3. Preferably a sound-isolated or acoustically treated room adequate for measuring 0 dB HL thresholds by air and by bone conduction

The main controls on a diagnostic audiometer include:

1. Stimulus selector (pure tone; warbled tone; pulsed or alternating tones; narrow-band, white, or speech noise; microphone)
2. Output selector (right, left, or both headphones; bone oscillator; right or left speaker; insert earphone)
3. Frequency dial (125 to 8000 Hz)
4. Attenuator dial (−10 to +110 dB HL) with maximum intensity limit indicator
5. Stimulus mode selector (tone or microphone—either continuously on or off)
6. Volume unit (VU) meter to monitor speech or external signal
7. Adjustment dials to maintain proper input levels of speech, noise, tape, and compact disc signals
8. Interrupter switch/bar to present or interrupt the stimulus
9. Talk-forward switch and dial enabling one to speak to the patient at a comfortable intensity level without needing to go into the microphone mode
10. Talk-back dial enabling one to hear the patient from the booth at a comfortable level

The immittance analyzer usually has the following minimum components:

1. Probe tip
2. Frequency selector (for acoustic reflex and reflex decay testing)
3. Intensity selector (for acoustic reflex and reflex decay testing)
4. Earphone (for stimulating the contralateral ear reflex)
5. Pressure control (to increase or decrease manually the pressure in the ear canal during tympanometry if there is no automatic pressure control)

A test will be valid only if the equipment used is appropriate and calibrated. Therefore, selection and maintenance of equipment, including care in use and at least annual calibrations, are vital.

Routine Test Battery

The purposes of the basic audiologic evaluation are to determine:

1. Degree and configuration of hearing loss (eg, moderate, flat hearing loss)
2. Site of lesion (conductive, sensorineural, or mixed)
3. Possible nonsurgical intervention, such as hearing aids, speech reading, and oral vs. sign language
4. Need for further testing

A test-battery approach allows cross-checking of results to judge reliability and validity. Inconsistencies may be due to nonorganic (functional) hearing loss, an inattentive or uncooperative patient, or a patient who does not understand the instructions. Results of a single test must be interpreted with caution.

A typical test battery for an audiologic evaluation includes:

1. Pure-tone audiometry (air conduction, and, if needed, bone conduction)
2. Speech audiometry (speech recognition/reception threshold and speech recognition/discrimination score)
3. Immittance/impedance measures (tympanometry and acoustic reflex)

Pure-Tone Audiometry

Pure-tone audiometry is the foundation of audiometric testing. Thus, its reliability and validity are paramount. Influencing factors include:

1. Test location (quiet enough to measure 0-dB thresholds; a sound-treated booth is usually required for both examiner and patient rooms; if ambient noise is excessive, a double-walled booth may be necessary)
2. Equipment calibration (complete calibration annually)
3. Personnel (audiologist vs. audiometric technician for proper use of equipment and testing procedures, including masking)
4. Clear instructions
5. Placement of headphones and bone oscillator
6. Patient comfort

Aspects of Pure-Tone Testing

*   Test of sensitivity to pure tones by air conduction; if there is hearing loss, by bone conduction.

- Determines thresholds: lowest levels at which patient responds at least 50% of time.
- Octave frequencies 250 to 8000 Hz; interoctave frequencies (eg, 1500 Hz) if 25 dB or more difference between octave frequencies.
- 6000 Hz for baseline audiograms—eg, persons exposed to high-level sound or receiving ototoxic medication.

Masking

- Noise introduced into nontest ear to prevent that ear from detecting signals intended for test ear.
- Necessary when signal to test ear strong enough to vibrate skull and travel to nontest ear: *crossover.*
- Reduction in sound energy from one side of skull to other is *interaural attenuation.*
- Interaural attenuation for air conduction with usual supraaural earphones 40 to 65 dB; for bone conduction, 0 to 10 dB.
- Therefore crossover in air conduction can occur as low as 45 dB HL and in bone conduction as low as 0 dB HL.
- For pure tones, masker is narrow-band noises; for speech, masker is speech-spectrum noise.
- Insert or tube earphones allow much higher interaural attenuation; thus, there is much less chance of crossover. Interaural attenuation may be 80 to 90 dB, which often eliminates the need for masking during air conduction testing.

Two rules of when to mask (pure-tone or speech audiometry):

1. Air conduction. Mask the nontest ear whenever the air conduction level to the test ear exceeds the bone conduction level of the nontest ear by 40 dB or more.
2. Bone conduction. Mask the nontest ear whenever there is an air–bone gap greater than 10 dB in the test ear. See examples in Figure 2-1.

Air–Bone Comparisons

- Air: earphones—hearing sensitivity from auricle to brain stem.
- Bone: bone oscillator on mastoid or forehead—hearing sensitivity only from cochlea to brain stem; bypasses outer and middle ears.
- Bone conduction results show degree of hearing loss due to inner ear or nerve damage; air conduction results show degree of hearing loss of any conductive or sensorineural disorder. The difference or gap reflects the loss due to reduced transmission or conduction of sound through outer and middle ears.

The thresholds for air and bone conduction are recorded on an audiogram, a graphic representation of a person's sensitivity to pure tones as a function of frequency. For each frequency, indicated by numbers across the top of the audiogram, the individual's threshold in decibels hearing level (dB HL), indicated by numbers along the side of the audiogram, is plotted where the two numbers intersect. The most commonly used audiogram symbols are shown in Table 2-6.[3]

Pure-tone testing yields one of several audiogram types:

1. *Normal hearing.* All air conduction thresholds in both ears are within normal limits (≤20 dB HL) (Figure 2-2).

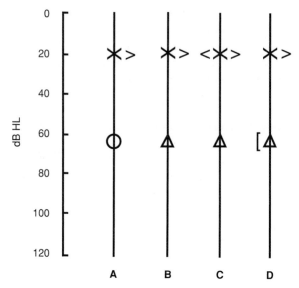

Figure 2-1. Examples of applying the rules that determine the need for masking and the results after having masked. A, Right air conduction threshold, unmasked, is 45 dB poorer than left bone conduction threshold and must be verified by masking. B, Right air conduction threshold masked (no change with masking). C, Right bone conduction threshold, unmasked, shows an air–bone gap greater than 10 dB. D, Right bone conduction threshold, masked (shifted with masking).

2. *Conductive hearing loss.* Hearing loss only by air conduction while bone conduction thresholds are normal, indicating outer or middle ear pathology (Figure 2-3).
3. *Sensorineural hearing loss.* Hearing loss by air and by bone conduction of similar degree, indicating pathology of the cochlea (sensory) or of the nerve (neural) (Figure 2-4).
4. *Mixed hearing loss.* Hearing loss by both air and bone conduction, but air conduction hearing is worse than bone conduction, indicating a combination of conductive pathology overlaid on sensorineural pathology (Figure 2-5).

When describing a hearing loss plotted on an audiogram, configuration of the loss is important information. The audiogram may be:

TABLE 2-6. COMMONLY USED AUDIOGRAM SYMBOLS

Left Ear	Interpretation	Right Ear
✕	Unmasked air conduction	◯
▯	Masked air conduction	△
>	Unmasked bone conduction	<
]	Masked bone conduction	[
↘	No response	↙
$	Soundfield	$

Adapted from American Speech-Language-Hearing Association. Guidelines for audiometric symbols. *ASHA.* 1990;20(Suppl 2): 25–30.

FREQUENCY IN HERTZ (Hz)

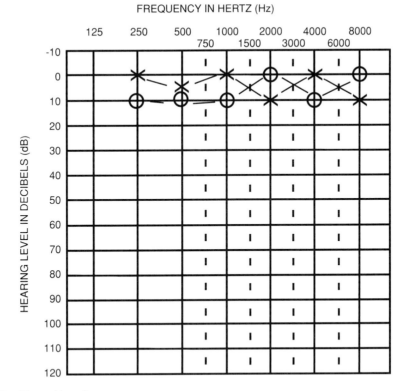

Figure 2-2. Normal hearing.

1. Flat (see Figure 2-5)
2. Rising (see Figure 2-3)
3. Sloping (see Figure 2-4)
4. Falling (Figure 2-6)
5. Notched (Figure 2-7)
6. Saucer-shaped (Figure 2-8)

Thus, pure-tone air and bone conduction threshold testing provides a good profile of an individual's hearing. However, pure-tone results should be interpreted in conjunction with speech audiometry, tympanometry, and acoustic reflexes.

Speech Audiometry

Routine speech audiometry measures speech recognition (reception) threshold (SRT) and speech recognition (discrimination) ability reflected in the speech recognition (discrimination) score (SRS/SDS). Speech may be presented by monitored live voice (MLV), cassette tape, or compact disc.

1. *Speech Recognition (Reception) Threshold*
   a. The SRT is the lowest level in dB at which a patient can repeat spondaic words (spondees) in 50% of presentations.

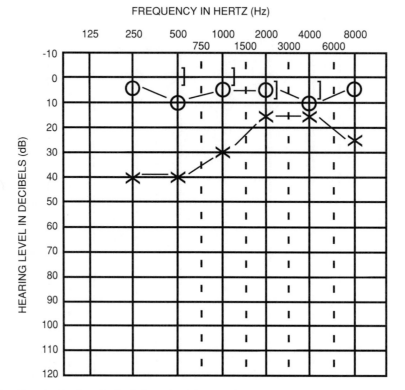

Figure 2-3. Conductive loss in the left ear in rising configuration.

    b.   A spondee is a two-syllable compound word that is pronounced with equal stress on both syllables (eg, railroad, sidewalk, and eardrum).

    c.   Measured primarily to confirm pure-tone thresholds, SRT should be within 10 dB of the pure-tone average (PTA, the average of air conduction thresholds at 500, 1000, and 2000 Hz). In a falling or rising hearing loss, a best two-frequency PTA may better corroborate the SRT.

2. *Speech Awareness/Detection Threshold (SAT/SDT)*

    a.   An SAT/SDT is the lowest level in dB at which an individual responds to the presence of speech.

    b.   An SAT/SDT is sometimes appropriate when assessing small children, persons with physical or mental disabilities, or those with a language barrier or any time an SRT cannot be obtained.

3. *Speech Recognition (Discrimination) Score*

    a.   This reflects how clearly a patient can hear speech.

    b.   The percentage of phonetically balanced (PB) words that a patient repeats correctly is the SRS/SDS.

    c.   A PB word list is a list of 50 monosyllabic words; the list contains the same proportion of phonemes as that which occurs in connected (American English) discourse; a half-list is composed of 25 PB words.

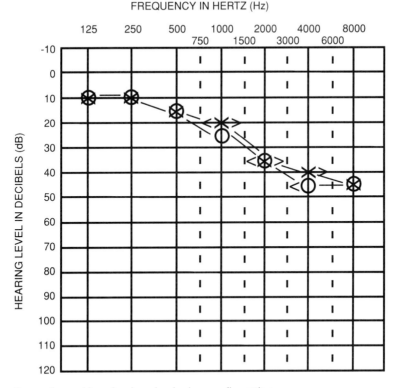

Figure 2-4.   Sensorineural hearing loss in sloping configuration.

d. The speech stimuli are presented at 30 to 40 dB SL re SRT in order to obtain the individual's maximum score. However, if a person has reduced loudness tolerance, the maximum score is sometimes obtained at a lower SL. Conversely, in sloping or falling configurations, a higher SL may yield one's maximum score.

e. Interpretation is as follows:

90 to 100% correct	Normal
76 to 88% correct	Slight difficulty
60 to 74% correct	Moderate difficulty
40 to 58% correct	Poor
40% correct	Very poor

Interpretation regarding communication difficulty must take into account not only the score but also the absolute presentation level of the stimuli. The level of average conversational speech is 50 dB HL. In a 25-dB hearing loss, 30 dB SL means that the test words are presented at 55 dB HL, a level we are likely to encounter in most situations. In a 45-dB loss, 30 dB SL means a presentation level of 75 dB HL, a higher level than we normally encounter. Therefore, two individuals with different degrees of hearing loss may have the same score but have marked differences in how well they understand daily conversation.

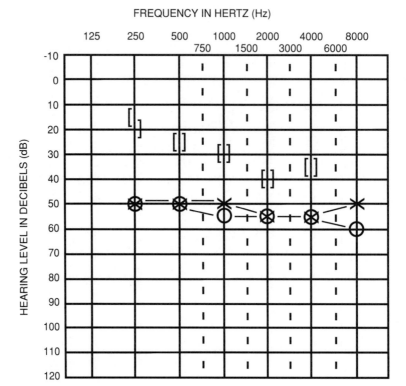

Figure 2-5.   Bilateral mixed hearing loss in flat configuration.

Immittance/Impedance Measures

Measures of middle ear function can be based on the amount of energy rejected (impedance) or the amount of energy accepted (admittance) by the middle ear. Impedance and admittance are opposite sides of the same phenomenon and yield the same information. The term *immittance* was coined to accommodate both approaches.

The tests performed on an immittance/impedance analyzer in a routine test battery are tympanometry and acoustic (stapedial) reflex.

Tympanometry is an objective test that measures the mobility (loosely termed *compliance*) of the middle ear at the tympanic membrane as a function of applied air pressure in the external ear canal. As the pressure (dekapascals, daPa) changes, the point of maximum compliance of the middle ear is identified as a peak on the tympanogram. The point of maximum compliance indicates the pressure at which the eardrum is most mobile and occurs when the pressure in the external ear canal equals the pressure in the middle ear.

There are five types of tympanograms. They are illustrated in Figure 2-9.

1. *Type A:* normal middle ear pressure and mobility. Peak is at 0 daPa; −100 to +100 daPa is considered normal (see Figure 2-9A).
2. *Type B:* flat or very low, rounded peak, but the indicated ear canal volume is within the normal range. This suggests little or no mobility and is consistent with fluid in the

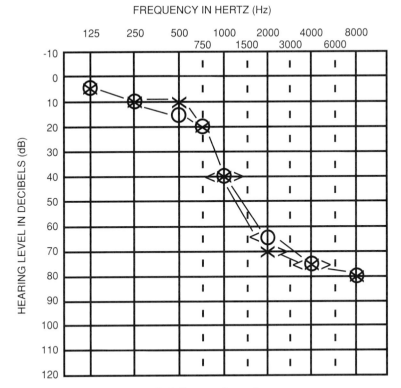

Figure 2-6. Sensorineural hearing loss in falling configuration.

middle ear. In contrast, when there is no or low peak but the indicated ear canal volume is large, there probably is a patent pressure equalizing (PE) tube or a perforation (see Figure 2-9B).

3. *Type C:* peak in region of negative pressure >−100 daPa; negative middle ear pressure. This is consistent with a retracted tympanic membrane and a malfunctioning eustachian tube (see Figure 2-9C).

4. *Type A$_s$:* type A with abnormally shallow or low peak; restricted mobility. This may be seen in otosclerosis, scarred tympanic membrane, or fixation of the malleus (see Figure 2-9D).

5. *Type A$_d$:* type A with abnormally deep or high peak; "loose" or hypercompliant middle ear system. This may be seen in flaccid tympanic membrane or in disarticulation, even partial, of the ossicular chain (see Figure 2-9E). In the case of flaccid eardrum, there is little or no hearing loss, while in the case of disarticulation, there is a substantial hearing loss and an air–bone gap.

Acoustic reflex testing is an objective measure of the lowest stimulus level that elicits the stapedial reflex. With the tympanic membrane held at its maximum compliance pressure, pure-tone stimuli are presented; the stapedial reflex occurs in response to loud sounds. Testing is performed with either ipsilateral or contralateral recording or both.

The acoustic reflex pathway is determined by the stimulation-recording arrangement.

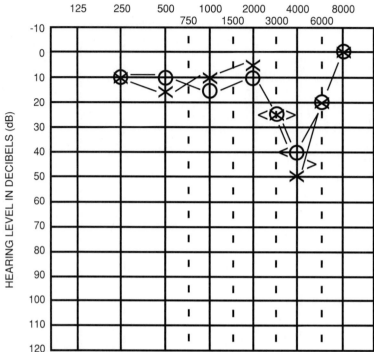

Figure 2-7. Sensorineural hearing loss in notched configuration.

1. *Ipsilateral recording*
    a. Acoustic nerve
    b. Ipsilateral ventral cochlear nucleus
    c. Trapezoid body
    d. Ipsilateral facial motor nucleus
    e. Ipsilateral facial nerve
    f. Ipsilateral stapedius muscle
    or
    a. Acoustic nerve
    b. Ipsilateral ventral cochlear nucleus
    c. Trapezoid body
    d. Ipsilateral medial superior olive
    e. Ipsilateral facial motor nucleus
    f. Ipsilateral facial nerve
    g. Ipsilateral stapedius muscle
2. *Contralateral recording*
    a. Acoustic nerve
    b. Ipsilateral ventral cochlear nucleus
    c. Contralateral medial superior olive
    d. Contralateral facial motor nucleus

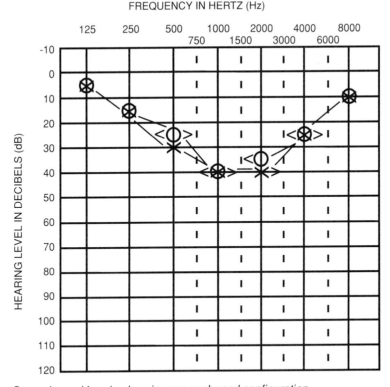

Figure 2-8. Sensorineural hearing loss in saucer-shaped configuration.

e. Contralateral facial nerve
f. Contralateral stapedius muscle

Stimulation of one side normally elicits a bilateral reflex. Normal findings are from 70 to 100 dB HL for pure tones. In the presence of any conductive pathology or hearing loss, the reflex will likely be absent; also if there is a sensorineural hearing loss greater than 65 dB HL, the reflex will likely be absent (Figure 2-10).

HEARING IMPAIRMENT AND DISORDERS OF HEARING

Hearing impairment due to an auditory disorder may be described by degree, type, and audiometric configuration.

Degree of Hearing Loss

Based on pure-tone thresholds, the hearing loss may be described according to various scales of hearing impairment. See Table 2-7 for an example of such a scale. It should be noted that depending on which scale is used, the same hearing loss may be described differently (eg, a 25-dB loss may be called "hearing within normal limits" on one scale and a "mild hearing loss" on another).

The degree of hearing impairment may also be described as a percentage of hearing impairment. Formulae for percentages of hearing loss are based on an individual's thresh-

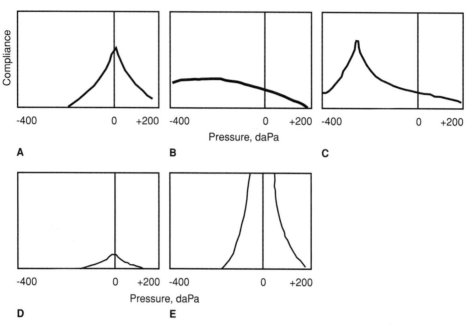

Figure 2-9. Five main types of tympanograms. **A.** Type A, normal middle ear function. **B.** Type B, poor middle ear compliance across pressures. **C.** Type C, abnormal negative middle ear pressure. **D.** Type A_s, abnormally low compliance. **E.** Type A_d, abnormally high compliance.

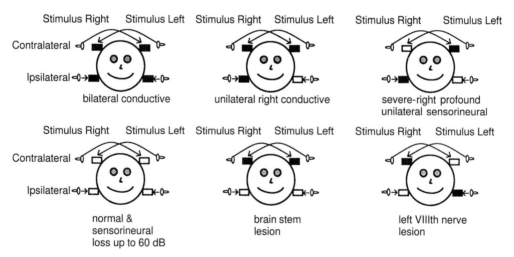

Figure 2-10. Acoustic reflex patterns. □, reflex present at normal level; ■, reflex absent/elevated.

TABLE 2-7. SCALE OF HEARING IMPAIRMENT

Threshold (dB HL)	Degree of Impairment
−10–20	Within normal limits
21–40	Mild hearing loss
41–55	Moderate hearing loss
56–70	Moderate to severe hearing loss
71–90	Severe hearing loss
>90	Profound hearing loss

olds at the speech frequencies of 500, 1000, 2000, and 3000 Hz. One such formula is used by the American Medical Association (Table 2-8). One advantage to using a percentage to describe a hearing loss is that it is a single number as opposed to a phrase, such as "mild sloping to severe." Its utility is in medicolegal cases. However, descriptive terminology is more useful in most other situations, such as communication. When describing a loss for the purpose of rehabilitation, for example, "mild, sloping to severe hearing loss" would be more useful than "40% loss" since a percentage is an absolute number that gives no indication of the configuration of the hearing loss.

Note: If a percentage score is used to describe degree of loss, it is important that the patient does not confuse the percentage hearing loss number with the SRS/SDS, which is often obtained at 40 dB above the SRT (not at the average conversational level, in which case the SRS would probably be poorer). Few comparisons can be made between percent of hearing loss and percent of a speech recognition score. For example, one patient may have a speech recognition score of 92% at 60 dB HL with an 17% hearing loss and another patient may have an SRS of 68% at 60 dB HL with a 4% hearing loss. The amount of difficulty that one may have for a given hearing loss is individual and cannot be generalized among patients.

The difference between "hearing impaired" and "deaf" should be noted. Whereas hearing impaired refers to anyone with a hearing loss, deaf applies only to those with profound, sensorineural hearing loss (usually greater than 90 dB HL and for whom hearing is nonusable even with a hearing aid). The term *hard-of-hearing* refers to the wide range of hearing ability between normal and deaf.

Types of Hearing Loss

Sample audiograms of the types of hearing loss—conductive, sensorineural, and mixed—can be found on pages 13–15.

Conductive

1. Caused by a disorder of external or middle ear.
2. Usually not exceeding 60 dB HL.

TABLE 2-8. AMA FORMULA FOR PERCENTAGE OF HEARING LOSS

For each ear
1. Average the thresholds at 500, 1000, 2000, and 3000 Hz. If a threshold is better than 0 dB, take the threshold as 0 dB; if the threshold is poorer than 100 dB, take the threshold as 100 dB.
2. Subtract 25 from this number.
3. Multiply by 1.5. This is the percentage of hearing loss for one ear.

For binaural hearing impairment
1. Multiply the percentage of hearing impairment for the better ear by 5.
2. Add to this number the percentage of hearing impairment for the poor ear.
3. Divide this sum by 6. This is the percentage of binaural hearing impairment.

3. Pathologies that increase middle ear stiffness—eg, effusion—primarily affect low frequencies.
4. Pathologies that decrease middle ear stiffness—e.g., ossicular interruption—produce a flat loss (exception: partial ossicular discontinuity produces a high-frequency loss).
5. Pathologies that alter only mass are infrequent and primarily affect high frequencies.
6. Sufficient effusion combines stiffness and mass, producing a loss in both low and high frequencies, often with a characteristic peak at 2000 Hz.

Sensorineural
1. Caused by a disorder of the cochlea or nerve VIII.
2. Can range from mild to total.
3. Great majority of cases are cochlear rather than retrocochlear, thus the term *sensorineural* is favored over *nerve* loss.

Mixed
1. Combination of conductive and sensorineural hearing losses

Central
1. Caused by a disorder of the auditory system in brainstem or higher.
2. Usually does not appear as hearing loss on pure-tone audiogram or yield abnormal results on conventional speech audiometric tests.
3. May cause patients to report disproportionate difficulty in understanding or processing speech relative to the audiogram.

SPECIAL AUDITORY TESTS: DIAGNOSTIC AUDIOLOGY

In cases of sensorineural hearing loss, certain tests can help identify whether the site of lesion is cochlear or retrocochlear. The classic example is a unilateral sensorineural impairment which, because of similar symptomatology, could be Ménière's disease (cochlear) or a vestibular schwannoma (retrocochlear). As in routine audiologic testing, site-of-lesion testing involves a battery approach.

There are both behavioral and physiologic tests of differential diagnosis, the latter being more efficient. Although largely of historical value, the behavioral tests still retain application. For example:

1. Conductive overlay
2. Severe degree of sensorineural hearing loss
3. Cost-effective screening for disorders of nerve VIII
4. Where advanced equipment is limited

As a general rule, for both behavioral and electrophysiologic procedures, tests that involve high signal levels are more effective because they "stress" the system more, thereby highlighting nerve VIII disorders. As in any test involving high intensity levels, one must consider the need for opposite ear masking.

Alternate Binaural Loudness Balance Test
Auditory phenomenon: Abnormally rapid loudness growth (recruitment)

Procedure
1. Requires one normal/near normal good ear and other ear at least 25 dB worse than better ear.

2. A tone is alternated between ears.
3. The intensity of the tone to the good ear is fixed.
4. The intensity of the tone to the poorer ear is varied until the patient judges the tones to be of equal loudness.
5. Usually performed at a few different reference levels from low to high intensity in the good ear to be balanced in the poorer ear, resulting in a "laddergram."

Interpretation

Loudness balanced at *same HL* (±10 dB) is recruitment and a cochlear sign.

Loudness balanced at the *same SL* (±10 dB) is absence of recruitment and a retro-cochlear sign. Sensitivity for cochlear site good (~90%), but sensitivity for site of nerve VIII poor (~59%).[4]

Short Increment Sensitivity Index

Auditory phenomenon: Ability to detect small changes in intensity

Procedure

1. In original form, steady 1000-Hz tone presented at 20 dB SL; in modified version, at 80 dB HL.
2. 20 momentary 1-dB increments superimposed on the steady tone every few seconds.
3. Patient indicates when detects the loudness "pips."

Interpretation

Originally, a high score was considered a cochlear sign. Later, it was found that normal and cochlear-impaired ears could detect the pips at high signal level—eg, 75 dB HL—whereas retrocochlear-impaired ears could not. Thus, the *absence of a high score* is a positive sign for a nerve VIII lesion.[5] Sensitivity to cochlear site good (90%), but sensitivity to nerve VIII site poor (69%).[4]

70–100%	Not nerve VIII
35–65%	Ambiguous
0–30%	Nerve VIII

Békésy Audiometry

Auditory phenomenon: Auditory adaptation or fatigue

Procedure

1. Using a Békésy audiometer, patient plots own threshold by pressing a button when a tone is just heard and releasing it when the tone is no longer heard.
2. Békésy audiometer automatically decreases and increases intensity according to patient's button responses while it sweeps across frequency.
3. Two tracings made, first for an interrupted (I) tone and then for a continuous (C) tone (time-consuming).
4. Alternatively, trace "most comfortable level" rather than threshold (Békésy Comfort Level or BCL)

Interpretation

Type I: I and C tracings overlap.
Type II: C drops 10 to 20 dB below I above 1000 Hz; cochlear site.

Type III: C drops steadily below I, beginning in low frequencies, by as much as 50 dB or to audiometer's limit; nerve VIII site.

Type IV: C drops below I tracing, beginning in low frequencies, by about 30 dB but courses parallel with I; nerve VIII site.

Type V: C is above I tracing, suggestive of nonorganic hearing loss.

Sensitivity for cochlear site good (93%), but sensitivity for nerve VIII poor (49%). BCL has greater sensitivity for nerve VIII (85%).[4] Tone Decay Test takes less time and is superior for assessing auditory fatigue; acoustic reflex decay even better.

Tone Decay Test

Auditory phenomenon: Auditory adaptation or fatigue

Procedure

1. Continuous tone presented at or slightly above threshold (20 dB SL more efficient because of less time).
2. Patient responds (eg, raises hand) as long as the tone is heard; lowers hand when tone fades (decays) to inaudibility.
3. If perception of the tone is not maintained for 60 seconds, add 5 dB and begin a new 1-minute timing period.
4. Continue until patient maintains perception of the tone for 1 minute (can be time-consuming)
5. Alternative for greater brevity is the Supra-Threshold Adaptation Test (STAT), in which tones 500 to 2000 Hz presented at ~ 105 dB HL for only 1 minute per frequency.

Interpretation

In conventional TDT, decay beyond 25 dB suggestive of nerve VIII lesion. In the STAT, failure to maintain perception for the 1 minute is positive for nerve VIII. Sensitivity of the TDT for cochlear site fairly good (87%), but sensitivity for nerve VIII site poor (70%).[4] Efficiency of the STAT hardly better. Tone decay tests useful as screen for nerve VIII lesion. Acoustic reflex decay superior test of auditory fatigue.

Performance-Intensity Function for Phonetically Balanced Words

Auditory phenomenon: Degradation in speech recognition at high levels

Procedure

1. Present half lists of PB words.
2. Construct a performance intensity function (PI-PB) by obtaining scores at successively higher intensities up to maximum of 90 dB HL.
3. Analyze portion of function beyond highest score for decrease in scores or rollover.
4. Rollover ratio = [PB max − PB min (beyond peak score)] / PB max.

Interpretation

Rollover is seen in sensorineural hearing losses. Although there is overlap, slight rollover is seen in cochlear lesions, whereas marked rollover is seen in nerve VIII lesions. Significant rollover ratio for nerve VIII depends on the speech material but is about 0.30 for the commonly used NU-6 test word list. Sensitivity to nerve VIII lesions is fair. However, PI-PB function can easily be added to conventional word recognition testing and requires no special equipment.

Acoustic Reflex Decay

The acoustic reflex decay test measures whether or not the stapedial reflex muscle contraction is maintained at 10 dB above acoustic reflex threshold for 10 seconds. As in the acoustic reflex test, both ipsilateral stimulation and contralateral stimulation are used. Inability to maintain the contraction (loss of half of the amplitude of the reflex in 5 seconds at 1000 Hz and especially at 500 Hz) is considered positive for retrocochlear involvement.

Glycerol Test for Ménière's Disease

The patient ingests 6 ounces of a mixture of 50% glucose and water. Prior to and 3 hours after ingestion, pure-tone thresholds and SRS are measured. In Ménière's patients, a temporary improvement in hearing occurs after ingesting the glycerol, which acts as a diuretic. The test is positive for Ménière's disease if there is a 15-dB improvement in threshold for at least one frequency between 250 and 8000 Hz, if there is a 12% improvement in SRS, or if the SRT improves by more than 10 dB.

Auditory Brain-Stem Response

Subject Variables

1. *Age.* The ABR is incomplete at birth; generally, only waves I, III, and V are observed; the absolute latencies of wave III and especially wave V are longer than those of adults, making their interpeak latency values (especially wave I–V) prolonged. The delay is due to the immaturity of the central auditory system. During the first 18 months, other wave components develop and the absolute latencies and resultant interpeak latencies of the waves shorten to adult values.

2. *Gender.* Females often have shorter latencies (0.2 millisecond) and larger amplitudes (waves IV and V) than males and may also have shorter interwave latencies.

3. *Temperature.* Temperatures exceeding +/– (below 36°C or above 38°C) may lengthen latencies. A temperature reading is necessary only on seriously ill patients. A correction factor of –0.2 millisecond for every degree of body temperature below normal and –0.15 millisecond for each degree of body temperature above normal can be used for the wave I to V interpeak latency.

4. *Medication and drugs.* The ABR is not affected by sedatives, barbiturates, anesthesia, or relaxants, but it is affected by phenytoin, lidocaine, and diazepam. A lower body temperature can be seen with alcohol intoxication; therefore, it is necessary to rule out the alcohol/temperature effect on an ABR.

5. *Attention and state of arousal.* Muscular (neck or jaw muscles) and movement artifacts are unwanted noise in an ABR assessment. It is important to encourage a natural sleep-like state or medically induce a drowsy or sleep state, if necessary, in order to obtain the best waveforms. Metabolic or toxic coma and sleep do not appear to affect the ABR.

6. *Hearing loss.* In conductive or mixed hearing losses, subtract the amount of the air–bone gap from the signal level and compare results to norms for that level. In cochlear impairments, low-frequency losses have negligible effect on the click ABR, and flat losses above 75 dB usually preclude the ABR. High-frequency cochlear losses yield essentially normal click ABRs provided that the loss is no more than moderate and that the signal is 20 dB above the pure-tone threshold at 4000 Hz. Otherwise, cochlear losses degrade waveform morphology, increase latency, and decrease amplitude, but not in a perfectly predictable way. When an ABR is abnormal, one must consider the type, degree, and configuration of hearing loss before presuming retrocochlear involvement.

Stimulus Variables

1. *Click polarity.* Rarefaction stimuli result in shorter latency, higher amplitude for early components, and a clearer separation of wave IV and V components than do condensation clicks.
2. *Rate.* Stimulus rates of over 30 clicks per second begin to increase latency of all components. Fast click rates >55 per second tend to reduce waveform clarity. Rate has more of an effect on premature than on term newborns, on children under 18 months than on older children, and on older children than on adults. Rate influences wave V the most and, therefore, the III–V and I–V intervals.
3. *Intensity.* As intensity increases, amplitude increases and latency decreases. As intensity decreases, amplitude decreases and latency increases. Wave V latency increases about 2 milliseconds when going from a high level (80 dB) to a low level (20 dB) (ie, the absolute latency may shift from 5.5 to 7.5 milliseconds).
4. *Stimulus frequency.* Higher-frequency stimuli, such as a click, result in shorter latencies than do lower-frequency stimuli, such as a 500-Hz tone pip.

Recording Parameters

1. *Electrode montage.* Waves IV and V are better separated in contralateral recordings; waves I and III are more prominent in ipsilateral recordings. A horizontal montage (ie, ear to ear as opposed to vertex to ear) results in an increase in wave I amplitude. Electrode placement on the earlobe results in less muscle potential and greater amplitude of wave I than does placement on the mastoid.
2. *Filter settings.* Up to 3000 Hz, high-frequency information results in increased amplitude and decreased latency. Below 1500 Hz, low-frequency information results in rounded peaks and longer latencies.

Otoacoustic Emissions

In a confirmed sensorineural hearing loss >40 dB, evoked otoacoustic emissions (OAE) are absent in cochlear lesions but present in neural lesions.

OTOACOUSTIC EMISSIONS

Otoacoustic emissions (OAEs):

1. Narrow-band tonal sounds generated within normal cochlea by outer hair cells.
2. Can be detected as acoustic energy within the external auditory canal.
3. Low-level sounds below 30 dB SPL, therefore, must be measured in a quiet environment with a sensitive microphone, spectral analysis, and computer averaging.
4. Pathway of energy transfer is outer hair cell, basilar membrane, cochlear fluids, oval window, ossicles, and tympanic membrane, which acts as a loudspeaker to external ear canal.
5. A sign that the cochlea has either normal function through the OHCs or has no more than approximately a 40-dB sensorineural hearing impairment.
6. OAEs are an epiphenomenon—ie, not a process of hearing but a byproduct of it.

Two classes of OAEs: spontaneous (SOAEs) and evoked (EOAEs):

A. SOAEs—occur spontaneously, ie, without an external stimulus
   1. Found in 35 to 60% of healthy normal-hearing ears.
   2. Absent when a cochlear hearing loss due to outer hair cell damage exceeds 40 dB.

3.   Usually not a basis for tinnitus.
4.   Little clinical utility.
B.   EOAEs—occur during or after an acoustic stimulus due to electromotile activity of OHCs in response to sound
    Three types according to method of measurement:
    1.   Transient evoked otoacoustic emissions (TEOAEs):
        *   Evoked by a click (transient) or tone pip approximately 4 to 15 milliseconds after the acoustic stimulus.
        *   Reflect the spectrum of stimulus.
        *   Therefore the response contains multiple frequencies.
    2.   Stimulus frequency otoacoustic emissions (SFOAEs):
        *   Evoked by a continuous pure tone.
        *   Produce a continuous tonal emission of the same frequency.
        *   Little clinical utility.
    3.   Distortion product otoacoustic emissions (DPOAEs):
        *   A single tone evoked by two simultaneously presented pure tones.
        *   Stimulus levels typically 55 to 65 dB SPL.
        *   Easiest to obtain a distortion product (DP) from the human cochlea when the stimulus (or primary) frequencies, f_2 and f_1, are separated by ratio of 1.2:1— eg, 2400 Hz and 2000 Hz.
        *   By using different combinations of primary tones, different distortion-product frequencies can be generated, thereby allowing objective assessment of a large portion of the basilar membrane.
        *   Of the several interactions of the stimulus tones, the interaction $2f_1$–f_2 (or the cubic difference tone) produces the most detectable distortion product, whose frequency is lower than that of either of the two stimulus frequencies.
        *   Reflects cochlear status near f_2 as opposed to f_1 or the DP.
        *   DPOAEs can be obtained in persons with a greater degree of outer hair cell loss and at higher frequencies than can TEOAEs.
        *   Help estimate presence of hearing loss, but not thresholds, in the 1000- to 8000-Hz range; absent DPOAEs with normal middle ear function indicate at least a 40-dB cochlear hearing loss.

Clinical Applications

1.   Efficient, objective, noninvasive "window" into cochlear function.
2.   Limited, but not precluded, by conductive hearing loss (inhibits sound energy from being transmitted both from external ear canal to cochlea and from cochlea to external ear canal); present OAEs indicate intact cochlea but absent OAEs do not indicate cochlear malfunction, unless normal middle ear status is confirmed.
3.   Neonatal ear-specific hearing screening via automated DPOAE instruments (although vernix in outer ear canal or mesenchyme in middle ear may preclude recording OAEs in first few days of extrauterine life).
4.   Part of test battery for *auditory neuropathy,* a rare condition in which there is sensorineural hearing loss, abnormal ABR, absent acoustic reflexes (ipsilateral and contralateral), and poorer word-recognition ability than expected based on the pure-tone audiogram, but OAEs are present.

5. Useful in patients who are difficult to test because they are unable or unwilling to respond validly during conventional audiometry; part of a test battery and the cross-check principle (see discussion of difficult-to-test patients, below).

6. Differentiating between cochlear and nerve VIII lesions in sensorineural hearing impairments (including idiopathic sudden loss and candidacy for cochlear implant). Because OAEs are preneural events, absent EOAEs in losses 40 dB or greater point to the cochlea as a site of lesion, whereas present OAEs support an nerve VIII site of lesion; part of a battery of tests.

7. Intraoperative monitoring of cochlear function during surgical removal of neoplasms involving nerve VIII.

8. Monitoring for ototoxicity or exposure to high sound levels; DPOAEs may be lost for high frequencies before there are changes in pure-tone thresholds.

9. In cases of suspected pseudohypacusis (nonorganic loss); presence of OAEs assures no significant conductive hearing loss and no cochlear loss greater than approximately 40 dB and probably less than 30 dB.

EVALUATION OF DIFFICULT-TO-TEST AND PEDIATRIC PATIENTS

Patients who are difficult to test, such as young children or persons with physical or cognitive limitations, require special testing techniques. Moreover, due to the nature of these populations, all testing techniques must be tailored to the patient. A major determinant of success, beyond the techniques themselves, is the clinician's flexibility, creativity, skills, and experience in working with these individuals. When behavioral testing is possible, even if incomplete, it is always preferable to electrophysiologic procedures. The former constitute true tests of hearing, whereas the latter are tests of some aspect of auditory functioning. The three behavioral techniques for eliciting responses are behavioral observation audiometry (BOA), visual reinforcement audiometry (VRA), and conditioned play audiometry (CPA). Modified speech audiometry and electrophysiologic procedures round out the battery approach.

Behavioral Observation Audiometry

1. Child seated on parent's lap (or older patient) placed in center of the sound field test room.

2. Speech, warbled tones/narrow-band noises, or other signals presented through loudspeaker(s) located off to the side rather than directly in front.

3. Responses observed, such as eye widening, eye blink, arousal from sleep, cessation of movement, cessation of vocalizing, cessation of crying, change in facial expression, movement of limbs, head turning, looking toward sound.

4. Intensity of the various signals is varied until lowest level of response obtained (often termed *minimum response level* rather than *threshold,* as these individuals may respond slightly above their true thresholds).

5. BOA should be avoided because responses fade quickly and reliability and validity are poor. The risk of a false-negative (missed hearing loss) is unacceptable.

Visual Reinforcement Audiometry

1. Child seated on parent's lap (or older patient) placed in center of the sound field test room.

2. Speech, warbled tones/narrow-band noises, or other signals presented through loudspeaker(s) located off to the side rather than directly in front.

3. When patient responds—typically a head turn toward the sound—a darkened toy on the same side as the loudspeaker lights up or moves.

4. If there is not a spontaneous head turn, the visual signal usually causes a head turn, or clinician prompts a head turn; in any case, the toy reinforces the behavior of looking in the direction of the sound; reinforcement converts the reflexive reaction into a conditioned response.

5. Conditioned orientation reflex (COR) is the variant of VRA that refers specifically to the orienting reflex of looking toward sound; reinforcement converts the orienting reflex into a conditioned response; it is usually not specified because it is subsumed under VRA.

6. Noting patient's localization ability permits some estimation of binaural hearing in the absence of testing with earphones, because to localize sound, hearing must be symmetrical within 30 dB.

7. Intensity of the various signals is varied until minimum response level obtained.

8. Lowest level of response to speech is speech awareness or detection thresholds (SAT/SDT).

9. VRA is appropriate for children of 6 to 30 months of age.

10. Nomative data are given in Table 2-9.

Conditioned Play Audiometry

1. Between 30 and 36 months, most children can be tested by more conventional methods.

2. In CPA, a game is made of listening for the "beeps"; each time a pure tone is presented, the child responds by playing the game—e.g., dropping blocks in a bucket or putting pegs in a board.

TABLE 2-9. NORMATIVE DATA AND EXPECTED RESPONSE LEVELS FOR INFANTS*

Age	Noisemakers (–SPL)	Warbled Pure Tones (dB HL)	Speech (dB HL)	Expected Response	Startle to Speech (dB HL)
0–6 wk	50–70	75	40–60	Eye widening, eye blink, stirring or arousal from sleep, startle	65
6 wk–4 mo	50–60	70	45	Eye widening, eye shift, eye blinking, quieting; beginning rudimentary head turn by 4 mo	65
4–7 mo	40–50	50	20	Head turn on lateral plane toward sound; listening attitude	65
7–9 mo	30–40	45	15	Direct localization of sounds to side, indirectly below ear level	65
9–13 mo	25–35	38	10	Direct localization of sounds to side, directly below ear level, indirectly above ear level	65
13–16 mo	25–30	30	5	Direct localization of sound on side, above and below	65
16–21 mo	25	25	5	Direct localization of sound on side, above and below	65
21–24 mo	25	25	5	Direct localization of sound on side, above and below	65

*Testing done in a sound room.

From Northern J, Downs M. *Hearing in Children*, 4th ed. Baltimore: Williams & Wilkins, 1991.

3. The game activity itself is the reinforcer.
4. By this age most children will wear earphones; therefore separate ear information regarding pure-tone thresholds can be obtained.

Note: It is erroneous to equate VRA with sound field testing and CPA with earphone testing. VRA and CPA are modes of eliciting a response; loudspeakers and earphones are means of presenting test signals. Some infants will tolerate earphones or bone conduction headband during VRA testing. Some 3-year-olds may reject any form of headset and must have CPA performed in a sound field.

Speech Audiometry

1. SRT may be obtained by using spondee picture cards or objects (eg, an airplane or toothbrush) for responses; the child points to the object or to the picture of the word presented.
2. SRS may be obtained using a picture-pointing task such as the Word Intelligibility by Picture Identification (WIPI) test. Rather than repeating words, the child points to a picture on a page. In the WIPI test, there are 25 words, and each word is worth 4%.
3. May be performed under earphones or in the sound field if the child will tolerate a headset.

Immittance Measures

1. Tympanometry and acoustic reflexes are objective measures and thus are very useful when testing persons who are difficult to test.
2. Immittance measures yield a good picture of middle ear status, although at least some cooperation is important. Struggling can complicate obtaining an acoustic seal or make recording and interpreting a tympanogram difficult; vigorous crying can induce high positive middle ear pressure and produce a valid peak at very positive pressures.
3. With infants below 6 months of age, the usual 220-Hz probe tone may produce false-normal tympanograms due to compliance of the external canal walls and may also underestimate the acoustic reflex; a higher probe tone of 660 Hz is preferable because it is more likely to produce valid results.
4. Gross impressions of hearing can be made on the basis of the tympanogram and reflexes. Given a normal tympanogram, a normal reflex suggests that hearing could range from normal to a severe sensorineural hearing loss, whereas absent reflexes suggest a severe–profound sensorineural hearing loss. A flat tympanogram suggests a slight to moderate conductive hearing loss regardless of sensorineural status.

Auditory Brain-Stem Response

1. Especially useful in evaluating persons who are difficult to test; behavioral procedures are always preferable to ABR, because they are direct tests of hearing whereas ABR is an indirect test.
2. Helps estimate hearing sensitivity for frequencies 1000 to 4000 Hz when usual click stimulus is used.
3. A 500-Hz toneburst stimulus helps estimate sensitivity in low frequencies.
4. Can be performed by bone conduction, if AC results abnormal.
5. Complicated by need for sedation and its requisite life support.

Otoacoustic Emissions

1. As with ABR, OAE testing can be particularly useful when evaluating persons who are difficult to test because it is a physiologic test.

2. Presence of OAE assures that hearing could not be worse than about 40 dB.
3. Takes much less time than ABR.
4. As with ABR, OAE testing requires that the patient be relatively still and quiet; sedation may be necessary, with its requisite life support.
5. A limitation is presence of a middle-ear disorder, which usually precludes recording the OAE.
6. In rare cases, persons may have hearing loss on behavioral testing, normal middle ear function, abnormal ABR, but present OAEs; this is *auditory neuropathy.*

History Interview

One of the most important and underrated components of evaluating the pediatric patient is the history interview. The following should be addressed:

1. What is the chief complaint?
2. How well does the child hear? Does the child respond as well as other children of the same age, ask "what?" excessively, or turn TV on loud? When was this behavior first noticed?
3. How well does the child talk? Is communication development as good as that of same-age children?
4. What is the birth history? Is there family history of hearing loss in early life other than that associated with ear infections?
5. What is the developmental history (ie, physical, cognitive, behavioral)?
6. Has the child had more than the usual number of childhood ear, nose, or throat problems? Does any hearing loss or speech or language lag seem disproportionate to the amount of the child's ear trouble? (The concern is that recurrent OME can mask a sensorineural hearing loss.)

IDENTIFICATION AUDIOMETRY: INFANTS

Early hearing detection and intervention (EHDI) in infants is an accepted health mandate.[6] Without early detection and intervention, children with hearing impairments will lag behind in communicative, cognitive, and social-emotional development and likely have lower educational and occupational levels later in life. Hence, universal neonatal hearing screening enjoys wide support, particularly because nearly 50% of congenital or early-life hearing losses have no associated risk indicator (many presumably recessive traits) or are late-onset conditions (see Table 2-10). The targeted hearing losses are permanent, unilateral or bilateral, sensorineural or conductive averaging 30 to 40 dB in the 500- to 4000-Hz range. In 2000, the Joint Committee on Infant Hearing endorsed these principles for an EHDI program[6]:

1. All neonates have hearing screening via a physiologic measure (ABR and/or OAE) during their birth admission; if not available then, before 1 month of age.
2. For those who do not pass the birth admission screen or subsequent rescreenings (either before discharge or as outpatients), appropriate audiologic and medical evaluations to confirm the presence of hearing loss should be in progress before 3 months of age.
3. Infants with confirmed permanent hearing impairment must receive intervention services before 6 months of age.
4. All infants who pass newborn screening but who have a risk indicator (see Table 2-10) for hearing loss or communicative delays should have ongoing audiologic and medical surveillance and monitoring. These include indicators associated with late-onset, progressive, or fluctuating hearing loss or auditory neural dysfunctions.

TABLE 2-10. INDICATORS ASSOCIATED WITH SENSORINEURAL AND/OR CONDUCTIVE HEARING LOSS (JOINT COMMITTEE ON INFANT HEARING, 2000)

Birth through 28 days (for use where universal hearing screening is not available)
An illness or condition requiring admission of 48 hours or greater to a NICU.
Stigmata or other findings associated with a syndrome known to include a sensorineural and or conductive hearing loss.
Family history of permanent childhood sensorineural hearing loss.
Craniofacial anomalies, including those with morphological abnormalities of the pinna and ear canal.
In utero infection such as cytomegalovirus, herpes, toxoplasmosis, or rubella.
**Neonates or infants 29 days through 2 years (indicators that place an infant at risk for progressive or
    delayed-onset sensorineural hearing loss and/or conductive hearing loss)**
Parental or caregiver concern regarding hearing, speech, language, and or developmental delay.
Family history of permanent childhood hearing loss
Stigmata of other findings associated with a syndrome known to include a sensorineural or conductive hearing loss
    or eustachian tube dysfunction.
Postnatal infections associated with sensorineural hearing loss, including bacterial meningitis.
In utero infections such as cytomegalovirus, herpes, rubella, syphilis, and toxoplasmosis.
Neonatal indicators—specifically hyperbilirubinemia at a serum level requiring exchange transfusion, persistent pul-
    monary hypertension of the newborn associated with mechanical ventilation, and conditions requiring the use of
    extracorporeal membrane oxygenation (ECMO).
Syndromes associated with progressive hearing loss such as neurofibromatosis, osteopetrosis, and Usher's syndrome.
Neurodegenerative disorders, such as Hunter syndrome, or sensory motor neuropathies, such as Friedreich's ataxia
    and Charcot-Marie-Tooth syndrome.
Head trauma.
Recurrent or persistent otitis media with effusion for at least 3 months.

PSEUDOHYPACUSIS

Pseudohypacusis (PHA) is the term used to describe hearing behaviors discrepant with audiologic test results, inconsistent/invalid test results, or an alleged loss of hearing sensitivity in the absence of organic pathology. The terms *functional* and *nonorganic* hearing loss
have been used synonymously with *pseudohypacusis,* although *functional* is now in less
favor. As with other diagnostic questions, a battery approach is paramount.

Pseudohypacusis can be conscious, unconscious, or a mix of the two, and the difference is not always clear. Thus, psychological labels, such as *malingering* or *hysteria,* and a
judgmental posture are best avoided.[7] The prevalence of PHA is probably underestimated
in children.[8] A typical age among children is 11 years.[8,9] Childhood PHA is twice as common in females as in males.[10] Pseudohypacusis ought not be dismissed lightly, particularly
in children, because it may be associated with a psychosocial disorder and require prompt
intervention.[9]

Signs of possible pseudohypacusis:

1. *Pretest interview.* Patient seems to have no difficulty understanding but presents a mod-
    erate, bilateral hearing loss during testing.
2. *Referral source.* A compensation case.
3. *Patient history.* Patient can name a specific incident that caused the hearing loss and
    stands to gain in some way as a result—eg, money, avoidance of some burdensome duty
    or task, or excuse for poor performance.
4. *Performance on routine tests.*
    a. Certain behaviors, such as leaning or cocking the head to the side of the signal,
        straining, looking confused or wondering, especially upon signal presentation,
        half-word responses during the SRT (*ear* for *eardrum*), and responding during
        speech audiometry with a questioning intonation as if uncertain.

b. Test–retest reliability worse than 5 dB. However, inattentiveness on the part of the patient must first be ruled out and reinstruction and retesting may be necessary. Factors affecting attention can be pain, mental confusion, advanced age, or other substantial psychomotor limitation.

c. Disparity between the PTA and the SRT >10 dB is one of the most common inconsistencies in pseudohypacusis. Agreement of the two measures should be within 10 dB. However, before pseudohypacusis is suspected, SRT–PTA disagreement due to audiogram configuration must be ruled out. In markedly rising or sloping patterns, the two-frequency average (the average of the two best/lowest thresholds of 500, 1000, and 2000 Hz) or even the one best speech frequency may better agree with the SRT.

d. An invalidly elevated SRT may be detected by obtaining a speech recognition score at or near the voluntary SRT (eg, SRT + 10 dB). If a good SRS is obtained, then the SRT was invalid.

e. Presence of acoustic reflexes with audiometric air–bone gaps.

f. Bone conduction thresholds >10 dB poorer than air conduction thresholds.

g. In unilateral or asymmetrical hearing losses, a difference greater than 65 dB between test ear and nontest ear results or absence of response or "shadow curve" (unmasked) in the poorer ear. In air conduction testing, cross-hearing (crossover) should occur at no worse than about 65 dB above opposite-ear bone conduction thresholds; in bone conduction testing, cross-hearing should occur at no worse than 10 dB above opposite-ear bone conduction thresholds.

Stenger Test

1. Excellent test for unilateral or asymmetrical hearing losses in which the difference between ears is at least 25 dB.

2. Based on the Stenger effect: when two tones of the same frequency are presented simultaneously to both ears, only the ear in which the tone is louder will perceive the tone.

3. To perform the Stenger test, simultaneously present a tone 5 dB above threshold to the good ear and an identical tone 5 dB below the voluntary threshold to the poor ear.

4. If the patient responds, the test is negative because the patient heard the tone in the good ear. If the patient does not respond, then the test is positive: The patient should respond, because the tone presented to the good ear is 5 dB above its threshold; if the patient does not respond, it must be because the tone was perceived in the poor ear and the patient chooses not to respond.

5. To help estimate thresholds, simultaneously present a tone at 5 dB SL to the good ear and 0 dB HL to the poor ear. The patient should respond. Increase the presentation level in the poor ear by 5-dB steps until the patient ceases to respond ("interference level"). This level should be within 15 dB of the patient's actual threshold in the poor ear.

6. A speech Stenger may be performed in the same manner using spondee (SRT) words in place of pure tones.

Lombard Test

1. Based on the phenomenon that one increases the volume of one's voice in the presence of loud background noise, because the noise interferes with self-monitoring.

2. To perform the test, the patient is seated in a sound-treated booth and wears headphones. Masking noise is introduced through the headphones as the patient reads aloud.

The tester monitors the volume of the patient's voice through the talkback of the audiometer on the VU meter.

3. With a true hearing loss, there is no change in the volume of the patient's voice.
4. If the loss is nonorganic—since the patient does not hear the masking noise—the volume of the patient's voice will increase.
5. Although applicable to monaural and binaural hearing losses, sensitivity is fair at best, and it affords only a rough estimate of the SRT; as a result, this test is infrequently used.

Delayed Auditory Feedback

1. Based on the principle that individuals monitor the loudness and rate of their speech by an auditory mechanism. Individuals presented with delayed auditory feedback will alter their speech, resulting in dysfluency.
2. To perform the test, record the patient reading aloud. The patient is asked to repeat the task while it is played back at a delay of 0.1 to 0.2 second at 0 dB HL. The task is repeated with an increase of 10 dB each time until a positive result is observed (eg, change in speed of reading, increase in vocal intensity, hesitations, prolongations, or stuttering).
3. Interpretation is similar to that of the Lombard test: If dysfluencies are noted, it is known that patients can hear themselves.
4. This test is applicable to monaural/binaural losses, has good sensitivity, and can provide an estimate of SRT. However, it requires proper tape recording and is seldom used.

Doerfler–Stewart Test

1. A confusion test used to detect monaural or bilateral pseudohypacusis.
2. Based on the principle that normal individuals and individuals with hearing loss can repeat words in the presence of masking noise that is as loud as the speech signal; those with pseudohypacusis may stop responding at lower masking noise levels.
3. An SRT is established. Spondaic words are presented through headphones with masking noise; the patient is asked to repeat the words. The intensity of the masking is increased with each word presentation.
4. The masking level at which the patient no longer responds is noted; this is the noise interference level.
5. A threshold for the masking noise is determined, as is a second SRT.
6. These measures are compared to normative data.
7. This procedure is involved and time-consuming and has only fair accuracy, hence it is rarely used. However, it is applicable to one- or two-ear hearing losses.

Békésy Audiometry

A type V Békésy tracing is suggestive of pseudohypacusis (see page 54). It can be used in either monaural or binaural losses. Even in modified Békésy versions, a type V pattern is fair at best both in sensitivity and in specificity. It is also a lengthy procedure. Audiologists infrequently use Békésy audiometry in cases of suspected pseudohypacusis.

Acoustic Reflex Testing

The presence of the acoustic reflex at a level 5 dB above voluntary auditory thresholds or less strongly suggests some degree of pseudohypacusis (see "Immittance Measures," under "Evaluation of Difficult-to-Test and Pediatric Patients," above).

Otoacoustic Emissions

The presence of OAEs indicates that cochlear hearing could not be worse than approximately 40 dB HL (see page 48).

Auditory Brain-Stem Response

Because it is an objective test, the ABR is a powerful tool for determining the presence or absence of hearing loss and for estimating degree of genuine hearing loss. However, it is far more time-consuming than most of the other procedures but can be helpful if the other approaches are not sufficient.

CENTRAL AUDITORY PROCESSING

Central auditory processing (CAP) is the active, complex set of operations performed by the central nervous system on auditory inputs. Auditory processing is not only central; auditory signals are acted upon throughout the auditory system, including the peripheral portion from the outer ear through the cochlea and nerve VIII. Certain behaviors are typical of persons, especially children, who have central auditory disorders. The behaviors associated with central auditory disorders overlap with those of peripheral hearing impairment. Examples include frequently misunderstanding or misinterpreting what is said; attention deficiency; difficulty discriminating among speech sounds, leading to reading, spelling, and other academic problems; unusual difficulty in background noise; reduced auditory memory; reduced receptive and expressive language skills; and in general difficulty learning through the *auditory* channel. History taking regarding hearing might well include consideration of these behaviors.

Before testing for a CAP disorder, one must rule out peripheral hearing impairment. Conventional audiologic assessment should include pure-tone audiometry (many CAP tests are presented at suprathreshold levels that are above the PTA) and speech audiometry, especially recognition ability. Additional procedures are the ipsilateral and contralateral acoustic reflexes and ABR, which help to assess the integrity of the brainstem. Since no single test can assess the several aspects of auditory processing, a battery of CAP tests is mandatory. Which tests to administer depends on a test's efficacy for the patient's symptomatology and age. The CAP tests are presented monotically (stimulation of one ear at a time) or dichotically (stimulation of both ears by different stimuli). The tests are designed to make demands on the auditory system: eg, understanding degraded speech (filtered; time-altered; competing speech or noise in the ipsilateral, contralateral, or each ear; part of the signal to one ear and another to the opposite ear), identifying auditory patterns, or requiring effective interaction of the two hemispheres.

If a CAP disorder is found, management should be based on the pattern of results from the test battery. In general, management includes optimizing the auditory experience: ie, good signal-to-noise ratio (signal well above noise), good acoustic environment (low noise and reverberation), enhanced speech input (strong, clear, and somewhat slowed). These are strategies that also are called for when there is peripheral hearing loss. In short, whether an auditory disorder is peripheral or central, intervention is most effective with a high-quality speech signal in quiet surroundings. Some patients may benefit from assistive listening devices (FM, infrared), which provide good signal vs. noise characteristics (see "Assistive Devices," page 61).

MANAGEMENT

There are a number of ways to help persons with permanent hearing loss. They include providing high-quality amplification, maximizing auditory skills, enhancing use of visual cues, counseling, appropriate education, and vocational assistance. The goal is to have the individual function to the best of his or her abilities and be a full, productive, independent, well-adjusted member of society.

Instrumentation

Hearing Aids

A. Function. The purpose of hearing aids is to amplify sound to make speech more audible without being uncomfortable. Hearing aids cannot restore normal or natural hearing; rather, they enable an individual to function better than he or she would without amplification. They cannot amplify only speech to the exclusion of all other sounds. Moreover, the finest hearing aid cannot nullify the distortion imposed by the patient's impaired auditory system. Generally, it is better to aid both ears binaurally; however, if only one ear is to be aided, the preferred ear is that which offers the greater speech recognition ability, loudness tolerance, and likelihood of providing audibility across the speech spectrum. In cases of marked asymmetry where one ear is to be selected, it is preferable to aid the ear whose hearing loss is in the 40- to 70-dB range, regardless of whether it is the better or worse ear. There is a rapidly growing and bewildering array of circuitry, controls, and features available in hearing aids. Some can be used only singly and others can be included in various combinations.

Terms of hearing aid function:

Gain: amplification or acoustic energy added to input sound, the difference between the input and output

Output: acoustic energy leaving the hearing aid receiver; combination of input and gain

Maximum power output: a hearing aid's limit in the sound level it can produce, no matter how high the input or gain; also known as saturation SPL (SSPL)

B. Components. All hearing instruments have a microphone, amplifier, and output receiver. Hearing aids may have additional components or features:

1. Screwdriver controls to adjust high-frequency or low-frequency gain, SSPL, and other aspects of a hearing aid's function.
2. Directional microphones that give relatively greater emphasis to sounds emanating from in front of the speaker. Since we usually face persons we talk to, there is greater gain for speech than for ambient noise, thereby improving *signal-to-noise ratio.*
3. A "telecoil" that detects and amplifies the magnetic field from a telephone; the microphone can be turned off, eliminating feedback while using a telephone.

C. Styles. There are five styles of hearing aids: body aid, behind-the-ear (BTE), in-the-ear (ITE), in-the-canal (ITC), and completely-in-canal (CIC) aids. Generally, BTEs are advisable for children. Size is not an indicator of sound quality or of the latest technology; rather, the larger the instrument, the greater the array of circuit capabilities that can be incorporated.

D. General Classes

1. *Peak clipping:* constant gain until the hearing aid's maximum power output is reached, at which point the amplitude peaks of the excess energy are "clipped off." For example, if a hearing aid's gain is 40 dB and its SSPL is 110 dB, any input up to 70 dB will have the 40 dB added. Inputs above 70 dB cannot have 40 dB added because the sum would exceed that capacity of the circuit; thus the signal's peaks are clipped. Peak clipping (PC) limits output to prevent amplified sound from being too loud, but it also results in distortion. Hence, linear-gain PC instruments are less commonly used nowadays.
2. *Compression limiting:* as with peak clipping aids, gain is linear, but output limiting is handled differently. Once a preset level is reached, gain is automatically reduced (com-

pressed) through a feedback circuit to an earlier stage in the electronic pathway of the hearing aid. The purpose of *automatic gain control* (AGC) is to limit the output without reaching saturation, thereby avoiding the distortion of peak clipping. There are two kinds of compression: (a) input compression at the microphone and (b) output compression at the output receiver.

3. *Wide dynamic range compression:* in contrast to compression-limiting hearing aids, compression is active over most of the operating range of the hearing aid, not just at high levels. In wide dynamic range compression (WDRC), gain decreases as input increases over a relatively wide range of sound input; for example, 30 dB gain for inputs up to 45 dB but only 10 dB of gain for inputs above 85 dB with proportionately varying amounts of gain in between. The purpose of WDRC is to compensate for the loss of OHCs. In normal ears, OHCs act as compressors to accommodate a large range of sound intensity; OHC damage curtails this "biologic compression" and results in loudness recruitment, the abnormally rapid loudness growth characteristic of cochlear hearing impairments. The concept of WDRC is to make soft sounds audible and keep loud sounds comfortable.

4. *Programmable.* Most WDRC hearing aids are "programmable"—ie, their characteristics are set by the dispenser using a digital programmer. Programmers have algorithms that specify gain and output according to the individual's threshold audiogram, but the dispenser can adjust those characteristics to meet the person's preferences. Most programmable instruments have multiband compression—ie, different gain and output for separate frequency bands—because degree of hearing loss often differs across frequencies. The programmer sets the differential gains for soft and loud inputs for the various frequency bands; the boundary between frequency bands is also adjustable. Thus, programmable instruments are highly flexible and more tunable to one's hearing loss than conventional instruments.

5. There are two types of programmable hearing aids: (a) programmable with analog (conventional) signal processing, also called digitally programmable, and (b) digital with entirely digital signal processing. Neither type of programmable instrument is inherently superior to the other or even to conventional instruments in speech intelligibility, although both types of programmables tend to be judged more comfortable at soft and loud input levels. Some digital instruments have more parameters that can be adjusted, making them even more flexible than analog programmable instruments. Also, digitals are particularly helpful for highly unusual audiometric configurations, and some devices may have an antifeedback feature. The term *digital* implies a technological superiority and hearing advantage that can be misleading. Further, programmable instruments, particularly digitals, are generally more expensive than conventional hearing instruments. Dispensers must consider the individual's listening needs and cost-benefit factors in selecting amplification devices.

E. ADDITIONAL CONSIDERATIONS

1. Acoustic modifications of a hearing aid's response:
   a. A vent (allowing sound in the ear canal to escape) reduces low frequencies, giving relatively more boost to high frequencies; reduces sense of pressure in the ear; and reduces the occlusion effect so the user's voice sounds more natural to him or her; a vent also increases the chance of feedback (whistling).
   b. Horn-shaped opening into the ear canal enhances high frequencies; conversely, a longer, narrowed opening or "reverse horn" attenuates high frequencies for hear-

ing losses with rising configurations; these are primarily in ear molds for BTE hearing aids.

c.   In BTE aids, an acoustic damper in the tubing smoothes the typical midfrequency peaks.

2.   For unaidable ears:

a.   CROS (Contralateral Routing of Signal) for unilateral, unaidable hearing losses. A CROS aid picks up the signal on the poor side and routes it to the normal hearing ear (via hardwire or FM transmission) to a nonoccluding ear mold. It is most effective when there is a slight high-frequency in the good ear. CROS aids are usually most helpful when the person is in a stationary position.

b.   BiCROS (Bilateral CROS) is for bilateral hearing loss when only one ear is aidable. In BiCROS, a CROS system on the poor side is combined with a conventional aid on the better side—ie, the aidable ear receives inputs from microphones on each side of the head. The ear mold is that used in a conventional fitting.

3.   Multimemory: different programs or settings stored in the hearing aid, from which the user can select for different listening situations by touching a switch or using a remote control.

4.   Bone conduction hearing aid: when air conduction aid not possible, such as atresia or chronic purulent otitis media or externa. A bone anchored hearing aid (BAHA) is a BC aid in which the output is connected to a metal post embedded through skin into the skull. BAHAs have slightly higher gain than conventional bone conduction hearing aid because of closer mechanical coupling. All BC hearing aids are limited to sensorineural hearing loss less than about 45 dB.

5.   FM: some hearing aids can include an FM receiver entirely within a hearing aid that is all at the ear. (For more information on FM, see "Assistive Devices," below.)

6.   Middle ear implant hearing aid: output driver connected to ossicles. A hearing aid is worn externally and coupled via magnet to a signal processor implanted under the skin and connected to output driver. As compared to conventional AC hearing aids, ME implant aids purport to provide greater gain for high frequencies and less distortion for mild and moderate sensorineural hearing losses, but they necessitate surgery.

7.   Disposable hearing aids: very low cost, preprogrammed with nonreplaceable battery; when the battery is exhausted after approximately 1 month of use, the entire unit is discarded and replaced with another instrument. Cost consideration should include expense of replacing these aids over the course of years.

8.   Tinnitus: for persons with tinnitus, a tinnitus masker (a noise generator in a hearing aid case) can drown out the tinnitus; once the masking sound is removed, some patients temporarily experience a reduction or elimination of tinnitus (residual inhibition). For persons with tinnitus and hearing loss, a hearing aid itself may help by masking the tinnitus. Also, there are masker hearing aids that combine a hearing aid and a separate noise generator and volume control. Unfortunately, tinnitus maskers are not very effective for long-term use.

F. REAL-EAR MEASUREMENTS AND FITTING FORMULAS.   The performance of a hearing aid in an analyzer chamber differs from that in an individual's ear canal. In real-ear measurements, a probe tube microphone measures sound very close to the tympanic membrane, thereby including the (real-ear) effects of the outer ear and canal and the loss of the natural gain produced by the ear canal resonance near 2700 Hz when a hearing aid is put in place. By making unaided and aided test runs, real-ear measurements help in assessing the suitability of a hearing aid, in setting controls for optimal output, and in finding the basis for a wearer's complaints. Real-ear instruments include fitting formulas or "prescriptions" of gain and output for maximum audibility of speech without being uncomfortable. The instruments display a formula's target of optimum gain and frequency response for a particular patient's hearing loss; then one can see if the desired target is reasonably well approximated with the hearing aid in place. The formulas have minor differences, and no one formula is best.

Cochlear Implants
This topic is covered in Chapter 6, "Cochlear Implantation."

Assistive Devices
1. A hearing-impaired individual's lifestyle may be helped by a variety of assistive devices, whether or not hearing aids are used. Some are auditory—assistive listening devices (ALDs)—and others are visual or vibratory devices.
2. Some of the major ALDs are
   a. Telephone amplifiers.
   b. FM or infrared television listening systems.
   c. FM systems for large areas (conference halls, houses of worship, theaters). The wearer receives an FM radio signal transmitted from a distance by a speaker who uses a small FM microphone. As a result, hearing at a distance is excellent. Also, the desired signal is far stronger than the background noise (favorable signal-to-noise ratio) and comprehension is much easier than without FM reception. FM systems are very helpful for persons in background noise, for communicating with others beyond several feet, and particularly for children in school.
3. Some visual or vibratory assistive devices are
   a. Alarm clocks, smoke detectors, security systems, baby-cry detectors, and doorbells with flashing lights or vibrator
   b. Closed-captioned television decoders (TV and videotaped and DVD movies)
   c. Text telephones (TT, also knows as TTD and TTY); persons who cannot use a telephone, even with amplification, can type and receive messages with a keyboard and monitor screen over telephone lines. TTs also allow access to many public services, medical care, governmental agencies, and businesses. TTs can be used by persons with severe voice or speech limitations as well as by those with severe hearing disorders.
   d. Although not specifically for the communicatively impaired, computers have tremendously broadened the social and communicative options available to those with communicative limitations.

Intervention, Training, and Education
At any age, the single most important element in hearing (re)habilitation is proper amplification. When hearing loss is present before communication is established, early and expert intervention is crucial to take advantage of the "sensitive" period of fastest communication growth. In the case of infants and toddlers, the approach is parent-centered, wherein trained teachers foster communication skills and show parents/caregivers how to do the same. From 3 to 21 years of age, federal and state mandates require that children have a "free, appropriate education" in the "least restrictive environment" (from regular class with support services to residential setting), and some areas mandate intervention from birth to age 3. (For more information, see Chapter 5, "Congenital Deafness.")

Communicative and educational options overlap and include auditory-oral, visual (sign and finger spelling), or a combination ("total communication"). The method of choice is controversial. Of equal importance is that any intervention be early and of high quality. Factors other than hearing loss must be considered (not "treat the audiogram"): family's communicative system and desires, psychosocial abilities, cultural values, and presence of other limiting conditions. Provided there is usable hearing, auditory training promotes listening skills, such as sound detection, recognition, and comprehension. Speech reading is the integrating of another's person's lip movements, facial expressions, body gestures, situational cues, and linguistic factors for visual comprehension. It is usually an adjunct to auditory input, although in some cases of extreme hearing loss, visual reception may be the lead linguistic input. School-age children can be taught specific speech (articulation, voice) and language (vocabulary, grammar) skills.

Adults who become hard of hearing may benefit from auditory training and speech reading lessons, although speech reading appears to be more an aptitude than a purely teachable ability. Adventitiously deafened adults can be helped to minimize the usual deterioration in speech and voice (due to absent auditory self-monitoring) and to become better users of visual cues.

Counseling and vocational guidance may be invaluable to individuals with hearing impairment. Counseling should not only give information (facts about communication, hearing loss, hearing aids, etc.) but also address psychosocial issues (acceptance of one's situation, parental guilt and anger, one's self-image, social adjustment, and so on). If left unresolved, such psychosocial concerns can limit how well adjusted or fulfilled a person may feel in spite of having achieved good communicative skills. Most states have agencies that can help individuals with hearing loss in career choices and preparation. Persons with substantial communicative difficulty may especially benefit from such services.

NOISE-INDUCED HEARING LOSS AND INDUSTRIAL AUDIOLOGY

Exposure to excessively strong sounds may destroy auditory cells, resulting in hearing loss. Such losses are often described as "noise-induced," but any sound—noise, speech, music— of sufficient intensity can damage hearing. Since noise is the most common cause of hearing loss due to exposure to high sound levels, the term *noise-induced hearing loss* (NIHL) is used in this context. The effects of noise on hearing may be classified as temporary threshold shift (TTS), permanent threshold shift (PTS), or acoustic trauma resulting from one or relatively few exposures to a very high sound level, such as an explosion. Typically, hearing loss from noise begins in a notch pattern in the 3000- to 6000-Hz region but with time broadens to the other frequency regions with a less steep slope.

Hazardous noise exposure can be occupational (eg, factory work, construction, farming, military service) and/or recreational (eg, performing music, shooting guns, and aviation). Occupational noise is not inherently more hazardous to hearing than is recreational noise. Since NIHL is the most common cause of sensorineural hearing loss after infancy and before old age, it is one of the prime examples of where the otolaryngologist can practice preventive medicine. The public tends to discount the dangers of noise, deny the degree of exposure, and disdain means to protect hearing. Shooters, in particular, are unaware of or minimize how much shooting they do and the risk involved. A sign of early damage in shooters is the asymmetrical 4000-Hz notch loss, which is worse in the ear opposite the shoulder from which the gun is fired. By informing, counseling, and motivating persons to protect their hearing, otolaryngologists can make an enormous impact on preventing hearing impairment.

Four prominent factors contribute to the effects of noise: sound level (in dB SPL), spectral composition, time distribution of the noise exposure during a working day, and cumulative noise exposure over days, weeks, or years. The *Occupational Health and Safety Administration* (OSHA) has established guidelines for permissible noise exposure levels for a working day, assuming constant, steady-state noise and a 20-year work life (Table 2-11). However, since occupational noise is not always constant, a time-weighted average takes into account level and duration and is a level that, if constant for an 8-hour day, would have the same effect as the measured dose.

A hearing conservation program has four main components:

1. Assess the level and cumulative dose of noise exposure in a given setting using a sound level meter and dosimeter.
2. Control the amount of overexposure in a given setting by reducing the amount of noise created by the source, reducing the amount of noise reaching an individual's ears by constructing barriers, or changing job procedures or schedule.
3. If sound cannot be brought within safe levels, provide ear protection devices and information to motivate their proper use.
4. Monitor hearing: preemployment testing with periodic follow-up tests, usually annually.

Ear protection devices act as barriers to sound. Earmuffs, custom-fitted earplugs, or disposable earplugs provide 20 to 40 dB of sound attenuation, more in high frequencies than in low frequencies. Proper fit, comfort, and motivation are just as important as type of protection, because no device is effective if it is not worn.

There are passive ear protection devices (non-electric) and active devices (electric). Some passive devices, such as valves, are amplitude-sensitive to allow relatively normal hearing. They pass moderate sound levels but reduce high sound levels, not, however, always to a safe level. A common misconception is that some devices "shut off" when sound is strong enough. In fact, they merely reduce sound level. For some individuals, notably musicians, the greater sound reduction for high frequencies of hearing protectors is objectionable because it alters sound quality. Thus, "musicians' plugs" have a uniform or flat attenuation across the sound spectrum. While effective, they do not assure complete protection against damage to hearing.

Active devices typically limit output to 85 dB SPL. However, to offset the blockage effect of the ear protectors, some units include slight amplification in order to hear usual conversation and environmental sounds. Nevertheless, the low level of peak clipping tends

TABLE 2-11. OSHA PERMISSIBLE NOISE EXPOSURES

Duration (hours/day)	SPL (on dBA scale, slow response)
8	90
6	92
4	95
2	100
1	105
0.5	110
≤0.25	115

to distort speech. Thus, the best application of active devices is brief use for intermittent and impulse noise (gunfire). Another strategy is "active noise reduction," in which the sound phase is inverted 180° to cancel the noise. ANR is effective below 1000 Hz. Combining the low-frequency attenuation of ANR with the high-frequency reduction of muffs provides a good overall result. ANR systems are advantageous in noisy communication situations (eg, for pilots) but give no better hearing protection than well-fitted earplugs or muffs.

References

1. American National Standard Specifications for Audiometers. ANSI S3.6-1996. New York: American National Standards Institute, Inc, 1996.
2. Durrant JD, Lovrinic JH. *Bases of Hearing Science,* 3rd ed. Baltimore: Williams & Wilkins, 1995.
3. American Speech-Language-Hearing Association. Guidelines for audiometric symbols. *ASHA* 1990;20(Suppl 2):225–230.
4. Turner RG, Shepard NT, Frazer GJ. Clinical performance of audiological and related diagnostic tests. *Ear Hear* 1984;5:187–194.
5. Sanders JW. Diagnostic audiology. In: Lass NJ, McReynolds LV, Northern JL, Yoder DE, eds. *Handbook of Speech-Language Pathology and Audiology.* Toronto: BC Decker, 1988, 1123–1143.
6. Year 2000 Position Statement: Principles and Guidelines for Early Hearing Detection and Intervention Programs. Joint Committee on Infant Hearing. *Am J Audiol* 2000;9:9–29.
7. Martin FN. Pseudohypacusis. In: Katz J, ed. *Handbook of Clinical Audiology,* 4th ed. Baltimore: Williams & Wilkins, 1994, 553–567.
8. Pracy JP, Walsh RM, Mepham GA, Dowdler DA. Childhood pseudohypacusis. *Int J Pediatr Otorhinolaryngol* 1996;37:143–149.
9. Aplin DY, Rowson VJ. Psychological characteristics of children with functional hearing loss. *Br J Audiol* 1990;24:77–87.
10. Aplin DY, Rowson VJ. Personality and functional hearing loss in children. *Br J Clin Psychol* 1986;25:313–314.

Bibliography

Campbell K. *Essential Audiology for Physicians.* San Diego, CA: Singular Publishing Group, 1998.

Gelfand SA. *Essentials of Audiology.* New York: Thieme Medical Publishers, 1997.

Goldenberg RA, ed. *Hearing Aids: A Manual for Clinicians.* Philadelphia: Lippincott-Raven Publishers, 1996.

Hall JW. *Handbook of Auditory Evoked Responses.* Boston: Allyn & Bacon, 1992.

Hall JW, Mueller HG. *Audiologists' Desk Reference.* Vol I. *Diagnostic Audiology Principles, Procedures, and Practices.* San Diego, CA: Singular Publishing Group, 1997.

Hall JW, Mueller HG. *Audiologists' Desk Reference.* Vol II. *Audiologic Management, Rehabilitation, and Terminology.* San Diego, CA: Singular Publishing Group, 1997.

Katz J, ed. *Handbook of Clinical Audiology,* 4th ed. Baltimore: Williams & Wilkins, 1994.

Martin FN. *Introduction to Audiology,* 6th ed. Boston: Allyn & Bacon, 1997.

Mendel LL, Danhauer JL, Singh S. *Singular's Illustrated Dictionary of Audiology.* San Diego, CA: Singular Publishing Group, 1999.

Northern JL, Downs MP: *Hearing in Children,* 4th ed. Baltimore: Williams & Wilkins, 1991.

Robinette MS, Glattke TJ, eds. *Otoacoustic Emissions: Clinical Applications.* New York: Thieme Medical Publishers, 1997.

Roeser RJ. *Roeser's Audiology Desk Reference.* New York: Thieme Medical Publishers, 1996.

Roeser RJ, Valente M, Hosford-Dunn H. *Audiology Diagnosis.* New York: Thieme Medical Publishers, 2000.

Stach BA. *Comprehensive Dictionary of Audiology Illustrated.* Baltimore: Williams & Wilkins, 1997.

Stecker NA: Central auditory processing: Implications in audiology. In: Katz J, Stecker NA, Henderson D, eds. *Central Auditory Processing: A Transdisciplinary View.* Boston: Mosby–Year Book, 1992, 117–126.

Electrical Response Audiometry 3

Electrical response audiometry (ERA), particularly brain stem audiometry, has become an important clinical tool for assessing auditory function. In this chapter, we review the basic principles of ERA and then describe the various techniques, emphasizing their clinical applications.

BASIC CONCEPTS OF ELECTRICAL RESPONSE AUDIOMETRY

The aim of ERA is to record the potentials that arise in the auditory system as a result of sound stimulation. The basic principles of recording the electrical potentials from the auditory system are the same for all potentials, although specific recording techniques vary depending on the potential being measured. Recording is difficult because auditory system potentials are minute compared with the background of electrical activity generated in other parts of the body, such as the brain, heart, and muscles.

The development of computers and other digital hardware to sample and average responses made it possible to extract the synchronous neural potentials arising from the auditory neural pathway in response to sound stimulation. The further development of small computer systems dedicated specifically to evoked potential averaging made it practical to record these potentials in a clinical setting. These commercially available systems can control the parameters of the stimuli and test procedures, perform simple averaging or more complex signal processing, as well as perform the normal functions of a microcomputer.

The basic equipment components for ERA are shown in a simplified block diagram in Figure 3-1. The stimulus generated depends on the types of responses that are to be recorded. For most types of recordings, the stimuli are short-duration acoustic signals. Variations of clicks, which are produced by applying short-duration (e.g., 0.1 millisecond) voltage pulses to a transducer (earphone or loudspeaker), and short duration pure tones called tone pips or bursts are the most commonly used stimuli. Such brief stimuli produce a synchronized discharge of neural elements in the auditory system. However, as reviewed later, amplitude- and/or frequency-modulated continuous tones are being used for an emerging ERA method.

The types and placement of electrodes to record the evoked potentials also vary with the types of responses that are to be recorded. Generally, the electrical activity is recorded differentially between one electrode placed either on the promontory, ear canal, scalp vertex, or forehead and a second electrode appropriately referenced to the first (eg, on the mastoid prominence or earlobe). A ground electrode may be placed anywhere on the scalp. The minute electrical activity these electrodes pick up is differentially amplified and filtered before being delivered to the computer for averaging or processing. In some systems, digital filtering can be performed in the computer after averaging to enhance the recording of the evoked potential. The simple response-averaging computer consists of a series of memory units, each receiving information a fraction of a second later than the one preceding it. Each point is like a small calculator capable of addition and subtraction.

The computer is triggered to begin a sweep (sequential processing of electrical activity over a period of time) each time a stimulus is delivered to the ear. The sweep length depends

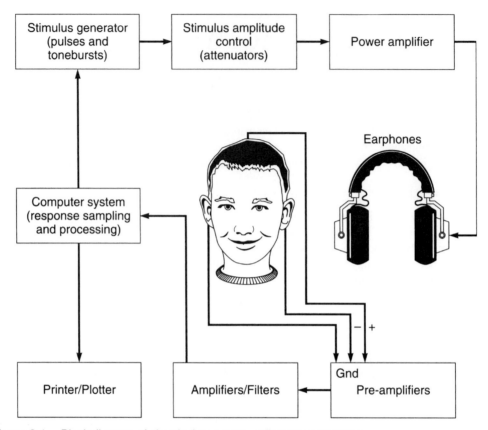

Figure 3-1. Block diagram of electrical response audiometry apparatus.

on the types of responses being recorded. A response to the stimulus is assumed to be time-locked to the stimulus and thus to the computer processing. Therefore, the response repeatedly occurs in the same group of memory locations. The electrical background noise that occurs during this response period is fairly random. Therefore, as more sweeps are averaged, the averaged residual noise in each memory location decreases.* By averaging many sweeps and reducing the background electrophysiologic noise, the auditory system response potentials that singly would be impossible to identify are extracted from the background electrical noise. The averaged response can be saved in a computer file, analyzed, and transferred to paper for inclusion in the patient's chart.

AUDITORY EVOKED POTENTIALS

Most of the important auditory evoked potentials and their probable sites of generation are outlined in Table 3-1. The actual sites of generation of some of these responses are not known, and there is still some controversy regarding these labels and the latencies. It is likely that there are multiple neural sites involved in the production of all of these responses. This table does not include the auditory steady-state evoked potentials (ASSEPs) that are

*For a description of averaging signals in noise, see Picton et al.[1]

TABLE 3-1. POTENTIALS EVOKED IN THE AUDITORY SYSTEM BY SHORT-DURATION SOUND STIMULATION: PROBABLE SITES OF ORIGIN, AND TYPICAL LATENCIES FOR MODERATELY HIGH LEVELS OF STIMULATION

  I. Cochlea (hair cells)
     Cochlear microphonic—immediate
     Summating potential—immediate
 II. Auditory nerve
     VIII nerve action potential (wave I) 2.0 msec
III. Brain stem
     Wave II—eighth nerve and cochlear nucleus 3.0 msec
     Wave III—cochlear nucleus and superior olive 4.1 msec
     Wave IV—lateral lemniscus 5.3 msec
     Wave V—inferior colliculus and fiber tracts 5.9 msec
 IV. Middle responses (auditory cortex)
     No—8 to 10 msec (variable)
     Po—13 msec
     Na—22 msec
     Pa—34 msec
     Nb—44 msec
  V. Vertex potential (auditory cortex)
     P1—50 msec (variable)
     N1—90 msec
     P2—180 msec
     N2—250 msec
     Mismatch negativity (MMN)—200 msec
     Sustained cortical potential
     Late positive component
     Contingent negative variation

Note: The basic principles for recording are the same in all electrical response audiometry. The techniques vary depending upon the response to be measured.

obtained with amplitude- and/or frequency-modulated continuous tones. ASSEPs are discussed later in the chapter. We cannot review all the potentials shown in Table 3-1. Measurements obtained from ERA methods are generally not measures of hearing per se. Hearing is a perceptual process that involves the entire auditory system and cannot be measured in terms of electrical responses unless those responses can be shown to relate directly to perception. The clinical value of ERA lies in the correlation of electrical responses with auditory pathology, performance, or both.

TYPES OF ELECTRICAL RESPONSE AUDIOMETRY

Three general techniques for recording the auditory evoked potentials have been described: electrocochleography, auditory brain stem response audiometry, and cortical electrical response audiometry. These techniques are compared in Table 3-2.

Electrocochleography

Electrocochleography (ECoG) measures the potentials arising within the cochlea and the auditory nerve: cochlear microphonic, summating, and the eighth nerve action potentials. The most sensitive recordings are obtained with a needle electrode placed through the tympanic membrane (transtympanic ECoG) on the bone of the promontory.[2]

Electrocochleography is the most accurate and sensitive of the ERA techniques by virtue of the close placement of the electrode to the generator sites. Accuracy also is enhanced because the peripheral auditory system is unaffected by sedation or general anesthesia.

TABLE 3-2.   [CE4]COMPARISON OF ELECTRICAL RESPONSE AUDIOMETRY TECHNIQUES

Technique	Electrode Placement	Effect of Anesthesia	Portion of Auditory System Tested	Reliability
Electrocochleography	Promontory or tympanic membrane or ear canal	None	Peripheral nerve and cochlea	Excellent
Auditory brain stem response	Surface	None	Brain stem and periphery	Good
Cortical evoked response	Surface	Marked	Entire, depending on response	Fair

An obvious disadvantage of this technique is the requirement for tympanic membrane penetration. Electrodes have been developed that can be placed into the ear canal or onto the tympanic membrane (extratympanic ECoG) with minimal discomfort; these avoid the need to penetrate the tympanic membrane. However, the amplitudes of the responses recorded from the ear canal are still greatly reduced in comparison to the transtympanic recordings. The tympanic membrane electrodes show better sensitivity and cause minimal or no discomfort to the patient. This electrode may circumvent this advantage of ECoG, although the amplitudes of the potentials are still much smaller than those recorded with the transtympanic electrode. Another limitation is that ECoG measures only the response of the most peripheral portion of the auditory system; therefore, it cannot be equated with hearing as such. Although relatively rare, there are cases in which the cochlea and auditory nerve function normally but brain stem or central defects produce hearing loss. Thus, it can be advantageous to use a technique that assesses only the peripheral end organ to localize the impaired part of the auditory system.

Auditory Brain Stem Response Audiometry

Auditory brain stem response (ABR) audiometry uses surface electrodes to measure the potentials arising in the auditory nerve and brain stem structures. Usually, one electrode is placed on the scalp vertex and one on the mastoid prominence or ear lobe of the test ear. The electrical activity is differentially recorded, amplified, and filtered from these two electrodes. The opposite mastoid is used as a ground. The events that occur during the first 10 to 15 milliseconds following sound stimulation are recorded. The advantage of ABR audiometry is that anesthesia is not required, because electrodes pasted on the surface of the scalp are used instead of an invasive penetrating electrode. In practice, however, either basal narcosis or anesthesia is often required in children to prevent excessive movement from interfering with accurate recordings. Auditory brain stem response audiometry, like ECoG, is not influenced by basal narcosis or general anesthesia.

Cortical Electrical Response Audiometry

Cortical electrical response (CER) audiometry measures the middle and slow potentials that arise in the auditory system above the brain stem. The simplest electrode configuration is the same as for auditory brain stem response audiometry. However, cortical potential studies often use arrays of 32 or more electrodes in a standard electroencephalography (EEG) configuration. Such studies are intended to determine the pattern of activity that is recorded at the surface of the head and/or where in the brain the neural activity is generated.

An advantage of CER audiometry is that, in measuring the most central responses, the entire auditory mechanism is tested. Responses can thus be best equated with clinical hearing. There are also some late potentials related to sound discrimination that may be important when there is a question of a central disturbance. A major disadvantage of this method is that the potentials are affected by sleep and sedation. Because of this, CER audiometry is less reliable for measuring threshold sensitivity in children and more difficult to perform in a clinical setting.

ELECTROCOCHLEOGRAPHY

Stimulation Techniques

The wide-band click is the stimulus most commonly used in ECoG. Acoustically the click is composed of many frequencies that stimulate the entire cochlea. In a flat hearing loss, the click is a good predictor of the audiometric threshold. In sloping or other configurations of hearing loss, however, one cannot predict the type of audiogram using click stimuli. Eggermont[2] has used tone bursts for ECoG and found them useful in predicting the behavioral audiogram quite accurately.

Recording Techniques

In the transtympanic approach, a standard Teflon insulated electromyographic recording needle is positioned onto the bone of the promontory after induction of anesthesia of the tympanic membrane by means of iontophoresis or topical phenol application. In the newest tympanic membrane approach, a small sponge connected to a wire and saturated with an electrolyte and a special catalyst is placed on the eardrum.[3,4] In most ear canal approaches, an electrolyte-saturated sponge is used. Responses are filtered below 30 Hz and above 3200 Hz. The computer is set to measure over a 10 millisecond window.

Measurable Potentials

Electrocochleography is a measure of the cochlear microphonic, summating, and eighth nerve action potential arising within the cochlea and the auditory nerve.

Cochlear Microphonic

The source of the cochlear microphonic (CM) is the hair-bearing surface of the hair cells. Its onset is immediate and it mimics the waveform of the acoustic stimulus. Because the response recorded from the promontory is diffuse and gives no definite information regarding specific populations of hair cells, most investigators do not find the CM clinically useful although its presence indicates stimulation of some functional hair cells. However, Gibson and Beagley[5] have used the CM to aid in differentiation of cochlear from retrocochlear lesions. They claim a tendency toward reduction in microphonics is associated with cochlear lesions, whereas in acoustic tumors the CM is often normal. Since the CM is not of primary interest in ECoG, recording of the other potentials free of the interfering CM can be obtained by alternating on each stimulus trial the phase of the click or tone burst. This results in phase cancellation of the CM as well as any electrical artifact that may contaminate the recordings.

Summating Potential

The summating potential (SP) also is generated by the hair cells and is a direct current (DC) shift of the baseline of the recording. It is almost always negative for all frequencies and intensity levels (Figure 3-2). This potential is thought to represent asymmetry in the basilar membrane movement resulting from a pressure difference between the scala tympani and the scala

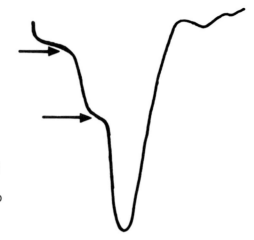

Figure 3-2. The summating potential is measured as the shift in the baseline recording superimposed on the descending limb of the compound action potential (arrows).

vestibuli during sound stimulation.[2] The source of this dc shift is also the hair cells. This potential may be a means of studying hair cells in Ménière's disease and other cochlear disorders.

Because the SP is superimposed on the eighth nerve action potential, its measurement is sometimes difficult. One technique for separating the SP from the eighth nerve action potential is to increase the click rate. As the rate of the click presentation increases, the eighth nerve action potential diminishes because the individual neurons do not have time to recover from their refractory period to respond again to the new stimulus. The SP is unaffected by the click rate. A recording is first done at a low click rate and the response, which comprises both the SP and the eighth nerve action potential, is stored in the computer. A second recording is then done with a high click rate. The response obtained represents primarily the SP. The second response can then be subtracted from the first response; the derived response will represent primarily the eighth nerve action potential devoid of the contaminating SP.

Compound Action Potential

The eighth nerve action potential is the averaged response of the discharge pattern of many auditory neurons. Cochlear dynamics, which influence the shape of the compound action potential, are complex and beyond the scope of this discussion.*

In most patients with normal hearing, an action potential can be elicited to within 5 to 10 dB of the patient's behavioral threshold. At high stimulus intensity, the potential is large, consistent, easily recordable, and reproducible. Action potentials are described by three parameters: latency, amplitude, and waveform. Latency is the time interval from the onset of the click to the maximal negative deflection in the action potential. Latency normally decreases systematically from approximately 4 milliseconds at threshold to 1.5 milliseconds at high intensity. Amplitude, on the other hand, characteristically increases in two steps: there is a gradual rise to the level of approximately 40 to 50 dB HL, where there is a plateau, followed by a second, more rapid increase in amplitude above that level.

By convention, latency and amplitude (as a percentage of maximal amplitude) are plotted in relation to stimulus intensity (Figure 3-3). The maximal amplitude and representative waveforms are plotted on the recording.

*See Eggermont, 1976,[2] for a comprehensive review of the subject.

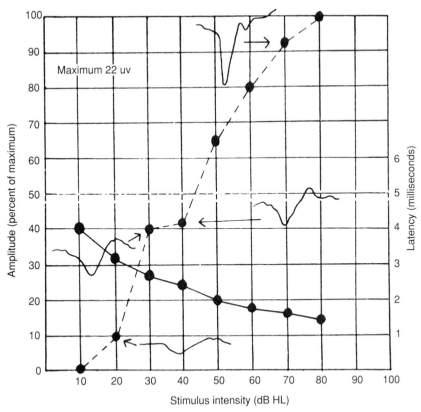

Figure 3-3.   Electrocochleographic input-output function graph. Amplitude as the percentage of maximal amplitude and latency are plotted against stimulus intensity. Representative waveforms are also shown.

Clinical Applications of Electrocochleography

There are three clinical uses for electrocochleography: threshold testing, the study of Ménière's disease, and the study of acoustic neurinomas.

Threshold Testing

Electrocochleography is the most accurate of the objective audiometric tests. Thresholds to the click are generally an indication of the audiometric threshold in the range of 3000 to 4000 Hz. The electrocochleographic threshold predicts the behavioral threshold to within 5 to 10 dB at this frequency in almost all cases. As stated before, however, one cannot predict the audiogram using clicks only; tone bursts produce a much better correlation to the subjective audiogram. The best correlation is found at frequencies of 1, 2, and 4 kHz, but correlation remains excellent at 500 and 8000 Hz. However, at high stimulus intensities, much of the cochlea can be activated by tone bursts, and correlations to the actual frequency regions of cochlear damage is problematic.

The disadvantage of using electrocochleography for threshold determination is the necessity for piercing the eardrum to place the needle electrode. It remains to be seen if recordings from the new tympanic membrane electrodes can provide sufficient electrocochleographic information. Recordings from canal electrodes may not provide sufficient sensitivity. At the House Ear Clinic in Los Angeles, ABR audiometry for threshold determination is used.

Ménière's Disease

The summating and compound action potentials may be useful in the study of Ménière's disease.

SUMMATING POTENTIAL   Eggermont[6] has found an increased negative summating potential during periods of hearing loss in the fluctuant hearing stage of Ménière's disease. He attributes this finding to either a mechanical displacement of the basilar membrane, which causes nonlinearities in its movement as a result of the presumed endolymphatic hydrops, or a metabolic disturbance resulting in a larger endolymphatic potential. As fixed hearing loss develops, the summating potential decreases, indicating a loss of hair cells. The summating potential may, therefore, be an indication of reversibility of the hearing impairment in Ménière's disease.

COMPOUND ACTION POTENTIAL   Compound action potentials in Ménière's disease are generally broad, most likely because of the contribution of a large negative summating potential. In a study of patients with Ménière's disease, approximately 50% demonstrated a distinctive type of eighth nerve action potential characterized by a tendency to form multiple negative responses.[7] We have not seen this type of response in other types of sensorineural hearing loss, and this may be a means of distinguishing endolymphatic hydrops. Some have suggested that special ABR recordings to clicks and high-pass noise masking may be correlated to Ménière's disease.[8]

Acoustic Neurinomas (Vestibular Schwannomas)

The compound action potential is of great interest in the study acoustic neurinomas or vestibular schwannomas. The compound action potential in acoustic neuromas is much broader than the normal potential. In our study by electrocochleography of 50 patients with acoustic neuromas, 85% had an abnormal action potential.[7] One of the major difficulties in using ECoG for tumor detection is that tumor patients often incur a cochlear loss as well, perhaps from vascular compromise by the tumor.[9] The conclusion derived from ECoG reflects only that there is cochlear involvement.

As observed in the following section, brain stem audiometry is a more accurate predictor of acoustic tumors, and we use it exclusively for this problem.

Future Applications of Electrocochleography

Because of the necessity of penetrating the tympanic membrane or the inconvenience of canal or tympanic membrane electrodes for ECoG, auditory brain stem response audiometry has replaced it in most clinics. However, if the tympanic membrane electrode can overcome the need for the transtympanic approach, there may be a renewed interest in ECoG. Threshold testing is nearly as accurate with auditory brain stem response audiometry as with ECoG provided that the auditory brain stem is normal. Auditory brain stem response audiometry is a more accurate predictor of retrocochlear pathology than is ECoG.

The future of ECoG lies in the study of cochlear and eighth nerve physiology and pathophysiology. Changes in cochlear microphonics and summating potentials indicate hair cell disease. As outlined earlier, study of the summating and compound action potentials are useful in assessing the state of the end organ in Ménière's disease.

Moffat et al.[10] has reported changes in these potentials during glycerol dehydration in patients with Ménière's disease. Gibson and colleagues[11] have demonstrated changes in these potentials with the administration of intravenous vasodilators. Electrocochleography is still, therefore, a useful tool in the study of cochlear disease.

AUDITORY BRAIN STEM RESPONSE AUDIOMETRY

Stimulation Techniques

As in ECoG, the stimulus most commonly used for ABR audiometry is a wide-band click. This stimulus presents the same limitations in brain stem audiometry as in ECoG in that the entire cochlea is stimulated, the audiogram cannot be predicted except in cases of flat hearing impairment. The majority of sensorineural losses are sloping with the loss greater in the higher frequencies. Therefore, errors might occur in predicting a more severe loss than is actually present because of preservation of low-tone hearing.

Relative frequency-specific stimuli, such as tone bursts, tone pips, filtered clicks, may also be used to elicit the brain stem responses. These stimuli give more frequency-specific information regarding the cochlea and may be used to estimate audiometric thresholds. However, moderate to high intensities can stimulate much of the cochlea, making it difficult to determine which parts of the cochlea are involved in the response.

The simultaneous addition of high-pass noise at various cut-off frequencies simultaneously and click stimulation is a means of assessing contributions from different areas of the cochlea. Using this technique, a good estimation of the audiogram based on place-specific cochlear function can be made. The principles of this and similar noise masking techniques are detailed later.

Recording Techniques

Standard electroencephalographic disc electrodes are attached to the vertex and both mastoids of the patient. The electrical activity over 10 to 15 milliseconds after stimulus onset is recorded differentially, usually from the vertex electrode (positive input to amplifier) and the mastoid electrode (negative input to amplifier) of the test ear. The mastoid of the non-test ear serves as the ground. The electrical activity is filtered with a passband from 100 Hz to 3 kHz, and this activity is amplified 100,000 times or more, because these potentials are generally less than a microvolt at the scalp surface.

Sedation is not used in adults or in small infants, who often sleep during the procedure. Uncooperative children weighing up to 25 lb are sedated with an intramuscular injection of a combination of meperidine (Demerol, 25 mg), promethazine (Phenergran, 6.25 mg), and chlorpromazine (Thorazine, 6.24 mg) per 1 mL; a maximum of 1 mL is used. Chloral hydrate (500 mg/5 mL) in an oral dose of 1 to 2 mL per 10 lbs may be used in place of injection.

Normal Brain Stem Responses

Transient Responses

A series of seven waves may be recorded from the vertex-mastoid electrode derivation during the first 10 to 15 milliseconds following moderately intense stimulation by transient signals such as clicks or tonebursts. These waves, labeled sequentially with Roman numerals, are thought to represent successive tracts, synapses, or both in the auditory pathway.[12] It is likely that there are multiple neural sites involved in the generation of these wave components. Generally, wave V is the largest and most consistent component observed at threshold intensities and is used in the clinical assessment of peripheral hearing (Figure 3-4).

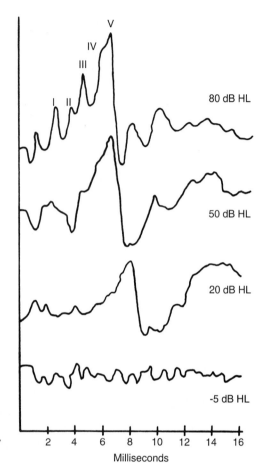

Figure 3-4. Normal brain stem responses (ABRs) to a broad-band click. Latency increases as click intensity decreases.

SN-10 Response

Davis and Hirsh[13,14] and Suzuki and coworkers[15,16] have described another response at around 10 millisecond after stimulus onset. Davis and Hirsh[13] have labeled this the SN-10 ("slow-negative") response and believe the generator is the primary auditory cortex.

Frequency-Following Responses

Like the cochlear microphonic response, the frequency following response follows the frequency of tonal stimulation.[17] It is distinguished from the cochlear microphonic by onset latency of about 6 milliseconds. This has led to the general consensus that its origin is in the region of the inferior colliculus. It is difficult to record the frequency-following response at frequencies above 2000 Hz.

Auditory Steady-State Evoked Potentials

Somewhat related to the frequency-following response, is the auditory steady-state evoked potential (ASSEP).* There are two main differences: (1) the amplitude and/or frequency of

*See brief review by Picton et al.[18]

the continuous tone is not constant but modulated at rates between 3 to 200 Hz and (2) the evoked response follows the frequency of modulation instead of the frequency of the tone. For example, if we present a continuous 1000 Hz tone amplitude modulated at a rate of 80 Hz, we will evoke neural activity that follows the 80 Hz modulation rate rather than the 1000 Hz carrier tone. Thus, unlike the frequency-following response, responses to high frequency tones can also be recorded by the ASSEP method. There have been several different names used in the early studies for this evoked potential. ASSEPs that originate in the brain stem can be obtained by using modulation rates 70 Hz or greater. Lower modulation rates will result in ASSEPs that represent both the brain stem and cortical areas. Widespread clinical use of this method will require the development of commercially available systems that will take care of the important and complex technical details concerned with stimulation, recording and analysis of ASSEPs.

Clinical Applications of Auditory Brain Stem Response Audiometry

There are several major clinical uses of brain stem audiometry: (1) screening neonates, in particular nursery intensive care unit infants who are at risk for hearing loss[19]; (2) threshold testing of infants, young children, and malingerers; (3) diagnosis of acoustic tumors (vestibular schwannomas); (4) diagnosis of peripheral neuropathies[20] and brain stem lesions; (5) intraoperatively monitoring of surgical procedures such as acoustic tumor removal, eighth nerve vascular decompression, vestibular nerve transections where the auditory nerve is at risk[21]; and (6) monitoring electrode placement of an auditory brain stem implant (ABI).[22]

Threshold Testing

Brain stem audiometry is used in cases in which standard behavioral audiometric techniques fail. This technique along with otoacoustic emissions (OAE) allows identification of hearing impairment in infancy so that rehabilitation can be started. As described above, wideband click stimuli stimulate the entire cochlea, and one cannot predict the audiogram except in cases of flat hearing impairment. Despite this deficiency, this is a valuable technique for early identification of hearing loss. If an error is made, it is usually in predicting a greater hearing loss than is actually present. In either case, early rehabilitation is begun.

Kodera et al.[23] and many subsequent investigators have claimed good correlation between the behavioral audiogram and brain stem audiometry using tone burst stimuli. As with the electrocochleography, the correlations are better for the high frequencies than the low. Use of these stimuli better predicts the pure tone audiogram than does use of broad-band click stimuli. This technique, however, is still deficient in accurately predicting low-frequency hearing.

Some studies have shown good correlation of the frequency following responses to low-frequency hearing thresholds. The disadvantage of the use of this response is that its amplitude is very small, especially for frequencies at 2 kHz and above, and it is difficult to separate artifact from the response. Instead, there has been a strong movement toward using ASSEPs. In particular, recent advancements have permitted the recording of SSEPs to eight different tonal stimuli presented simultaneously.[24] The simultaneous testing of eight different frequencies is accomplished by modulating each of the eight tones with a different modulation rate. Using eight frequencies simultaneously allows for more rapid data acquisition that should reduce test time.

As with the frequency-following response, there is still some question regarding the area(s) of the cochlea from which this response is initiated at moderate to high levels of stimulation. Nonetheless, reasonable estimates of the pure tone behavioral audiogram have been obtained.

We have applied a technique using clicks and high-pass masking noise in the same ear, which reasonably reconstructs the pure-tone audiogram.[25] This technique was first introduced in animal work by Teas et al.[26] and was later applied to ECoG by Elberling.[27]

The High-Pass Masking Technique

Don and Eggermont[28] and Parker and Thornton[29] have demonstrated that the entire basilar membrane contributes to the brain stem response to a broad-frequency click. The technique for deriving the contribution initiated from each portion of the basilar membrane is illustrated in Figure 3-5. In this figure, the cochlea is rolled out flat and marked off in sections A through F. Section A represents the area of the cochlea whose maximum sensitivity is 8 kHz and above; section B, from 4 to 8 kHz; section C, from 2 to 4 kHz; section D, from 1 to 2 kHz; section E, from 0.5 to 1 kHz; and section F, below 500 Hz.

A click stimulus presented at or above moderate hearing levels and above will stimulate the entire cochlea because of its broad-band spectral nature. The brain stem response R1, (line 1 of Figure 3-5), represents the sum of brain stem activity initiated by stimulation of the whole cochlea (ie, from sections A through F). Next, as seen in line 2, the level of continuous broad-band noise sufficient to desynchronize and thereby obliterate the response to the click is determined. This masked activity is denoted as MR.

After the appropriate noise level has been determined, the noise is steeply high-pass filtered at 8 kHz (the high-frequency components of the noise above 8 kHz is allowed to pass), and the clicks are presented in this noise. As seen in line 3 of Figure 3-5, the brain stem response, R2, obtained under these conditions results from click-synchronous activity initi-

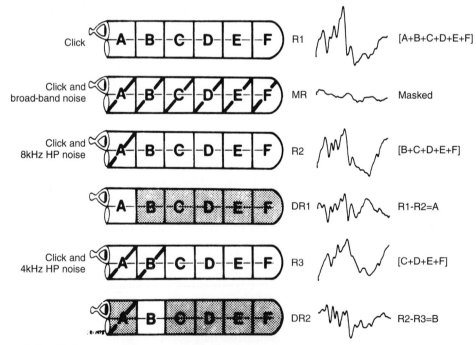

Figure 3-5. High-pass masking technique. See text for details.

ated from the unmasked region below 8 kHz. The subtraction of R2 from R1 results in the derived narrow-band response, DR1, seen in line 4. This subtraction procedure eliminates the common contributions from regions below 8 kHz (stippled area in line 4) and results in the contribution from the cochlea masked by the 8 kHz high-pass noise (section A). Next the high-pass cutoff of the noise is lowered by an octave to 4 kHz, and the clicks are presented in this noise. The brain stem response, R3, is recorded and is shown in line 5 of Figure 3-5. It results from click-evoked synchronous activity from the unmasked portion of the cochlea, that is, the region below 4 kHz. Subtraction of the response R3 from that obtained with the 8 kHz high-pass noise (R2) eliminates the common contribution from the region below 4 kHz (stippled area, line 6). The response derived from this subtraction (DR2) is initiated from the narrow-band region of the cochlea not masked by 8 kHz high-pass noise, but masked by the 4 kHz high-pass noise (section B). In similar fashion, by successive high-pass masking and subtraction of the responses, one obtains the derived narrow-band contribution to the brain stem response for the other sections of the cochlea. This procedure is repeated for different click intensities, and, in this manner the contribution from each portion of the basilar membrane at each intensity is derived.

In patients with normal hearing, contributions to the brain stem response to the click can be detected down to the 30 dB sensation level for the 8 kHz and above region and 500 Hz and below regions of the cochlea. Contributions to the brain stem response from octave-wide mid-frequency (1–6 kHz) regions can be detected down to at least the 10 dB sensation level. Differences in the threshold levels for a hearing-impaired patient and for individuals with normal hearing for each of the derived frequency regions are used as the estimate of hearing loss for estimating the audiogram.[25] The major advantage of this technique is that it provides information as to the place in the cochlea where losses occur, which is not always the case for techniques using tonal stimuli of moderate to high sound levels. The major disadvantages are that it requires more time than most other procedures, special filters for the masking noise, and equipment capable of storing and subtracting waveforms. However, these disadvantages are minor because most newer equipment employs hardware and/or software with these capabilities. The slight increase in testing time is offset by the accurate assessment of peripheral hearing function in very young or difficult-to-test patients made possible with this technique.

Other ABR techniques can be used in estimating the audiogram; some of these use noise-masking strategies. The advantages and disadvantages of these alternative techniques are reviewed elsewhere.[30] Also, there have been attempts to use ABR recordings to help fit hearing aids in children.[31]

Use of a Combination of Techniques

Another approach for estimating the pure tone audiogram is to combine various techniques. Davis and Hirsh[14] have proposed using ABRs to 2 and 4 kHz tone pips to estimate the audiogram at those frequencies. The later SN-10 response to 1 and 0.5 kHz tone pips is used to estimate the peripheral hearing at those frequencies. Moushegian et al.[17] have proposed using the ABRs to assess the more basal portions of the cochlea and the frequency-following response to assess the apical region.

Response Detection at Threshold

One of the major problems in threshold estimation is the recognition of a response near threshold. The need to interpret visually the presence of a response means that the method is neither entirely objective nor based on the parameters of the response only. There are methods to detect responses quantitatively to permit a truly objective definition of ABR threshold[32–36] and methods to form weighted averages that favor sweeps with good signal-to-noise ratios.[37,38] Although they must be clinically verified, combinations of these techniques promise objective, accurate prediction of the pure-tone audiogram.

Acoustic Neurinoma Diagnosis

Auditory brain stem response audiometry has proved to be the best audiometric test for acoustic tumor detection.[39] The success of ABR depends upon the fact that acoustic tumors stretch or compress the auditory nerve, producing a delay in the response latency that ABR can detect. This delay may occur in an ear with normal hearing. Conversely, cochlear lesions have little effect on the brain stem response latencies for high-intensity stimuli until the hearing loss becomes severe.[39]

There are several methods used to detect a delayed ABR caused by an acoustic tumor. The simplest method is to compare the suspected latency with a normal standard. This procedure will only detect delays that are greater than the normal latency differences among individuals, which can vary substantially. This limitation makes the measure too insensitive to detect the smaller acoustic tumors, which produce small time shifts. A better method is to compare the suspected latency with the latency of the opposite ear. This interaural difference in wave V latency, called IT5, will normally be 0 +/– 0.2 milliseconds (allowing for observational error). A typical data reporting form is shown in Figure 3-6.

False-positive findings are minimized by adjusting each observed wave V latency (T5) for delay caused by conductive hearing losses and the severe cochlear losses. In such cases we use an empirically derived formula for latency adjustment. For responses to our standard 80 dB nHL broad-band click, we deduct 0.1 millisecond for each 10 dB that the 4 kHz hearing loss exceeds 50 dB.

Conductive hearing losses increase ABR latency by reducing the physical stimulation to the cochlea. The stimulation to both cochleae should be equal for IT5 to be zero. By altering the stimulus levels to the two ears, thus equalizing the stimulation to the cochleae, one can use IT5 (though less reliably when there is a conductive component to the hearing loss associated with a suspected acoustic tumor).

A third method of using the ABR avoids the complications of cochlear and conductive loss delays but introduces other complications. This method focuses on the interval between the first and fifth waves. Prolongation of the I to V wave interval should reflect only the delay of propagation in the auditory nerve secondary to tumor compression. As with T5, this measure, T1-5, has greater significance when it is compared to the T1-5 of the opposite ear than when compared to a normal standard. We call this interaural difference IT1-5 and presume that for normal ears the expected value should be 0 milliseconds, just as for IT5. The +/– 0.2 millisecond variation from 0 that we accept as normal for IT5 will be exceeded more often because computation of IT1-5 requires four latency readings (and more observational errors) instead of the two needed for IT5. As a result, more false positive findings can be expected with IT1-5. Furthermore, sometimes a tumor will delay all waves I through V. Then IT1-5 can be normal while IT5 shows the delay.

A practical difficulty with IT1-5 occurs when wave I from surface electrodes cannot be recorded in patients with tumors or advanced hearing losses. To enhance the recording of wave I, electrodes may be placed on the earlobe, in the ear canal[40] on the eardrum[3,4] and on the promontory,[9] listed in order from least to greatest enhancement of wave I. Of these four

LATENCIES IN MS		BERA	THRESHOLDS	
	R	L		R	L

Panel 1

LATENCIES IN MS   BERA   THRESHOLDS

	R	L		R	L
T5	5.3	5.3	P5	20	20
Adj.	0	0	4kHz		
Net	5.3	5.3	A C	10	10
IT5	0		A/B Gap	0	0
T5-3	2.0	2.0			

Panel 2

LATENCIES IN MS   BERA   THRESHOLDS

	R	L		R	L
T5	5.3	5.9	P5	20	70
Adj.	0	.1	4kHz		
Net	5.3	5.8	A C	10	60
IT5	0.5		A/B Gap	0	0
T5-3	2.4	CNT			

Panel 3

LATENCIES IN MS   BERA   THRESHOLDS

	R	L		R	L
T5	5.3	5.5	P5	20	70
Adj.	0	.1	4kHz		
Net	5.3	5.4	A C	10	60
IT5	0.1		A/B Gap	0	0
T5-3	2.0	2.1			

Figure 3-6. Typical clinical ABR data reporting form for patient's chart.

positions, the eardrum may prove to be the best choice, since the promontory placement involves surgical procedures.

In general, we believe IT5 is the better single measure for acoustic tumor detection, except possibly when a conductive loss exists. Combination of the IT5 and IT1-5 can enhance detection.[9] A comparison of ABR with other standard neuro-otologic tests are shown in Table 3-3.

Tumor Size and Detection

Large acoustic tumors press against the brain stem. If significant pressure is exerted on the auditory tracts in the brain stem, abnormalities in the brain stem response are detectable when testing the opposite (nontumor) ear. This effect is best detected by measuring the interval

TABLE 3-3. FOUR SCREENING TESTS' FAILURES LISTED AS PERCENTAGES OF TEST PERFORMED

	Tests			
Results	ABR	X-ray	ENG	ART
Percent false-negative (tumor missed)	4	11	23	30
Percent false-positive (false alarm)	8	27	28	28

ABR, auditory brain stem response; ENG, electronystagmography; ART, acoustic reflex test.

between waves III and V. Normally, this interval, T_{3-5}, will be 1.9 ± 0.1 milliseconds; T_{3-5} of 2.1 to 2.8 milliseconds has been found on 71% of 55 patients with tumors larger than 3 cm. Thus, brain stem audiometry may predict not only the presence of an acoustic tumor, but also the general size of the tumor. Again, this is dependent on the location of the tumor and the extent of compression on the eighth nerve. There is some indication that derived ABRs using the high-pass noise-masking technique can sometimes help predict whether the tumor is in the internal auditory meatus or in the pontine angle.[41]

Until recently, these standard ABR measures were an important component of the clinical test battery for acoustic neuromas. In early studies, reported detection rates were in the range of 90 to 98%,[39,42–44] but these tumors were typically fairly large. Using estimates from computed tomography (CT) scans and surgical reports, Eggermont, et al.[9] examined the impact of tumor size on detection and concluded that tumors smaller than 1.0 cm (typically intracanalicular) often go undetected by the above standard clinical ABR methodologies. This conclusion is now supported by more recent, extensive studies comparing the sensitivity of this ABR methodology with gadolinium- (Gd-DTPA) enhanced magnetic resonance imaging (MRI).[45–51] Using standard peak and inter-peak latency measures, waveform morphology, or presence of waves, the ABR tests detected nearly 100% of all extra- and intracanalicular tumors larger than 1.0 cm. However, these standard latency measures detected 63 to 93% of intracanalicular tumors smaller than 1.0 cm. This wide range of detection rates is due to the different criteria selected.[44,45,47,48,50,52,53] Since many studies have demonstrated the inadequacy of standard ABR measures in the detection of tumors smaller than 1.0 cm, clinical practice has shifted to using MRI. Gd-DTPA MRI has now replaced contrast CT as the "gold standard" in the diagnosis of acoustic tumors. However, three major drawbacks of MRI compared to ABR are (1) current high cost, (2) poorer availability, and (3) patient comfort.

Recently, a new ABR measure, the stacked derived-band ABR amplitude, was shown to be sensitive to the presence of small intracanalicular tumors in patients and has excellent specificity for the absence of tumors in normal-hearing individuals.[54] Derived narrow-band responses, as described earlier, are required. The stacked ABR is constructed by (1) time shifting the derived narrow-band waveforms so the peak latencies of wave V in each derived narrow-band coincide and (2) adding together these shifted waveforms. Figures 3-7 and 3-8 illustrate the construction of the stacked ABR from the derived narrow-band ABRs. Figure 3-7 shows a series of derived narrow-band ABRs. The top trace is the unmasked response to the clicks. Notice that the successive responses from the basal to apical regions of the cochlea show a shift in latency. In Figure 3-8, the derived narrow-band responses are shifted to align the wave V peaks. The bottom trace is the stacked ABR representing the sum of the temporally aligned waveforms shown above it. Aligning the peak activity initiated from each segment of the cochlea synchronizes the total activity. Thus, as a first approximation, the

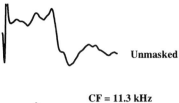

Unmasked

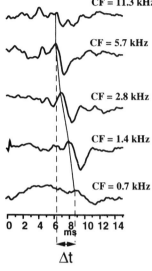

CF = 11.3 kHz

CF = 5.7 kHz

CF = 2.8 kHz

CF = 1.4 kHz

CF = 0.7 kHz

0 2 4 6 8 10 12 14
ms

Δt

Figure 3-7. The unmasked response (top trace) and a series of derived narrow-band ABRs obtained with the high-pass noise masking method using clicks. The unmasked response is essentially the sum of these derived bands. The theoretical center frequency (CF) of each band is also indicated. Note the time delay increases as the CF for the derived bands becomes lower.

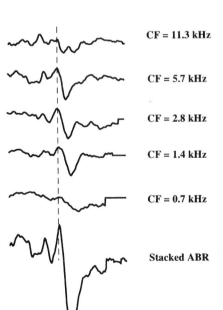

CF = 11.3 kHz

CF = 5.7 kHz

CF = 2.8 kHz

CF = 1.4 kHz

CF = 0.7 kHz

Stacked ABR

0 2 4 6 8 10 12 14
ms

Figure 3-8. Construction of the stacked ABR: The derived narrow-bands in Figure 3-7 are shifted so that the wave V peaks are aligned. The shifted waveforms are then added together to produce the stacked ABR (bottom trace). This better reflects the total activity than does the standard unmasked response and is more sensitive to the loss of neural activity.

amplitude (peak-succeeding trough) of the stacked ABR wave V reflects more directly the total amount of cochlear activity. As we have demonstrated,[54] small intracanalicular tumors 1 cm or less are detected. This method, in combination with standard ABR measures, appears promising both as a cost-effective approach to reducing the number of non-tumor patients imaged and as a method for acoustic tumor screening when MRI scans are unavailable, not appropriate because of patient comfort, or need to be justified because of their cost.

Conductive Hearing Losses

Conductive hearing impairments produce latency shifts that mimic acoustic tumors; standard audiometric tests to rule out conductive losses should first be performed. There have been efforts to record ABRs using bone-conducted signals to assess the extent of the conductive impairment. Although the techniques and interpretation are still problematic, there have been claims of useful clinical information derived from such recordings. Further research is still needed.

Use of ABR in the Neuro-otologic Evaluation

Our routine evaluation of suspected tumors includes petrous pyramid x-rays and ABR. If the x-rays show definite enlargement of the internal auditory canal on the suspect side or ABR is abnormal, a definitive study is obtained. We use MRI with Gd-DPTA as our primary definitive test for tumor diagnosis. If MRI is not available, CT with intravenous contrast is used. If the intravenously enhanced CT is normal, air contrast CT is necessary to exclude a small acoustic neurinoma. Occasionally, a small-dose Pantopaque study is necessary when air contrast CT is not diagnostic.

Nonacoustic Cerebellopontine Angle Tumors

In an early study of 28 patients with cerebellopontine angle tumors, brain stem audiometry identified the tumor in cases where there was pressure on the cochlear nerve. Because some nonacoustic lesions of the angle do not produce pressure on the cochlear nerve, the detection rate for non-acoustic tumors is not as good as that for acoustic neurinomas (Table 3-4).

Brain Stem Lesions

Brain stem audiometry is of distinct value in the diagnosis and localization of brain stem lesions. Intra-axial pontine masses that impinge on the auditory tracts cause loss of brain stem responses. The level of the mass can be predicted on the basis of the presence or absence of succeeding brain stem responses.[55] A number of studies have demonstrated that patients with multiple sclerosis often have abnormal ABRs.[56] For example, absence of brain stem responses may be an early indication of multiple sclerosis in a large percentage of those patients.[57] Lesions in the auditory tract produce desynchronization of the responses, which make them undetectable despite the presence in many cases of normal pure tone and speech audiometry.

TABLE 3-4.   DETECTION RATE FOR 28 NONACOUSTIC CEREBELLOPONTINE ANGLE TUMORS

Wave V: Normal, 25%
Wave V: Absent or delayed, 75%
      Meningiomas, 7 of 10
      Cholesteatomas, 4 of 5
      Facial nerve neurinomas, 2 of 4
      Arachnoid cyst, 1 of 1

It should be remembered that a given ABR abnormality is often found in many types of neuropathies such that a particular neuropathy cannot usually be diagnosed from the ABR abnormality alone.

CORTICAL ELECTRICAL RESPONSE AUDIOMETRY

At the present time, we do not use cortical responses in our clinical practice. Nevertheless, a brief review of possible clinical applications of these potentials is warranted.

Slow and Late Potentials

Initially, the vertex potentials were explored for threshold testing. Some reasons for recording these potentials are that (1) they represent activity of higher central levels and, therefore, are apt to reflect more of the "hearing process"; (2) stimuli more frequency-specific than clicks (eg, tone bursts) can be used to elicit a response; and (3) the responses are relatively large and require only a small number of trials. However, after a few years of research and application, it was evident that vertex potentials do not result in accurate threshold testing. They correlate well (within 10 dB of threshold) with the audiogram in waking adults, but are affected by the patient's physiologic state and by medications and anesthesia. More important, these responses are not reliable in children, the population most in need of an ERA technique. In general, the slow and late cortical potentials may be reliable in waking adults; in children these responses are unreliable for threshold estimation. Thus, these responses can occasionally be used for gross testing but must be interpreted with great caution. ABRs (clicks, tonebursts, modulated tones) are more appropriate for threshold testing.

The late potentials that signal cognition have been studied extensively[58]; in particular, the mismatch negativity (MMN) which can be evoked by physical differences in the acoustic or electrical stimuli.[59] The MMN is used to study acoustic and speech discrimination in a variety of patient populations. Currently, there is much interest in studying these potentials using brain-mapping techniques (topographical distributions and dipole source analyses). These analyses coupled with other brain-imaging techniques (functional MRI and positron emission tomography) may eventually be useful in understanding how and where in the brain sounds are processed and discriminated.

Middle Components

The use of slow and late cortical responses to measure threshold sensitivity was superseded by electrical responses in the range of 12 to 50 milliseconds. These middle-latency responses (MLRs) were thought to be more stable than the slow and late cortical responses and thus better for predicting thresholds of various frequencies when using clicks and filtered-tone pips. The long latencies of the MLR components do not generally allow stimulus rates greater than 10 per second. A special way of recording MLRs was developed that presents the stimuli at a faster rate, nearly 40 per second. At this rate, the MLR to one stimulus is not over before the next stimulus arrives. But the spacing of the stimuli is such that an early wave component of the MLR to a succeeding stimulus coincides with a late wave of the MLR to the previous stimulus. This superimposition of two response components results in a large amplitude component in the resultant recording and is called the 40 Hz response.[60] Research on the middle latency 40 Hz response indicates that, like the late and slow responses, it is sensitive to the subject's state.[61] Thus, threshold estimation using MLRs in sedated children is problematic.

Another major disadvantage of responses in this middle time domain is contamination by the myogenic responses. For threshold testing, whether the response is myogenic or neurogenic may be irrelevant as long as both responses are mediated by the auditory pathway. However, at high stimulus levels, some of these myogenic responses from the scalp muscles are thought to be mediated by other portions of the labyrinth.

Perhaps MLRs can be used to provide information on some level of processing and thereby aid in assessing central problems. Because of the difficulties in recording these later responses, the earlier surface-recorded brain stem responses are of much greater clinical usefulness.

EVOKED POTENTIALS TO ELECTRICAL STIMULATION

The advent of cochlear implants and their potential application in children has emphasized the need for studying evoked potentials to electrical stimulation. Both ABRs and MLRs and late cortical potentials including the MMN have been recorded to electrical stimulation[62–66] and may provide valuable diagnostic information about the potential value and functioning of the cochlear implant. Also, some cochlear implant systems, in addition to stimulation, allow recordings of the eighth nerve activity using the electrodes in the implant. The technique, referred to as neural response telemetry (NRT), is used to evaluate peripheral electrical stimulation by the implant.

CONCLUSIONS

Electrical response audiometry is an exciting field with broad implications in the otology, audiology, and neurology disciplines. At the present time, it is the best objective audiometric test for predicting hearing thresholds in infants or difficult-to-test patients.

Electrocochleography offers a means to study the function of the inner ear and to differentiate types of sensorineural hearing impairment. Auditory brain stem response audiometry is a valuable addition to the audiologic test battery for acoustic tumor diagnosis as well as threshold screening. It also offers a means of studying brain stem function in a variety of neurologic disorders including auditory neuropathy. Cortical potentials seem promising for studying hearing and cognition. Evoked potentials monitored during surgical procedures that may compromise the auditory nerve appear helpful and evoked potentials to electrical stimulation may provide additional information for assessing the value and performance of cochlear and brain stem implants. Finally, evoked potentials provide additional information that may be very useful in the otologic practice.

References

1. Picton TW, Hink RF, Perez-Abalo M, et al. Evoked Potentials: How Now? *J Electrophysiol Technol* 10:177, 1984.
2. Eggermont, JJ. Electrocochleography. In: Keidel WD, Neff WD, eds. *Handbook of Sensory Physiology*. Vol. V: *Auditory System*. Part 3: *Clinical and Special Topics*. Berlin: Springer-Verlag, 1976.
3. Stypulkowski P, Staller SJ: Clinical evaluation of a new ECoG recording electrode. *Ear and Hearing* 8:304, 1987.
4. Ferraro JA, Ferguson, R. Tympanic EcochG and conventional ABR: A combined approach for the identification of wave I and I-V interwave interval. *Ear and Hearing* 10:161–166, 1989.
5. Gibson WPR, Beagley HA. Transtympanic electrocochleography in the investigation of the retrolabyrinthine disorders. *Rev Laryngol* 97: 507, 1976.
6. Eggermont JJ. Summating Potentials in Meniere's Disease. *Arch Otorhinolaryngol* 22: 63, 1979.

7. Brackmann DE, Selters WA. Electrocochleography in Meniere's disease and acoustic neuromas. In: Ruben RJ, Elberling C, Salomon G, eds. *Electrocochleography.* Baltimore: University Park Press, 1976, 315.

8. Thornton ARD, Farrell G. Apparent travelling wave velocity changes in cases of endolymphatic hydrops. *Scand Audiol* 20:13, 1991.

9. Eggermont JJ, Don M, Brackmann DE. Electrocochleography and auditory brainstem electric responses in patients with pontine angle tumors. *Ann Otol Rhinol Laryngol* 89 (Suppl 75): 1–19, 1980.

10. Moffat DA, Gibson WPR, Ramsden RT, et al. Transtympanic electrocochleography during glycerol dehydration. *Acta Otolaryngol* 85:158, 1978.

11. Gibson WPR, Ramsden RT, Moffat DA. The immediate effects of naftidrofuryl on the human electrocochleogram in Meniere's disorder—preliminary findings. *J Laryngol Otol* 91:679, 1977.

12. Jewett DL, Romano MN, Williston JS. Human auditory evoked potentials: Possible brain stem components detected on scalp. *Science* 167:1517, 1970.

13. Davis H, Hirsh SK. A slow brain stem response for low-frequency audiometry. *Audiology* 18: 445, 1979.

14. Davis H, Hirsh SK. The audiometric utility of brain stem responses to low-frequency sounds. *Audiology* 15:181, 1976.

15. Suzuki T, Hirai Y, Horiuchi K. Auditory brain stem responses to pure tone stimuli. *Scand Audiol* 6:51, 1977.

16. Suzuki T, Horiuchi K. Effect of high-pass filter on auditory brain stem responses to tone pips. *Scand Audiol* 6:123, 1977.

17. Moushegian G, Allen RL, Stillman RD. Evaluation of frequency-following potentials in man: Masking and clinical studies. *EEG Clin Neurophysiol* 45:711, 1978.

18. Picton TW, Skinner CR, Champagne SC, et al. Potentials evoked by the sinusoidal modulation of the amplitude or frequency of a tone. *J Acoust Soc Am* 82:165, 1987.

19. Fria TJ. Identification of congenital hearing loss with the auditory brainstem response. In: Jacobson J, ed. *The Auditory Brainstem Response.* San Diego, CA: College Hill Press, 1985, 317.

20. Starr A, Sininger YS, Pratt H. The varieties of auditory neuropathy. *J Basic Clin Physiol Pharmacol,* 11(3):215, 2000.

21. Kileny P, McIntyre JWR. The ABR in intraoperative monitoring. In: Jacobson J, ed. *The Auditory Brainstem Response.* San Diego, CA: College Hill Press, 1985, 237.

22. Waring MD. Intra-operative electrophysiological monitoring to assist placement of auditory brainstem implant. *Ann ORL* 104(Suppl 166): 33–36, 1995.

23. Kodera K, Yamane H, Yamada O, et al. Brain stem response audiometry at speech frequencies. *Audiology* 16:469, 1977.

24. Lins OG, Picton TW, Boucher BL, et al. Frequency-specific audiometry using steady-state responses. *Ear and Hearing,* 1976:81, 1996.

25. Don M, Eggermont JJ, Brackmann DE. Reconstruction of the audiogram using brain stem responses and high-pass noise masking. *Ann Otol Rhinol Laryngol* 88(Suppl 57):1, 1979.

26. Teas DC, Eldredge DH, Davis H. Cochlear responses to acoustic transients: An interpretation of whole-nerve action potentials. *J Acoust Soc Am* 34:1483, 1962.

27. Elberling C. Action potentials along the cochlear partition recorded from the ear canal in man. *Scand Audiol* 3:13, 1974.

28. Don M, Eggermont JJ. Analysis of the click-evoked brain stem potentials in man using high-pass noise masking. *J Acoust Soc Am* 63:1084, 1978.

29. Parker DJ, Thornton ARD. Frequency-specific components of the cochlear nerve and brain stem evoked responses of the human auditory. *Scand Audiol* 7:53, 1978.

30. Stapells DR et al. Frequency specificity in evoked potential audiometry. In: Jacobson J, ed. *The Auditory Brainstem Response.* San Diego, CA: College Hill Press, 1985, 147.

31. Mahoney TM. Auditory brainstem response hearing aid applications. In: Jacobson J, ed. *The Auditory Brainstem Response.* San Diego, CA: College Hill Press, 1985, 349.

32. Elberling C, Don M. Quality estimation of auditory brainstem responses. *Scand Audiol* 13:187, 1984.

33. Don M, Elberling C, Waring M. Objective detection of the human auditory brainstem response. *Scand Audiol* 13:219, 1984.

34. Mason SM. On-line computer scoring of the auditory brainstem response for estimation of hearing threshold. *Audiology* 24:288, 1984.

35. Friedman J, Zapulla R, Bergelson M, et al. Application of phase spectral analysis for brainstem auditory evoked potential detection in normal subjects and patients with posterior fossa tumors. *Audiology* 23:99, 1984.

36. Dobie RA, Wilson MJ. Analysis of auditory evoked potentials by magnitude-squared coherence. *Ear and Hearing* 10:2, 1989.

37. Elberling C, Wahlgreen O. Estimation of auditory brainstem response, ABR, by means of Bayesian inference. *Scand Audiol* 14:89, 1985.

38. Hoke M, Ross B, Wickesberg R, et al. Weighted averaging-theory and application to electric response audiometry. *EEG Clin Neurophysiol* 57:484, 1984.

39. Selters WA, Brackmann DE. Acoustic tumor detection with brain stem electric response audiometry. *Arch Otolaryngol* 103:181, 1977.

40. Coats AC. Human auditory nerve action potential and brain stem evoked response latency-intensity functions in detection of cochlear and retrocochlear pathology. *Arch Otolaryngol* 104:709, 1978.

41. Eggermont JJ, Don M. Mechanisms of central conduction time prolongation in brain stem auditory evoked potentials. *Arch Neurol* 43:116, 1986.

42. Barrs DM, Brackmann DE, Olson JE, et al. Changing concepts of acoustic neuroma diagnosis. *Arch Otolaryngol* 111:17, 1985.

43. Bauch CD, Olsen WO, Harner SG. Auditory brain-stem response and acoustic reflex test. *Arch Otolaryngol* 109:522, 1983.

44. Josey AF, Jackson CG, Glasscock ME. Brainstem evoked response audiometry in confirmed eighth nerve tumors. *Am J Otol* 1:285, 1980.

45. Chandrasekhar SS, Brackmann DE, Devgan KK. Utility of auditory brainstem response audiometry in diagnosis of acoustic neuromas. *Am J Otol* 16:63, 1995.

46. Selesnick SH, Jackler RK. Atypical hearing loss in acoustic neuroma patients. *Laryngoscope* 103:437, 1993.

47. Kotlarz JP, Eby TL, Borton TE. Analysis of the efficiency of retrocochlear screening. *Laryngoscope* 102:1108, 1992.

48. Wilson DF, Hodgson RS, Gustafson MF, et al. The sensitivity of auditory brainstem response testing in small acoustic neuromas. *Laryngoscope* 102:961, 1992.

49. Levine SC, Antonelli PJ, Le CT, et al. Relative value of diagnostic tests for small acoustic neuromas. *Am J Otol* 12:341, 1991.

50. Josey AF, Glasscock ME, Musiek FE. Correlation of ABR and medical imaging in patients with cerebellopontine angle tumors. *Am J Otol* 9(suppl):12, 1988.

51. Ferguson MA, Smith PA, Lutman ME, et al. Efficiency of tests used to screen for cerebellopontine angle tumors: A prospective study. *Br J Audiol* 30:159–176, 1996.

52. Gordon ML, Cohen NL. Efficacy of auditory brainstem response as a screening test for small acoustic neuromas. *Am J Otol* 16:136, 1995.

53. Dornhoffer JL, Helms J, Hoehmann DH. Presentation and diagnosis of small acoustic tumors. Otolaryngol Head Neck Surg 111:232, 1994.

54. Don M, Masuda A, Nelson RA, et al. Successful detection of small acoustic tumors using the stacked derived-band ABR amplitude. *Am J Otol* 18:608, 1997.

55. Starr A, Achor J. Auditory brain stem responses in neurological disease. *Arch Neurol* 32:761, 1975.

56. Keith RW, Jacobson JT. Physiological responses in multiple sclerosis and other demyelinating diseases. In: Jacobson JT, ed. *The Auditory Brainstem Response*. San Diego, CA: College Hill Press, 1985, 219.

57. Stockard JJ, Stockard JE, Sharbrough FW. Detection and localization of occult lesions with brain stem auditory responses. *Mayo Clin Proc* 52:761, 1977.

58. Picton TW, Hillyard SA. Endogenous event-related potentials. In: *Handbook of Electroencephalography and Clinical Neurophysiology*. Vol. 3. *Human Event-Related Potentials*. Amsterdam-New York-Oxford: Elsevier, 1988, 361.

59. Näätänen R. The mismatch negativity: A powerful tool for cognitive neuroscience. *Ear and Hearing* 16:6, 1995.

60. Galambos R, Makeig S, Talmachoff PJ. A 40 Hz auditory potential recorded from the human scalp. *Proc Nal Acad Sci USA* 78:2643, 1981.

61. Shallop JK, Osterhammel PA. A comparative study of measurements of SN-10 and the 40/sec middle latency responses in newborns. *Scand Audiol* 12:91, 1983.

62. Starr A, Brackmann DE. Brainstem potential evoked by electrical stimulation of the cochlea in human subjects. *Ann Otol* 88:550, 1979.
63. van den Honert C, Stypulkowski PH. Characterization of the electrically evoked auditory brainstem response (ABR) in cats and humans. *Hear Res* 21:109, 1986.
64. Waring MD, Don M, Brimacomb JA. Assessment of stimulation in induction coil implant patients. In: Schindler RA, Merzenich MM, eds.

Cochlear Implants. New York: Raven Press, 1985, 375.
65. Kileny PR, Kemink JL. Electrically evoked middle-latency auditory Potentials in cochlear implant candidates. *Arch Otolaryngol Head Neck Surg* 113:1072, 1987.
66. Ponton CW, Don M. The mismatch negativity in cochlear implant users. *Ear and Hearing* 16:131, 1995.

The Vestibular System and Its Disorders

4

To understand the vestibular system and its disorders is to comprehend its applied anatomy, physiology, and biochemistry. The analysis of pathology and pathophysiology of the vestibular system leads to a diagnosis, but even today the most important aspect of that and of the management of patients with disequilibrium is the clinical history.

PHYSIOLOGY OF THE VESTIBULAR SYSTEM

The paired membranous vestibular portion of the inner ear consists of three semicircular canals at approximately right angles to each other: the lateral, where there is no medial; the superior, where there is no inferior; and the posterior, where there is no anterior. In addition there are two otolithic organs, the utricle and the saccule.

The neuroepithelium of the utricle and the saccule is found in a specialized region called the macula. The macula contains the otolithic membrane, an irregular and complex membrane composed in part of calcium carbonate crystals. *The otolithic membrane is sensitive to changes of motion relative to gravity, while the utricle is sensitive to linear acceleration.*

The three canals sit at right angles to each other, allowing response to angular acceleration in all planes. *They sense head rotation acceleration.* They are commonly referred to as the vertical canals and include the superior and posterior canals and the horizontal or lateral canal. Within the membranous ducts, a dilated portion contains the neuroepithelium responsible for the translation of mechanical stimuli into electrical neural stimuli. These dilated regions are referred to as the ampullae.

The crista is supported within an ampulla at right angles to its long axis. This bow- or saddle-shaped organ supports the mechanically sensitive hair cells that are responsible for initiation of the neural message from the vestibular apparatus. Suspended above the crista is a gel-like network called the cupula that extends across the ampulla. *This sail-like structure is exquisitely sensitive to motion.*

The hair cells that subserve the semicircular canals, the saccule, and the utricle are of two anatomic types. Type I hair cells are described as chalice-shaped, whereas type II cells demonstrate a boutonniere-shaped ending. Both types of hair cells contain numerous stereocilia embedded in a surrounding cuticular plate. Juxtaposing the tallest of the stereocilia but not fixed in the cuticle is a singular kinocilium. The kinocilium, in contact with the basal body of the hair cell cytoplasm, is semiflexible and is the ultimate determinant of the direction of polarization.

There is a resting basal discharge rate from the hair cells within the ampullae of the vestibular apparatus. When the kinocilium is deflected *away* from the stereocilia, the resting discharge rate is *increased.* Conversely, when the kinocilium is directed *toward* the stereocilia, the resting discharge rate is *decreased.* Therefore, in the lateral semicircular canal, ampullopetal (utriculopetal) endolymphatic flow causes displacement of the kinocilium toward the utricle and away from the stereocilia, thus increasing the discharge rate. Conversely, ampullofugal (utriculofugal) endolymphatic flow directs the kinocilium toward the stereocilia in the horizontal canal, resulting in a decrease in the basal firing rate of the responsive hair cells. Because of the orientation of the kinocilia and stereocilia in the vertical canals, ampullofugal movement results in an increase in the resting hair cell firing rate, and ampullopetal endolymphatic flow causes a decrease in the basal firing rate within the ampullae.

CLINICAL PRESENTATION OF VESTIBULAR SYSTEM DISORDERS

Patients with "dizziness" may have a multitude of presenting symptoms.

1. To some patients the symptoms of *dizziness* may mean any nonpainful discomfort related to the head, which could be cerebral, visual, gastrointestinal, or vestibular in origin.
2. *Vertigo* is an hallucination of movement of the patient's body or the patient's environment. The direction of motion is rotary or tumbling. The etiology is felt to be mainly vestibular but could be central.
3. *Unsteadiness* is a loss of equilibrium in relation to one's environment. It is described by the patient as "bumping into things" or the feeling of "almost falling." The etiology could be cerebral, cerebellar, vestibular, posterior columns, or pyramidal tract. A pure labyrinthine etiology seldom gives rise to unsteadiness without vertigo.
4. *Light-headedness* is a loss of equilibrium within one's head. It is poorly described by the patient, since the feeling defies the average vocabulary. Some describe it as a feeling of faintness. The etiology can be vestibular, cerebral, cardiovascular, or metabolic.
5. *Drop attack*. The patient loses extensor powers and falls to the ground suddenly, severely, and with no warning. There is no loss of consciousness and complete recovery occurs almost immediately. This is a variant of Ménière's syndrome called crisis of Tumarkin.

With problems of disequilibrium, the ability to give clear-cut historical information depends on the patient's vocabulary and previous experience with vestibular stimulation. Some may express being "just dizzy"; others may feel a rotational experience. With yet others there is an illusion of movement of the environment without rotation. The sensation of walking on a cloud or a floating feeling are other expressions of symptoms that are often referable to abnormalities in the vestibular system. A pure labyrinthine disorder rarely if ever causes loss of consciousness.

The main step in evaluating the patient with dizziness is to obtain a good history, including past illnesses, family, allergy, medication, dietary, and smoking histories. If the dizziness occurs in spells, then it is important to ascertain the elements of the spells.

Onset	First spell: date and time of day
	Frequency at this time
	Was there a change in frequency and when?
Duration	First spell
	Current spells
	Was there a change in duration and when?
Severity	Includes a description of the symptom in understanding the severity
	Was there a change in severity and when?

| What makes the symptom worse? | Sitting, lying, standing, moving, rolling in bed, getting up, food, medications, anxiety, stress |
| What makes the symptom better? | Sitting, lying, standing, food, medication |

If the dizziness is not in spells, then the elements need to be documented in the patient's words.

A complete ear, nose, throat, and neurologic examination that includes observation for spontaneous nystagmus in three directions of gaze, either through Frenzel glasses (+20 lenses) or other methods, may be followed by other studies, such as audiometric tests, mastoid and internal acoustic meatus view, caloric tests, or electronystagmography (ENG). Positional testing is performed if the symptoms are questionably induced or provoked when the patient assumes a particular position. One should note that a sudden change of position may aggravate the symptoms in any type of dizziness without necessarily implying a disease of labyrinthine origin or positional vertigo. A feeling of light-headedness upon rapidly assuming an upright position does not indicate a labyrinthine or vestibular disorder.

Gaze Nystagmus

First-degree gaze nystagmus is present when the nystagmus beats in the direction of the gaze. Second-degree nystagmus is present on straight gaze and on gaze in the direction of the fast component. Third-degree nystagmus is in all three directions of gaze.

When testing for gaze nystagmus, one does not bring the patient to a complete lateral gaze, as it induces fatigue or "endpoint" nystagmus. The patient is tested with the eyes in a straight gaze, 20 to 30° to the left and 20 to 30° to the right.

Vestibular or labyrinthine nystagmus has slow and quick components. The slow phase of nystagmus is the direction of the flow of the endolymph and is vestibular in origin. Since the excursion of the eyes is limited by the anatomy, the *reticular formation corrects the slow phase* by quickly returning the eyes to the last field of gaze. By convention, *the direction of the nystagmus is determined by the fast component.*

Nystagmus is classified into four categories:

Gaze	Nystagmus present when looking to the left or right
Induced	Nystagmus elicited by stimulation (eg, caloric, rotation, head-shaking)
Positional	Nystagmus elicited by assuming a specific position as during positional testing
Spontaneous	Nystagmus present without positional or other labyrinthine stimulation

Nystagmus can be pendular. *Pendular nystagmus eye movements are of an equal velocity in each direction.* These eye movements are seen with central or oculomotor abnormalities, such as congenital nystagmus, albinism, miner's nystagmus, and multiple sclerosis.

Labyrinthine spontaneous nystagmus can be suppressed by fixation. Thus, it is more pronounced when the eyes are closed. Central spontaneous nystagmus is not suppressed by fixation. In fact, central spontaneous nystagmus that is present during fixation may be eliminated during eye closure. *Failure to have fixation suppression is a central sign.*

In vestibular physiology, the word *central* means central nervous system (CNS). An acoustic neuroma or vestibular neuronitis affects the acoustic nerve. They are classified as peripheral problems unless the acoustic neuroma is so large that it affects the brain stem or cerebellum. On the other hand, in auditory brain stem response (ABR) terminology, *retrocochlear* includes the acoustic neuroma, which is retro to the labyrinth.

When a pathology causes "less function" of the peripheral system, it is called a *paralytic* situation. In this situation, the spontaneous nystagmus beats away from the involved side. Examples of this include acoustic neuroma and vestibular neuronitis. In Ménière's disease, it is an irritative phenomenon, and the spontaneous nystagmus is toward the diseased ear. In the case of a patient with bilateral chronic otitis media with cholesteatoma and severe vertigo, it is paralytic. Therefore, the spontaneous nystagmus beats away from the ear, thereby causing the vertigo.

Dix-Hallpike Positional Testing

Positional nystagmus is nystagmus elicited clinically during positional testing with the eyes open or under ENG monitoring with the eyes closed.

Test Technique

1. Sit the patient on a bench in an upright position with arms folded.
2. Reassure the patient that he or she is not going to fall regardless of sense of direction. Insist that it is of utmost importance to keep the eyes open during the clinical test so that the tester can observe the eyes. The eyes are closed during ENG monitoring.
3. Bring the patient backward swiftly with head hanging. Watch for nystagmus induced by assuming this position. Notice (1) the latency between assuming the position and the onset of nystagmus, (2) the character and direction of nystagmus, (3) the duration of the nystagmus. (If the nystagmus has a rotary component, it is classified as clockwise or counterclockwise, as illustrated in Figure 4-1. If performing an ENG, measure the slow-phase velocity.)
4. Bring the patient back to the upright position after the nystagmus has stopped and observe (1) the direction of the nystagmus, (2) the duration of the nystagmus, and, in ENG testing, (3) determine the slow-phase velocity.
5. Repeat steps 3 and 4 except that now the patient's head is positioned with the left ear down in step 3.
6. Repeat steps 3 and 4 again except that now the patient's head is positioned with the right ear down in step 3.

This test has many implications; however, the only practical clinical application to date is separation of positional vertigo of the benign paroxysmal type from positional vertigo

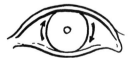
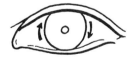

Clockwise rotatory nystagmus

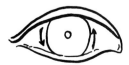
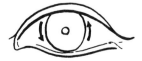

Counterclockwise rotatory nystagmus

Figure 4-1. Rotatory nystagmus.

secondary to CNS disease (Table 4-1). Characteristics of positional vertigo of the benign paroxysmal type are:

1. The nystagmus elicited is rotary.
2. If the left ear is the pathologic ear, the patient manifests a clockwise rotary nystagmus when assuming the left-ear-down position.
3. There is a latency of 5 to 15 seconds between assuming that position and the onset of nystagmus.
4. The nystagmus fatigues out (stops after a while).
5. Upon resumption of the upright position, the patient may manifest a nystagmus in the opposite direction.
6. On repeat testing without rest in between, the positional nystagmus can no longer be elicited.

Positional Testing

In simple positional testing, the patient is placed in a supine position, then on the left side with the left ear down, the head *NOT* hanging; then on the right side with the right ear down, the head *NOT* hanging.

The nystagmus can be seen clinically with the eyes open or recorded under ENG monitoring with the eyes closed. The nystagmus elicited can be classified according to Nylen's classification or as modified by Aschan.

Nylen's Classification

Type I   The direction of nystagmus varies with the position of the head during positional testing.

Type II   The direction of nystagmus remains fixed regardless of the position of the head during positional testing. When present in different head positions, the nystagmus is stronger in a particular position.

Type III   The nystagmus is irregular, characterized by variations in its behavior. Thus, it is sometimes direction-changing or direction-fixed, or it changes its direction with the same head position. Type III is used to label all forms of positional nystagmus that cannot be classified under type I or type II.

Clinical Correlation

Type I   Implies a CNS disorder (eg, multiple sclerosis or cerebellar tumor).
Type II   Implies a possible peripheral lesion.
Type III   Nonlocalizing significance.

TABLE 4-1. COMPARISON OF THE FEATURES OF PERIPHERAL AND CENTRAL NYSTAGMUS

Feature	Peripheral	Central Eliminate
Latency	5–15 sec	No latency
Persistence	Disappears within 50 sec	Lasts >1 min
Fatigability	Disappears on repetition	Repeatable
Position	Present in one head position	Present in multiple head positions
Vertigo	Always present	Occasionally absent
Direction of nystagmus	One direction	Changing with different head positions
Incidence	85% of all positional vertigo	10–15% of all positional vertigo

Aschan's Classification

Type I   The nystagmus is nonfatigable and persistent; its direction changes with head position.

Type II   The nystagmus is nonfatigable and persistent; its direction remains fixed with a change of head position.

Type III   All varieties of transitory positional nystagmus with latency and fatigue are included.

Clinical Correlation

Type I   Mostly CNS disorders.

Type II   Possible end-organ lesion, but mainly CNS disorders.

Type III   Peripheral disease; usually indicating positional vertigo of the benign paroxysmal type.

Fistula Test

In the presence of fistula, stimulation of the ear with positive pressure causes a nystagmus whose fast component is directed to that ear, whereas negative pressure brings about a nystagmus whose fast component is directed away from that ear. The presence of nystagmus may be accompanied by vertigo. It is the presence of nystagmus that is significant in this test. If the patient is experiencing vertigo without nystagmus of the type mentioned, he or she could be undergoing a cool caloric stimulation without a positive fistula test.

Example: When a fistula is present in the right ear, stimulation of this ear with positive (+) pressure produces nystagmus to the right and negative pressure produces nystagmus to the left.

STIMULATION TESTS USED TO TEST FOR PATHOLOGY OF THE VESTIBULAR SYSTEM

Cool Caloric Test of the Right Ear

The results of caloric stimulation of the right lateral semicircular canal (SCC) must be examined. A caloric stimulus cooler than body temperature is applied to the right external auditory canal with the lateral SCC placed vertically. Placing the lateral SCC in a vertical plane, elevating the head 30° from the supine position, or tilting the head back 60° in the upright position causes a flow of endolymph in an ampullofugal or utriculofugal direction. The lateral SCC hair cell electrical discharge is decreased or abolished, which reduces the electrical potential of the ipsilateral vestibular nuclear cells. The vestibular nuclear cells sampled on the contralateral side of the brain stem show a corresponding increase in electrical potential. When this electrical potential difference occurs across the brain stem, the medial longitudinal fasciculus (MLF) is stimulated. This, in turn, stimulates the oculomotor nuclei, particularly the III and VI cranial nerves, for lateral SCC stimulation and horizontal eye movement (nystagmus).

Similar to the resting discharge of the hair cells, the extraocular muscles of the eyes have a constant group of muscle fibers in contraction. By altering the extraocular muscles in contraction and in relaxation, the eye will move. Thus, with increased potential on the left side of the brain stem, there is relaxation of the medial rectus of the right eye and lateral rectus of the left eye. This has a corresponding increase in contraction of the lateral rectus of the right eye and medial rectus of the left eye that results in slow eye movement to the right. When the eyes reach a critical deviation to the side, a feedback input (probably through the oculomotor motor system to the prepontine reticular formation) evokes the rapid corrective fast component of nystagmus. By convention *nystagmus is named by its fast component.* As the head is rotated to the right, the endolymph rotates to the left, which is manifest as the slow phase of the nystagmus. When the eye snaps back, it is recorded as the fast phase of the nystagmus.

When the right ear is stimulated with cool water, the fluid contracts and becomes heavier. When the patient's head is elevated 30° from the supine position, the lateral SCC is in the vertical plane, causing the fluid to drop and displace away from the ampulla. This action corresponds to the slow phase of the nystagmus. *Stimulating the right ear with warm water will cause the opposite reaction to occur.*

Cool Caloric Test of the Left Ear

If the left ear is stimulated with water cooler than body temperature, a right beating nystagmus is produced. Stimulating the right ear with water warmer than body temperature results in an ampullopetal or utriculopetal movement of the endolymph. This endolymph flow deflects the stereocilia toward the kinocilia. This action increases the electrical discharge of the lateral SCC hair cell population over the resting potential. In the brain stem, there is an increase in the potential of the ipsilateral vestibular nuclear cells receiving input from the SCC and a corresponding decrease in the potential of the contralateral vestibular nuclei. The situation reproduces the events of the brain stem similar to a cool water stimulus in the left ear. Thus, the right-beating nystagmus produced by cool water in the left ear is the same as that produced by warm water in the right ear.

If water of 30°C or 44°C is irrigated simultaneously into both ears and if the response in both sets of hair cells is equal, no nystagmus occurs. The change in the output from the hair cells on each side is transmitted to the brain stem and summated by the vestibular nuclear cells, resulting in equal electric activity across the brain stem vestibular nuclei; therefore, the MLF is not stimulated and no nystagmus is produced.

Simple Caloric Test

The caloric tests have been recognized as the most beneficial in vestibular diagnosis. Each ear should be stimulated by water warmer and cooler than body temperature. A bithermal stimulus (30°C and 40°C) applied to the same ear can stimulate and produce an opposite direction of beating of nystagmus. The cool stimulus will produce nystagmus whose fast phase is away from the stimulated ear. The warm stimulus will produce nystagmus whose fast phase is toward the stimulated ear.

The simple caloric test may be performed by different methods. It is a qualitative test measuring the response between the right and left ears. It does not matter which method is used provided that the physician is familiar with the method and its clinical implications and limitations. It is important that the irrigating fluid reaches the tympanic membrane and is not just reflected by the anterior osseous canal or impacted cerumen. This is an especially crucial point if small amounts of water are used.

To determine the function of the vestibular apparatus, one can measure the duration of the nystagmus or the number of beats per unit time. For an ENG test, calculate the velocity of the slow phase of the nystagmus.

The test, as devised by Kobrak (Kobrak test) to measure the latency and duration of nystagmus, uses 0.2 to 5.0 mL of ice water instilled against the tympanic membrane of the patient in a sitting position with the head tilted 60° back. Other tests include Veit's minimal caloric test, Linthicum's minimal caloric test, Bárány's mass caloric test, and Dundas-Grant's cold air test for patients with perforated tympanic membranes.

Laboratory Methods of Testing the Vestibular System

Any test of the vestibular system without an electrical recording of nystagmus behind closed eyes may mislead the clinician in the proper management of the patient.

Electronystagmography (ENG) is an electronic method of producing a permanent record of eye movement. It is an objective means of studying the vestibulo-ocular reflex based on the difference in potential between the cornea (+) and the retina (−). Movement of the corneoretinal potential (an electrical potential between the cornea and the retina) in the recording field of the electrodes allows for the measurement of eye movement. The electronic recording of the nystagmus is the ENG value.

As with any procedure, the technician or physician should explain all aspects of the procedure as it progresses to relieve apprehension and act as a form of constant alerting for the patient.

1. The patient is seated on the ENG table, and the ears are examined for obstructing cerumen, tympanic membrane perforations, or the presence of prior mastoid surgery.
2. Electrodes are placed as shown in Figure 4-2 (A–E). The grounding electrode is placed above the bridge of the nose. To record horizontal nystagmus, place the electrodes at points B and E, as close as possible to the outer canthus of each eye. To record vertical nystagmus, place the electrodes at points A and C, above and below an eye.
3. By convention and calibration, an upward swing of the pen indicates eye movement to the right, and a downward swing indicates eye movement to the left.
4. The patient lies supine with the head elevated 30°. The patient is 8.5 feet from the wall and gazes at points A, B, and C for calibration (Figure 4-3). Once calibrated, the cor-

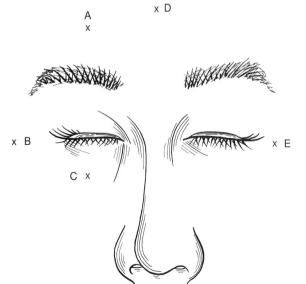

Figure 4-2. Electrode placement for ENG. AC, vertical axis; BE, horizontal axis; D, grounding.

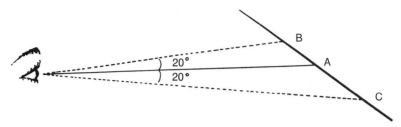

Figure 4-3.   Points of gaze for ENG calibration.

neoretinal potential may vary with the amount of light stimulation to the eyes. Thus, it may be necessary to periodically recalibrate the gain during the test. The effect of the corneoretinal change can be circumvented by having the patient regularly open the eyes during the test to "recharge" the potential.

5.   *During calibration, if a patient has more than 50% overshoot, it suggests a cerebellar or brainstem lesion.*

6.   Recordings are then taken with the eyes open and closed to check for spontaneous nystagmus.

7.   ENG recordings can be obtained from the rotation test, positional test, and so on. The patient is moved into various positions to determine if nystagmus can be recorded. Nystagmus may occur in only one position, in combinations of positions, or in all of the positions. The nystagmus may be beating in the same direction or may change in one or more positions. The velocity of the nystagmus may change significantly from one position to the other. Turning the head on the body (neck torsion) may also produce nystagmus, turn off or change the direction of pre-existing nystagmus, or enhance any nystagmus already present by lying on that side. The presence of nystagmus in any of these positions is abnormal. The significance as to the site or cause of the abnormality is not clear. Any form of spontaneous, positional, or positioning nystagmus that is present is abnormal. It may not represent a serious problem or it may be the only clue to substantiate an organic vestibular disorder.

8.   *In alternate binaural bithermal stimulation* the patient is then irrigated with 250 mL of water at 30°C and 250 mL of water at 44°C in turn in each ear, as outlined in the Fitzgerald and Hallpike test.

When interpreting an ENG, one can compare the following:

1.   The duration of nystagmus present
2.   The number of beats per unit time
3.   The velocity of the slow phase

The velocity of the slow phase is considered to be the most accurate predictor as to the etiology of the disease, and directional preponderance can give further diagnostic clues. In order to have a significant classification, the velocity of the slow phase needs to be at least 8° per second. If the total of the slow phase velocity of all alternate binaural bithermal caloric stimulations is less than 30° per second, there is bilateral weakness. A *hyperactive caloric response* has no diagnostic value.

Directional Preponderance Test

Directional preponderance is believed to be toward the side of a central lesion and away from the side of a peripheral lesion. To determine directional preponderance, Fitzgerald and Hallpike used the following system.

The patient is placed supine with the head elevated 30°. Each ear is douched in turn with no less than 250 mL of water at exactly 30°C (86°F) and 44°C (112°F). At least 5 minutes must elapse between each douche. Directional preponderance is calculated as follows:

1. Right ear irrigated with cold H_2O: duration of nystagmus to (L) = a
2. Right ear irrigated with warm H_2O: duration of nystagmus to (R) = b
3. Left ear irrigated with cold H_2O: duration of nystagmus to (R) = c
4. Left ear irrigated with warm H_2O: duration of nystagmus to (L) = d

If a + b is less than c + d, the right ear is hypoactive. If a + d is less than b + c, there is directional preponderance to the right.

Another method of calculating directional preponderance is by comparison of the velocity of the slow phases of the right- and left-beating nystagmus.

Right-beating	Left cold + right warm / total $\times$ 100% = x%
Left-beating	Right cold + left warm / total $\times$ 100% = y%

If x% is greater than y%, there is a right directional preponderance. According to Jongkee's formula, to be significant, the difference between the right-beating nystagmus and the left-beating nystagmus needs to be 25 to 30% or more.

Massive Caloric Test

Symptomatic patients after destructive inner ear surgery or with apparent absent caloric function on bithermal testing may require further testing. A search is made for any residual function, and a massive caloric stimulus may demonstrate this function. Two temperatures of water are used: ice water and water at 46 to 48°C. The recorder remains on during the entire stimulus time. The volume delivered is about 300 mL in about 30 seconds for each stimulus. A search is made for the production and reversal of nystagmus as a demonstration of residual caloric function. Since only the integrity of the lateral SCC is examined, when the massive test fails to stimulate any residual function, any further management decisions require information from other tests.

Ocular Fixation Suppression/Failure of Fixation Suppression

When the caloric-induced nystagmus is intense, opening the eyes should reduce or eliminate the nystagmus by ocular fixation or attempted fixation. This occurs with a normal vestibular system or in one with a peripheral vestibular disorder. In some central lesions, the caloric-induced nystagmus does not appear until the eyes are opened. The nystagmus may also significantly increase when the eyes are opened or show no signs of suppression of the already present induced nystagmus. The test should be performed on all four caloric responses to the alternate binaural bithermal stimulus. When present, failure of ocular fixation suppression is a reliable sign of a central disorder.

TRACKING TESTS

An asymmetrical *optokinetic tracking* suggests a central lesion. An abnormal *sinusoidal tracking* (ie, one with jerks and saccades), implies a central lesion. However, there is a high rate of false-positive results. A *normal gaze accompanied by asymmetrical optokinetic nystagmus* suggests a cerebral hemisphere lesion. The predominant optokinetic response beats toward the side of the lesion. An *abnormal gaze accompanied by asymmetrical optokinetic nystagmus* suggests a brainstem or cerebellar lesion.

ROTATIONAL TESTING

Harmonic Acceleration Testing

Since it is less accurate than it is sensitive, harmonic acceleration testing should be used in conjunction with conventional vestibular evaluation. It monitors the progression of the central compensatory mechanism, which is responsible for the reduction or elimination of dizziness symptoms. It also aids in the discovery of an abnormally functioning vestibular system unrecognized by conventional vestibular testing. Caloric testing mainly assesses the horizontal semicircular canal. The harmonic acceleration test increases diagnostic sensitivity in about 1 to 2% of patients who may have formally been classified as "psychogenic vertigo." Patients in this group show abnormalities of phase, symmetry, or both.

Testing is performed in a darkened enclosure. The sinusoidal harmonic rotational stimulus stimulates several frequencies in the range of 0.01 to 1.0 Hz. The peak velocity is in the range of 50° to 60°/sec. Three parameters are derived by the computer: the gain, the phase, and the symmetry.

The gain is a ratio of the peak amplitude of the chair speed compared to eye speed. The gains are expected to be within a normal range in an adequately functioning vestibular system. When the gains are insufficient at all frequencies and the alerting was adequate, then an ototoxic or central processing abnormality explains the findings. The phase is the relationship of the peak response of the slow component eye movement compared to the peak velocity of the chair. The phase can lead or lag. At the lower frequencies, the normal response is to lead; while at the higher frequencies, there is no lead or lag. Abnormal phases occur when they deviate from the norm. Abnormal phase leads at the low frequencies are seen with peripheral vestibular disorders. Abnormal phase leads for all the frequencies are common indicators of central lesions. Lags occur in peripheral vestibular disorders or in the presence of poor gains.

Because the abnormalities found on conventional vestibular tests remain the same over a period of time regardless of the course of the symptoms, the symmetry of the rotational response has become important. The symmetry of the response is examined for direction of the nystagmus. When there is a more than normal preponderance of nystagmus in one direction, this is considered abnormal symmetry. When the abnormal symmetry is present at the outset of treatment, it can be used as a monitor of the changing vestibular function. As the patient improves, the symmetry may be less abnormal or revert to normal. If there is no benefit from a treatment, then the symmetry may remain unchanged or become more abnormal.

There are two possible explanations for normal symmetry with significant symptoms. The first occurs where the location of the vestibular symptoms in a vestibulo-ocular reflex arc does not include the lateral semicircular canals and their central connections. The second explanation is found where there is a greater metabolic factor in the production of the symptoms.

Vestibular Autorotational Testing/Head Autorotational Test

There appears to be diagnostic and monitoring information available in higher-frequency rotational testing. The head can comfortably shake at higher frequencies. An accelerometer attached to a headband senses the head velocity while electro-oculography measures the eye movement and a computer program analyzes the head sensor and eye movement information. The resulting information is expressed in gains, phases, and symmetry. As more clinical data are accumulated and compared to the other investigative modalities, the indications for this testing are being consolidated.

Dynamic Posturography

Dynamic posturography is a correlative systemic balance function test. It assesses the patient's balance capabilities in challenging visual and support surface environments similar to those encountered in daily life. The test cannot stand alone as a vestibular testing modality; however, it can correlate with caloric tests in some vestibular conditions. It is an objective technique that measures the proprioceptive and ocular inputs concurrently with the vestibular input. The undisputed role for posturography is in the rehabilitative management of patients—that is, in determining which patients suffering from dizziness, imbalance, or both would benefit from physical therapy and aiding in the design and monitoring of physical therapy protocol.

Separate protocols evaluate sensory and motor components of balance. There are six sensory conditions.

1. Eyes open, horizon stable, platform stable
2. Eyes closed, horizon stable, platform stable
3. Eyes open, horizon swayed, platform stable
4. Eyes open, horizon stable, platform swayed
5. Eyes open, horizon swayed, platform swayed
6. Eyes closed, horizon stable, platform swayed

In the case of central vestibular and extravestibular CNS pathology, posturography may be the only positive test. The pattern of results seen in dynamic posturography can also document the presence of nonphysiologic elements contributing to imbalance.

CLINICAL ENTITIES

The clinical entities presenting with vertigo or disequilibrium have been named by their mode of presentation. As more information becomes available about clinical entities, the emphasis is shifting toward finding an etiology for the symptoms. When evaluating a patient with vertigo, one should try to differentiate between vertigo of peripheral origin and that of central origin (see Table 4-1). The following list of differential diagnoses constitutes the more common etiologies of the dizzy patient:

1. Acoustic neuroma
2. Presbystasis and cardiovascular causes
3. Cogan syndrome
4. Benign paroxysmal positional vertigo
5. Internuclear ophthalmoplegia
6. Intracranial tumors
7. Ménière's disease
8. Metabolic vertigo
9. Multiple sclerosis
10. Oscillopsia

11. Otitis media
12. Otosclerosis
13. Ototoxic drugs
14. Perilymph fistula
15. Posttraumatic vertigo
16. Syphilis
17. Temporal bone fracture
18. Vascular insufficiency
19. Vestibular neuronitis
20. Vertiginous epilepsy
21. Vertigo due to whiplash
22. Vertigo with migraine

Acoustic Neuroma (Vestibular Schwannoma)

Acoustic neuroma, a benign, slow-growing tumor, has its origin most commonly in the vestibular division of the eighth cranial nerve. Most patients with acoustic neuromas complain of unsteadiness rather than episodic vertigo. As the enlarging tumor spills over into the cochlear division of the eighth nerve or compromises the artery to the inner ear, hearing symptoms become manifest. These symptoms include unilateral tinnitus, hearing loss, or both. Initially the findings may be indistinguishable from Ménière's syndrome. With time, there is a progressive hearing loss, with a disproportionate loss of speech discrimination occurring long before a total hearing loss occurs. Acoustic neuroma accounts for 80% of tumors of the cerebellopontine (CP) angle.

Even though the facial nerve is in close proximity, visible signs of facial (seventh) nerve palsy occur only rarely in advanced cases. More commonly, the first modality effected by the pressure on the fifth (trigeminal) nerve is demonstrated by altered corneal sensation. Later there may be symptoms of numbness in any or all divisions of the trigeminal nerve. On rare occasions, trigeminal neuralgia has been a presenting symptom.

The audiologic evaluation may vary from normal pure-tone hearing with poor speech discrimination to a pure-tone sensorineural hearing loss and poor or absent speech discrimination. A search for the acoustic stapedial reflexes with the impedance bridge may show reflexes present at normal levels without evidence of decay in about 18% of the tumors. The reflexes are helpful when they are absent or show evidence of decay when the behavioral pure tones are in the normal range. Auditory brain stem response is the most sensitive test in detecting acoustic neuromas, being abnormal in 82% of small intracanalicular tumors.

When there is an absent caloric response in the suspect ear with no history of disequilibrium, the vestibular evaluation heightens one's suspicion.

Magnetic resonance imaging (MRI) with intravenous contrast (gadolinium-DPTA) is a reliable and cost-effective method of identifying tumors and may be selected as the first or only imaging technique. Tumors as small as 2 mm may be enhanced and identified.

Presbystasis (Dysequilibrium of Aging) and Cardiovascular Causes

Age-related decline in peripheral vestibular function, visual acuity, proprioception, and motor control has a cumulative effect upon balance and is the most common cause of disequilibrium.

Arrhythmias usually produce disequilibrium. They rarely present to the otologist but are seen in consultation with the cardiologist. However, consideration must be given when seeing a new patient with disequilibrium.

Cogan Syndrome

See Chapter 9.

Benign Paroxysmal Positional Vertigo (BPPV)

The symptoms include sudden attacks of vertigo precipitated by sitting up, lying down, or turn-ing in bed. These attacks have been reported to be prompted by sudden movement of the head to the right or left or by extension of the neck when looking upward. The sensation of vertigo is always of short duration even when the provocative position is maintained. Diagnosis can be confirmed by positional testing (Dix-Hallpike test), which indicates positional nystagmus with latency and fatigability.

Etiologies include degenerative changes, otitis media, labyrinthine concussion, previ-ous ear surgery, and occlusion of the anterior vestibular artery. The cause is thought to involve abnormal sensitivity of the semicircular canal ampullae, specially the posterior, to gravitational forces stimulated by free-floating abnormally dense particles (canaliths). These particles can be repositioned and the symptoms resolved in a high percentage of cases by the canalith repositioning procedure.

To effectively carry out the procedure, one should be able to envision the ongoing orien-tation of the SCCs while carrying out the head maneuvers. Figure 4-4 illustrates the position-ing sequence for the left posterior semicircular canal as viewed by the operator (behind patient).

Internuclear Ophthalmoplegia

Internuclear ophthalmoplegia is a disturbance of the lateral movements of the eyes charac-terized by a paralysis of the internal rectus on one side and weakness of the external rectus on the other. In testing, the examiner has the patient follow his or her finger, first to one side and then to the other, as when testing for horizontal nystagmus. Internuclear ophthalmople-gia is recognized when the adductive eye (third nerve) is weak and the abducting eye (sixth nerve) moves normally and displays a coarse nystagmus (involvement of the vestibular nuclei?). The pathology is in the MLF. When the disorder is bilateral, it is pathognomonic of multiple sclerosis. When it is unilateral, one should consider a tumor or vascular process.

Intracranial Tumors

There is a small but definite number of patients that present with disequilibrium associated with primary or secondary intracranial tumors. The use of CT and MRI scanning, without and with intravenous contrast, in selected patients helps to identify these otherwise silent lesions.

Ménière's Disease

The symptoms, when complete and classically present, include fluctuating sensorineural hearing loss, fluctuating tinnitus, and fluctuating fullness in the affected ear. In addition, as the tinnitus, fullness, and hearing loss intensify, an attack of episodic vertigo follows, lasting 30 minutes to 2 hours. The process may spontaneously remit, never occur again, and leave no residual or perhaps a mild hearing loss and tinnitus. In 85% of the patients, the disease affects only one ear. However, should the second ear become involved, it usually happens within 36 months. The natural history is final remission occurs in about 60% of the patients.

Cochlear hydrops, vestibular hydrops, or Lermoyez syndrome have aural fullness as the common denominator. *Cochlear hydrops* is characterized by the fluctuating sensorineural hearing loss and tinnitus. *Vestibular hydrops* has episodic vertigo as well as the aural full-ness. *Lermoyez syndrome is* characterized by increasing tinnitus, hearing loss, and aural

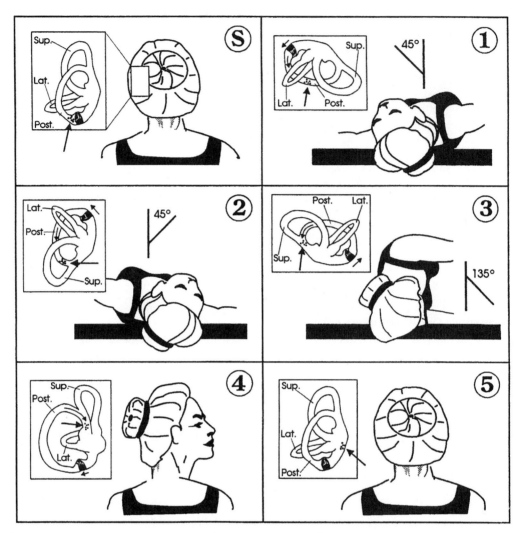

Figure 4-4. Positioning sequence for left posterior semicircular canal as viewed from behind the patient. *Box.* Exposed view of the labyrinth, showing migration of particles (large arrow). S, Start—patient seated (oscillator applied). 1, Place head over end of table, 45 degrees to left. 2, Keeping head tilted downward, rotate to 45 degrees right. 3, Rotate head and body until facing downward 135 degrees from supine. 4, Keeping head turned right, bring patient to seated position. 5, Turn head forward, chin down 20 degrees. Pause at each position until induced nystagmus approaches termination or for T (latency + duration) seconds if no nystagmus. Keep repeating entire series (1–5) until no nystagmus in any position. (*From Eppley JM. Particle repositioning for BPPV.* Otolaryngol Clin North Am *1996;29:323–331.*)

fullness that is relieved after an episodic attack of vertigo. Recurrence of this phenomenon can be expected. *Crisis of Tumarkin or drop attack* is another variant of Ménière's syndrome, in which the patient loses extensor powers and falls to the ground suddenly and severely. There is no loss of consciousness and complete recovery occurs almost immediately. This occurs late in the disease process with no warning.

Audiometric tests show a fluctuating low-tone sensorineural hearing loss and little to no tone decay. The ENG findings commonly show very little between the initial episodes. During the attack there may be active spontaneous nystagmus with direction changing components even in the midst of caloric testing.

Because the stage at which a spontaneous remission occurs cannot be predicted, several medical and surgical therapies have evolved to alter the natural history. The medical therapies are aimed at the symptoms and include vestibular suppressants, vasodilators, and diuretics. The surgical therapies are either destructive or preservative of residual hearing. The first includes labyrinthectomy or translabyrinthine eighth nerve section when there is no useful hearing. Procedures when there is useful hearing include selective (middle cranial fossa, retrolabyrinthine, or retrosigmoid) vestibular nerve section or gentamicin or streptomycin application to the inner ear. Conservative procedures include those performed on the endolymphatic sac. They range from sac decompression to endolymphatic–mastoid shunts. The latter appears directed at correcting the resultant mechanical or production-reabsorption changes seen in the histopathology of endolymphatic hydrops in the temporal bone. Cochleosacculotomy is indicated in elderly patients with disabling vertigo, poor hearing, and residual vestibular function under local anesthesia.

Glycerol Test

It is speculated that the administration of glycerol in an oral dose of 1.2 mL/kg of body weight with the addition of an equal amount of physiologic saline to a patient with Ménière's syndrome may have diagnostic value in clinical management. Within 1 hour of administration, the patient may sense an improvement in the hearing loss, tinnitus, and sensation of fullness in the ear, with maximum effects occurring within 2 to 3 hours. After 3 hours, the symptoms slowly return.

Metabolic Vertigo

There are no clinical symptoms that separate metabolic from other forms of vertigo. A prerequisite may be an abnormally functioning vestibular system. In this instance the metabolic factor exaggerates or interferes with the compensatory mechanisms and brings about the symptoms. Dietary modification often results in a striking improvement in symptoms.

Hypothyroidism is an extremely rare but definite cause. Many times the patients are not otherwise clinically hypothyroid.

Allergic causes are very elusive in the management of the dizzy patient, but the screening immunoglobulin E (IgE) assay may give a clue. Radioallergosorbent test (RAST) or skin testing may provide more precise findings about an allergic cause and its treatment. When there is no clear-cut history and in the absence of any other clearly defined cause, an allergic management should be undertaken.

Multiple Sclerosis

Multiple sclerosis is one of the more common neurologic diseases encountered in a clinical practice. Vertigo is the presenting symptom of multiple sclerosis in 7 to 10% of the patients or eventually appears during the course of disease in as many as one-third of the cases. The patient usually complains of unsteadiness along with vertigo. Vertical nystagmus, bilateral internuclear ophthalmoplegia, and ataxic eye movements are other clues to this disease. *Charcot triad* (nystagmus, scanning speech, and intention tremor) may be present. Electronystagmography may show anything from normal findings to peripheral findings to central findings. Auditory brain stem evoked potentials may show delay of central conduction. More likely, there is a significant delay of the visually evoked potentials. Research into an etiology for this disorder is pointing to an autoimmune disorder of the myelin.

Oscillopsia (Jumbling of the Panorama): Dandy's Syndrome

Since our heads bob up and down while walking, the otolithic system controls eye movement to maintain a constant horizon when walking. When there is bilateral absent vestibular function as seen with ototoxic drug use, *the loss of otolithic function results in oscillopsia,* which is the inability to maintain the horizon while walking.

Otitis Media

Suppurative or serous otitis media may have associated vestibular symptoms. In serous otitis media, the presence of fluid in the middle ear restricting the round window membrane, serous labyrinthitis, may be responsible for the vestibular symptoms. Removal of the serous fluid either medically or surgically gives rise to remission of the dizziness.

In the presence of suppuration, there may be reversible serous labyrinthitis or irreversible suppurative labyrinthitis and the more extensive sequestrum, with a dead ear and facial nerve palsy. In this instance, judgment about the disease and its effects determines the proper treatment.

Otosclerosis (Otospongiosis)

There appear to be three areas where otosclerosis may bear relation to disequilibrium. The first occurs in relation to the fixed footplate. There may be a change in the fluid dynamics of the inner ear, giving rise to vestibular symptoms. In a large number of patients, the symptoms are cleared by stapedectomy.

Sometimes vertigo begins after stapedectomy. It may occur with a perilymph fistula that requires revision and repair. A total, irreversible loss of hearing with vertigo may also occur. A destructive surgical procedure of labyrinthectomy with or without eighth nerve section is indicated if the vestibular suppressants fail to control the disequilibrium. The coexistence of otosclerotic foci around the vestibular labyrinth with elevated blood fats or blood glucose abnormalities may give rise to vestibular symptoms. Effective treatment requires fluoride therapy.

There is also evidence that an otosclerotic focus may literally grow through the vestibular nerve. In this instance, a reduced vestibular response (RVR) is found on ENG testing. This clinical presentation may look like vestibular neuronitis in the absence of a hearing loss.

Ototoxic Drugs

Ototoxic drugs, predominantly aminoglycoside antibiotics, are usually used in lifesaving situations where no other antibiotics are judged to be as effective. The main symptom is oscillopsia and results from lack of otolithic input to allow the eyes to maintain a level horizon. This is found while the head is bobbing up and down as the individual walks. The use of rotational testing, especially at the higher frequencies, may reveal function that is not evident on caloric testing. The presence of this rotational function indicates intact responses in other areas of vestibular sensitivity. This intact function may separate the patient who will benefit from vestibular rehabilitation from the patient who will not. This may also explain the difference in the degree of disability between patients.

Sometimes the usual vestibular suppressants aid the patient. In other instances, one is frustrated by an inability to adequately treat this condition.

Perilymph Fistula

In the absence of hearing loss, perilymph fistula is a cause of vertigo. The history should be straightforward for impulsive trauma or barotrauma, and the resultant symptoms clearly follow. However, this is not always the case, as a sneeze or vigorous blowing of the nose may be the inciting event. The resultant vertigo may not occur for some time. The clue in the history is one of an episodic nature usually related to exertion. Many patients are asymptomatic on awakening in the morning only to have symptoms appear once they are up and around. A positive fistula sign with or without ENG results is helpful, although a negative sign does not rule out a fistula.

Associated symptoms of ear fullness, tinnitus, and mild or fluctuating hearing loss help to localize the problem to the ear. Many patients demonstrate nystagmus with the affected ear down; however, this finding alone is not a reliable sign to determine the pathologic ear. The definitive diagnosis occurs at surgery, but there are instances where there are equivocal findings at surgery.

Posttraumatic Vertigo

Posttraumatic vertigo comprises a history of head trauma followed by a number of possible symptoms, such as disequilibrium. If there is a total loss of balance and hearing function, the use of vestibular suppressants may result in a cure that is sustained after cessation of the suppressants. In some instances when there is no cure, a labyrinthectomy or eighth nerve section ameliorates the symptoms. Occasionally, there is a progressive hearing loss.

After trauma, delayed Ménière's syndrome may develop. This may be resistant to medical therapy and require surgery. In this instance, endolymphatic sac surgery can improve the symptoms if there is no fracture displacement through the endolymphatic duct.

The statoconia of the otolithic system may have become dislodged by the trauma. With head movement, they roll toward the ampullated end of the posterior SCC. Their weight deflects the ampullary contents, producing a gravity stimulus that stimulates a positional vertigo of a posttraumatic type. The nystagmus is said to occur with the affected ear down. The most effective treatment is with habituation exercises. Vestibular neurectomy is also a recommended therapy.

Syphilis: Congenital and Acquired

The neurotologic findings associated with syphilis usually present with bilateral Ménière's syndrome. There is a significant hearing loss and usually bilateral absent caloric function. Another common clinical manifestation is the presence of interstitial keratitis. The patients, as a rule, are in their mid-40s; however, when the onset occurs during childhood, the hearing loss is abrupt, bilaterally symmetrical, and more severe.

These patients usually have a positive Hennebert's sign (ie, positive fistula test without any demonstrable fistula along with a normal external auditory canal and tympanic membrane). The positive fistula test indicates an abnormally mobile footplate or an absence or softening of the bony plate covering the lateral SCC. The patient also may demonstrate Tullio phenomenon (see Chapters 9 and 23).

Histopathologically, the soft tissue of the labyrinth may demonstrate mononuclear leukocyte infiltration with obliterative endarteritis, inflammatory fibrosis, and endolymphatic hydrops. Osteolytic lesions are often seen in the otic capsule. The treatment consists of an intensive course of penicillin therapy for an adequate interval. Patients allergic to penicillin should be desensitized to this drug in the hospital and given 20 million units of penicillin intravenously daily for 10 days. The use of steroids may result in a dramatic improvement in hearing and a reduction of vestibular symptoms. Usually, the steroids must be maintained indefinitely to retain the clinical improvement.

Temporal Bone Fracture and Labyrinthine Concussion

Transverse Fracture

Because a transverse fracture destroys the auditory and vestibular function, the patient has no hearing or vestibular response in that ear. Initially, the patient is severely vertiginous and demonstrates a spontaneous nystagmus whose fast component is away from the injured side. The severe vertigo subsides after a week, and the patient may remain mildly unsteady for 3 to 6 months. The patient may also have labyrinthine concussion of the contralateral side, and facial nerve palsy is not uncommon.

Longitudinal Fracture

Longitudinal fractures constitute 80% of the temporal bone fractures. With this type of fracture, there is usually bleeding into the middle ear with perforation of the tympanic membrane and disruption of the tympanic ring. Thus, there may be a conductive hearing loss from the middle ear pathology and a sensorineural high-frequency hearing loss from a concomitant labyrinthine concussion. There may also be evidence of a peripheral facial nerve palsy. Dizziness may be mild or absent except during positional testing.

Labyrinthine Concussion

Labyrinthine concussion is secondary to head injury. The patient complains of mild unsteadiness or light-headedness, particularly with a change of head position. Audiometric testing may reveal a high-frequency hearing loss. The ENG may show a spontaneous or positional nystagmus, a reduced vestibular response, or both. As the effects of the concussion reverse, the symptoms and objective findings also move toward normal.

Vascular Insufficiency and Its Syndromes

Vascular insufficiency can be a common cause of vertigo among people over the age of 50 as well as patients with diabetes, hypertension, or hyperlipidemia. The following syndromes have been recognized among patients with vascular insufficiency.

Labyrinthine Apoplexy

Labyrinthine apoplexy is due to thrombosis of the internal auditory artery or one of its branches. The symptoms include acute vertigo with nausea and vomiting. Hearing loss and tinnitus may also occur.

Wallenberg Syndrome

Wallenberg syndrome (see also Chapter 9) is also known as the lateral medullary syndrome secondary to infarction of the medulla, which is supplied by the posterior inferior cerebellar artery. This syndrome is believed to be the most common brainstem vascular disorder. The symptoms include:

1. Vertigo, nausea, vomiting, nystagmus
2. Ataxia, falling toward the side of the brain

3. Loss of the sense of pain and temperature sensations on the ipsilateral and contralateral body
4. Dysphagia with ipsilateral palate and vocal cord paralysis
5. Ipsilateral Horner syndrome

Subclavian Steal Syndrome

Subclavian steal syndrome is characterized by intermittent vertigo, occipital headache, blurred vision, diplopia, dysarthria, pain in the upper extremity, loud bruit or palpable thrill over the supraclavicular fossa, a difference of 20 mmHg in systolic blood pressure between the two arms, and a delayed or weakened radial pulse. The blockage can be surgically corrected.

Anterior Vestibular Artery Occlusion

This symptom complex, first described by Lindsay and Hemenway in 1956, includes:

1. A sudden onset of vertigo without deafness
2. A slow recovery followed by months of positional vertigo of the benign paroxysmal type
3. Signs of histologic degeneration of the utricular macula, cristae of the lateral and superior SCCs, and the superior vestibular nerve

Vertebrobasilar Insufficiency

The symptoms of vertebrobasilar insufficiency include vertigo, hemiparesis, visual disturbances, dysarthria, headache, and vomiting. These symptoms are a result of a drop in blood flow to the vestibular nuclei and surrounding structures. The posterior and anterior inferior cerebellar arteries are involved. Tinnitus and deafness are unusual symptoms.

Drop attacks without loss of consciousness and precipitated by neck motion are characteristic of vertebrobasilar insufficiency.

Cervical Vertigo

Cervical vertigo can be caused by cervical spondylosis as well as by other etiologies. Cervical spondylosis can be brought about by degeneration of the intervertebral disc. As the disc space narrows, approximation of the vertebral bodies takes place. With mobility, the bulging of the annulus is increased, causing increased traction on the periosteum to which the annulus is attached and stimulating proliferation of bone along the margins of the vertebral bodies to produce osteophytes.

Barre believed that the symptoms of cervical spondylosis (including vertigo) are due to irritation of the vertebral sympathetic plexus, which is in close proximity to the vertebral artery. Laskiewicz claimed that spondylosis irritates the periarterial neural plexus in the wall of the vertebral and basilar arteries, leading to contraction of the vessels. Temporary ischemia then gives rise to vertigo. Others claimed that the loss of proprioception in the neck can give rise to cervical vertigo. Emotional tension, rotation of the head, and extension of the head can cause the neck muscle (including the scalenus anticus) to be drawn tightly over the thyrocervical trunk and subclavian artery, compressing these vessels against the proximal vertebral artery. In elderly individuals, a change from the supine to the upright position may give rise to postural hypotension, which in turn may cause vertebrobasilar insufficiency. The aortic arch syndrome and subclavian steal syndrome may also cause cervical vertigo.

Symptoms include:

1. Headache, vertigo
2. Syncope
3. Tinnitus and loss of hearing (usually low frequencies)
4. Nausea and vomiting (vagal response)
5. Visual symptoms, such as flashing lights (not uncommon), due to ischemia of the occipital lobe, supplied by the posterior cerebral artery, a branch of the basilar artery
6. Supraclavicular bruit seen by physical examination in one-third of the patients

Each of these symptoms usually appears when the head or neck assumes a certain position or change of position.

Proper posture, neck exercises, cervical traction, heat massage, anesthetic infiltration, and immobilization of the neck with a collar temporarily are all good therapeutic measures. If traction is required, it can be given as a few pounds horizontally for several hours at a time. For cervical spondylosis without acute root symptoms, heavy traction (100 lbs) for 1 to 2 minutes continuously or 5 to 10 minutes intermittently is considered by some to be more effective.

Vertiginous Epilepsy

Disequilibrium as a symptom of epilepsy is seen in two forms. The first is an aura of a major jacksonian seizure. The second is the momentary, almost petit mal seizure whose entire brief moment is experienced as disequilibrium. The diagnosis of the latter form may require a sleep electroencephalogram. These patients respond to usual seizure control therapy.

Cortical vertigo either can be as severe and episodic as Ménière's disease or may manifest itself as a mild unsteadiness. It is usually associated with hallucinations of music or sound. The patient may exhibit daydreaming and purposeful or purposeless repetitive movements. Motor abnormalities—such as chewing, lip smacking, and facial grimacing—are not uncommon. The patient may experience an unusual sense of familiarity (déjà vu) or a sense of strangeness (jamais vu). Should the seizure discharge spread beyond the temporal lobe, grand mal seizures may ensue.

Vertigo Due to Whiplash Injury

Patients often complain of dizziness following a whiplash injury. In some cases, there is no physiologic evidence for this complaint. In others, ENG has documented objective findings, such as spontaneous nystagmus. The onset of dizziness often occurs 7 to 10 days following the accident, particularly with head movements toward the side of the neck most involved in the whiplash. The symptoms may last months or years after the accident.

Otologic examination is usually normal. Audiometric studies are normal unless there is associated labyrinthine concussion. Vestibular examination can reveal spontaneous nystagmus or positional nystagmus with the head turned in the direction of the whiplash. The use of ENG is essential for evaluation of these patients.

Vertigo with Migraine

Vertebrobasilar migraine is due to impairment of circulation of the brain stem. The symptoms include vertigo, dysarthria, ataxia, paresthesia, diplopia, diffuse scintillating scotomas, or homonymous hemianopsia. The initial vasoconstriction is followed by vasodilatation, giving rise to an intense throbbing headache, usually unilateral. A positive family history is obtained in more than 50% of these patients. Treatment of migraine includes butalbital (Fiorinal), ergot derivatives, and methysergide (Sansert). The latter has the tendency to cause retroperitoneal fibrosis.

Vestibular Neuronitis

Occasionally referred to as viral labyrinthitis, vestibular neuronitis begins with a nonspecific viral illness followed in a variable period of up to 6 weeks by a sudden onset of vertigo, with nausea, vomiting, and the sensation of blacking out accompanied by severe unsteadiness. The patient, however, does not lose consciousness. The severe attack can last days to weeks. Cochlear symptoms are absent and without associated neurologic deficits. When seen initially, the patient has spontaneous nystagmus to the contralateral side, and ENG demonstrates a unilaterally reduced caloric response. The remainder of the evaluation is negative for a cause. In most patients, vestibular compensation clears the symptoms in time. The remission may be hastened by the effective use of vestibular suppressant medication for a period of up to 6 weeks. After the acute episode has subsided, which may take weeks, the patient continues to experience a slight sensation of light-headedness for some time, particularly in connection with sudden movements. The acute episode may also be followed by a period of positional vertigo of the benign paroxysmal type.

A small percentage of afflicted patients do not respond to vestibular suppression or to vestibular compensation. In these patients, an evaluation for metabolic, otosclerotic, or autoimmune factors is indicated. If these other factors are identified and the appropriate treatment is initiated, the symptoms may disappear. If, after an appropriate treatment and observation period, incapacitating symptoms persist, a retrolabyrinthine vestibular nerve section is indicated. Abnormal myelination has been found in some of these nerve specimens.

Bibliography

Ahistrom P, Thalmann I, Thalmann R, et al. Cyclic AMP and adenylate cyclase in the inner ear. *Laryngoscope* 1975;85:1241–1258.

Alpers BJ. Vertiginous epilepsy. *Laryngoscope* 1960; 70:631.

Alpert JN. Failure of fixation suppression: A pathologic effect of vision on caloric nystagmus. *Neurology* 1974;24:891–896.

Althaus SR. Perilymph fistulas. *Laryngoscope* 1981;91:538–562.

Anantaa E, Riekkinen PJ, Frey HJ. Electronystagmographic findings in multiple sclerosis. *Acta Otolaryngol* 1973;75:1–5.

Anthony PF. Partitioning the labyrinth for BPPV: Clinical and histologic findings. *Am J Otol* 14; 334–342: 1993.

Arnold W, Altermatt H, Gebbers JP. Demonstration of immunoglobulins in the human endolymphatic sac. *Laryngol Rhinol Otol* 1984;63: 464–467.

Aschan G, Stahle J. Vestibular neuritis. A nystagmographical study. *J Laryngol* 1956;70:497–511.

Aschan G. The pathogenesis of positional nystagmus. *Acta Otolaryngol* 1961;(Suppl 159):90.

Aschan G, Bergstedt M, Stahle J. Nystagmography. *Acta Otolaryngol* 1956;(Suppl 129):1–103.

Baloh RW, Honrubia V. Childhood onset of benign positional vertigo. *Neurology* 1998;50:1494–1496.

Baloh RW, Honrubia V, eds. *Clinical Neurophysiology of the Vestibular System,* 2nd ed. Philadelphia: Davis, 1990.

Barber HO, Wright G. Release of nystagmus suppression in clinical electronystagmography. *Laryngoscope* 1967;72:1016–1027.

Barber HO, Wright G, Demanuele F. The hot caloric test as a clinical screening device. *Arch Otolaryngol* 1971;94:335–337.

Barratt H, et al. Testing the vestibular-ocular reflexes: Abnormalities of the otolith contribution in patients with neuro-otological disease. *J Neurol Neurosurg Psychiatry* 1987;50:1029–1035.

Beck C, Schmidt CL. Ten years of experience with intratympanal streptomycin in the therapy of morbus Meniere. *Arch Otorhinolaryngol* 1978; 221:149–152.

Becker GD, Clemis JD. Monothermal upright inverted caloric test. *Am Otol* 1979;1:100–102.

Behramm S. Vestibular epilepsy. *Brain* 1955;78: 471–486.

Behrman S, Wyke B. Vestibulogenic seizures. *Brain* 1958;81:529.

Bergan JJ. Vascular implications of vertigo. *Arch Otolaryngol* 1967;85:78–83.

Bernstein P, McCabe BF, Ryu JH. The effect of diazepam on vestibular compensation. *Laryngoscope* 1974;84:267–272.

Bhansali SA, Honrubia V. Current status of ENG testing. *Otolaryngol Head Neck Surg* 120:416–426, 1999

Biemond A, de Jong JMBV. On cervical nystagmus and related disorders. *Brain* 1969;92:437–458.

Bos JH, Oosterveld WJ, Philipszoon AJ, et al. On pathological spontaneous and positional nystagmus. *Pract Otol Rhinol Laryngol* 1963; 25:282–290.

Bosher SK, Warren RL. Very low calcium content of cochlear endolymph, an extracellular fluid. *Nature* 1978;273:377–378.

Boyles JHJ. Allergy testing in otology. *Am J Otol* 1984;5:450–455.

Brackmann DE, Nissen RL. Meniere's disease: Results of treatment with the endolymphatic subarachnoid shunt compared with endolymphatic mastoid shunt. *Am J Otol* 1987;8:275–282.

Brandt Y, Daroff RB. Physical therapy for benign paroxysmal positional vertigo. *Arch Otolaryngol* 1980;106:484–485.

Brightwell DR, Abramson M. Personality characteristics in patients with vertigo. *Arch Otolaryngol Head Neck Surg* 1975;101:364–366.

Bronstein A. Oscillopsia of peripheral vestibular origin. *Acta Otolaryngol (Stockh)* 1987;104: 307–314.

Brookes GB. Circulating immune complexes in Meniere's disease. *Arch Otolaryngol* 1986;112: 536–540.

Brookler KH. Directional preponderance in clinical electronystagmography. *Laryngoscope* 1970;80: 747–754.

Brookler KH. Identification of inferior vestibular nerve lesions. *Equil Res* 1973;3:1.

Brookler KH. Meniere's disease: Role of otospongiosis and metabolic disorders. *Acta Otolaryngol* 1984;(Suppl 406):31–36.

Brookler KH. The clinical and practical aspects of electronystagmography. In: Lee KJ, ed. *Ambulatory Surgery and Office Procedures in Head and Neck Surgery.* New York: Grune & Stratton, 1986, 247–266.

Brookler KH. Electronystagmography 1990. *Neurol Clin* 1990;8:235–259.

Brookler KH. Benign paroxysmal positional vertigo. *Am J Otol* 1990;11:233–234.

Brookler KH, Rubin W. The dizzy patient: Etiologic treatment. *Otolaryngol Head Neck Surg* 1990; 103(5 (Pt 1)):677–80. Review.

Brookler KH, Baker AH, Grams G. Closed loop water irrigator system. *Otolaryngol Head Neck Surg* 1979;87:364–365.

Brown J. A systematic approach to the dizzy patient. *Neurol Clin North Am* 1990;8:209–224.

Buckley RE. Vertiginous temporal lobe seizures stimulated by functional hyperinsulinism. *JAMA* 1963;186:726–727.

Busis SN. A guide to neuro-otological diagnosis for the practicing otolaryngologist. *Acta Otolaryngol* 1965;(Suppl 209):1–65.

Buttner U, et al. Cerebellar control of eye movements. *Prog Brain Res* 1986;64:225–233.

Causse J, Bel J, Mischaux P, et al. Vertiges et otospongiose. *Ann Otolaryngol Chir Cervicofac* 1970;87:145–166.

Cawthorne T. Labyrinthectomy. *Ann Otol* 1960;69: 1170.

Cawthorne T. The physiological basis for head exercises. *J Chart Soc Physiother* 1994;30:106–107.

Cawthorne TE, Fitzgerald G, Hallpike CS. Studies in human vestibular function. II. Observations on the directional preponderance of caloric nystagmus ("Nystagmusbereitschaft") resulting from unilateral labyrinectomy. *Brain* 1942;65: 138–160.

Claussen CF, Schlachta IV. Butterfly chart for caloric nystagmus evaluation. *Arch Otolaryngol* 1972; 96:371–375.

Clemis JD. Allergy of the inner ear. *Ann Allergy* 1967;34:23–31.

Coats AC. Vestibular neuronitis. *Acta Otolaryngol* 1969;(Suppl 251):1–32.

Cody D. The tack operation. *Arch Otolaryngol* 1973;97:109–111.

Cogan DG. Syndrome of nonsyphilitic interstitial keratitis and vestibuloauditory symptoms. *Arch Ophthalmol* 1945;33:144.

Collins WE. Effects of mental set upon vestibular nystagmus. *J Exp Psychol* 1962;63:191–197.

Cooksey FS. Rehabilitation in vestibular injuries. *Proc R Soc Med* 1946;39:273.

Cope S, Ryan GMS. Cervical and otolith vertigo. *J Laryngol* 1959;73:113.

Currier WD. Dizziness related to hypoglycemia: Role of adrenal steroids and nutrition. *Laryngoscope* 1971;81:18–35.

Cyr DG, Moore GF, Moller CG. Clinical application of computerized dynamic posturography. *ENTechnology* 1988;(September):36–47.

Dandy WE. Meniere's disease. Its diagnosis and methods of treatment. *Arch Surg* 1928;16:1127.

Daspit CR, Churchill D, Linthicum FHJ. Diagnosis of perilymph fistula using ENG and impedance. *Laryngoscope* 1980;90:217–223.

Dayal VS, Farkashidy J, Kuzin B. Clinical evaluation of the hot caloric test as screening. *Laryngoscope* 1973;83:1433–1439.

Dayal VS, Tarantino L, Farkashidy J, et al. Spontaneous and positional nystagmus: A reassessment of clinical significance. *Laryngoscope* 1974;84:2033–2044.

de la Cruz A, McElveen JT Jr. Hearing preservation in vestibular neurectomy. *Laryngoscope* 1984;94(7):874–877.

Derebery MJ. The diagnosis and treatment of dizziness. *Med Clin North Am* 1999;83(1): 163–177.

DeRosier DJ, Tilney LG, Engehnan E. Actin in the inner ear: The remarkable structure of the stereocilium. *Nature* 1980;287:291–296.

Diener HC. Long loop reflexes in a standing subject and their use for clinical diagnosis. *Proceedings of the VII International Symposium: Vestibular and Visual Control on Posture and Locomotor Equilibrium* Houston Karger publishing, 1986.

Dieringer N, Precht W. Modification of synaptic input following unilateral labyrinthectomy. *Nature* 1977;269:431–433.

Dix MR. Rehabilitation of vertigo. In: Dix MR, Hood JD, eds. *Vertigo.* New York: John Wiley & Sons, 1984, 467–479.

Dohlman GF. The attachment of the cupulae, otolith and tectorial membranes to the sensory cell area. *Acta Otolaryngol* 1971;71:89–105.

Drachman D, Hart CW. An approach to the dizzy patient. *Neurology* 1972;22:323–334.

Eldredge DH, et al. The electrical polarization of the semicircular canals. *Ann Otol* 1961;70:1024–1036.

Epley JM: The canalith repositioning procedure: For treatment of benign paroxysmal positional vertigo. *Otolaryngol Head Neck Surg* 1992;107:399–404.

Evans RW, Baloh RW. Episodic vertigo and migraine. *Headache* 2001;41:604–605.

Fee WEJ. Aminoglycoside otoxicity in the human. *Laryngoscope* 1980;(Suppl 24):1–19.

Fetter M. Assessing vestibular function: Which tests, when? *J Neurol* 2000;247:335–342.

Fisch U. Vestibular nerve section for Meniere's disease. *Am J Otol* 1984;5:543–545.

Fitzgerald DC. Perilymphatic fistula and Meniere's disease. Clinical series and literature review. *Ann Otol Rhinol Laryngol* 2001;110:430–436.

Fitzgerald G, Hallpike CS. Studies in human vestibular function 1. Observations on directional preponderance of caloric nystagmus resulting from cerebral lesions. *Brain* 1942;65:115–137.

Flock A, Cheung H. Actin filaments in sensory hairs of inner ear receptor cells. *J Cell Biol* 1977;75:339–343.

Fluur E. Vestibular compensation after labyrinthine destruction. *Acta Otolaryngol* 1960;52:360–374.

Fluur E, Siegborn J. Interaction between the utricles and the horizontal semicircular canals. I. Unilateral selective sectioning of the horizontal ampullar nerve followed by tilting around the longitudinal axis. *Acta Otolaryngol* 1973;75:17–20.

Fowler EPJ. Streptomycin treatment of vertigo. *Trans Am Acad Ophthalmol Otolaryngol* 1948;52:293–301.

Frederic MW. Central vertigo. *Otolaryngol Clin North Am* 1973;6:267–285.

Frederickson JM, Fernandez C. Vestibular disorders in fourth ventricle lesions. *Arch Otolaryngol* 1964;80:521–540.

Freeman J. Otosclerosis and vestibular dysfunction. *Laryngoscope* 1980;90:1481–1487.

Freeman P, Edmonds C. Inner ear barotrauma. *Arch Otolaryngol* 1972;95:556–563.

Friedland DR, Wackym PA. A critical appraisal of spontaneous perilymphatic fistulas of the inner ear. *Am J Otol* 1999;20:261–276.

Fuchs AF. Role of the vestibular and reticular nuclei in control of gaze. In: Baker R, Berthoz A, eds. *Control of Gaze by Brain Stem Neurons, Developments in Neuroscience.* New York: Elsevier/North-Holland Biomedical Press, 1977, 341–348.

Furman JM. Role of posturography in the management of vestibular patients. *Otolaryngol Head Neck Surg* 1995;112:8–15.

Garcia-Ibanez E, Garcia-Ibanez JL. Middle fossa vestibular neurectomy: A report of 373 cases. *Otolaryngol Head Neck Surg* 1980;88:486–490.

Ghorayeb BY, Linthicum FHJ. Otosclerotic inner ear syndrome. *Ann Otol Rhinol Laryngol* 1978; 87:85–90.

Goebel JA, Paige GD. Dynamic posturography and caloric test results in patients with and without vertigo. *Otolaryngol Head Neck Surg* 1989; 100:553.

Grad A, Baloh RW. Vertigo of vascular origin. *Arch Neurol* 1989;46:281–284.

Graham MD. Titration streptomycin therapy for bilateral Meniere's disease. *J Otolaryngol Head Neck Surg* 1984;92:440–447.

Gresty MA, Hess K, Leech J. Disorders of the vestibulo-ocular reflex producing oscillopsia and mechanisms compensating for loss of labyrinthine function. *Brain* 1977;100:693–716.

Haid TC, et al. Head-shaking nystagmus in patients with unilateral peripheral vestibular lesions. *Am J Otolaryngol* 1987;8:36–47.

Hamid MA, Hughes GB, Kinney SE. Specificity and sensitivity of dynamic posturography. *Acta Otolaryngol Suppl (Stockh)* 1991;481:596–600.

Hart CW. The Quix test. *Laryngoscope* 1983;93: 1160–1161.

Healy GB. Hearing loss and vertigo secondary to head injury. *N Engl J Med* 1982;306:1029–1031.

Hecker HC, Haug CO, Herndon JW. Treatment of the vertiginous patient using Cawthorne's vestibular exercises. *Laryngoscope* 1974;84:2065–2072.

Henriksson NG, Pfaltz CR, Torok N, Rubin W. *A Synopsis of the Vestibular System* Basel: Sandoz, 1972.

Herdman S, Tusa R, Zee D, et al: Single treatment approaches to benign paroxysmal positional vertigo. *Arch Otolaryngol Head Neck Surg* 1993; 119:450–454.

Herdman SJ, ed. *Vestibular Rehabilitation.* Philadelphia: Davis, 1994.

Hine T. Compensatory eye movements during active head rotation for near targets: Effects of imagination, rapid head oscillation and vergence. *Vision Res* 1987;27:1639–1657.

Honrubia V. Contemporary vestibular function testing: Accomplishments and future perspectives. *Otolaryng Head Neck Surg* 1995;112: 64–77.

Hood JD, Korres S. Vestibular suppression in peripheral and central vestibular disorders. *Brain* 1979; 102:785–804.

House WF. Subarachnoid shunt drainage of hydrops. *Arch Otolaryngol* 1964;79:338.

House WF. Surgical exposure of the internal auditory canal and its contents through the middle cranial fossa. *Laryngoscope* 1961;71:1363.

Huizing EH. Deafness and vertigo after gentamicin. *Ned Tijdschr Geneeskd* 1972;116:1261–1264.

Igarashi M. Vestibular compensation: An overview. *Acta Otolaryngol (Stockh)* 1984;406:78–82.

Igarashi M, Alford B, Watanabe T, Maxian PM. Role of neck proprioceptors for the maintenance of dynamic bodily equilibrium in the squirrel monkey. *Laryngoscope* 1969;79:713.

Janetta PJ, Moller MB, Moller AR. Disabling positional vertigo. *N Engl J Med* 1984;310: 1700–1705.

Johnstone BM. *Ion Pumps and Hair Cells in the Inner Ear* Huntsville, AL: Strode Publishers, 1981, 216–218.

Jongkees LBW. Cervical vertigo. *Laryngoscope* 1969;79:1473–1484.

Jongkees LBW. Value, origin, preferable method of performing the caloric test of the labyrinth. *Arch Otolaryngol* 1949;49:594–608.

Juhn SK, Youngs JN. Changes in perilymph glucose concentration. *Arch Otol* 1972;96:556–558.

Juhn SK, Youngs JN. The effect of perilymph of the alteration of serum glucose or calcium concentration. *Laryngoscope* 1976;86:273–279.

Katsarkas A, Outerbridge J. Compensation of unilateral vestibular loss in vestibular neuronitis. *Ann N Y Acad Sci* 1981;374:784–793.

Kohut RI, Hinojosa R, Ryu JH. Update on idiopathic perilymphatic fistula. *Otolaryngol Clin North Am* 1996;29:343–352.

Lachman J, Stahle J. Vestibular neuritis. A clinical and electronystagmographic study. *Neurology* 1967;17:376–380.

Ledoux A, Demanez JP. "Ocular fixation index" in the caloric test. Contribution to the nystagmographic diagnosis of central diseases. In: Stahle J, ed. *Vestibular Function on Earth and in Space.* New York: Pergamon Press, 1970, 177–185.

Lehrer JF. Vertigo from perilymphatic fistulas. *JAMA* 1986;256:1002–1003.

Linthicum FH, Alonso A, Denia A. Traumatic neuroma: A complication of transcanal labyrinthectomy. *Arch Otolaryngol* 1979;105:654.

Linthicum FH Jr, Waldorf R, Luxford WM, Caltogirone S. Infrared/video ENG recording of eye movements to evaluate the inferior vestibular nerve using the minimal caloric test. *Otolaryngol Head Neck Surg* 1988;98:207–210.

Liston LS, Paparella MM, Anderson HJ. Otosclerosis and endolymphatic hydrops. *Laryngoscope* 1984;94(8):1003–1007.

Mathog RH. Testing of the vestibular system by sinusoidal angular acceleration. *Acta Otolaryngol* 1972;74:96–103.

McCabe BF. The quick component of nystagmus. *Laryngoscope* 1965;75:1619–1646.

McCabe BF, Ryu JH. Experiments on vestibular compensation. *Laryngoscope* 1969;79:1728–1736.

Mccabe B, Gantz B. Vascular loop as a cause of incapacitating dizziness. *Am J Otol* 1989; 10(2):117–120.

McElveen M, Shelton C, Hitselberger WE, et al. Retrolabyrinthine vestibular neurectomy: A re-evaluation. *Laryngoscope* 1988;98:502–506.

Molnar EM, Torok N. The effect of ocular fixation on the caloric nystagmus. *ORL J Otorhinolaryngol Relat Spec* 1974;36(2):76–84.

Money KE, Myles WS. Heavy water nystagmus and effects of alcohol. *Nature* 1974;247:404–405.

Money KE, Myles WS, Hoffert BM. The mechanism of positional alcohol nystagmus. *Can J Otolaryngol* 1974;3:302–313.

Montandon PB, Hausler R, Kimura RS. Treatment of endolymphatic hydrops with cochleosacculotomy. *Otolaryngol Head Neck Surg* 1985;93: 615–621.

Mowrer OH, Ruch TC, Miller NE. The comeoretinal potential difference as the basis of the galvanometric method of recording eye movements. *Am J Physiol* 1936;114:423–428.

Nashner LM. Analysis of movement control in man using the movable platform. *Adv Neurol* 1983; 39:607–619.

Nashner LM, McCollum G. The organization of human postural movements: A formal basis and experimental synthesis. *Behav Brain Sci* 1985; 8:135–172.

Norre ME. The importance of rotatory tests in the evaluation of the dizzy patient. *Acta Otorhinolaryngol* 1977;31:89–98.

Norre ME, DeWeerdt W. Treatment of vertigo based on habituation. Technique and results of habituation training. *J Laryngol Otol* 1980;94:971–977.

Norre ME, DeWeerdt W. Treatment of vertigo based on habituation treatment. Physiopathological basis. *J Laryngol Otol* 1980;94:689–696.

Norris CH. Application of streptomycin to the lateral semicircular canal. *Trans Am Otol Soc* 1988; 75:84–88.

Nylen COS. A clinical study on positional nystagmus in cases of brain tumors. *Acta Otolaryngol Suppl (Stockh)* 1931;15:1–113

O'Leary DP, Davis LL. Spectral analysis of low-frequency, active-head vestibulo-ocular reflex responses. *J Vestib Res* 1998;8:313–324.

O'Leary DP, Davis LL. Vestibular autorotation testing of Meniere's disease. *Otolaryngol Head Neck Surg* 1990;103:66–71.

O'Leary D, Davis LL, Kitsigianis GA. Analysis of vestibulo-ocular reflex using sweep frequency active head movements. *Adv Otol Rhinol Laryngol* 1988;41:179–183.

Odkvist LM, Moller CG, Larsby B, et al. Vestibular compensation measured by the broad frequency band rotatory test. In: Graham MD, Kemink JL, eds. *The Vestibular System: Neurophysiologic and Clinical Research.* New York: Raven Press, 1987, 287–291.

Palacios E, Valvassori G. Vestibular aqueduct syndrome. *Ear Nose Throat J* 1999;78:676.

Paparella MM, Mancini F. Trauma and Meniere's syndrome. *Laryngoscope* 1983;93:1004–1012.

Parnes LS, McClure JA. Posterior semicircular canal occlusion for intractable benign paroxysmal positional vertigo. *Ann Otol Rhinol Laryngol* 1990;99:330–334.

Parnes LS, McClure JA: Free-floating endolymph particles: A new operative finding during posterior canal occlusion. *Laryngoscope* 1992;102: 988–992.

Parnes LS. Update on posterior canal occlusion for BPPV. *Otolaryngol Clin North Am* 1996;29: 33–342.

Parnes LS. Further observations during the particle repositioning maneuver for BPPV. *Otolaryngol Head Neck Surg* 1997;116:238–243.

Pensak ML, Keith RWJ. Vestibular physiology and clinical testing. In: Lee KJ, ed. *Textbook of Otolaryngology and Head and Neck Surgery.* New York: Elsevier Science, 1989, 31–39.

Pillsbury HC. Metabolic causes of hearing loss and vertigo. *Otolaryngol Clin North Am* 1981;14: 347–354.

Powers WH. Metabolic aspects of Meniere's disease. *Laryngoscope* 1972;82:1716–1725.

Powers WH. Allergic factors in Meniere's disease. *Trans Am Acad Ophthalmol Otolaryngol* 1973; 77:22–29.

Rock EH. Vascular dizziness and transcranial Doppler ultrasonography. *Ann Otol Rhinol Laryngol* 1989;98(Suppl 141):3–24.

Rubenstein RL, Norman DM, Schindler RA, et al. Cerebellar infarction—A presentation of vertigo. *Laryngoscope* 1980;90:505–514.

Rubin W. How do we use state of the art vestibular testing to diagnose and treat the dizzy patient? An overview of vestibular testing and balance system integration. *Neurol Clin* 1990;8(2):225–234.

Rubin W. Differential diagnosis of disorders causing dizziness. *Am J Otol* 1993;14:309–312.

Rubin W. Rotation vestibular testing. *Am J Otolaryngol* 1984;5:441.

Rubin W. The SHA test in vestibular diagnosis. *Laryngoscope* 1981;81:1702–1704.

Rubin W. Symposium on low frequency harmonic acceleration, the rotary chair, SHA as a modality for monitoring patient progress. *Laryngoscope* 1981;91:1282–1284.

Rubin W. Vestibular suppressant drugs. *Arch Otolaryngol* 1973;97:135–138.

Sandstrom J. Cervical syndrome with vestibular symptoms. *Acta Otolaryngol* 1962;54:207.

Sato Y, Kato L, Kawasaki T, et al. Failure of fixation suppression of caloric nystagmus and ocular motor abnormalities. *Arch Neurol* 1980;37: 35–38.

Schuknecht HF. Cochleosacculotomy for Meniere's disease: Theory, technique and results. *Laryngoscope* 1982;92:853–858.

Schuknecht HF. Behavior of vestibular neurons following labyrinthectomy. *Ann Otol Rhinol Laryngol* 1987;96(2 Pt 1):238.

Schuknecht HF. Pathophysiology of endolymphatic hydrops. *Arch Otorhinolaryngol* 1976;212(4): 253–262.

Schuknecht HF. Cupulolithiasis. *Arch Otolaryngol* 1969;90:765–768.

Schumacher GA. Demyelinating diseases as a cause for vertigo. *Arch Otol* 1967;85:93–94.

Semont A, Freyss G, Vitte E: Curing the BPPV with a liberator maneuver. *Adv Otorhinolaryngol* 1988;42:290–293.

Shea JJ. Perfusion of the inner ear with streptomycin. *Am J Otol* 1989;10(2):150–155.

Shea JJ. Endolymph pressure in Meniere's disease. *Otolaryngol Head Neck Surg* 1990;103(5 (Pt 1)): 695–696.

Sidorov JE, Benkovic GW, Greenfield LS, et al. Metabolic abnormalities and vertigo. *Arch Intern Med* 1987;147:197.

Silverstein H, Norrell H. Retrolabyrinthine vestibular neurectomy. *Otolaryngol Head Neck Surg* 1982;90:778–782.

Silverstein H et al. Direct round window membrane application of gentamicin in the treatment of Meniere's disease. *Otolaryngol Head Neck Surg* 1999;120:649–655.

Sismanis A, Hughes GB, Abedi E. Coexisting otosclerosis and Meniere's disease: A diagnostic and therapeutic dilemma. *Laryngoscope* 1986;96: 9–13.

Slepecky N, Chamberlain S. Actin in cochlear hair cells. Implications for stereocilia movement. *Arch Otol Rhinol* 1982;234:131–134.

Spencer JTJ. Hyperlipoproteinemia, hyperinsulinism, and Meniere's disease. *South Med J* 1981; 74:1194–1198.

Spencer JT. Hyperlipoproteinemia in the etiology of inner ear disease. *Laryngoscope* 1974;83: 639–678.

Staller SJ et al. Pediatric vestibular evaluation with harmonic acceleration. *Otolaryngol Head Neck Surg* 1987;95:471–476.

Stroud M, Newman NM, Keltner JL, et al. Abducting nystagmus in the medial longitudinal fasciculus syndrome. *Adv Otol Rhinol Laryngol* 1973;19: 367–376.

Syms CA III, House JW. Idiopathic Dandy's syndrome. *Otolaryngol Head Neck Surg* 1997; 116:75–78.

Takemori S. Visual suppression of vestibular nystagmus after cerebellar lesions. *Ann Otol Rhinol Laryngol* 1975;84:318–326.

Takemori S. Visual suppression test. *Ann Otol Rhinol Laryngol* 1977;86:80–85.

Takemori S, Aiba T, Shizawa R. Visual suppression of caloric nystagmus in the brainstem lesions. *Ann N Y Acad Sci* 1981;374:846–854.

Telian SA, Shepard NT. Update on vestibular rehabilitation therapy. *Otolaryngol Clin North Am* 1996;29(part 1):359–372.

Telischi FF, Luxford WM. Long-term efficacy of endolymphatic sac surgery for vertigo in Meniere's disease. *Otolaryngol Head Neck Surg* 1993;109(1):83–87.

Thalmann R. Metabolic features of auditory and vestibular systems. *Laryngoscope* 1971;81: 1245–1260.

Tilney LG, DeRosier DJ, Mulroy MJ. The organization of actin filaments in the stereocilia of cochlear hair cells. *J Cell Biol* 1980;86: 244–259.

Torok N. The culmination phenomenon and frequency pattern of thermic nystagmus. *Acta Otolaryngol* 1957;48:530–535.

Valli P, Zucca G, Casella C. Ionic composition of the endolymph and sensory transduction in labyrinthine organs. *Acta Otolaryngol* 1979;87: 466–471.

Wall CI. The sinusoidal harmonic acceleration rotary chair test. *Neurol Clin North Am* 1990;8(2): 269–285.

Welling DB et al. Endolymphatic sac occlusion for the enlarged vestibular aqueduct syndrome. *Am J Otol* 1998;19:145–151.

Wiet RJ, Schramm DR, Kazan RP. The retro-labyrinthine approach and vascular loop. *Laryngoscope* 1989;99:1035–1039.

Wilson VJ, Melvill-Jones G, eds. *Mammalian Vestibular Physiology*. New York: Plenun Press, 1979.

Wilson WR, Schuknecht HF. Update on the use of streptomycin therapy for Meniere's disease. *Am J Otol* 1980;2:108–111.

Wolfe JW, Engelken EJ, Kos CM. Low frequency harmonic acceleration as a test of labyrinthine function: Basic methods and illustrative cases. *Trans Am Acad Ophthalmol Otolaryngol* 1978; 86:130–142.

Wolfe JW, Engelken EJ, Olson JW. Vestibular responses to bithermal caloric and harmonic acceleration. *Ann Otol Rhinol Laryngol* 1978; 87:861–867.

Zalzal GH, Tomaski SM, Vezina LG, et al. Enlarged vestibular aqueduct and sensorineural hearing loss in childhood. *Arch Otolaryngol Head Neck Surg* 1995;121:23–28.

Zee DS. Adaptative control of eye movements: Clinical implications. *Can J Neurol Sci* 1994;21: 177–184.

Zee DS. Afternystagmus and headshaking nystagmus. *Equil Res* 1993;52:442–447.

Congenital Deafness 5

One person in eight carries a recessive gene for deafness; hereditary deafness appears in 1:4000 live births. One percent of hereditary hearing loss is sex-linked, 9% is due to an autosomal dominant inheritance, and 90% is the result of autosomal recessive transmission. Hereditary deafness constitutes 15% of all congenital deafness. Dominant hearing loss usually progresses, whereas the recessive type is nonprogressive.

Hereditary deafness can be classified as follows:

1. Hereditary (congenital) deafness without associated abnormalities (autosomal dominant, autosomal recessive, or sex-linked)
2. Hereditary congenital deafness associated with integumentary system disease (autosomal dominant, autosomal recessive, or sex-linked)
3. Hereditary congenital deafness associated with skeletal disease (autosomal dominant, autosomal recessive, or sex-linked)
4. Hereditary congenital deafness associated with other abnormalities (autosomal dominant, autosomal recessive, or sex-linked)

Each category can be subdivided along three kinds of hearing impairment: sensorineural, conductive, and mixed.

Otologists have attempted to classify inner ear development anomalies. Some of the classifications are as follows:

1. *Michel:* Complete failure of development of the inner ear (bony and membranous aplasia). The middle ear and external auditory canal may be normal.
2. *Mundini–Alexander:* Incomplete development of the bony and membranous labyrinth. The cochlea may be represented by a single curved tube, and the vestibular labyrinth is not developed.
3. *Scheibe:* Membranous cochlea-saccular aplasia (pars inferior). The bony labyrinth is normal, as are the utriculus and semicircular canals (pars superior).
4. *Alexander:* Partial aplasia of the cochlear duct giving rise to high-frequency hearing loss.
5. *Bing–Siebenmann:* The membranous vestibular apparatus is maldeveloped. The membranous cochlea may or may not be normal.

Scheibe's type of inner ear anomaly is the one most commonly encountered. It is believed to be autosomally recessive. The next most common is the Mundini–Alexander type, which is believed to be autosomally dominant.

The rubella syndrome includes congenital cataract, cardiovascular anomalies, mental retardation, retinitis, and deafness. It has been reported that 5 to 10% of mothers with rubella during the first trimester give birth to children with deafness. Alford[1] reported that 90 of 141 rubella-syndrome children presented with deafness. The eye is the most commonly affected organ, followed by the ears, and then the heart. Histologically, middle ear as well as inner ear anomalies have been described. Confirmatory tests for the rubella syndrome include identification of fluorescent antibody, serum hemagglutination, and viral cultures from stool and

116

throat. Deafness of a viral etiology shows (1) degeneration of the organ of Corti, (2) adhesions between the organ of Corti and Reissner's membrane, (3) rolled up tectorial membrane, (4) partial or complete stria atrophy, and (5) scattered degeneration of neural elements (cochlea-saccule degeneration).

Twenty percent of kernicteric babies have severe deafness secondary to damage to the dorsal and ventral cochlear nuclei as well as the superior and inferior colliculi nuclei. Clinically, bilateral sensorineural loss, especially in high frequencies, is manifested. The most accepted indication for exchange transfusion is a serum bilirubin of more than 20 mg/dL.

Syphilitic deafness occurs. Tamari and Itkin[2] estimated that hearing loss occurred in:

17% of early congenital syphilis
18% of late congenital syphilis
25% of late latent syphilis
29% of asymptomatic patients with congenital syphilis
39% of symptomatic neurosyphilis

Karmody and Schuknecht[3] reported 25 to 38% of patients with *congenital* syphilis have hearing loss. There are two forms of congenital syphilis: early (infantile) and late (tardive). The infantile form is often severe and bilateral. These children usually have multisystem involvement and hence a fatal outcome.

Late congenital syphilis has progressive hearing loss of varying severity and time of onset. Hearing losses that have their onset during early childhood are usually bilateral, sudden, severe, and associated with vestibular symptoms. The symptom complex is similar to that of Ménière disease. The late-onset form (sometimes as late as the 5th decade of life) has mild hearing loss. Karmody and Schuknecht[3] also pointed out that the vestibular disorders of severe episodic vertigo are more common in the late-onset group than in the infantile group. Histopathologically, osteitis with mononuclear leukocytosis, obliterative endarteritis, and endolymphatic hydrops is noticed. Serum and cerebrospinal fluid (CSF) serology may or may not be positive. Treatment with steroids and penicillin seems to be of benefit. Other sites of congenital syphilis are:

1. Nasal cartilaginous and bony framework
2. Periostitis of the cranial bones (bossing)
3. Periostitis of the tibia (saber shin)
4. Injury to the odontogenous tissues (Hutchinson's teeth)
5. Injury to the epiphyseal cartilages (short stature)
6. Commonly, interstitial keratitis (cloudy cornea)

Two signs are associated with congenital syphilis: *Hennebert's sign* consists of a positive fistula test without clinical evidence of middle ear or mastoid disease, or a fistula. It has been postulated that the vestibular stimulation is mediated by fibrous bands between the footplate and the vestibular membranous labyrinth. Hennebert's sign also may be present in Ménière disease. Another explanation is that the vestibular response is due to an excessively mobile footplate. The nystagmus in Hennebert's sign usually is more marked upon application of a negative pressure (see "Hennebert's Sign," Chapter 9).

Tullio's phenomenon consists of vertigo and nystagmus on stimulation with high-intensity sound, such as the Bárány noise box. This phenomenon occurs not only in congenital syphilis patients with a semicircular canal fistula but also in postfenestration patients if the footplate is mobile and the fenestrum patent. It also can be demonstrated in chronic otitis media should the patient have an intact tympanic membrane, ossicular chain, and a fistula—a rare combination.

For Tullio's phenomenon to take place, a fistula of the semicircular canal and intact sound transmission mechanism to the inner ear (ie, intact tympanic membrane, intact ossicular chain, and mobile footplate) must be present. The pathophysiology is that the high-intensity noise energy transmitted through the footplate finds the course of least resistance and displaces toward the fistula instead of toward the round window membrane.

Hearing loss may occur in the secondary or tertiary forms of *acquired syphilis.* Histopathologically, osteitis with round cell infiltration is noticed. With tertiary syphilis, gummatous lesions may involve the auricle, mastoid, middle ear, and petrous pyramid. These lesions can cause a mixed hearing loss. Because penicillin and other antibiotic therapies are quite effective in treating acquired syphilis, this form of deafness is now rare.

Cretinism, which consists of retarded growth, mental retardation, and mixed hearing loss, is seen in conjunction with congenital deafness.

HEREDITARY DEAFNESS WITHOUT ASSOCIATED ABNORMALITIES

Stria Atrophy (Hereditary, Not Congenital)

1. Autosomal dominant
2. The sensorineural hearing loss begins at middle age and is progressive
3. Good discrimination is maintained
4. Flat audiometric curve
5. Positive Short Increment Sensitivity Index (SISI) test
6. Bilaterally symmetrical hearing loss
7. Patient never becomes profoundly deaf

Otosclerosis (Hereditary, Not Congenital)

See Chapter 31.

HEREDITARY CONGENITAL DEAFNESS ASSOCIATED WITH INTEGUMENTARY SYSTEM DISEASE

Albinism with Blue Irides

1. Autosomal dominant or recessive
2. Sensorineural hearing loss

Ectodermal Dysplasia (Hidrotic)

Note that anhidrotic ectodermal dysplasia is sex-linked recessive, with a mixed or conductive hearing loss.

1. Autosomal dominant
2. Small dystrophic nails
3. Coniform teeth
4. Elevated sweat electrolytes
5. Sensorineural hearing loss

Forney Syndrome

1. Autosomal dominant
2. Lentigines

3. Mitral insufficiency
4. Skeletal malformations
5. Conductive hearing loss

Lentigines
1. Autosomal dominant
2. Brown spots on the skin, beginning at age 2 years
3. Ocular hypertelorism
4. Pulmonary stenosis
5. Abnormalities of the genitalia
6. Retarded growth
7. Sensorineural hearing loss

Leopard Syndrome
1. Autosomal dominant with variable penetrance
2. Variable sensorineural hearing loss
3. Ocular hypertelorism
4. Pulmonary stenosis
5. Hypogonadism
6. Electrocardiographic (ECG) changes with widened QRS or bundle branch block
7. Retardation of growth
8. Normal vestibular apparatus
9. Lentigines
10. Skin changes progressively over the 1st and 2nd decades

Piebaldness
1. Sex-linked or autosomal recessive
2. Blue irides
3. Fine retinal pigmentation
4. Depigmentation of scalp, hair, and face
5. Areas of depigmentation on limbs and trunk
6. Sensorineural hearing loss

Tietze Syndrome
1. Autosomal dominant
2. Profound deafness
3. Albinism
4. Eyebrows absent
5. Blue irides
6. No photophobia or nystagmus

Waardenburg Disease
1. Autosomal dominant with variable penetrance
2. Contributes 1 to 7% of all hereditary deafness
3. Widely spaced medial canthi (present in all cases)
4. Flat nasal root in 75% of cases
5. Confluent eyebrow
6. Sensorineural hearing loss—unilateral or bilateral (present in 20% of cases)
7. Colored irides
8. White forelock

9. Areas of depigmentation (10% of patients)
10. Abnormal tyrosine metabolism
11. Diminished vestibular function (75% of patients)
12. Cleft lip and palate (10% of patients)

HEREDITARY CONGENITAL DEAFNESS ASSOCIATED WITH SKELETAL DISEASE

Achondroplasia

1. Autosomal dominant
2. Large head and short extremities
3. Dwarfism
4. Mixed hearing loss (fused ossicles)
5. Saddle nose, frontal and mandibular prominence

Apert Disease (Acrocephalosyndactyly)

1. Autosomal dominant
2. Syndactylia
3. Flat conductive hearing loss secondary to stapes fixation
4. Patent cochlear aqueduct histologically
5. Frontal prominence, exophthalmos
6. Craniofacial dysostosis, hypoplastic maxilla
7. Proptosis, saddle nose, high-arched palate, and occasionally spina bifida
8. Occurs in about 1 : 150,000 live births

Atresia Auris Congenital

1. Autosomal dominant
2. Unilateral or bilateral involvement
3. Middle ear abnormalities with VII nerve anomaly
4. Internal hydrocephalus
5. Mental retardation
6. Epilepsy
7. Choanal atresia and cleft palate

Cleidocranial Dysostosis

1. Autosomal dominant
2. Absent or hypoplastic clavicle
3. Failure of fontanelles to close
4. Sensorineural hearing loss

Crouzon Disease (Craniofacial Dysostosis)

1. Autosomal dominant
2. Hearing loss in one-third of cases
3. Mixed hearing loss in some cases
4. Cranial synostosis
5. Exophthalmos and divergent squint
6. Parrot-beaked nose
7. Short upper lip
8. Mandibular prognathism and small maxilla
9. Hypertelorism

10. External auditory canal sometimes atretic
11. Congenital enlargement of the sphenoid bone
12. Premature closure of the cranial suture lines, sometimes leading to mental retardation

Engelmann Syndrome (Diaphyseal Dysplasia)
1. Autosomal dominant; ? recessive
2. Progressive mixed hearing loss
3. Progressive cortical thickening of diaphyseal regions of long bones and skull

Hand–Hearing Syndrome
1. Autosomal dominant
2. Congenital flexion contractures of fingers and toes
3. Sensorineural hearing loss

Klippel–Feil (Brevicollis; Wildervanck) Syndrome
1. Autosomal recessive or dominant
2. Incidence in female subjects greater than in male subjects
3. Sensorineural hearing loss along with middle ear anomalies
4. Short neck due to fused cervical vertebrae
5. Spina bifida
6. External auditory canal atresia

Madelung Deformity (Related to Dyschondrosteosis of Leri–Weill)
1. Autosomal dominant
2. Short stature
3. Ulna and elbow dislocation
4. Conductive hearing loss secondary to ossicular malformation with normal tympanic membrane and external auditory canal
5. Spina bifida occulta
6. Female to male ratio of 4:1

Marfan Syndrome (Arachnodactyly, Ectopia Lentis, Deafness)
1. Autosomal dominant
2. Thin, elongated individuals with long spidery fingers
3. Pigeon breast
4. Scoliosis
5. Hammer toes
6. Mixed hearing loss

Mohr Syndrome (Oral-Facial-Digital Syndrome II)
1. Autosomal recessive
2. Conductive hearing loss
3. Cleft lip, high-arched palate
4. Lobulated nodular tongue
5. Broad nasal root, bifid tip of nose
6. Hypoplasia of the body of the mandible
7. Polydactyly and syndactyly

Osteopetrosis (Albers–Schonberg Disease; Marble Bone Disease)
1. Autosomal recessive (rare dominant transmission has been reported)
2. Conductive or mixed hearing loss
3. Fluctuating facial nerve paralysis
4. Sclerotic, brittle bone due to failure of resorption of calcified cartilage
5. Cranial nerves II, V, VII involved sometimes
6. Optic atrophy
7. Atresia of paranasal sinuses
8. Choanal atresia
9. Increased incidence of osteomyelitis
10. Widespread form: may lead to obliteration of the bone marrow, severe anemia, and rapid demise
11. Hepatosplenomegaly possible

Oto-Facial-Cervical Syndrome
1. Autosomal dominant
2. Depressed nasal root
3. Protruding narrow nose
4. Narrow elongated face
5. Flattened maxilla and zygoma
6. Prominent ears
7. Preauricular fistulas
8. Poorly developed neck muscles
9. Conductive hearing loss

Oto-Palatal-Digital Syndrome
1. Autosomal recessive
2. Conductive hearing loss
3. Mild dwarfism
4. Cleft palate
5. Mental retardation
6. Broad nasal root, hypertelorism
7. Frontal and occipital bossing
8. Small mandible
9. Stubby, clubbed digits
10. Low-set small ears
11. Winged scapulae
12. Malar flattening
13. Downward obliquity of eye
14. Down-turned mouth

Paget Disease (Osteitis Deformans)
1. Autosomal dominant with variable penetrance
2. Mainly sensorineural hearing loss but mixed hearing loss as well
3. Occasional cranial nerve involvement
4. Onset usually at middle age, involving skull and long bones of the legs
5. Endochondral bone (somewhat resistant to this disease)

Pierre Robin Syndrome (Cleft Palate, Micrognathia, and Glossoptosis)

1. Autosomal dominant with variable penetrance (possibly not hereditary but due to intra-uterine insult)
2. Occurs in 1:30,000 to 1:50,000 live births
3. Glossoptosis
4. Micrognathia
5. Cleft palate (in 50% of cases)
6. Mixed hearing loss
7. Malformed auricles
8. Mental retardation
9. Hypoplastic mandible
10. Möbius syndrome
11. Subglottic stenosis not uncommon
12. Aspiration a common cause of death

Pyle Disease (Craniometaphyseal Dysplasia)

1. Autosomal dominant (less often autosomal recessive)
2. Conductive hearing loss can begin at any age. It is progressive and secondary to fixation of the stapes or other ossicular abnormalities. Mixed hearing loss also possible
3. Cranial nerve palsy secondary to narrowing of the foramen
4. Splayed appearance of long bones
5. Choanal atresia
6. Prognathism
7. Optic atrophy
8. Obstruction of sinuses and nasolacrimal duct

Roaf Syndrome

1. Not hereditary
2. Retinal detachment, cataracts, myopia, coxa vara, kyphoscoliosis, retardation
3. Progressive sensorineural hearing loss

Dominant Proximal Symphalangia and Hearing Loss

1. Autosomal dominant
2. Ankylosis of proximal interphalangeal joint
3. Conductive hearing loss early in life

Treacher–Collins Syndrome (Mandibulofacial Dysostosis; Franceschetti–Zwahlen–Klein Syndrome)

1. Autosomal dominant or intrauterine abuse
2. Antimongoloid palpebral fissures with notched lower lids
3. Malformation of ossicles (stapes usually normal)
4. Auricular deformity, atresia of external auditory canal
5. Conductive hearing loss
6. Preauricular fistulas
7. Mandibular hypoplasia and malar hypoplasia
8. "Fishmouth"
9. Normal IQ
10. Usually bilateral involvement

11.   May have cleft palate and cleft lip
12.   Arrest in embryonic development at 6 to 8 weeks to give the above findings

Van Buchem Syndrome (Hyperostosis Corticalis Generalisata)
1.   Autosomal recessive
2.   Generalized osteosclerotic overgrowth of skeleton including skull, mandible, ribs, and long and short bones
3.   Cranial nerve palsies due to obstruction of the foramina
4.   Increased serum alkaline phosphatase
5.   Progressive sensorineural hearing loss

Van der Hoeve Syndrome (Osteogenesis Imperfecta)
1.   Autosomal dominant with variable expressivity
2.   Fragile bones, loose ligaments
3.   Blue or clear sclera, triangular facies, dentinogenesis imperfecta
4.   Blue sclera and hearing loss are seen in 60% of cases and are most frequently noted after age 20. The hearing loss is conductive and is due to stapes fixation by otosclerosis. Hearing loss also can be due to ossicular fracture. (Some use the term van der Hoeve syndrome to describe osteogenesis imperfecta with otosclerosis. Others use the term interchangeably with osteogenesis imperfecta regardless of whether or not otosclerosis is present.)
5.   The basic pathologic defect is "abnormal osteoblastic activity"
6.   When operating on such a patient, it is important to avoid fracture of the tympanic ring or the long process of the incus. It is also important to realize that the stapes footplate may be "floating"
7.   The sclera may have increased mucopolysaccharide content
8.   These patients have normal calcium, phosphorus, and alkaline phosphatase in the serum
9.   Occasionally, capillary fragility is noted

HEREDITARY CONGENITAL DEAFNESS ASSOCIATED WITH OTHER ABNORMALITIES
Acoustic Neurinomas (Inherited)
1.   Autosomal dominant
2.   Progressive sensorineural hearing loss during the 2nd or 3rd decade of life
3.   Ataxia, visual loss
4.   No *café au lait* spots

Alport Syndrome
1.   Autosomal dominant
2.   Progressive nephritis and sensorineural hearing loss
3.   Hematuria, proteinuria beginning the 1st or 2nd decade of life
4.   Men with this disease usually die of uremia by age 30. Women are less severely affected
5.   Kidneys are affected by chronic glomerulonephritis with interstitial lymphocytic infiltrate and foam cells
6.   Progressive sensorineural hearing loss begins at age 10. Although it is not considered sex-linked, hearing loss affects almost all male but not all female subjects. Histologically, degeneration of the organ of Corti and stria vascularis is observed
7.   Spherophalera cataract

8. Hypofunction of the vestibular organ
9. Contributes to 1% of hereditary deafness

Alström Syndrome
1. Autosomal recessive
2. Retinal degeneration giving rise to visual loss
3. Diabetes, obesity
4. Progressive sensorineural hearing loss

Cockayne Syndrome
1. Autosomal recessive
2. Dwarfism
3. Mental retardation
4. Retinal atrophy
5. Motor disturbances
6. Progressive sensorineural hearing loss bilaterally

Congenital Cretinism
Congenital cretinism must be distinguished from Pendred syndrome.

1. About 35% present with congenital hearing loss of the mixed type (irreversible)
2. Goiter (hypothyroid)
3. Mental and physical retardation
4. Abnormal development of the petrous pyramid
5. This disease is not inherited in a specific mendelian manner. It is restricted to a certain geographic locale where a dietary deficiency exists

Duane Syndrome
1. Autosomal dominant (some sex-linked recessive)
2. Inability to abduct eyes, retract globe
3. Narrowing of palpebral fissure
4. Torticollis
5. Cervical rib
6. Conductive hearing loss

Fanconi Anemia Syndrome
1. Autosomal recessive
2. Absent or deformed thumb
3. Other skeletal, heart, and kidney malformations
4. Increased skin pigmentation
5. Mental retardation
6. Pancytopenia
7. Conductive hearing loss

Fehr Corneal Dystrophy
1. Autosomal recessive
2. Progressive visual and sensorineural hearing loss

Flynn–Aird Syndrome
1. Autosomal dominant
2. Progressive myopia, cataracts, retinitis pigmentosa

3. Progressive sensorineural hearing loss
4. Ataxia
5. Shooting pains in the joints

Friedreich Ataxia
1. Autosomal recessive
2. Childhood onset of nystagmus, ataxia, optic atrophy, hyperreflexia, and sensorineural hearing loss

Goldenhar Syndrome
1. Autosomal recessive
2. Epibulbar dermoids
3. Preauricular appendages
4. Fusion or absence of cervical vertebrae
5. Colobomas of the eye
6. Conductive hearing loss

Hallgren Syndrome
1. Autosomal recessive
2. Retinitis pigmentosa
3. Progressive ataxia
4. Mental retardation in 25%
5. Sensorineural hearing loss
6. Constitutes about 5% of hereditary deafness

Hermann Syndrome
1. Autosomal dominant
2. Onset of photomyoclonus and sensorineural hearing loss during late childhood or adolescence
3. Diabetes mellitus
4. Progressive dementia
5. Pyelonephritis and glomerulonephritis

Hurler Syndrome (Gargoylism)
1. Autosomal recessive
2. Abnormal mucopolysaccharides are deposited in tissues (when mucopolysaccharides are deposited in the neutrophils they are called Adler bodies); middle ear mucosa with large foamy gargoyle cells staining PAS-positive
3. Chondroitin sulfate B and heparitin in urine
4. Forehead prominence with coarsening of the facial features and low-set ears
5. Mental retardation
6. Progressive corneal opacities
7. Hepatosplenomegaly
8. Mixed hearing loss
9. Dwarfism
10. Cerebral storage of three gangliosides: GM_3, GM_2, and GM_1
11. Beta-galactosides-deficient

Hunter Syndrome
Signs are the same as for Hurler syndrome, except they are sex-linked.

Jervell and Lange–Nielsen Syndrome

1. Autosomal recessive
2. Profound bilateral sensorineural hearing loss (high frequencies more severely impaired)
3. Associated with heart disease (prolonged QT interval on ECG) and Stokes–Adams disease
4. Recurrent syncope
5. Usually terminates fatally with sudden death
6. Histopathologically, PAS-positive nodules in the cochlea

Laurence–Moon–Bardet–Biedl Syndrome

1. Autosomal recessive
2. Dwarfism
3. Obesity
4. Hypogonadism
5. Retinitis pigmentosa
6. Mental retardation
7. Sensorineural hearing loss

(Recessive) Malformed Low-Set Ears and Conductive Hearing Loss

1. Autosomal recessive
2. Mental retardation in 50%

(Dominant) Mitral Insufficiency, Joint Fusion, and Hearing Loss

1. Autosomal dominant with variable penetrance
2. Conductive hearing loss, usually due to fixation of the stapes
3. Narrow external auditory canal
4. Fusion of the cervical vertebrae and the carpal and tarsal bones

Möbius Syndrome (Congenital Facial Diplegia)

1. Autosomal dominant, ? recessive
2. Facial diplegia
3. External ear deformities
4. Ophthalmoplegia
5. Hands or feet sometimes missing
6. Mental retardation
7. Paralysis of the tongue
8. Mixed hearing loss

(Dominant) Saddle Nose, Myopia, Cataract, and Hearing Loss

1. Autosomal dominant
2. Saddle nose
3. Severe myopia
4. Juvenile cataract
5. Sensorineural hearing loss that is progressive, moderately severe, and of early onset

Norrie Syndrome

1. Autosomal recessive
2. Congenital blindness due to pseudotumor retini
3. Progressive sensorineural hearing loss in 30%

Pendred Syndrome

1. Autosomal recessive
2. Variable amount of bilateral hearing loss secondary to atrophy of the organ of Corti. A U-shaped audiogram is often seen
3. Patients are euthyroid and develop diffuse goiter at the time of puberty. It is said that the metabolic defect is faulty iodination of tyrosine
4. Positive perchlorate test
5. The goiter is treated with exogenous hormone to suppress thyroid-stimulating hormone (TSH) secretion
6. Normal IQ
7. Unlike congenital cretinism, the bony petrous pyramid is well developed
8. Constitutes 10% of hereditary deafness

Refsum Disease (Heredopathia Atactica Polyneuritiformis)

1. Autosomal recessive
2. Retinitis pigmentosa
3. Polyneuropathy
4. Ataxia
5. Sensorineural hearing loss
6. Visual impairment usually beginning in the 2nd decade
7. Ichthyosis often present
8. Elevated plasma phytanic acid levels
9. Etiology: neuronal lipid storage disease and hypertrophic polyneuropathy

(Recessive) Renal, Genital, and Middle Ear Anomalies

1. Autosomal recessive
2. Renal hypoplasia
3. Internal genital malformation
4. Middle ear malformation
5. Moderate to severe conductive hearing loss

Richards–Rundel Syndrome

1. Autosomal recessive
2. Mental deficiency
3. Hypogonadism (decreased urinary estrogen, pregnanediol, and total 17-ketosteroids)
4. Ataxia
5. Horizontal nystagmus to bilateral gazes
6. Sensorineural hearing loss beginning during infancy
7. Muscle wasting during early childhood and absent deep tendon reflexes

Taylor Syndrome

1. Autosomal recessive
2. Unilateral microtia or anotia
3. Unilateral facial bone hypoplasia
4. Conductive hearing loss

Trisomy 13–15 (Group D); Patau Syndrome

1. Low-set pinnae
2. Atresia of external auditory canals

3. Cleft lip and cleft palate
4. Colobomas of the eyelids
5. Micrognathia
6. Tracheoesophageal fistula
7. Hemangiomas
8. Congenital heart disease
9. Mental retardation
10. Mixed hearing loss
11. Hypertelorism
12. Incidence is 0.45 : 1000 live births
13. Usually die early in childhood

Trisomy 16–18 (Group E)
1. Low-set pinnae
2. External canal atresia
3. Micrognathia, high-arched palate
4. Peculiar finger position
5. Prominent occiput
6. Cardiac anomalies
7. Hernias
8. Pigeon breast
9. Mixed hearing loss
10. Incidence is 0.25:1000 to 2:1000 live births
11. Ptosis
12. Usually die early in life

Trisomy 21 or 22 (Down Syndrome; G Trisomy)
1. Extra chromosome on No. 21 or No. 22
2. Mental retardation
3. Short stature
4. Brachycephaly
5. Flat occiput
6. Slanted eyes
7. Epicanthus
8. Strabismus, nystagmus
9. Seen in association with leukemia
10. Subglottic stenosis not uncommon
11. Decreased pneumatized or absent frontal and sphenoid sinuses
12. Incidence is 1:600 live births

Turner Syndrome
1. Not inherited; ? due to intrauterine insult
2. Low hairline
3. Webbing of neck and digits
4. Widely spaced nipples
5. XO; 80% sex-chromatin negative
6. Gonadal aplasia
7. Incidence is 1:5000 live births (Klinefelter syndrome is XXY)

8. Ossicular deformities
9. Low-set ears
10. Mixed hearing loss
11. Large ear lobes
12. Short stature
13. Abnormalities in the heart and kidney
14. Some with hyposmia

(Dominant) Urticaria, Amyloidosis, Nephritis, and Hearing Loss

1. Autosomal dominant
2. Recurrent urticaria
3. Amyloidosis
4. Progressive sensorineural hearing loss due to degeneration of the organ of Corti; ossification of the basilar membrane and cochlear nerve degeneration
5. Usually die of uremia

Usher Syndrome (Recessive Retinitis Pigmentosa with Congenital Severe Deafness)

1. Autosomal recessive
2. Retinitis pigmentosa giving rise to progressive visual loss. The patient is usually completely blind by the 2nd or 3rd decade
3. These patients usually are born deaf secondary to atrophy of the organ of Corti. Hearing for low frequencies is present in some patients
4. Ataxia and vestibular dysfunction are common. Usher syndrome, among all congenital deafness syndromes, is the most likely to include vestibular symptoms
5. It constitutes 10% of hereditary deafness
6. Gorlin and coworkers[4] classified Usher syndrome into four types:

   Type I: Profound congenital deafness with the onset of retinitis pigmentosa by age 10; has no vestibular response; constitutes 90% of all cases of Usher syndrome

   Type II: Moderate to severe congenital deafness with the onset of retinitis pigmentosa in late teens or early twenties; normal or decreased vestibular response; constitutes 10% of all cases

   Type III: Progressive hearing loss; retinitis pigmentosa begins at puberty; constitutes less than 1% of all cases (types I, II, and III are autosomal recessive)

   Type IV: X-linked inheritance; phenotype similar to that of type II

Well Syndrome

1. Nephritis
2. Hearing loss
3. Autosomal dominant

MIDDLE AND EXTERNAL EAR CONGENITAL DEFORMITIES

Middle and external ear congenital deformities have been classified into class I, II, and III. However, the classification is less commonly used than that for inner ear developmental anomalies.

Class I

1. Normal auricle in shape and size
2. Well-pneumatized mastoid and middle ear

3. Ossicular problem
4. Most common type

Class II

1. Microtia
2. Atretic canal and abnormal ossicles
3. Normal aeration of mastoid and middle ear

Class III

1. Microtia
2. Atretic canal and abnormal ossicles
3. Middle ear and mastoid poorly aerated
   a. The external deformity does not correlate necessarily with the middle ear abnormality
   b. Patients with a congenitally fixed footplate have the following characteristics that differentiate them from patients with otosclerosis:
      (1) Onset during childhood
      (2) Nonprogressive
      (3) Negative family history
      (4) Flat 50 to 60 dB conductive hearing loss
      (5) Carhart's notch not present
      (6) Schwartze's sign not present

References

1. Alford BR. Rubella—la bete noire de la medecine. *Laryngoscope* 1968;78:1623.
2. Tamari M, Itkin P. Penicillin and syphilis of the ear. *Eye Ear Nose Throat Monthly* 1951; 30:252, 301, 358.
3. Karmody C, Schuknecht HF. Deafness in congenital deafness. *Arch Otolaryngol* 1966; 83:18.
4. Gorlin RJ, et al. Usher's syndrome type III. *Arch Otolaryngol* 1979;105:353.

Bibliography

Farrior J. Congenital aural atresia and hearing loss: Evaluation and management. In: Lee KJ, ed. *Textbook of Otolaryngology and Head and Neck Surgery.* New York: Elsevier Science Publishing Co., Inc., 1989.

Hemenway WG, Bergstrom L. Symposium on congenital deafness. *Otolaryngol Clin North Am* 1971;4(2).

Hemenway WG, et al. Temporal bone pathology following maternal rubella. *Arch Ohr Nas Kehlkopfheilk* 1969;193:287.

Hennebert C. Un syndrome nouveau dans la labyrinthite heredo-syphilitique. *Presse Med* 1911; 63:467.

Lindsay J, et al. Inner ear pathology following maternal rubella. *Ann Otol Rhinol Laryngol* 1953;62: 1201.

Noyek A, Maniglia A. Congenital disorders in otolaryngology. *Otolaryngol Clin North Am* 1981;14.

Noyek A, Maniglia AJ, eds. Symposium on congenital disorders in otolaryngology. *Otolaryngol Clin North Am* 1981;14:1.

Page JM, ed. Symposium on central auditory disorders. *Otolaryngol Clin North Am* 1985;18:2.

Perlman H, Leek J. Late congenital syphilis of the ear. *Laryngoscope* 1952;62:1175.

Schucknecht HF. *Pathology of the Ear,* 2nd ed. Philadelphia: Lea & Febiger, 1993.

Tietz W. A syndrome of deafmutism associated with albinism showing dominant autosomal inheritance. *Am J Hum Genet* 1963;15:259.

Cochlear Implantation 6

Cochlear implants are electronic devices that convert sound energy into electrical signals to stimulate ganglion cells and the cochlear nerve, thus transmitting information to the brain. These devices are indicated for patients with severe to profound sensorineural hearing loss who receive little or no benefit from hearing aids. These patients have either a lack of hair cell development (in the case of congenital hearing loss) or acquired damage to the hair cells. The cochlear implant basically takes over the function of the hair cells by stimulating the cochlear ganglion cells and cochlear nerve. A normal cochlea has 30,000 spiral ganglion cells (the cell bodies of the auditory nerve fibers) arranged in a spiral around the modiolus of the cochlea. In patients with severe hearing loss due to hair cell damage, many of the spiral ganglion cells survive and can be stimulated directly by a cochlear implant. A cochlear implant neither eliminates the underlying disease nor restores normal function to the end organ of hearing, but it is now the standard rehabilitative option for patients with severe sensorineural hearing loss. Although an implant does not provide normal hearing, recent advances in technology have allowed the majority of cochlear implant users to achieve some degree of speech understanding, including use of the telephone with varying degrees of proficiency.

The first description of direct auditory nerve stimulation was by Djourno and Eyries from France in 1957.[1] This early work stimulated William House to develop a cochlear implant, which was first implanted in 1961. Other early pioneers in the development of cochlear implants included Simmons, Michaelson, Banfai, Chouard, Clark, Eddington, and the Hochmairs. The first wearable implant was a single-electrode, single-channel device developed by House, which became available in 1973. The electrode was 6 millimeters long and was inserted into the scala tympani through the round window. More than 1000 were implanted. A later version of this single-electrode implant was approved by the *U.S. Food and Drug Administration* (FDA) for use in adults in 1984. The first pre-school-aged child was implanted with this device in 1981.[2]

Clark implanted a multiple-electrode, multichannel implant in 1978, which began widespread clinical trials in 1985 as the Nucleus Multichannel Cochlear Implant. The FDA approved it for use in adults in 1987 and for children over the age of 2 years in 1990. Over the years, more than 30 various cochlear implant designs have been tried. These include transcutaneous (through intact skin) or percutaneous (a direct connector protruding through the skin) transmission, single or multiple electrodes, extracochlear or intracochlear placement of electrodes, and different types of signal processing schemes. There are now more than 30,000 implanted patients worldwide. There are currently three major device manufacturers with multichannel cochlear implants either in commercial use or clinical trials in the United States (Nucleus, Clarion, Med-El). There is also currently one manufacturer of a single-electrode cochlear implant with an FDA-approved clinical trial in progress (AllHear).

In addition to cochlear implantation, electrodes may be placed directly on the brain stem at the cochlear nucleus in patients with neurofibromatosis 2 (NF2).[3] The first patient was implanted with a single electrode placed on the brain stem, and later, an eight-electrode system was used.[4] The current technology includes 21 electrodes placed on the cochlear nucleus.

NEURAL RESPONSES TO SOUND

There are two ways in which auditory information is coded into neural responses: place coding and temporal coding. *Temporal coding* refers to the temporally varying aspect of the neural responses that convey the temporal properties of sound. Temporal coding of information appears to be limited to frequencies below 500 Hz and is similar at all cochlear locations. *Place coding* refers to the specific perceptual quality of sound (pitch and timbre) that comes from the cochlear location of the neurons. Both single and multiple electrode implants allow temporal coding, but only multiple electrode systems are designed specifically to take advantage of place coding. The pitch percept associated with electrical stimulation of an electrode is determined by a combination of the electrode's tonotopic (place) location and the stimulation rate. Electrodes each typically have a characteristic pitch that changes from a high pitch near the base of the cochlea to a low pitch near the apex. Recognition of speech may require at least four channels of pitch information.[5] As more electrodes have been added to cochlear implants over the years, performance has improved steadily, partly due to the additional electrodes and partly due to improved signal processing. Different cochlear implant devices take different approaches to signal processing, using different speech coding strategies, number of channels of information, and stimulation modes.

Speech Coding Strategies

1. Feature extraction: Analysis of speech signal and extraction of certain key features (ie, voicing, intensity, and format frequencies).
2. Analog: A filter bank separates the speech into frequency bands, transmitting the full speech waveform, not just extracted features.

Number of Channels

The number of channels has to do with the amount and type of information transfer and is not necessarily equal to the number of electrodes.

1. A single-channel system represents all sound information as one electrical signal applied to a single electrode or to all electrodes simultaneously. If one electrode or one pair is selected for all stimulation, there is no place coding of the signal.
2. Multiple-channel systems send different electrical signals to different sites in the cochlea. This requires multiple active electrodes and can take advantage of the tonotopic organization of the cochlea.

Stimulation Mode (Multichannel Stimulation)

1. Simultaneous: stimulating several electrodes at a given time.
2. Sequential: a continuous series of electrodes being activated either in succession or as determined by the dominant spectral energy of choice in the speech signal, one electrode at a time.

COMPONENTS OF THE COCHLEAR IMPLANT

Microphone
External processor (body or over the ear)
External transmitter (in current devices, transcutaneous)
Internal receiver-stimulator
Electrode array (1 to 24 electrodes)

Sound enters the microphone and is transmitted to the external processor, where it is processed into components to be sent to various electrodes. The signal is transmitted across the skin at radio frequencies in coded form as an analog or pulsatile waveform. The internal receiver decodes the signal and routes it along the implanted wires across the mastoid to the cochlea. The various electrodes, in turn, stimulate the cells of the spiral ganglion and auditory nerve.

PATIENT SELECTION

Etiology of Deafness

Etiology of deafness is usually not a factor in selection of patients for implantation so long as the auditory nerve is not completely absent. Results of a recent multicenter study by Cochlear Corporation revealed the following distribution of etiologies for adults and children receiving the Nucleus 24 Contour cochlear implant[*]:

	Adults	Children
Unknown	64.3%	61.7%
Hereditary	21.4%	21.7%
Meningitis	1.8%	8.3%
Ménière's disease	1.8%	—
Otosclerosis	1.8%	—
Ototoxicity	1.8%	—
Viral	1.8%	1.7%
Mondini deformity	—	3.3%
Other	5.4%	3.3%

*Nucleus 24 Contour (C124R (CS)) Cochlear Implant System IDE #990110
Final Report. Personal communication, 2001.

Other etiologies included bacterial labyrinthitis, Cogan syndrome, congenital syphilis, and trauma.

Patient Evaluation

One of the most important aspects of the cochlear implant process is the patient's pre-evaluation to determine suitability for a cochlear implant. Because the cochlear implant can destroy residual hearing, it is imperative to establish that the patient is likely to perform better with an implant than with an appropriately fitted hearing aid. This evaluation is performed by specially trained audiologists who have experience working with implant patients.

The criteria for implant candidacy are evolving and changing as implant technology improves. The early cochlear implants were indicated only for patients with total sensorineural hearing loss. Technology has improved so that now patients with residual hearing may gain considerable benefit from cochlear implants.

Sample of Current Criteria for Selection of Adult Candidates

Nucleus

Aided HINT (Hearing in Noise Test) sentences ≤50% correct in the implant ear
Aided HINT sentences ≤60% correct in nonimplant ear

Med-El
> Moderate to profound SNHL (sensorineural hearing loss) in low frequencies
> 90 dB or greater SNHL in middle and high frequencies
> Aided HINT sentences ≤40%

Clarion
> Pure-tone average >70 dB
> Aided HINT sentences ≤40%

Typical Criteria for Selection of Pediatric Candidates

1. 12 months of age for most devices.
2. Bilateral profound hearing loss for 12- to 18-month-olds, severe to profound for those older than 18 months.
3. Little to no benefit from hearing aids (for youngest children, plateau in auditory development; for children above age 5, minimal open-set word recognition despite appropriately fitted hearing aids and therapeutic intervention over a trial period of 3 to 6 months) (the trial period is waived for postmeningitis children with radiographic evidence of ossification).
4. No medical contraindications.
5. Enrollment in an educational program that emphasizes auditory development.
6. Appropriate family support and expectations.

Tests Commonly Performed

The basic evaluation includes audiological tests and the medical evaluation.

1. Pure-tone air and bone conduction thresholds and speech discrimination.
2. Distortion Product Otoacoustic Emissions (DPOAES).
3. Immitance audiometry.
4. ABR for thresholds if indicated.
5. Soundfield testing for warble-tone thresholds and speech perception measures with hearing aids. These include tests of speech discrimination for monosyllabic words and sentences presented in an open-set (no answer list) format. Commonly used tests include the hearing in noise test (HINT) for sentence discrimination in adults and age-appropriate tests of pattern perception, closed-set word discrimination, and open-set speech understanding for children such as the Early Speech Perception Test (ESP), Meaningful Auditory Integration Scale (MAIS), Lexical Neighborhood Test (LNT), Multisyllabic Lexical Neighborhood Test (MLNT), and Phonetically Balanced Kindergarten (monsyllabic word lists) (PBK).
6. CT scan to look for cochlear ossification, inner ear deformities, internal auditory symmetry, mastoid pneumatization, and status of the middle ear.[6]

A meeting is conducted with the otologist, audiologist, patient, and family in order to review the findings and discuss options.

Counseling

An important aspect of the pre-evaluation is the counseling of the patient. It is important to counsel the patient and his or her family regarding appropriate expectations for the implant. The counseling includes:

1. Case history and hearing aid history.
2. Expectations—what the implant will and will not do for the patient.
3. Commitment to attend all scheduled appointments during the first year.
4. Highly recommend that they attend at least one Cochlear Implant support group meeting. At these meetings they have the opportunity to talk to cochlear implant patients and their families, see them functioning in a group setting and learn about the realities of the implant.
5. The risks and complications of surgery. This should also be reviewed with the surgeon. It is a good idea to give the patient a printed sheet with the risks and complications listed.
6. Discuss the various devices available and explain the features of each. Explain how they differ from each other. We do not favor any particular device and allow the patient to decide on the device he or she prefers.

A final step in the preoperative management of the implant patient is, if necessary, to obtain insurance authorization for the surgery and authorization for the postoperative rehabilitation. There are specific guidelines for Medicare patients. These need to be stated in the operative note in order for Medicare to pay for the procedure.

SURGICAL TECHNIQUE

The surgery is performed under general endotracheal anesthesia with continuous intraoperative facial nerve monitoring. The postauricular incision begins inferiorly following around the auricle, extending anterior, superior and curving posterior at its superior pole. It is important that the internal receiver is not placed in the incision line (1–2 cm wider than the internal processor-stimulator). It needs to be located far enough superior and posterior from the auricle to allow room for a postauricular processor. Good vascular supply to the flap must be maintained to minimize the chance of wound healing failure. The temporalis muscle and fascia are exposed, the periosteum is elevated from the mastoid cortex, and the wound is held open in a self-retaining retractor. The mastoidectomy differs from standard mastoid surgery in that an overhang of bone is retained. This allows the electrode to be tucked under the overhang to help prevent extrusion. The facial recess is opened, exposing the pyramidal process and round window. In order to visualize the round window, it is necessary to remove bone inferiorly and posteriorly. Using a small diamond burr with continuous irrigation, the lip of the round window niche is removed to expose the round window membrane. Damage to the facial nerve is avoided by not rotating the burr while passing through the facial recess to the round window area. In some cases (especially post-meningitis) the round window niche is replaced by bony growth, necessitating a "drill out" of the basal turn.[7]

A small portion of temporalis muscle is removed and a seat is formed for the internal receiver. Suture tunnel holes are drilled adjacent to the seat to secure the internal receiver with silk ties. The cochleostomy is performed at the round window. It has to be large enough to admit the electrode array. The Clarion requires a larger opening than does the Nucleus or Med-El devices. The electrode array is carefully advanced into the scala tympani. The wound is closed in layers, a head dressing is applied, and most patients can be discharged on the same day as surgery. The dressing is removed the day following surgery.

COMPLICATIONS

Potential complications are the same as those for chronic otitis media surgery.[8]

1. Facial weakness or paralysis (rare)

    Prevention: Facial nerve monitoring.
                     Leave bony covering on bone in facial recess.
                     Avoid advancing or removing turning drill through facial recess while
                     creating cochleostomy.
    Treatment: Steroids
                     Exploration; possible decompression, repair or graft

2. Wound infection

    Treatment: Appropriate antibiotics

3. Cerebrospinal fluid drainage

    Prevention: Muscle packing into cochleostomy
    Treatment: Middle ear packing with muscle
                     Spinal drain

4. Meningitis

    Treatment: Appropriate antibiotics

5. The usual risks of anesthesia

    Complications unique to cochlear implants include the following:

1. Extrusion or device failure (2–5%) requiring explantation and reimplantation.

    Prevention: The internal receiver is placed 1 to 2 cm from the wound.
    Treatment: Rotation flap may be necessary to cover internal receiver.
                     At reimplantation internal receiver repositioned.

2. Loss of residual hearing—unavoidable and must be discussed with patient preoperatively.

INITIAL FITTING OF THE COCHLEAR IMPLANT

The patient returns to the audiologist for the initial fitting of the external processor and transmitter approximately 1 month after surgery. A month is adequate time for the operative edema to subside over the internal receiver. At this visit the audiologist will spend 1 to 2 hours working with the patient, perhaps longer with children.

Steps in First Fitting

1. Determine magnet strength for the transmitter.
2. Measure electrical threshold levels.
3. Measure electrical comfort levels.
4. Sweep electrode array and determine appropriate pitch percept.
5. Balance volume of comfort levels across array in pairs or groups.
6. Create "map" (depending on device maps are created with different strategies—ie, CIS (Continuous Interleaved Sampler Strategy), MPS (Multiple Pulsatile Sampler Strategy),

SAS (Simultaneous Analog Stimulation), ACE (Advanced Combination Encoder), or Speak (this is not an acronym but the actual name of the speech coding strategy).

7. Manipulate map for comfort, for example:
    a. Global change in comfort levels.
    b. Remove electrodes which produce nonauditory stimulation.
    c. Decrease gains on basal/middle/apical electrodes depending on complaint.
8. Discuss and demonstrate speech processor controls.
    a. Volume control.
    b. Sensitivity control.
    c. Program selector.
    d. On/off switch.
    e. Changing batteries.
9. Demonstrate and dispense items in accessory kit.
10. Warranty information.
11. Aural rehabilitation.
    a. Exercises practiced during sessions and take home activities.
    b. Handouts on making the most of the cochlear implant.
    c. Learning to listen through the implant.
    d. Discuss adaptation and expectations.
    e. Include significant others and family members in adjustment process.
    f. Troubleshooting the device when there is a malfunction.

Subsequent Appointments

Subsequent appointments with the audiologist are the next day, in 2 weeks, 1 month, and 3 months. During each of these visits the audiologist spends time reviewing progress, answering questions, and making adjustments in the settings. Medical follow- up is included in some of these visits and includes inspection of the wound, ear, and skin over the internal receiver. It is important to watch for possible skin breakdown or extrusion (these are rare).

RESULTS

Most deaf patients can detect medium to loud sounds and hear speech at a comfortable listening level. They can learn to recognize familiar sounds. Patients who are postlingually deafened and who have been deaf for a short time learn to use the auditory information provided by the implant more quickly and effectively than those who are born with profound hearing loss or lose their hearing early in life. Many adult patients are able to gain open-set speech discrimination and use the telephone with their implant. Children implanted at a young age can develop significant open-set speech discrimination, with resultant improvements in oral/aural communication skills (speech and language). Results of implantation have been extensively presented in the literature for different devices and different population groups.[9–20]

SUMMARY

1. Cochlear implants are not experimental.
2. Cochlear implants are not hearing aids.
3. Candidates are those patients who have bilateral severe to profound sensorineural hearing loss and do not benefit from hearing aids.

4. Complications are rare.

5. Implants improve auditory cues and, therefore, improve speech understanding and speech production.

6. The best candidates are postlingually deafened adults with a short duration of deafness or children implanted at a young age.

7. Postlingually deafened children in aural programs progress more rapidly with cochlear implants. Those children who are prelingually deaf show substantial benefit when they are implanted early, but they may not achieve maximum benefits if implanted at an older age.

References

1. Brackmann DE: The cochlear implant: basic principles. *Laryngoscope* 86:373–388, 1976.

2. Luxford WM, Brackmann DE: The history of cochlear implants. In Gray RF, ed *Cochlear Implants.* London, Croom Helm, 1985; p 1–26.

3. Brackmann DE, Hitselberger WE, Nelson RA, et al: Auditory brainstem implant I. Issues in surgical implantation. *Otolaryngol Head Neck Surg* 108:624–633, 1993.

4. Otto SR, Shannon RV, Brackmann DE, et al: The multichannel auditory brainstem implant: performance in twelve patients. *Otolaryngol Head Neck Surg* 118:291–303, 1998.

5. Shannon RV, Zeng FG, Kamath V, et al: Speech recognition with primarily temporal cues. *Science* 270:303–304, 1995.

6. Gray RF, Evans RA, Freer CEL, et al: Radiology for cochlear implants. *J Laryngol Otol* 105:85–88, 1991.

7. Balkany T, Gantz B, Nadol JB Jr.: Multichannel cochlear implants in partially ossified cochleas. *Ann Otol Rhinol Laryngol Suppl* 135:3–7, 1988.

8. Cohen NL, Hoffman RA: Complications of cochlear implant surgery in adults and children. *Ann Otol Rhinol Laryngol* 100:708–711, 1991.

9. Parkin JL, Randolph LJ: Auditory performance with simultaneous intracochlear multichannel stimulation. *Laryngoscope* 101:379–383, 1991.

10. Geier L, Barker M, Fisher L, et al: The effect of long-term deafness on speech recognition in postlingually deafened adult CLARION cochlear implant users. *Ann Otol Rhinol Laryngol Suppl* 177:80–83, 1999.

11. Osberger MJ, Fisher L: SAS-CIS preference study in postlingually deafened adults implanted with the CLARION cochlear implant. *Ann Otol Rhinol Laryngol Suppl* 177:74–79, 1999.

12. Cheng AK, Grant GD, Niparko JK: Meta-analysis of pediatric cochlear implant literature. *Ann Otol Rhinol Laryngol Suppl* 177:124–128, 1999.

13. Brown C, McDowall DW: Speech production results in children implanted with the CLARION implant. *Ann Otol Rhinol Laryngol Suppl* 177:110–112, 1999.

14. Palmer CS, Niparko JK, Wyatt JR, et al: A prospective study of the cost-utility of the multichannel cochlear implant. *Arch Otolaryngol Head Neck Surg* 125:1221–1228, 1999.

15. Young NM, Grohne KM, Carrasco VN, et al: Speech perception of young children using nucleus 22-channel or CLARION cochlear implants. *Ann Otol Rhinol Laryngol Suppl* 177:99–103, 1999.

16. Osberger MJ, Zimmerman-Phillips S, Barker M, et al: Clinical trial of the CLARION cochlear implant in children. *Ann Otol Rhinol Laryngol Suppl* 177:88–92, 1999.

17. Tyler RS, Gantz BJ, Woodworth GG, et al: Initial independent results with the Clarion cochlear implant. *Ear Hear* 17:528–536, 1996.

18. Kelsay DM, Tyler RS: Advantages and disadvantages expected and realized by pediatric cochlear implant recipients as reported by their parents. *Am J Otol* 17:866–873, 1996.

19. Zwolan RA, Kileny PR, Ashbaugh C, et al: Patient performance with the Cochlear Corporation "20 + 2" implant: bipolar versus monopolar activation. *Am J Otol* 17:717–723, 1996.

20. Staller S, Menapace C, Domico E, et al: Speech perception of adult and pediatric nucleus implant recipients using the Spectral Peak (SPEAK) Coding Strategy. *Otolaryngol Head Neck Surg* 117:236–242, 1997.

Skull Base Surgery 7

Probably the greatest advance in the management of malignant and benign tumors of the head and neck in the last two decades is the development of skull base surgery. This entails the combined expertise of the otolaryngologist/head-and-neck surgeon and the neurologic surgeon in a preoperatively planned and well-coordinated way to remove tumors that transgress the calvarium from the upper aerodigestive tract and neck into the intracranial space. Prior to the advent of cranial base surgery, the malignant tumors that invaded the skull base were uniformly considered to be inoperable and were almost always fatal.

ANATOMY[1–3]

An intimate and detailed knowledge of the anatomy of the undersurface of the skull and the immediate intracranial contents juxtaposed to it, as well as the structures of the head and neck at these same sites, is essential for the proper execution of the skull base procedures. The procedures are largely grouped according to the cranial fossae to which the surgery is directed. They are classified as anterior, middle, and posterior approaches, corresponding to those cranial fossae thus named; central for access to those lesions located in the central midline, in the region of the sella turcica and clivus; and finally the far lateral, for those in the region of the brain stem and medulla, where the approach is through the lateral mass of C1, the occipital condyle, and the basiocciput (Fig. 7-1).

ANTERIOR SKULL BASE

The orbital roofs, fovea ethmoidalis, planum sphenoidale, and cribriform plate make up the bony floor of the anterior cranial fossa. On the intracranial side, the gyri of the frontal lobes of the brain overlie the majority of the fossa floor. The ocular gyri are located more laterally and the gyrus rectus lies just lateral to the midline. On the undersurface of the gyrus rectus is the olfactory bulb, which sends the olfactory filaments through the cribriform plate. There are, on average, 43 olfactory foramina through each plate.[4] A dural sleeve encases each olfactory filament as it passes from its intracranial to its extracranial course.

ANTERIOR SKULL BASE (ANTERIOR CRANIAL FOSSA)

Anterior:	Frontal crest and posterior wall of the frontal sinus
Posterior:	Lesser wing of the sphenoid bone
Medial:	Cribriform plate extending along the line of the planum sphenoidale to the tuberculum sellae
Lateral:	Frontal bone
Superior:	Frontal lobes, olfactory bulb, and olfactory tract
Inferior:	Orbital plates of the frontal bone, with the medial portion of the floor being formed by the roof of the ethmoid sinus. The cribriform plate is the thinnest portion and transmits the first cranial nerve to the olfactory fossa. The crista galli, a vertical plate of bone, defines the midline.

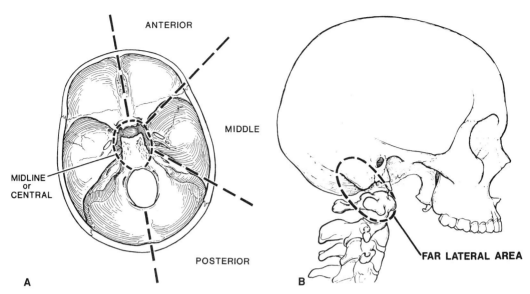

Figure 7-1.   **A.** Diagram outlining the various regions of cranial base surgery. [*From Donald PJ: Presentation and preparation of patients with skull base lesions, in Donald PJ, ed:. Surgery of the Skull Base. Philadelphia: Lippincott-Raven, 1998:74, with permission.*] **B.** The far lateral approach.

MIDDLE CRANIAL AND INFRATEMPORAL FOSSAE

The infratemporal fossa is the area just inferior to the temporal fossa in which resides the bulk of the temporalis muscle. The temporalis muscle inserts on the coronoid process and a variable distance down the mandibular ramus. As the distal part of the temporalis muscle traverses deep to the zygomatic arch, it forms the lateral wall of the infratemporal fossa. The roof of the fossa is the floor of the middle cranial fossa.

The middle cranial fossa houses the temporal lobe of the brain, whose anterior horn extends for a variable distance under the anterior cranial fossa floor underneath the lesser wing of the sphenoid. This portion of the temporal lobe lies just lateral to the orbital apex. The superior orbital fissure and the optic canal penetrate the anterior wall of this fossa medially. Most of the floor of the middle cranial fossa is made up by the temporal bone and only to a small part by the lesser wing of the sphenoid. Both petrous pyramids meet medially at their articulation with the body of the sphenoid bone, which is aerated by the sphenoid sinus and is indented superiorly by the sella turcica.

The key anatomic structures in the middle fossa floor are the gasserian ganglion. situated in Meckel's cave, and the mandibular branch of the trigeminal nerve exiting the foramen ovale. Just posterior to this foramen is the foramen spinosum, through which the middle meningeal artery passes.

The internal carotid artery runs in the longitudinal axis of the petrous temporal bone. It enters the carotid canal through the undersurface of the bone encircled by the fibrous ring, ascends anteriorly to the hypotympanum, then turns anteromedially, running medial to the eustachian tube, where it indents the tube's posterior wall. It runs under the gasserian ganglion, which sits on the floor of the middle fossa and is separated from it by only a thin plate of bone. The artery then ascends through the foramen lacerum and begins its serpiginous course through the cavernous sinus.

The cavernous sinus is located laterally to the sphenoid sinus and is a highly vascular structure, containing venous structures and vascular sinusoids. The third, fourth, and sixth nerves pass through the cavernous sinus—the former two in a double fold of dura in its lateral wall and the latter in the sparse adventitia of the lateral wall of the internal carotid artery (Fig. 7-2). Until only a few decades ago, this was considered to be a surgeon's no-man's land; but with modern techniques and instrumentation, it is amenable to excision even when invaded by some head-and-neck carcinomas. Numerous extracranial veins and dural venous sinuses connect in the cavernous sinus. The superior and inferior petrosal sinuses posteriorly and the sphenoparietal sinus anteriorly, as well as bridging veins from the anterior and middle cerebral hemispheres, drain into the sinus. The circular sinus around the pituitary stalk and the basilar plexus across the clivus connect each cavernous sinus to that on the opposite side.

Middle Cranial Fossa

Anterior:	Greater and lesser wings of the sphenoid bone. The wings are separated by the superior orbital fissure.
Posterior:	Petrous portion of the temporal bone.
Medial:	Foramen rotundum—V_2 to the pterygopalatine fossa.
	Foramen ovale—V_3 to the infratemporal fossa.
	Foramen spinosum—middle meningeal artery.
	Foramen lacerum—a fibrocartilaginous canal juxtaposing the internal carotid artery and formed by the petrous apex, body of the sphenoid bone, and basiocciput.
Superior:	Temporal lobe.
Inferior:	Medially, the floor is formed by the petrous portion of the temporal bone and the greater wing of the sphenoid. The upper surface houses the sellae turcica. The sphenoid sinus lies below, with the cavernous sinus sitting laterally. Posterior and lateral to this lies the trigeminal ganglion in Meckel's cave.

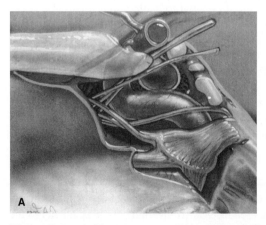 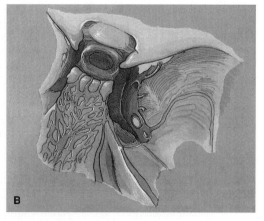

Figure 7-2. A. The cavernous sinus showing the cranial nerves and the internal carotid artery. **B.** The venous connections to the cavernous sinus.

Cervical Cranial Junction

This region is important anteriorly for approaches to the clivus and the anterior aspects of the upper cervical vertebrae but also laterally in the region of the atlantooccipital joint. The important structures laterally are the vertebral artery and the hypoglossal nerve (Fig. 7-3). Anteriorly, the basipharyngeal fascia inserts onto the pharyngeal tubercles of the clivus; posterior to that is the tough fascia overlying the sphenoid and occipital contributions to the claval bone.

Infratemporal Fossa

This complex space lies below the middle cranial fossa and behind the infraorbital fissure. Anteromedial to the infratemporal fossa, natural pathways lead to the pterygopalatine foramen, which opens into the nasopharynx.

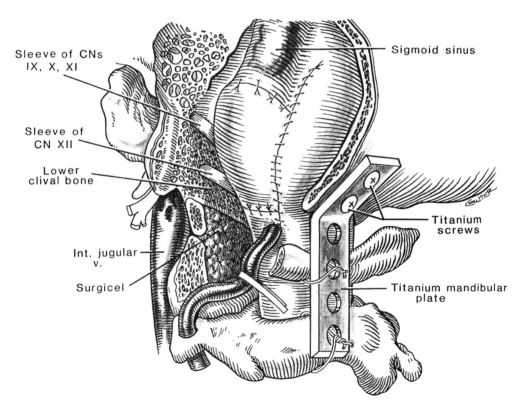

Figure 7-3. The craniocervical junction and the position of the vertebral artery and hypoglossal nerve. Following extradural tumor removal, note the skeletonized nerves of the hypoglossal and jugular foramina, occluded jugular bulb, and titanium plate fixation after complete removal of the occipital condyle. This fixation allows relatively artifact-free imaging and maintains the normal distance between occiput and C1-C2. [*From Sen C, Sekhar L: Extreme lateral transcondylar and transjugular approaches, in Sekhar L, Janecka I, eds:* Surgery of Cranial Base Tumors. *New York: Raven Press, 1993:397, with permission.*]

Temporal Bone

The four constituent parts of the temporal bone are as follows:

1. Mastoid
2. Squamosa
3. Tympanic
4. Petrous

The petrous portion is directed anteromedially, with its base lying laterally. The three surfaces formed are directed anteriorly, posteriorly, and inferiorly.

Posterior Surface of Temporal Bone

1. Bounded superiorly and inferiorly by the superior and inferior petrosal sinuses, respectively.
2. Midway across its surface lies the internal auditory canal, which carries the seventh and eighth cranial nerves.
3. The endolymphatic duct lies on the posteroinferior face of the temporal bone. The vestibular aqueduct enters the temporal bone deep to the operculum and travels to the vestibule's inferior surface.

Inferior Surface of Temporal Bone (Lateral to Medial)

1. Mastoid tip.
2. Digastric ridge, which runs sagitally medial to the mastoid tip and intersects with the stylomastoid foramen.
3. Styloid process, which is anterior to the stylomastoid foramen.
4. Temporomandibular fossa, which is directly anterior to the styloid process.
5. Jugular foramen, which is medial to the styloid process.
   a. The medial compartment contains cranial nerves IX, X, and XI.
   b. The jugular bulb rests in the lateral compartment. The mastoid canaliculus enters the lateral wall of the jugular foramen and transmits Arnold's nerve (a branch of cranial nerve X).
6. The cochlear aqueduct enters medially between the jugular fossa and the carotid canal anteriorly.
7. Jacobson's nerve (a branch of cranial nerve IX) enters inferiorly in the crotch between the jugular and the carotid canal.
8. The carotid canal is anterior to the jugular foramen and medial to the styloid process. It proceeds superiorly to the petrous apex then turns 90 degrees, angling anteromedially. At the anterior aspect of the apex, the carotid artery proceeds superiorly once again.
9. The spine of the sphenoid is anterior to the vertical segment of the carotid canal.
10. The cartilaginous portion of the eustachian tube begins medial to the spine of the sphenoid.
11. The hypoglossal canal is medial and inferior to the jugular foramen.
12. Crescent-shaped occipital condyles lie medial to the hypoglossal canal and form the lateral wall of the foramen magnum.
13. The basioccipital synostosis forms the anterior limit of the foramen magnum.

Anterosuperior Surface of the Temporal Bone

1. Arcuate eminence is a bulge on the superior surface of the petrous bone overlying the superior semicircular canal

2. Facial hiatus transmitting the greater superficial petronal nerve exits anteromedial to the arcuate eminence

Posterior Skull Base (Posterior Fossa)

Anterior: The superior angle of the posterior surface of the petrous ridge forms the anterolateral boundary of the fossa; the tentorium cerebelli and superior petrosal sinus are attached to this.

Posterior: Occipital and parietal bones.

Medial: Foramen magnum, vermion fossa, and internal occipital crest and protuberance.

Lateral: Parietal bone.

Superior: Cerebellar hemisphere lodged in the inferior occipital fissures.

Inferior: Cerebellar fossa, jugular and hypoglossal foramina.

CLINICAL INVESTIGATION

History and Physical Examination

Review of past records is absolutely essential. Past operative and pathology reports, the results of other laboratory tests, and records of the previous clinical examinations must be read in detail.

Many different pathologic processes involve the region of the skull base. Attention in this chapter is principally paid to the management of tumors, especially malignancies. The commonest malignant tumor found invading the skull base is squamous cell carcinoma, followed closely by adenocarcinoma, including adenoid cystic carcinoma. Many of these tumors arise in the paranasal sinuses, but a significant number arise primarily in the skin, parotid salivary gland, naso- and oropharynx, and orbit. These are extensive tumors; as such, their presenting signs and symptoms are those of advanced cancer at these sites. Since one of the mechanisms of intracranial spread is through neural foramina, cranial nerve symptoms are very common. The commonest symptoms are anosmia in advanced nasal and paranasal carcinomas, blindness or diplopia when the orbit or cavernous sinus is involved, facial numbness when branches of the trigeminal nerve are invaded and the jugular foramen is involved; as well as symptoms of dysphagia and hoarseness.

Headache is an uncommon presenting symptom unless there is sinus obstruction and secondary infection; it is usually seen only when there is extensive intracranial involvement. Similarly, a leak of cerebrospinal fluid (CSF) is rarely seen on presentation. Facial pain is commensurate with that of the advanced paranasal sinus or other diseases of the head and neck, from which many of these tumors arise and then extend intracranially.

Trismus is common in the posterior extension of sinus malignancy or pharyngeal carcinoma into the pterygoid region. In these instances, perineural spread of tumor along nerve V_3 to the foramen ovale is suspected.

RADIOGRAPHY

The radiographic examination should include computed tomography (CT); magnetic resonance imaging (MRI); angiography, possibly including a balloon test occlusion (BTO); and single photon emission computed tomography (SPECT); finally, positron emission tomography (PET) may be indicated. A PET scan is most useful in an attempt to establish a local recurrence or distant metastatic disease. It is especially helpful in differentiating between tumor and fibrosis in patients in whom a recurrence of disease is suspected. MRI and CT scans are essential in every case. They should be done in the axial, coronal, and sagittal planes. Gadolinium contrast should be used and fat-suppression software employed if, on MRI, the differentiation of fat from tumor is difficult. Fine-cut CT scans will detect bone erosion in most instances. An angiogram, BTO, and SPECT scans are done only if, on the scans, there is suspicion of carotid artery invasion. A blood flow differential of greater than 92% between the cerebral hemispheres will usually predict that a stroke will not occur if the internal carotid is sacrificed. A word of caution is that despite the sophistication of our modern scans, there are a significant number of false-positives and false-negatives.

Any past histologic material is reviewed. An examination of the patient under anaesthesia and multiple biopsies secure the pathologic diagnosis as well as establishing the subcranial limits of the tumor.

PREPARATION

Once the preoperative evaluation has been completed, the patient is presented to the multidisciplinary skull-base tumor board. The neurosurgeon, the head-and-neck surgeon, and the plastic surgeon plan the details of the procedure and the timing of each individual's intervention.

First the decision is made as to the candidate's operability. The general criteria of inoperability are (1) distant metastasis, (2) patient fragility, and (3) lack of patient cooperation or reluctance to have the surgery. The tumor-specific criteria are (1) invasion of the brain stem; (2) involvement of both internal carotid arteries; (3) involvement of both cavernous sinuses; (4) invasion of a portion of the brain that, if removed, will give a poor quality of life; and (5) invasion of the spinal cord. Invasion of the optic chiasm is a relative contraindication, and usually patients choose to die rather than lose their sight in both eyes.

The informed consent is a long and tedious affair discussing all options, possibilities of complications, and projected prognosis.

The preparation for surgery usually entails the placement of a tracheostomy, a lumbar subarachnoid drain, temporary tarsorrhaphy sutures in the eyelids, anesthetic vascular monitoring equipment, and, finally, if carotid sacrifice is anticipated, the installation of scalp electrodes to monitor the brain waves during carotid clamping. To do this, the patient's head is placed on a horseshoe-shaped Mayfield head rest.

SURGERY OF THE ANTERIOR FOSSA

If the amount of brain invasion brings into question the patient's operability, the neurosurgeon opens first with a low anterior craniotomy. In most cases this is not an issue, and the head-and-neck surgeon approaches the tumor first. Most cases are approached through a lateral rhinotomy (Fig. 7-4).[5] An anterior wall maxillary ostectomy is done, initially registering osseous fixation plates where the osteosynthesis will be done at the end of the case (Fig. 7-5). Ethmoidectomy and medial maxillectomy are done at this point; at the same time as the tumor is debulked. The debulking does not imply that the tumor will be removed piecemeal; it will eventually be completely removed in a modified en bloc fashion. An excellent view is now obtained of the posterior wall of the maxilla, sphenoid rostrum, anterior clivus, and nasopharynx. If tumor invades the posterior wall, the wall is removed along with a margin of healthy bone. The pterygomaxillary space may be invaded; if so, the pterygoid plates are drilled away and the soft tissue is removed with a good margin. Extensive invasion of the

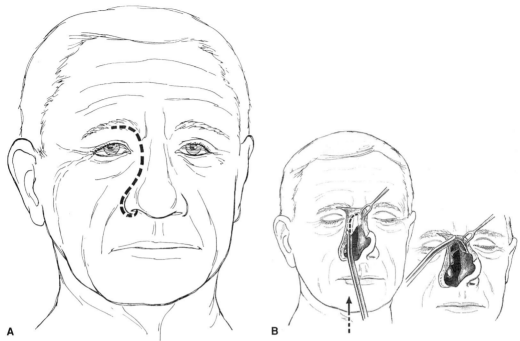

Figure 7-4.   **A.** Lateral rhinotomy skin incision. [*From Donald PJ: Transfacial approach, in Donald PJ, ed:* Surgery of the Skull Base. *Philadelphia: Lippincott-Raven, 1998:169, with permission.*] **B.** Curved osteotome used to create bony lateral rhinotomy incision. [*From Donald PJ: Transfacial approach, in Donald PJ, ed:* Surgery of the Skull Base. *Philadelphia: Lippincott-Raven, 1998:169, with permission.*]

pterygoid muscle mandates a different, more elaborate approach that will entail removal of the ramus and condyle of the mandible.

The anterior wall of the sphenoid sinus is drilled away. Tumor that has invaded the sinus floor is removed with a drill. The interior of the sinus is exteriorized in its entirety so that any vestige of tumor can be removed (Fig. 7-6). Small portions of the lateral sphenoid wall can be removed, as can small areas of the medial cavernous sinus as long as it is away from the internal carotid artery. Hemostasis is secured at this site with the use of hemostatic gauze or cotton.

Inferiorly, the palatal muscles and the cartilaginous eustachian tube can be removed if invaded by tumor. If the bony canal is involved, the middle fossa–infratemporal fossa approach will be employed at a second sitting.

All tumors are removed with a sufficient margin of surrounding healthy tissue and the margins checked by frozen section. The only area in which residual tumor remains is on the extracranial part of the anterior fossa floor. The neurosurgical portion of the operation now begins.

A bicoronal scalp flap is raised without cutting the pericranium. Once the scalp flap has been elevated, the scalp posterior to the initial incision is lifted as far as necessary to create

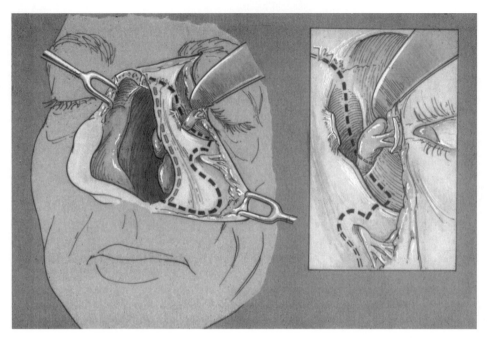

Figure 7-5. Anterior maxillary ostectomy.

a pericranial flap of adequate length. This flap is created by making two parallel incisions in the calvarial periosteum on either side of the frontal skull; the length of the scalp flap extending to just above the origin of the temporalis muscles. These are connected across the vertex posterior to the scalp incision and the flap is elevated down to the brows, where it is pedicled on the supraorbital and supratrochlear vessels (Fig. 7-7). A low, small craniotomy is done that is extensive enough to allow for the safe extirpation of the intracranial extent of the tumor. The dura and superior sagittal sinus are dissected free and the intracranial extent of the tumor is exposed. The tumor in dura is cleared by a margin of about 5 mm. Any invasion into the brain will be suspected preoperatively by the appearance of an area of rarefaction on the MRI, which represents a halo of necrosis surrounding the area of tumor involvement. The brain is excised with a margin of similar width to that of the dura, with frequent checks by frozen section. Fortunately brain involvement by tumor is uncommon, as the dura provides a stout barrier to penetration by cancer.

Delineation of the circumference of tumor penetrating the anterior fossa floor is done by the neurosurgeon from above, aided by the head-and-neck surgeon from below. The bony margins are clearly visualized through the exenteration cavity left by the resection of the sinuses. As the involved anterior fossa floor is cleared by a margin of 5 to 10 mm, the vital structures at the undersurface of the brain are protected by the neurosurgeon (Fig. 7-8).

Once multiple frozen sections have ensured clearance of the malignancy, reconstruction begins. The dura is replaced by temporalis fascia, fascia lata, lyophilized dura, or bovine pericardium. The pericranial flap is swung under the dural reconstruction, placed across the defect in the anterior fossa floor, and sandwiched between the healthy dura beyond the

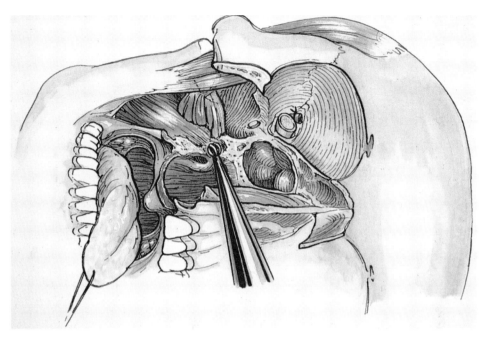

Figure 7-6.   View of the posterior wall of the pterygomaxillary space and nasopharynx after the posterior wall maxillectomy. Note: burr removing pterygoid plates. [*From Donald PJ. Extended transfacial surgical approach, in Donald PJ, ed:* Surgery of the Skull Base. *Philadelphia: Lippincott-Raven, 1998:299, with permission.*]

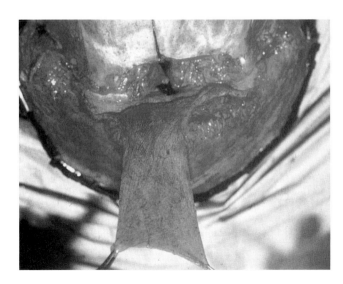

Figure 7-7.   Pericranial flap. [*From Donald PJ: Transfacial approach, in Donald PJ, ed:* Surgery of the Skull Base. *Philadelphia: Lippincott-Raven, 1998:184, with permission.*]

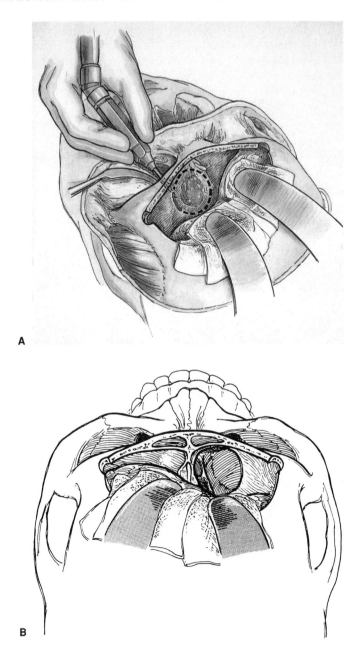

Figure 7-8. **A.** The neurosurgeon protects the brain from above while the head-and-neck surgeon outlines the amount of bone resection from below. [*From Donald PJ: Transfacial approach, in Donald PJ, ed:* Surgery of the Skull Base. *Philadelphia: Lippincott-Raven, 1998:188, with permission.*] **B.** Defect after anterior fossa resection for carcinoma of the ethmoid sinuses with intracranial invasion.

posterior extremity of the defect and the residual anterior fossa floor at this site. The exenteration cavity is lined with split-thickness skin and the previously saved bony maxillary wall is anchored in place with micro- and miniplates. If the nasolacrimal duct has been severed during the resection, a dacryocystorhinostomy is done and a silastic stent placed through the lacrimal puncta and through the duct into the nose.

If the tumor is more extensive, a total maxillectomy is required. An attempt is always made to preserve the orbit. If the globe or orbital apex is invaded by the neoplasm, the orbit must be exenterated. When a high-grade tumor invades the periorbita but spares the orbital fat or ocular muscles, the eye is saved. In low-grade tumors, even the involvement of these structures does not necessarily spell doom for the eye. Table 7-1 is a treatment algorithm describing the relative indications for orbital sparing and exenteration.

SURGERY OF THE MIDDLE CRANIAL FOSSA

This approach combines the infratemporal fossa approach, originally described by Fisch,[6] with a small, low, middle fossa craniotomy. The incision begins near the midline of the calvarium about 2 cm behind the hairline. It is carried inferiorly in front of the ear for lesions originating in the parotid, sinuses, or upper neck or behind the ear for lesions beginning in the temporal bone or clivus. It continues into the upper aspect of the neck, like the incision used for parotidectomy (Fig. 7-9).[7] The flap is elevated from the level of the lateral orbital rim superiorly to the angle of the jaw inferiorly. The external auditory canal is cut across at the junction of bone and cartilage. The skin flap is dissected in the same plane as a face-lift to the orbital rim and the mandibular angle. Care is taken to avoid injury to the facial nerves, especially the temporal branch. The latter is avoided by elevating a patch of temporal fascia deep to the branch during the skin elevation. The main trunk of the facial nerve is not exposed.

The internal carotid artery (ICA) and internal jugular vein are identified in the neck and isolated with vascular loops. An incision is made in the pericranium about 2 cm outside the periphery of the origin of the temporalis muscle, and the entire body of the muscle is dissected from the temporal and infratemporal fossae down to its insertion in the coronoid process of the mandible (Fig. 7-10). The arch of the zygoma and the condyle of the mandible are removed. The condyle is discarded but the zygoma preserved for replacement at the end of the procedure (Fig. 7-11).

The dissecting microscope is brought in and a tympanomeatal flap is raised in the skin of the external auditory canal. The middle ear is entered anteriorly and the opening of the eustachian tube exposed. Cuts within the tympanic annulus are made at about 2 and 7 o'clock,

TABLE 7-1. TREATMENT ALGORITHM FOR ORBITAL EXENTERATION/ORBITAL PRESERVATION WITH ORBITAL INVOLVEMENT WITH CARCINOMA

	Malignancy		
	Well Diff	**Poorly Diff**	**Sq Cell Ca**
1. Orbital base	P	P	P
2. Periorbita	P	±P	P
3. Orbital fat	P	E	E
4. Muscle	E	E	E

Key: P, preservation; E, exenteration.

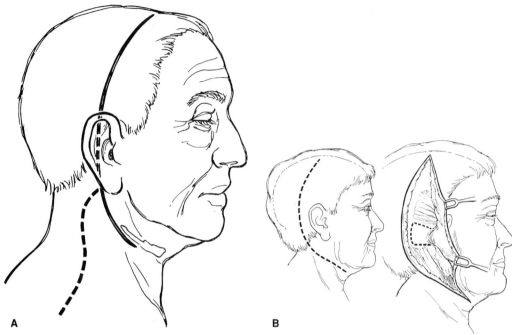

A   B

Figure 7-9.   Incision for the infratemporal fossa middle fossa approach. **A.** Line drawing of anterior incision. Lazy "S" incision added if neck dissection is required. [*From Donald PJ: Craniofacial surgery for head-and-neck cancer, in Johnson JT, Blitzer A, Ossoff RH, Thomas JR, eds:* AAO-HNS Instructional Courses. *Vol. 2. St. Louis: Mosby, 1989:244, with permission.*] **B.** Line drawing of posterior incision. [*From Donald PJ: Infratemporal fossa-middle cranial fossa approach, in Donald PJ, ed:* Surgery of the Skull Base. *Philadelphia: Lippincott-Raven, 1998:314, with permission.*]

Figure 7-10.   Temporalis elevated, but further dissection impeded by the presence of the zygomatic arch. [*From Donald PJ: Infratemporal fossa-middle cranial fossa approach, in Donald PJ, ed:* Surgery of the Skull Base. *Philadelphia: Lippincott-Raven, 1998:319, with permission.*]

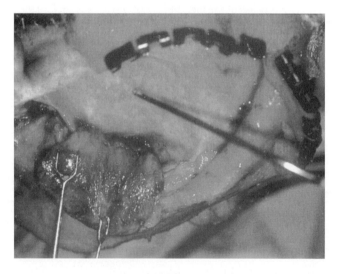

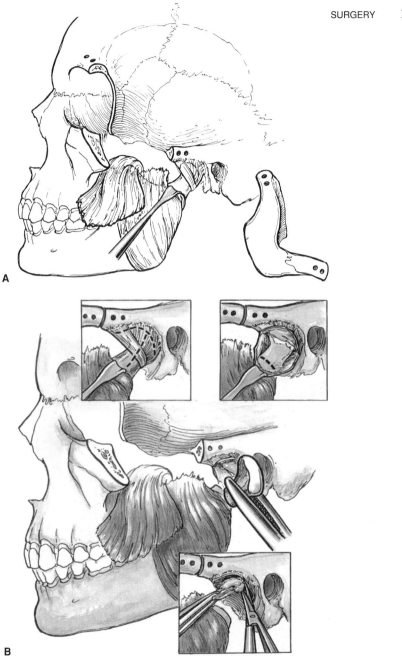

Figure 7-11.   **A.** Bony excision complete. [*From Donald PJ: infratemporal fossa-middle cranial fossa approach, in Donald PJ, ed:.* Surgery of the Skull Base. *Philadelphia: Lippincott-Raven, 1998:324, with permission.*] **B.** Condylectomy: Lateral aspect of the temporomandibular joint capsule is opened and connected to the mandibular neck. The condylar neck is transected and the condyle removed. The meniscus and attached soft tissue are removed. [*From Donald PJ: Infratemporal fossa-middle cranial fossa approach, in Donald PJ, ed:* Surgery of the Skull Base. *Philadelphia: Lippincott-Raven, 1998:325, with permission.*]

respectively, with a small cutting bur. The superior cut is directed superiorly into the bone of the middle ear, across the tensor tympani canal anterior to the cochleariform process, into the superior part of the protympanum; the inferior cut extends from the inferior annulus across the hypotympanum into the mouth of the eustachian tube at about 7 o'clock. The bony external canal is now cut down to the level of the dura out onto the squamosal part of the temporal bone superiorly and then inferiorly through the thickness of the external canal into the glenoid fossa. Although the cuts through the bony external auditory canal are full-thickness cuts, those in the glenoid fossa are only about 1 to 2 mm thick. The cut through the glenoid fossa is directed toward the foramen spinosum, at which site the middle meningeal artery is ligated. The foramen spinosum cut is connected to the foramen ovale and is deepened to the level of the middle fossa dura (Fig. 7-12). This osseous incision is carried across the middle fossa floor and to the level just above the pterygoid plates.

The neurosurgeon continues at this point, creating a small craniotomy through the greater wing of the sphenoid and squamosal portion of the temporal bone and connecting the cut in the external auditory canal posteriorly to the area near the base of the pterygoid plates anteriorly. The dura is dissected away and the bone flap removed (Fig. 7-13). A greenstick fracture will occur such that the protympanum is fractured across and the internal carotid artery (ICA) exposed as it indents the posterior wall of the bony eustachian tube. If the tumor approximates or invades the artery, the vessel is dissected from the fibrous ring at the opening of the carotid canal through the vertical and horizontal course of the artery all the way to the cavernous sinus. The tumor is removed in a modified en bloc method, frequently checking frozen sections until total removal has been effected. Involved dura and brain are removed, as are the cavernous sinus and the ICA. The artery is grafted if it has been invaded by the cancer.

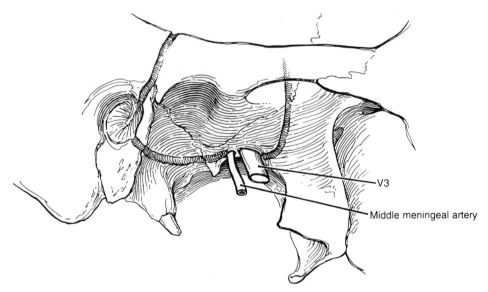

Figure 7-12.   Close-up view of inferior aspect of cut through the external auditory canal and glenoid fossa, and connecting the foramen spinosum to the foramen ovale. [*From Donald PJ: Skull base surgery for sinus neoplasms, in Donald PJ, Gluckman JL, Rice DH, eds:* The Sinuses. *New York: Raven Press, 1995:483, with permission.*]

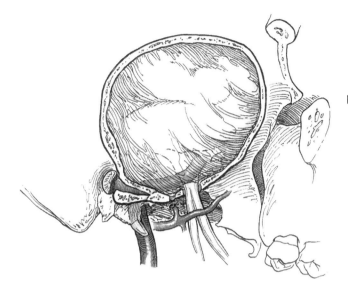

Figure 7-13. Flap removed. Note the bone flap has been fractured across the eustachian tube. [*From Donald PJ: Infratemporal fossa-middle cranial fossa approach, in Donald PJ, ed:* Surgery of the Skull Base. *Philadelphia: Lippincott-Raven, 1998:330, with permission.*]

Subcranially, the eustachian tube is removed and the nasopharynx exposed. Since many of these tumors take their origin in the nasopharynx, the entire tube and part of the clivus require excision.

Once the tumor is completely excised, closure of the dura is done using fascia grafts, and the nasopharynx is isolated from the intracranial cavity with either a temporalis muscle flap or with a free flap, usually of the rectus abdominis muscle. The craniotomy bone flap and the zygomatic arch are returned and plated into position.

THE FAR LATERAL APPROACH

The far lateral approach is usually reserved for those tumors taking origin in the clivus or the upper posterior neck or those extending posteroinferiorly from the temporal bone. The incision is in a question-mark configuration that begins high in the occiput, courses around the postauricular area, and descends into the upper neck (Fig. 7-14). The muscles of the posterior skull base—the trapezius, splenius capitis, semispinalis capitis, and longissimus capitis—are separated from the basiocciput and the upper cervical spine is exposed. The vertebral artery is exposed and the foramina transversaria in the region involved with tumor are identified. The bone of the spinous processes is drilled away, with care taken not to injure the vertebral artery. If the artery is invaded by tumor, it is usually safe to sacrifice the vessel. A preoperative balloon test occlusion and SPECT scan will establish the safety in removing this artery.

The artery is mobilized up to the foramen magnum and the atlantooccipital joint exposed.[8] The lateral mass of the atlas is drilled away, keeping in mind the position of the occipital emissary vein and the hypoglossal canal. At least half of the joint can be removed without destabilizing the spine.

The neurosurgeon does an occipital craniotomy of sufficient size to resect the tumor. This resection can extend as far as the temporal bone; a mastoidectomy with exposure of the jugular bulb may be necessary in order to encompass the tumor. Occipital-spinal fusion is a decision made by the neurosurgeon on the basis of assumed spinal instability. The com-

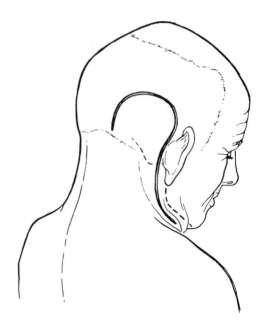

Figure 7-14. "Question mark" incision used for the far lateral approach.

monest means of stabilizing the atlantooccipital joint is with a plate placed along the lamina of the upper cervical vertebrae and fixed to the unresected occiput. The dura is closed primarily or grafted with fascia, the occipital bone flap is restored, the muscles are approximated, and skin is closed.

APPROACHES TO THE INTERNAL AUDITORY CANAL, CEREBELLOPONTINE ANGLE, AND SKULL BASE

Ninety-one percent of cerebellopontine angle tumors are vestibular schwannomas. The remaining 10% of tumors comprise meningiomas, arachnoid cysts, cholesteatomas, facial neuromas, and metastatic lesions.[9] Vestibular schwannomas typically begin in the internal auditory canal at the junction of the Schwann cells and astrocytes. They have an average growth rate of 1 to 2 mm per year.[10] When monitored longitudinally, one-third of tumors do not grow.[10,11] Hearing loss is generally of insidious onset with gradual progression; however, 10 to 22% will present with sudden onset sensorineural hearing loss.[12–13] The incidence of vestibular schwannomas in patients who present with sudden sensorineural hearing loss is 1.5%.[14] Up to 70% of patients with vestibular schwannomas complain of tinnitus. The motor function of the facial nerve is resilient to compression by the tumors, but subtle deficits are observed in 10% of patients.[15] Sensory fibers are less resilient, with up to 85% of patients having some hypesthesia (Hitselberger's sign).[16] Workup for vestibular schwannomas has changed over the past decade due to the relatively low sensitivity and specificity of auditory brain stem responses (ABRs) and the declining costs and increased availability of MRI scans. An MRI with gadolinium is now the preferred first-line investigation.

The differential diagnosis of cerebellopontine angle (CPA) lesions with MRI is shown in Table 7-2.

TABLE 7-2. DIFFERENTIAL DIAGNOSIS OF CEREBELLOPONTINE ANGLE LESIONS WITH MRI

Tumor	T_1	T_1-Gad	T_2
Vestibular schwannoma	↓	↑	↑
Meningioma	↓	↑	↑
Cholesteatoma	↓	+/−	↑
Arachnoid cyst	↓	↓	↑
Lipoma	↑	↑	+/−
Cholesterol granuloma	↑	↓	↑

Key: T_1, weighted sequence; T_1-Gad, weighted sequence with gadolinium; T_2, weighted sequences.

There are three main approaches to the internal auditory canal (IAC) and CPA. Each approach has advantages and disadvantages.[17]

1. Translabyrinthine approach
    a. Advantages
        (1) Minimized cerebellar retraction and potential subsequent atrophy
        (2) Fewer postoperative headaches
        (3) Visualizes facial nerve prior to tumor dissection
    b. Disadvantages
        (1) Up to 21% incidence of CSF fistula
        (2) Loss of residual hearing
2. Retrosigmoid approach
    a. Advantages
        (1) Quicker approach
        (2) 50% hearing preservation in tumors less than 2 cm
    b. Disadvantages
        (1) 23% incidence of postoperative headache
        (2) Requires cerebellar retraction with possible subsequent atrophy
        (3) 7 to 21% incidence of CSF fistula
        (4) In larger tumors, dissection precedes identification of the facial nerve
3. Middle cranial fossa approach
    a. Advantages
        (1) 50 to 75% chance of hearing preservation
        (2) Minimal risk of CSF fistula
    b. Disadvantages
        (1) Slightly increased risk to facial nerve if tumor originates on inferior vestibular nerve
        (2) Requires some temporal lobe retraction, which could pose additional risks in the elderly

Translabyrinthine Approach

This approach was first introduced in 1904 by Panse but did not become a standard approach until its reintroduction by William House.[18]

Technique

1. A curved postauricular incision is made 3 cm behind the postauricular crease.
2. A complete mastoidectomy is performed.

3. The sigmoid sinus is skeletonized and only a very thin wafer of bone is left covering the sinus (Bill's island).
4. The dura is explored anterior and 2 cm posterior to the sinus, allowing compression of the sinus for improved exposure.
5. A complete labyrinthectomy is performed.
6. The internal auditory canal is skeletonized 180 degrees.
7. All bone covering the dura from the sigmoid sinus to the porus acusticus is removed, as well as the bone covering the middle fossa dura.
8. The jugular bulb is skeletonized.
9. The intralabyrinthine segment of the facial nerve is identified, together with the vertical crest (Bill's bar), which separates the facial nerve from the superior vestibular nerve in the lateralmost aspect of the IAC.
10. The dura over the IAC and posterior fossa is incised.
11. The superior vestibular nerve together with the tumor is reflected off of the facial nerve.
12. Tumor debulking proceeds with bipolar cautery, CO_2 laser, or Cavatron ultrasonic surgical aspiration (CUSA) together with microdissection.
13. Temporalis fascia is placed over the dural incision and aditus ad antrum.
14. The mastoid cavity is packed with abdominal fat.
15. Incision is closed in three layers.
16. Pressure dressing is applied for 5 days.

Transotic Approach

The transotic approach as described by Fisch is a modification of the translabyrinthine approach.[19] It adds additional exposure anterior to the IAC and decreases the risk of a postoperative CSF fistula. In addition to the steps of a translabyrinthine approach, the following components are added:

Technique

1. Complete resection of the skin of the medial external auditory canal and tympanic membrane.
2. Evert skin of lateral external auditory canal and suture closed.
3. Complete two-layer closure of external auditory canal with an anterior pedicled periosteal flap raised from the mastoid cortex.
4. Resect the posterior canal wall down to the facial nerve.
5. Drill through the cochlea, skeletonizing the IAC anteriorly. This increases circumferential skeletonization of the IAC from 180 degrees with the translabyrinthine approach to 300 degrees.
6. Close the eustachian tube by inverting the mucosa and plugging the orifice with a piece of muscle and the incus.

Middle Fossa Approach

This approach is reserved for small intracanalicular tumors where hearing preservation is a consideration. Other applications include facial nerve decompression, vestibular nerve section, part of a total temporal bone resection, and approach to the petrous apex.

Technique

1. A lazy-S skin incision extending from the preauricular crease toward the vertex is created.

2. The temporalis muscle is split vertically and retracted, exposing the squamosal portion of the temporal bone.
3. Create a 4- by 4-cm bone window with a cutting bur beginning at the level of the root of the zygoma. Two-thirds of the window is located anterior to the vertical plane of the external auditory canal and one-third is posterior.
4. Elevate the temporal lobe extradurally and retract it with a middle fossa retractor. The foramen spinosum containing the middle meningeal artery is the anterior limit of exposure.
5. Blue-line the superior semicircular canal under the arcuate eminence.
6. The internal auditory canal lies within the meatal plane, which is formed by a 60 degree angle anterior to the superior semicircular canal.
7. The internal auditory canal is skeletonized 180 degrees over the superior aspect of the canal back to the porus acusticus.
8. The facial nerve is identified at the geniculate and intralabyrinthine segment. The greater superficial petrosal nerve can be traced posteriorly back through the facial hiatus to the geniculate ganglion. "Bill's bar," the vertical crest, separates the facial nerve anteriorly from the superior vestibular nerve posteriorly.
9. The tumor is dissected off of the facial nerve.
10. Bone wax is applied to any exposed air cells.
11. Temporalis fascia is placed over the internal auditory canal.
12. The bone plate is returned to the skull and the temporalis and scalp reapproximated.

Retrosigmoid Approach

This approach is the current modification of the suboccipital approach, which has been the standard neurosurgical approach for much of the twentieth century. The modification involves more anterior placement of the craniectomy and with a smaller window.

Technique

1. The patient is placed in the three-quarters lateral or park bench position with the head in a Mayfield head rest.
2. A lazy-S incision is created 4 cm behind the postauricular crease.
3. A 4- by 4-cm craniotomy is performed immediately posterior to the sigmoid sinus.
4. A dural flap is created and retracted.
5. Arachnoid is incised and CSF is drained from the cisterna magna.
6. The cerebellum is covered with a cottonoid and retracted posteriorly with a flat-blade retractor.
7. The cerebellopontine angle is now visualized.
8. At this point, tumor can be excised, the vestibular nerve sectioned, or the trigeminal, facial, or vestibular nerve decompressed.
9. The tumor is debulked with bipolar cautery, Cavitron ultrasonic aspirator, or CO_2 laser.
10. Once adequate exposure of the posterior face of the petrous bone and operculum is exposed, the dura overlying the internal auditory canal is incised and elevated.
11. The internal auditory canal is skeletonized posterosuperiorly.
12. The operculum is an important landmark, which identifies the entry point of the endolymphatic duct.
13. By remaining anteromedial to the endolymphatic duct while approaching the internal auditory canal, one decreases the risk of entry into the labyrinth and the resultant deafness.

14. In general, up to 7 mm of bone can be removed safely from the medial aspect of the internal auditory canal.
15. Once the facial nerve is identified, the remainder of the tumor is peeled off the nerve and excised.
16. All exposed air cells are occluded with bone wax.
17. Fascia is placed over the internal auditory canal.
18. The dural flap over the CPA is closed.
19. The craniotomy defect is filled with bone chips or a cranioplasty is performed with hydroxyapatite cement and the wound closed.

Retrolabyrinthine Approach

This approach was originally described by Hitselberger and Pulec in 1972 for section of the fifth nerve; its use has since been expanded.[20] At present it is limited to vestibular nerve sections and management of hemifacial spasm by microvascular decompression. There are minimal advantages to this approach and a significant disadvantage of limited visualization.

Technique

1. A postauricular incision is made and a layered flap created.
2. A cortical mastoidectomy is performed.
3. The dura is skeletonized along the posterior fossa and superiorly along the middle fossa dura.
4. The facial nerve, labyrinth, and incus are identified.
5. The sigmoid sinus is decorticated and retrosigmoid air cells are removed to expose the retrosigmoid dura.
6. A dural flap is made parallel to the sigmoid sinus (behind the endolymphatic sac) up to the level of the superior petrosal sinus.
7. The cerebellum is retracted and the arachnoid incised, exposing the seventh- to eighth-nerve complex.
8. The vestibular nerve is sectioned or a nerve decompression is performed.
9. The tumor is removed or the nerve sectioned.
10. The wound is closed with silk sutures on the dura; abdominal fat may be used to obliterate the surgical defect prior to layered closure.

THE PETROUS APEX

Evaluation of the patient with pathology at the petrous apex must include consideration of lesions involving the clivus, pituitary, nasopharynx, sphenoid, temporal bone, and meninges.

Lesions of the Petrous Apex

1. Cholesteatoma
   a. Arises from the foramen lacerum from the epithelial elements congenitally included in Sessel's pocket of the cephalic flexure of the embryo.
   b. Some 94% of cases present with hearing loss.
2. Mucocele.
3. Metastatic tumor.
4. Mesenchymal tumor (chondroma).
5. Osteomyelitis, including malignant external otitis and mastoiditis.
6. Clival tumor (chordoma).

7. Glomus tumor.
8. Nasopharyngeal tumors.
9. Meningioma.
10. Neurinoma (trigeminal or acoustic).
11. Aneurysm of the ICA.
12. Lesions involving the cavernous sinus.
13. Cholesterol granuloma.
14. Histiocytosis X.

Symptoms

1. Cranial neuropathy
   a. Nerves III, IV, V, VI, VII, and VIII
   b. Jugular foramen syndrome of nerves IX, X, and XI
   c. Hypoglossal foramen XII
2. Headache (often retroorbital or vertex)
3. Tinnitus, hearing loss
4. Eustachian tube dysfunction; serous effusion
5. Meningitis
6. Gradenigo's syndrome (otorrhea, lateral rectus palsy, trigeminal pain)

Evaluation

1. Audiometry
2. Contrast-enhanced CT scanning with bone density windows
3. MRI with gadolinium
4. Arteriography, including digital subtraction arteriography

Goals of Surgical Management

1. Provide exposure or permit easy access for exteriorization.
2. Preserve residual hearing.
3. Preserve facial function.
4. Preserve the ICA.
5. Protect the brain stem.
6. Prevent CSF leakage.

Approaches

1. Middle cranial fossa
2. Retrosigmoid
3. Transsphenoid
4. Transcochlear
5. Infratemporal fossa
6. Infracochlear

The Transcochlear Approach

This approach[21] provides access to the skull base medial to the porus acusticus and anterior to the petrous apex and brain stem.

Technique

1. An extended postauricular incision is made.
2. A cortical mastoidectomy is performed.

3. The facial nerve is skeletonized from the stylomastoid foramen to the geniculate ganglion.
4. Bone covering the posterior fossa dura, sigmoid sinus, and middle fossa dura is removed.
5. A labyrinthectomy is performed.
6. The chordae tympani and greater superficial petrosal nerves are divided and the facial nerve is mobilized posteriorly.
7. The stapes and incus are removed and the cochlea is drilled out.
8. The dissection is bounded by the carotid artery anteriorly, the superior petrosal sinus above, the jugular bulb below, and the sigmoid sinus posteriorly; the medial extent is the petrous apex just below Meckel's cave.
9. Following tumor removal, the wound may be filled with harvested fat and closed in layers.

The Infratemporal Fossa Approach

Fisch describes three approaches or modifications[22]:

Type A: Access to the temporal bone (infralabyrinthine and apical compartments and inferior surface)

Type B: Access to clivus

Type C: Access to the parasellar region and nasopharynx

Indications

TYPE A

1. Glomus tumors
2. Adenoid cystic carcinoma, acinus cell carcinoma, and mucoepidermoid carcinoma
3. Squamous cell carcinoma
4. Cholesteatoma
5. Neurinoma (nerves IX and X)
6. Meningioma
7. Rhabdomyosarcoma, myxoma, teratoma

TYPE B

1. Chordoma
2. Chondroma
3. Squamous cell carcinoma
4. Dermoid and epidermoid cysts
5. Meningioma, craniopharyngioma, plasmacytoma, arachnoid cyst, and craniopharyngeal fistula

TYPE C

1. Squamous cell carcinoma (failed radiation therapy)
2. Adenoid cystic carcinoma developing around the eustachian tube
3. Advanced juvenile nasopharyngeal angiofibroma

Technique

There have been a number of modifications in approaches to the infratemporal fossa. The technique described below is the approach employed by the authors.

1. A C-shaped incision is made from the temporal region extending 4 cm postauricularly and then down into the neck.

2. The anteriorly based flap exposes the parotid and neck region.
3. The external auditory canal is transected at the bony cartilaginous junction.
4. Neck dissection exposes nerves IX, X, XI, and XII as well as the ICA and internal jugular vein (IJV).
5. The seventh nerve is identified at the stylomastoid foramen.
6. Wide-field mastoidectomy is performed; the mastoid tip, entire bony external auditory canal (EAC), and middle ear contents are removed.
7. The seventh nerve is removed from its canal and translocated anteriorly.
8. The mandibular condyle or entire ramus is mobilized forward to expose the glenoid fossa.
9. The ICA is traced from the neck along the skull base and below the labyrinth to the region proximal to the cavernous sinus.
10. The dura over the posterior and middle fossae is exposed and opened for intracranial extension.
11. The labyrinth and cochlea may be sacrificed to expose the internal auditory canal, petrous apex, clivus, and anterior brain stem.
12. Abdominal fat may be used to fill the wound or, following tumor removal, an anteriorly based rotated temporalis muscle-fascia flap may be used to fill the wound.
13. A layered closure is performed and compression dressing is applied.

Complications of Infratemporal Fossa Surgery
1. Circulatory collapse, cardiac arrythmia, and hemorrhage
2. Meningitis
3. CSF leak
4. Wound breakdown
5. Cerebral edema
6. Hydrocephalus
7. Cranial neuropathy
8. Aspiration, dysfunction of speech, and deglutition problems
9. Hearing loss
10. Facial paralysis
11. Depression and psychological disability

These approaches to the infratemporal fossa are used most effectively for glomus tumors.

GLOMUS TUMORS

Glomus tumors are from the family of paragangliomas and have the following characteristics:

1. They arise from normally occurring neuroectocrine cells found in the jugular bulb adventitia or along Jacobson's or Arnold's nerve.
2. Onset is insidious.
3. Early symptoms include hearing loss, pulsatile tinnitus, unsteady gait, or true vertigo.
4. Late symptoms reflect other cranial neuropathies of nerves V, VI, VII, IX, X, XI, and XII. Nerves VII and X are the most frequently affected.
5. Glomus tumors may be associated with a paraneoplastic syndrome of vasoactive catecholamine release and/or other neuropeptide secretion, including serotonin (1–5%).[23]
6. Some 3 to 10% are synchronous or of multicentric origin.[24–25]
7. Glomus tumors are the most common neoplasms affecting the middle ear.

8. A familial tendency is noted and the majority of patients are women, by nearly a 5:1 ratio.
9. Metastatic change is rare (3 to 4%).[25,26]
10. Radiation has mixed results, as the cells of this tumor are generally considered radio-resistant.

Classification of Glomus Tumors

Fisch[27]

Type A: Tumors confined to the middle ear space

Type B: Tumors confined to the mastoid and middle ear: no intralabyrinthine involvement

Type C: Tumors extending to the infralabyrinthine region of the temporal and petrous apex

Type D: Tumors with intracranial extension of less than 2-cm diameter.

Glasscock/Jackson[28]

1. Glomus tympanicum
   a. Small mass limited to the promontory
   b. Tumor completely filling the middle ear space
   c. Tumor filling the middle ear, extending into the mastoid or through the tympanic membrane to fill the EAC; may also extend anterior to the IAC
2. Glomus jugulare
   a. Small tumors involving the jugular bulb, middle ear, and mastoid
   b. Tumor extending under the IAC; may have intracranial extension
   c. Tumor extending into the petrous apex; may have intracranial extension
   d. Tumor extending beyond the petrous apex into the clivus or infratemporal fossa; may have intracranial extension

Evaluation

1. Physical examination including:
   a. Full neurologic examination
   b. Otomicroscopic evaluation
2. Laboratory workup including:
   a. 24-h urine evaluation for vanillylmandelic acid, metanephrine, and normetanephrine
   b. Complete blood count (CBC)
3. Audiogram
4. Radiographic examination including:
   a. CT scanning
      (1) Density resolution to differentiate tumor types
      (2) Describe good bone window and identify tumor destruction
   b. Arteriography
      (1) Define primary and subordinate feeding vessels
      (2) Determine relative size and extent of tumor
      (3) Contralateral filling, which occurs when cross-compression applied
      (4) Identify multiple tumors
   c. MRI with gadolinium
      (1) In the absence of bone windows, soft tissue masses are well defined
      (2) Identify flow voids by examining vascular plane of study

Treatment

The primary treatment is surgical removal of the entire tumor mass. This may be done as a single or multistage procedure. Embolization has been used to decrease the vascularity of these lesions. Radiation may be used as an adjunct modality but should not be relied upon for cure.

CLIVAL LESIONS

These lesions are frequently insidious in their growth pattern until they encroach upon regional neural or vascular structures. Included in the differential diagnosis of clival lesions are the following:

1. Chordoma
2. Meningioma
3. Neuroma
4. Craniopharyngioma
5. Chondrosarcoma
6. Brain stem neoplasm

Neither MRI nor CT scanning are uncommon; both may be employed in the assessment of these lesions. Generally, approaches to these lesions are dictated by both the site and size of the lesion as well as the attendant morbidity.

SURGERY FOR VERTIGO

Surgery pays a limited role in the management of vertigo. Only in persistent incapacitating vertigo that has failed medical management is surgical intervention considered.

1. Meniere's disease
    A. Symptoms, signs, medical treatment
        (1) Fluctuating hearing loss.
        (2) Episodic vertigo.
        (3) Tinnitus.
        (4) Aural pressure.
        (5) 15 to 30% bilateral.
        (6) Medical management includes low-salt diet (<2000 mg/day), diuretics, stress reduction, vestibular rehabilitation therapy.
        (7) Other possible medical therapies include corticosteroids, Meniett therapy,[29] treatment of allergies.
        (8) Differential diagnosis includes autoimmune inner ear disease, tertiary syphilis, vestibular schwannoma, perilymphatic fistula.
    B. Surgical options
        (1) Endolymphatic shunt or sac decompression 60 to 75% success rate drops to 50% at 5 years[30]; 1 to 3% sensorineural hearing loss (SNHL).
        (2) Intratympanic gentamicin (3/4 mL gentamicin 40 mg/mL mixed with 1/4 mL of bicarbonate 0.6M). 90% success rate.[31,32] Limit use to unilateral disease. Two to six treatments, up to 20% incidence of SNHL.[31,32]
        (3) Labyrinthectomy used in patients with unilateral disease with nonserviceable hearing in the affected ear. There is an 80% success rate.
        (4) Vestibular neurectomy used in patients with unilateral disease and serviceable hearing bilaterally. There is a 90% success rate and a 10% incidence of SNHL.

2. Benign paroxysmal positional vertigo
   A. Signs, symptoms, medical treatment
      (1) Vertigo induced by head motion.
      (2) Vertigo lasts for less than 1 min.
      (3) Resolves over weeks to months.
      (4) Frequently recurrent.
      (5) Hallpike maneuver demonstrating rotatory nystagmus with 5- to 10-s latency; 10- to 30-s duration is pathognomonic.
      (6) Vertigo is secondary to debris in the posterior semicircular canal.
      (7) Canalith repositioning maneuver is effective 74 to 91% of the time.[33–35]
   B. Surgical options
      (1) Singular neurectomy: 90% success rate with 25% risk of complete or partial hearing loss.[36,37]
      (2) Posterior occlusion of the semicircular canal[38]: 90% success rate with 20% risk of hearing loss.[39]
3. Perilymphatic fistula
   A. Signs, symptoms, medical treatment
      (1) Sensorineural hearing loss.
      (2) Vertigo.
      (3) Symptoms exacerbated with Vasalva or loud noises.
      (4) Site of leak around stapes footplate and round window.
      (5) Treat initially with bed rest and stool softeners.
   B. Surgical options
      (1) Exploratory tympanotomy and closure of fistula by denuding surrounding mucosa and sealing small pieces of fascia
4. Unilateral labyrinthine injury (trauma, vascular, viral, tumor)
   A. Signs, symptoms, medical treatment
      (1) Manage with vestibular rehabilitation therapy
   B. Surgical options
      (1) Labyrinthectomy.
      (2) Vestibular neurectomy via retrosigmoid, middle cranial fossa or translabyrinthine approaches; 85% success rate.
5. Superior canal dehiscence syndrome
   A. Signs, symptoms, medical treatment
      (1) Vertigo and oscillopsia in response to Vasalva or loud noises
      (2) Chronic disequilibrium
   B. Surgical options[40]
      (1) Plug superior semicircular canal via middle cranial fossa approach.
      (2) Resurface superior semicircular canal via the middle cranial fossa approach.

COMPLICATIONS AND RESULTS

The development of complications in skull base surgery, especially for malignancy, is common. Most series quote a 50% complication rate when all complications, both medical and surgical, are included.[41–43] The most serious complication, perioperative death, most commonly results from cerebrovascular compromise, especially in those series in which the ICA has been sacrificed. In our practice we have eliminated the sacrifice of the ICA without grafting. This has resulted in a precipitous drop in the perioperative mortality rate. Myocardial infarction, pulmonary embolism, and cerebral edema make up the remainder of the commonest causes of perioperative death.

The commonest surgical complications are CSF leaks, almost half of which stop spontaneously; meningitis; tension pneumocephalus; and wound infection. CSF leaks that do not spontaneously heal in 7 to 10 days should be reexplored and closed surgically. The efficacy of antibiotic prophylaxis remains unclear, but common practice is the use of perioperative antibiotics that continues until any CSF leak stops. Tension pneumocephalus is only rarely seen if a tracheostomy is done. However, postoperative pneumocephalus is a common finding. The air will be absorbed and there should be no adverse side effects. On the other hand, tension pneumocephalus is life-threatening and must be relieved by tapping of the air, followed by closure of the dural defect responsible for the leak. It is essential to maintain the integrity of the flap that separates the upper aerodigestive tract from the intracranial space, especially in an irradiated bed. The use of free vascularized flaps diminishes wound complications dramatically.

The overall 5-year tumor-free survival rate for skull base malignancies at our institution is 40%. Tumors invading the anterior cranial fossa have a better survival rate than those that involve the other sites. Involvement of dura produces a significantly lower survival rate at 2 years, but there is no statistically significant difference at 5 years. For patients with brain invasion the 2- and 5-year tumor-free survival rate is 33%. Invasion of the cavernous sinus and ICA portends a poor prognosis.

References

1. Anson B, Donaldson J: *Surgical Anatomy of the Temporal Bone and Ear.* Philadelphia: Saunders, 1983.
2. Hughes GB: *Textbook of Clinical Otology.* New York: Thieme-Stratton, 1985.
3. Shambaugh GE, Glasscock ME: *Surgery of the Ear.* Philadelphia: Saunders, 1990.
4. Lange J: *Clinical Anatomy of the Nose, Nasal Cavity and Paranasal Sinuses.* New York, Thieme, 1989:121.
5. Donald PJ: Transfacial approach, in Donald PJ, ed: *Surgery of the Skull Base.* Philadelphia: Lippincott-Raven, 1998:168–175.
6. Fisch U: Infratemporal fossa approach for extensive tumors of the temporal bone and base of the skull, in Silverstein H, ed:. *Neurological Surgery of the Ear.* Birmingham, AL: Aesculapius, 1997:4–53.
7. Donald PJ: Infratemporal fossa-middle cranial fossa approach, in Donald PJ, ed. *Surgery of the Skull Base.* Philadelphia: Lippincott-Raven, 1998:314.
8. George B: Management of the vertebral artery, in Donald PJ, ed: *Surgery of the Skull Base.* Philadelphia: Lippincott-Raven, 1998:537–541.
9. Brackman DE, Bartels LJ: Rare tumors of the cerebellopontine angle. *Otolaryngol Head Neck Surg* 1980;88:555–559.
10. Nedzelski JM et al: Conservative management of acoustic neuromas. *Otolaryngol Clin North Am* 1992;25:691–705.
11. Strasnick B, Glasscock ME, Haynes D, et al: The natural history of untreated acoustic neuromas. *Laryngoscope* 1994;104:1115–1119.
12. Pensak ML, Glasscock ME, Josey AF, et al: Sudden hearing loss and cerebellopontine angle tumors. *Laryngoscope* 1985;95:1188–1193.
13. Berenholz LP, Eriksen C, Hirsch FA: Recovery from repeated sudden hearing loss with corticosteroid use in the presence of an acoustic neuroma. *Ann Otol Rhinol Laryngol* 1992;101:827–831.
14. Saunders JE, Luxford WM, Devgan KK, Fetterman BL: Sudden hearing loss in acoustic neuroma patients. *Otolaryngol Head Neck Surg* 1995;113:23–31.
15. Selesnick SH, Jackler RK, Pitts LW: The changing clinical presentation of acoustic tumors in the MRI era. *Laryngoscope* 1993;103:431–436.

16. Hitselberger WE: External auditory canal hypesthesia. *Ann Surg* 1966;32:741–743.

17. Brodie HA, Bohrer PB: Evaluation and management of vestibular schwannomas, in Donald PJ, ed: *Surgery of the Skull Base*. Philadelphia: Lippincott-Raven, 1998:443–472.

18. House WF: Evolution of the transtemporal bone removal of acoustic tumors. *Arch Otolaryngol* 1964;80:731–742.

19. Jenkins HA, Fisch U: The transotic approach to resection of difficult acoustic tumors of the cerebellopontine angle. *Am J Otol* 1980;2(2):70–76.

20. Hitselberger WE, Pulec JL: Trigeminal nerve retrolabyrinthine selective section. *Arch Otolaryngol* 1972;96:412.

21. House WF, Hitselberger WE: The transcochlear approach to the skull base. *Arch Otolaryngol* 1976;102:334.

22. Fisch U: Infratemporal fossa approach to tumours of the temporal bone and base of the skull. *J Laryngol Otol* 1978;92:949–967.

23. Brodie HA, Roche JPD: Paraneoplastic syndromes, in Jackler RK, Driscoll CLW, eds: *Tumors of the Ear and Temporal Bone*. Philadelphia: Lippincott Williams & Wilkins, 2000: 20–28.

24. Alford BR, Guilford FR: A comprehensive study of tumors of the glomus jugulare. *Laryngoscope* 1962;72:765.

25. Spector GJ, Ciralsky R, Maisel RH, et al: Multiple glomus tumors in the head and neck. *Laryngoscope* 1975;85:1066.

26. Spector GJ, Sobol S, Thawley SE, et al: Glomus jugulare tumors of the temporal bone. Patterns of invasion in the temporal bone. *Laryngoscope* 1979;89:1628.

27. Oldring D, Fisch U: Glomus tumors of the temporal region: surgical therapy. *Am J Otol* 1979; 1(1):7–18.

28. Jackson CG, Glasscock ME III, Harris PF: Glomus tumors. diagnosis, classification, and management of large lesions. *Arch Otolarngol* 1982; 108(7):401–410.

29. Densert B, Sass K: Control of symptoms in patients with Ménière's disease—using middle ear pressure applications: two years follow-up. *Acta Otolaryngol* 2001;121:616–621.

30. Hughes GB: A new decade of surgery for vertigo. *Am J Otol* 1981;4(2):391–401.

31. Nedzelski JM, Chiong CM, Fradet G, et al: Intratympanic gentamicin instillation as treatment of unilateral Meniere's disease: update of an ongoing study. *Am J Otol* 1993;14:278–282.

32. Odkvist LM: Middle ear ototoxic treatment for inner ear disease. *Acta Otolaryngol Suppl (Stockh)* 1988;457:83–86.

33. Epley JM: Human experience with canalith repositioning maneuvers. *Ann NY Acad Sci* 2001; 942:179–191.

34. Ruckenstein MJ: Therapeutic efficacy of the Epley canalith repositioning manuever. *Laryngoscope* 2001;111(6):940–945.

35. Nunez RA, Cass SP, Furman JM: Short- and long-term outcomes of canalith repositioning for benign paroxysmal positional vertigo. *Otolaryngol Head Neck Surg* 2000;122(5):647–652.

36. Gacek RR: Singular neurectomy update, II: review of 102 cases. *Laryngoscope* 1991;101: 855–862.

37. Silverstein H, White DW: Wide surgical exposure for singular neurectomy in the treatment of benign positional vertigo. *Laryngoscope* 1990; 100:701–706.

38. Parnes LS, McClure JA: Posterior semicircular canal occlusion in the normal hearing ear. *Otolaryngol Head Neck Surg* 1991;104:52–57.

39. Hawthorne M, El-Nagger M: Fenestration and occlusion of the posterior semicircular canal for patients with intractable benign paroxysmal positional vertigo. *J Laryngol Otol* 1994;108: 935–939.

40. Minor LB: Superior canal dehiscence syndrome. *Am J Otol* 2000;21(1):9–19.

41. Donald PJ. Complications in skull base surgery for malignancy. *Laryngoscope* 1999;109:1959–1966.

42. Dias FL, Sa GM, Kligerman J, et al: Complications of anterior craniofacial resection. *Head Neck* 1998;20:1–9.

43. Kraus DH, Shah JP, Arbit E, et al: Complications of craniofacial resection for tumors involving the anterior skull base. *Head Neck* 1994;16(4): 307–312.

Facial Nerve Paralysis 8

EMBRYOLOGY

A discussion of the facial nerve and the disorders commonly affecting it should begin with a brief description of its development. During the 3rd week of gestation, the fascioacoustic primordium appears and eventually gives rise to the VII and VIII cranial nerves. By the 4th week, the facial nerve splits into two parts: the chorda tympani, which courses ventrally to enter the first (mandibular) arch, and the main trunk, which disappears into the mesenchyme approaching the epibranchial placode. It is not until the beginning of the 5th week that the geniculate ganglion, the nervus intermedius, and the greater superficial petrosal nerve are visible. The muscles of facial expression develop within the second (hyoid) arch during the 6th and 7th weeks of gestation. During this time the facial nerve courses across the region that will become the middle ear toward its destination to provide innervation to these muscles. By the 11th week, the facial nerve has branched extensively, and the majority of anastomoses have occurred. At term, the anatomy of the facial nerve approximates that of the adult, with the exception of its superficial location within a poorly formed mastoid (Figure 8-1). Development of the mastoid occurs between ages 1 and 3 and displaces the facial nerve medially and inferiorly until the time of puberty.[1]

The development of the external ear correlates with that of the nerve. Because the facial nerve is the nerve to the second branchial arch, any malformations in the derivatives of Reichert's cartilage makes the nerve suspect for variation. By the 6th week of gestation, the first and second arches give rise to small condensations of mesoderm known as hillocks of His. These will eventually coalesce to form the auricle around the 12th week. During the 8th week of development the first pharyngeal groove begins to invaginate and grow toward the middle ear. The external auditory canal (EAC) and tympanic membrane do not appear until the 28th week. At birth, the shape of the auricle is complete, the tympanic ring is small, and the EAC has yet to ossify.

Understanding the development of the facial nerve and how it correlates with the external ear is crucial for the otologic surgeon. The presence of a congenitally malformed external ear warns the physician of the possibility of additional abnormalities. The physician may be able to predict the anomalous course of the nerve by determining the age at which development arrested.[1] Other findings that alert the physician to possible facial nerve abnormalities include ossicular anomalies, craniofacial anomalies, and the presence of a conductive hearing loss.

ANATOMY

The facial nerve, like most of the cranial nerves, is a mixed nerve containing motor, sensory, and parasympathetic fibers. It can be divided into four functional components, two efferent and two afferent.[2] One group of efferent fibers arises from the motor nucleus and innervates the posterior belly of the digastric muscle, the stylohyoid muscle, the stapedius muscle, and the muscles of facial expression. The upper motor neuron tracts to the upper face cross and recross in the pons, sending bilateral innervation to the superior part of the motor nucleus. However, tracts to the lower face only cross once. This has diagnostic sig-

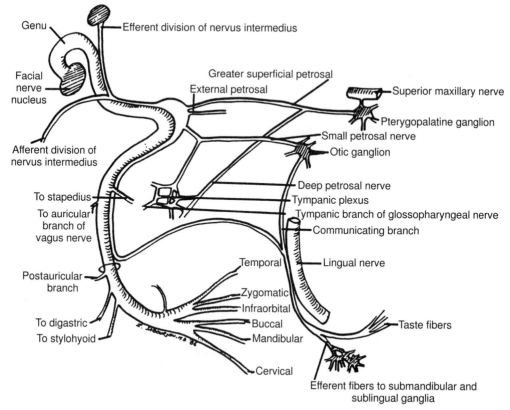

Figure 8-1.   Branches of the facial nerve. *(From Sataloff RT, ed.* Embryology and Anomalies of the Facial Nerve and Their Surgical Implications. *New York: Raven Press, 1991, 26.)*

nificance, as lesions proximal to the nucleus spare the upper face of the involved side where distal lesions produce complete paralysis of the affected side. The second efferent component consists of parasympathetic fibers responsible for lacrimation and salivation. These fibers constitute the *greater superficial petrosal nerve* and *chorda tympani,* respectively. The sensation of taste from the anterior two-thirds of the tongue is transmitted by afferent fibers to the nucleus tractus solitarius. This complex path is by way of the lingual nerve, the chorda tympani, and eventually the nervus intermedius, the sensory root of the facial nerve. A second set of afferent fibers conducts sensation from specific areas of the face, including the concha, external auditory canal, and earlobe.

The course of the facial nerve is divided into six segments (Figure 8-2):

1. *Intracranial segment:* 23 to 24 mm long from the brain stem to the internal auditory canal (IAC).
2. *Meatal segment:* 8 to 10 mm, from the fundus of the IAC to the meatal foramen. Throughout this segment the nerve runs anterior to the acoustic nerve.
3. *Labyrinthine segment:* 3 to 5 mm long from the meatal foramen to the geniculate ganglion. Within this segment the facial nerve gives rise to its first branch, the greater

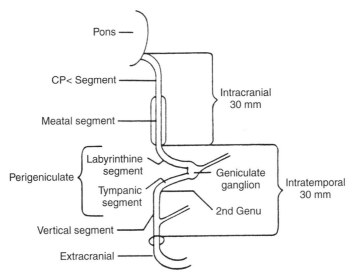

Figure 8-2.   Segments of the facial nerve. *(From Adkins WY, Osguthorpe JD. Management of trauma of the facial nerve. Otolaryngol Clin North Am 1991;24:587–611.)*

    superficial petrosal nerve. Also of significance, the fallopian canal (the bony conduit through which the facial nerve travels). It is narrowest within the labyrinthine segment.

4. *Tympanic segment:* 8 to 11 mm, at the geniculate ganglion the nerve makes a 40 to 80° turn to proceed posteriorly across the tympanic cavity to the pyramidal eminence. The majority of intratemporal facial nerve injuries resulting from trauma occur in the post-geniculate region.[3]

5. *Mastoid (vertical) segment:* 10 to 14 mm long from the pyramidal process to the stylomastoid foramen. Fascicular arrangement is thought to occur in this segment.

6. *Extratemporal segment:* from the stylomastoid foramen to the muscles of innervation.

    After emerging from the stylomastoid foramen, the nerve courses anteriorly and slightly inferiorly to enter the posterior surface of the parotid gland. At this point the nerve lies on the posterior belly of the digastric muscle. Once it enters the substance of the parotid gland it almost immediately begins to divide. Branching within the gland is variable, but an upper *temporozygomatic* and a lower *cervicofacial division* are common. The extensive network of anastomoses that develops between the various limbs is called the *pes anserinus.* By the time it exits the anterior border of the parotid, the ultimate components of the facial nerve can be identified: the temporal, zygomatic, buccal, marginal mandibular, and cervical branches (Figure 8-3).

SURGICAL ANATOMY

Surgical exposure of the extratemporal facial nerve is accomplished a number of different ways, and each has its advantages. The most commonly used methods include identification of the tragal pointer, identification of the tympanomastoid fissure (the facial nerve can be identified at 6–8 mm below the inferior "drop off" of the fissure), and retrograde dissec-

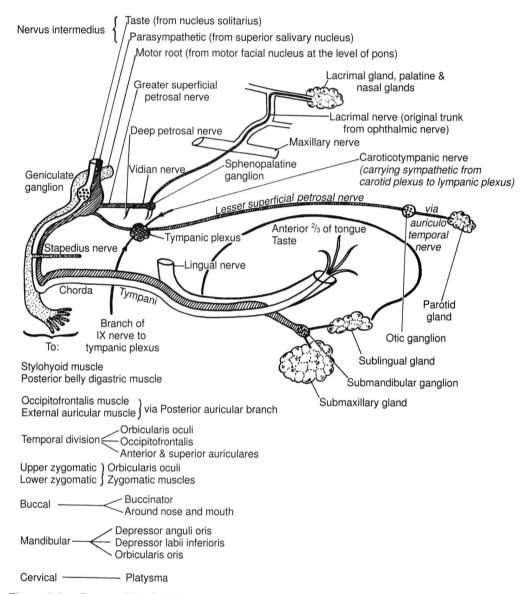

Nervus intermedius { Taste (from nucleus solitarius)
Parasympathetic (from superior salivary nucleus)
Motor root (from motor facial nucleus at the level of pons)

Lacrimal gland, palatine & nasal glands

Greater superficial petrosal nerve

Lacrimal nerve (original trunk from ophthalmic nerve)

Deep petrosal nerve

Maxillary nerve

Caroticotympanic nerve (carrying sympathetic from carotid plexus to tympanic plexus)

Geniculate ganglion

Vidian nerve

Sphenopalatine ganglion

Lesser superficial petrosal nerve

via auriculo temporal nerve

Tympanic plexus

Anterior 2/3 of tongue Taste

Stapedius nerve

Lingual nerve

Chorda Tympani

Parotid gland

Otic ganglion

Branch of IX nerve to tympanic plexus

To:

Sublingual gland

Submandibular ganglion

Submaxillary gland

Stylohyoid muscle
Posterior belly digastric muscle

Occipitofrontalis muscle } via Posterior auricular branch
External auricular muscle

Temporal division ⟨ Orbicularis oculi
Occipitofrontalis
Anterior & superior auriculares

Upper zygomatic) Orbicularis oculi
Lower zygomatic } Zygomatic muscles

Buccal ⟨ Buccinator
Around nose and mouth

Mandibular ⟨ Depressor anguli oris
Depressor labii inferioris
Orbicularis oris

Cervical ——— Platysma

Figure 8-3. Course of the facial nerve.

tion along the posterior belly of the digastric muscle to its insertion on the mastoid process. Identification of the facial nerve trunk is at times difficult, especially in cases of parotid neoplasia with distorted anatomy. In these cases, peripheral identification of one or more branches allows the surgeon to follow their course proximally through the parotid gland.

Identification of the facial nerve within the temporal bone or tympanic cavity during middle ear or mastoid surgery is important to prevent iatrogenic injury. Within the mastoid cavity and middle ear the short process of the incus (fossa incudis), the cochleariform process, the horizontal and posterior canals, and the digastric ridge mark their courses.[3] A prominence of the nerve posterior and lateral to the horizontal canal (pyramidal turn) makes the nerve more susceptible to injury in this area. This is the most common site of facial nerve injury during mastoid surgery.[4] Dehiscence of the fallopian canal is extremely common, with a reported incidence of 50%.[5] The most common location of dehiscence, and also the most common site of iatrogenic injury during middle ear surgery, is the tympanic segment over the oval window.[3]

EVALUATION

Evaluation of a patient with facial nerve paresis/paralysis requires a thorough understanding of facial nerve function and the numerous conditions that may lead to its involvement. It should include a detailed history, review of systems, physical examination, audiometry, and possibly radiographic or electrophysiologic studies. Crucial to appropriate management is early presentation and close follow-up to document the evolution of nerve involvement. The common causes of facial paralysis are listed in Table 8-1.

The history serves to narrow the differential diagnosis and allows the clinician to choose the appropriate laboratory and diagnostic tests. The typical scenario is unilateral facial weakness over the course of 2 to 3 weeks. Often a specific event or day of onset is unknown. Any palsy demonstrating progression beyond a 3-week period or lack of improvement after 6 months should be considered a neoplasm until proven otherwise. The coexistence of this indolent course with facial twitching, additional cranial nerve involvement, or

TABLE 8-1. COMMON CAUSES OF FACIAL PARALYSIS

Idiopathic	**Neoplasia**
Bell's palsy	Cholesteatoma
Recurrent facial palsy	Carcinoma (primary or metastatic)
Congenital	Acoustic neuroma
Möbius syndrome	Meningioma
Congenital unilateral lower lip paralysis	Facial neuroma
Melkersson–Rosenthal syndrome	Glomus jugulare or tympanicum
Dystrophic myotonia	Schwannoma of lower cranial nerves
Traumatic	Leukemia
Temporal bone fractures	Hemangioblastoma
Intrauterine compression	Osteopetrosis
Birth trauma	Histiocytoses
Facial contusions/lacerations	Rhabdomyosarcoma
Penetrating wounds to the face or temporal bone	**Metabolic/Systemic**
Iatrogenic injury	Diabetes mellitus
Infection	Hyperthyroidism
Herpes zoster oticus (Ramsay Hunt syndrome)	Pregnancy
Otitis media with effusion	Autoimmune disorders
Acute mastoiditis	**Neurologic**
Malignant otitis externa	Guillain–Barré syndrome
Acute suppurative otitis media	Multiple sclerosis
Tuberculosis	Millard–Gubler syndrome
Lyme disease	
Acquired immunodeficiency syndrome	
Infectious mononucleosis	
Influenza infection	
Encephalitis	
Sarcoidosis	

sensorineural hearing loss is also highly suggestive of a tumor. Numbness in the middle and lower face, otalgia, hyperacusis, diminished tearing, and an altered taste are common findings in Bell's palsy and herpes zoster oticus. Herpes zoster oticus (Ramsay Hunt syndrome) will also manifest as vesicular eruptions of the face and ear as well as sensorineural hearing loss and vertigo. A previous history or family history of facial paralysis is also helpful in establishing a diagnosis. The patient should be questioned in detail regarding other medical conditions, including sarcoidosis, carcinoma, diabetes mellitus, and pregnancy; previous ear disease, hearing loss, or otologic surgery; and present medications. Exposure to tick-borne disease and risk factors for HIV should also be addressed.

The physical examination focuses on the motor function of the facial nerve. The initial evaluation should determine if the lesion is complete or partial. In an attempt to standardize the description of partial nerve involvement, House and Brackmann devised a grading system[6] (Table 8-2). This delineation significantly impacts the remainder of the examination and the course of therapy. A common mistake is to interpret upper eyelid movement as partial facial nerve integrity. Remember that the levator palpebrae muscle is innervated by the oculomotor nerve and will remain intact despite a total facial nerve paralysis. An assessment of central vs. peripheral involvement should also be performed. Central unilateral facial paralysis usually involves only the lower face, as the innervation of the upper face is derived from

TABLE 8-2.   HOUSE–BRACKMANN FACIAL NERVE GRADING SYSTEM

Grade	Characteristics
I. Normal	Normal facial function in all areas
II. Mild dysfunction	**Gross**
	Slight weakness noticeable on close inspection. May have very slight synkinesis. At rest, normal symmetry and tone.
	Motion
	Forehead: moderate-to-good function
	Eye: complete closure with minimal effort
	Mouth: slight asymmetry
III. Moderate dysfunction	**Gross**
	Obvious, but not disfiguring difference between the two sides. Noticeable but not severe synkinesis, contracture, or hemifacial spasm. At rest, normal symmetry and tone.
	Motion
	Forehead: slight-to-moderate movement
	Eye: complete closure with effort
	Mouth: slightly weak with maximum effort
IV. Moderately severe dysfunction	**Gross**
	Obvious weakness and/or disfiguring asymmetry. At rest, normal symmetry and tone.
	Motion
	Forehead: none
	Eye: incomplete closure
	Mouth: asymmetric with maximum effort
V. Severe dysfunction	**Gross**
	Only barely perceptible motion. At rest, asymmetry.
	Motion
	Forehead: none
	Eye: incomplete closure
	Mouth: slight movement
VI. Total paralysis	No movement

crossed and uncrossed fibers. Lesions of the peripheral nerve involve the upper and lower face. In addition, the presence of emotional facial expression as well as lacrimation, taste, and salivation on the ipsilateral side suggest a central lesion. These functions are not governed by the motor cortex of the precentral gyrus and, therefore, would be unaffected by a lesion of this area.[2] Further evaluation including a meticulous otologic examination, an evaluation of remaining cranial nerves, and an assessment of cutaneous involvement, signs of trauma, or associated systemic findings should be performed (Table 8-3).

Radiologic Tests

The need for radiologic evaluation is based on the history and clinical course of each individual case. High-resolution computed tomography (CT) is the study of choice for bone assessment, and it provides the best assessment of the integrity of the fallopian canal. A CT scan adds additional information regarding disease of the mastoid, middle ear, and bony detail of the temporal bone. A magnetic resonance imaging (MRI) scan is the best means of evaluating soft tissues and can be instrumental in detecting neuronal enhancement from infection or neoplasia. The MRI is also necessary to evaluate the facial nerve at the level of the cerebellopontine angle. Interest in using MRI in the evaluation of Bell's palsy and Ramsay Hunt syndrome has not proven advantageous.[7,8] While most agree that the increased signal intensity observed in both conditions is similar, there is no correlation between the level of enhancement and the severity of the paralysis, the electrophysiologic and intraoperative findings, and the prognosis of the facial paralysis.[8,9] There are few indications for mastoid roentgenograms, as they provide limited data and can be difficult to interpret.

Prognostic Tests

An understanding of the pathophysiology of nerve injury is crucial to the clinician's understanding of the course of disease and the determination of prognosis. The classic description divides neural lesions into one of three categories depending on the mechanism of injury. *Neuropraxia* is the blockage of axonal transport due to local compression. The nerve does not sustain permanent damage and no wallerian degeneration occurs. Normal function will

TABLE 8-3.   DIAGNOSIS OF LESIONS FROM LEVEL OF IMPAIRMENT

Level of Impairment	Signs	Diagnosis
Supranuclear	Good tone, intact upper face, presence of spontaneous smile, neurologic deficits	Cerebrovascular accident, trauma
Nuclear	Involvement of the VI and VII cranial nerves, corticospinal tract signs	Vascular or neoplastic, poliomyelitis, multiple sclerosis, encephalitis
Angle	Involvement of vestibular and cochlear portions of the VIII cranial nerve (facial nerve, particularly taste, lacrimation, and salivation may be altered); the V and later IX, X, and XI cranial nerves may become impaired	Neurinoma, meningioma, fracture cholesteatoma, arachnoid cyst
Geniculate ganglion	Facial paralysis, hypercusis, alteration of lacrimation, salivation, and taste	Herpes zoster oticus, fracture, Bell's palsy, cholesteatoma, neurinoma, arteriovenous malformation, meningioma
Tympanomastoid	Facial paralysis, alteration in salivation and taste, lacrimation intact	Bell's palsy, cholesteatoma, fracture, infection
Extracranial	Facial paralysis (usually a branch is spared), salivation and taste intact, deviation of jaw to normal side	Trauma, tumor, parotid carcinoma, pharyngeal carcinoma

be restored when the compression is removed. All electrophysiologic tests will be within normal limits. In *axonotmesis*, the axonal integrity has been disrupted, but endoneurial sheaths are preserved. Wallerian degeneration distal to the lesion occurs. Electrophysiologic tests will reveal rapid and complete degeneration. As long as the endoneurium is preserved there will be complete recovery with return of normal function. Finally, *neurotmesis* describes the destruction of the axon and surrounding support cells. It is characterized by wallerian degeneration, an unpredictable regeneration potential, and the likelihood of significant resultant dysfunction. Early electrophysiologic testing mimics that of axonotmesis.

Any significant injury to the facial nerve that results in nerve regeneration is at risk of developing errors during reinnervation. *Synkinesis* is defined as the loss of discrete facial movements after facial nerve injury. It is the result of a single axon or a small group of axons innervating motor end units of numerous and separated muscles. When fibers originally destined for the submaxillary gland innervate the lacrimal gland, the result is profuse lacrimation during eating, also known as *Bogorad syndrome* (or crocodile tear syndrome).

Topodiagnostic testing is the concept of testing specific neuronal function corresponding to the numerous branches of the facial nerve in an attempt to isolate the site of damage and to predict outcome. Commonly used examples include the Schirmer test, the submandibular flow test, and the stapedial reflex test. Experience has shown, however, that these manipulations have little correlation with the site of injury and fail to serve as a useful measurement of prognosis. While they are included in this discussion, they should only be performed if information about a specific function is required.

Not all patients with facial paralysis require prognostic tests because the outcome may already be predictable (acoustic tumor surgery) or because the underlying cause is the indication for treatment (chronic otitis media with facial nerve paralysis). Testing is indicated for acute total facial palsies (that is, while the nerve is in the degenerative phase) and for following the course of disease in situations of persistent paralysis. The tests provide no pertinent information during paresis. The mere existence of facial activity portends an excellent chance of complete recovery. The most common causes of acute facial paralysis (Bell's palsy, trauma, and infection) produce nerve degeneration in the first 3 weeks following onset.

Nerve Excitability Test (NET)

The NET was first described by Hilger in 1964.[11] It compares the current thresholds required to elicit minimal muscle contraction on the normal side of the face to those of the paralyzed side. The current, measured in milliamperes (mA), is delivered percutaneously with a DC current while the face is monitored for the slightest movement. The electrodes are then placed in corresponding locations on the involved side, and the same procedure is performed. A difference of 3.5 mA or greater is considered significant and suggests degeneration.

Maximum Stimulation Test (MST)

The MST is similar to the NET except that it uses maximal rather than minimal stimulation. The main trunk as well as each major portion of the distal branches of the nerve on the normal and abnormal sides are stimulated at an intensity that produces maximal stimulation of the nonparalyzed side without discomfort. The results of the test are expressed as a difference in facial muscle movement between the normal and paralyzed sides. May[12] and others found that a maximal stimulus elicits a response from the entire nerve and, therefore, serves as a better prognostic indicator of impending denervation. However, this test is difficult to quantitate and is more subject to interobserver variation.[13]

Electroneurography (ENoG)

Unlike the NET and MST, ENoG provides quantitative analysis of the extent of degeneration without being dependent on observer qualification. It is thought of as the most accurate prognostic indicator of all the electrodiagnostic tests,[14] and is similar in principle to the MST. Instead of visual observation of the degree of response, there is a recording of the summation potential on an instrument similar to an electromyography recording device. The normal side is compared to the involved side, and the degree of degeneration is directly proportional to the difference between the amplitudes of the measured summation potentials. It is commonly believed that surgical decompression should be performed when 90% degeneration has occurred. In Bell's palsy, patients exceeding 95% degeneration within the first 14 days fall into the guarded prognostic category.[15]

Electromyography (EMG)

This test determines the activity of the muscle itself. A needle electrode is inserted into the muscle, and recordings are made during rest and voluntary contraction. Degeneration of a lower motor nerve is followed in 14 to 21 days by spontaneous activity called fibrillation potential. However, at 6 to 12 weeks prior to clinical return of facial function, polyphasic reinnervation potentials are present and provide the earliest evidence of nerve recovery. Alone, EMG is of limited clinical value; however, in combination with ENoG, EMG may detect active motor units that would not have been detected otherwise, perhaps resulting in unnecessary surgery.

Lacrimation (Schirmer's Test)

This test evaluates greater superficial petrosal nerve function (ie, tear production). Paper strips are placed in the conjunctival fornix of both eyes. After 5 minutes the length of paper moistened is compared. Significant abnormalities include unilateral reduction of greater than 30% of the total amount of lacrimation of both eyes or reduction of total lacrimation to less than 25 mm after a 5-minute period. The latter criterion is significant because a unilateral transgeniculate lesion may produce bilateral reduction of lacrimation. The Schirmer's II test is a modification of this test with the addition of nasal mucosal stimulation. The significance of these tests is not in their topographic information but in their evaluation of the protective mechanism of the eye.

Stapedial Reflex

The stapedius muscle contracts reflexively when the contralateral ear is stimulated with a loud tone. This alters the reactive compliance of the middle ear, which can be measured with impedance audiometry. If the lesion involves the nerve proximal to the branch to the stapedius muscle, the muscle will not contract and no change in impedance will be recorded.

Trigeminofacial (Blink) Reflex

Percutaneous electrical stimulation of the supraorbital nerve elicits a blink reflex that is recorded by electrodes placed over the orbicularis oculi muscle. Due to the trigeminal–facial arc it measures central lesions and may prove to be a beneficial diagnostic tool in the future.

Salivary Flow Testing

By cannulating Wharton's papillae, a measurement of salivary flow to gustatory stimulation can be obtained. A reduction of 25% as compared to the uninvolved side is considered abnormal. This test is difficult to perform and is subject to a significant level of inaccuracy.

Electrogustometry

The tongue is stimulated electrically to produce a metallic taste, and the two sides of the tongue are compared. This test is rarely performed.

Magnetic Evoked Neuromyography (MNoG)

This is a relatively new technique that was designed to stimulate the facial nerve intra-cranially (ie, proximal to the site of injury). With the use of varying magnetic fields, neural depolarization can be initiated. The potentials can then be measured as muscular responses using surface electrodes. This test remains experimental.

IDIOPATHIC FACIAL PARALYSIS (BELL'S PALSY)

The most common form of facial paralysis is idiopathic facial paralysis, also referred to as Bell's palsy. The annual estimated incidence ranges from 15 to 40 per 100,000. It can occur in any age group but is most prevalent in the 3rd decade.[16] There is no sexual or racial predilection, and both sides of the face are affected in equal proportions. The presentation is recurrent in approximately 10 to 12% of patients. A positive family history is reported in up to 14% of cases.

Despite the fact that Bell's palsy is idiopathic by definition, numerous attempts have been made to explain its etiology. The most prevalent theories include ischemic neuronitis, viral infection, polyneuropathy, and entrapment neuropathy. The most likely explanation is that numerous factors can lead to the characteristic signs and symptoms. There is a significant amount of evidence, however, to suggest a common pathophysiology of nerve damage regardless of the precipitating event. An external stimulus results in inflammation of the nerve within a nonforgiving bony canal. The resultant swelling leads to entrapment and eventual ischemia. This ischemia results in further inflammation and edema, creating a cycle of injury.

Originally documented by Sir Charles Bell in 1821, the description of idiopathic facial paralysis has remained relatively unchanged over the last 2 centuries. It is a unilateral facial weakness of sudden onset that resolves spontaneously. The diagnosis is generally considered one of exclusion. However, May and coworkers[12] emphasized that, based on specific clinical features, it is a positive diagnosis. Minimum diagnostic criteria include: (1) paralysis or paresis of all muscle groups of one side of the face; (2) sudden onset; and (3) absence of signs of central nervous system disease, ear disease, or cerebellopontine angle disease.[17] Paralysis is complete in two-thirds of patients, but denervation is uncommon. In addition to the typical facial weakness, Bell's palsy also appears to have certain characteristics: a viral prodrome (60%); numbness or pain of the ear, face, or neck (60%); dysgeusia (57%); hyperacusis (30%); and decreased tearing (17%).[18,19] "In all cases of Bell's palsy," describes May and Klein, "the process is self-limiting, nonprogressive, nonlife-threatening, and spontaneously remitting, with typical Bell's palsy improving within 4 to 6 months, and always by 12 months after onset."[18]

The initial evaluation for someone with facial paralysis is described in detail in a previous section. It is important to remember that a thorough history and physical examination is the cornerstone of establishing a diagnosis. An audiogram is obtained to provide a good general screening of the auditory system. If complete paralysis is identified, electrophysiologic tests should be performed to document the status and prognosis of the neural lesion. Under normal circumstances, when Bell's palsy is suspected, a CT or MRI scan is not indicated.

However, in cases of total paralysis with sensorineural hearing loss, recent facial paralysis, or recent trauma, a complete radiologic workup is mandated. The clinical follow-up of these patients is also dependent on consistent physical evaluations and appropriate testing.

The treatment of Bell's palsy is extremely controversial and is guided as much by personal experience as by scientific data. We know from Peitersen's landmark paper that the prognosis is very good regardless of the extent of intervention.[20] He documented the 1-year clinical course of 1011 patients who received neither steroid nor surgical therapy. All of those with incomplete paralysis had excellent recovery, with only 6% having slight residual weakness. Of those with complete paralysis, 71% had a complete recovery and 13% had a good clinical recovery with mild residual palsy. Other studies have confirmed these results.[16,21,22] The remaining 16% had a fair to poor recovery and is the group that would benefit most from aggressive medical or surgical intervention. Unfortunately, it is extremely difficult to predict which patients fall into this category.

The effectiveness of medical management is controversial. Trials of adrenocorticotropic hormones, corticosteroids, vasodilators, vitamins, and cromolyn sodium have all been reported. However, none have been shown to be effective in altering the natural course of the disease. After reviewing 92 articles on this subject, Stankiewicz concluded that steroid treatment is beneficial.[23] "While not affecting the etiology of the disease or preventing partial denervation or contracture, steroids may be helpful in preventing denervation, autonomic dyskinesis, and progression of incomplete to complete paralysis." Recent studies have upheld these findings and suggest that improved outcomes are associated with earliest possible initiation of steroid therapy.[24] In addition, another recent double-blind study suggests improved outcome with concomitant treatment with acyclovir.[25] In addition, most authors agree that steroids early in the course of the disease help shorten the recovery time and serve as an analgesic. There are virtually no side effects of short course steroid management. Gastrointestinal complaints are the most common side effects associated with acyclovir.

Surgical decompression has been advocated for cases of total paralysis with evidence of extensive nerve degeneration. Clinical experience has shown that when the number of motor fibers falls to less than 10% of normal (as documented by serial ENoG), the recovery rate falls substantially. In cases of facial paralysis with greater than 90% loss of motor fibers and normal hearing, a middle cranial fossa approach is used for facial nerve decompression. In cases associated with prior deafness, a translabyrinthine approach allows for a more complete decompression. It should be pointed out, however, that surgical intervention remains controversial and scientific studies to support this are limited.[26] Critics of this algorithm argue that the risk of iatrogenic injury from surgical decompression outweighs the advantages since the majority of patients recover without intervention.

TRAUMA

Second only to idiopathic disease, traumatic injury is the most significant cause of facial nerve paralysis. Unlike Bell's palsy, its diagnosis is usually easy due to the mechanism of injury, related injuries, or recent surgical history. The facial nerve's arduous tract through the internal auditory canal, middle ear, mastoid, and eventually the parotid gland makes it vulnerable to traumatic injury. It is not surprising that it is the most commonly injured cranial nerve. Traumatic injuries of the facial nerve are subdivided into iatrogenic and non-iatrogenic causes. Each has its typical presentation and management objectives.

Iatrogenic Injury

Facial nerve injury during mastoid or middle ear surgery is relatively uncommon (approximately 1%) but warrants discussion. As mentioned previously, the most common area of iatrogenic injury in middle ear surgery is the tympanic segment. Extratemporal resections, including parotid or neck tumors, may necessitate the sacrifice of part of the nerve. Usually, these injuries are identified at the time of surgery and appropriate repair (ie, end-to-end anastomosis or neural grafting) is performed. The difficult management problem arises when there is unexpected postoperative facial paralysis. Local anesthetics (ie, lidocaine) may result in residual weakness or paralysis and should be given appropriate time to wear off. If paralysis persists, mastoid packing that may be compressing a dehiscent section of the nerve should be removed. The decision to explore the nerve is dependent on the surgeon's confidence of the status of the nerve. If the nerve was not identified during the procedure or if injury is felt to be a possibility, the nerve should be explored and repaired as soon as possible. If, on the other hand, the surgeon is convinced that the nerve was not compromised, it is safe to follow the paralysis with electrical tests and explore only if there are signs of significant degeneration. A postoperative paresis is almost always the result of minor trauma and edema and rarely progresses to paralysis.

Intratemporal Injury

Noniatrogenic injury to the facial nerve is most commonly the result of automobile accidents and blunt trauma to the head and face. Intratemporal injuries occur as a result of temporal bone fractures, which are classified as longitudinal or transverse with respect to the temporal bone. Adequate evaluation of the injury must include both coronal and axial CT scans. Eighty to ninety percent of temporal bone fractures are *longitudinal* and usually result from trauma to the temporoparietal area. They almost always involve the middle ear, but only 20% will have concomitant facial nerve injury.[27] Common presentation includes bleeding from the middle ear, laceration of the tympanic membrane, and conductive hearing loss. Facial nerve injury, if present, is usually the result of compression and ischemia as opposed to neural disruption.[28] *Transverse* fractures account for a much smaller proportion of temporal bone injuries, but an associated facial nerve injury is present in up to half of the cases. It is usually the result of trauma to the occipitomastoid area. Common presentation includes hemotympanum, vestibular symptoms, and a dead ear. Nerve severance is the typical form of injury. Gunshot wounds make up a much smaller proportion of intratemporal injuries but are equally challenging. When the nerve is injured, it is usually in the tympanic and mastoid segments and is often the result of thermal and compression injury as opposed to disruption. Even with decompression, recovery is often incomplete. In addition, it is often accompanied by significant central nervous system or vascular injury.

Regardless of the type of trauma, when an associated facial nerve injury is present, a simple algorithm is used for management decision making. If paralysis is incomplete, conservative management is indicated since most will resolve spontaneously. Serial examinations as well as electrical testing are important to ensure that degeneration does not occur. The use of steroids remains controversial. As long as there are no contraindications to short-course steroid use, there is some evidence to suggest that this may assist in shortening the recovery phase. Complete paralysis or progressing injuries should be evaluated with a coronal and axial CT, audiometry, ENoG, and, in cases of penetrating injury, arteriography. If degeneration of greater than 90% of motor end units (as tested by ENoG) is identified within 6 days after the injury, complete surgical decompression should be performed. Paralysis reaching 90% degeneration after 6 days has a better prognosis than that of other conditions causing degeneration and does not require surgical intervention.[29] The only other indication for surgery (albeit controversial) is persistent symptoms of paralysis for greater than 4 months despite a lack of degeneration as documented by electrical testing.

More than 90% of temporal bone fractures with complete facial paralysis involve the region of the geniculate ganglion, especially the labyrinthine segment.[30] If surgical exploration of the facial nerve is undertaken, therefore, the decompression should extend beyond this region.[30] The surgical approach is dependent on the hearing status of the patient. A middle cranial fossa approach must be employed in a patient with intact hearing. Often this procedure can be combined with a transmastoid approach. In the case of a nonhearing ear, a translabyrinthine approach is much easier and results in less morbidity. Decompression of the nerve, including internal neurolysis, is adequate in cases where obvious impingement was present and the nerve is otherwise intact; however, if the injury to the nerve is significant, despite its apparent continuity, resection and reanastomosis or nerve grafting will offer a better surgical result than decompression alone. In cases of complete transection, the decision to reanastomose should be based on the ability to approximate the nerve edges with negligible tension. The greater auricular nerve is well suited for facial nerve grafting based on its size and location. If a longer segment of nerve is required, the sural nerve is the graft of choice.

Extratemporal Injury

The extracranial nerve is also susceptible to trauma, especially penetrating injuries, and an immediate assessment should be done to evaluate the status of nerve function, the extent of soft-tissue injury, and the amount of contamination. Electrical testing can be of significant value in evaluating peripheral injuries of the facial nerve. A transected or severely injured nerve will show no response to stimulation proximal to the injury. In addition, electrical testing is instrumental in identifying nerve branches intraoperatively. An extensive exam should also include a survey of surrounding soft tissues, including the globe, the parotid duct, and the mouth.

Injuries to the trunk or main branches of the facial nerve are extremely debilitating. Due to the extensive network of branching and anastomoses, peripheral injuries are associated with much less morbidity. Nonetheless, evidence suggests that all facial nerve injuries associated with loss of function should be explored and repaired as soon as possible. In the past, injuries occurring distal to the lateral canthus and the oral facial crease were left to recover spontaneously. May argues that immediate repair, when possible, offers a better chance of complete recovery without synkinesis. Once again, the decision to repair the nerve primarily vs. nerve grafting depends on the tension placed on the nerve. Two exceptions to immediate repair are cases of significant soft tissue loss and extensive gross contamination. Under these circumstances, immediate exploration with wound debridement and tagging of the nerve branches is initially performed. A second-stage procedure for nerve repair can be achieved safely within 30 days from the time of the injury.

INFECTION

Viral

Of the infectious agents known to cause facial nerve paralysis, herpes zoster is the most common. It is distinguishable from Bell's palsy because of its associated findings. These are intense otalgia, vesicular eruptions (occasionally extending onto the tympanic membrane), sensorineural hearing loss, tinnitus, and vertigo. The combination of vesicular eruption and facial paralysis is referred to as *Ramsay Hunt syndrome*. Its incidence increases dramatically after age 60, presumedly because of decreased cell-mediated immunity in this age group. Serologic and epidemiologic data suggest that the reactivation of a latent virus, as opposed to a reinfection, is the mechanism of infection. The diagnosis is rarely in question but can be confirmed by rising titers of antibodies to the varicella zoster virus. Enhancement patterns of the facial nerve by gadolinium MRI are similar to those observed in Bell's palsy, but again there is no correlation between the level of enhancement and the severity of the paralysis, the electrophysiologic and intraoperative findings, and the prognosis of the facial paralysis.[8,9] Compared to idiopathic facial paralysis, nerve degeneration tends to be more significant and, therefore, its prognosis for recovery is worse.[31] The treatment of herpes zoster oticus is fraught with the same controversy as that of other causes of facial nerve paralysis. Systemic corticosteroids are thought to relieve the acute pain, reduce vertigo, and minimize postherpetic neuralgia despite their questionable role in reversing the disease process. Acyclovir, steroids, or the combination of the two has been reported to improve outcome. Postherpetic neuralgia is known to occur and can be prolonged and incapacitating. It is treated with oral analgesics and topical capsiacin.

Bacterial

Infections involving the ear may also result in facial nerve paralysis. Acute suppurative otitis media, chronic otitis media, mastoiditis, and malignant otitis externa have all been implicated and appear to have the same etiology. A dehiscence in the fallopian canal serves as a portal of entry for direct bacterial invasion. The treatment for acute otitis is oral antibiotic coverage for gram-positive cocci and *Haemophilus* and wide myringotomy for middle ear evacuation. In cases of chronic otitis media, complete eradication of the disease warrants tympanomastoidectomy and decompression of the nerve.

Malignant otitis externa (MOE) is a condition that represents a true otologic emergency requiring rapid, aggressive management. It usually affects older patients with a long-standing history of diabetes and can result in cranial nerve palsies. The clinical picture most consistent with this diagnosis is severe, painful inflammation of the EAC with purulent otorrhea, decreased hearing, and fleshy granulation tissue at the inferior aspect of the EAC. *Pseudomonas aeruginosa* is the most common pathogen, accounting for up to 98% of documented cultures.[32] The nidus of disease originates in the EAC but spreads into adjacent tissues. The temporal bone, parotid gland, and cranial nerves may become involved. The diagnosis is made by physical findings and can be confirmed with a *technetium radioisotope scan*, which identifies increased osteogenic activity. Once positive the bone scan will remain positive for an indefinite period. A *gallium scan* detects inflammatory response (granulocyte binding) and is useful in following the treatment course. Improvement of the gallium scan correlates with clinical improvement. Treatment consists of localized surgical debridement and an extended antipseudomonal antibiotic regimen.[33] Ciprofloxacin is becoming the drug of choice.[34]

Lyme Disease

Lyme disease has gained attention and has been suggested by some to be the etiologic agent of at least part of the patients diagnosed with Bell's palsy. Facial nerve palsy occurs in only

10% of infected patients but remains the most common neurologic sign of Lyme disease.[35] It can be distinguished from Bell's palsy due to its flu-like symptoms and characteristic cutaneous manifestations, erythema chronicum migrans. It is a rash that starts as a flat reddened area and extends with central clearing. Antibody titers are unreliable and offer little to the diagnostic workup. The prognosis of facial paralysis is excellent, with almost 100% achieving a complete recovery.[36] Treatment with antibiotics is mandatory to prevent late complications of the infection.

Systemic Diseases

Various systemic diseases may result in facial nerve paralysis but should remain relatively low in the differential diagnosis. *Guillain–Barré syndrome* should be considered when facial paralysis accompanies a generalized weakness, autonomic dysfunction, or central nervous system involvement. Along with Lyme disease, it is a common cause of facial diplegia. *Mononucleosis* is characterized by a prodrome of headache, malaise, myalgia, and lymphadenopathy and may eventually result in facial nerve paralysis.[18] *Sarcoidosis* is an idiopathic, chronic non-caseating granulomatous disease. Facial nerve paralysis is present in 50% of patients with a variant of sarcoidosis, also referred to as *uveoparotid fever* or *Heerfordt's disease*. Facial nerve paralysis may occur in any stage of *HIV infection*; however, it must be emphasized that this is a rare sequela of the disease.[37] Palsy may be a direct result of the virus itself, or it may be secondary to the immunodeficiency. The palsy often mimics that of Bell's and has the same general recovery pattern.[38]

NEOPLASIA

Tumors resulting in facial nerve paralysis may involve the facial nerve itself or may originate from surrounding structures and eventually compromise nerve function. Of patients presenting with new-onset paralysis, only 5% are due to a neoplastic process. Features of facial nerve paralysis that suggest the possibility of tumor involvement include:

1. A slowly evolving paresis/paralysis
2. Persistent facial paralysis of greater than 4 months' duration
3. Ipsilateral recurrence of a facial paralysis
4. Facial paralysis with concurrent sensorineural hearing loss
5. The presence of multiple cranial nerve deficits
6. History of carcinoma

Intracranial lesions resulting in facial nerve paralysis are generally benign but can be extremely debilitating due to the mass effect on surrounding structures. Facial neurinomas are rare, slow-growing tumors that arise from the facial nerve at any point along its course, but most frequently involve the geniculum.[39] Facial paralysis is the most common presenting complaint. Other intracranial processes include acoustic neuromas (91%), meningiomas (2.5%), congenital cholesteatomas (2.5%), hemangiomas, adenoid cystic carcinomas, and arachnoid cysts.[40] A suspicion of tumor requires an extensive otologic workup, including audiometry and imaging. In situations where tumor is suspected, an MRI is the best means of assessing neural structures and continuity. The treatment, despite the histologic diagnosis, is surgical excision. The approach is dependent on the hearing status of the involved side and the location of the tumor.

Extracranial masses resulting in facial nerve paralysis are almost exclusively of parotid origin. They can be classified into benign vs. malignant lesions. Benign neoplasms constitute approximately 85% of parotid masses, of which pleomorphic adenomas make up the vast majority. The typical presentation is that of a slowly growing, nontender mass in the parotid region. Although uncommon, benign lesions may cause compression of surrounding soft tissues, resulting in facial nerve dysfunction and salivary flow obstruction. Fine-needle aspiration biopsies are an acceptable and commonly used method to evaluate salivary gland neoplasms. Treatment consists of surgical excision with a cuff of normal salivary gland tissue. This is best accomplished with a superficial or total parotidectomy, depending on the nature and extent of the neoplasm. Great care must be taken to preserve the facial nerve, as the normal anatomy may be somewhat altered due to the mass effect and surrounding inflammation from the tumor.

Malignant neoplasms involving the facial nerve may be of parotid origin or more rarely may arise from the facial nerve itself. These lesions are often indistinguishable from benign masses and must be confirmed by fine-needle aspiration. Approximately 12 to 15% of malignant parotid neoplasms have associated facial nerve paralysis. Mucoepidermoid carcinoma is the most common malignancy of the parotid gland; however, adenoid cystic carcinoma has a higher predilection for facial nerve involvement. Despite the histologic type, facial nerve paralysis is a poor prognostic sign. Malignancy involving the nerve requires excision for a tumor-free margin. Reconstruction of the nerve should take place during the initial procedure and often requires a nerve graft. The remainder of cases are treated with surgical excision of the gland with sparing of the nerve. Adjunctive radiotherapy and chemotherapy also may be indicated.

PEDIATRIC

The incidence of facial nerve paralysis in the newborn is approximately 1 in 2000 deliveries.[41] Birth trauma accounts for the majority of cases and is characterized by unilateral complete facial nerve dysfunction, a complicated delivery, ecchymosis of the face or temporal region, and hemotympanum. While the use of forceps is still considered to be the most common insulting agent, often paralysis is present after an uncomplicated low or outlet forceps delivery. As discussed previously, the mastoid tip is poorly formed in the newborn infant, and the stylomastoid process lies just beneath the skin. This makes the facial nerve vulnerable to compression and injury.

Congenital paralysis makes up the remainder of cases and is typically associated with other findings, including contralateral facial paralysis, additional cranial nerve deficits, and other congenital aberrances. The most common developmental anomalies affecting facial muscle function are *Möbius syndrome* and *agenesis of the depressor anguli oris muscle*.[42] Möbius syndrome is a congenital facial diplegia that is associated with the inability to abduct one or both eyes. Other cranial nerve motor functions may be weak, and skeletal abnormalities may also be present. Controversy exists as to the specific site of lesion.[43] Agenesis of the depressor anguli oris muscle, also termed *congenital unilateral lower lip paralysis (CULLP)*, is thought to be a brain stem lesion that results in a lack of development of the depressor anguli oris muscle. It usually affects one side, is noted by the asymmetry of the face during crying, and is associated with other congenital anomalies, notably otologic or cardiovascular anomalies.

In any neonate where facial nerve paralysis is identified, a complete physical examination should be performed, including an assessment of partial vs. complete paralysis, an otoscopic evaluation, and a survey of other traumatic sequelae, additional anomalies, or both. Electrophysiologic testing is extremely important in documenting the extent of the lesion and in following the clinical course. Tests that attempt to localize the site of disruption are usually of limited value in the neonate.

Regardless of the etiology of neonatal facial nerve paralysis, the spontaneous recovery rate approaches 90%[44,45] and is usually complete. The prognosis is worse, however, for congenital lesions.[41] Smith and coworkers recommend following patients with congenital lesions for at least 2 years to determine the degree of residual dysfunction.[41] Many of these children will have persistent asymmetrical function, but most will adapt well and not require surgical intervention.

The treatment approach for traumatic neonatal facial nerve paralysis is considerably more controversial. Some authors argue that evidence of significant facial nerve injury (increasing facial nerve excitability thresholds, fibrillation potentials on EMG, or evidence of intratemporal facial nerve injury by radiographic examination) is an indication for immediate exploration.[41] Bergman and others argue that, in light of the excellent spontaneous recovery rate and the risk of iatrogenic injury, a more conservative approach is indicated.[42] Their criteria for surgical intervention is limited to:

1. Unilateral complete paralysis at birth
2. Hemotympanum with displaced temporal bone fracture
3. Electrophysiologic studies demonstrating complete absence of voluntary and evoked motor unit responses in all muscles innervated by the facial nerve by 3 to 5 days
4. No return of facial nerve function clinically or electrophysiologically by 5 weeks of life

Children are subject to the same etiologic factors that result in adult facial nerve paralysis. Infection, trauma, and systemic disease have all been implicated in pediatric cases. Consistent with adult series, Bell's palsy is the most common diagnosis. It has a characteristic prodrome of an upper respiratory illness and presents as unilateral facial paralysis associated with pain, altered taste, and reduced tearing. The prognosis is excellent. Prescott reported a 96% overall recovery rate in his series of 228 children. He also noted that steroids had no effect on the extent or time period of recovery. Treatment consists of supportive care, eye protection, and close observation. If there is no evidence of recovery by 6 months, the diagnosis of Bell's palsy should be reconsidered.

EYE CARE

The most common complication of facial nerve paralysis, regardless of cause, is corneal desiccation. In addition to complete paralysis and diminished lacrimation, there is often altered corneal reflex. The result is significant risk of corneal ulceration, scarring, and permanent damage. Treatment consists of liberal application of "artificial tears," wearing protective eye bubbles at night, and using protective eye wear, especially outdoors. If recurrent ophthalmologic conditions warrant treatment, gold-weight implants, palpebral spring procedure, or tarsorrhaphy may be required, with the two former procedures preferred. Tarsorrhaphy gives limited vision, incomplete corneal coverage, and adds to the cosmetic deformity.

FACIAL REANIMATION

A complete discussion of the principles and techniques of facial reanimation is beyond the scope of this section, but the basic concepts and treatment approaches will be addressed. Complete recovery of facial motor function is the goal for all patients with facial nerve paralysis; however, many will be left with significant dysfunction and will require further intervention. Knowledge of the etiology of the paralysis, as well as the status of the nerve and distal musculature, is crucial for appropriate management decision making.

The ideal rehabilitative procedure for facial nerve injuries provides symmetrical appearance at rest and selective movement of all facial musculature, both voluntary and involuntary. In addition, it eliminates or prevents mass movement and other motor deficits. The most successful outcome is obtained with direct neural anastomosis, *neurorrhaphy*, or using interpositional grafts when tension-free primary anastomosis is not possible. This procedure requires early recognition of the injury and assumes that the distal portion of the nerve and facial musculature are intact. The best surgical results are obtained when an epineural anastomosis is performed.[46]

Nerve crossover anastomosis is an excellent technique to provide neural input to an intact distal facial nerve. It is most often employed in situations where damage to the proximal aspect of the nerve precludes primary neurorrhaphy or when a conservative treatment approach has failed to obtain reasonable long-term results (less than 18 months). The procedure requires intact facial musculature that is documented by EMG or muscle biopsy. The hypoglossal facial anastomosis provides the best result and is the only crossover anastomosis that has been reproducible.[46] Resting muscle tone and protection are recovered in up to 95% of patients. Facial hypertonia and synkinesis are expected shortcomings of the surgery.

In situations of irreversible atrophy of facial musculature, alternative procedures are necessary to protect the eye and provide improved facial function. *Neuromuscular transfers* and *facial slings* are used. They confer static as well as dynamic support to oppose the activity of the contralateral facial musculature. The results are usually cosmetically inferior to that of neural reconstitution but provide important protective function to the eye and mouth.

As mentioned earlier, protection of the eye is the primary concern in someone with facial nerve paralysis. In addition to the procedures already described, gold-weight implants, spring implants, and tarsorrhaphy procedures are often employed to ensure complete closure of the eye. Gold weights and spring implants provide better protection, are easily reversible, and have become the procedures of choice. Spring procedures are technically more difficult than gold-weight implants.

Finally, hemifacial spasm and hyperkinetic blepharospasm are common side effects of facial nerve injury that can be extremely debilitating. Investigation has shown promise in the use of an injectible agent. *Clostridium botulinim* toxin is a potent neurotoxin that interferes with acetylcholine release from terminal ends of motor nerves. Also employed for patients with spastic dysphonia, botulinim toxin has shown promise in alleviating symptoms for short intervals.[47] Its long-term applicability is still under investigation.

MISCELLANEOUS

1. Blood supply of the facial nerve
   External carotid artery (ECA) → Postauricular artery → Stylomastoid artery
   ECA → Middle meningeal artery → Greater superficial petrosal artery

2. Pons to internal auditory meatus (IAM) = 23–24 mm

   IAM   = 8–10 mm
   Labyrinthine   = 3–5 mm
   Tympanic   = 8–11 mm
   Mastoid   = 10–14 mm
   Parotid before branching = 15–20 mm

3. In parotid surgery, the facial nerve can be identified at 6 to 8 mm below the inferior "drop off" of the tympanomastoid fissure. This was described by HG Tabb.
4. The chorda tympani branches off at about 5 to 7 mm before the stylomastoid foramen.
5. *Bell's phenomenon:* The globe turns up and out during an attempt to close the eyes.
6. Facial paralysis of central origin is characterized by:
   a. Intact frontalis and orbicularis oculi
   b. Intact mimetic function
   c. Absence of Bell's phenomenon
7. Bilateral simultaneous facial paralysis is a sign of central generalized disease and should not be confused with Bell's palsy. The most common cause of bilateral facial paralysis is Guillain–Barré syndrome.
8. Facial nerve paralysis not involving the greater superficial petrosal nerve would give a "tearing" eye because of:
   a. Paralysis of Horner's muscle that dilates the nasolacrimal duct orifice
   b. Ectropion that produces malposition of the puncta
   c. Absence of blinking (ie, lack of the pumping action)
9. Patients with partial or total slowly progressive facial paralysis of more than 3 weeks' duration and those with no evidence of recovery after 6 months should be suspected of having a neoplasm involving the facial nerve. Remember that progression of Ramsay Hunt syndrome may continue for 14 to 21 days.
10. Nearly 100% of patients with Ramsay Hunt syndrome as the cause of facial paralysis have associated pain, and 40% have sensorineural hearing loss. Vertigo, a red pinna, and vesicles in the area of sensory distribution of the facial nerve (pinna, face, neck, or oral cavity) are other signs and symptoms seen with herpes zoster oticus (Ramsay Hunt syndrome); however, the presence of pain does not rule out Bell's palsy, as 50% of these patients will also complain of pain.
11. Hitselberger's sign, involving decreased sensitivity in the posterior-superior aspect of the concha corresponding to the sensory distribution of the VII nerve, suggests a space-occupying lesion in the internal auditory canal.
12. The incidence of severe degeneration with Bell's palsy approximates 15%, whereas with herpes zoster the incidence approximates 40%.
13. 10% of patients with Bell's palsy have a positive family history. Recurrent facial paralysis is seen in 12% of patients with Bell's palsy and is equally common on the ipsilateral and on the contralateral side. Recurrent facial paralysis is also seen in Melkersson–Rosenthal syndrome.
14. Tumors occur in 30% of patients with recurrent ipsilateral facial paralysis.
15. 25% of longitudinal fractures involve the facial nerve; 50% of transverse fractures involve the facial nerve.

16. Korczyn reported that among 130 patients with Bell's palsy, 66% had either frank diabetes or an abnormal glucose tolerance test. It has also been stated that the percentage of denervation in Bell's palsy is higher in diabetics.[48]

17. The most likely areas of compression in Bell's palsy have been noted to be in the stylomastoid area and around the pyramidal eminence.

18. *Melkersson–Rosenthal syndrome:* Recurrent unilateral or bilateral facial palsy of unknown etiology. It is associated with chronic or recurrent edema of the face with fissured tongue. The peak age group is the 20s. Histologically, dilated lymphatic channels, giant cells, and inflammatory cells are seen.

19. *Crocodile tears:* Regenerating fibers innervate the lacrimal gland instead of the submaxillary gland.

20. The facial nerve regenerates at 3 mm/day.

TREATMENT OF BELL'S PALSY

Before one can specifically advocate one mode of treatment over another, it is imperative to realize that the great majority of Bell's palsy patients have either partial paralysis or total paralysis without degeneration (ie, maintaining the neuropraxia state). It is also fairly well recognized that, unless denervation has occurred, the patient more than likely will recover spontaneously with little synkinesis. Hence, surgical treatment, if proposed, is reserved for those with total paralysis that have shown signs of denervation. There is no conclusive evidence to date that surgical decompression is of definite benefit. Some protocols treat Bell's palsy of all severities with steroids, or steroids plus acyclovir, while others treat only cases of total facial palsy with these medications. Some clinicians believe that if the nerve is allowed to degenerate completely, the prognosis is poor and synkinesis is common.

A GUIDELINE FOR THE MANAGEMENT OF FACIAL NERVE PARALYSIS

Bell's Palsy

A complete otologic, audiometric, and radiographic workup is needed.

Partial: No treatment
Total: Determine level of involvement
          Daily electrical test until
          1. Threshold of the involved side increases to 4 mA greater than the normal side
          2. There is evidence of some return of facial function

If (1) is found, decompression of the facial nerve from the stylomastoid foramen to the level of blockage should be considered. A middle fossa decompression should be done if the greater superficial petrosal nerve is involved.

Post Ear Surgery

Rule out effects of local anesthetics and an overly tight mastoid packing.

1. Delayed onset (partial or complete): Follow plan for Bell's palsy
2. Immediate onset (partial or complete): Explore the nerve before the "sun sets"

Traumatic (Head Injury)

1. Delayed onset (partial or complete): Follow plan for Bell's palsy
2. Immediate onset (partial or complete): Explore the nerve when the patient is stabilized

Herpes Zoster Oticus

The most common motor nerve involved is the VII nerve, the next are III, IV, and VI. Treat with acyclovir or acyclovir plus steroids.

Chronic Otitis Media

Partial or complete: Mastoidectomy and facial nerve decompression; ? tympanoplasty

Acute Otitis Media

1. ? Treat like Bell's palsy
2. ? Simple mastoidectomy
3. ? Myringotomy

Acute Mastoiditis with Facial Paralysis

Treatment includes simple mastoidectomy and decompression of the facial nerve and myringotomy or simple mastoidectomy and myringotomy.

References

1. Sataloff RT. *Embryology and Anomalies of the Facial Nerve and Their Surgical Implications.* New York: Raven Press, 1991.
2. Miehlke A. *Surgery of the Facial Nerve.* Philadelphia: WB Saunders, 1973.
3. Coker NJ, Fisch U. Disorders of the facial nerve. In: English GM, ed. *Otolaryngology.* Philadelphia: Harper and Row, 1990, 1–43.
4. Fowler EP. Variations in the temporal bone course of the facial nerve. *Laryngoscope* 1961; 71:937–946.
5. Dietzel VK. Ueber die dehiszenzen des facialiskanals. *Z Laryngol Rhinol Otol* 1961;40: 36–379.
6. House JW, Brackmann DE. Facial nerve grading system. *Otolaryngol Head Neck Surg* 1985;93: 146–147.
7. Schwaber MK. Gadolinium-enhanced magnetic resonance imaging in Bell's palsy. *Laryngoscope* 1990;100:1264.
8. Jonsson L, Tien R, Engstrom M, Thuomas K. GdDPTA enhanced MRI in Bell's palsy and herpes zoster oticus: An overview and implications for future studies. *Acta Otolaryngol* 1995;115: 577–584.
9. Brandle P, Satoretti-Schefer S, Bohmer A, et al. Correlation of MRI, clinical, and electroneuronographic findings in acute facial nerve palsy. *Am J Otol* 1996;17: 154–161.
10. Fisch U, Esslen E. Total intratemporal exposure of the facial nerve. *Arch Otolaryngol* 1972;95: 335–341.
11. Hilger JA. Facial nerve stimulator—New instrument. *Trans Am Acad Ophthalmol Otolaryngol* 1964;68:74–76.
12. May M, Harvey JE, Marovitz WF. The prognostic accuracy of the maximal stimulation test compared with that of the nerve excitability test in Bell's palsy. *Laryngoscope* 1971;81: 63–70.
13. Manni JJ, Stennert E. Diagnostic methods in facial nerve pathology. *Adv Otol Rhinol Laryngol* 1984;34:202.
14. May M, Klein SR, Taylor FH. Idiopathic (Bell's) palsy: Natural history defies steroid or surgical treatment. *Laryngoscope* 1985;95:406.
15. Fisch U. Prognostic value of electrical tests in acute facial paralysis. *Am J Otolaryngol* 1984; 5:494.
16. Moore GF. Facial nerve paralysis. *Primary Care* 1990;17:437–460.
17. Tavener D. The prognosis and treatment of spontaneous facial palsy. *Proc R Soc Med* 1959;52: 1077.

18. May M, Klein SR. Differential diagnosis of facial nerve palsy. *Otolaryngol Clin North Am* 1991;24:613–645.

19. Adour KK, et al. The true nature of Bell's palsy: Analysis of 1000 consecutive patients. *Laryngoscope* 1978;88:787–801.

20. Peitersen E. The natural history of Bell's palsy. *Am J Otolaryngol* 1982;4:107–111.

21. Adour KK, Hilsinger JRL, Callan EJ. Facial paralysis and Bell's palsy: A protocol for differential diagnosis. *Am J Otolaryngol* 1985;(Suppl):68–73.

22. Katusic SK. Incidence, clinical features and prognosis in Bell's palsy, Rochester, Minnesota, 1968–1982. *Ann Neurol* 1986; 20:622.

23. Stankiewicz JA. Steroids and idiopathic facial paralysis. *Otolaryngol Head Neck Surg* 1983; 91:672–677.

24. Shafshak TS, Essa AY, Bakey FA. The possible contributing factors for the success of steroid therapy in Bell's palsy: A clinical and electrophysiological study. *J Laryngol Otol* 1994;108: 940–943.

25. Adour KK, et al. Bell's palsy treatment with acyclovir and prednisone compared with prednisone alone: A double-blind, randomized, controlled trial. *Ann Otol Rhinol Laryngol* 1996;105: 371–378.

26. Hughes GB. Practical management of Bell's palsy. *Otolaryngol-Head Neck Surg* 1990;102: 658–663.

27. McHugh HE. Surgical treatment of facial paralysis and traumatic conductive deafness in fractures of the temporal bone. *Ann Otol Rhinol Laryngol* 1959;68:855.

28. Lathrop FD. Facial paralysis of traumatic origin: Prevention and treatment. In: English GM, ed. *Otolaryngology*. Philadelphia: Harper and Row, 1990, 1–31.

29. McKennan KX, Chole RA. Facial paralysis in temporal bone trauma. *Am J Otol* 1992; 13:167–172.

30. Adkins WY, Osguthorpe JD. Management of trauma of the facial nerve. *Otolaryngol Clin North Am* 1991;24:587–611.

31. Adour KK, Wingerd J. Idiopathic facial paralysis (Bell's palsy): Factors affecting severity and outcome in 446 patients. *Neurology* 1974;24: 1112.

32. Cohen D, Friedman P, Eilon A. Malignant external otitis versus acute external otitis. *J Laryngol Otol* 1987;101:211–215.

33. Rubin J, Yu VL. Malignant external otitis: Insights into pathogenesis, clinical manifestations, diagnosis, and therapy. *Am J Med* 1988; 85:391–398.

34. Brody T, Pensak ML. The fluoroquinolones. *Am J Otol* 1991;12:477–479.

35. Clark JR, Carlson RD, Sasaki CT. Facial paralysis in Lyme disease. *Laryngoscope* 1985;95: 1341–1345.

36. Lesser TH, Dort JC, Simmen DP. Ear, nose and throat manifestations of Lyme disease. *J Laryngol Otol* 1990;104:301–304.

37. Murr AH, Benecke JE. Association of facial paralysis with HIV positivity. *Am J Otol* 1991; 12:450–451.

38. Belec L. Peripheral facial paralysis and HIV infection: Report of four African cases and review of the literature. *J Neurol* 1989;236:411.

39. Fisch U, Ruttner J. Pathology of intratemporal tumors involving the facial nerve. In: Fisch U, ed. *Facial Nerve Surgery*. Birmingham, AL: Aesculapius Publishers, Inc., 1977, 448–456.

40. Brackmann DE, Bartels LJ. Rare tumors of the cerebellopontine angle. *Otolaryngol Head Neck Surg* 1980;88:555–559.

41. Smith JD, Crumley RL, Harker LA. Facial paralysis in the newborn. *Otolaryngol Head Neck Surg* 1981;89:1021–1024.

42. Bergman I, May M, Wessel HB, Stool SE. Management of facial palsy caused by birth trauma. *Laryngoscope* 1986;94:381–384.

43. Orobello P. Congenital and acquired facial nerve paralysis in children. *Otolaryngol Clin North Am* 1991;24:647–652.

44. Manning JJ, Adour KK. Facial paralysis in children. *Pediatrics* 1972;49:102–109.

45. Alberti PW, Biagioni E. Facial paralysis in children. A review of 150 cases. *Laryngoscope* 1972;82:1013–1020.

46. Spector JG. Mimetic surgery for the paralyzed face. *Laryngoscope* 1985;95:1494–1522.

47. May M, Croxson GR, Klein SA. Bell's palsy: Management of sequellae using EMG rehabilitation, botulinim toxin, and surgery. *Am J Otol* 1989;10:220–229.

48. Korczyn A. Bell's palsy and diabetes mellitus. *Lancet* 1971;1:108–109.

Bibliography

Aoyagi M, Koike Y, Ichige A. Results of facial nerve decompression. *Acta Otolaryngol (Stockh)* 1988;446(Suppl):101–105.

Burres SA. Objective grading of facial paralysis. *Ann Otol Rhinol Laryngol* 1986;95:238–241.

Cramer HB, Kartush JM. Testing facial nerve function. *Otolaryngol Clin North Am* 1991;24: 555–570.

Graham MD, Kartush JM. Total facial nerve decompression for recurrent facial paralysis: An update. *Otolaryngol-Head Neck Surg* 1989; 101:442–444.

Inamura H, Aoyagi M, Tojima H, Koike Y. Effects of aciclovir in Ramsay Hunt syndrome. *Acta Otolaryngol (Stockh)* 1988;446(Suppl):111–113.

Marsh MA, Coker NJ. Surgical decompression of idiopathic facial palsy. *Otolaryngol Clin North Am* 1991;24:675–689.

Mattox DE. *Clinical Disorders of the Facial Nerve*, 2nd ed. New York: Mosby-Year Book, 1993.

May M, SM S, Mester SJ. Managing segmental facial nerve injuries by surgical repair. *Laryngoscope* 1990;100:1062–1067.

Melkersson E. Et fall ay recidiverande facilspares i samband med angioneurotiskt öden. *Hygiea* 1928;90:737.

Prescott CA. Idiopathic facial nerve palsy: The effect of treatment with steroids. *J Laryngol Otol* 1988;102:403–407.

Rosenthal C. Klinischerbiologischer beitrag zur Konstitutionspathologie. Gemeinsames auftreten von (rezidivierender familiärer) Facialislähmung, Angioneurotischem Gesichtsödem und Lingua Plicata in Arthritismus-Familien. *Z Neurol Psychiatry* 1931;131:475.

Sunderland S. *Nerve and Nerve Injuries*, 2nd ed. New York: Churchill Livingstone, 1978.

Tabb HG. Exposure of the facial nerve in parotid surgery. *Laryngoscope* 1970;80:559–567.

Tani M, et al. Medical treatment of Bell's palsy. *ACTA Otolaryngol (Stockh)* 1988;446 (Suppl): 114–118.

Zimmer WM, Rogers RS, Reeve CM, Sheridan PJ. Orofacial manifestations of Melkersson–Rosenthal syndrome. *Oral Surg Oral Med Oral Pathol* 1992;74:610–619.

Syndromes and Eponyms

9

SYNDROMES AND DISEASES

Adult Respiratory Distress Syndrome

Adult respiratory distress syndrome (ARDS) is characterized by a delay in onset (12–24 hours) following injury, shock, and/or successful resuscitative effort. Septic shock, extrathoracic trauma, central nervous system (CNS) pathology, fat embolism, oxygen toxicity, head and facial injuries, and massive blood transfusions can lead to ARDS. It is characterized by hypoxia and pulmonary infiltrates secondary to increased pulmonary vascular permeability, microvascular hemorrhage, or both.

Aide Syndrome

Aide syndrome is characterized by decreased pupillary reaction and deep tendon reflex. The etiology is unknown.

Alagille Syndrome

Marked by cardiovascular abnormalities, characteristic facial appearance, chronic cholestasis, growth retardation, hypogonadism, mental retardation, vertebral arch defect, temporal bone anomalies in the cochlear aqueduct, ossicles, semicircular canals, and subarcuate fossa. Liver transplantation is a possible treatment.

Albers–Schönberg Disease

Also known as osteopetrosis. A genetic disorder, this disease results in progressive increase in the density (but also increase in weakness) of the bones in the skeletal system. Vascular nutrition to affected bones is also decreased by this disease. Broken down into three categories, there is osteopetrosis with precocious manifestations, osteopetrosis with delayed manifestations, and pyknodysostosis. In the mandible, long-term antibiotic therapy, multiple debridements, sequestrectomies, or even resection are possible treatments.

Albright Syndrome

Polyostotic fibrous dysplasia usually manifests early in life as multicentric lesions involving the long bones and bones of the face and skull with scattered skin lesions similar to melanotic *café au lait* spots and precocious puberty in female patients. Frequently, there is an elevation of serum alkaline phosphatase as well as endocrine abnormalities.

Aldrich Syndrome

Thrombocytopenia, eczema, and recurrent infections occur during the first year of life. It is inherited through a sex-linked recessive gene. The bleeding time is prolonged, the platelet count is decreased, and the bone marrow megakaryocytes are normal in number.

Amalric Syndrome

Granular macular pigment epitheliopathy (foveal dystrophy) is associated with sensorineural hearing loss. Visual acuity is usually normal. This syndrome may be a genetic disorder, or it may be the result of an intrauterine rubella infection.

Aortic Arch Syndrome

See Takayasu disease.

Apert Syndrome

Not to be confused with Pfeiffer syndrome, which has different types of hand malformations.

Ascher Syndrome

This syndrome is a combination of blepharochalasis, double lip, and goiter.

Auriculotemporal Syndrome (Frey Syndrome)

This syndrome is characterized by localized flushing and sweating of the ear and cheek region in response to eating. It usually occurs after parotidectomy. It is assumed that following parotidectomy the parasympathetic fibers of the IX nerve innervate the sweat glands. It has been estimated that 20% of the parotidectomies in children result in this disorder.

Avellis Syndrome

Unilateral paralysis of the larynx and velum palati, with contralateral loss of pain and temperature sensitivity in the parts below the larynx characterize Avellis syndrome. The syndrome is caused by involvement of the nucleus ambiguus or the vagus nerve along with the cranial portion of the XI nerve.

Babinski–Nageotte Syndrome

This syndrome is caused by multiple or scattered lesions, chiefly in the distribution of the vertebral artery. Ipsilateral paralysis of the soft palate, larynx, pharynx, and sometimes tongue occurs. There is also ipsilateral loss of taste on the posterior third of the tongue, loss of pain and temperature sensation around the face, and cerebellar asynergia. Horner syndrome with contralateral spastic hemiplegia, and loss of proprioceptive and tactile sensation may also be present.

Baelz Syndrome

Painless papules at the openings of the ducts of the mucous glands of the lips with free exudation of mucus are characteristic. Congenital and familial forms are precancerous. Acquired forms are benign and caused by irritating substances.

Bannwarth Syndrome (Facial Palsy in Lymphocytic Meningoradiculitis)

A relatively benign form of acute unilateral or bilateral facial palsy that is associated with lymphocytic reactions and an increased protein level in the cerebrospinal fluid (CSF) with minimal, if any, meningeal symptoms is known as Bannwarth syndrome. Neuralgic or radicular pain without facial palsy and unilateral or bilateral facial palsy of acute onset are symptoms of this syndrome. A virus has been suggested as a possible etiology. Males are more often affected than females, with the greatest number of cases occurring in the months of August and September.

Barany Syndrome

This syndrome is a combination of unilateral headache in the back of the head, periodic ipsilateral deafness (alternating with periods of unaffected hearing), vertigo, and tinnitus. The syndrome complex may be corrected by induced nystagmus.

Barclay–Baron Disease

Vallecular dysphagia is present.

Barre–Lieou Syndrome

Occipital headache, vertigo, tinnitus, vasomotor disorders, and facial spasm due to irritation of the sympathetic plexus around the vertebral artery in rheumatic disorders of the cervical spine are characteristic. It is also known as cervical migraine.

Barrett Syndrome

Barrett syndrome is characterized by esophagitis due to change in the epithelium of the esophagus.

Barsony–Polgar Syndrome

A diffuse esophageal spasm—caused by disruption of the peristaltic waves by an irregular contraction resulting in dysphagia and regurgitation—is evidence of this syndrome. It most commonly affects excitable elderly persons.

Basal Cell Nevoid Syndrome

This familial syndrome, nonsex-linked and autosomal dominant with high penetrance and variable expressivity, manifests early in life. It appears as multiple nevoid basal cell epitheliomas of the skin, cysts of the jaw, abnormal ribs and metacarpal bones, frontal bossing, and dorsal scoliosis. Endocrine abnormalities have been reported and it has been associated with medulloblastoma. The cysts in the jaw, present only in the maxilla and mandible, are destructive to the bone. The basal cell epitheliomas are excised as necessary, and the cysts in the jaw rarely recur after complete enucleation.[1]

Bayford–Autenrieth Dysphagia (Arkin Disease)

Dysphagia lusoria is said to be secondary to esophageal compression from an aberrant right subclavian artery.

Beckwith Syndrome

This is a congenital disorder characterized by macroglossia, omphalocele, hypoglycemia, pancreatic hyperplasia, noncystic renal hyperplasia, and cytomegaly of the fetal adrenal cortex.

Behçet Syndrome

Of unknown etiology, this disease runs a protracted course with periods of relapse and remission. It manifests as indolent ulcers of the mucous membrane and skin, and stomatitis, as well as anogenital ulceration, iritis, and conjunctivitis. No definitive cure is known, though steroids help.

Besnier–Boeck–Schaumann Syndrome

Sarcoidosis is present.

Bloom Syndrome

An autosomal recessive growth disorder, this syndrome is associated with chromosomal breaks and rearrangements. It is also associated with an unusually high rate of cancer at an early age. Associated with facial erythema, growth retardation, immunodeficiency, infertility, and sun sensitivity, diagnosis is confirmed by chromosome analysis. Anomalous numbers of digits or teeth, asymmetric legs, heart malformation, hypopigmented spots in blacks, protruding ears, sacral dimple, simian line, and urethral or meatal narrowing are less common characteristics. For head and neck tumor patients, there is an increased chance of secondary and primary tumors.

Bogorad Syndrome

This syndrome also is known as the syndrome of crocodile tears, characterized by residual facial paralysis with profuse lacrimation during eating. It is caused by a misdirection of regenerating autonomic fibers to the lacrimal gland instead of to the salivary gland.

Bonnet Syndrome

Sudden trigeminal neuralgia accompanied by a Horner syndrome and vasomotor disorders in the area supplied by the trigeminal nerve are manifestations of this syndrome.

Bonnier Syndrome

This syndrome is caused by a lesion of Deiters' nucleus and its connection. Its symptoms include ocular disturbances (eg, paralysis of accommodation, nystagmus, diplopia), deafness, nausea, thirst, and anorexia, as well as other symptoms referable to involvement of the vagal centers, cranial nerves VIII, IX, X, and XI, and the lateral vestibular nucleus. It can simulate Ménière disease.

Bourneville Syndrome

This is a familial disorder whose symptoms include polyps of the skin, harelip, moles, spina bifida, and microcephaly.

Bowen Disease

This is a precancerous dermatosis characterized by the development of pinkish or brownish papules covered with a thickened horny layer. Histologically, it shows hyperchromatic acanthotic cells with multinucleated giant cells. Mitoses are frequently observed.

Branchio-Oto-Renal Syndrome

This is an autosomal disorder characterized by anomalies of the external, middle, and inner ear in association with preauricular tissues, branchial cleft anomalies, and varying degrees of renal dysplasia, including aplasia. Many of the following symptoms (but not necessarily all) are present:

1. Conductive or mixed hearing loss
2. Cup-shaped, anteverted pinnae with bilateral preauricular sinuses
3. Bilateral branchial cleft fistulas or sinuses
4. Renal dysplasia

This syndrome is among a group of syndromes characterized by deformities associated with the first and second branchial complexes. The precise incidence of the disorder is unknown.

Briquet's Syndrome

Briquet's syndrome is characterized by a shortness of breath and aphonia due to hysteric paralysis of the diaphragm.

Brissaud–Marie Syndrome

Unilateral spasm of the tongue and lips of an hysteric nature are characteristic.

Brown Syndrome

This syndrome is a congenital or acquired abnormality of the superior oblique muscle tendon characterized by vertical diplopia and the inability to elevate the eye above midline or medial gaze. There are two types of Brown syndrome, true and simulated. True Brown syndrome is always congenital. Simulated Brown syndrome is either congenital or acquired. The congenital simulated type may be caused by thickening of an area in the posterior tendon or by the firm attachment of the posterior sheath to the superior oblique tendon. The acquired simulated type may be caused by inflammation extending from the adjacent ethmoid cells to the posterior sheath and tendon, an orbital floor fracture, frontal ethmoidal fracture, crush fracture of nasal bones, sinusitis, frontal sinus surgery, or surgical tucking of the superior oblique tendon.

Brun Syndrome

Vertigo, headache, vomiting, and visual disturbances due to an obstruction of CSF flow during positional changes of the head are seen. The main causes of this syndrome include cysts and cysticercosis of the fourth ventricle as well as tumors of the midline cerebellum and third ventricle.

Burckhardt Dermatitis

This dermatitis appears as an eruption of the external ear. It consists of red papules and vesicles that appear after exposure to sunlight. The rash usually resolves spontaneously.

Caffey Disease (Infantile Cortical Hyperostosis)

Of familial tendency, its onset is usually during the first year of life. It is characterized by hyperirritability, fever, and hard nonpitting edema that overlies the cortical hyperostosis. Pathologically, it involves the loss of periosteum with acute inflammatory involvement of the intratrabecular bone and the overlying soft tissue. Treatment is supportive, consisting of steroids and antibiotics. The prognosis is good. The mandible is the most frequently involved site.

Caisson Disease

This symptom complex occurs in men and women who work in high air pressures and are returned too suddenly to normal atmospheric pressure. Similar symptoms may occur in fliers when they suddenly ascend to high altitudes unprotected by counterpressure. It results from the escape from solution in the body fluids of bubbles (mainly nitrogen) originally absorbed at higher pressure. Symptoms include headache; pain in the epigastrium, sinuses, and tooth sockets; itchy skin; vertigo; dyspnea; coughing; nausea; vomiting; and sometimes paralysis. Peripheral circulatory collapse may be present. Nitrogen bubbles have been found in the white matter of the spinal cord. It also can injure the inner ear through necrosis of the organ of Corti. There is a question of rupture of the round window membrane; hemotympanum and eustachian tube obstruction may occur.

Camptomelic Syndrome

The name is derived from a Greek word meaning "curvature of extremities." The syndrome is characterized by dwarfism, craniofacial anomalies, and bowing of the tibia and femur, with malformation of other bones. The patient has cutaneous dimpling overlying the tibial bend. Respiratory distress is common, and the patient has an early demise in the first few months of life. In the otolaryngologic area the patient exhibits a prominent forehead, flat facies with a broad nasal bridge and low-set ears, cleft palate, mandibular hypoplasia, and tracheobronchial malacia that contributes to the respiratory distress and neonatal death. Histologically, two temporal bone observations showed defective endochondral ossification with no cartilage cells in the endochondral layer of the otic capsule. The cochlea was shortened and flattened, presenting a scalar communis. The vestibule and the semicircular canal were deformed by bone invasion.

This syndrome is often of unknown etiology, although some believe it is autosomal recessive. Others believe it may be due to an exogenous cause.

This syndrome is not to be confused with Pierre Robin syndrome, which presents with very similar clinical features.

Cannon Nevus

This is an autosomal dominant disorder characterized by spongy white lesions of the oral and nasal mucosa. The lesions are asymptomatic and may be found from the newborn period with increasing severity until adolescence. The histologic picture is that of keratosis, acanthosis, and parakeratosis.

Carcinoid Syndrome

The symptoms include episodic flushing, diarrhea, and ascites. The tumor secretes serotonin. Treatment is wide excision. The tumor may give a positive DOPA reaction.

Carotid Sinus Syndrome (Charcot–Weiss–Barber Syndrome)

When the carotid sinus is abnormally sensitive, slight pressure on it causes a marked fall in blood pressure due to vasodilation and cardiac slowing. Symptoms include syncope, convulsions, and heart block.

Castleman Disease

This disease was first described by Castelman et al in 1954. It is a benign lymphoepithelial disease that is most often mistaken for lymphoma. It is also known as localized nodal hyperplasia, angiomatous lymph node hyperplasia, lymphoid hamartoma, and giant lymph nodal hyperplasia. Symptoms include tracheobronchial compression, such as cough, dyspnea, hemoptysis, or dysphagia. Masses in the neck are also not uncommon. There are two histologic types—the hyaline vascular type and the plasma cell type. Follicles in the hyaline vascular type are traversed by radially oriented capillaries with plump endothelial cells and collagenous hyalinization surrounding the vessels. The follicles in the plasma cell type are normal in size without capillary proliferation or hyalinization. Intermediate forms exist but are rare. Treatment entails complete excision of the mass. Etiology is unknown.

Cavernous Sinus Syndrome

The cavernous sinus receives drainage from the upper lip, nose, sinuses, nasopharynx, pharynx, and orbits. It drains into the inferior petrosal sinus, which in turn drains into the internal jugular vein. The cavernous sinus syndrome is caused by thrombosis of the cavernous intracranial sinus, 80% of which is fatal. The symptoms include orbital pain (V_1) with venous congestion of the retina, lids, and conjunctiva. The eyes are proptosed with exophthalmos. The patient has photophobia and involvement of nerves II, III, IV, and V_1. The treatment of choice is anticoagulation and antibiotics. The most common cause of cavernous sinus thrombosis is ethmoiditis. The ophthalmic vein and artery are involved as well. (The nerves and veins are lateral to the cavernous sinus, and the internal carotid artery is medial to it.)

Cestan–Chenais Syndrome

This is caused by occlusion of the vertebral artery below the point of origin of the posteroinferior cerebellar artery. There is paralysis of the soft palate, pharynx, and larynx. Ipsilateral cerebellar asynergia and Horner syndrome are also present. There is contralateral hemiplegia and diminished proprioception and tactile sensation.

Champion–Cregah–Klein Syndrome

This is a familial syndrome consisting of popliteal webbing, cleft lip, cleft palate, lower lip fistula, syndactyly, onychodysplasia, and pes equinovarus.

Chapple Syndrome

This disorder is seen in the newborn with unilateral facial weakness or paralysis in conjunction with comparable weakness or paralysis of the contralateral vocal cord, the muscles of deglutition, or both. The disorder is secondary to lateral flexion of the head in utero, which compresses the thyroid cartilage against the hyoid or cricoid cartilages or both, thereby injuring the recurrent or superior laryngeal nerve, or both.

Charcot–Marie–Tooth Disease

This is a hereditary and degenerative disease that includes the olivopontocerebellar, cerebello-parenchymal, and spinocerebellar disorders and the neuropathies. This disease is characterized by chronic degeneration of the peripheral nerves and roots, and distal muscle atrophy in feet, legs, and hands. Deep tendon reflexes are usually nil. It is also associated with hereditary cerebellar ataxia features, optic atrophy, and other cranial involvement. Some suggest that this disease is linked to auditory dysfunction and that it is also linked to other CNS dysfunctions. This disease can be progressive, and it can also spontaneously arrest.

Chédiak–Higashi Syndrome

This syndrome is the result of an autosomal recessive trait. It is characterized by albinism, photophobia, nystagmus, hepatosplenomegaly, anomalous cellular granules, and development of lymphoma. These patients usually die during childhood of fulminant infections.

Cleft Lip Palate and Congenital Lip Fistulas

This syndrome is transmitted in an autosomal dominant manner with 80% penetrance; it occurs in 1:100,000 live births. Usually bilateral, symmetrically located depressions are noted on the vermilion portion of the lower lip and communicate with the underlying minor salivary glands. The lip pits may be an isolated finding (33%) or be found with cleft lip palate (67% of cases). Associated anomalies of the extremities may include talipes equinovarus, syndactyly, and popliteal pterygia. Congenital lip pits have also been seen in association with the oral-facial-digital syndrome.

Cockayne Syndrome

Autosomal recessive, progressive bilateral sensorineural hearing loss, associated with dwarfism, facial disharmony, microcephaly, mental deficiency, retinitis pigmentosa, optic atrophy, intracranial calcification, and multiple dental caries. Patients succumb to respiratory or genitourinary infection in the teens or twenties.

Cogan Syndrome

Nonsyphilitic interstitial keratitis and vestibuloauditory symptoms are characteristics of this syndrome. Interstitial keratitis gives rise to rapid visual loss. Symptoms include episodic severe vertigo accompanied by tinnitus, spontaneous nystagmus, ataxia, and progressive sensorineural hearing loss. There are remissions and exacerbations. It is believed to be related to periarteritis nodosa. Eosinophilia has been reported in this entity. Pathologically, it is a degeneration of the vestibular and spiral ganglia with edema of the membranous cochlea, semicircular canals, and inflammation of the spiral ligament. Treatment with steroids has been advocated.

Cyclophosphamide and azathioprine have been used in addition to prednisone (40 mg daily). This syndrome is not to be confused with Ménière disease despite vertiginous symptoms and fluctuating hearing loss. Vogt–Koyanagi–Harada syndrome is also similar but involves alopecia, poliosis, and exudative uveitis. Syphilis is also confused with this syndrome, but in syphilis, the interstitial keratitis is old and usually does not demonstrate active inflammatory changes. Syphilitic involvement of the cornea is often centrally located. Follow-up treatment of patients must be thorough in order to detect more extensive involvement, such as systemic vasculitis or aortitis.

Collet–Sicard Syndrome

The IX, X, XI, and XII nerves are involved with normal sympathetic nerves. The etiology is usually a meningioma or other lesion involving the nerves in the posterior cranial fossa.

Conradi–Hünerman Syndrome

The most common variant of chondrodysplasia punctata, this syndrome is characterized by punctate epiphyseal calcifications. Clinical features include saddle nose deformity, micromelia, rhizomelia, short stature, flexion contractures, and dermatoses. This syndrome is also known as chondrodystrophia epiphysialis punctata, stippled epiphysis disease, dysplasia epiphysialis punctata, chondroangiopathia calcarea punctata, and Conradi disease. Some cases point to sporadic mutations and others to autosomal dominant patterns of inheritance. The clinical features of this syndrome are so varied from case to case that only a complete workup can exclude other versions of this syndrome.

Costen Syndrome

Costen syndrome is a temporomandibular joint (TMJ) abnormality, usually due to impaired bite and characterized by tinnitus, vertigo, and pain in the frontal, parietal, and occipital areas with a blocked feeling and pain in the ear. After a careful workup to rule out other abnormalities, the patient is treated with aspirin, heat, and slow exercise of the joint. An orthodontist may help the patient. The TMJ differs from other joints by the presence of avascular fibrous tissue covering the articulating surfaces with an interposed meniscus dividing the joint into upper and lower compartments. The right and left TMJs act as one functional unit. The condyle is made up of spongy bone with marrow and a growth center. The condyle articulates with the glenoid fossa of the temporal bone (squamosa). The squamotympanic fissure separates the fossa from the tympanic bone. The joint is a ginglymoarthrodial joint with hinge and transverse movements. The key supporting ligament of the TMJ is the temporomandibular ligament. The boundaries of the glenoid fossa are:

Anterior:	Margins of the articular eminence
Posterior:	Squamosotympanic fissure
Lateral:	Zygomatic process of the temporal bone
Medial:	Temporal spine

The TMJ derives its nourishment from the synovial membrane, which is richly vascularized and produces a mucinous-like substance. The joint has a gliding motion between the meniscus and the temporal bone (upper compartment). It has a hinge motion between the disk and the condyle (lower compartment). It is innervated by the auriculotemporal nerve, masseter nerve, lateral pterygoid nerve, and temporal nerve. It is supplied by the superficial temporal artery and the anterior tympanic branch of the internal maxillary artery. The lateral pterygoid muscle protracts the jaw, and the masseter, medial pterygoid, and temporalis muscles act as elevators. All these muscles are innervated by V_3 (see Chapter 37 for muscles of the mandible). The sphenomandibular and stylomandibular ligaments have no function in TMJ articulation.

Cowden Syndrome

This is a familial syndrome characterized by adenoid facies, hypoplasia of the mandible and maxilla, high-arched palate, hypoplasia of the soft palate and uvula, microstomia, papillomatosis of the lips and pharynx, scrotal tongue, multiple thyroid adenomas, bilateral breast hypertrophy, pectus excavatum, and liver and CNS abnormalities.

Cri du Chat Syndrome

A condition caused by a B group chromosome with a short arm, its symptoms are mental retardation, respiratory stridor, microcephaly, hypertelorism, midline oral clefts, and laryngomalacia with poor approximation of the posterior vocal cords.

Crouzon Disease

See Chapter 5.

Curtius Syndrome

This is a form of hypertrophy that may involve a single small part of the body or an entire system (ie, muscular, nervous, or skeletal systems). It is also known as congenital hemifacial hypertrophy.

Dandy Syndrome

Oscillopsia or jumbling of the panorama common in patients after bilateral labyrinthectomy is characteristic of this syndrome. These patients are unable to focus while walking or moving.

Darier Disease (Keratosis Follicularis)

Autosomal dominant, this skin disorder of the external auditory canal is characterized by keratotic debris in the canal. Some investigators have advocated the use of vitamin A or steroids.

De'Jean Syndrome

Exophthalmos, diplopia, superior maxillary pain, and numbness along the route of the trigeminal nerve are found with lesions of the orbital floor in this syndrome.

Déjérine Anterior Bulbar Syndrome

This syndrome is evidenced by thrombosis of the anterior spinal artery resulting in either an alternating hypoglossal hemiplegia or an alternating hypoglossal hemianesthetic hemiplegia.

Dermarquay–Richet Syndrome

This syndrome is a congenital orofacial disorder characterized by cleft lip, cleft palate, lower lip fistulas, and progeria facies. Defective dentition, heart defects, dwarfism, and finger abnormalities may be seen.

Didmoad Syndrome

This syndrome is an autosomal recessive disorder associating diabetes insipidus, diabetes mellitus, optic atrophy, and deafness. Diabetes mellitus is usually juvenile in onset and insulin-dependent. The diabetes insipidus has a varied time of onset and is vasopressin-sensitive, indicative of degeneration of the hypothalamic cells or of the supraopticohypophyseal tract. The hearing loss is sensorineural and progressive, and primarily affects the higher tones.

Urinary tract abnormalities ranging from atonic bladder to hydronephrosis and hydroureter have been reported with this disorder.

DiGeorge Syndrome

Lischaneri reported three categories of this syndrome:

1. Third and fourth pharyngeal pouch syndrome, characterized by cardiovascular and craniofacial anomalies as well as abdominal visceral abnormalities
2. DiGeorge syndrome (thymus agenesis)
3. Partial DiGeorge syndrome (thymic hypoplasia in which the thymus gland weighs less than 2 g)

The patients have small malformed pinnae with narrow external auditory canals and abnormal ossicles. The patients also have shortened cochlea of the Mundini type as well as an absence of hair cells in the hook region, hypertelorism with nasal cleft, shortened philtrum, and micrognathia. Other middle ear anomalies include an absence of stapedial muscle, hypoplastic facial nerve, and absent oval window. Most of the findings are symmetrical.

Down Syndrome

See "Trisomy" in Chapter 5.

Dysphagia Lusoria

Dysphagia lusoria is secondary to an abnormal right subclavian artery. The right subclavian arises abnormally from the thoracic aorta by passing behind or in front of the esophagus, thus compressing it.

Eagle Syndrome

The patient has elongation of the styloid process or ossification of the stylohyoid ligament causing irritation of the trigeminal, facial, glossopharyngeal, and vagus nerves. Symptoms include recurrent nonspecific throat discomfort, foreign body sensation, dysphagia, facial pain, and increased salivation. Carotidynia may result from impingement of the styloid process on the carotid artery, producing regional tenderness or headaches. The only effective treatment for Eagle syndrome is surgical shortening of the styloid process.

Ectodermal Dysplasia, Hidrotic

See Chapter 6.

Ectodermal Dysplasia, Hypohidrotic

This syndrome consists of hypodontia, hypotrichosis, and hypohidrosis. Principally, the structures involved are of ectodermal origin. Eyelashes and especially eyebrows are entirely missing. Eczema and asthma are common. Aplasia of the eccrine sweat glands may lead to severe hyperpyrexia. The inheritance is X-linked recessive.

18q Syndrome

This syndrome consists of psychomotor retardation, hypotonia, short stature, microcephaly, hypoplastic midface, epicanthus, ophthalmologic abnormalities, cleft palate, congenital heart disease, abnormalities of the genitalia, tapered fingers, aural atresia, and conductive hearing loss.

Eisenlohr Syndrome

Numbness and weakness in the extremities; paralysis of the lips, tongue, and palate; and dysarthria are evidenced.

Elschnig Syndrome

Extension of the palpebral fissure laterally, displacement of the lateral canthus, ectopion of the lower lid, and lateral canthus are observed. Hypertelorism, cleft palate, and cleft lip are frequently seen.

Empty Sella Syndrome

The patient has an enlarged sella, giving the appearance of a pituitary tumor. An air encephalogram shows an empty sella. The syndrome consists of the abnormal extension into the sella turcica of an arachnoid diverticulum filled with CSF, displacing and compressing the pituitary gland. Four causal theories of this syndrome exist: (1) rupture of an intrasellar or parasellar cyst; (2) infarction of a pituitary adenoma; (3) pituitary hypertrophy and subsequent involution; and (4) the most common theory, the syndrome is due to CSF pressure through a congenitally deficient sella diaphragm leading to the formation of an intrasellar arachnoidocele. A transseptal or transsphenoidal route to the sella is a treatment to consider.

The primary empty sella syndrome is due to congenital absence of the diaphragm sella, with gradual enlargement of the sella secondary to pulsations of the brain. Secondary empty sella syndrome may be due to necrosis of an existing pituitary tumor after surgery, post-irradiation directed at the pituitary, or pseudotumor cerebri.

Face–Hand Syndrome

This syndrome is a reflex sympathetic dystrophy that is seen after a stroke or myocardial infarction. There may be edema and erythema of the involved parts along with persistent burning.

Fanconi Anemia Syndrome

Patients have aplastic anemia with skin pigmentation, skeletal deformities, renal anomalies, and mental retardation. Death due to leukemia usually ensues within 2 years. The disorder rarely occurs in adults. (A variant is congenital hypoplastic thrombocytopenia, which is inherited as an autosomal recessive trait.) It is characterized by spontaneous bleeding and other congenital anomalies. The bleeding time is prolonged, the platelet count is decreased, and the bone marrow megakaryocytes vary from decreased to absent.

It is associated with unrepaired chromosome breakage. Congenital anomalies of the inner, middle, and external ear could be causes of the deafness that accompanies this syndrome.

Felty Syndrome

Felty syndrome is a combination of leukopenia, arthritis, and enlarged lymph nodes and spleen.

First and Second Branchial Arch Syndromes (Hemifacial Microsomia, Lateral Facial Dysplasia)

This disorder consists of a spectrum of craniofacial malformations characterized by asymmetric facies with unilateral abnormalities. The mandible is small with hypoplastic or absent ramus and condyle. Aural atresia, hearing impairment, tissue tags from the tragus to the oral commissure, coloboma of the upper eyelid, malar hypoplasia, and cleft palate also may be present. Cardiovascular, renal, and nervous system abnormalities have been noted in association with this disorder.

Fish Odor Syndrome

Clinical symptoms of this peculiar syndrome consist of a fish odor emanating from the mucus, particularly in the morning. A challenge test with either choline bitartrate or trimethylamine is diagnostic of this disease. Eating noncholine-containing foods usually helps. No long-term effects are known.

Fordyce Disease

This disease is characterized by pseudocolloid of the lips, a condition marked by the presence of numerous, small yellowish white granules on the inner surface and vermilion border of the lips. Histologically, the lesions appear as ectopic sebaceous glands.

Foster Kennedy Syndrome

Patients with this disorder show ipsilateral optic atrophy and scotomas and contralateral papilledema occurring with tumors or other lesions of the frontal lobe or sphenoidal meningioma. Anosmia may be seen.

Fothergill Disease

The combination of tic douloureux and anginose scarlatina is characteristic of this disease.

Foville Syndrome

Facial paralysis with ipsilateral paralysis of conjugate gaze and contralateral pyramidal hemiplegia are diagnostic. Tinnitus, deafness, and vertigo may occur with infranuclear involvement. Loss of taste of the anterior two-thirds of the tongue with decreased salivary and lacrimal secretions is seen with involvement of the nervus intermedius.

Frey Syndrome

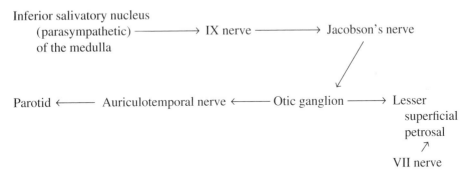

In the normal person, the sweat glands are innervated by sympathetic nerve fibers. After parotidectomy, the auriculotemporal nerve sends its parasympathetic fibers to innervate the sweat glands instead. The incidence of Frey syndrome after parotidectomy in children has been estimated to be about 20%.

Also called preauricular gustatory sweating, parotidectomy is considered the most common etiology.

Friedreich Disease

The disease consists of facial hemihypertrophy involving the eyelids, cheeks, lips, facial bones, tongue, ears, and tonsils. It may be seen alone or in association with generalized hemihypertrophy.

Garcin Syndrome

Paralysis of cranial nerves III through X, usually unilateral or occasionally bilateral, is observed. It may be the result of invasion by neoplasm, granulomas, or infections in the retropharyngeal space.

Gard–Gignoux Syndrome

This syndrome involves paralysis of the XI nerve and the X nerve below the nodose ganglion. The cricothyroid function and sensation are normal. The symptoms include vocal cord paralysis and weakness of the trapezius and sternocleidomastoid muscles.

Gardner Syndrome

An autosomal-dominant disease whose symptoms include fibroma, osteoma of the skull, mandible, maxilla, and long bones, with epidermoid inclusion cysts in the skin and polyps in the colon. These colonic polyps have a marked tendency toward malignant degeneration.

Gargoylism (Hurler Syndrome)

See Chapter 6.

Gaucher Disease

As an autosomally recessive inherited disorder of lipid metabolism, this syndrome results in a decrease in activity of the glucocerebrosidase. This leads to an increased accumulation of glucocerebrosides, particularly in the retroendothelial system. There are three classifications of the disease: (1) the chronic nonneuronopathic form, characterized by joint pain, aseptic necrosis, pathologic fractures, hepatosplenomegaly, thrombocytopenia, anemia, and leukopenia; (2) the acute neuronopathic Gaucher disease (infantile form), causing increased neurologic complications that often end in death before the first 2 years of life; and (3) the juvenile and less severe forms than the infantile form.

Gerlier Disease

With the presence of vertigo and kubisagari, it is observed among cowherds. It is marked by pain in the head and neck with visual disturbances, ptosis, and generalized weakness of the muscles.

Giant Apical Air Cell Syndrome

This syndrome, first described in 1982, consists of giant apical air cells, spontaneous CSF rhinorrhea, and recurrent meningitis. It is caused by the constant pounding of the brain against the dura overlying the giant apical air cell, which leads to dural rupture and CSF leak.

Gilles de la Tourette Syndrome

Characterized by chorea, coprolalia, and tics of the face and extremities, it affects children (usually boys 5 to 10 years old). Repetitive facial grimacing, blepharospasms, and arm and leg contractions may be present. Compulsive grunting noises or hiccupping subsequently become expressions of frank obscenities.

Goldenhar Syndrome

A rare, nonhereditary congenital variant of hemifacial microsomia, this is a congenital syndrome of the first and second arch. It is characterized by underdevelopment of craniofacial structures, vertebral malformations, and cardiac dysfunction. Clinical features of this syndrome are malar and maxillary hypoplasia, poor formation of external auditory canal, supernumerary ear tags and antetragal pits, orbit, enlarged mouths, renal anomalies, and missing growth centers in the condyle, causing delayed eruption of teeth and teeth crowding. Intelligence is usually normal or mildly retarded. Maxillofacial reconstruction in young patients demands consideration of future growth and development. It is also recommended for psychologic reasons as well as reasons involving the proper expansion of the skin that will later aid in further reconstruction. This syndrome is not to be confused with Treacher–Collins, Berry, or Franceschetti–Zwahlen–Klein syndromes. These tend to show well-defined genetic patterns (irregular but dominant), whereas Goldenhar syndrome does not.

Goodwin Tumor (Benign Lymphoepithelial Lesion)

This syndrome is characterized by inflammatory cells, lymphocytes, plasma cells, and reticular cells.

Gradenigo Syndrome

This syndrome is due to an extradural abscess involving the petrous bone. The symptoms are suppurative otitis, pain in the eye and temporal area, abducens paralysis, and diplopia.

Grisel Syndrome

This syndrome, also known as nasopharyngeal torticollis, is the subluxation of the atlanto-axial joint and is usually associated with children. It is associated with pharyngitis, nasopharyngitis, adenotonsillitis, tonsillar abscess, parotitis, cervical abscess, and otitis media. This syndrome has been known to occur after nasal cavity inflammation, tonsillectomy, adenoidectomy, mastoidectomy, choanal atresia repair, and excisions of a parapharyngeal rhabdomyosarcoma. Proposals for etiology include overdistention of the atlantoaxial joint ligaments by effusion, rupture of the transverse ligament, excessive passive rotation during general anesthesia, uncoordinated reflex action of the deep cervical muscles, spasm of the prevertebral muscles, ligamentous relaxation from decalcification of the vertebrae, and weak lateral ligaments. Clinical features include spontaneous torticollis in a child, a flexed and rotated head with limited range of motion, flat face, and Sudeck's sign (displacement of the spine of the axis to the same side as the head is turned). Treatment includes skeletal skull traction under fluoroscopic control to realign the odontoid process within the transverse ligament sling, followed by 6 to 12 weeks of immobilization. Timely treatment is usually successful.

Guillain–Barré Syndrome

This is infectious polyneuritis of unknown etiology (? viral) causing marked paresthesias of the limbs, muscular weakness, or a flaccid paralysis. Cerebrospinal fluid protein is increased without an increase in cell count.

Hallerman–Streiff Syndrome

This syndrome consists of dyscephaly, parrot nose, mandibular hypoplasia, proportionate nanism; hypotrichosis of scalp, brows, and cilia; and bilateral congenital cataracts. Most patients exhibit nystagmus or strabismus. There is no demonstrable genetic basis.

Hanhart Syndrome

A form of facial dysmorphia, this syndrome is characterized by (1) bird-like profile of face caused by micrognathia, (2) opisthodontia, (3) peromelia, (4) small growth, (5) normal intelligence, (6) branchial arch deformity resulting in conductive hearing loss, (7) tongue deformities and often a small jaw, and (8) possibly some limb defects as well. Ear surgery should be carefully considered because of the abnormal course of the facial nerve due to this syndrome.

Heerfordt Syndrome or Disease

In this syndrome, the patient develops uveoparotid fever. Heerfordt syndrome is a form of sarcoidosis (see Chapter 39).

Hick Syndrome

This is a rare condition characterized by a sensory disorder of the lower extremities resulting in perforating feet and by ulcers that are associated with progressive deafness due to atrophy of the cochlear and vestibular ganglia.

Hippel–Lindau Disease

This disease consists of angioma of the cerebellum, usually cystic, associated with angioma of the retina and polycystic kidneys.

Hollander Syndrome

With this syndrome there is appearance of a goiter during the 3rd decade of life related to a partial defect in the coupling mechanism in thyroxine biosynthesis. Deafness due to cochlear abnormalities is usually related to this.

Homocystinuria

This is a recessive hereditary syndrome secondary to a defect in methionine metabolism with resultant homocystinemia, mental retardation, and sensorineural hearing loss.

Horner Syndrome

The presenting symptoms are ptosis, miosis, anhidrosis, and enophthalmos due to paralysis of the cervical sympathetic nerves.

Horton Neuralgia

Patients have unilateral headaches centered behind or close to the eye accompanied or preceded by ipsilateral nasal congestion, suffusion of the eye, increased lacrimation, and facial redness and swelling.

Hunt Syndrome

1. Cerebellar tumor, an intention tremor that begins in one extremity gradually increasing in intensity and subsequently involving other parts of the body
2. Facial paralysis, otalgia, and aural herpes due to disease of both motor and sensory fibers of the VII nerve
3. A form of juvenile paralysis agitans associated with primary atrophy of the pallidal system

Hunter Syndrome

A hereditary and sex-linked disorder, this incurable syndrome involves multiple organ systems through mucopolysaccharide infiltration. Death, usually by the 2nd decade of life, is often caused by an infiltrative cardiomyopathy and valvular disease leading to heart failure. Physical characteristics include prominent supraorbital ridges, large flattened nose with flared nares, low-set ears, progressive corneal opacities, generous jowls, patulous lips and prognathism, short neck, abdominal protuberance, hirsutism, short stature, extensive osteoarthritis (especially in the hips, shoulders, elbows, and hands), TMJ arthritis, pseudopapilledema, and low-pressure hydrocephalus. Chondroitin sulfate B and heparitin in urine, mental retardation, beta-galactoside deficiency, and hepatosplenomegaly are also features of this syndrome. There is cerebral storage of three gangliosides: GM_1, GM_2, and GM_3. Compressive myelopathy may result from vertebral dislocation. High spinal cord injury is a great complication in surgery. Neurologic development is often slowed or never acquired. Abdominal abnormalities, respiratory infections, and cardiovascular troubles plague the patient.

Immotile-Cilia Syndrome

This syndrome appears to be a congenital defect in the ultrastructure of cilia that renders them incapable of movement. Both respiratory tract cilia and sperm are involved. The clinical picture includes bronchiectasis, sinusitis, male sterility, situs inversus, and otitis media. Histologically, there is a complete or partial absence of dynein arms, which are believed to be essential for cilia movement and sperm tail movement. Also no cilia movements were observed in the mucosa of the middle ear and the nasopharynx.

Inversed Jaw-Winking Syndrome

When there are supranuclear lesions of the V nerve, touching the cornea may produce a brisk movement of the mandible to the opposite side.

Jackson Syndrome

Cranial nerves X, XI, and XII are affected by nuclear or radicular lesion. There is ipsilateral flaccid paralysis of the soft palate, pharynx, and larynx with weakness and atrophy of the sternocleidomastoid and trapezius muscles and muscles of the tongue.

Jacod Syndrome

This syndrome consists of total ophthalmoplegia, optic tract lesions with unilateral amaurosis, and trigeminal neuralgia. It is caused by a middle cranial fossa tumor involving the II through VI cranial nerves.

Job Syndrome

This syndrome is one of the group of hyperimmunoglobulin E (IgE) syndromes that are associated with defective chemotaxis. The clinical picture includes fair skin, red hair, recurrent staphylococcal skin abscesses with concurrent other bacterial infections and skin lesions, as well as chronic purulent pulmonary infections and infected eczematoid skin lesions. This syndrome obtained its name from the Biblical passage referring to Job being smitten with boils. It is of interest to the otolaryngologist because of head and neck infections.

Jugular Foramen Syndrome (Vernet Syndrome)

Cranial nerves IX, X, and XI are paralyzed, whereas XII is spared because of its separate hypoglossal canal. Horner syndrome is not present because the sympathetic chain is below the foramen. This syndrome is most often caused by lymphadenopathy of the nodes of Krause in the foramen. Thrombophlebitis, tumors of the jugular bulb, and basal skull fracture can cause the syndrome. The glomus jugulare usually gives a hazy margin of involvement, whereas neurinoma gives a smooth, sclerotic margin of enlargement. The jugular foramen is bound medially by the occipital bone and laterally by the temporal bone. The foramen is divided into anteromedial (par nervosa) and posterolateral (par vasculara) areas by a fibrous or bony septum. The medial area transmits nerves IX, X, and XI as well as the inferior petrosal sinus. The posterior compartment transmits the internal jugular vein and the posterior meningeal artery. The right foramen is usually slightly larger than the left foramen.

Kallmann Syndrome

This syndrome consists of congenital hypogonadotropic eunuchoidism with anosmia. It is transmitted via a dominant gene with variable penetrance.

Kaposi Sarcoma

Patients have multiple idiopathic, hemorrhagic sarcomatosis particularly of the skin and viscera. Radiotherapy is the treatment of choice.

Kartagener Syndrome

The symptoms are complete situs inversus associated with chronic sinusitis and bronchiectasis. It is also called Kartagener triad.

Cilia and flagella of patient lack normal dynein side arms of ciliary A-tubes. Deficient mucociliary transport causes sterility in both sexes.

Keratosis Palmaris et Solaris

This disorder is an unusual inherited malformation. If these people live to 65 years of age, 50 to 75% of them develop carcinoma of the esophagus.

Kimura's Disease

This was first described by Kimura et al in 1949 as a chronic inflammatory condition occurring in subcutaneous tissues, salivary glands, and lymph nodes. Etiology is unknown. Histologically, there is dense fibrosis, lymphoid infiltration, vascular proliferation, and eosinophils. This is different from angiolymphoid hyperplasia with eosinophilia (ALHE). It is much more prevalent in people of Oriental descent. Laboratory studies show eosinophilia and elevated IgE. Differential diagnosis includes ALHE, eosinophilic granuloma, benign lymphoepithelial lesion, lymphocytoma, pyogenic granuloma, Kaposi sarcoma, harmartoma, and lymphoma. Treatment includes corticosteroids, cryotherapy, radiation, and surgery.

The differences between Kimura's disease and ALHE are as follows:

Kimura's   Age: 30–60   (ALHE age 20–50)
            Sex: male   (ALHE female)
            Larger lesions   (ALHE less than 1 cm)
            Deep   (ALHE superficial)
            More lymphoid follicles than ALHE
            Fewer mast cells than ALHE
            Less vascular hyperplasia than ALHE
            More fibrosis than ALHE
            More eosinophilia than ALHE
            More IgE than ALHE

Kleinschmidt Syndrome

Symptoms include influenzal infections resulting in laryngeal stenosis, suppurative pericarditis, pleuropneumonia, and occasionally meningitis.

Klinefelter Syndrome

This syndrome is a sex chromosome defect characterized by eunuchoidism, azoospermia, gynecomastia, mental deficiency, small testes with atrophy, and hyalinization of seminiferous tubules. The karyotype is usually XXY.

Klinkert Syndrome

Paralysis of the recurrent and phrenic nerves due to a neoplastic process in the root of the neck or upper mediastinum is evidenced. The sympathetics may be involved. (Left side involvement is more common than right side involvement.) It can be a part of Pancoast syndrome.

Lacrimoauriculodentodigital Syndrome

Autosomal dominant, occasional middle ear ossicular anomaly with cup-shaped ears, abnormal or absent thumbs, skeletal forearm deformities, sensorineural hearing loss, and nasolacrimal duct obstruction.

Large Vestibular Aqueduct Syndrome

The large vestibular aqueduct as an isolated anomaly of the temporal bone is associated with sensorineural hearing loss. It is more common in childhood than in adulthood. In this syndrome the rugose portion of the endolymphatic sac is also enlarged. Endolymphatic sac procedures to improve hearing are not often successful.

Larsen Syndrome

Larsen syndrome is characterized by widely spaced eyes, prominent forehead, flat nasal bridge, midline cleft of the secondary palate, bilateral dislocation of the knees and elbows, deformities of the hands and feet, and spatula-type thumbs; sometimes tracheomalacia, stridor, laryngomalacia, and respiratory difficulty are present. Therapy includes maintaining adequate ventilation.

Lermoyez Syndrome

This syndrome is a variant of Ménière disease. It was first described by Lermoyez in 1921 as deafness and tinnitus followed by a vertiginous attack that relieved the tinnitus and improved the hearing.

Lethal Midline Granuloma Syndrome

Destroying cartilage, soft tissue, and bone, this disease manifests itself by a number of entities, including idiopathic midline destructive disease, Wegener granulomatosis, polymorphic reticulosis, nasal lymphoma, and non-Hodgkin's lymphoma. High-dose local radiation totaling 5000 rads is the treatment of choice for localized cases. Chemotherapy involving an alkylating agent (cyclophosphamide) is recommended for disseminated cases.

Löffler's Syndrome

This syndrome consists in pneumonitis characterized by eosinophils in the tissues. It is possibly of parasitic etiology.

Loose Wire Syndrome

This syndrome occurs in patients with stapedectomy and insertion of a prosthesis that attaches to the long process of the incus by means of a crimped wire. It is a late complication, occurring on the average 15 years after surgery. A triad of symptoms are present that improve temporarily with middle ear inflation: auditory acuity, distortion of sound, and speech discrimination. Treatment in revision surgery involves finding the loose wire attachment at the incus and tightening that wire to allow the incus and prosthesis to move as one.

Louis–Bar Syndrome

This autosomal-recessive disease presents as ataxia, oculocutaneous telangiectasia, and sinopulmonary infection. It involves progressive truncal ataxia, slurred speech, fixation nystagmus, mental deficiency, cerebellar atrophy, deficient immunoglobulin, and marked frequency of lymphoreticular malignancies. The patient rarely lives past age 20.

Maffucci Syndrome

This syndrome is characterized by multiple cutaneous hemangiomas with dyschondroplasia and often enchondroma. The origin is unknown, and it is not hereditary. Signs and symptoms of this syndrome usually appear during infancy. It equally affects both sexes and has no racial preference. The dyschondroplasia may cause sharp bowing or an uneven growth of the extremities as well as give rise to frequent fractures. Five to ten percent of Maffucci syndrome patients have head and neck involvement giving rise to cranial nerve dysfunction and hemangiomas in the head and neck area. The hemangiomas in the nasopharynx and larynx could cause airway compromise as well as deglutition problems. Fifteen to twenty percent of these patients later undergo sarcomatous degeneration in one or more of the enchondromas. The percentage of malignant changes is greater in older patients, with the percentage of malignant degeneration approaching 44% in patients over age 40.

This syndrome is not to be confused with Klippel–Trenaunay syndrome, which causes no underdeveloped extremities, Sturge–Weber syndrome, or von Hippel–Lindau syndrome. No treatment is known for this syndrome, although surgical procedures to treat the actual deformities are sometimes necessary.

Marcus Gunn Syndrome (Jaw-Winking Syndrome)

This syndrome results in an increase in the width of the eyelids during chewing. Sometimes the patient experiences rhythmic elevation of the upper eyelid when the mouth is open and ptosis when the mouth is closed.

Marie–Strümpell Disease

This disease is rheumatoid arthritis of the spine.

Masson's Tumor

Intravascular papillary endothelial hyperplasia caused by excessive proliferation of endothelial cells. It is a benign condition. Differential diagnosis includes angiosarcoma, Kaposi's sarcoma, pyogenic granuloma.

Melkersson–Rosenthal Syndrome

This is a congenital disease of unknown etiology, it manifests as recurring attacks of unilateral or bilateral facial paralysis (see Chapter 8), swelling of the lips, and furrowing of the tongue. It is associated with high serum levels of angiotensin-converting enzyme during affliction.

Treatment should focus on facial paralysis and edema. Steroids and facial nerve decompression have had limited success.

Middle Lobe Syndrome

This syndrome is a chronic atelectatic process with fibrosis in one or both segments of the middle lobe. It is usually secondary to obstruction of the middle lobe bronchus by hilar adenopathy. The hilar adenopathy may be transient, but the bronchiectasis that resulted persists. Treatment is surgical resection.

Mikulicz Disease

The symptoms characteristic of Mikulicz disease (swelling of the lacrimal and salivary glands) occur as complications of some other disease, such as lymphocytosis, leukemia, or uveoparotid fever (see Chapter 25).

Millard–Gubler Syndrome

Patients present with ipsilateral paralysis of the abducens and facial nerves with contralateral hemiplegia of the extremities due to obstruction of the vascular supply to the pons.

Möbius Syndrome

This syndrome is a nonprogressive congenital facial diplegia (usually bilateral) with unilateral or bilateral loss of the abductors of the eye, anomalies of the extremities, and aplasia of the brachial and thoracic muscles. It frequently involves other cranial nerves. Saito showed evidence that the site of nerve lesions is in the peripheral nerve. The etiology could be CNS hypoplasia, primary peripheral muscle defect with secondary nerve degeneration, or lower motor neuron involvement.

Morgagni–Stewart–Morel Syndrome

This syndrome occurs in menopausal women and is characterized by obesity, dizziness, psychological disturbances, inverted sleep rhythm, and hyperostosis frontalis interna. Treatment is supportive.

Multiple Endocrine Adenomatosis (MEA)

MEA Type IIA (Sipple Syndrome)

Sipple syndrome is a familial syndrome consisting of medullary carcinoma of the thyroid, hyperparathyroidism, and pheochromocytoma.

MEA Type IIB

This MEA variant consists of multiple mucosal neuromas, pheochromocytoma, medullary carcinoma of the thyroid, and hyperparathyroidism. This syndrome is inherited in an autosomal dominant pattern. Mucosal neuromas principally involve the lips and anterior tongue. Numerous white medullated nerve fibers traverse the cornea to anastomose in the pupillary area.

Münchausen Syndrome

This syndrome was named after Baron Hieronymus Karl Freidrich von Münchausen (1720–1791) by Asher in 1951. The integral features of this syndrome are:

1. A real organic lesion from the past that has left some genuine signs but is causing no organic symptoms
2. Exorbitant lying with dramatic presentation of nonexistent symptoms
3. Traveling widely with multiple hospitalizations
4. Criminal tendencies
5. Willingness to undergo painful and dangerous treatment
6. Presenting challenging illnesses for treatment
7. Unruly behavior during hospital stays and early self-discharge without prior approval
8. Patients often inflict pain on their own children and forcibly create symptoms to indirectly receive hospital treatment

The patients usually go from one medical center to another to be admitted with dramatic presentations of nonorganic symptoms related to a real organic lesion on the past medical history.

Myenburg Syndrome (Familial Myositis Fibrosa Progressiva)

This syndrome is a disease in which the striated muscles are replaced by fibrosis. Fibrosarcoma rarely originates from this disease.

Nager Syndrome (Acrofacial Dysostosis)

Acrofacial dysostosis patients have facies similar to those seen with Treacher–Collins syndrome. They also present with preaxial upper limb defects, microtia, atresia of the external auditory canals, and malformation of the ossicles. Conductive and mixed hearing losses may occur.

Nager–de Reynier Syndrome

Hypoplasia of the mandible with abnormal implantation of teeth associated with aural atresia characterize this syndrome.

Neurofibromatosis (von Recklinghausen Disease)

Salient Features

1. Autosomal dominant
2. Mental retardation common in families with neurofibromatosis
3. Arises from neurilemmal cells or sheath of Schwann and fibroblasts of peripheral nerves
4. Café au lait spots—giant melanosomes (presence of six or more spots > 1.5 cm is diagnostic of neurofibromatosis even if the family history is negative)
5. Of all neurofibromatosis, 4 to 5% undergo malignant degeneration with a sudden increase in growth of formerly static nodules. These nodules may become neurofibrosarcomas, and they may metastasize widely

External Features

1. Café au lait spots
2. Fibromas

Internal Features

1. Pheochromocytoma
2. Meningioma
3. Acoustic neurinoma: often bilateral
4. Gastrointestinal bleeding
5. Intussusception bowel
6. Hypoglycemia (intraperitoneal fibromas)
7. Fibrous dysplasia
8. Subperiosteal bone cysts
9. Optic nerve may be involved, causing blindness and proptosis
10. May present with macroglossia
11. May involve the parotid or submaxillary gland
12. The nodules may be painful
13. Nodules may enlarge suddenly if bleeding of the tumor occurs or if there is malignant degeneration

The treatment is only to relieve pressure from expanding masses. It usually does not recur if the tumor is completely removed locally.

Nothnagel Syndrome

The symptoms include dizziness, a staggering and rolling gait with irregular forms of oculomotor paralysis, and nystagmus often is present. This syndrome is seen with tumors of the midbrain.

Oculopharyngeal Syndrome

This is characterized by hereditary ptosis and dysphagia and is an autosomal dominant disease having equal incidence in both sexes. It is related to a high incidence of esophageal carcinoma. Age of onset is between 40 and 50 years, and it is particularly common among French Canadians. Marked weakness of the upper esophagus is observed together with an increase in serum creatinine phosphokinase. It is a myopathy and not a neuropathy. Treatment includes dilatation and cricopharyngomyotomy.

Ollier Disease

This consists of multiple chondromatosis, 10% of which is associated with chondrosarcoma.

Ondine Curse

Failure of respiratory center automaticity with apnea, especially evident during sleep, is symptomatic. Also known as the alveolar hypoventilation syndrome, it may be associated with increased appetite and transient central diabetes insipidus. Hypothalamic lesions are thought to be the cause of this disorder.

Oral-Facial-Digital Syndrome I

See Chapter 6 for oral-facial-digital syndrome II.

A lethal trait in men, it is inherited as an X-linked dominant trait limited to women. Symptoms include multiple hyperplastic frenula, cleft tongue, dystopia canthorum, hypoplasia of the nasal alar cartilages, median cleft of the upper lip, asymmetrical cleft palate, digital malformation, and mild mental retardation. About 50% of the patients have hamartoma between the lobes of the divided tongue. This mass consists of fibrous connective tissue, salivary gland tissue, few striated muscle fibers, and rarely cartilage. One-third of the patients present with ankyloglossia.

Orbital Apex Syndrome

This syndrome involves the nerves and vessels passing through the superior sphenoid fissure and the optic foramen with paresis of cranial nerves III, IV, and VI. External ophthalmoplegia is associated with internal ophthalmoplegia with a dilated pupil that does not react to either light or convergence. Ptosis as well as periorbital edema are due to IV nerve paresis. Sensory changes are secondary to the lacrimal frontal nasal ciliary nerves as well as the three branches of the ophthalmic nerve. The optic nerve usually is involved.

Ortner Syndrome

Cardiomegaly associated with laryngeal paralysis secondary to compression of the recurrent laryngeal nerve is observed with this syndrome.

Osler–Weber–Rendu Disease (Hereditary Hemorrhagic Telangiectasia)

This is an autosomal-dominant disease in which the heterozygote lives to adult life, whereas the homozygous state is lethal at an early age. The patient has punctate hemangiomas (elevated, dilated capillaries and venules) in the mucous membrane of the lips, tongue, mouth, gastrointestinal tract, etc. Pathologically, they are vascular sinuses of irregular size and shape lined by a thin layer of endothelium. The muscular and elastic coats are absent. Because of their thin walls these vascular sinuses bleed easily, and because of the lack of muscular coating the bleeding is difficult to control. The patient has normal blood elements and no coagulation defect. The other blood vessels are normal. If a person with this disease marries a normal person, what are the chances that the offspring will have this condition?

Because the patient with this disease is an adult, we can assume that he is heterozygous, as the homozygote dies early in life. Therefore, the child will have a 50% chance of having this hereditary disease.

Otopalatodigital Syndrome

This syndrome is characterized by skeletal dysplasia, conductive hearing loss, and cleft palate. Middle ear anomalies are also associated with this syndrome. Although the mode of inheritance is not known, some suggest that X-linked recessive inheritance is possible. Symptoms tend to be less severe in females than in males. The diagnosis of otopalatodigital (OPD) syndrome is sometimes based on characteristic facies and deformities of hands and feet. Physical features include mild dwarfism, mental retardation, broad nasal root, frontal and occipital bossing, hypertelorism, small mandible, stubby, clubbed digits, low-set and small ears, winged scapulae, malar flattening, downward obliquity of the eye, and down-turned mouth. The inner ear has been known to display deformities likened to a mild type of Mondini dysplasia. Surgical attempts to improve hearing loss are not always recommended since certain deformities, such as a missing round window, make such attempts unsuccessful.

Paget Disease (Osteitis Deformans)

See Chapter 5.

This term also is used to characterize a disease of elderly women who have an infiltrated, eczematous lesion surrounding the nipple and areola associated with subjacent intraductal carcinoma of the breast.

Paget Osteitis

This disorder is related to sarcomas.

Pancoast Syndrome

See Chapter 13.

Pelizaeus–Merzbacher Disease

This disease is an X-linked recessive sudanophilic leukodystrophy. The CNS myelin forms improperly and never matures, sometimes ending in death by the age of 2 or 3 years. Nystagmoid eye movements are characteristic at age 4 to 6 months, followed by a delay in motor development. Prenatal amniocentesis is not useful in detecting this disease. Neonatal stridor, a specific genealogy combined with a characteristic auditory brain stem response (ABR) wave can lead to early diagnosis. Characteristic waves have been known to be missing rostral waves and normal wave I latency. Males are afflicted, whereas females are unknowing carriers.

Peutz–Jegher Syndrome

The patient has pigmentation of the lips and oral mucosa and benign polyps of the gastrointestinal tract. Granulosa theca cell tumors have been reported in female patients with this syndrome.

Pheochromocytoma

Pheochromocytoma is associated with neurofibromatosis, cerebellar hemangioblastoma, ependymoma, astrocytoma, meningioma, spongioblastoma, multiple endocrine adenoma, or medullary carcinoma of the thyroid. Pheochromocytoma with or without the tumors may be inherited as an autosomal-dominant trait. Some patients have megacolon, others suffer neurofibromatosis of Auerbach and Meissner plexuses.

Pierre Robin Syndrome

This syndrome consists of glossoptosis, micrognathia, and cleft palate. There is no sex predilection. The etiology is believed to be intrauterine insult at the 4th month of gestation, or it may be hereditary. Two-thirds of the cases are associated with ophthalmologic difficulties (eg, detached retina or glaucoma), and one-third are associated with otologic problems (eg, chronic otitis media and low-set ears). Mental retardation is present occasionally. If the patient lives past 5 years, he or she can lead a fairly normal life (see Chapter 5). The symptoms are choking and aspiration as a result of negative pressure created by excessive inspiratory effort. Passing a NA tube may alleviate the negative pressure. Aerophagia has to be treated to prevent vomiting, airway compromise, and aspiration. Tracheotomy may not be the answer.

A modification of the Douglas lip–tongue adhesion has helped prevent early separation of the adhesion. One theory explains that the cause may be that the fetus's head is flexed, preventing forward growth of the mandible, forcing the tongue up and backward between the palatal shelves, and producing the triad of micrognathia, glossoptosis, and cleft palate.

Plummer–Vinson Syndrome (Paterson–Kelly Syndrome)

Symptoms include dysphagia due to degeneration of the esophageal muscle, atrophy of the papillae of the tongue, as well as microcytic hypochromic anemia. Achlorhydria, glossitis, pharyngitis, esophagitis, and fissures at the corner of the mouth also are observed. The prevalence of this disease is higher in women than in men, and usually presents in patients who are in their 4th decade. Treatment consists of iron administration, with esophagoscopy for dilatation and to rule out carcinoma of the esophagus, particularly at the postcricoid region. Pharyngoesophageal webs or stenosing may be noted.

This disease is to be contrasted with pernicious anemia, which is a megaloblastic anemia with diarrhea, nausea and vomiting, neurologic symptoms, enlarged spleen, and achlorhydria. Pernicious anemia is secondary to failure of the gastric fundus to secrete intrinsic factors necessary for vitamin B_{12} absorption. Treatment consists of intramuscular vitamin B_{12} (riboflavin).

Folic acid deficiency also gives rise to megaloblastic anemia, cheilosis, glossitis, ulcerative stomatitis, pharyngitis, esophagitis, dysphagia, and diarrhea. Neurologic symptoms and achlorhydria are not present. Treatment is the administration of folic acid.

Potter Syndrome

One of every 3000 infants is born with Potter syndrome. Most of them die during delivery and the rest die shortly after birth. Potter syndrome is characterized by severely malformed, low-set ears bilaterally, a small lower jaw, and extensive deformities of the external and middle ear (eg, an absence of auditory ossicles, atresia of the oval window, and abnormal course of the facial nerve). The cochlear membranous labyrinth is normal in its upper turn but contains severe hypoplasia in its basal turn, a rare cochlear anomaly.

One cause for this syndrome that has been proposed is fetal compression caused by oglioamnios.

Pseudotumor Cerebri Syndrome

Also known as benign intracranial hypertension, this syndrome is characterized by increased intracranial pressure without focal signs of neurologic dysfunction. Obstructive hydrocephalus, mass lesions, chronic meningitis, and hypertensive and pulmonary encephalopathy should be ruled out and not confused with this syndrome. The patient is typically a young, obese female with a history of headaches, blurring of vision, or both. Facial pain and diplopia caused by unilateral or bilateral abducens nerve paralysis are less common symptoms. The CSF opening pressure on a patient lies between 250 and 600 mm of water. Cerebrospinal fluid composition, electroencephalogram (EEG), and computed tomography (CT) scans of the head are typically normal. X-rays of the skull may reveal enlargement of the sella turcica or thinning of the dorsum sellae. This simulates a pituitary tumor, but pituitary function is normal. This syndrome is self-limited and spontaneous recovery usually will occur within a few months. Auscultation of ear canal, neck, orbits, and periauricular regions should be performed for diagnosis, as well as fundoscopic examination to identify papilloma. Complete audiologic evaluations, electronystagmography (ENG), and radiographic examinations should also be made. Occlusion of the ipsilateral jugular vein by light digital pressure should make the hum disappear by cessation of blood flow in this structure.

Purpura-like Syndrome

This syndrome is autoimmune thrombocytopenic purpura, which can be accompanied by systemic lupus erythematosus, chronic lymphocytic leukemia, or lymphoma. There seems to be a strong association between syndromes resembling autoimmune thrombocytopenia and nonhematologic malignancies.

Pyknodysostosis

This is a syndrome consisting of dwarfism, osteopetrosis, partial agenesis of the terminal phalanges of the hands and feet, cranial anomalies (persistent fontanelles), frontal and occipital bossing, and hypoplasia of the angle of the mandible. The facial bones are usually underdeveloped with pseudoprognathism. The frontal sinuses are consistently absent, and the other paranasal sinuses are hypoplastic. The mastoid air cells often are pneumatized. Toulouse-Lautrec probably had this disease.

Raeder Syndrome

This relatively benign, self-limiting syndrome consists of ipsilateral ptosis, miosis, and facial pain with intact facial sweating. Pain exists in the distribution of the ophthalmic division of the V cranial nerve. It results from postganglionic sympathetic involvement in the area of the internal carotid artery or from a lesion in the anterior portion of the middle cranial fossa.

Reichert Syndrome

Neuralgia of the glossopharyngeal nerve, usually precipitated by movements of the tongue or throat, is present.

Reiter Syndrome

Arthritis, urethritis, and conjunctivitis are evident.

Reye Syndrome

This syndrome is an often fatal disease primarily afflicting young children during winter and spring months. Its cardinal pathologic features are marked encephalopathy and fatty metamorphosis of the liver. Though its etiology is unclear, Reye syndrome has been known to occur after apparent recovery from a viral infection, primarily varicella or an upper respiratory tract infection. In some patients there is also structural damage in cochlear and vestibular tissues of the membranous labyrinth.

Intracranial pressure monitoring and respiratory support may limit brain edema. Tracheal diversion and pulmonary care may be necessary.

Riedel Struma

This disorder is a form of thyroiditis seen most frequently in middle-aged women manifested by compression of surrounding structures (ie, trachea). There is loss of the normal thyroid lobular architecture and replacement with collagen and lymphocyte infiltration.

Rivalta Disease

This disease is an actinomycotic infection characterized by multiple indurated abscesses of the face, neck, chest, and abdomen that discharge through numerous sinus tracts.

Rollet Syndrome (Orbital Apex–Sphenoidal Syndrome)

Caused by lesions of the orbital apex that cause paralysis of cranial nerves III, IV, and VI, this syndrome is characterized by ptosis, diplopia, ophthalmoplegia, optic atrophy, hyperesthesia or anesthesia of the forehead, upper eyelid, and cornea, and retrobulbar neuralgia. Exophthalmos and papilledema may occur.

Romberg Syndrome

This syndrome is characterized by progressive atrophy of tissues on one side of the face, occasionally extending to other parts of the body that may involve the tongue, gums, soft palate, and cartilages of the ear, nose, and larynx. Pigmentation disorders, trigeminal neuralgia, and ocular complications may be seen.

Rosai–Dorfman Disease

Benign, self-limiting lymphadenopathy. Has no detectable nodal involvement. Histiocytosis, plasma cell proliferation, and lymphophagocytosis may all be present.

Rutherford Syndrome

A familial oculodental syndrome characterized by corneal dystrophy, gingival hyperplasia, and failure of tooth eruption.

Samter Syndrome

Samter syndrome consists of three symptoms in combination:

1. Allergy to aspirin
2. Nasal polyposis
3. Asthma

Scalenus Anticus Syndrome

The symptoms for scalenus anticus syndrome are identical to those for cervical rib syndrome. In scalenus anticus syndrome, the symptoms are caused by compression of the brachial plexus and subclavian artery against the first thoracic rib, probably as the result of spasms of the scalenus anticus muscle bringing pressure on the brachial plexus and the subclavian artery. Any pressure on the sympathetic nerves may cause vascular spasm resembling Raynaud disease.

Schafer Syndrome

Hereditary mental retardation, sensorineural hearing loss, prolinemia, hematuria, and photogenic epilepsy are characteristic. This syndrome is due to a deficiency of proline oxidase with a resultant buildup of the amino acid proline.

Schaumann Syndrome

This syndrome is generalized sarcoidosis.

Schmidt Syndrome

Unilateral paralysis of a vocal cord, the velum palati, the trapezius, and the sterno-cleidomastoid muscles is found. The lesion is located in the caudal portion of the medulla and is usually of vascular origin.

Scimitar Syndrome

This congenital anomaly of the venous system of the right lung gets its name from the typical shadow formed on a thoracic roentgenogram of patients afflicted with it. (The scimitar is a curved Turkish sword that increases in diameter toward its distal end.) The most common clinical features are dyspnea and recurrent infections. The cause of scimitar syndrome is abnormal development of the right lung bed. The syndrome may be the result of vascular anomalies of the venous and arterial system of the right lung, hypoplasia of the right lung, or drainage of part of the right pulmonary venous system into the inferior vena cava, causing the scimitar sign on the thoracic roentgenogram.

The syndrome occurs between the 4th and 6th weeks of fetal life. Clinical features include displacement of heart sounds as well as heart percussion shadow toward the right. When dextroposition of the heart is marked, tomography can also help in diagnosis. Bronchography and angiography also aid in diagnosis and in providing exact information for surgical correction.

Seckel Syndrome

This is a disorder that consists of dwarfism associated with a bird-like facies, beaked nose, micrognathia, palate abnormalities, low-set lobeless ears, antimongoloid slant of the palpebral fissures, clinodactyly, mental retardation, and bone disorders.

Secretion of Antidiuretic Hormone Syndrome

Also referred to as the Syndrome of Inappropriate Secretion of Antidiuretic Hormone (SIADH). Antidiuretic hormone helps maintain constant serum osmolality by conserving water and concentrating urine. This syndrome involves low serum osmolality, elevated urinary osmolality less than maximally dilute urine, and hyponatremia. This can lead to lethargy, anorexia, headache, convulsions, coma, or cardiac arrhythmias. Increased CSF and intracranial pressure are possible etiologies. Fluid restriction can help prevent this condition.

Sheehan Syndrome

Ischemic necrosis of the anterior pituitary associated with postpartum hypotension characterize this syndrome. It is seen in menopausal women and is associated with rheumatoid arthritis, Raynaud phenomenon, and dental caries. Changes in the lacrimal and salivary glands resemble those of Mikulicz disease. Some physicians attribute this syndrome to vitamin A deficiency. A positive lupus erythematosus (LE) preparation, rheumatoid factor, and an abnormal protein can be identified in this disorder.

Shy–Drager Syndrome

Usually presented in late middle age, this syndrome is a form of neurogenic orthostatic hypotension that results in failure of the autonomic nervous system and signs of multiple systems atrophy affecting corticospinal and cerebellar pathways and basal ganglia. Symptoms include postural hypotension, impotence, sphincter dysfunction, and anhidrosis with later progression to panautonomic failure. Such autonomic symptoms are usually followed by atypical parkinsonism, cerebellar dysfunction with debilitation, or both, and then death. Shy–Drager syndrome (SDS) should always be considered when the patient displays orthostatic hypotension, laryngeal stridor, restriction in range of vocal cord abduction (unilaterally or bilaterally), vocal hoarseness, intermittent diplophonia, and slow speech rate. This syndrome is often compared with Parkinson disease. However, Shy–Drager syndrome involves the nigrostriatal, olivopontocerebellar, brain stem, and intermediolateral column of the spinal cord. It is a multiple system disorder, whereas Parkinson disease involves only the nigrostriatal neuronal system. The symptoms, such as autonomic failure, pyramidal disease, and cerebellar dysfunction, have been associated with pathology of the pigmented nuclei and the dorsal motor nucleus of the vagus.

Sjögren Syndrome (Sicca Syndrome)

This syndrome is often manifested as keratoconjunctivitis sicca, dryness of the mucous membranes, telangiectasias or purpuric spots on the face, and bilateral parotid enlargement. It is a chronic inflammatory process involving mainly the salivary and lacrimal glands and is associated with hyperactivity of the B lymphocytes and with autoantibody and immune complex production. One of the complications of this syndrome is the development of malignant lymphoma. Computed tomography aids in the diagnosis.

Sleep Apnea Syndrome

The definition of apnea is a cessation of airflow of more than 10 seconds in duration. The conditions for sleep apnea syndrome are said to be met when at least 30 episodes of apnea occur within a 7-hour period or when 1% of a patient's sleeping time is spent in apnea. The cause of sleep apnea is unclear. Some people believe it is of central origin; others think that it may be aggravated by hypertrophied and occluding tonsils and adenoids. Some investigators classify sleep apnea into central apnea, upper airway apnea, and mixed apnea. Monitoring of the EEG and other brain stem–evoked response measurements may help identify central apnea.

Sluder Neuralgia

The symptoms are neuralgia of the lower half of the face, nasal congestion, and rhinorrhea associated with lesions of the sphenopalatine ganglion. Ocular hyperemia and increased lacrimation may be seen.

Stevens–Johnson Syndrome

This syndrome is a skin disease (erythema multiforme) with involvement of the oral cavity (stomatitis) and the eye (conjunctivitis). Stomatitis may appear as the first symptom. It is most common during the 3rd decade of life. Treatment consists largely of steroids and supportive therapy. It is a self-limiting disease but has a 25% recurrence rate. The differential diagnosis includes herpes simplex, pemphigus, acute fusospirochetal stomatitis, chickenpox, monilial infection, and secondary syphilis.

Still Disease

Rheumatoid arthritis in children is sometimes called Still disease (see a pediatric textbook for more details).

Sturge–Weber Syndrome

This syndrome is a congenital disorder that affects both sexes equally and is of unknown etiology. It is characterized by venous angioma of the leptomeninges over the cerebral cortex, ipsilateral port wine nevi, and frequent angiomatous involvement of the globe, mouth, and nasal mucosa. The patient may have convulsions, hemiparesis, glaucoma, and intracranial calcifications. There is no specific treatment.

Subclavian Steal Syndrome

Stenosis or occlusion of the subclavian or innominate artery proximal to the origin of the vertebral artery causes the pressure in the vertebral artery to be less than that of the basilar artery, particularly when the upper extremity is in action. Hence the brain receives less blood and may be ischemic. The symptoms consist of intermittent vertigo, occipital headache, blurred vision, diplopia, dysarthria, and pain in the upper extremity. The diagnosis, made through the patient's medical history, can be confirmed by the difference in blood pressure in the two upper extremities, by a bruit over the supraclavicular fossa, and by angiography.

Superior Orbital Fissure Syndrome (Orbital Apex Syndrome; Optic Foramen Syndrome; Sphenoid Fissure Syndrome)

There is involvement of cranial nerves III, IV, V_1, and VI, the ophthalmic veins, and the sympathetics of the cavernous sinus. The syndrome can be caused by sphenoid sinusitis or any neoplasia in that region. Symptoms include paralysis of the upper eyelid, orbital pain, photophobia, and paralysis of the above nerves. The optic nerve may be damaged as well.

Superior Vena Cava Syndrome

This syndrome is characterized by obstruction of the superior vena cava or its main tributaries by bronchogenic carcinoma, mediastinal neoplasm, or lymphoma. Rarely, the presence of a substernal goiter causes edema and engorgement of the vessels of the face, neck, and arms, as well as a nonproductive cough and dyspnea.

Takayasu Disease

Also called "pulseless disease" and aortic arch syndrome, this disease involves narrowing of the aortic arch and its branches. Possibly an autoimmune disorder, the etiology is unknown. Symptoms often originate in the head and neck area. Sensorineural hearing loss is often an associated symptom. An association has also been found with B-cell alloantigens DR4 and MB3. Steroid treatment and cyclophosphamide have been known to help, as does surgery, although operating during a relatively inactive phase of the disease is recommended.

Tapia Syndrome

Unilateral paralysis of the larynx and tongue is coupled with atrophy of the tongue; the soft palate and cricothyroid muscle are intact. The syndrome is usually caused by a lesion at the point where the XII and X nerves, together with the internal carotid artery, cross one another.

Trauma is the most common cause of Tapia syndrome. Pressure neuropathy due to inflation of the cuff of an endotracheal tube within the larynx, rather than within the trachea, is associated with the palsy of the laryngeal nerve.

Tay–Sachs Disease

An infantile form of amaurotic familial idiocy with strong familial tendencies, it is of questionably recessive inheritance. It is more commonly found among those of Semitic extraction. Histologically, the nerve cells are distorted and filled with a lipid material. The juvenile form is called Spielmeyer–Vogt disease, and the patient is normal until after 5 to 7 years of age. The juvenile form is seen in children of non-Semitic extraction as well.

Tietze Syndrome

Tietze syndrome is a costal chondritis chondropathia tuberosa of unknown etiology. Its symptoms include pain, tenderness, and swelling of one or more of the upper costal cartilages (usually the second rib). Treatment is symptomatic.

Tolosa–Hunt Syndrome

It is a cranial polyneuropathy usually presenting as recurrent unilateral painful ophthalmoplegia. Cranial nerves II, III, IV, V_1, and VI may be involved. The etiology is unknown, and there is a tendency for spontaneous resolution and for recurrence. An orbital venogram may show occlusion of the superior ophthalmic vein and at least partial obliteration of the cavernous sinus. The clinical course often responds well to systemic steroids.

Erroneous diagnoses include inflammation, tumor, vascular aneurysm, thrombus involving the orbit, superior orbital fissure, anterior cavernous sinus, parasellar area, or posterior fossa. An extension of nasopharyngeal carcinoma, mucocele, or contiguous sinusitis must also be ruled out. Sources of infection in the head and neck region, such as the tonsils, can be treated, relieving the pain of ophthalmoplegia.

Tourette Syndrome

This syndrome is a disorder of the CNS, characterized by the appearance of involuntary tic movements, such as rapid eye blinking, facial twitches, head jerking, or shoulder shrugging. Involuntary sounds, such as repeated throat clearing, "nervous" coughing, or inappropriate use of words, sometimes occur simultaneously. Tourette syndrome in many cases responds to medication. It has a higher rate of absorption, or binding at D2 dopamine receptors on cells in the caudate nucleus. The etiology of this syndrome is unknown.

Toxic Shock Syndrome

Cases of toxic shock syndrome have been found related to nasal packing and to staphylococcal infection of surgical wounds. Although the pathogenesis of the disease is incompletely understood, it is believed that packing left too long can cause bacterial overgrowth, leading to toxic shock syndrome. Symptoms include fever, rash, hypotension, mucosal hyperemia, vomiting, diarrhea, laboratory evidence of multiorgan dysfunction, and desquamation during recovery. It has been found that although antibiotic impregnation into the packing material may reduce bacterial overgrowth, it does not provide absolute protection against toxic shock syndrome.

Single-dose antimicrobial prophylaxis has proven highly effective as a treatment. Additionally, screening for TSST-1–producing *S. aureus* is helpful in pointing out high-risk patients for this syndrome.

Treacher–Collins Syndrome

See Chapter 5.

Trigeminal Trophic Syndrome

Trigeminal trophic syndrome, also called trigeminal neurotrophic ulceration or trigeminal neuropathy with nasal ulceration, involves ulceration of the face, particularly ala nasi, and histologic features, such as chronic, nonspecific ulceration and crusting, erythema, tendency to bleed easily, and predominant granulation tissue. Whether caused by self-induced trauma, surgery, or any process involved with the trigeminal nerve or its connections, the etiologies of nasal ulceration to be excluded with this syndrome are basal cell carcinoma, blastomycosis, leishmaniasis, leprous trigeminal neuritis, lethal midline granuloma, paracoccidioidomycosis, postsurgical herpetic reactivation, pyoderma gangrenosum, and Wegener's granulomatosis. Treatment should focus on prevention of trauma to lesion and prevention of secondary infection.

Trotter Syndrome (Sinus of Morgagni Syndrome)

Neuralgia of the inferior maxillary nerve, conductive hearing loss secondary to eustachian tube blockage, preauricular edema caused by neoplastic invasion of the sinus of Morgagni, ipsilateral akinesia of the soft palate, and trismus are observed in this syndrome.

Tube-Feeding Syndrome

See Chapter 39.

Turner Syndrome

See Chapter 5.

Turpin Syndrome

Patients have congenital bronchiectasis, megaesophagus, tracheoesophageal fistula, vertebral deformities, rib malformations, and a heterotopic thoracic duct.

Vail Syndrome

This syndrome consists of unilateral, usually nocturnal, vidian neuralgia that may be associated with sinusitis.

VATER Syndrome

This syndrome is a nonrandom association of vertebral defects, anal atresia, tracheoesophageal fistula with esophageal atresia, renal defects, and radial limb dysplasia. Vascular anomalies, such as ventricular septal defect and single umbilical artery, have also been associated with this syndrome. Vertebral anomalies consist of hypoplasia of either the vertebral bodies or the pedicles, leading to secondary scoliosis in children. Anal and perineal anomalies consist of hypospadias, persistent urachus, female pseudohermaphroditism, imperforate anus, and genitourinary fistulas. Gastrointestinal anomalies include duodenal atresia, esophageal atresia, and tracheoesophageal fistula. Radial anomalies include supernumerary digiti, hypoplastic radial rays, and preaxial lower extremity anomalies. Renal anomalies include aplasia or hypoplasia of the kidneys with ectopia or fusion as well as congenital hydronephrosis and hydroureter. Hold–Oram syndrome is often confused with this syndrome, but VATER syndrome is random whereas Hold–Oram is inherited. This syndrome is suggested to be formed prior to the 5th week of fetal life during organogenesis.

Vernet Syndrome

See "Jugular Foramen Syndrome" (page 207).

Villaret Syndrome

This syndrome is the same as the jugular foramen syndrome except that Horner syndrome is present here, suggesting more extensive involvement in the region of the jugular foramen, the retroparotid area, and the lateral pharyngeal space.

Vogt–Koyanagi–Harada Syndrome

Spastic diplegia with athetosis and pseudobulbar paralysis associated with a lesion of the caudate nucleus and putamen, bilateral uveitis, vitiligo, deafness, alopecia, increased CSF pressure, and retinal detachment are evidenced.

Von Hippel–Lindau Disease

Associated with cerebellar, medullary, and spinal hemangioblastoma, retinal angiomata, pheochromocytoma, and renal cell carcinoma, this sometimes fatal disease is predisposed to papillary adenoma of the temporal bone. The etiology is unknown.

Wallenberg Syndrome

Also called syndrome of the posterior-inferior cerebellar artery thrombosis or lateral medullary syndrome, this syndrome is due to thrombosis of the posteroinferior cerebellar artery giving rise to ischemia of the brain stem (lateral medullary region). Symptoms include vertigo, nystagmus, nausea, vomiting, Horner syndrome, dysphagia, dysphonia, hypotonia, asthenia, ataxia, falling to the side of the lesion, and loss of pain and temperature sense on the ipsilateral face and contralateral side below the neck.

Weber Syndrome

This syndrome is characterized by paralysis of the oculomotor nerve on the side of the lesion and paralysis of the extremities, face, and tongue on the contralateral side. It indicates a lesion in the ventral and internal part of the cerebral peduncle.

Whistling Face Syndrome

Also known as craniocarpotarsal dysplasia, this syndrome is mostly transmitted through autosomal dominant genes (although heterogenic transmission is not unknown). The main physical features are antimongoloid slant of the palpebral fissures, blepharophimosis, broad nasal bridge, convergent strabismus, enophthalmos, equinovarus with contracted toes, flat midface, H-shaped cutaneous dimpling on the chin, kyphosis–scoliosis, long philtrum, mask-like rigid face, microglossia, microstomia, protruding lips, small nose and nostrils, steeply inclined anterior cranial fossa on roentgenogram, thick skin over flexor surfaces of proximal phalanges, ulnar deviation, and flexion contractures of fingers.

Wildervack (Cervico-Oculo-Acoustic) Syndrome

This syndrome consists of mixed hearing loss, Klippel–Feil anomalad (fused cervical vertebrae), and bilateral abducens palsy with retracted bulb (Duane syndrome). Occurring in more female than male subjects, in almost a 75:1 ratio, it has sex-linked dominance with lethality in the homozygous male subject.

Wilson Disease (Hepatolenticular Degeneration)

There are two chief types of Wilson disease, one rapidly progressive that occurs during late childhood, and the other slowly progressive occurring in the 3rd or 4th decades. Familial, its symptoms are cirrhosis with progressive damage to the nervous system and brown pigmentation of the outer margin of the cornea, called Kayser–Fleischer ring. It can present with hearing loss as well.

Winkler Disease (Chondrodermatitis Nodularis Chronica Helicis)

Arteriovenous anastomosis and nerve ending accumulation at the helical portion of the ear are evident. It presents with pain and is characterized by hard, round nodules involving the skin and cartilage of the helix. Ninety percent of all cases occur in men. The treatment is to excise the nodules or administer steroids.

Xeroderma Pigmentosum (Autosomal-Recessive)

This disorder presents as photosensitive skin with multiple basal cell epitheliomas. Squamous cell carcinoma or malignant melanoma can result from it. The condition occurs mainly in children. These children should be kept away from the sun.

EPONYMS

Abrikossoff's tumor (granular cell myoblastoma). Causes pseudoepithelial hyperplasia in the larynx, the site most favored in the larynx being the posterior half of the vocal cord. Three percent of granular cell myoblastoma progress to malignancy. In order of decreasing frequency of involvement the granular cell myoblastoma occurs in tongue, skin, breast, subcutaneous tissue, and respiratory tract.

Adenoid facies. Crowded teeth, high-arched palate, underdeveloped nostrils.

Adler bodies. Deposits of mucopolysaccharide found in neutrophils of patients with Hurler syndrome.

Antoni's type A and type B. See Chapter 39.

Arnold–Chiari malformation

Type I: Downward protrusion of the long, thin, cerebellar tonsils through the foramen magnum.

Type II: Protrusion of the inferior cerebellar vermis through the foramen.

Type III: Bony occipital defect with descent of the entire cerebellum.

Type IV: Cerebellar hypoplasia.

Arnold's ganglion. Otic ganglion.

Aschoff body. Rheumatic nodule found in rheumatic disease.

Ballet's sign. Paralysis of voluntary movements of the eyeball with preservation of the automatic movements. Sometimes this sign is present with exophthalmic goiter and hysteria.

Bechterew syndrome. Paralysis of facial muscles limited to automatic movements. The power of voluntary movement is retained.

Bednar's aphthae. Symmetrical excoriations of the hard palate in the region of the pterygoid plates due to sucking of the thumb, foreign objects, or scalding.

Bezold's abscess. Abscess in the sternocleidomastoid muscle secondary to perforation of the tip of the mastoid by infection.

Blandin, gland of. A minor salivary gland situated in the anterior portion of the tongue.

Brooke's tumor (epithelioma adenoides cysticum). Originates from the hair follicles in the external auditory canal and auricle and of basal cell origin. Treatment is local resection.

Broyle's ligament. Anterior commissure ligament of the larynx.

Brudzinski's sign. With meningitis, passive flexion of the leg on one side causes a similar movement to occur in the opposite leg. Passive flexion of the neck brings about flexion of the legs as well.

Brunner's abscess. Abscess of the posterior floor of the mouth.

Bruns' sign. Intermittent headache, vertigo, and vomiting, especially with sudden movements of the head. It occurs in cases of tumor of the fourth ventricle of the brain.

Bryce's sign. A gurgling is heard in a neck mass. It suggests a laryngocele.

Carhart's notch. Maximum dip at 2000 kHz (bone conduction) seen in patients with otosclerosis.

Charcot–Leyden crystals. Crystals in the shape of elongated double pyramids, composed of spermine phosphates and present in the sputum of asthmatic patients. Synonyms are Charcot–Newman crystals and Charcot–Robin crystals. Also found in fungal infection.

Charcot triad. The nystagmus, scanning speech, and intention tremor seen in multiple sclerosis.

Cherubism. Familial, with the age of predilection between 2 and 5 years. It is characterized by giant cell reparative granuloma causing cystic lesions in the posterior rami of the mandible. The lesions are usually symmetrical. It is a self-limiting disease with remissions after puberty. The maxilla also may be involved.

Chvostek's sign. It is the facial twitch obtained by tapping the distribution of the facial nerve. It is indicative of hypocalcemia and is the most reliable test for hypocalcemia.

Curschmann's spirals. Spirally twisted masses of mucus present in the sputum of bronchial asthmatic patients.

Dalrymple's sign. Upper lid retraction with upper scleral showing is a clinical manifestation of Grave's orbitopathy (exophthalmos).

Demarquay's sign. Absence of elevation of the larynx during deglutition. It is said to indicate syphilitic induration of the trachea.

Di Sant'Agnese test. It measures the elevated sodium and chloride in the sweat of cystic fibrotic children.

Dupre's sign. Meningism.

Ebner, gustatory glands of. These glands are the minor salivary glands near the circumvallate papillae.

Escherich's sign. In hypoparathyroidism, tapping of the skin at the angle of the mouth causes protrusion of the lips.

Flexener–Wintersteiner rosettes. True neural rosettes of Grade III and IV esthesio-neuroblastoma.

Galen's anastomosis. An anastomosis between the superior laryngeal nerve and the recurrent laryngeal nerve.

Goodwin's tumor. Benign lymphoepithelioma.

Griesinger's sign. Edema of the tip of the mastoid in thrombosis of the sigmoid sinus.

Guttman's test. In the normal subject, frontal pressure on the thyroid cartilage lowers the tone of voice produced, whereas lateral pressure produces a higher tone of voice. The opposite is true with paralysis of the cricothyroid muscle.

Guyon's sign. The XII nerve lies directly upon the external carotid artery, whereby this vessel may be distinguished from the internal carotid artery. (The safer way prior to ligation of the external carotid artery is to identify the first few branches of the external carotid artery.)

Henle, glands of. They are the small glands situated in the areolar tissue between the buccopharyngeal fascia anteriorly and the prevertebral fascia posteriorly. Infection of these glands can lead to retropharyngeal abscess. Because these glands atrophy after age 5, retropharyngeal abscess is less likely to occur after that age.

Hennebert's sign. See Chapter 5. The presence of a positive fistula test in the absence of an obvious fistula is called Hennebert's sign. The patient has a normal-appearing tympanic membrane and external auditory canal. The nystagmus is more marked upon application of negative pressure. This sign is present with congenital syphilis and is believed to be due to an excessively mobile footplate or caused by motion of the saccule mediated by fibrosis between the footplate and the saccule.

Hering–Breuer reflex. A respiratory reflex from pulmonary stretch receptors. Inflation of the lungs sends an inhibitory impulse to the CNS via the vagus nerve to stop inspiration. Similarly, deflation of the lungs sends an impulse to stop expiration. This action is the Hering–Breuer reflex.

Homber–Wright rosettes. Pseudorosette pattern seen in grade I esthesioneuroblastoma.

Kernig's sign. When the subject lies on the back with the thigh at a right angle to the trunk, straightening of the leg (extending the leg) elicits pain, supposedly owing to the pull on the inflamed lumbosacral nerve roots. This sign is present with meningitis.

Kiesselbach's plexus. This area is in the anterior septum where the capillaries merge. It is often the site of anterior epistaxis and has also been referred to as Little's area.

Koplik's spot. Pale round spots on the oral mucosa, conjunctiva, and lacrimal caruncle that are seen in the beginning stages of measles.

Krause's nodes. Nodes in the jugular foramen.

Lhermitte's sign. A rare complication of radiation to the head and neck region causing damage to the cervical spinal cord. Symptoms consist of lightning-like electrical sensation spreading to both arms, down the dorsal spine, and to both legs upon neck flexion.

Lillie–Crowe test. Used in the diagnosis of unilateral sinus thrombophlebitis. Digital compression of the opposite internal jugular vein causes the retinal veins to dilate.

Little's area. See Kiesselbach's plexus.

Luschka's pouch. See Thornwaldt's cyst.

Marcus Gunn phenomenon. Unilateral ptosis of the eyelid with exaggerated opening of the eye during movements of the mandible.

Marjolin's ulcer. A carcinoma that arises at the site of an old burn scar. It is a well-differentiated squamous cell carcinoma that is aggressive and metastasizes rapidly.

Meckel's ganglion. Sphenopalatine ganglion.

Mikulicz's cells. These cells are macrophages in rhinoscleroma. (Russell bodies, which are eosinophilic, round structures associated with plasma cells, are also found with rhinoscleroma.)

Mollaret–Debre test. This test is performed for cat-scratch fever.

Morgagni, sinus of. A dehiscence of the superior constrictor muscle and the buccopharyngeal fascia where the eustachian tube opens.

Morgagni, ventricle of. It separates the quadrangular membrane from the conus elasticus in the larynx.

Nikolsky's sign. Detachment of the sheets of superficial epithelial layers when any traction is applied over the surface of the epithelial involvement in pemphigus is characteristic of Nikolsky's sign. Pemphigus involves the intraepithelial layer, whereas pemphigoid involves the subepithelial layer. The former is a lethal disease in many instances.

Oliver–Cardarelli sign. Recession of the larynx and trachea is synchronous with cardiac systole in cases of aneurysm of the arch of the aorta or in cases of a tumor in that region.

Parinaud's sign. Extraocular muscle impairment with decreased upward gaze and ptosis seen in association with pinealomas and other lesions of the tectum.

Paul–Bunnel test. Measures the elevated heterophile titer of infectious mononucleosis.

Physaliferous cells. "Soap-bubbles" cells of chordoma.

Psammoma bodies. Found with papillary carcinoma of the thyroid.

Rathke's pouch. See Thornwaldt's cyst.

Reinke's tumor. A "soft" tumor variant of lymphoepithelioma in which the lymphocytes predominate. (With the hard tumor the epithelial cells predominate; it is called Schmincke's tumor).

Rhomberg's sign. If a patient standing with feet together "falls" when closing the eyes, then the Rhomberg test is positive. It is indicative of either abnormal proprioception or abnormal vestibular function. It does not necessarily distinguish central from peripheral lesions. Cerebellar function is not evaluated by this test.

Rosenbach's sign. Fine tremor of the closed eyelids seen in hyperthyroidism and hysteria.

Rouvier's node. Lateral retropharyngeal node. It is a common target of metastases in nasopharyngeal carcinoma.

Russell's bodies. Eosinophilic, round structures, associated with plasma cells found in rhinoscleroma.

Santorini's cartilage. Corniculate cartilage of the larynx, composed of fibroelastic cartilage.

Santorini's fissures. Fissures in the anterior bony external auditory canal leading to the parotid region.

Schaumann's bodies. Together with asteroids, they are found in sarcoid granuloma.

Schmincke's tumor. The "hard" variant of lymphoepithelioma in which the epithelial cells predominate (see Reinke's tumor).

Schneiderian mucosa. Pseudostratified ciliated columnar mucosa of the nose.

Seeligmüller's sign. Contraction of the pupil on the affected side in facial neuralgia.

Semon's law. A law stating that injury to the recurrent laryngeal nerve results in paralysis of the abductor muscle of the larynx (cricoarytenoid posticus) before paralysis of the adductor muscles. During recovery, the adductor recovers before the abductor.

Straus's sign. With facial paralysis the lesion is peripheral if injection of pilocarpine is followed by sweating on the affected side later than on the normal side.

Sudeck's sign. It is sometimes associated with Grisel syndrome and is recognized by the displacement of the spine of the axis to the same side as the head is turned.

Sulkowitch's test. It determines an increase in calciuria.

Thornwaldt's cyst. A depression exists in the nasopharyngeal vault that is a remnant of the pouch of Luschka. When this depression becomes infected, Thornwaldt's cyst results. In the early embryo, this area has a connection between the notochord and entoderm. Thornwaldt's cyst is lined with respiratory epithelium with some squamous metaplasia. Anterior to this pit, the path taken by Rathke's pouch sometimes persists as the craniopharyngeal canal, running from the sella turcica through the body of the sphenoid to an opening on the undersurface of the skull.

Tobey–Ayer–Queckenstedt test. Used in the diagnosis of unilateral and bilateral sinus thrombophlebitis. In cases where the lateral sinus is obstructed on one side, compression of the jugular vein on the intact side causes a rise in CSF pressure, whereas compression of the obstructed side does not raise the CSF pressure.

Toynbee's law. When CNS complications arise in chronic otitis media, the lateral sinus and cerebellum are involved in mastoiditis, whereas the cerebrum alone is involved in instances of cholesteatoma of the attic.

Trousseau's sign. With hypocalcemia a tourniquet placed around the arm causes tetany.

Tullio phenomenon. See Chapter 5. This phenomenon is said to be present when a loud noise precipitates vertigo. It can be present in congenital syphilis, with a semicircular canal fistula, or in a postfenestration patient if the footplate is mobile. The tympanic membrane and ossicular chain must be intact with a mobile footplate.

Wartenberg's sign. Intense pruritus of the tip of the nose and nostril indicates cerebral tumor.

Warthin–Finkelday giant cells. They are found in the lymphoid with measles.

Warthin–Starry stain. To identify cat-scratch bacillus.

Weber's glands. These glands are minor salivary glands in the superior pole of the tonsil.

Wrisberg's cartilage. It is the cuneiform cartilage of the larynx, composed of fibroelastic cartilage.

Xeroderma pigmentosa. Hereditary precancerous condition that begins during early child-hood. These patients die at puberty.

Zaufal's sign. Saddle nose.

Zellballen. Nest of cells surrounded by sustentacular cells in paraganglioma tumors.

Reference

1. Maddox WD, et al. Multiple nevoid basal cell epitheliomas, jaw cysts, and skeletal defects. *JAMA* 1964;188:106.

Bibliography

Afzelius LE, Elmqvist D, et al. Sleep apnea syndrome—An alternative treatment to tracheostomy. *Laryngoscope* 1981;91:285.

Arasi R, McKay M, et al. Trigeminal trophic syndrome. *Laryngoscope* 1988;98:1330.

Baker S, Ross L, Arbor A. Sleep apnea syndrome and supraglottic edema. *Arch Otolaryngol Head Neck Surg* 1980;106:486.

Ballard R, Cummings C. Job's syndrome. *Laryngoscope* 1980;90:1367.

Batsakis JG. Lymphoepithelial lesion and Sjögren's syndrome. *Ann Otol Rhinol Laryngol* 1987;96:354.

Begstrom L. Pendred's syndrome with atypical features. *Ann Otol Rhinol Laryngol* 1980; 89:135.

Berkower AS, Biller HF. Head and neck cancer associated with Bloom's syndrome. *Laryngoscope* 1988;98:746.

Black FO, Spanier SS, et al. Aural abnormalities in partial DiGeorge's syndrome. *Arch Otolaryngol Head Neck Surg* 1975;101:129.

Blanchard CL, et al. Acquired inflammatory superior oblique tendon sheath (Brown's) syndrome. *Arch Otolaryngol Head Neck Surg* 1984; 110:120.

Bomholt, A. Facial palsy in lymphocytic meningoradiculitis (Bannwarth's syndrome). *Arch Otolaryngol Head Neck Surg* 1984;110:763.

Borovik HR, Kveton JF. Pierre Robin syndrome combined with unilateral choanal atresia. *Otolaryngol Head Neck Surg* 1987;96:67.

Breda SD, et al. Toxic shock syndrome in nasal surgery: A physiochemical and microbiologic evaluation of Merocel® and NuGauz® nasal packing. *Laryngoscope* 1987;97:1388.

Brown JS, Moster ML, et al. The Tolosa–Hunt syndrome: A case report. *Otolaryngol Head Neck Surg* 1990;102:402.

Burstein F, et al. Kawasaki disease in adults. *Arch Otolaryngol Head Neck Surg* 1984;110:543.

Chandra-Sekhar HK, et al. Hanhart's syndrome with special reference to temporal bone findings. *Ann Otol Rhinol Laryngol* 1987;96:309.

Cremers WRJ, et al. Hearing loss in the cervico-oculo-acoustic (Wildervanck) syndrome. *Arch Otolaryngol Head Neck Surg* 1984;110:54.

Crockett DM, et al. Osteomyelitis of maxilla in patients with osteopetrosis (Albers–Schönberg disease). *Otolaryngol Head Neck Surg* 1986; 95:117.

Day TA, et al. Treatment of Kimura's disease: A therapeutic enigma. *Otolaryngol Head Neck Surg* 1995;112:333.

Denenberg S, Levine PA. Castleman's disease—the lymphoma imposter. *Laryngoscope* 1984; 94:601.

Ensink RJH, et al. Congenital conductive hearing loss in the lacrimoauriculodentodigital syndrome. *Arch Otolaryngol Head Neck Surg* 1997;123:97.

Feldman J Jr, Kearns DB, et al. The otolaryngologic manifestations of Pelizaeus–Merzbacher disease. *Arch Otolaryngol Head Neck Surg* 1990; 116:613.

Folsom R, Widen JE, et al. Auditory brainstem response in infants with Down's syndrome. *Arch Otolaryngol Head Neck Surg* 1983;109:607.

Frable MAS, Myer EC. Tolusa–Hunt syndrome. A resolution of a 12 year course after tonsillectomy. *Laryngoscope* 1987;97:334.

Gelmers H. Tapia's syndrome after thoracotomy. *Arch Otolaryngol Head Neck Surg* 1983; 109:622.

Goodman R. Frey's syndrome secondary to condylar fracture. *Laryngoscope* 1986;96:1397.

Gorlin RF, Tilsner TJ, et al. Usher's syndrome type III. *Arch Otolaryngol Head Neck Surg* 1979;105:353.

Gray WC, Sakman M. CSF rhinorrhea associated with the empty-sella syndrome. *Arch Otolaryngol Head Neck Surg* 1980;106:302.

Hanson DG. Vocal fold paresis in Shy–Drager syndrome. *Ann Otol Rhinol Laryngol* 1983;92:85.

Harada T, Sando I. Temporal bone histopathologic features in Fanconi's anemia syndrome. *Arch Otolaryngol Head Neck Surg* 1980;106:275.

Harada T, Sando I. Temporal bone histopathologic findings in Down's syndrome. *Arch Otolaryngol Head Neck Surg* 1981;107:96.

Hochman M, et al. Conradi–Hunerman syndrome. *Ann Otol Rhinol Laryngol* 1987;97:565.

Hull HF, et al. Toxic shock syndrome related to nasal packing. *Arch Otolaryngol Head Neck Surg* 1983;109:624.

Jackler RK, de la Cruz A. The large vestibular aqueduct syndrome. *Laryngoscope* 1989;99:1238.

Jacobson J, Stevens M. Evaluation of single dose cefazolin prophylaxis for toxic shock syndrome. *Arch Otolaryngol Head Neck Surg* 1988;114:326.

Jahrsdoerfer R, Feldman PS, et al. Otitis media and the immotile cilia syndrome. *Laryngoscope* 1979;89:769.

Johnson LG, Arenberg IK. Cochlear abnormalities in Alport's syndrome. *Arch Otolaryngol Head Neck Surg* 1981;107:340.

Jubelirer SJ, Goodloe-Greens L, Dreykin D. Autoimmune thrombocytopenic purpura-like syndrome in a patient with head and neck cancer. *Laryngoscope* 1981;91:408.

Keipper VL, Chikes PG. Surgical correction of the snout suffocation syndrome. *Arch Otolaryngol Head Neck Surg* 1990;116:460.

Kenyon GS, et al. Stridor and obstructive sleep apnea in Shy–Drager syndrome treated by laryngofissure and cord lateralization. *Laryngoscope* 1984;94:1106.

Koch WM, McDonald GA. Stevens–Johnson syndrome with supraglottic laryngeal obstruction. *Arch Otolaryngol Head Neck Surg* 1989; 115:1381.

Kraus EM, McCabe BF. The giant apical air cell syndrome: A new entity. *Ann Otol Rhinol Laryngol* 1982;91:237.

Kumar A, et al. Vestibular and auditory function in Usher's syndrome. *Ann Otol Rhinol Laryngol* 1984;93:600.

Leopold PA, Preti G, et al. Fish odor syndrome presenting as dysosmia. *Arch Otolaryngol Head Neck Surg* 1990;116:354.

Levenson MJ, et al. Melkersson–Rosenthal syndrome. *Arch Otolaryngol Head Neck Surg* 1984;110:540.

Levenson MJ, Parisier SC, et al. The large vestibular aqueduct syndrome in children: A review of 12 cases and the description of a new clinical entity. *Arch Otolaryngol Head Neck Surg* 1989;115:54.

Lowell S, Mathog R. Head and neck manifestations of Maffucci's syndrome. *Arch Otolaryngol Head Neck Surg* 1979;105:427.

Marasovich WA, Mazaheri M, et al. Otolaryngologic findings in whistling face syndrome. *Arch Otolaryngol Head Neck Surg* 1989;115:1373.

March DE, Rao V, et al. Computed tomography of salivary glands in Sjögren's syndrome. *Arch Otolaryngol Head Neck Surg* 1989;115:105.

Mathog R, Leonard M. Surgical correction of Goldenhar's syndrome. *Laryngoscope* 1980; 90:1137.

McDonald TJ, et al. Cogan's syndrome: Audiovestibular involvement and prognosis in 18 patients. *Laryngoscope* 1985;95:650.

McGee TM. The loose wire syndrome. *Laryngoscope* 1981;91:1478.

Medina JE, et al. Oat cell carcinoma of the larynx and Eaton–Lambert syndrome. *Arch Otolaryngol Head Neck Surg* 1984;110:123.

Musiek FE, Weider DJ, et al. Audiologic findings in Charcot–Marie–Tooth disease. *Arch Otolaryngol Head Neck Surg* 1982;108:595.

Nolph M, Dion M. Raeder's syndrome associated with internal carotid artery dilation and sinusitis. *Laryngoscope* 1982;92:1144.

Ohtani I, Schuknecht HF. Temporal bone pathology in DiGeorge's syndrome. *Ann Otol Rhinol Laryngol* 1984;93:220.

Okamura H, Tsotsumi S, et al. Esophageal web in Plummer–Vinson syndrome. *Laryngoscope* 1988;98:994.

Okumo T, Takahashi H, et al. Temporal bone histopathologic findings in Alagille's syndrome. *Arch Otolaryngol Head Neck Surg* 1990; 116:217.

Orlando MR, Atkins JS Jr. Melkersson–Rosenthal syndrome. *Arch Otolaryngol Head Neck Surg* 1990;116:728.

Ozünlü A, et al. Rosai–Dorfman disease involving the nasal septum. *Ear Nose Throat J* 1995;74:831.

Palmer JM, et al. Papillary adenoma of the temporal bone in von-Hippel–Lindau disease. *Otolaryngol Head Neck Surg* 1989;100:64.

Pender DJ, Pender VB. Otolaryngologica prevarica: Munchausen's syndrome update and report of a case. *Laryngoscope* 1980; 90:657.

Phillips SG, Miyamoto RT. Congenital conductive hearing loss in Apert syndrome. *Otolaryngol Head Neck Surg* 1986;95:429.

Pickens JP, Modica L. Current concepts of lethal midline granuloma syndrome. *Otolaryngol Head Neck Surg* 1989;100:623.

Rarey KE, et al. Effects of influenza infection, aspirin, and an arginine-deficient diet on the inner ear in Reye's syndrome. *Ann Otol Rhinol Laryngol* 1984;93:551.

Richardson MA, et al. Evaluation of tonsils and adenoids in sleep apnea syndrome. *Laryngoscope* 1980;90:1106.

Saito H, Kishimoto S, Furuta M. Temporal bone findings in a patient with Möbius' syndrome. *Ann Otol Rhinol Laryngol* 1981;90:80.

Saito R, Takata N, et al. Anomalies of the auditory organ in Potter's syndrome. *Arch Otolaryngol Head Neck Surg* 1982;108:484.

Sakai N, et al. Temporal findings in VATER syndrome. *Arch Otolaryngol Head Neck Surg* 1986;112:416.

Sasaki CT. Development of laryngeal function: Etiologic significance in the sudden infant death syndrome. *Laryngoscope* 1979;89:1964.

Sasaki C, Ruiz R, et al. Hunter's syndrome: A study in airway obstruction. *Laryngoscope* 1987;97:280.

Schachern PA, Shea DA, Papparella MM. Mucopolysaccharidosis I-H (Hurler's syndrome) and human temporal bone histopathology. *Ann Otol Rhinol Laryngol* 1984; 93:65.

Schwartz MR, et al. Gaucher's disease involving the maxillary sinuses. *Arch Otolaryngol Head Neck Surg* 1988;114:203.

Sculerati N, Ledesma-Medina J, et al. Otitis media and hearing loss in Turner syndrome. *Arch Otolaryngol Head Neck Surg* 1990;116:704.

Shi S. Temporal bone findings in a case of otopalatodigital syndrome. *Arch Otolaryngol Head Neck Surg* 1985;111:119.

Shinkawa H, Nadol JB. Histopathology of the inner ear in Usher's syndrome as observed by light and electron microscopy. *Ann Otol Rhinol Laryngol* 1986;95:313.

Siglog TJ. Sensorineural hearing loss associated with Takayasu's disease. *Laryngoscope* 1987; 97:797.

Sismanis A, et al. Otologic symptoms and findings of pseudotumor cerebri syndrome. *Otolaryngol Head Neck Surg* 1985;93:398.

Smith JD. Treatment of airway obstruction in Pierre Robin syndrome. *Arch Otolaryngol Head Neck Surg* 1981;107:419.

Smith PG, et al. Clinical aspects of branchio-otorenal syndrome. *Otolaryngol Head Neck Surg* 1984;92:468.

Smith RJH. A DNA linkage study of Usher's syndrome excluding much of chromosome 4. *Laryngoscope* 1989;99:940.

Strauss M, Zohar Y, et al. Elongated styloid process syndrome: Intraoral versus external approach for styloid surgery. *Laryngoscope* 1985; 95:976.

Strome M. Down's syndrome: A modern oto-rhinolaryngological perspective. *Laryngoscope* 1981; 91:1581.

Sukerman S, Healy GB, et al. Sleep apnea syndrome associated with upper airway obstruction. *Laryngoscope* 1979;89:878.

Tachibana M, et al. Duane's syndrome associated with crocodile tear and ear malformation. *Arch Otolaryngol Head Neck Surg* 1984;110:761.

Tag A, Mitchell F, et al. Toxic shock syndrome: Otolaryngologic presentations. *Laryngoscope* 1982; 92:1070.

Thompson JW, Rosenthal P, et al. Vocal cord paralysis and superior laryngeal nerve dysfunction in Reye's syndrome. *Arch Otolaryngol Head Neck Surg* 1990;116:46.

Tokita N, Chandra-Sekhar HK. The campomelic syndrome. *Arch Otolaryngol Head Neck Surg* 1979;105:449.

Van den Broek P, Kersing W. Laryngeal problems in the scimitar syndrome. *Arch Otolaryngol Head Neck Surg* 1983;109:705.

Walby AP, Schuknecht HF. Concomitant occurrence of cochleosaccular dysplasia and Down's syndrome. *Arch Otolaryngol Head Neck Surg* 1984;110:477.

Walter RF, Danielson JR, et al. Characterization of a chemotactic defect in patients with Kartagener syndrome. *Arch Otolaryngol Head Neck Surg* 1990;116:465.

Wenig BL, et al. The syndrome of inappropriate secretion of antidiuretic hormone (SIADH) following neck dissection. *Laryngoscope* 1987; 97:467.

Wilson BC, et al. Nontraumatic subluxation of the atlantoaxial joint: Grisel's syndrome. *Ann Otol Rhinol Laryngol* 1987;96:705.

Windle-Taylor PC, Emery PJ. Ear deformities associated with the Klippel–Feil syndrome. *Ann Otol Rhinol Laryngol* 1981;90:210.

Zohar Y, et al. Otolaryngologic cases of Munchausen's syndrome. *Laryngoscope* 1987; 97:201.

Embryology of Clefts and Pouches

10

CORRELATION BETWEEN AGE AND SIZE OF EMBRYO

Weeks	Millimeters
2.5	1.5
3.5	2.5
4	5
5	8
6	12
7	17
8	23
10	40
12	56
16	112
5–10 months	160–350

DEVELOPMENT OF THE BRANCHIAL ARCHES

The first 8 weeks constitutes the period of greatest embryonic development of the head and neck. There are five arches that are named either pharyngeal or branchial. Between these arches are the grooves or clefts externally and the pouches internally. Each pouch has a ventral or dorsal wing. The derivatives of the arches are usually of mesoderm origin. The groove is lined by ectoderm, and the pouch is lined by entoderm (Figure 10-1).

Each arch has an artery, nerve, and cartilage bar. These nerves are anterior to their respective arteries, except in the fifth arch where the nerve is posterior to the artery. (Embryologically, the arch after the fourth is called the fifth or sixth arch depending on the theory one follows. For simplicity in this synopsis, it is referred to as the fifth arch.) Caudal to all the arches lies the XII nerve. The sternocleidomastoid muscles are derived from the cervical somites posterior and inferior to the above arches.

There are two ventral and two dorsal aortas in early embryonic life. The two ventral aortas fuse completely, whereas the two dorsal ones only fuse caudally (Figure 10-2A). During the course of embryonic development, the first and second arch arteries degenerate. The second arch artery has an upper branch that passes through a mass of mesoderm, which later chondrifies and ossifies as the stapes. This stapedial artery usually degenerates during late fetal life but occasionally persists in the adult. The third arch artery is the precursor of the carotid artery in both left and right sides. The left fourth arch artery becomes the arch of the aorta. The right fourth arch artery becomes the proximal subclavian. The rest of the right subclavian and the left subclavian are derivatives of the seventh segmental arteries. The left fifth arch artery becomes the pulmonary artery and ductus arteriosus. The right fifth arch artery becomes the pulmonary artery with degeneration of the rest of this arch vessel (Figure 10-2B).

232

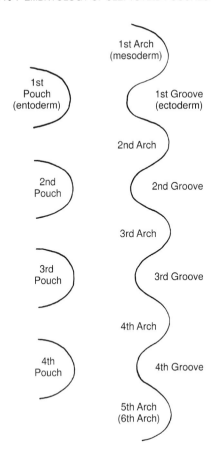

Figure 10-1.   Pouches and grooves.

Should the right fourth arch artery degenerate and the right subclavian arise from the dorsal aorta instead, as shown in Figure 10-2C, the right subclavian becomes posterior to the esophagus, thus causing a constriction of the esophagus without any effect on the trachea (dysphagia lusoria). The innominate artery arises ventrally. Hence when it arises too far from the left, an anterior compression of the trachea results (anomalous innominate).

The fifth arch nerve is posterior and caudal to the artery. As the connection on the right side between the fifth arch artery (pulmonary) and the dorsal aorta degenerates, the nerve (recurrent laryngeal nerve) loops around the fourth arch artery, which subsequently becomes the subclavian. On the left side, the nerve loops around the ductus arteriosus and the aorta. Table 10-1 lists the branchial arches and their derivatives.

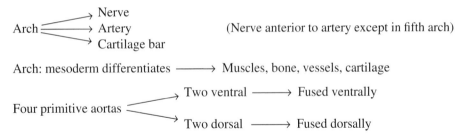

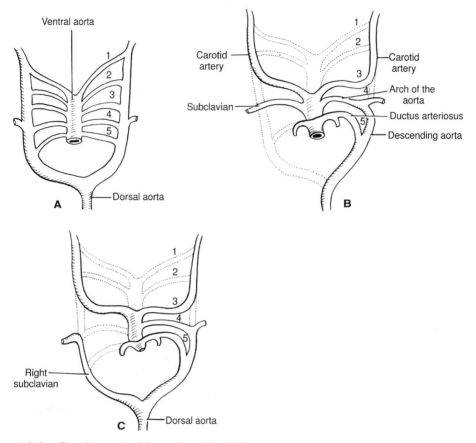

Figure 10-2.   Development of the embryonic arteries.

DERIVATIVES OF THE POUCHES

1. Each pouch has a ventral and a dorsal wing. The fourth pouch has an additional acces-
    sory wing. The entodermal lining of the pouches proliferates into glandular organs.

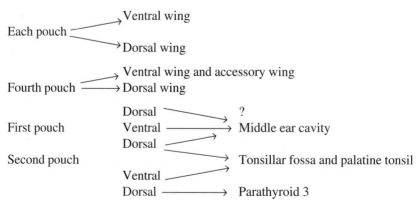

TABLE 10-1. BRANCHIAL ARCHES AND THEIR DERIVATIVES

Arch	Ganglion or Nerve	Derivatives
First (mandibular)	Semilunar ganglion V₃	Mandible Head, neck, manubrium of malleus Body and short process of incus Anterior malleal ligament Sphenomandibular ligament Tensor tympani Mastication muscles, mylohyoid Anterior belly of digastric muscle Tensor palati muscle
Second (hyoid)	Geniculate ganglion VII	Manubrium of malleus Long process of incus All of stapes except vestibular portion of footplate and annular ligament Stapedial artery Styloid process Stylohyoid ligament Lesser cornu of hyoid Part of body of hyoid Stapedius muscle Facial muscles Buccinator, posterior belly of digastric muscle Styloid muscle Part of pyramidal eminence Lower part of facial canal
Third	IX	Greater cornu of hyoid and rest of hyoid Stylopharyngeus muscle, superior and middle constrictors; common and internal carotid arteries
Fourth	Superior laryngeal nerve	Thyroid cartilage, cuneiform, inferior pharyngeal constrictor, cricopharyngeus, cricothyroid muscles, aorta on the left, proximal subclavian on the right
Fifth*	Recurrent laryngeal nerve	Cricoid, arytenoids, corniculate, trachea, intrinsic laryngeal muscles, inferior constrictor muscle, ductus arteriosus

*Often called the *sixth arch* from the standpoint of evolution and comparative anatomy.

Third pouch   Ventral $\longrightarrow$ Thymus

Dorsal $\longrightarrow$ Parathyroid 4

Fourth pouch   Ventral $\longrightarrow$?

Accessory $\longrightarrow$ Ultimobranchial body

2. During embryonic development the thymus descends caudally, pulling with it parathyroid 3. Consequently, parathyroid 3 is inferior to parathyroid 4 in the adult.

3. The ultimobranchial body becomes infiltrated by cells of neutral crest origin, giving rise to the interfollicular cells of the thyroid gland. These cells secrete thyrocalcitonin.

4. As these "out-pocketing" pouches develop into glandular elements, their connections with the pharyngeal lumen, referred to as pharyngobranchial ducts, become obliterated. Should obliteration fail to occur, a branchial sinus (cyst) is said to have resulted.

5. The second pharyngobranchial duct (between the second and third arches) is believed to open into the tonsillar fossa, the third pharyngobranchial duct opens into the pyriform sinus, and the fourth opens into the lower part of the pyriform sinus or larynx. An alternative school of thought believes that branchial sinuses and cysts are not remnants of patent pharyngobranchial ducts but, rather, are remnants of the cervical sinus of His.[1]

6. The cutaneous openings of branchial sinuses, if present, are always anterior to the anterior border of the sternocleidomastoid muscle. The tract always lies deep to the platysma muscle, which is derived from the second arch (Figure 10-3).
   a. Course of a second arch branchial cyst
      (1) Deep to second arch derivatives and superficial to third arch derivatives
      (2) Superficial to the XII nerve and anterior to the sternocleidomastoid
      (3) In close relation with the carotid sheath but superficial to it
      (4) Superficial to the IX nerve, pierces middle constrictor, deep to stylohyoid ligament, opens into tonsillar fossa

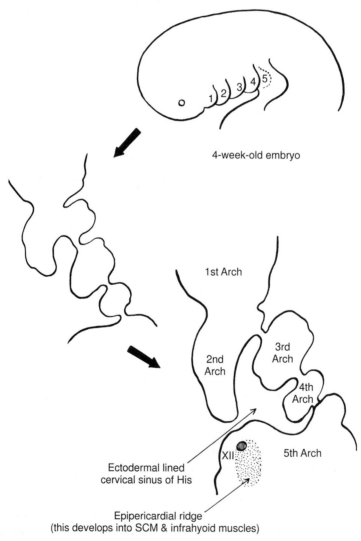

Figure 10-3. Pharyngobranchial ducts.

    b.   Course of a third arch branchial cyst
- (1) Again, subplatysmal and opens externally anterior to the sternocleidomastoid muscle
- (2) Superficial to the XII nerve, deep to the internal carotid artery and the IX nerve
- (3) Pierces the thyrohyoid membrane above the internal branch of the superior laryngeal nerve and opens into the pyriform fossa

    c.   Course of a fourth arch branchial cyst
- (1) Right
  - (a) The tract lies low in the neck beneath the platysma and anterior to the sternocleidomastoid muscle.
  - (b) It loops around the subclavian and deep to it, deep to the carotid, lateral to the XII nerve, inferior to the superior laryngeal nerve; opens into the lower part of the pyriform sinus or into the larynx.
- (2) Left
  - (a) Because the fourth arch vessel is the adult aorta, the cyst may be intra-thoracic, medial to the ligamentum arteriosus and the arch of the aorta.
  - (b) It is lateral to the XII nerve, inferior to the superior laryngeal nerve.
  - (c) It opens into the lower pyriform sinus or into the larynx.

ARCHES
First Arch (Mandibular Arch)

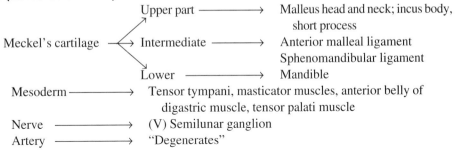

Meckel's cartilage
- Upper part ⟶ Malleus head and neck; incus body, short process
- Intermediate ⟶ Anterior malleal ligament / Sphenomandibular ligament
- Lower ⟶ Mandible

Mesoderm ⟶ Tensor tympani, masticator muscles, anterior belly of digastric muscle, tensor palati muscle

Nerve ⟶ (V) Semilunar ganglion

Artery ⟶ "Degenerates"

Second Arch (Hyoid Arch)

Reichert's cartilage ⟶
- Manubrium of malleus
- Long process of incus
- Lenticular process
- Stapes (except vestibular part of footplate)
- Styloid process, pyramidal eminence
- Stylohyoid ligament
- Lesser cornu of the hyoid
- Part of the body of the hyoid
- Lower half of facial canal

Mesoderm ⟶ Platysma, stapedius muscle and tendon, facial muscles, auricular muscle, posterior belly, stylohyoid muscle

Nerve ⟶ (VII) Geniculate ganglion

Artery ⟶ "Degenerates" (stapedial artery)

Third Arch

Cartilage bar $\longrightarrow$ Greater cornu of the hyoid, part of body of the hyoid
Mesoderm $\longrightarrow$ Stylopharyngeus muscle
Nerve $\longrightarrow$ (IX) Superior and inferior ganglia
Artery $\longrightarrow$ Common and internal carotid arteries

Fourth Arch

Cartilage bar $\longrightarrow$ Thyroid cartilage, cuneiform cartilage
Mesoderm $\longrightarrow$ Inferior pharyngeus constrictor muscle, cricothyroid muscle, cricopharyngeus muscle
Nerve $\longrightarrow$ Superior laryngeal nerve (jugular and nodose ganglion)
Artery: Left $\longrightarrow$ Aorta
Right $\longrightarrow$ Proximal subclavian (the rest derived from seventh segmental artery)

Fifth Arch (? Sixth)

Cartilage bar $\longrightarrow$ Cricoid, arytenoid, corniculate
Mesoderm $\longrightarrow$ Intrinsic muscles of larynx (except cricothyroid); trachea
Artery: Left $\longrightarrow$ Pulmonary $\longrightarrow$ Ductus arteriosus
Right $\longrightarrow$ Pulmonary
Nerve $\longrightarrow$ Recurrent laryngeal nerve

EMBRYOLOGY OF THE THYROID GLAND

In a 4-week-old embryo, a ventral (thyroid) diverticulum of endodermal origin can be identified between the first and second arches on the floor of the pharynx. It also is situated between the tuberculum impar and the copula. (The tuberculum impar together with the lingual swellings becomes the anterior two-thirds of the tongue, and the copula is the precursor of the posterior one-third of the tongue.) The ventral diverticulum develops into the thyroid gland. During development it descends caudally within the mesodermal tissues. At 4.5 weeks the connection between the thyroid diverticulum and the floor of the pharynx begins to disappear. By the 6th week it should be obliterated and atrophied. Should it persist through the time of birth or thereafter, a thyroglossal duct cyst is present. This tract travels either superficial to, through, or just deep to the hyoid and reaches the foramen cecum (Figure 10-4).

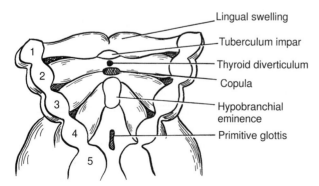

Figure 10-4. Four-week-old embryo.

EMBRYOLOGY OF THE TONGUE

The tongue is derived from ectodermal origin (anterior two-thirds) and entodermal origin (posteriorly). At the 4th week, two lingual swellings are noted at the first arch, and a swelling, the tuberculum impar, appears between the first and second arches. These three prominences develop into the anterior two-thirds of the tongue. Meanwhile, another swelling is noted between the second and third arches, called the copula. It develops into the posterior one-third of the tongue. At the 7th week the somites from the high cervical areas differentiate into voluntary muscle of the tongue. The circumvallate papillae develop between the 8th and 20th weeks and the filiform and fungiform papillae develop at the 11th week (Table 10-2).

EMBRYOLOGY OF TONSILS AND ADENOIDS

1. Palatine tonsil (8 weeks) develops from the second pouch (ventral or dorsal).
2. Lingual tonsil (6.5 weeks) develops from between the second and third arches ventrally.
3. Adenoids (16 weeks) develop as a subepithelial infiltration of lymphocytes.

EMBRYOLOGY OF SALIVARY GLANDS

1. Parotid gland (5.5 weeks) is of ectodermal origin derived from the first pouch.
2. Submaxillary gland (6 weeks) is of ectodermal origin derived from the first pouch.
3. Sublingual gland (8 weeks) is of ectodermal origin derived from the first pouch.

EMBRYOLOGY OF THE NOSE

The nasal placode is of ectodermal origin and appears between the middle of the 3rd and 4th weeks of gestation (Figure 10-5A). It is of interest to note that at this stage the eyes are laterally placed, the auricular precursors lie below the mandibular process, and the primitive mouth is wide. Hence abnormal embryonic development at this stage may result in these characteristics in postnatal life.

At the 5th week, the placodes become depressed below the surface and appear as invaginated pits. The nasal pit extends backward into the oral cavity but is separated from it by the bucconasal membrane (Figure 10-5B). This membrane ruptures at the 7th to 8th week of gestation to form the posterior nares. Failure in this step of development results in choanal atresia. The nasal pit extends backward as well as upward toward the forebrain area. Epithelium around the forebrain thickens to become specialized olfactory sensory cells.

Anteriorly, the maxillary process fuses with the lateral and medial nasal processes to form the anterior nares. The fusion between the maxillary process and the lateral nasal

TABLE 10-2. EMBRYONIC DEVELOPMENT OF THE TONGUE

Age (weeks)	Structure
4	Tuberculum impar, lingual swellings, copula
7	Voluntary muscles, nerve XII, papillae, tonsillar tissues
8–20	Circumvallate papillae
11	Filiform and fungiform papillae

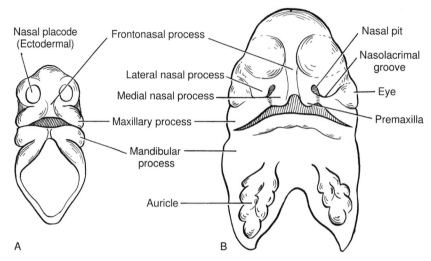

Figure 10-5. Development of the nasal placode. **A,** Four-week-old embryo; **B,** Five-week-old embryo.

process also creates a groove called the nasolacrimal groove. The epithelium over the groove is subsequently buried, and, when the epithelium is resorbed, the nasolacrimal duct is formed, opening into the anterior aspect of the inferior meatus. The duct is fully developed at birth.

The frontonasal process (mesoderm) is the precursor of the nasal septum (Figure 10-6). The primitive palate (premaxilla) located anteriorly is also a derivative of the frontonasal process (mesoderm). Posteriorly (Figure 10-7), the septum lies directly over the oral cavity until the 9th week, at which time the palatal shelves of the maxilla grow medially to fuse with each other and with the septum to form the secondary palate. The hard palate is formed by the 8th to 9th week (Figure 10-8), and the soft palate and the uvula are completed by the 11th to 12th week.

From the 8th week to the 24th week of embryonic life, the nostrils are occupied by an epithelial plug. Failure to resorb this epithelium results in atresia or stenosis of the anterior nares.

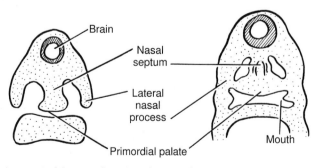

Figure 10-6. Development of the nasal septum (see text).

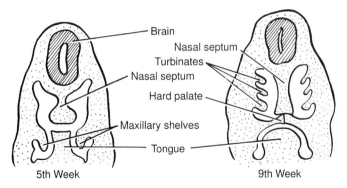

Figure 10-7. Further development of the nasal septum (see text).

Along the lateral wall of the nasal precursor, the maxilloturbinal is the first to appear, followed by the development of five ethmoturbinals and one nasoturbinal. Table 10-3 gives the derivatives of each embryonic anlage, and Table 10-4 gives a timetable of their development.

EMBRYOLOGY OF THE LARYNX

Figure 10-9 depicts the embryonic development of the larynx between the 8th and 28th weeks of fetal life.

The entire respiratory system is an outgrowth of the primitive pharynx. At 3.5 weeks, a groove called the laryngotracheal groove develops in the embryo at the ventral aspect of the foregut. This groove is just posterior to the hypobranchial eminence and is located closer to the fourth arch than to the third arch. During embryonic development, when a single tubal structure is to later become two tubal structures, the original tube is first obliterated by a proliferation of lining epithelium, then as resorption of the epithelium takes place, the second tube is formed and the first tube is recannulized. Hence any malformation involves both tubes. This process of growth accounts for the fact that more than 90% of tracheoesophageal fis-

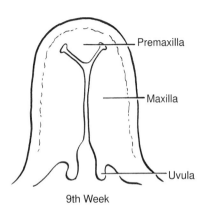

Figure 10-8. Parts of the palate.

TABLE 10-3. EMBRYONIC ANLAGEN AND THEIR DERIVATIVES

Anlagen	Derivatives
Maxilloturbinal	Inferior concha
First ethmoturbinal	Middle concha
Second and third ethmoturbinals	Superior concha
Fourth and fifth ethmoturbinals	Supreme concha
Nasoturbinal	Agger nasi area

tulas are associated with esophageal atresia. During development the mesenchyme of the foregut grows medially from the sides, "pinching off" this groove to create a separate opening. With further maturation, two separate tubes, the esophagus and the laryngotracheal apparatus, are formed.

This laryngotracheal opening is the primitive laryngeal aditus and lies between the fourth and fifth arches. The sagittal slit opening is altered to become a T-shaped opening by the growth of three tissue masses. The first is the hypobranchial eminence, which appears during the 3rd week. This mesodermal structure gives rise to the furcula, which later develops into the epiglottis. The second and third growths are two arytenoid masses, which appear during the 5th week. Later, each arytenoid swelling shows two additional swellings that eventually mature into the cuneiform and corniculate cartilages.

As these masses grow between the 5th and 7th weeks, the laryngeal lumen is obliterated. At the 9th week the oval shape lumen is re-established. Failure to recannulize may result in atresia or stenosis of the larynx. The true and false cords are formed between the 8th and 10th weeks. The ventricles are formed at the 12th week.

The two arytenoid masses are separated by an "interarytenoid notch," which later becomes obliterated. Failure of this obliteration to occur results in a posterior cleft up to the cricoid cartilage, and opening into the esophagus. This is a culprit of severe aspiration in the newborn.

Table 10-5 outlines the muscular and cartilaginous development of the larynx.

The laryngeal muscles are derivatives from the mesoderm of the fourth and fifth arches and hence are innervated by the X nerve. The infant larynx is situated at a level between the second and third cervical vertebrae. In the adult it lies opposite the body of the fifth cervical vertebra.

Table 10-6 outlines the development of the paranasal sinuses.

TABLE 10-4. TIMETABLE OF NASAL DEVELOPMENT

Structures	Time of Development (week)
Inferior concha formed	7
Middle concha formed	7
Uncinate process formed	7
Superior concha formed	8
Cartilage laid down	10
Vomer formed and calcified	12
Ethmoid bone calcified	20
Cribriform plate calcified	28
Perpendicular plate, crista galli calcified	After birth

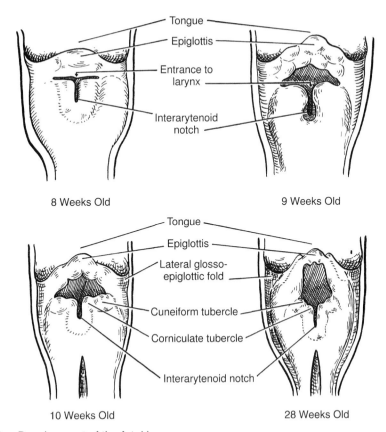

Figure 10-9. Development of the fetal larynx.

TABLE 10-5. LARYNGEAL MUSCULAR AND CARTILAGINOUS DEVELOPMENT WITH EMBRYONIC AGE

Development	Age (weeks)
Muscular	
Inferior pharyngeal constrictor and cricothyroid muscles formed	4
Interarytenoid and postcricoarytenoid muscles formed	5.5
Lateral cricoarytenoid muscle formed	6
Cartilaginous	
Development of epiglottis (hypobranchial eminence)	3
Thyroid cartilage (fourth arch) and cricoid cartilage (fifth arch) appear	5
Chondrification of these two cartilages begins	7
Development and chondrification of arytenoid (fifth arch) and corniculate (fifth arch) (vocal process is the last to develop)	12
Chondrification of the epiglottis	20
Development of the cuneiform cartilage (fourth arch)	28

TABLE 10-6.   DEVELOPMENT OF PARANASAL SINUSES

Sinus	Characteristics	Age
Maxillary	Arises as a prolongation of the ethmoid infundibulum	12 wk
	Pneumatizes	At birth
	Reaches stable size	18 yr
Frontal	Arises from the upper anterior area of the middle meatus	Starts at late fetal life or even after birth
	Pneumatizes	After 1 yr
	Full size	20 yr
Sphenoid	Arises from the epithelial outgrowth of the upper posterior region of the nasal cavity in close relation with the sphenoid bone	Starts at 3rd fetal mo
	Pneumatizes	During childhood
	Full size	15 yr
Ethmoid	Arises from the evagination of the nasal mucosa into the lateral ethmoid mass	6th fetal mo
	Pneumatization completed	7 yr
	Full size	12 yr

OSSIFICATION OF LARYNGEAL SKELETON

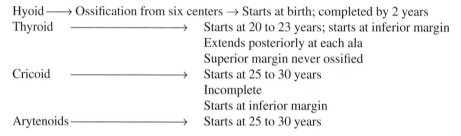

Hyoid ⟶ Ossification from six centers → Starts at birth; completed by 2 years

Thyroid ⟶ Starts at 20 to 23 years; starts at inferior margin
Extends posteriorly at each ala
Superior margin never ossified

Cricoid ⟶ Starts at 25 to 30 years
Incomplete
Starts at inferior margin

Arytenoids ⟶ Starts at 25 to 30 years

MIDDLE EAR CLEFT
Embryology of the Ear and Congenital Deformities (Tables 10-7A and B)

1. Embryology of the ear
   a. External ear
   b. Middle ear
   c. Inner ear
   d. Facial nerve
2. Congenital deformities
   a. Incidents
   b. Congenital hearing loss
   c. Common syndromes
   d. Microtia, atresia, grading
   e. External ear deformities
   f. Evaluation of congenital hearing loss
   g. Audiology
3. Radiology
4. Management
   a. Reconstruction of the pinna
   b. Atresia
   c. Alternative treatments

TABLE 10-7A. EMBRYOLOGY OF THE EAR

Week	External Ear	Middle Ear	Inner Ear	Facial Nerve
3–5	Ectoderm—first branchial groove Endoderm—first branchial pouch	2nd branchial pouch—middle ear space, 2nd mesenchymal arch—stapes arch	Neuroectoderm + ectoderm—otic placode evolves to otic pit, vesicle, and endolymphatic duct and sac; ventral—vestibule; dorsal—cochlea, acoustic ganglion; superior—vestibular; inferior—cochlear, otic capsule from mesenchyme tissue	Primoridal facial–acoustic—sensory fibers: chordae tympani n., nervus intermedius, geniculate ganglion, greater superficial petrosal n.
6–9	1st–2nd arch form hillocks of His 1st arch 1 tragus 2 helical crus 3 helix 2nd arch 4 antihelix 5 antitragus 6 loblule	Malleus & incus—single mesenchymal mass, mesenchymal stapes footplate; Meckel's cartilage—head & neck of malleus, body & short process of incus; Reichert's cartilage—manubrium of malleus, long process of incus, stapes arch	Semicircular canals, macula divides: upper—utricle, lower—saccule; cochlea—2½ turns wks. 6–8.5	VII & VIII separate, extends to facial muscles, fallopian canal evolves as sulcus 9th wk. and fuses with Reichert's cartilage
10–14	Hillocks fuse—auricle	Stapes arch formed, 4 mucosal pouches formed: anterior—ant. pouch of von Trolch; medius—petrous & epitympanium; superior—post. pouch of von Trolch, mastoid; posterior—oval & round window niche, sinus tympani	Vestibular end-organs formed, otolithic membrane, macula, cochlea tectorial membrane, scala tympani, fissula ante fenestram, fossula post fenestram	Extensive facial branching, location anterior in relation to external ear
15–20	Auricle recognizable, tympanic ring formed	Ossicles adult size, ossification begins	Membranous labyrinth complete without end-organs, ossification begins at 14 sites	Located anterior & superficial, migration posterior
21–28	EAC Epithelial core reabsorbs, complete 28th wk.	Drum formed 28th wk.; ectoderm–squamous; mesoderm—fibrous; entoderm—mucosal	Ossification complete 23rd wk.; last to ossify fissula ante fenestram, fossula post fenestram; cochlea structures formed	Fallopian canal closes and ossifies
30–Birth	Auricle and ear canal continued to grow to age 9 yrs.	Middle ear air space formed; tympanic ring ossifies by age 3 yrs.; eustachian tube grows 17–36 mm.	Membranous and bony labyrinth adult size; endolymphatic sac grows until adulthood	Facial n. lateral until mastoid tip formed at age 3 yrs.; 25% fallopian canals dehiscent

From Sataloff RT, *Embryology and Anomalies of the Facial Nerve and Their Surgical Implications.* New York: Raven Press, 1991.

TABLE 10-7A. *Continued*

Grade	Microtia	Atresis
I	Slight deformity of pinna	EAC normal—atretic, ossicles–deformed or fixed, abnormal course of facial n.
II	Deformed cartilage framework of pinna	Atresia, absent tympanic bone, small middle ear space, deformed ossicles, facial n. anterior & lateral
III	Soft tissue remnant of pinna	Middle and inner ear deformities
IV	Anotia	Severe inner ear deformities: Shibe—collapse of cochlear duct, deformed organ of Corti; Michelle—absent inner ear

Congenital deformities incidence: Microtia 0.13–6 per 1000 live births; atresia 1.2–5.5 per 1000 births; ossicular abnormalities 2% of patients having stapes surgery; bilateral deformities 10%

Congenital hearing loss: Sensorineural 85%; conductive 15% with external deformities in 50%.

Common syndromes associated with conductive hearing loss: Mandibulofacial dysostosis (Treacher Collins); hemifacial microsomia; oculoauricular vertebral dysplasia (Goldenhar); craniofacial dysostosis (Crouzon's disease)

TABLE 10-7B. MICROTIA–ATRESIA

External ear deformities:

  Preauricular pits & sinuses:
    Etiology: failure of complete closure 1st & 2nd branchial arch hillock
    Incidence: white 0.18%, black 1.49%
    Pathology: epithelial lined tract, may be associated with chronic inflammation, may extend to tragus or scaphoid fossa
    Management: observation unless infected; excision of complete fistula tract

  Auricular deformities:
    Microtia grade I–IV often associated with atresis grade I–IV; protruding ear–cupped ear–deep conchal bowl; helical & antihelical rim deformities
    Management: dependent on severity of deformity; otoplasty—reconstruction

  Evaluation Congenital Hearing Loss & Deformities:
    Audiology: Birth—Otoacoustic Emissions (OAE); Brain stem Evoked Response Audiometry (BERA); play audiometry 1½ yrs. of age
    Atresia: 60–70 dB conductive loss
    Stapes fixation: 50–65 dB conductive loss; presence of a Carhart notch may suggest abnormal course of facial nerve and need for a fenestration
    Ossicular abnormalities: 25–50 dB conductive loss
    Facial nerve impinging on stapes: 20–35 dB conductive loss

  Radiology: Computed Tomography (CT) thin 0.75–1.5-mm sections, axial and coronal views; sensorineural hearing loss—early childhood; conductive hearing loss—prior to reconstruction

Management
    Amplification: 6 mo. of age hearing aids, sound stimulation
    Cochlear implant: age 2–3 yrs with profound sensorineural hearing loss
    Bone anchored hearing device considered for nonsurgical patients—age 6 yrs
    Surgical Reconstruction:
    Reconstruction of pinna prior to EAC and middle ear; age 5–8 yrs, depending on size of opposite ear. Four stages: 1. Bury carved rib cartilage skeleton of pinna. 2. Construct lobule. 3. Elevate helical rim and graft postauricular sulcus. 4. Construct conchal bowl and tragus, may be combined with atresia surgery.

    Atresia, middle ear reconstruction: Indications—conductive hearing loss >30 dB, bone conduction <20 dB, aerated and accessible middle ear space. Reconstruction 70% tympanoplasty—ear canal, drum, and ossicular chain, stapes and oval window 17%, 60% have additional ossicular abnormalities, facial nerve covers the oval window 13% requiring fenestration of the horizontal canal.

    Alternative treatment: Bone anchored auricular prosthesis and hearing aid; no treatment with normal or aidable opposite ear.

References

1. Goodwin WJ, Godley F. Developmental anatomy and physiology of the nose and paranasal sinuses. In: Lee KJ, ed. *Textbook of Otolaryngology and Head and Neck Surgery* New York: Elsevier Science Publishing Co., Inc., 1989.

2. Smith HW. The atlas of cleft lip and cleft palate surgery. In: Lee KJ, ed. *Comprehensive Surgical Atlases in Otolaryngology and Head and Neck Surgery* New York: Grune & Stratton, 1983.

3. Sataloff RT. *Embryology and Anomalies of the Facial Nerve and Their Surgical Implications* New York: Raven Press, 1990.

4. Jafek BW, Nager GT, Strife J, et al. Congenital Atresia of the Ear and Analysis of 311 Cases and Transactions American Academy Ophthalmol., Otolaryngol., 1975;80:588–595.

5. Anson BJ, Donaldson JA. *The Ear: Developmental Anatomy and Surgical Anatomy of the Temporal Bone.* 3rd ed.; Philadelphia: WB Sanders Company, 1981, 23–57.

6. Lambert PR. Congenital aural atresia. In: Bailey ed. *Head & Neck Surgery–Otolaryngology* Philadelphia: Lippincott–Raven, 1998, 1997–2010.

7. Hough JVD. Malformations and anatomical variations seen in the middle ear during operation for mobilization of the stapes. *Laryngoscope* 1958;68:1337–1379.

8. De la Cruz A, Linthicum FH, Luxford W. Congenital atresia of the external auditory canal, *Laryngoscope* 1985;95:421–27.

9. Schuknecht HF. Mondini dysplasia. *Ann Otol Rhinol Laryngol* 1980;89(Suppl 65):1–23.

10. Farrior J. Management of congenital hearing loss. *Adv Plast Reconstr Surg* 1989:217–236.

11. Belluci RJ. Congenital aural malformations, diagnosis and treatment. *Otolaryngol Clin North Am* 1981;14:95–124.

12. Jahrsdoerfer R. Congenital malformations of the ear. *Ann Otolaryngol* 1980;89:348–53.

13. Farrior J, Rophie S. Fenestration of the horizontal semicircular canal and congenital conductive deafness. *Laryngoscope* 1985;95:1025–1036.

14. Miyamoto RT, Myres WA, Pope ML, et al. Cochlear implants for deaf children. *Laryngoscope* 1986;96:990–996.

15. Bauer BS. Management and therapy of congenital malformations and traumatic deformities of the ear. In: Alberti PW, Reuben RJ, eds. *Otologic Medicine and Surgery.* Vol. 2. New York: Churchill Livingstone: 1988, 1025–1072.

16. Reuben RJ. Management and therapy of congenital malformations of the external and middle ear. In: Alberti PW, Reuben LJ, eds. *Otologic Medicine and Surgery.* Vol. 2. New York: Churchill Livingstone: 1988, 1135–1151.

17. Bardach J. Surgery for congenital and acquired malformations of the auricle. *Otolaryngology Head and Neck Surgery.* Vol. 4. *Ear and Skull Base.* Edited by Cummings, Fredrickson, Harker, Krause, Schuller, St. Louis: Mosby, 1986, 2861–2898.

Cleft Lip and Palate 11

INCIDENCE AND EPIDEMIOLOGY

Cleft Lip −/+ Palate (see Table 11-1)

1. The incidence of cleft lip/palate (CL +/− P) is approximately 1 per 1000 live births.
2. The incidence of CL +/− P varies considerably according to race:

American Indians	3.6:1000
Japanese	2.1:1000
Chinese	1.7:1000
Caucasians	1:1000
Blacks	0.7:1000

3. 14% of CL +/− P defects are associated with syndromes.
4. Two-thirds of the CL +/− P defects occur in males; the more severe the defect, the more males are affected.
5. Cleft defects are unilateral in 80% of patients and bilateral in 20%.
6. Cleft palate is associated with 70% of unilateral defects and 80% of bilateral defects.
7. Cleft defects are left-sided in two-thirds of patients and right sided in one-third.

Cleft Palate

1. The incidence of cleft palate (CP) alone is 1 per 2500 live births.
2. The incidence of CP is greater in females (three-quarters).
3. 33% of CP defects are associated with syndromes.
4. More than 300 genetic conditions have been associated with cleft palate, including

   Stickler's syndrome
   Velocardiofacial syndrome
   Pierre Robin sequence

5. The incidence of submucous cleft palate is 1 per 1600 births.
6. The incidence of bifid uvula is 1 per 80 live births.

ETIOLOGY

1. Development of CL +/− P and CP is strongly dependent on genetic factors.
2. Clefting is heterogeneous and results also from environmental insults.
3. Environmental factors likely capable of inducing clefting:

   Fetal alcohol exposure
   Cigarette smoking
   Folic acid deficiency or antagonists
   Phenytoin
   Retinoic acid derivatives
   Amniotic band syndrome
   Maternal diabetes

4. Multivitamins with folic acid likely reduce the incidence of clefting.

248

TABLE 11-1. WHAT ARE THE NEXT CHILD'S CHANCES OF A CLEFTING DEFECT?

	Cleft Lip +/− Cleft Palate (%)	Cleft Palate (%)
Parents normal, first child affected		
No affected relatives	4	2
Affected relatives	4	7
Parents normal, two affected relatives	9	10
One parent, no affected children	4	6
One parent, one affected child	17	15

EMBRYOLOGY (SEE FIGURE 11-1)

1. The critical period of palatal development is from 8 to 12 weeks.
2. The critical period for CL +/− P development is from 4 to 6 weeks.
3. The five facial primordia appear around the stomodeum (primitive mouth) early in the fourth week.

    Frontonasal prominence—proliferation of mesenchyme ventral to the forebrain
    Paired *maxillary prominences*—first branchial arch structures forming sides
    Paired *mandibular processes*—first branchial arch structures forming caudal boundary

4. The *nasal placodes* form inferior to the frontonasal prominence and develop into *medial and lateral nasal prominences.*
5. At 6 to 7 weeks, the medial nasal prominences merge with each other and the lateral maxillary processes to form the *intermaxillary segment,* which gives rise to the

    Philtrum
    Premaxilla
    Primary palate (median palatine process)
    Nasal tip

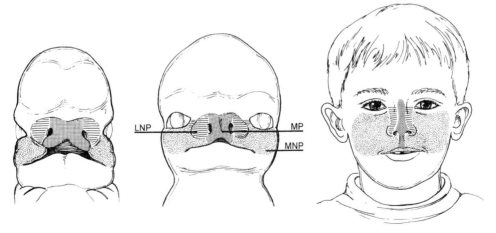

Figure 11-1. Embryologic development of the midface demonstrating the contributions of the maxillary prominence (MP) and medial nasal prominence (MNP) to the lip and the contributions of the medial nasal prominence and lateral nasal prominence (LNP) to the nose.

6. The lateral maxillary prominences form the

    Lateral lip
    Lateral maxilla
    Secondary palate
    Lateral nasal ala

7. The lateral maxillary prominences form the shelf-like *lateral palatine processes.* As the tongue moves inferiorly, the processes elongate and move horizontally to fuse and form the secondary palate.
8. The nasal septum grows inferiorly from the fused median nasal prominences and fuses ventrally to dorsally with the palate from 9 to 12 weeks.
9. The palatine processes fuse about a week later in girls, which may explain the increased incidence of CP in females.
10. Failure of fusion of the medial nasal prominences with the maxillary prominences results in minimal to complete CL +/– P.
11. Failure of fusion of the lateral palatine processes results in CP.
12. The precise mechanism of abnormal development leading to clefting (deficient mesenchymal proliferation, disrupted flow of neural crest cells, altered programmed cell death) is incompletely understood.

CLASSIFICATION

1. Multiple classification systems exist to describe cleft lip and cleft palate anomalies.
2. Basic classification methods divide clefts into

    CL +/– P
    CP
    Unilateral
    Bilateral
    Complete
    Incomplete

3. Because of the myriad possibilities, diagrams and photographic documentation should be included in cleft descriptions.

MANAGEMENT
General Philosophy

1. The care of cleft patients is complex and should be coordinated by a cleft team. Team members should include a

    Cleft surgeon
    Orthodontist
    Oral surgeon
    Audiologist
    Speech language pathologist
    Otolaryngologist
    Geneticist
    Pediatrician
    Social worker/psychologist

2. Feeding difficulties need early assessment and management to optimize infant growth at 5 to 8 oz per week. Minimal accepted weight gain is $\frac{1}{2}$ oz per day with the help of

   A modified nipple
   A compressible feeder
   Alteration of feeding position
   Concentrated formula

3. Airway issues may require early management.
4. Speech problems are found in 25% of cleft patients.
5. Cleft palate is associated with COME (chronic otitis media with effusion) in 95% of patients.
6. Psychological issues of grief, guilt, anger, and inadequacy necessitate early intervention with the parents and family.
7. Patients with CL +/− P will require multiple surgical procedures throughout their childhood and into adolescence. (See Table 11-2.)

Unilateral Cleft Lip (See Figure 11-2)

Defect

1. The orbicularis muscle is oriented upward, parallel to cleft margins, and the orbicularis sphincter is disrupted.
2. The maxilla is hypoplastic on the cleft side.
3. The nasal ala on the cleft side is inferiorly, posteriorly, and laterally displaced.
4. The columella is displaced to the noncleft side.
5. The medial crus is shorter and the lateral crus is longer on the cleft lower lateral cartilage (LLC).
6. The dome on the cleft side is lower, resulting in alar flattening and horizontal nostril shape.
7. The alveolar defect passes through the developing dentition.
8. The nasal floor is absent.
9. The caudal septum is deviated to the noncleft side, and there is an obstructing septal spur on the cleft side.

Surgical Repair (See Figure 11-3)

1. The goals of primary repair of CL include

   Correct alignment of the orbicularis oris muscle
   Correct alignment of the vermilion and Cupid's bow

TABLE 11-2. TIMING OF CLEFT SURGERY

Procedure	Age
Primary lip repair	3 months
Tip rhinoplasty	3 months
Tympanostomy tubes	3 months
Palatoplasty	9–18 months
Speech evaluation	3–4 years
VPI evaluation and repair (if necessary)	4–6 years
Alveolar bone grafting	7–11 years
Nasal reconstruction	14–18 years
Orthognathic surgery	> 16 years

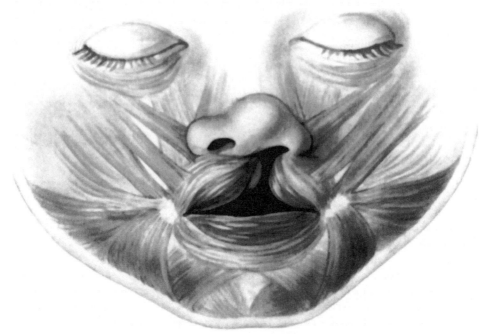

Figure 11-2. Muscles of the unilateral cleft lip deformity. Note the dehiscence of the orbicularis muscle sphincter and the insertion of the muscle along the edges of the cleft. In addition, the columella is deviated away from the cleft side, and the ala on the side of the cleft is displaced laterally and inferiorly. (From Ref. 9, with permission.)

> Creation of a nasal floor and sill
> Symmetric placement of the alar base and columella
> Camouflage and minimization of scarring

2. Assessment of the lip defect with the pinch test may indicate the need for lip adhesion or taping prior to definitive repair.
3. The Millard rotation advancement repair rotates the medial lip segment downward and advances the lateral lip segment. (See Figure 11-2.)

> Most common repair in the United States.
> Advantages include creation of scar that simulates philtral column, allows primary correction of cleft nasal deformity, and flexibility of repair.
> Disadvantages include difficulty with wide clefts and creation of a small nostril.

4. The Tennison-Randall triangular flap repair utilizes a lateral, inferiorly based triangular flap and z-plasty transposition.

> Advantages include utility with wide clefts and minimal discarding of tissue.
> Disadvantages include z-shaped scar and lack of flexibility with need for precise measurements.

5. Initial treatment of the nasal deformity should occur at the time of primary cleft repair (primary rhinoplasty).

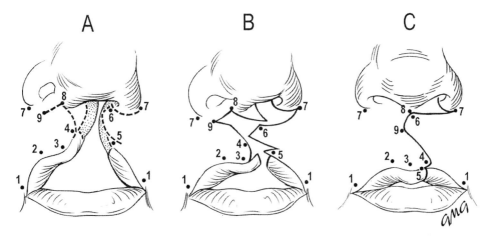

Figure 11-3. The Millard repair of cleft lip consists of a rotation of the noncleft side and advancement of the cleft side. A. Points are drawn on the patient to plan the rotation and advancement. The distance 1–2 equals the distance 1–5, and the distance 2–3 equals the distance 3–4. B. A back cut is made to point 9 to allow for rotation of the noncleft side. C. The flaps are then brought into correct anatomic position and closed in layers with meticulous closure of the orbicularis muscle and vermilion border.

Bilateral Cleft Lip (See Figure 11-4)

Defect
1. Muscle fibers are absent in the prolabial segment.
2. The levator palatini muscle is primarily responsible for elevating the palate.
3. The vermilion is absent in the prolabial segment.
4. The prolabial segment has diminished blood supply.
5. The prolabium is underdeveloped vertically and overdeveloped horizontally.
6. The columella is short.
7. The nasal floor and sill are absent bilaterally.
8. The central portion of alveolar arch is displaced anteriorly and superiorly.
9. The premaxilla is mobile.
10. The nasal tip is widened.

Surgical Repair
1. The goals of surgical repair in bilateral cleft are identical to those in unilateral cleft.
2. The bilateral cleft can be closed in a single procedure, which offers the following advantages:

   Increased lip and nasal symmetry
   Mucosa lined labial sulcus
   Good orbicularis oris muscle function

3. The bilateral defect can be repaired in stages:

   Widest cleft repaired first.
   Second cleft repaired several months later.

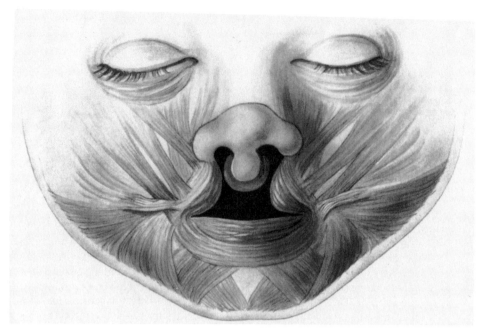

Figure 11-4.   Musculature of the bilateral cleft lip deformity. Note the absence of orbicularis muscle in the prolabial segment and the shortened columella. (From Ref. 9, with permission.)

Staged repair results in poor orbicularis oris muscle function.
Lip can eventually be too long.
Trifurcation scar beneath columella is difficult to camouflage.

Cleft Palate (See Figure 11-5)

Defect
1.   The velopharyngeal sling is disrupted; the muscles insert into the medial margins of the cleft and the posterior hard palate.
2.   The cleft may involve only the soft palate, the hard palate (secondary palate), or the complete primary and secondary palate.
3.   The nasal and oral cavities communicate freely, resulting in velopharyngeal insufficiency.
4.   A submucous cleft palate may be difficult to diagnose. The classic physical findings are

Zona pellucida (hyperlucent gray area in midline soft palate).
Bifid uvula.
Notch in posterior hard palate.
Nasopharyngoscopy during speech is the most sensitive diagnostic tool.

Surgical Repair
1.   The surgical goals of palate repair are

Separation of the oral and nasal cavities
Construction of a levator sling that results in velopharyngeal valving and adequate eustachian tube function

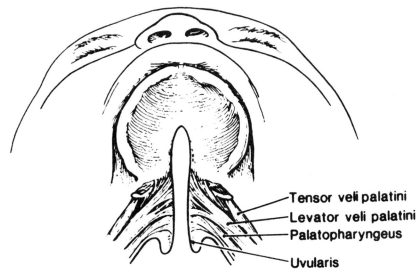

Figure 11-5. Schematic diagram of a cleft of the secondary palate indicating the abnormal muscles of the soft palate. Note the abnormal insertion of the muscles along the edge of the cleft. (From Ref. 9, with permission.)

> Preservation of midfacial growth
> Development of functional dentition

2. Early and aggressive palatal repair can result in abnormal midfacial growth.
3. Delayed palatal closure can result in significant speech disorders.
4. *Von Langenbeck's palatoplasty* advances bipedicled mucoperiosteal flaps.

> Easy to perform
> Decreased denuded palatal bone
> Does not provide increased palatal length

5. *V-Y push-back palatoplasty* retrodisplaces two posteriorly based mucoperiosteal flaps by a V-to-Y closure technique.

> Lengthens the palate
> Leaves a large, raw palatal surface

6. *Two-flap palatoplasty* utilizes two posteriorly placed mucoperiosteal flaps that extend to the alveolar cleft.

> Good for complete clefts of palate/alveolus

7. The *Schweckendiek two-stage repair* closes the soft palate cleft and leaves the hard palate cleft for obturation with a prosthesis until delayed closure at 4 to 5 years.

> Minimal disturbance of facial growth
> Requires frequent changes of prosthesis
> Results in significant speech disorders if not properly obturated
> Not frequently used

8. A successful palatoplasty relies on the creation of a levator muscular sling. The *intervelar veloplasty* completely dissects the veli palatini muscle to recreate the velopharyngeal sling.

9. The *Furlow palatoplasty* utilizes a double reversing Z-plasty of musculomucosa and mucosa only flaps to repair the palatal cleft.

Usually used for submucosal or soft-palate clefts.
Good speech results with proper muscle alignment.
Difficult for wide clefts.

ASSOCIATED PROBLEMS

Otologic Disease

1. Virtually all patients with cleft palate have middle ear disease.
2. The incidence of middle ear disease decreases with age.
3. Factors contributing to eustachian tube dysfunction in cleft patients include

Ineffective tubal dilation of tensor veli palatini secondary to muscular hypoplasia and malposition
Nasopharyngeal reflux and contamination of the eustachian tube orifice

4. Ventilation tubes are placed in cleft palate patients at the time of primary lip repair.

Speech

Diagnosis of Velopharyngeal Insufficiency

1. Velopharyngeal insufficiency (VPI) results in hypernasal speech and nasal escape in CP patients often even after cleft repair.
2. Hypernasal speech is due to the conspicuous amount of nasal cavity resonance that results from inappropriate acoustic coupling of the nasopharynx and oropharynx during sounds other than /m/, /n/, and /ng/.
3. Nasal escape is the audible passage of air through an incompetent sphincter. This will fog a mirror held beneath the nostril during speech.
4. VPI evaluation includes:

History and physical
Speech evaluation
Nasopharyngoscopy
Multiview videofluoroscopy
Audiometry

Treatment of Velopharyngeal Insufficiency

1. The defect in closure during speech will direct the surgical or prosthetic management. Lateral, anteroposterior (AP) or posterior (Passavant's ridge) wall motion is noted.
2. Initial treatment of VPI consists of speech therapy.
3. Failure of speech therapy to improve VPI in 6 to 12 months indicates the need for more aggressive therapy.
4. Dental obturator prostheses can improve VPI.

Indicated in poor surgical candidates and surgical failures.
Requires frequent resizing and modification.

5. Pharyngeal implants and rolls can create an artificial Passavant's ridge.

6. Orticochea sphincteroplasty utilizes lateral pharyngeal flaps to narrow the pharynx and augment the posterior wall.

   Ideal in patients with good AP motion and poor lateral wall motion.

7. A pharyngeal flap utilizes a posterior pharyngeal mucosa/muscle flap to create two lateral ports.

   Ideal in patients with good lateral wall motion and poor AP motion.

References

1. Cotton RT, Meyers ET III, eds: *Practical Pediatric Otolaryngology.* Philadelphia: Lippincott-Raven, 1999.
2. Millard DR Jr: *Cleft Craft, the Evolution of Its Surgery.* Boston: Little Brown, 1980.
3. Mosher G: Genetic counseling in cleft lip and palate. *Ear Nose Throat J* 65:330–336, 1986.
4. Myer CM III, Cotton RT, Wiatrak BJ: Cleft lip and palate. In Lee KJ, ed. *Essential Otolaryngology,* 6th ed. New Hyde Park, NY: Medical Examination Publishing Co., 1995.
5. Ness JA, Sykes JM: Basics of the Millard rotation-advancement technique for repair of the unilateral cleft lip deformity. In: *Facial Plastic Surgery.* New York: Thieme, 1993.
6. Wardill WEM: Techniques of operation for cleft palate. *Br J Surg* 25:117, 1937.
7. Kilner TP: Cleft lip and palate repair technique. *St Thomas Hosp Rep* 2:127, 1937.
8. Furlow LT Jr: Cleft palate repair by double opposing Z-plasty. *Plast Reconstr Surg* 78:724, 1986.
9. Sykes JM, Senders CW: Pathologic anatomy of cleft lip and palate. *Biol Basis Fac Plast Surg* 5:57–71, 1993.

Immunology and Allergy   12

The immune system is composed of a complex set of elements designed to distinguish "self" from "nonself." This system protects against foreign pathogens while not responding adversely to self components. This distinction is made possible by an elaborate, specific recognition system that is composed of receptors on T and B lymphocytes—the *only immunologically specific components* of the immune apparatus. There are also nonspecific effector mechanisms that include phagocytes, leukocytes, and complement.

The immune system has distinct features that help serve its function:

Specificity: Mediated through the antigen-specific receptors on the surfaces of T and B lymphocytes and antibodies.

Memory: The initial immune response to an antigen stimulus usually leaves the immune system changed. A second exposure to antigen results in an amplified response.

Mobility: The elements of the immune system can circulate. This includes T and B cells, immunoglobulins (Ig), complement, hematopoietic cells, and cytokines.

Replicability: The cellular components of the immune system can replicate or clone. This feature allows for greater amplification of responses.

Specificity and memory are so crucial in immunologic responses that they may be used as criteria for defining what is and is not immunologic. For example, reactions to sulfites and aspirin seem neither to be specific nor to have memory; therefore, they are not immunologic.

SPECIFIC IMMUNITY

T and B lymphocytes and immunoglobulins generate specific immunity. This specificity is mediated through the antigen-specific receptors on the surfaces of T and B lymphocytes and through antibodies. The T and B lymphocytes are the *only* immunologically specific components of the immune apparatus.

Specific immunity is the second line of defense, after the nonspecific response of macrophages, natural killer cells, and polymorphonuclear leukocytes. This type of recognition of foreign antigens is specific and has memory. It is mediated by the action of the following proteins:

Antigen: Originally named as the *anti*body and *gen*erator molecule to which antibody and T-cell antigen receptor bind; any molecule that can be specifically recognized by the specific immune system (T cells, B cells, or both).

Antibody: A specific immunoglobulin (Ig) produced by a specific B cell that recognizes and binds to specific molecules (antigens) recognized as nonself.

T-cell antigen receptor: A specific protein on T-cell surfaces that binds to specific antigens. Memory for a specific antigen results from memory T and B cells that are generated after initial contact with a foreign antigen. They produce either a faster and more vigorous response during the next encounter with the foreign substance (anamnestic response, positive immunologic memory), a lesser response, or a non-response (acquired tolerance, negative immunologic memory).

NONSPECIFIC IMMUNITY

This type of foreign antigen recognition is nonspecific and the organism has no memory of previous contacts. This is in contrast to lymphocytes, which are the unique bearers of immunologic specificity. The full development of an immune response requires that non-lymphoid cells and molecules act primarily as amplifiers and modifiers.

Examples of nonspecific immune amplifiers and modifiers include

1. Polymorphonuclear leukocytes and monocytes
2. Antigen-presenting cells
3. Complement
4. Interleukins
5. Interferons
6. Other cytokines (ie, tumor necrosis factor)
7. Many other biologic systems—skin- and surface-lining barriers, stomach acid, lysozyme, and commensal organisms that prevent overgrowth by pathogens.

ORGANS AND TISSUES OF THE IMMUNE SYSTEM

The cellular immune system is classified into two parts based on the two lines of differentiation from stem cells: the lymphoid and the myeloid (Table 12-1, Figure 12-1).

Lymphoid System

The Primary Lymphoid System

This includes the major sites of lymphopoiesis (proliferation and differentiation): the thymus and the bone marrow. They produce about 10^9 lymphocytes a day.

1. THYMUS   The thymus is a compound organ. It develops from the third and fourth pharyngeal pouches. Thymus cells are believed to be critical for the development of major histocompatibility complex (MHC) restriction, which is imposed on lymphoid precursors that arise from the yolk sac, fetal liver, and bone marrow. The thymus exercises control over the entire immune system by modifying lymphocytes that pass through it. It produces fully immunocompetent "thymus derived" cells or T lymphocytes.

TABLE 12-1. CELLULAR IMMUNE SYSTEM

Lymphoid (Produces Lymphocytes)	Myeloid (Produces Phagocytes)
T-helper and suppressor cytotoxic cells	Platelets
	Eosinophils
B cells and plasma cells	Neutrophils
Null cells (large granular lymphocytes),	Basophils and mast cells
includes cytotoxic lymphocytes	Monocytes and macrophages

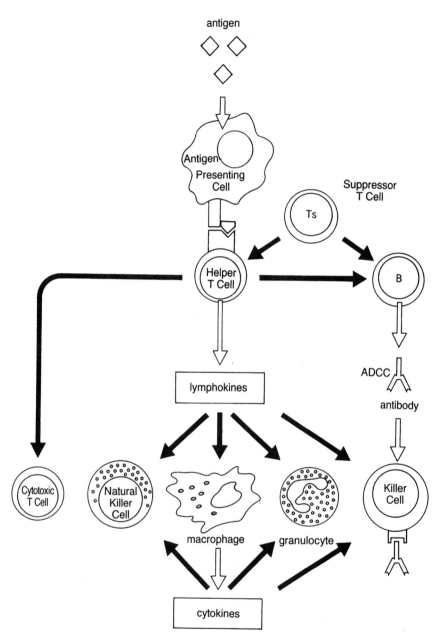

Figure 12-1.   Major cells of the immune response.

2. Bone marrow   Generates precursors of both T and B lymphocytes and other hematopoietic precursors—i.e., granulocytes, erythrocytes, and megakaryocytes.

The Secondary Lymphoid System

This system provides the environment that enhances antigen-effector cell interactions and includes Waldeyer's ring, lymph nodes, spleen, and mucosa-associated lymphoid tissue (MALT—i.e., Peyer's patches). The secondary lymphoid system is a rich source of memory T cells that can respond quickly to subsequent antigen challenges.

Lymph nodes (LNs) have both afferent and efferent lymphatics.

1. Cortex: B cells
2. Paracortex: T cells, antigen-presenting cells
3. Medulla: T and B cells, plasma cells

LN act like lymphoid filters in the vascular tree and are important sites of antibody production.

1. **Lymph nodes:** Act like lymphoid filters within the lymphatic circulatory system. Regional lymph nodes respond to antigens introduced proximally.
2. **Thoracic duct:** A rich source of mature T cells. A chylous fistula can cause T-cell depletion and immunosuppression.

Mucosa-Associated Lymphoid Tissue (MALT)   MALT consists of dispersed aggregates of nonencapsulated lymphoid tissue found in the lamina propria and submucosa of the gastrointestinal, respiratory, and urogenital tracts. It includes the tonsils and adenoids and comprises the bulk of the body's immune tissue. Important for the local immune response at mucosal surfaces, MALT produces secretory IgA and may promote differentiation of precursor B cells into B lymphocytes. MALT has efferent lymphatics only.

Tonsils and Adenoids   These organs are important in IgA production. A system of channels or clefts covered by specialized epithelium allows intimate contact between antigens in the upper aerodigestive tract and immune-competent cells. M cells in the specialized epithelium transport the antigens into a tubovesicular system that allows lymphocytes to approach to within 1 μm of the lumen. Antigen-presenting cells include macrophages, dendritic cells, endothelial cells, and epithelial cells. Beneath the specialized epithelium lie many lymphoid follicles and germinal centers. The extrafollicular space surrounding the follicles contains abundant vasculature, including postcapillary venules, through which circulating lymphocytes gain access to the tonsils (Figure 12-2). The major immune function of the tonsils is generation of antigen-specific B cells in the follicles. The B cells then produce specific secretory IgA within the tonsil or after they migrate to surrounding structures, including, probably, the major and minor salivary glands.

Cluster of Differentiation (CD) Classification System

Cell surface antigens vary depending on lineage (lymphoid, myeloid), stage of maturation, or degree of immune activation. Patterns of cell surface antigens can be correlated with the function of the cells. The CD system is used to describe antigens on the surface of immune system cells. This system is based on computer correlations of groups of monoclonal antibodies that recognize specific cell surface antigens (Table 12-2).

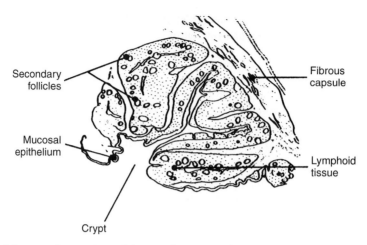

Figure 12-2.   Microscopic structure of the tonsil.

Major Cell Types of the Immune Response: T, B, and Null

T Cells

1.   T cells are classified into many different subsets, depending on the pattern of cell surface antigens. The most important antigens are

    a.   CD2, CD3 (all T cells)

    b.   CD4 (helper/inducer)

       (1)   60% of peripheral T cells

       (2)   Augment T-T, T-B, and T-macrophage interactions

TABLE 12-2. SELECTED CELL DIFFERENTIATION ANTIGENS

Antigen	Previous Designations	Distribution	Comments
CD2	T-11, Leu-5, LFA 2	All T, NK	Receptor for sheep RBCs; accessory molecule for T-APC interaction
CD3	T3, Leu-4	All mature T	Associated with TcR for antigen
CD4	T4, Leu-3	50–70% mature T	Associated with class II HLA-restricted response; often called a marker for helper T cells; receptor for HIV
CD8	T8, Leu-2	30–40% mature T	Associated with class I HLA-restricted responses; often called a marker for "cytotoxic-suppressor" T cells; reciprocal with CD4
CD11b	Leu-15, OKMI	Monocytes, NK, granulocytes, some T	Part of complement receptor No. 3; associated with CD18
CD16	Leu-11	NK, granulocytes	FcγIII
CD19 and 20	B4, B1	B	. . .
CD21	B2	B, dendritic cells	Complement receptor No. 2; EBV receptor
CD29	4B4	Some CD4+ and CD8+	"Memory" T-cell marker
CD35	. . .	All B, a few T, monocytes granulocytes	Complement receptor No. 1

(3)　Induce cytotoxic/suppressor cells (CD8+ cells)
(4)　Allergic inflammation is characterized by emphasis of T_H2 response over the T_H1 response (Figure 12-3).
(5)　T_H1 cells
　　(a)　Produce interleukin-2 (IL-2) and interferon gamma (IFN-γ) when activated
　　(b)　Produce cytotoxicity, local inflammation
　　(c)　Inhibit B cells
(6)　T_H2 cells
　　(a)　Produce IL-4, 5, 6, and 10
　　(b)　Stimulate B cells
c.　CD8 (cytotoxic/suppressor)
　(1)　20 to 30% of peripheral T cells
　(2)　Specific killing of target cells
　(3)　Inhibit the response of B cells and other T cells
　(4)　Important in immunologic tolerance

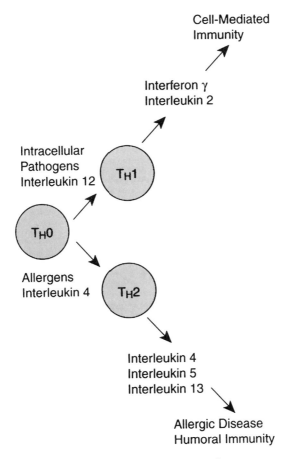

Figure 12-3. T_H1 and T_H2 effector cells.

Antigen specificity is conferred by the T-cell receptor, a cell surface polypeptide heterodimer associated with CD3 that is similar to Ig. T cells require that the antigen be presented in close association with a major histocompatibility complex (MHC) molecule on the antigen-presenting cell (class II MHC for T-helper cells, class I MHC for T-cytotoxic cells).

INTERLEUKINS   T cells produce IL-2 when activated; IL-1 induces proliferation of both T and B cells. T cells may need interleukin-1 (IL-1) produced by macrophages to become sensitive to the effects of IL-2 (Figure 12-4).

B Cells

B cells carry endogenously produced Igs on their surfaces, which act as antigen receptors. When activated by contact with an antigen, B cells differentiate into plasma cells and produce the specific Ig that they are genetically programmed to produce. B cells may be stimulated directly by an antigen, especially antigens with multiple repeating antigenic sequences, or they may require help from T cells and macrophages (Figures 12-1 and 12-4). B-cell characteristics include

1. They comprise 5 to 15% of circulating lymphocytes.
2. Their surface Ig is mostly IgM.
3. They are positive for CD19, 20, and 22.
4. They carry MHC class II antigens on their surface.

Null Cells

These cells are large, granular lymphocytes that are neither T nor B cells (Figure 12-1). They function as

1. Natural killer cells—nonspecific lymphoid cells that are able to eliminate cells which spontaneously become malignant. Characteristics:
   a. 15% of blood lymphocytes
   b. Positive for CD16, 56

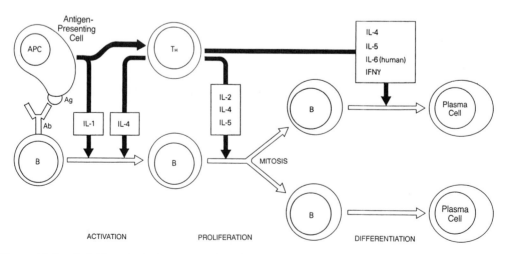

Figure 12-4. Cytokines in the immune response.

c.   Also cytotoxic for virus-infected cells

d.   Have IgG receptors

2.   K (killer) cells in antibody-dependent cytotoxicity (ADCC); they have cell surface Fc receptors for IgG.

Immune Response

The binding of a specific antigen in the presence of accessory cells (i.e., macrophages or helper T cells) activates lymphoid cells. Proliferation of specific clones of antigen-sensitive cells produces large populations of mature effector cells—i.e., plasma cells, cytotoxic T cells, and memory cells.

Myeloid Cells

There are three major myeloid cell types: macrophages, antigen-presenting cells (APCs), and polymorphonuclear (PMNs) granulocytes. The myeloid cells function mainly in phagocytic immunity and antigen presentation. Phagocytes include PMNs (neutrophils, basophils, eosinophils, and other granulocytes) (Table 12-3). APCs include cells of the macrophage/monocyte lineage.

Major Histocompatibility Complex (MHC) Proteins

The MHC is crucial in the immune response. MHC products control not only transplantation reactions but also the detailed regulation of all immune responses. The MHC molecule is a cell surface glycoprotein that is encoded in each species by the MHC gene complex.

The principal function of MHC molecules is to bind fragments of foreign protein, thereby forming complexes that are recognized by T lymphocytes (Figures 12-5 and 12-6). The MHC in humans is called the HLA complex, and its genes are on the short arm of chromosome 6. Class I MHC antigens include HLA-A, HLA-B, HLA-C. Class II MHC antigens include HLA-DP, HLA-DQ, HLA-DR.

Class I MHC molecules are membrane-associated glycoproteins present on nearly all nucleated cells. Class II MHC molecules are normally expressed only on B lymphocytes, macrophages of dendritic cells, endothelial cells, and a few other cells. The molecules of classes I and II have a general configuration similar to that of a typical Ig molecule; i.e., they

TABLE 12-3. POLYMORPHONUCLEAR GRANULOCYTES

Cells	% of Circulating Granulocytes	Substances Released When Activated	Function
Neutrophils	9%		Phagocytosis
Eosinophils	2–5%	Histaminase and aryl sulphatase inhibit histamine and leukotriene C4+D4 (slow reacting substance of anaphylaxis, SRS-A) released by mast cells; many cytokines	Probably involved in helminth infections. Potent release of mediators of the allergic inflammatory response
Basophils and mast cells	Basophils are 0.2%, probably related to mast cells	Histamine, heparin, leukotriene C4+D4 (SRS-A), eosinophil chemotactic factor of anaphylaxis (ECF-A), neutrophil chemotactic factor (NCF)	Granules are released usually by contact with an allergen that cross-links specific IgE on the cell surface

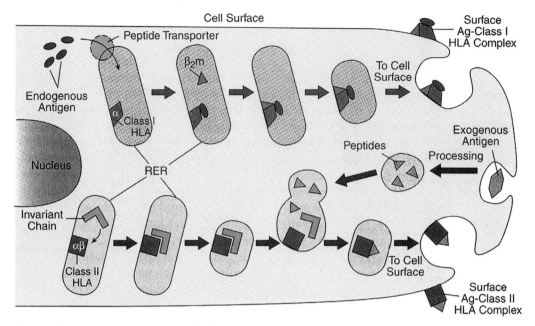

Figure 12-5. Antigen processing. Endogenous antigens are processed through the rough endo-plasmic reticulum and associated with class I molecules and B2 microglobulin, to be expressed on the cell surface. Exogenous antigens are hydrolyzed and associated with class II molecules on the cell surface.

are composed of polypeptide chains joined by disulfide bonds and have variable and common regions (Figure 12-6).

Cytokines—Soluble Mediators of the Immune Response

These immunoactive peptides were originally thought to be lymphocyte-derived and were called lymphokines. However, they are produced by virtually any cell type and are more appropriately termed *cytokines*. They modulate the function of virtually all cell types and help regulate immune responses. Cytokines are not antigen-specific but may be antigen-stimulated.

Types of Cytokines

1. Interferons (IFNs)—potent antiviral activity. A group of unrelated classes of polypep-tides that are released from cells in response to viral infection, double-stranded RNA, endotoxin, mitogens, and various antigens.
    a. Alpha
        (1) Made by leukocytes
        (2) Decreases viral replication, increases cell membrane proteins, and decreases lymphocyte mitogenesis
    b. Beta
        (1) Made by fibroblasts and epithelial cells
        (2) Functions are similar to alpha

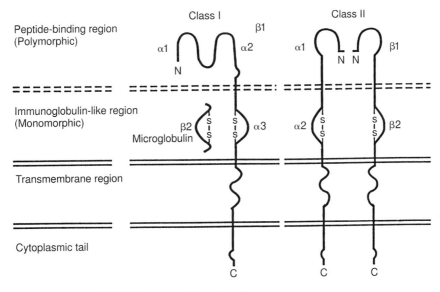

Figure 12-6. Structure of MHC class I and II molecules.

    c.   Gamma
        (1)   Made by activated T and NK cells
        (2)   Increases expression of cell membrane antigens, including class I and II HLA
             and Fc receptors
        (3)   Potent activator of eosinophils
  2.   Colony-stimulating factors (CSFs)—induce maturation of bone marrow precursor cells
      into circulating cells.
  3.   Tumor necrosis factors (TNFs)—have the capacity to destroy tumor cells by inducing
      hemorrhagic necrosis.
  4.   Interleukins—Largest, most heterogeneous, and *most important group* of cytokines.
      They deliver signals between cells and mediate action between cells of the immune sys-
      tem as well as between other cells.

      Cytokines are soluble glycoproteins released by cells in a highly regulated manner and act nonenzymatically to regulate host-cell functions. Together with cell- or matrix-mediated signals, cytokines form part of a complex cellular signaling language. Cytokines are involved in every aspect of immunity, including cellular differentiation, cellular activation and recruitment, antigen presentation, and adhesion molecule expression as well as acute- and late-phase allergic responses.

      Clinically significant allergen-induced reactions are generally characterized by an IgE-dependent biphasic response. Following exposure to allergens, atopic patients have an immediate reaction that is caused primarily by mast cell release of mediators and proteases. This phenomenon occurs within 15 to 60 minutes of allergen challenge and subsides within 30 to 90 minutes.

      Some 3 to 4 hours later, an intense inflammatory reaction, defined as the "late-phase response," occurs. During this period, the predominant cellular infiltration includes eosinophils, mononuclear cells, and, to a lesser extent, neutrophils. Eosinophils and neutro-phils reach their peak cellular accumulation in 6 to 8 hours. About 24 to 48 hours after a single allergen challenge, the cellular infiltration consists predominately of T cells and monocytes/macrophages. These T cells have been demonstrated by in situ hybridization to primarily express mRNA for interleukin (IL-4, IL-5) and granulocyte/macrophage colony-stimulating factor (GM-CSF).

The IgE-mediated late-phase response is thought to play an important role in the trig-gering of allergic diseases such as asthma, atopic dermatitis, and allergic rhinitis.

It has been demonstrated that IgE cross-linking on mast cells and basophils induces the synthesis and release of a variety of cytokines, including IL-1, IL-3, Il-4, IL-5, Il-6, GM-CSF, and TNF-α. These cytokines play a critical role in inducing the late-phase response, regulating IgE synthesis, promoting eosinophil differentiation and survival, and sustaining chronic allergic inflammation by modulating leukocyte effector function and expression of cellular adhesion molecules (Tables 12-4 and 12-5).

Cytokines may have different activities on various cell types, and several cytokines have related functions on the same cell (Table 12-6). The major cytokines involved in aller-gic inflammation are IL-4, IL-13, and IL-5.

IL-4   IL-4 induces switch recombination to IgG4 and IgE synthesis. IL-4 also enhances B-cell growth, antigen presentation of B cells by the stimulation of (MHC) class II antigen, B7-1 (CD80), B7-2 (CD86), CD40, surface IgM, and low-affinity IgE receptor (CD23) expression.

In addition to these effects on B cells, IL-4 also induces T-cell proliferation. IL-4 induces differentiation of uncommitted T-cell precursors toward T-helper 2 (T_H2)-like phe-notype and also induces adhesion molecules such as vascular-cell adhesion molecule-1 (VCAM-1). In addition to T_H lymphocytes, IL-4 may be secreted by NK cells, mast cells, and basophils.

IL-13   IL-13 has IL-4-like activities on B cells and monocytes but not on T cells. IL-12 stimulates human B-cell growth and induces IgE isotype switching in allergic inflammation. Moreover, IL-13 also induces adhesion molecules such as VCAM-1 at sites of allergic inflammation, contributing to the selective accumulation of eosinophils and lymphocytes.

IL-5   IL-5 is a potent proliferation and differentiation factor for eosinophils. In addition to stimulating eosinophil production, IL-5 is a chemotactic factor for eosinophils and activates mature eosinophils, induces eosinophil secretion, and prolongs eosinophil survival by reducing apoptosis.

TABLE 12-4. SOURCES OF CYTOKINES IN ALLERGIC INFLAMMATION

Cell Type	Cytokines
Macrophage	IL-1, IL-6, IL-8, IL-10, GM-CSF
T_H1 cell	IL-2, IFN-γ, GM-CSF, lymphotoxin, inhibits IgE synthesis
T_H2 cell	IL-4, IL-5, Il-6, IL-9, IL-10, IL-12, GM-CSF, stimulates IgE synthesis
Mast cell	IL-4, IL-5, IL-8, IL-10, TNF, GM-CSF
Eosinophils	GM-CSF, IL-3, IL-5, IL-4, IL-8, TGF, β1
Airway epithelium or skin keratinocytes	IL-1β, IL-6, GM-CSF, TNF-α, eotaxin, RANTES

TABLE 12-5. KEY CYTOKINES IN ALLERGIC INFLAMMATION

	Origins	Some Functions
IL-1	Macrophages, keratinocytes, etc.	Proinflammatory = endogenous pyrogen; activation of fibroblasts, granulocytes, osteoclasts; makes T cells responsive to signals
IL-2	T cells	Proliferation of T, B, and NK cells
IL-3	T cells	Proliferation of early hematopoietic cells (multi-CSF)
IL-4	T cells, mast cells	Governs B-cell isotype switching to IgG_1 and IgE, encourages T_H2 cell production
IL-5	T cells, mast cells, ? B cells	Eosinophil differentiation and proliferation; IgA production
IL-6	Macrophages, T cells, fibroblasts	Proinflammatory; B-cell differentiation; thymocyte growth
IL-7	BM stroma	B-cell differentiation and maturation
IL-8	Keratinocytes, fibroblasts, monocytes	Neutrophil chemotaxis and activation
IL-9	T cells	Proliferation of T cells; thymocytes, mast cells
IL-10	T cells, mast cells, ? B cells	Inhibition of cytokine synthesis in various cells; proliferation of mast cells
IL-13	Activated T cells	Stimulates B-cell growth; IgE isotype switching; similar to IL-4

CSF, colony-stimulating factor; BM, bone marrow.

Examples of Cytokine Activity

1. The excessive production of IgE antibodies is the result of the opposing actions of IL-4 and IFN-γ. IFN-γ specifically inhibits the IL-4 isotype switch to IgE. The capacity of T-cell clones to support IgE production is inversely proportional to the production of IFN-γ.
2. Eosinophils—Eosinophilia is a T-cell-mediated response. IL-5 is essential for the development of eosinophilia.
3. Mast cells—IL-3, IL-9, IL-10 stimulate proliferation of mast cells.
4. The chronic atopic diseases—allergic rhinitis, asthma, and eczema (atopic)—are characterized by inflammation. All classes of cytokines participate in the induction of allergen-induced inflammation.

Cell Mediated Immune System

Antigen-Presenting Cells (APCs)

T cells respond to antigens presented *by other cells* in the context of the MHC proteins. Such APCs are usually macrophages, endothelial cells, or glial cells. These are often dendritic

TABLE 12-6. ROLE OF CYTOKINES IN ALLERGIC RESPONSES

	Cytokines	Activity
IgE regulation	IL-4, IL-13, IL-2, IL-5, IL-6	IgE isotype switch, synergize with IL-4
	IFN-γ, IL-12	Inhibits IL-4 actions and T_H2 cell differentiation
	IL-12	Enhances IFN-γ production and T_H1 cell differentiation
Eosinophilia	IL-3, Il-5, GM-CSF	Eosinophil differentiation, function, and survival
Mast cell development and activation	IL-3, IL-9, IL-10, stem cell factor	Mast cell growth factors
	CTAP-III, NAP-2, MCP-1, RANTES	Histamine-releasing factors and chemokines
Inflammation	IFN-γ, TNFs, IL-1, IL-4, IL-13	Induction of adhesion molecules
	GM-CSF, TNFs, IL-1, IL-3, IL-5	Eosinophil activating factors
	IFN-γ, GM-CSF, M-CSF, TNF, IL-1, IL-4	Macrophage activating factors
	RANTES, eotaxin, MCP-2, MIP-1α	Eosinophil chemoattractants

cells found in the skin and mucosa (Langerhans' cells), lymph nodes, spleen, and thymus. After ingesting and processing the antigen, they migrate to the lymph nodes to induce a reaction to the antigen. They present the antigen in association with class II MHC molecules. When present in the spleen and thymus, they may be important in recognizing self antigens. Glia, endothelial cells, and activated B cells may also act as APCs.

T-Cell Activation

When resting T cells are activated by the proper signals, they carry out one of several functions: i.e., proliferation, differentiation, production of cytokines, and various effector functions. T-cell activation is a complex reaction involving transmembrane signaling and intracellular activation steps.

The molecules of T-receptor sites have a general configuration similar to that of a typical Ig molecule—i.e., they are composed of polypeptide chains joined by disulfide bonds and have variable and common regions (Figure 12-7).

The B cells mature from precursors in both prenatal and postnatal life. They can be stimulated to enlarge, divide, mature, and secrete antibody. Efficient antibody production in response to complex protein antigens requires T-cell help. First an APC, usually a macrophage, presents the antigen to the T cell. This activated T cell secretes a variety of cytokines that trigger the B cell to develop into an antibody-secreting cell—a plasma cell (Figure 12-4).

The Macrophage

This is the major antigen-processing and antigen-presenting cell.

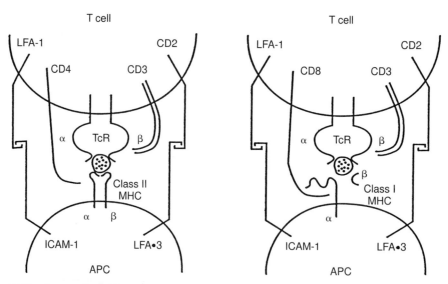

Figure 12-7. Interaction of T cells with antigen and antigen-presenting cells (APCs). Left, CD4 T (helper) cell where the T-cell receptor (TcR) interacts with antigen (stippled area) and class II MHC on the APC. Accessory molecules LFA-1, ICAM-1, CD2, and LFA-3 facilitate the interaction. Right, CD8 T (cytotoxic-suppressor) cell where the TcR interacts with antigen and class I MHC on the APC.

1. It responds to antigen exposure by secreting (IL-1); lymphocyte activation factor stimulates precursor helper (H) T cell → mature T_H.
2. Mature T_H cells secrete IL-2.
3. IL-2 promotes clonal expansion of B cells into antigen-specific antibody-secreting plasma cells.
4. IgE antibodies are specific and combine through their Fab fragment only with the antigen that stimulated their synthesis. These IgE antibodies travel through two different IgE antibody pathways.
    a. Traverse into adjacent lymphoid tissues and encounter mast cells and combine with the mast cell Fc receptor sites.
    b. IgE antibodies transported into the blood serum. The antibodies similarly bind to Fc binding sites on blood basophilic leukocytes and distant lymphoid tissues and their associated mast cells.

It is now clear that the T-cell product IL-4 controls the switch to IgE production and that IFN-γ, from other T cells, inhibits IgE production.

Humoral Immune System

Specificity for antigens is determined by immunoglobulins (Ig)—polypeptides produced by B cells. There are five major classes (isotypes) of Ig as well as subclasses (Figure 12-8, Tables 12-7 and 12-8).

Features of an Ig Molecule

1. Chains
    a. Four polypeptide chains connect with disulfide bonds
    b. Two identical light polypeptide chains (25,000 MW)
    c. Two identical heavy polypeptide chains (50,000–77,000 MW)
2. Constant region (C-terminal end of the Ig molecule) or Fc fragment
    a. The heavy chain binds to host tissues and complement (Cq) and determines Ig class.
    b. The light chain determines light chain class: kappa or lambda.

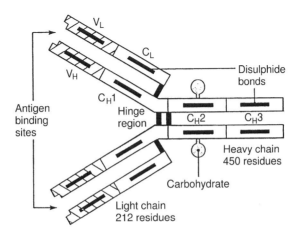

Figure 12-8.   Structure of immunoglobulin molecule.

TABLE 12-7. FEATURES OF THE CLASSES OF IMMUNOGLOBULINS

Ig	Form	Heavy Chain	MW	Adult Serum Conc., mg/dL	% of Ig	Complement Fixation	Placental Transfer
IgG	Monomer	Gamma	146,000	1150 ± 300	70–75%	. . .	. . .
IgG$_1$				615 ± 200		++	Yes
IgG$_2$				295 ± 180		+	Yes
IgG$_3$				35 ± 14		+++	Yes
IgG$_4$				18 ± 16		0	Yes
IgM	Pentamer	Mu	970,000	100 ± 25	10%	+++	No
IgA	Dimer	Alpha	385,000	200 ± 60	15–20%	0	No
IgD	Monomer	Delta	184,000	3	<1%	0	No
IgE	Monomer	Epsilon	188,000	0.005	Trace	0	No

0, none; +, weak; ++, intermediate; +++, strong.

3. Variable region (N-terminal end) or Fab fragment
   a. Binds to antigen
4. IgA
   a. Predominant Ig in seromucous secretions (saliva, tracheobronchial secretions)
   b. Dimer associated with "secretory component" (prevents proteolysis by digestive enzymes) and a "J" chain
5. IgD
   a. Found in large quantities on circulating B cells
   b. May be involved in antigen-induced lymphocyte proliferation
6. IgE

The IgE class contains the classic skin-sensitizing, anaphylactic antibodies important in type I hypersensitivity (the Gell and Coombs classification, Table 12-9). Most of its unique biological properties depend on the fact that the Fc portion of the chain binds this molecule with high avidity to Fc I receptors on mast cells and basophils. When these cell-associated IgE molecules of a particular antigenic specificity are cross-linked by their appropriate antigen, the cells degranulate and the pharmacologic mediators of anaphylaxis and type I reactions are released. IgE is present in small quantities in plasma and tissue, but because of its extraordinary affinity for basophils and mast cells, it is an antibody class of potent biological abilities.

TABLE 12-8. FUNCTION OF Ig CLASSES

IgG: Major antibody of secondary (anamnestic) responses
   Important activity against viruses, bacteria, parasites, and some fungi
   Only Ig class that crosses the placenta (provides 3–6 months immunity after birth)
   Fixes complement by classic pathway
IgM: Predominant antibody in early immune response
   Pentamer in association with a "J" chain
   Fixes complement by classic pathway
IgA: Predominant Ig in seromucous secretions (saliva, tracheobronchial secretions)
   Dimer associated with "secretory component" (prevents proteolysis by digestive enzymes) and a "J" chain
IgD: Found in large quantities on circulating B cells
   May be involved in antigen-induced lymphocyte proliferation
IgE: Found on basophils and mast cells
   Involved in response to helminthic infections and immediate hypersensitivity

TABLE 12-9. CHARACTERISTICS OF THE GELL AND COOMBS ALLERGIC REACTIONS

	Type	Inciting Agents	Biological Consequences

I	IgE on mast cells	Inhalants (dust, mold, pollens)
		Some foods
		Insect sting
		Drugs (penicillin)
			Immediate, symptoms apparent
			  within minutes
			Upper respiratory: rhinorrhea,
			  sneezing, conjunctivitis
			Lower respiratory: asthma
			Urticaria, angioedema,
			  anaphylaxis

II	Cytotoxic, IgG or IgM reacts
	  with antigen on cell surface,
	  activates complement
		Uncertain	Uncertain allergic manifestations,
			  can lead to hemolytic anemias,
			  transfusion reactions, hyper-
			  acute graft rejection, Good-
			  pasture's syndrome,
			  myasthenia gravis

III	Immune complex, usually IgG;
	  activates complement;
	  complex precipitates in
	  tissue, inciting inflammation
		Possibly foods
		Drugs
			May be delayed for up to days
			Bronchial tree: cough, wheezing
			Skin: angioedema
			Joints: arthritis
			Gastrointestinal: cramps,
			  diarrhea
			Can lead to allergic alveolitis in
			  the lung, glomerulonephritis,
			  serum sickness

IV	Cell-mediated	Poison ivy
		Cosmetics
		Various metals and chemicals
			Acute and chronic dermatitis;
			  involved in formation of granu-
			  lomas (tuberculosis, sarcoid)

ALLERGIES

About 17% of the population suffers from an allergic disease. An allergen is an antigen that causes an allergic reaction. An allergic reaction is an immune response with a deleterious effect on the host. The Gell and Coombs classification (1975) divided allergic reactions into four types (Figure 12-9, Table 12-10). An antibody mediates the first three, T cells and macrophages, the fourth.

Mechanism of Allergic Reactions

Type I

On first exposure, the allergen enters through mucosa, is processed by APCs, and is then presented to T and B cells. The resulting immune response produces a proliferation of cell populations specific for the antigen and results in the development of memory cells and plasma cells. IgE specific for the allergen is produced and binds to mast cells throughout the body. On second exposure, the allergen again enters through mucosa and then cross-links IgE on mast cells. Degranulation of mast cells releases mediators such as heparin and histamine. Activation of arachidonic acid metabolism produces prostaglandins and leukotrienes (SRS-A). These mediators produce symptoms. Memory cells exposed to the allergen produce more IgE.

Type II

On first exposure, the allergen induces a B-cell response with production of antibodies. On second exposure, the antibodies bind to cell surfaces expressing the allergen. Then, either complement is activated and the cell is lysed or the attached antibody acts as an opsonin and phagocytic cells are attracted. Damage is tissue-specific, depending on the distribution of

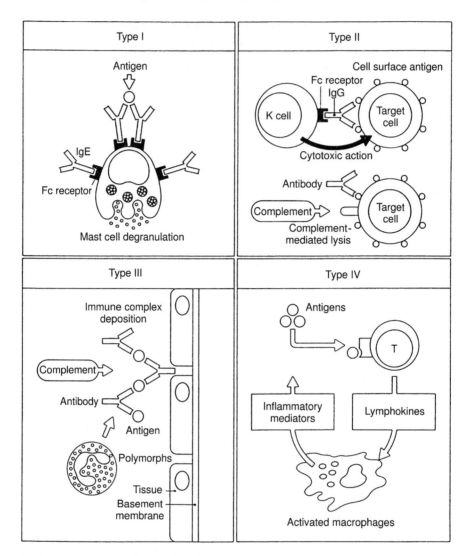

Figure 12-9.   Gell and Coombs classification.

the cell surface allergens. It is unclear if type II reactions are involved in producing allergic symptoms.

Type III

On first exposure, the allergen induces a B-cell response with production of antibodies. On second exposure, the allergen circulating in the blood binds to the antibody to create an immune complex. When large quantities of antigen are present, the complexes become numerous, large, and irregular, and they cannot be removed quickly enough by the reticuloendothelial system. The complexes attach to the endothelium of small blood vessels and initiate an inflammatory response (edema, cellular infiltrates) through complement activation. The site of damage depends on the tissues where the complexes are deposited.

TABLE 12-10. PATTERSON'S SYSTEM FOR SCORING SKIN TESTS

Reaction	Symbol	Criteria
Negative	–	No reaction or no different from control
One plus	+	Erythema smaller than a nickel in diameter (21 mm)
Two plus	++	Erythema larger than a nickel in diameter with no wheal
Three plus	+++	Wheal with surrounding erythema
Four plus	++++	Wheal with pseudopods and surrounding erythema

Type IV Delayed Hypersensitivity

On first exposure, the allergen sensitizes T cells. On second exposure, the allergen is detected on a target cell surface. Previously sensitized T cells then lyse the target cell and an inflammatory response is initiated.

Atopy

Although the normal function of the immune system is protection of the host from foreign antigens, abnormal immune responses (hypersensitivity) can lead to tissue injury and disease. A genetic contribution is seen in the atopic constitution. This may be called isotype-specific immunodysregulation, as atopic individuals tend to overproduce Igs of the IgE class isotype.

The immune system has many antibody-mediated effector mechanisms. The type I immediate hypersensitivity subset consists of the reactions primarily mediated by IgE. Although Prausnitz and Kustner, in 1921, first demonstrated the presence of a serum "reagin" in allergic persons that was capable of transferring the allergic wheal-and-flare reaction, it was not until 45 years later that Ishizaka and then Johannson and Bennich demonstrated the identity of *reagin or skin-sensitizing antibody* as a new class of immunoglobulin, termed IgE.

These reactions produce the atopic diseases via the immediate hypersensitivity response.

The final expression of immediate hypersensitivity results from the culmination of the following sequence of events:

1. Exposure to antigen (allergen).
2. Development of an IgE antibody response to antigen.
   a. The production of antigen-specific IgE antibodies requires active collaboration between macrophages, T lymphocytes, and B lymphocytes. An allergen—i.e., ragweed or Bermuda grass pollen, introduced through the respiratory tract, gastrointestinal tract, or skin—reacts with macrophages that "process" this antigen and present it to the appropriately responsive (sensitized) T lymphocytes. The B lymphocytes, in the presence of the APC, antigen, and sensitized T lymphocytes, are stimulated to develop into plasma cells, which synthesize and secrete antigen-specific IgE.

   The IgE-producing plasma cells are located mainly in the lamina propria of the skin, the respiratory tract, and the gastrointestinal tract.
3. Binding of the IgE to mast cells.
   a. IgE antibodies have the unique property of being able to bind to mast cells. They bind to receptors on the mast cell that are specific for the Fc region of the epsilon heavy chain. By *passive transfer* into the serum, these IgE-laden mast cells are distributed all over the body.

  b. Mast cell characteristics:
      (1) A perivascular connective tissue cell found in all tissues.
      (2) Migrates into the vascular system as a basophil (really the same cell).
      (3) May have from 5000 to 500,000 antigen-specific IgE antibodies on its surface.
      (4) Serum level of the IgE is a reflection of the amount of cell-bound IgE.
      (5) The mast cell or basophil contains potent mediators of immediate hyper-sensitivity.
4. Reexposure to antigen.
  a. The binding of IgE antibody to mediator-cell receptors is directly related to serum IgE concentration. The higher the IgE serum level, the greater the binding of IgE to mast cells and basophils. The greater the patient's sensitivity, the fewer antigens are required to initiate an allergic response.
5. Antigen interaction with antigen-specific IgE bound to the surface membrane of mast cells. Repeat allergen stimulation by *the same specific allergen* initiates the cross-linking of two or more mast cell bound IgE molecules. This stimulus transmits a signal to the cell's interior that initiates a molecular response, particularly:
  a. Increased ratio of cyclic GMP:AMP
      (1) Fc receptors are linked to a transmembrane coupling protein and adenylate cyclase. The coupling protein activates adenylate cyclase when cross-linking of antigen to two IgE antibodies occurs.
      (2) Adenylate cyclase reduces ATP→cGMP/AMP.
      (3) AMP decreased by kinase enhances mediator release.
      (4) The formation of cytoplasmic granules that migrate to the cell's surface membrane, fuse with each other and the cell membrane, and then extrude through the membrane into the cell's external microenvironment.
  b. Enhances the influx of Ca^{2+} from the extracellular space. This results in the release of mediators of type I anaphylaxis and the production of leukotrienes and prostaglandins via the activation of arachidonic acid metabolism (Figure 12-10).

Mast Cell Degranulation
1. When triggered by an antigen, the mast cell membrane allows calcium influx, which triggers degranulation and the release of granule-associated preformed mediators (Figure 12-11).
2. Releases arachidonic acid, which is then metabolized by the lipoxygenase pathway to leukotrienes, such as LTD4 + LTD5 (Figure 12-10), or the cyclo-oxygenase pathway to prostaglandins and thromboxanes.

Granule-Associated Preformed Mediators
HISTAMINE
1. Main mediator of immediate allergic reaction, but also found in late reaction
2. Vasodilatation
3. Increased capillary permeability
4. Bronchoconstriction
5. Tissue edema
6. Two types of tissue receptors
  a. H_1: Smooth muscle of vessels, bronchi, goblet cells, and GI mucosa
  b. H_2: Suppressor T cells, basophils, mast cells, neutrophils, and gastric cells

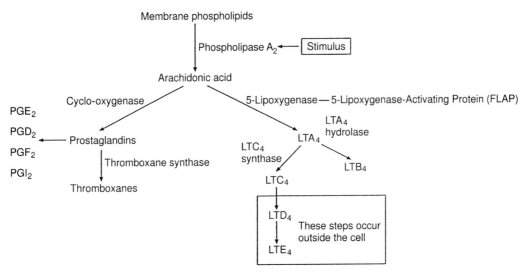

Figure 12-10. Arachidonic acid metabolism.

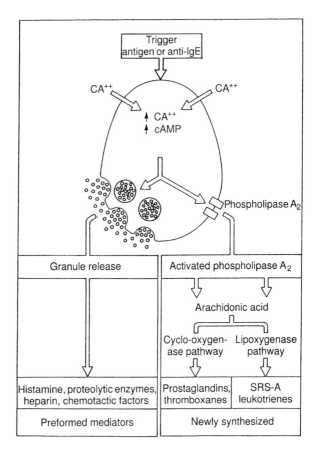

Figure 12-11. Mast cell degranulation.

HEPARIN
1. Anticoagulant
2. Suppresses histamine production
3. Enhances phagocytosis

TRYPTASE, BETA-GLUCOSAMINIDASE
1. Proteolytic enzymes

EOSINOPHIL AND NEUTROPHIL CHEMOTACTIC FACTORS
1. TAME (tosyl-L-arginine methyl ester esterase)
2. Degradative enzyme
3. Kininogenase: Causes vasoactive mucosal edema

Newly Formed Mediators
LEUKOTRIENES D4 AND E4   (Formed from arachidonic acid by the lipoxygenase pathway)
1. Vasoactive
2. Chemotaxis
3. Bronchoconstriction

PROSTAGLANDINS AND THROMBOXANES   (Formed from arachidonic acid by the cyclo-oxygenase pathway.)
1. Bronchoconstriction
2. Platelet aggregation
3. Vasodilatation

PLATELET ACTIVATING FACTOR
1. Chemotactic for eosinophils
2. Stimulates other cells to release mediators

Allergic Signs and Symptoms
Eyes
1. Allergic shiners
2. Long, silky eyelashes
3. Dennie's lines: fine horizontal lines in the lower lids
4. Conjunctivitis, burning, and itching
5. Lymphoid aggregates on the palpebral conjunctiva
6. Injection of the bulbar conjunctiva

Nose
1. Itching
2. Allergic salute and supratip crease, associated with itching and rubbing
3. Facial grimace
4. Nasal obstruction secondary to mucosal edema and excess mucus
5. Sneezing

Mouth
1. Chronic mouth breathing secondary to nasal obstruction
2. Palatal itching
3. Nocturnal tooth grinding

Pharynx
1. Dry, irritated, frequently sore throat secondary to allergen exposure, chronic mouth breathing, or both
2. Repeated throat clearing
3. Lymphoid aggregates or patches on the posterior pharyngeal wall

Larynx and Lungs
1. Hoarseness
2. Asthma—with cough, wheezing, and expiratory slowing
3. Wet cough, especially with mold allergy

Inhalant Allergy
Perennial Allergens
These are present year round and can be difficult to avoid.

HOUSE DUST
1. Composite allergen—mites, cockroach, cotton particles, human scales, etc.
2. Airborne allergen is >10 μm and settles quickly; usually comes from disturbance of bedding and upholstered furniture
3. Most noticeable in enclosed buildings

DUST MITES
1. Most allergic component is feces of the dust mite (an arachnid) *Dermatophagoides pteronyssimus* and *D. farinae*
2. Feed on human skin scales
3. Prefer 70 to 80°F and 35 to 70% relative humidity
4. Absent at higher than 5000 feet of altitude

ANIMAL DANDERS
1. Cats:
   a. Fel D1 antigen is produced in sebaceous glands in the skin and found on cat skin scales that are shed
   b. 2- to 4-μm particles remain airborne for long periods
2. Dogs: Allergen is not well understood

MOLDS
1. Indoors and out
2. Grow best in damp areas on decaying matter: basements, old newspapers, firewood, indoor green plants
3. Leading offenders: *Alternaria, Aspergillus, Pullularia, Hormodendrum, Penicillium,* and *Cephalosporium*

COCKROACH
1. Allergen is secreted by the insect, found on body and wings
2. Difficult to eradicate
3. More common in low-income housing

Seasonal Allergens

These are usually plant pollens.

Thommen's postulate states that to be an effective allergen, the pollen must be:

1. Windborne
2. Light enough to be carried long distances (generally less than 38 μm in diameter)
3. Produced in large quantities
4. Abundantly distributed
5. Allergenic

Types include

1. Trees: Winter and spring; February to May
2. Grasses: Spring, summer, and fall; April to frost
3. Weeds: Summer and fall; July to frost

Diagnosis of Allergy

Nasal Cytology

Nasal cytology is a simple office procedure helpful in differential diagnosis. Sampling should be done before any manipulation, such as vasoconstrictor spray, is done. Scraping the midportion of the inferior turbinate, blowing into a plastic bag, or both provides an adequate specimen. Wright-Giemsa adequately stains the inflammatory cells of interest, bacteria, and epithelial cells.

DIAGNOSTIC SIGNIFICANCE

1. Goblet cells: Increased in allergy and infections, acute and chronic
2. Eosinophils: Increased in inhalant allergy (diagnostic if eosinophils are >20% of granulocytes), nonallergic eosinophilic rhinitis, and aspirin sensitivity syndrome
3. Mast cells and basophils: Increased in food allergy (>5/hpf) and nasal mastocytosis
4. Neutrophils: Often seen with bacteria, suggest bacterial infection
5. Ciliocytophoria: Result of viral damage to ciliated epithelial cells; apical ciliated portion of cell separates from basal nucleated portion. Ciliated portion resembles "bear's foot"—that is, it has cilia at one end and a pointed heel at the other.

Specific Allergen Testing

A major aid in the diagnosis of inhalant allergy is in vivo or in vitro testing for allergy to specific allergens. Testing should indicate not only what the patient is allergic to but also the degree of each specific allergy. Testing for inhalants is relatively simple, since the mechanism is well understood (IgE-mediated type I reaction) and inhalant allergic reactions usually occur within minutes. However, one can have a positive test without clinical symptoms. Therefore, one should always correlate the test result with patient symptoms prior to treatment with hyposensitization.

SKIN TESTING   This test is based on the observable response to an allergen challenge on/in the skin—that is, wheal formation.

Scratch: Epicutaneous This is the original technique first described by Charles Blackley in 1873. It consists of making tiny 2-mm superficial lacerations in the patient's skin followed by the application of a drop of concentrated antigen.

ADVANTAGES
1. Safe, rarely causes systemic reaction
2. Lack of delayed skin reaction
3. Concentrates are used; economical, long shelf life

DISADVANTAGES
1. False-positive (irritation of skin rather than allergic reaction)
2. More painful
3. Not as reproducible as intradermal skin test

Because of limited reproducibility and other drawbacks, this form of testing is no longer a recommended diagnostic procedure according to the Allergy Panel of the AMA Council of Scientific Affairs.

Prick: Epicutaneous Lewis and Grant first described the technique of the prick test in 1926. As currently performed, a single drop of antigen concentrate is placed on the skin. A sterile 26-gauge needle is passed through this drop and inserted into the skin in a superficial manner so that no bleeding is caused. A variant of this test is the "multitest," in which a sterile, disposable applicator with eight puncture heads is utilized, which allows for the simultaneous testing of six antigens and a positive (histamine) and negative (glycerine) control. Grading of skin reactivity is done on a subjective 0-to-4+ basis (Table 12-10).

ADVANTAGES
1. Rapid
2. Better correlation with intradermal tests
3. Relatively safe

DISADVANTAGES
1. Gives qualitative measure of allergy only
2. Will miss low degree of allergy (false-negative)
3. Grading of skin test is subjective

The prick test is a rapid way to screen for multiple antigens. If the skin test is positive, then the patient is almost certainly allergic, but the converse is not true. If the patient has a positive history and a negative prick test, the physician is obliged to proceed with intradermal testing.

Intradermal Tests Robert Cooke gave the first description of the intradermal skin test in 1915. The technique has undergone few modifications since that time. As described today, the procedure is to use a #26-gauge needle to inject intradermally a small amount of antigen, variously reported to range from 0.01 to 0.05 mL. The concentration of the extract ranges from 1:500 to 1:1000. The tests are read at 10 to 15 minutes. The erythema and whealing are measured and graded on a subjective scale of 0 to 4+.

ADVANTAGES

1. Highly sensitive (low degree of allergy detected)
2. Reproducible within one office

DISADVANTAGES

1. Qualitative, not quantitative
2. Grading of response is subjective
3. No standardization as to the amount or concentration of test dose
4. Variable results between offices
5. May have false-positives due to high sensitivity

The intradermal test is a good test, sensitive and highly reproducible. Accuracy is clearly improved by testing with various dilutions of extract, but lack of standardization of testing protocol, as to volume and concentration of test dose, as well as degree of subjectivity in grading the skin response are serious drawbacks to this original technique.

Serial Dilution Endpoint Titration (SDET)   The development of SDET is a natural outgrowth and refinement of the single-dilution intradermal skin test. In fact, the Office of Biologic Research and Review (a part of the Food and Drug Administration) uses a form of SDET to standardize allergic extracts. The technique of SDET was first developed by Hansel and subsequently refined by Herbert Rinkel (1962), who introduced the concept of the 1:5 dilutions.

The actual technique of SDET entails mixing fivefold dilutions of the allergenic extracts. These are labeled dilutions #1 through #6. The #1 dilution is five times weaker than the concentrate (1:20 in most cases), so the weight per volume designation of the #1 dilution would be 1:100. The same procedure is followed to make the remaining dilutions (Figure 12-12).

The test material, starting with the #6 dilution, is injected intradermally; 0.01 mL of the extract is utilized, which will make a 4-mm wheal that enlarges (without reaction) to a 5-mm wheal. If there is no significant growth of the wheal after 10 minutes, the next stronger dilution (#5) is similarly injected. In the allergic individual, a progression of the whealing response will be observed. The endpoint is defined as that dilution which initiates progressive positive whealing.

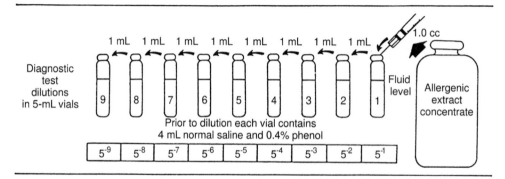

Figure 12-12.   Serial dilution titration.

THE WHEALING RESPONSE   Injection of 0.01 mL of any liquid (antigen, diluent, saline) produces a wheal of approximately 4 mm diameter, which soon grows to about 5 mm by local tissue infiltration. Positive responses enlarge beyond this by the production of a "wheal and flare" response. Such a response requires that skin mast cells (normally about 10,000 per mm^3 of skin) have antigen-specific IgE on the cell surface. Chemical mediators (i.e., histamine) are released, thereby producing a Gell and Coombs type I hypersensitivity reaction. The immediate response phase of this reaction produces the wheal and accompanying flare (surrounding redness). The wheal begins to grow within 2 to 5 minutes, and enlarges to maximum size at 10 to 15 minutes. (Later wheal enlargement is often due to a Gell and Coombs type III reaction and has a different significance than the acute reaction. Such a late reaction is most often associated with mold hypersensitivity.) Local vasodilatation produces the accompanying flare response, but although erythema should be noted in reading skin tests, only the diameter of the palpable induration at 10 to 15 minutes determines the reaction.

POSITIVE WHEALING AND SERIAL DILUTION ENDPOINT TITRATION   If a hypersensitivity ("allergic") reaction is present, a positive wheal will enlarge at least an additional 2 mm beyond the size of the "negative" (5-mm) wheal within 10 minutes. Rinkel showed that if progressively stronger (fivefold) concentrations of antigen were applied, each succeeding positive wheal would be at least 2 mm larger than the preceding one. He defined the "endpoint" as the dilution that initiates progressive positive whealing. In other words, the first dilution that yields a wheal at least 2 mm larger than the preceding negative wheal and is followed by a wheal at the next stronger dilution that is at least 2 mm larger still. This second positive wheal is called a "confirming wheal" and is very important in defining a true endpoint. This method of determining the level of positive reaction is termed "skin endpoint titration."

EXAMPLES (ENDPOINT UNDERLINED)
- 5-5-7-9 (if carried further, -11-12, etc.)
- 5-5-7-7-9 (plateau reaction)
- 5-8-11 (variable increment)

Once the endpoint is determined, the individual treatment vials are made, taking into account the quantitative as well as the qualitative aspect of that patient's allergic disease.

ADVANTAGES
1. Quantitative as well as qualitative measure of allergy
2. Highly reproducible
3. Very sensitive
4. Safe

DISADVANTAGES
1. Time-consuming test procedure
2. Possible false-positives in low degree of allergy
3. More supplies needed in office (syringes, needles, etc.)

SDET has been approved by the Allergy Panel of the AMA Council of Scientific Affairs as being both useful and effective in the diagnosis of allergy. To encourage standardization in use of this procedure, the American Academy of Otolaryngic Allergy (AAOA) has developed a protocol to be closely followed by physicians using this technique.

CONCURRENT MEDICATION WITH SDET   Antihistamines suppress the wheal-and-flare response. With almost all common antihistamines, this effect has effectively ceased within 24 hours or less of the delivery of the last medication to the body, and skin testing may thus be carried out if the patient has taken no such drugs for 36 hours. Short-acting antihistamines such as diphenhydramine and triprolidine can often be given the day before testing without affecting skin responses (Table 12-11).

Antihistamines are also contained in or include some soporifics, cough syrups, "cold" remedies, antipruritics, and anxiolytics.

Tricyclic antidepressants have been observed to suppress skin test responses for from 2 to 4 days.

Decongestants, cromolyn, corticosteroids, and bronchodilators do not affect skin test results and need not be discontinued before testing.

Patients who have undergone previous treatment may have altered skin test responses as compared to pretreatment levels, due to the production of IgG4 blocking antibodies as well from a lowered level of allergen-specific IgE.

IN VITRO ALLERGY TESTING

Radioallergosorbent Test (RAST)
The original Phadebas RAST assay was modified in 1979 because of insufficient sensitivity. While the Phadebas RAST, with its excellent specificity, is still the most widely used assay outside the United States, the Modified RAST Test (MRT) has replaced it in the United States as the most widely used in vitro allergy diagnostic assay. The MRT assay, whether using enzyme immunosorbent assay (EIA) or radioactive immunosorbent assay (RIA) technology, still provides the most reliable balance between sensitivity and specificity as well as intratest allergen-to-allergen consistency, and it is considered by many to be the gold standard against which all such assays are compared.

The RAST measures the level of allergen-specific IgE in the serum. The classic technique is based on a paper disc with antigen bound to the surface. The disc is placed in a test tube to which the patient's serum is added. Allergen-specific IgE that may be present in the serum binds to antigen on the disc; excess nonspecific IgE is then washed away. Radiolabeled anti-IgE antibody is added and binds to the patient's IgE bound to the antigen on the disc; the excess anti-IgE is washed away. The amount of bound radiolabel is then measured in a gamma counter (Figure 12-13). Proper controls must be used for best sensitivity and specificity of the test.

TABLE 12-11. DRUGS AFFECTING SKIN WHEALING

Drug	Comment
Antihistamines	All antihistamines are capable of inhibiting immediate skin responses. Hydroxyzine is the most potent and prolonged inhibitor.
Epinephrine and other beta-adrenergic agonists	Variable inhibiting ability.
Theophylline	Variable inhibiting ability.
Steroids	Inhibit type IV delayed skin reactions. May interfere with immediate skin test in massive doses.
Cromolyn	Theoretically capable of inhibiting immediate skin responses.
Dimethyl carbamazine	Interferes with SRS-A. Not used clinically.
Phenothiazine	Antihistaminic activity.
Imipramine	Antihistaminic activity.

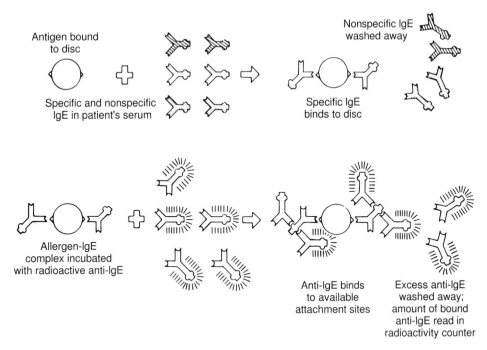

Figure 12-13.   RAST: basic mechanism.

ADVANTAGES AND DISADVANTAGES OF IN VITRO TESTING

Advantages

1. Eliminates variability of the skin response
2. Eliminates drug effects (antihistamines)
3. Can be done in one blood test; eliminates lengthy skin testing
4. Is more specific than skin testing
5. Provides a quantitative assessment of degree of allergy and can be used as a basis for determining starting doses for immunotherapy
6. Is safe for patients on beta blockers

Disadvantages

1. May be more expensive
2. Requires specialized laboratory equipment and technician training
3. May be less sensitive than skin testing

Initially the measurement of total IgE had been employed as a screening test for atopic or type I hypersensitivity allergy reactions, but it was soon noted that a number of symptomatic patients with so-called "normal" total IgE levels had elevated levels of specific IgE.

As a result, other schemes using total IgE together with specific IgE levels were proposed for a more efficient diagnosis. It was implied that an individual with a total IgE level of less than 25 IU with only RAST class 1 scores would be unlikely to have atopic allergies, whereas one with a high total IgE level together with a RAST score of class 2 and above was likely to have atopic allergy.

Indications and Contraindications for in Vitro Testing

INDICATED

> In patients not responding to environmental control and conservative medical management
>
> In apprehensive children and infants in whom atopic sensitization seems likely
>
> In symptomatic patients with conditions in which in vivo skin testing is contraindicated (dermatographism, eczema, etc.)
>
> In patients unable to stop medication adversely affecting skin testing
>
> In patients doing poorly on immunotherapy
>
> In evaluating individual sensitivities when initiating specific immunotherapy in atopic patients
>
> In transfer allergic patients on immunotherapy
>
> In venom sensitivity
>
> In the diagnosis of IgE-mediated food sensitivity

CONTRAINDICATED

> In patients with positive histories of sensitivity in whom nonspecific therapy is effective in alleviating symptoms
>
> In asymptomatic atopic patients currently on immunotherapy
>
> In symptomatic patients with negative skin tests
>
> In patients with total IgE levels below 10 U/ml
>
> In the diagnosis of non-IgE-mediated disorders

Treatment of Inhalant Allergy

Treatment for inhalant allergy involves environmental control, pharmacotherapy, and immunotherapy.

Environmental Control

This involves decreasing the allergen load by altering the patient's environment. Environment control for pollens is difficult because of airborne spread. It is limited to the elimination of offending plants from the immediate surroundings and the addition of filtered, air-conditioned ventilation.

Decreasing growth of molds includes

1. Avoid living near damp places
2. Avoid dense landscaping and mulch near house
3. Preventing moisture accumulation indoors around pipes, air conditioners

Dust precautions include

1. Use of synthetic carpets or elimination of carpets
2. Regular and frequent vacuuming
3. Regular changes of filters on air conditioners and regular changes for various types of mechanical or electrical filters
4. Avoiding large amounts of stored papers, clothing in the house

Animal danders are most effectively handled by removal or avoidance of pets; however, this may be traumatic for the patient and family. Weekly washing of cats in warm water and removal from the bedroom may help.

Pharmacotherapy

Pharmacotherapy of inhalant allergy is most often indicated for

1. Mild to moderate symptoms for only 3 to 4 months of the year
2. Temporary relief of symptoms when immunotherapy is started
3. Occasional breakthrough symptoms while on immunotherapy

Drug therapy for allergic rhinitis is not for cure but to control symptoms. Antihistamines, decongestants, mast cell stabilizers, and corticosteroids have been the drug armamentarium used to provide symptomatic relief of allergic rhinitis. The first-line drug approach for the management of allergic rhinitis consists of antihistamines to control the rhinorrhea, itching, and sneezing as well as the ocular symptoms. The newer preparations need be given only once or twice daily and have reduced sedation and anticholinergic side effects.

The nasal challenge model shows that inflammation is responsible for allergic rhinitis. Intranasally inhaled allergens in contact with the nasal mucosa provoke an IgE-mediated early-phase immunologic response. The early phase activates mast cells, leading to the release of inflammatory mediators such as histamine, leukotrienes (LTC_4, LTD_4, LTE_4), prostaglandins D_2 (PGD_2), platelet activating factor (PAF), and chemotactic factors such as PAF, leukotriene (LTB_4), hydroxyeicosatetraenoic acids ($HETE_5$), and cytokines. The chemotactic factors released are responsible for recruiting eosinophils, neutrophils, and basophils and for the late-phase reaction in the nasal mucosa. The late phase starts after 5 to 7 hours, with a return of symptoms, and peaks 6 to 8 hours after the allergen challenge.

ANTIHISTAMINES. These are H_1 receptor antagonists that act mainly by dose-related competitive binding of the H_1 receptors on target cells. They work best on symptoms of the immediate allergic response (itching, mild congestion, sneezing, rhinorrhea) but do little to relieve marked congestion, which is a result of a late-phase allergic reaction.

First-generation (or sedating) antihistamines (Table 12-12) are lipophilic and cross the blood-brain barrier, attaching to H_1 receptors on brain cells and resulting in sedation or hypnotic effects. They are anticholinergic and may result in drying of mucous membranes, blurry vision, constipation, urinary retention, and impotence. They are degraded by the P450 microsomal system in the liver. Tachyphylaxis occurs due to a class-specific induction of degradative enzymes in the liver. If tachyphylaxis occurs, change to a different class of traditional antihistamines.

Second-generation (nonsedating) antihistamines (Table 12-13) have the ability to inhibit the release of inflammatory mediators and reduce eosinophil migration, probably by their effect on intercellular adhesion molecules (ICAM). Therefore, they not only have become simple histamine receptor antagonists but also tend to dampen the entire allergic inflammatory cascade.

The ability of an agent to cross the blood-brain barrier and penetrate central nervous system (CNS) tissue easily is directly related to its effect on a patient's alertness and performance. This ability is related to a molecule's size in addition to other properties such as its polarity, lipophilic nature, and charge. Sedating antihistamines can have a detrimental

TABLE 12-12. FIRST-GENERATION ANTIHISTAMINES

Agent	Brand Name	Other Actions
Diphenhydramine	Benadryl	Anticholinergic
	Many others	Sedative
Chlorpheniramine	Chlor-Trimeton	Anticholinergic
	Many others	Weakly sedative
Promethazine	Phenergan	Anticholinergic
		Highly sedative
		Antiemetic
		α-adrenergic blocking
Hydroxyzine	Atarax	Anticholinergic
	Vistaril	Highly sedative

Note: Second-generation (or nonsedating) antihistamines (Table 12-13) are lipophobic, pass the blood-brain barrier less readily, and have little affinity for brain H_1 receptors. They have little or no anticholinergic effects and little if any tachyphylaxis.

effect on quality of life and performance; therefore, recognition of the side effects in susceptible individuals is important.

Cardiovascular Effects of Antihistamines   Astemizole and terfenadine can, at high plasma levels, act directly on cardiac cells to slow repolarization, prolong the QT interval, and predispose patients to torsades de pointes, a life-threatening ventricular arrhythmia. Drugs and conditions that inhibit or compete for the CYP3A4 isoenzyme of the hepatic cytochrome P450 system, which is responsible for metabolism of terfenadine and astemizole, can increase serum levels (C_{max}) of these drugs and thus prolong cardiac repolarization. Important CYP3A3/4 inhibitors include certain newer antidepressants, macrolide antibiotics, and imidazole antifungal agents.

Astemizole and terfenadine also have the ability to block cardiac potassium channels. Increased serum levels of terfenadine and astemizole may result from overdose, drug interaction, or patient characteristics. Numerous agents are known to inhibit or compete for the CYP3A4 isoenzyme of the cytochrome P450 hepatic system, which is responsible for metabolism of terfenadine and astemizole.

Agents known to increase serum levels of terfenadine and astemizole by inhibiting CYP3A4 include specific macrolide antibiotics, oral antifungals, flavonoids, lovastatin, and certain antidepressants such as fluvoxamine and nefazodone.

TABLE 12-13. SECOND-GENERATION ANTIHISTAMINES

Agent	Brand Name	Other Actions
Terfenadine	Seldane—no longer available in the USA	Weak H_2 antagonist
		Nonsedative
		Mast cell inhibition
Astemizole	Hismanal—no longer available in the USA	Nonsedative
Loratadine	Claritin	Nonsedative
		Mast cell inhibition
		Inhibits eosinophils
Certirizine	Zyrtec	Mildly sedative
		Affects late phase
Fexofenadine	Allegra	Nonsedative

Other 3A4 substrates may possibly compete with astemizole and terfenadine and therefore lead to increased serum levels.

Patient-related conditions that may increase serum levels of terfenadine and astemizole include drug overdose and hepatic dysfunction secondary to alcohol or exposure to hepatotoxins.

Hepatic impairment is an important consideration in antihistamine dosing. Due to extensive hepatic metabolism (P450-CYP34A) of terfenadine and astemizole, administration of these agents in patients with hepatic impairment is contraindicated. Dosing adjustment of cetirizine is also necessary in patients with moderate to severe renal impairment and in patients on dialysis. Astemizole should be used with caution in patients with renal impairment. The potential for increasing the incidence of adverse reactions can become greater when patients increase their dosage to achieve optimal symptom relief (Tables 12-14 and 12-15). Due to the cardiovascular effects of terfenadine and astemizole, these drugs are no longer available in the United States.

Systemic Decongestants   Nasal decongestants administered orally decrease nasal obstruction but have minimal effects on rhinorrhea, itching, and sneezing.

These are often combined with traditional antihistamines to counteract sedation. They are used extensively in prescription and nonprescription combinations. All systemic decongestants act as alpha-adrenergic agonists and can raise the blood pressure in hypertensive patients.

TABLE 12-14. ANTIHISTAMINE SELECTION CRITERIA

	Astemizole	Cetirizine	Chlorpheniramine	Hydroxyzine	Loratadine	Terfenadine
Clinical efficacy						
SAR	+++	+++	++	+++	+++	+++
PAR	++	++	?	++	++	++
Urticaria	+++	+++	+++	+++	+++	+++
Onset of action	>1 h	<1 h	<1 h	?	<1 h	<1 h
Duration	24 h	24 h	12–24 h	12–36 h	24 h	18–24 h
Somnolence	No	Yes	Yes	Yes	No	No
Alcohol sedation potentiation	No	Yes	Yes	Yes	No	No
CV side effects with						
Ketoconazole	Yes	No	?	No	No	Yes
Erythromycin	Yes	No	?	No	No	Yes
Cimetidine (weak)	?	No	?	No	No	Yes
Potential drug interactions						
Theophylline	?	Yes	?	?	?	No
Weight gain	Yes	No	?	No	No	?
Dose reduction						
Renal dysfunction	?	Yes	?	Yes	No	No
Liver dysfunction	*	Yes	—	Yes	Yes	*

Key: CV, cardiovascular; SAR, seasonal allergic rhinitis; PAR, perennial allergic rhinitis.
*Use should be avoided.

TABLE 12-15. FORMULATIONS AND DOSAGES OF REPRESENTATIVE H₁-RECEPTOR ANTAGONISTS

H₁-Receptor Antagonist	Formulation	Recommended Dose
First generation		
Chlorpheniramine maleate (Chlor-Trimeton)	Tablets: 4 mg, 8 mg, 12 mg Syrup: 2.5 mg/5 mL Parenteral solution: 10 mg/mL	Adult: 8–12 mg 2×/day Child: 0.35 mg/kg/24 h
Hydroxyzine hydrochloride (Atarax)	Capsules: 10 mg, 25 mg, 50 mg Syrup: 10 mg/5 mL	Adult: 25–50 mg 2×/day (or once a day, at bedtime) Child: 2 mg/kg/24 h
Diphenhydramine hydrochloride (Benadryl)	Capsules: 25 mg, 50 mg Elixir: 12.5 mg/5 mL Syrup: 6.25 mg/5 mL Parenteral solution: 50 mg/mL	Adult: 25–50 mg 3×/day Child: 5 mg/kg/24 h
Second generation		
Terfenadine (Seldane)	Tablets: 60 mg, 120 mg Suspension: 30 mg/5 mL	Adult: 60 mg 2×/day or 120 mg/day Child: 3–6 yr, 15 mg 2×/day; 7–12 yr, 30 mg 2×/day
Astemizole (Hismanal)	Tablets: 10 mg Suspension: 10 mg/5 mL	Adult: 10 mg/day Child: 0.2 mg/kg/day
Loratadine (Claritin)	Tablets: 10 mg Syrup: 1 mg/mL	Adult: 10 mg/day Child: 2–12 yr, 5 mg/day; >12 yr and >30 kg, 10 mg/day
Cetirizine hydrochloride (Reactine)	Tablets: 10 mg	Adults: 5–10 mg/day
Acrivastine (Semprex)	Tablets: 8 mg	Adult: 8 mg, 3×/day
Ketotifen fumarate (Zaditen)	Tablets: 1 mg, 2 mg Syrup: 1 mg/5 mL	Adult with urticaria: 4 mg/day Child >3 yr: 1 mg 2×/day or 2 mg/day
Azelastine hydrochloride (Astelin)	0.1% Nasal solution: 0.127 mg/spray	Topical: 2 sprays/nostril/day or 2×/day
Levocabastine hydrochloride (Livostin)	Microsuspension: 0.5 mg/mL	Topical: 2 sprays (50 µg each) nostril 2–4×/day or 1 drop (0.15 µg) in each eye 2–4×/day

They can also decrease appetite and produce cardiac symptoms, such as tachycardia and palpitations. Vasoconstriction in the nasal mucosa decreases hyperemia, congestion, edema, and nasal congestion.

1. Pseudoephedrine: Isomer of ephedrine that produces less central stimulation.
2. Phenylpropanolamine: No longer available in the United States due to risk of intracerebral hemorrhage.

TOPICAL DECONGESTANTS Topical decongestants are potentially addicting due to rebound congestion caused by mucosal anoxia and neurotransmitter depletion (rhinitis medicamentosa): They should not be used for more than 3 days at a time.

Phenylephrine	4- to 6-hour duration (Neo-Synephrine, Dristan)
Oxymetazoline	12-hour duration (Afrin, Duration)
Naphazoline	6-hour duration (Privine)
Xylometazoline	10-hour duration (Otrivin)
Tetrahydrozoline	(Tyzine)

CORTICOSTEROID THERAPY Corticosteroids block the generation and release of mediators and the influx of inflammatory cells. Corticosteroids have a wide range of effects on multiple cell types (mast cells, eosinophils, neutrophils, macrophages, and lymphocytes) and mediators (histamine, eicosanoids, leukotrienes, and cytokines) involved in inflammation; they are presently the most effective anti-inflammatory agents. They are available in parenteral, oral, and topical forms.

Parenteral Steroids   May be given as intramuscular injections of a depot formulation. This may be helpful for patients with a single 2- to 3-month allergy season. Turbinate injection may provide relief of symptoms for up to 6 weeks at a time. However, to minimize the risk of blindness (from retinal embolization and vasospasm), use cocaine as a vasoconstrictor, a gentle injection technique, and small particle size (i.e., triamcinolone acetonide) formulation.

Oral Steroids   The time necessary for corticosteroids to be biologically effective is in the range of hours, depending on the formulation.

Types of Medication	Equivalence
Short-acting:	
Cortisone	25 mg
Hydrocortisone	25 mg
Intermediate-acting:	
Prednisone	5 mg
Prednisolone	5 mg
Methylprednisolone	4 mg
Triamcinolone	4 mg
Long-acting:	
Dexamethasone	0.75 mg
Betamethasone	0.75 mg

TOPICAL STEROIDS   Over the past two decades, a number of highly active intranasal steroids have been developed for topical application in order to minimize systemic toxicity and side effects. These can be used safely for years without significant risk of adrenal suppression. The patients should be advised of the need for regular use and altering the dosage depending on the season.

1. Dexamethasone: Not widely used due to problems with systemic absorption.
2. Beclomethasone: Single-pass steroid; absorbed systemically but eliminated quickly in the circulation; aqueous forms may cause less nasal irritation than powder forms in a Freon propellant. (Vancenase, Beconase)
3. Flunisolide: Effective, but propylene glycol base may cause irritation and burning, which are usually transient. (Nasalide, Nasarel)
4. Fluticasone: Aqueous-base spray shown to be effective in 12 hours after initial usage. (Flonase)
5. Budesonide: Aqueous-base spray. (Rhinocort)
6. Triamcinolone acetate. (Nasacort)
7. Mometasone. (Nasonex)

All of these have a similar clinical efficacy when used for the treatment of allergic rhinitis. Also, the efficacy of topical intranasal corticosteroids is equivalent to that of systemic corticosteroids in the treatment of allergic rhinitis.

Intranasal topical corticosteroids should now be considered first-line therapy for the treatment of allergic rhinitis, nonallergic rhinitis (NARES), rhinitis medicamentosa, and nasal polyps.

CROMOLYN SODIUM (4% SPRAY)   In animal experiments, it acts by preventing mast cell degranulation; the mechanism of action in humans is less clear. It is lipophobic and not absorbed systemically; thus it produces no side effects.

Available in both a nasal form and an ophthalmic form, cromolyn is effective but must be used prophylactically three to four times a day. It has a significant compliance problem. For patients with significant eye symptoms, a new mast cell stabilizer, lodoxamide, is available.

LEUKOTRIENE INHIBITORS   Leukotriene receptor antagonists and synthesis inhibitors useful in the treatment of asthma may prove to be helpful in allergic rhinitis. Studies are in progress to evaluate this prospect. The medications used at present are zafirlukast, pranlukast, and zileuton.

Immunotherapy

Allergen immunotherapy is the process by which increasing doses of allergen are injected subcutaneously over time as a treatment to reduce allergic symptoms. This therapy, using the nasal challenge model, correlates with a reduction in mediator (histamine, kinins, leukotrienes, prostaglandins) release, antigen-induced eosinophil migration, and clinical symptoms, in both the immediate-phase and the late-phase reaction.

Other specific changes with immunotherapy include (1) a rise in serum IgG–blocking antibody levels; (2) a suppression of the annual seasonal rise in IgE antibody levels, followed by a decline in the level of specific IgE over the course of immunotherapy; and (3) an increase in IgA and IgG antibody levels in nasal secretions.

A satisfactory response to immunotherapy requires (1) identifying the allergen; (2) correlating it to the clinical picture; (3) providing an adequate therapeutic dose; and (4) treating for an adequate period of time (3–5 years or longer).

Standardization of allergen extracts has been a significant problem, but it is improving. Currently extracts from most licensed laboratories have comparable potencies. Allergen extracts are supplied in 50% glycerine to maintain potency of the allergen while in storage.

DILUENTS   Several diluents are used for making allergen concentrations suitable for skin testing or immunotherapy:

Saline
1. Inexpensive
2. Allergens lose potency within 6 weeks, refrigeration helps only a little

Human Serum Albumin in Saline
1. Inexpensive
2. Helps prevent adherence of allergen to walls of vials, which would result in a loss of potency
3. Allergens keep potency for 12 weeks with refrigeration
4. Heat-treated to inactivate viruses

Glycerin

1. Irritating to skin
2. Skin reactions are marked at 50%, rare at 2%
3. 10% will preserve antigens for about 3 months

STARTING DOSES   Starting doses should be high enough to initiate an immunologic response but low enough to avoid significant local or systemic reactions.

SET	0.05 mL of endpoint (dilution that produced the first positive reaction)
RAST	0.05–0.10 mL of 1:200,000 for high-sensitivity allergens (>8000 counts)
	0.05–0.10 mL of 1:20,000 for low-sensitivity allergens (<8000 counts)

ADVANTAGES OF QUANTITATIVE TESTING   There are two major advantages of quantitative testing over single-dilution skin testing. First, since the starting dose for a specific antigen is usually higher than the arbitrary dose chosen after single-dilution testing, progressive increases result in reaching the maintenance dose with fewer injections, with faster improvement in symptoms, and at lower cost. Second, the potency of each allergen in a multiallergen vial is adjusted to minimize the risk of a local or systemic reaction. This is done either by varying the potency of each allergen in a multiallergen treatment vial or by dividing high- and low-sensitivity allergens into separate vials. Therefore, the maintenance concentrations of low-sensitivity allergens can be much higher than if they were included along with high-sensitivity allergens. If all allergens are included in a vial at the same dose, as is done with systems based on single-dilution testing, the high-sensitivity allergens limit the maintenance dose of the vial and also the dose of the low-sensitivity antigens. Such therapy may cause clinically important but less reactive allergens to fail in achieving a dose that will relieve symptoms.

DOSE ESCALATION   The maintenance dose should be high enough to control symptoms but low enough to avoid local or systemic reactions. After starting immunotherapy, the dose should be increased as quickly as possible. Generally, increasing by 0.05 mL each week is very safe. Increases of 0.10 mL each week may be used for weaker dilutions if well tolerated. Increases of 0.20 mL each week may be used for weaker dilutions if shots are given outside of the blooming season. If unexpected reactions are encountered, look for developing upper respiratory infection, massive allergen exposure, or concomitant food allergy.

The plateau of clinical improvement is limited by the maintenance dose; hopefully control of symptoms for at least 1 week can be achieved. Local reaction of 2 to 3 cm that lasts for more than 48 hours also limits the maintenance dose. No arbitrary level can be set for all patients.

EXCESSIVE LOCAL REACTIONS   Vial division based on antigen sensitivity can avoid these; that is, the high-sensitivity allergen in one vial and the low-sensitivity allergen in another. If a local reaction occurs before clinical improvement, one or two antigens may be at fault; identify them by history or by splitting the allergens into two vials.

DOSING INTERVAL   This interval can be increased from weekly to every 2 or 3 weeks after the first full year of well-controlled symptoms.

BREAKTHROUGH SYMPTOMS   These are caused by heavy allergen exposure, such as a change in home environment or a new pet. Treat with environmental controls, steroids, or antihistamines.

STOPPING IMMUNOTHERAPY   Many patients can stop immunotherapy after 3 to 5 years of maintenance. If symptoms recur, the patient should be retested and further immunotherapy considered.

INDICATIONS FOR IMMUNOTHERAPY
- Symptoms initiated by IgE antibodies
- Respiratory allergy—perennial nasal allergy, seasonal hay fever, bronchial asthma
- Severe symptoms—not controlled by medications and avoidance
- Long seasons
- Multiple seasons
- Perennial symptoms
- Complications:
  Recurrent infections
  Serous otitis media or hearing loss
  Asthma
  Increased morbidity
  Increased absenteeism
  Decreased quality of life
  Intolerance to antiallergenic drugs

CONTRAINDICATIONS FOR IMMUNOTHERAPY
- Nonimmune mechanism responsible for symptoms
- IgE-mediated mechanism
- Mild symptoms—readily controlled by simple methods
- Easily avoidable allergen
- Atopic dermatitis
- Gastrointestinal food allergies
- Very short seasons
- Noncompliant patients
- Food allergy
- Patient taking beta-blocking agents.

RELATIVE CONTRAINDICATIONS FOR IMMUNOTHERAPY
- Infants and children under 2 years of age
- IgE-mediated drug and chemical sensitivity

COMPLICATIONS OF IMMUNOTHERAPY   These are caused by
1. Inadvertent use of the wrong antigen
2. Giving a treatment dose from the wrong vial
3. Too rapid escalation of dose
4. Unrelated stimulation of immune system, such as upper respiratory infection
5. Unrecognized food allergy

Local Reactions
1. Are defined as erythema larger than 3.0 cm, are accompanied by induration, and last more than 24 hours
2. Are often due to a single antigen because of a blooming season
3. Appear as maximum tolerated dose is reached
4. Do not predict susceptibility to systemic reactions

Worsening of allergic symptoms after a shot may actually be psychological. However, such symptoms may represent a true systemic reaction if they appear shortly after the dose. Doses in the vials may need to be rechecked.

Urticaria or Angioedema   When this occurs soon after injection, it may indicate early stages of anaphylaxis. Give subcutaneous epinephrine and antihistamines (IV Benadryl) acutely. Reduce the treatment dosage and then slowly escalate.

Anaphylactic Shock   A massive, acute, IgE-mediated allergic reaction causes this. Life-threatening complications include laryngeal edema, bronchospasm, and cardiovascular collapse. Anaphylaxis is usually apparent within seconds or minutes.

SYMPTOMS OF ANAPHYLAXIS
1. Flare of allergic symptoms
2. Congestion, heaviness in chest
3. Cough, dysphagia, stridor
4. Warm skin, rapid pulse
5. Initial elevation of blood pressure, then decrease
6. Itching, urticaria
7. Feeling of impending doom (angor animi)
8. Nausea, vomiting

TREATMENT OF ANAPHYLAXIS
1. Lay patient down; take vital signs
2. Ammonia ampoule for nasal stimulation
3. Tourniquet proximal to injection site
4. Oxygen
5. Airway support with suction and intubation, if necessary
6. Intravenous line for fluids, medication
7. Epinephrine: 0.3 mg (range 0.2 to 0.5 mg) IM or SC; repeat PRN every 10 to 15 minutes, up to a total of 1 mg
8. Dopamine drip for hypotension
9. Heparin, 10,000 units SC or slow IV
10. Diphenhydramine 50 mg IV
11. Cimetidine 300 mg IM or slow IV
12. Dexamethasone 4 mg IV
13. Intensive care unit observation as soon as possible

Food Allergy
Food allergy is classified into two general types:

Cyclic: 60 to 95% of Cases

1. Severity depends on frequency and dose of ingestion
2. Symptoms may not be apparent for 4 to 48 hours
3. Little if any IgE mediation
4. In part an IgG-mediated, immune complex disease

Noncyclic: 5 to 40% of Cases

1. Severity is fixed
2. Usually does not depend on dose or frequency of ingestion
3. Onset of symptoms within minutes
4. IgE-mediated

Symptoms

Symptoms are related to the tissues containing sensitized mast cells (shock organ) and usually involve the upper aerodigestive tract. Occasionally the lower digestive tract is involved.

Food Allergens

- Cow's milk protein: casein
- Wheat: cross-reacts with all cereal grains
- Corn and corn derivatives
- Soy: Can produce allergic problems when used as a substitute for cow's milk
- Yeast: Baked goods, fermented beverages, cheese, mushrooms, skins of fresh fruit
- Egg: Baked goods, dairy substitute in creamers and toppings

Diagnosis of Cyclic Food Allergy

Diagnosis of cyclic food allergy is relatively difficult because there is a lack of understanding of the mechanism; probably all four Gell and Coombs types are involved. Allergic reactions are often delayed for hours to days, and allergic symptoms are dose- and frequency-related. Many methods are used to diagnose cyclic food allergy.

HISTORY   A history is taken and is combined with a 1-week food diary.

ORAL CHALLENGE   After 4 days of not eating the food, evaluate for symptoms if a large amount is eaten.

1. Time-consuming
2. Disruptive to lifestyle
3. Very subjective
4. Difficult to eliminate common foods, such as corn

SCRATCH AND PRICK

1. Many false-positive and false-negative results
2. Cyclic food allergy is not IgE-mediated

INTRADERMAL PROGRESSIVE DILUTION FOOD TESTING (IPDFT)   The IPDFT depends on a potent dose of the food antigen extract to produce a positive skin wheal. Consequently one should never test a patient for a food that historically has caused an anaphylactic reaction or test patients who are "brittle" or highly sensitive and suffer severe reactions to inhalant or food allergens. Test only for foods that are eaten twice a week or more. As with inhalant skin testing, avoid antihistamines for 48 hours prior to testing. Testing may provoke signs and symptoms of allergy. However the skin response or wheal is the most important measure of hypersensitivity. A positive test is 2 mm larger than the glycerine control wheal. Once a positive wheal is produced, one neutralizes this wheal with a neutralizing dose. The neutralizing dose is considered the next weaker dose that gives a negative reaction. The neutralizing dose is the endpoint of reaction and becomes the beginning point of immunotherapy.

The IDPFT has 79.7% sensitivity and 72.4% specificity.

Treatment of Cyclic Food Allergy

Treatment is based on the elimination of the food. Omission for 3-month intervals with challenge test feedings can be used to test for tolerance. Omission of the food until tolerance develops (may take up to 18 months) will then usually allow gradual reintroduction of the food into the diet (starting with weekly ingestions and working up to every other day).

Patients with multiple food sensitivities can use rotation of specific foods in the diet. The rotary diversified diet includes eating a variety of foods, with a specific food eaten only once every 4 days. Limiting the number of foods but increasing the amount of each at mealtime is a practical approach.

Allergic Fungal Sinusitis

Clinical Features

1. Persistent sinusitis despite antibiotics and surgery
2. Normal immune system
3. Pathology: allergic mucin with eosinophils, Charcot-Leyden crystals, fungal hyphae
4. Usually *Aspergillus,* but also *Bipolaris, Alternaria, Curvularia*

Radiographic Features

1. Hypercalcified speckling of sinus opacity
2. Thickening of sinus walls
3. Bone erosion

Diagnosis

1. Still uncertain; disease was first described in 1983, and experience is limited.
2. Elevated total IgE, peripheral eosinophilia.
3. Cultures positive for known pathogens
4. Histologic evidence of hyphae on fungal stains

Treatment

1. Surgical drainage, either external or endoscopic
2. Postoperative systemic steroids; prednisone 80 to 90 mg/day for 2 weeks, then slowly taper

IMMUNODEFICIENCY

Genetically determined immunodeficiency is rare. Infection is the most prominent manifestation of immunodeficiency (Table 12-16).

Types of Infection

Immunoglobulin (B cell) or neutrophil defect: Bacterial
T-cell defect: Fungal, viral, protozoal

TABLE 12-16. IMMUNODEFICIENCY DISORDERS

Disease	Dysfunction	Cause	Problems	Treatment
B-Cell Disorders				
Congenital agamma-globulinemia	Low Ig after maternal Ig is catabolized	Sporadic or X-linked (Bruton's)	Otitis media, sinusitis, sepsis; encapsulated pyogenic organisms; hypoplastic tonsils and adenoids	Prophylactic antibiotics, replacement of Ig
Selective IgA deficiency (incidence of 0.03–0.97%)	Low IgA; any age	Unknown	Atopy; sinusitis, otitis media; pneumonia	Antibiotics prn (high incidence of anaphylaxis with attempted IgA replacement)
Selective IgG subclass	IgG1, 2, 3, or 4; IgG4 is most common	Unknown	Otitis media, sinusitis, pneumonia	Ig replacement
Common variable	Low IgG, IgA, IgM; any age; abnormal G-cell differentiation	Low B or helper T; excessive suppressor T	Sinopulmonary infections, malignancy, normal tonsils and adenoids	Ig replacement
T-Cell Disorders				
DiGeorge (thymic hypoplasia)	T cells	Dysgenesis of pharyngeal pouches III and IV (includes thymus)	Hypertelorism, mandibular hypoplasia, bifid uvula, short philtrum, thrush, diarrhea, viral illnesses, pneumocystis pneumonia	Fetal thymus transplantation is experimental
Mucocutaneous candidiasis	T cells	Defect specific to *Candida*	Thrush, infection of nails and skin	Antifungals
AIDS	T-cell function	Human immunodeficiency virus (HIV)	*Pneumocystis carinii* pneumonia, candidiasis, Kaposi's sarcoma	Zidovudine, sulfa antibiotics, Ara-C, pentamidine
Combined Disorders				
Severe combined	Severe T and B cell	Multiple: X-linked, recessive	Otitis, pneumonia, *Pneumocystis carinii, Candida,* diarrhea; death by age 2	Transplanted bone marrow, fetal thymus or liver; gnotobiotic isolation; Ig replacement
Wiskott-Aldrich	Abnormal humoral response to polysaccharide antigens	X-linked recessive	Triad: thrombocytopenia, eczema, progressively severe recurrent infections	Antibiotics; platelets; high-dose Ig replacement; bone marrow transplantation
Ataxia-telangiectasia	IgA, T-cell function	Obscure	Recurrent sinopulmonary infections, oculocutaneous telangiectasia, progressive cerebellar ataxia, high incidence of malignancy	Antibiotics prn

Basic Laboratory Screen for Immunodeficiency

Cellular

1. Total lymphocyte count
2. Delayed hypersensitivity skin tests

Humoral

1. Total protein electrophoresis
2. Quantitative immunoglobulins

AUTOIMMUNITY

Systemic Lupus Erythematosus

Larynx

1. Thickening of vocal cords; hoarseness
2. Perichondritis, chondritis; loss of laryngeal or tracheal cartilage support, obstruction
3. Cricoarytenoid joint arthritis; airway obstruction

Nose

1. Butterfly rash over nose and cheeks, often triggered by exposure to sun
2. Dryness, nasal septal ulcers
3. Nasal septal perforation, probably as a result of vasculitis and infarct

Oral Cavity

1. Superficial ulcers with surrounding erythema, especially on cheeks and palate
2. Petechiae and hemorrhagic bullae if thrombocytopenia develops

Other Clinical Features

1. Vasculitis that predominantly affects small blood vessels
2. Antinuclear antibodies in 95% of patients
3. Antibodies to double-stranded DNA
4. Possible viral etiology
5. Predilection for young women

Sjögren's Syndrome

Eyes

1. Keratoconjunctivitis sicca
2. Grittiness, itching
3. Schirmer test is 85% sensitive, 85% specific

Mouth

1. Oral dryness (xerostomia)
2. Difficulty swallowing
3. Painful tongue
4. Dental caries

Other Clinical Features

1. Disorder of exocrine glands that occurs alone (primary) or with other autoimmune diseases (secondary), usually rheumatoid arthritis
2. Nine times more common in women

3. Also affects skin, esophagus, genitals
4. Often have antinuclear antibodies (ANA) and antibodies to extractable nuclear proteins, SS-A and SS-B

Rheumatoid Arthritis
Temporomandibular Joint Arthritis

Larynx
1. Cricoarytenoid joint arthritis
2. Vocal cord thickening

Cervical Spine
1. Subluxation; carefully evaluate before endoscopy

Ears
1. Synovitis of ossicular chain; leads to erosion of ossicles rather than fixation
2. Autoimmune inner ear disease

Other Clinical Features
1. Involves both cell-mediated and humoral immunity

Bibliography

Anonymous. Primer on allergic and immunologic diseases. *JAMA* 1997;278(22):1803–2030.

Barbey JT, Meltzer EO, Weinreb L. *Antihistamine Update.* Amherst, MA: University of Massachusetts Medical Center, 1996, 1–5.

Bellanti JA, ed. *Immunology III.* Philadelphia: Saunders, 1985.

Bennich HH, Ishizaka K, Johansson SGO, et al. Immunoglobulin E. A new class of immunoglobulin. *Bull WHO* 1968;38:151.

Breneman JC. *Basics of Food Allergy,* 2nd ed. Springfield, IL: Charles C Thomas, 1984.

Emanuel IA. *New Horizons in Otolaryngic Allergy. In Vitro Allergy Testing:* March 1990.

Fadal RG, Nalebuff DJ, eds. *RAST in Clinical Allergy.* Chicago: Yearbook, 1981.

Frank MM, Austen KF, eds. *Samter's Immunologic Diseases,* 5th ed. Boston: Little, Brown, 1995.

Ishizaka K, Ishizaka T. Identification of E antibodies as carrier of reaginic activity. *J Immunol* 1967; 99:1187.

Jirapongsananuruk O, Leung DY. Clinical applications of cytokines: New directions in the therapy of atopic diseases. *Ann Allergy Asthma Immunol* 1997;79(1):5–16.

King HC. *An Otolaryngologist's Guide to Allergy.* New York: Thieme, 1990.

King WP et al: Provocation—neutralization: A two-part study. Part I, The intracutaneous food test: A multi-center study; Part II, Subcutaneous neutralization therapy: A multi-center study. *Otolaryngol Head Neck Surg* 1988;99: 263–277.

Krause HF, ed. *Otolaryngic Allergy and Immunology.* Philadelphia: Saunders, 1989.

Lawlor GJ Jr, Fischer TJ. *Manual of Allergy and Immunology: Diagnosis and Therapy,* 3rd ed. Boston: Little Brown, 1994.

Male D, Champion B, Cooke A, Owen M. *Advanced Immunology,* 3rd ed. London; Gower, 1996.

Nathan RA: Changing strategies in the treatment of allergic rhinitis. *Ann Allergy Asthma Immunol* 1996;77:255–259.

Otolaryngic allergy, in Mabry RL, ed: *Otolaryngol Clin North Am* 1992;25(1):61–70.

Perelmutter L, Emanuel I. Assessment of in vitro IgE testing to diagnose allergic disease. *Ann Allergy* 1985;55(6):762–765.

Radford ER, Becker GD. *The Diagnosis and Management of Inhalant Allergy: A Self-Instructional Package.* Washington DC: American Academy of Otolaryngology—Head and Neck Surgery Foundation, 1986.

Rinkle HJ, Randolph TG, Zeller M. *Food Allergy.* Springfield, IL: Charles C. Thomas, 1951.

Rinkel HJ. The management of clinical allergy. Part I. *Arch Otolaryngol* 1962;76:491–508.

Rinkel HJ. The management of clinical allergy. Part II. *Arch Otolaryngol* 1963;77:42–75.

Rinkle HJ. The management of clinical allergy. Part III. *Arch Otolaryngol* 1963;77:205–225.

Rinkle HJ. The management of clinical allergy. Part IV. *Arch Otolaryngol* 1963;77:302–326.

Roitt IM, Brostoff J, Male DK. *Immunology,* 6th ed. St Louis: Mosby, 2001.

Trevino RJ, Dixon HS. *Food Allergy.* New York: Thieme, 1997; 67–70.

Williams RI. *The Management of Clinical Allergy.* Cheyenne, WY: Frontier Printing, 1983.

Willoughby JW. Serial dilution titration skin tests in inhalant allergy. *Otolaryngol Clin North Am* 1974;7(3):579–615.

The Chest 13

Many view pulmonary physiology as a discipline that is so complex that only physicians specializing in pulmonary medicine and critical care need be familiar with its principles. In actual fact, however, all physicians should have a basic understanding of the fundamentals of lung function. Otolaryngologists, in particular, need to be well acquainted with the basics of pulmonary function because a significant number of patients treated by the otolaryngologist have concomitant disease involving the lungs.

DEFINITIONS

Lung volumes can be divided into primary volumes and capacities.

1. Primary volumes
   a. *Tidal volume:* the volume of gas that is either inspired or expired during each normal respiratory cycle.
   b. *Residual volume:* the amount of gas that remains in the lungs at the end of a maximal expiratory effort.
2. Capacities
   a. *Total lung capacity:* the amount of gas contained in the lung at the end of a maximal inspiratory effort.
   b. *Vital capacity:* the maximum volume of gas exhaled when a patient makes a forceful exhalation after inspiring to the total lung capacity.
   c. *Functional residual capacity:* the volume of gas that remains in the lung at the end of quiet exhalation.

Dynamic lung volumes are as follows:

1. Forced expiratory volume in 1 second (FEV_1): the volume of gas exhaled from the lung after initiation of a forceful exhalation following a maximal inspiration.
2. Forced expiratory volume in 1 second/forced vital capacity (FEV_1/FVC) ratio: the ratio of the volume of gas exhaled from the lungs during the first second after forceful exhalation divided by the total volume of gas exhaled after forceful exhalation.

BASIC TESTS OF PULMONARY FUNCTION

Spirometry

The spirometer is widely used in pulmonary function laboratories because it and a nitrogen or helium analyzer allow the physician to obtain data concerning lung volumes, capacities, and dynamic lung volumes. By analyzing data obtained with a spirometer, the physician is able to determine whether a patient has normal or abnormal lung function. In addition, the spirometer enables the physician to assess the abnormalities of function and place the individual into one of two major pulmonary disease categories: chronic airflow limitation (diseases such as asthma, chronic bronchitis, and pulmonary emphysema) or restrictive lung disease (diseases such as pulmonary fibrosis).

302

Flow Volume Loops

The maximal expiratory flow volume curve has been widely used by pulmonary laboratories for the past several years. In a spirometer tracing, volume is plotted against time (FEV_1 is the volume of gas exhaled during the first second after exhalation from a maximal inspiration). If the volume–time relation is normal, the flow rate is presumed to be normal; flow is never actually measured. In the flow volume loop, however, instantaneous flow is measured by means of a pneumotachygraph, and flow is plotted against lung volume. Conditions that produce airflow limitation cause a reduction in measured flow rates throughout the patient's FVC maneuver.

Figure 13-1 illustrates a normal flow volume loop and a flow volume loop from a patient with chronic airflow limitation (such as chronic obstructive pulmonary disease, COPD). Note that the shape of the curve is concave in the normal patient but convex in the patient with limited flow. Note also that the flow volume loop characterizes the relations between flow and volume during the inspiratory portion of the respiratory cycle. The uses of this portion of the curve are discussed in a subsequent section of this chapter.

As with patients whose spirometry tracings indicate airflow limitation, bronchodilator medication is administered to patients with abnormal flow volume loops compatible with airflow limitation. Patients with reversible disease demonstrate a 15 to 20% improvement in the flow volume loop after bronchodilator administration. Patients with restrictive lung

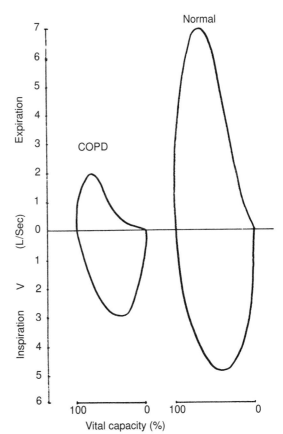

Figure 13-1. Flow volume loop. Note the reduction in flow.

diseases have abnormal flow volume loops, but because they do not have an abnormality of the airways, their FEV_1/FVC ratio is usually normal. The slope of the expiratory loop in these patients is normal, in keeping with their normal airways.

Additional Uses of the Flow Volume Curve

As noted, the flow volume curve can be used to evaluate inspiration as well as exhalation. This feature enables the pulmonary physiologist to evaluate the upper airway and assess the presence or absence of upper airway obstruction; this can also be a useful test for an otolaryngologist.

The ability of the flow volume loop to detect upper airway obstruction is based on the following physiologic principle: On inspiration, pleural pressure becomes more negative than the intraluminal pressure in the intrathoracic airways.

Consequently, on inspiration the caliber of the airways located within the chest increases. In the extrathoracic airways, such as the trachea, however, inspiration leads to a reduction in the intraluminal pressure, making atmospheric pressure greater than the pressure within the tracheal lumen. As a result, during inspiration the caliber of the tracheal lumen tends to diminish because atmospheric pressure exceeds intratracheal pressure.

In patients with variable extrathoracic (upper airway) obstruction, the obstruction tends to narrow the tracheal lumen. On inspiration, this narrowing becomes more pronounced by the effect of inspiration, which also causes a reduction in the size of the tracheal lumen. Hence, on inspiration, patients with variably obstructing lesions of the upper airway show a reduction in inspiratory flow, so that the inspiratory curve often appears flattened. On exhalation, intratracheal pressure becomes greater than atmospheric pressure, which causes the tracheal lumen to expand. This expansion tends to negate the effect of a variably obstructing tracheal lesion, and the expiratory portion of the flow volume curve appears normal even if there is a variably obstructing lesion present. Thus, in a patient with a variably obstructing lesion of the upper airway, the inspiratory curve is flattened whereas the expiratory curve appears normal. Figure 13-2 illustrates the curve produced by variably obstructing extrathoracic (upper airway) lesions.

Lung Compliance

The compliance of the lung refers to the elastic properties of that organ. Compliance is a measure of the distensibility, or elasticity, of the lung parenchyma. Many physicians are confused by the term elasticity. Elasticity refers to the ability of a structure to resist deformation. A rubber band is often referred to as an "elastic band"; it is an elastic structure not because it can be stretched but because it reverts to its original length when released. Hence, elasticity is the property whereby the original shape is preserved.

Distensibility, on the other hand, is the ease with which shape can be altered. An elastic structure is not distensible, whereas a distensible structure does not possess elastic qualities. In the lung, distensibility refers to the ease with which changes in distending pressure change lung volume. A lung in which small distending pressures produce large changes in volume is a highly distensible (or highly compliant) lung. A lung in which high distending pressures are required to produce even small changes in lung volume is poorly distensible and poorly compliant. It is also a highly elastic (or "stiff") lung. Clinical examples are (1) the emphysematous lung, which is highly distensible, highly compliant, and poorly elastic secondary to the destruction of the elastic structures of the lung, and (2) the fibrotic lung, which is poorly compliant, poorly distensible, and very elastic or stiff owing to the increased deposition of collagen. Figure 13-3 illustrates compliance curves in patients with normal, highly compliant (emphysematous), or "stiff" (fibrotic) lungs.

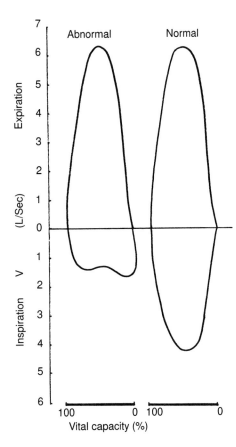

Figure 13-2.   Extrathoracic obstruction.

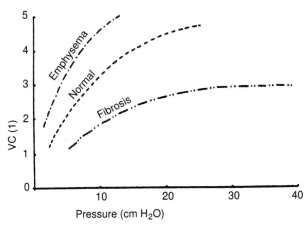

Figure 13-3.   Compliance curve: pressure–volume relation.

Diffusing Capacity

The diffusing capacity refers to the quantity of a specific gas that diffuses across the alveolar–capillary membrane per unit of time. The diffusing capacity is often used to assess the size of the pulmonary capillary blood volume. A full discussion of the methods employed to measure the diffusing capacity is beyond the scope of this text. In most pulmonary function laboratories, carbon monoxide is used to measure the diffusing capacity. This gas avidly binds to hemoglobin. In clinical practice, the diffusing capacity is thought to represent the volume of capillary blood into which carbon monoxide can dissolve. Diseases such as emphysema, which are characterized by a reduction in capillary blood volume, are associated with a low diffusing capacity.

Blood Gases

Alveolar ventilation refers to the volume of gas in each breath that participates in gas exchange times the respiratory frequency. Alveolar ventilation determines the level of arterial carbon dioxide; in the clinical setting, the adequacy of alveolar ventilation is assessed by measuring the arterial partial pressure of carbon dioxide (Pco_2).

In clinical practice, the most common causes of hypoxemia are simple hypoventilation and ventilation–perfusion inequality. Other causes of hypoxemia include anatomic shunts and abnormalities of diffusion, but these problems are rarely found in clinical hypoxemia.

The otolaryngologist is often confronted with a patient whose blood gas measurements reveal hypoxemia, and it is important that the attending physician be able to distinguish patients who have intrinsic pulmonary disease from those with simple hypoventilation (such as may be produced by anesthetic administration) and normal lungs. One useful technique for evaluating the presence or absence of intrinsic lung disease is the determination of the alveolar–arterial (A–a) gradient. A simple way to calculate the A–a gradient is to assume that the alveolar oxygen tension is $148 - $ arterial $Pco_2 \times 1.2$. If the alveolar oxygen tension is calculated and the arterial Po_2 measured, the A–a gradient can be estimated. If there is less than a 20-mm Hg gradient between alveolar and arterial oxygen tensions, it is likely that the lungs are normal and that alveolar hypoventilation is the sole abnormality producing the hypoxemia. Patients with normal lungs who have primary alveolar hypoventilation exhibit normal oxygen tensions when the cause of the alveolar hypoventilation is removed. A patient with a sedative overdose has normal oxygenation when the effects of the sedative on respiratory drive wear off.

Diseases that produce widened A–a gradients produce hypoxemia that cannot be corrected by simply increasing the level of alveolar ventilation. As stated, the most common cause of hypoxemia in these patients is maldistribution of alveolar ventilation and pulmonary blood flow. Diseases such as asthma, bronchitis, and emphysema impair ventilation because of abnormal airway flow. The reduction in flow produces abnormal ventilation–blood flow relations, which creates the observed hypoxemia.

The rationale for the treatment of hypoxemia produced by ventilation–perfusion abnormalities is illustrated in Figure 13-4. If alveolus 1 has a reduction in ventilation due to airway narrowing, the alveolar oxygen tension in alveolus 1 falls. The saturation of red blood cells (RBCs) in blood vessel I supplying alveolus 1 also falls. Alveolus 2, which receives normal ventilation, has a normal alveolar oxygen tension. RBCs in blood vessel II supplying alveolus 2 are normally saturated. Blood vessel III, which receives blood from vessels I and II, thus holds partially and fully saturated RBCs, so that the saturation of RBCs in III

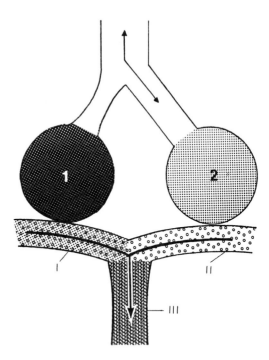

Figure 13-4. Ventilation perfusion mismatch. 1, 2, alveoli; I, II, III, blood vessels.

is reduced. Ventilation–perfusion abnormalities cannot be corrected by simple hyperventilation because hyperventilation does not increase the alveolar oxygen tension in alveolus 1 enough to increase the saturation of RBCs in vessel I. Hyperventilation may slightly increase the alveolar oxygen tension in alveolus 2, but the RBCs in blood vessel II are already fully saturated, and, therefore, the increase in alveolar oxygen tension cannot improve the saturation in the blood vessels supplying the alveolus. Thus vessel III, supplied by vessels I and II, remains with less than optimal RBC saturation. On the other hand, if the inspired oxygen tension delivered to the patient is increased, the alveolar oxygen tension in alveolus 1 can be improved and the saturation of RBCs will increase. Samples of blood from vessel III will show an increase in saturation as well.

As shown in Figure 13-5, the shape of the oxyhemoglobin dissociation curve is such that small increments in oxygen tension may be associated with significant improvement in oxygen saturation if the increments occur on the steep slope of the dissociation curve. A higher inspired oxygen tension creates a situation in which the alveolar oxygen tension in alveolus 1 rises, thus raising the RBC saturation in vessel I. As already noted, RBCs in vessel II are fully saturated, but now vessel III has improved RBC saturation in RBCs emanating from vessel I plus normally saturated blood from vessel II. It is evident that if the inspired oxygen tension delivered to the patient is increased, the alveolar oxygen tension in alveolus 1 can be improved and the saturation of RBCs will increase. Samples of blood drawn from vessel III will demonstrate an increase in saturation as well.

It is for these reasons that diseases characterized by ventilation–perfusion mismatching show improvement in hypoxemia when treated with higher inspired oxygen tensions. However, if there is a true anatomic shunt present in alveolus 1, so that blood vessel I does

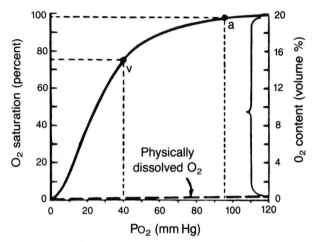

Figure 13-5. Oxyhemoglobin dissociation curve. O_2 saturation is given by the vertical axis on the left and O_2 content by the vertical axis on the right. Note the S shape of the curve and the location of the arterial point on the flat part of the dissociation curve and the venous point on the steep portion of the curve. The hemoglobin content of this blood is 15 g/dL, and the amount of O_2 carried in physical solution is much less than that bound to hemoglobin, as indicated by the bracket on the O_2 content axis.

not come into contact with the alveolus, raising the inspired oxygen tension will have no effect on the hypoxemia because the RBC saturation in vessel I cannot be increased. True anatomic shunts do not respond to increases in inspired oxygen tension.

PULMONARY VOLUMES AND CAPACITIES

Tidal volume (TV): depth of breathing; volume of gas inspired or expired during each normal respiratory cycle; 0.5 L (average).

Inspired reserve volume (IRV): maximum that can be inspired from end-inspiratory position; 3.3 L (average).

Expired reserve volume (ERV): maximum volume that can be expired from end-respiratory level; 0.7 to 1.0 L (average).

Residual volume (RV): volume left in lungs after maximum expiration; 1.1 L (average).

Forced expiratory volume in 1 second (FEV_1): should be 80% or more of predicted value from a normative chart.

Forced vital capacity (FVC): should be 80% or more of predicted value from a normative chart. The FEV_1/FVC ratio should be more than 0.75 for younger patients and 0.70 for older individuals.

Total lung capacity (6 L for men; 4.2 L for women): IRV + TV + ERV + RV (total volume contained in the lungs after maximum inspiration).

Vital capacity (4.8 L for men; 3.1 L for women): IRV + TV + ERV (maximum volume that can be expelled from the lungs for effort following maximum inspiration).

Functional residual capacity (2.2 L for men; 1.8 L for women): RV + ERV (volume in the lungs at resting expiratory level).

Physiologic dead space (dead space of upper airway bypassed by tracheotomy, 70–100 mL): anatomic dead space + the volume of gas that ventilates the alveoli that have no capillary blood flow + the volume of gas that ventilates the alveoli in excess of that required to arteriolize the capillary blood.

MEAN NORMAL BLOOD GAS AND ACID-BASE VALUES

	Arterial Blood	*Mixed Venous Blood*
pH	7.40	7.37
P_{CO_2}	41 mm Hg	46.5 mm Hg
P_{O_2}	95 mm Hg	40 mm Hg
O_2 sat	97.1%	75.0%
HCO_3	4.0 mEq/L	25.0 mEq/L

MISCELLANEOUS INFORMATION

1. Silo-filler disease (bronchiolitis obliterans) is a pathologic entity consisting of a collection of exudate in the bronchioles obliterating the lumen. This complication often follows inhalation of nitrogen dioxide, exposure to open bottles of nitric acid, and exposure to silos. The diagnosis is based on a history of exposure, dyspnea, cough, and x-ray findings similar to those of miliary tuberculosis. Treatment is symptomatic. Prognosis is poor; most patients eventually succumb to this disease.

2. Bronchogenic cysts are congenital, arise from the bronchi, and are lined with epithelial cells. Furthermore, their walls may contain glands, smooth muscles, and cartilage. In the absence of infection, they may remain asymptomatic; otherwise, they give a productive cough, hemoptysis, and fever. The recommended treatment is surgical excision.

3. Blebs or bullae are air-containing structures resembling cysts, but their walls are not epithelium-lined.

4. Anthracosilicosis is also called coal miner's pneumoconiosis.

5. Berylliosis is characterized by an infiltration of the lungs by beryllium. It often is found in workers at fluorescent lamp factories.

6. Bagassosis is characterized by an infiltration of the lungs by sugar cane fibers.

7. Byssinosis is characterized by an infiltration of the lungs by cotton dust.

8. Adenocarcinoma of the bronchus is the leading primary pulmonary carcinoma in women, and bronchogenic (squamous cell) is most common in men.

9. Pancoast syndrome (superior sulcus tumor) is caused by any process of the apex of the lung that can invade the pleural layers and infiltrate between the lower cords of the brachial plexus, and may involve the cervical sympathetic nerve chain, phrenic, and recurrent laryngeal nerves. It is usually secondary to a benign or malignant tumor; however, a large inflammatory process may cause this syndrome as well. The symptoms are:

   a. Pain in shoulder and arm, particularly in the axilla and inner arm

   b. Intrinsic hand muscle atrophy

   c. Horner syndrome (enophthalmos, ptosis of the upper lid, constriction of the pupil with narrowing of the palpebral fissure, and decreased sweating homolaterally)

10. Congenital agenesis of the lung has been classified by Schneider as follows:
    Class I: total agenesis
    Class II: only the trachea is present
    Class III: trachea and bronchi are present without any pulmonary tissue.

11. Apnea after tracheotomy is due to carbon dioxide narcosis causing the medulla to be depressed. Prior to the tracheotomy, the patient was breathing secondary to the lack of oxygen. After the tracheotomy this oxygen drive is removed, and hence the patient remains apneic. Treatment is to ventilate the patient until the excess carbon dioxide level is reduced. Mediastinal emphysema and pneumothorax are the most common complications of tracheotomy. (For other complications, see Chapter 31.)

12. Hypoxemia is defined as less than 75% oxygen saturation or less than 40 mm Hg Po_2. A methemoglobin level of more than 5 mg/dL produces cyanosis.

13. Bronchogenic cyst is a defect at the 4th week of gestation. It constitutes less than 5% of all mediastinal cysts and tumors.

14. The bronchial tree ring is cartilaginous until it reaches 1 mm in diameter. These small bronchioles without cartilaginous rings are held patent by the elastic property of the lung. The bronchial tree is lined by pseudostratified columnar ciliated epithelium as well as nonciliated cuboidal epithelium.

15. The adult trachea measures 10 to 12 cm and has 16 to 20 rings. The diameter is approximately 20×15 mm.

16. The larynx descends on inspiration and ascends on expiration. It also ascends in the process of swallowing and in the production of a high-pitched note.

17. The esophageal lumen widens on inspiration.

18. The total lung surface measures 70 m². The lung contains 300 million aveoli. It secretes 200 mL of fluid per day.

19. During inspiration, the nose constitutes 79% of the total respiratory resistance, the larynx, 6%, and the bronchial tree, 15%. During expiration, the nose constitutes 75% of the resistance, the larynx, 3%, and the bronchial tree, 23%.

20. Tracheopathia osteoplastica is a rare disease characterized by growths of cartilage and bone within the walls of the trachea and bronchi that produce sessile plaques that project into the lumen. There is no specific treatment other than supportive. It is of unknown etiology. The serum calcium is normal, and there are not other calcium deposits.

21. Calcification found in a pulmonary nodule implies that it is a benign nodule.

22. Middle lobe syndrome (see Chapter 39) may be present.

23. The right upper lobe and its bronchus is the lobe that is most susceptible to congenital anomaly.

24. Cystic fibrosis (mucoviscidosis) is familial and may be autosomal-recessive. The patient presents with multiple polyps, pulmonary infiltration with abscesses, and rectal prolapse. The pancreas is afflicted with a fibrocystic process and produces no enzymes. Trypsin is lacking in the gastric secretion. Ten to fifteen percent of the patients pass trypsin in the stool. There is general malabsorption of liposoluble vitamins. Treatment consists of a high-protein, low-fat diet with water-soluble vitamins and pancreatic extracts. Many patients die of pulmonary abscesses.

25. A person ventilated with pure oxygen for 7 minutes is cleared of 90% of the nitrogen and can withstand 5 to 8 minutes without further oxygenation.

MEDIASTINUM

1. Suprasternal fossa has these characteristics:
   a. It is the region in which the sternocleidomastoid muscles converge toward their sternal attachments. Bound inferiorly by the suprasternal notch, they have no superior boundary.
   b. The deep cervical fascia splits into an anterior and a posterior portion. These portions are attached, respectively, to the anterior and posterior margins of the manubrium.
   c. The space between these fascial layers is the small suprasternal space containing (1) anterior jugular veins and (2) fatty connective tissues.
   d. Behind this space lies the pretracheal fascia.
   e. Laterally on each side are the medial borders of the sternohyoid and sternothyroid muscles.
2. In the adult the innominate artery crosses in front of the trachea, behind the upper half of the manubrium. In the child it crosses over the level of the superior border of the sternum.
3. The trachea enters the mediastinum on the right side.
4. The trachea bifurcates at T4-T5 or about 6 cm from the suprasternal notch. As a person approaches 65 years of age or more, it is possible that the trachea bifurcates at T6.
5. To the left of the trachea are the aorta, left recurrent laryngeal nerve, and left subclavian artery. To the right of the trachea are the superior vena cava, azygos vein, right vagus, and right lung pleura.
6. The innominate and left carotid arteries lie anterior to the trachea near their origin. As they ascend, the innominate artery lies to the right of the trachea.
7. The pulmonary artery passes anterior to the bronchi and assumes a position superior to the bronchi at the hilus, with the exception that the right upper lobe bronchus is superior to the right pulmonary artery.
8. The left main bronchus crosses in front of the esophagus. It presses on the esophagus and together with the aorta forms the bronchoaortic constriction. The first part of the aorta is to the left of the esophagus. As it descends it assumes a left posterolateral position to the esophagus.
9. The course of the esophagus is as shown in Figure 13-6. The esophagus has four constricting points:
   a. Cricopharyngeus muscle
   b. Aorta crossing
   c. Left main stem bronchus crossing
   d. Diaphragm (a < b = c < d). At the level of c the esophagus passes from the superior mediastinum to the posterior mediastinum.
10. The following structures are found within the concavity of the aorta:
    a. Left main stem bronchus
    b. Left recurrent laryngeal nerve
    c. Tracheobronchial nodes
    d. Superficial part of the cardiac plexus
11. The right main stem bronchus is wider, shorter, and follows a more vertical course than the left one.

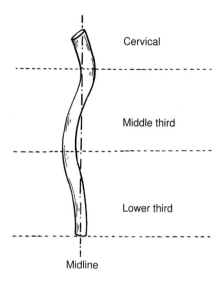

Cervical

Middle third

Lower third

Midline

Figure 13-6.   Course of the esophagus.

12. The interior thyroid vein is immediately in front of the trachea in its infraisthmic portion.
13. Ten percent of the population has a thyroidea ima artery. It arises from either the innominate artery or the aorta and passes upward along the anterior aspect of the trachea.

Course of the Vagus
Left Side
1. It passes inferiorly between the left subclavian and the left carotid.
2. It follows the subclavian to its origin.
3. It passes to the left of the arch of the aorta.
4. It gives off the recurrent laryngeal nerve, which passes superiorly along the left border of the tracheoesophageal groove (between the esophagus and trachea).
5. The main vagus continues to descend behind the left main stem bronchus.

Right Side
1. It descends anterior to the subclavian where it gives off the recurrent laryngeal nerve that loops around the subclavian artery and ascends posteromedial to the right common carotid artery to reach the tracheoesophageal groove (between the esophagus and the trachea).
2. The main trunk descends posteriorly along the right side of the trachea, between the trachea and right pleura.
3. It descends posterior to the right bronchus.

Fascia of the Mediastinum
The space between the various mediastinal organs is occupied by loose areolar tissues. The fascial layers of the mediastinum are a direct continuation of the cervical fascia. A portion of the cervical fascia, the perivisceral fascia, encloses the larynx, pharynx, trachea, esophagus, thyroid, thymus, and carotid sheath contents. This space enclosed by this perivisceral fascia extends to the bifurcation of the trachea. Anteriorly it is bound by the pretracheal fascia. The

pretracheal fascia is an important landmark in mediastinoscopy in that dissection should be done only beneath this layer.

Boundaries of the Mediastinum

See Figure 13-7.

Lateral: parietal pleura
Anterior: sternum
Posterior: vertebrae
Inferior: diaphragm
Superior: superior aperture of the thorax

Superior Mediastinum

The boundaries are:

Superior: superior aperture of the throat
Anterior: manubrium with sternothyroid and sternohyoid muscles
Posterior: upper thoracic vertebrae
Inferior: manubrium to fourth vertebra

Structures of the superior mediastinum are the thymus, innominate veins, aorta, vagus, recurrent laryngeal nerve, phrenic nerve, azygos vein, esophagus, and thoracic duct.

Anterior Mediastinum

It lies between the body of the sternum and the pericardium and contains

1. Loose areolar tissues
2. Lymphatics
3. Lymph nodes
4. Thymus gland

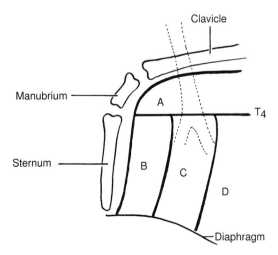

Figure 13-7. Various chambers of the mediastinum. **A,** Superior mediastinum; **B,** Anterior mediastinum; **C,** Middle mediastinum; **D,** Posterior mediastinum.

Middle Mediastinum

It contains the heart, ascending aorta, superior vena cava, azygos vein, bifurcation of the main bronchus, pulmonary artery trunk, right and left pulmonary veins, phrenic nerves, and the tracheobronchial lymph nodes.

Posterior Mediastinum

Anteriorly lie the bifurcation of the trachea, the pulmonary vein, the pericardium, and the posterior part of the upper surface of the diaphragm. Posteriorly lies the vertebral column from T4 to T12. Laterally lies the mediastinal pleura.

The posterior mediastinum contains the thoracic aorta, azygos vein, hemizygous vein, cranial nerve X, splanchnic nerve, esophagus, thoracic duct, posterior mediastinal lymph nodes, and the intercostal arteries.

LYMPH NODES OF THE THORAX

See Figure 13-8.

1. Parietal nodes are inconsequential clinically. They are grouped into intercostal, sternal, and phrenic nodes.
2. Visceral nodes are of greater clinical importance. They are grouped as follows:

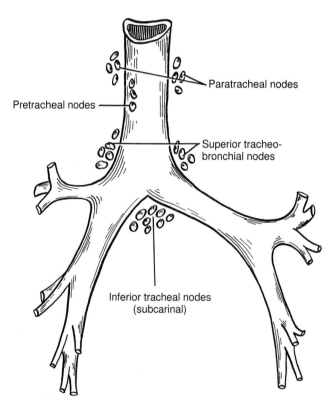

Figure 13-8. Thoracic lymph nodes.

a. Peritracheobronchial
    (1) Paratracheal
    (2) Pretracheal
    (3) Superior tracheobronchial
    (4) Inferior tracheobronchial
b. Bronchopulmonary (hilar nodes)
c. Anterior mediastinal or prevascular
d. Pulmonary
e. Posterior mediastinal

Lymphatic Drainage of the Lung
Right Side
1. Superior area (anteromedial area of the right upper lobe): right paratracheal nodes
2. Middle area (posterolateral area of right upper lobe, right middle lobe, and superior right lower lobe): right paratracheal nodes and inferior tracheobronchial nodes
3. Inferior area (lower half of right lower lobe): inferior tracheobronchial nodes and posterior mediastinal nodes

Left Side
1. Superior area (upper left upper lobe): left paratracheal, anterior mediastinal, and subaortic nodes.
2. Middle area (lower left upper lobe and upper left lower lobe): left paratracheal, inferior tracheobronchial, and anterior mediastinal nodes.
3. Inferior area (inferior part of the left lower lobe): inferior tracheobronchial nodes. (Inferior tracheobronchial nodes drain into the right paratracheal nodes.)

Right upper lung:	right neck
Right lower lung:	right neck
Left lower lung:	right neck
Left upper lung:	left neck
Lingular lobe:	both sides of the neck

PURPOSES OF MEDIASTINOSCOPY

(Barium swallow and tracheogram are usually obtained before mediastinoscopy if indicated.)

1. Histologic diagnosis
2. To determine which nodes are involved
3. To make the diagnosis of sarcoidosis

MEDIASTINAL TUMORS

One-third of all mediastinal tumors are malignant. Among the malignant ones, lymphoma is most commonly encountered.

1. Superior mediastinum: thyroid, neurinoma, thymoma, parathyroid
2. Anterior mediastinum: dermoid, teratoma, thyroid, thymoma
3. Low anterior mediastinum: pericardial cyst
4. Middle mediastinum: pericardial cyst, bronchial cyst, lymphoma, carcinoma
5. Posterior mediastinum: neurinoma, enterogenous cyst

SUPERIOR VENA CAVA SYNDROME

1. Etiology: malignant metastasis, mediastinal tumors, mediastinal fibrosis, vena cava thrombosis
2. Signs and symptoms: edema and cyanosis of the face, neck, and upper extremities; venous hypertension with dilated veins; normal venous pressure of lower extremities; visible venous circulation of the anterior chest wall

ENDOSCOPY

Size of Tracheotomy Tubes and Bronchoscopes

Age	Tracheotomy Tubes	Bronchoscope (mm)
Premature	No. 000 × 26 mm to No. 00 × 33 mm	3
6 months	No. 0 × 33 mm to No. 0 × 40 mm	3.5
18 months	No. 1 × 46 mm	4
5 years	No. 2 × 50 mm	5
10 years	No. 3 × 50 mm to No. 4 × 68 mm	6
Adult		7

Esophagoscopy

Size of Esophagoscope

Child	5 × 35 mm or 6 × 35 mm
Adult	9 × 50 mm

Average Distance from Incisor Teeth to Other Areas During Esophagoscopy

See Figure 13-9.

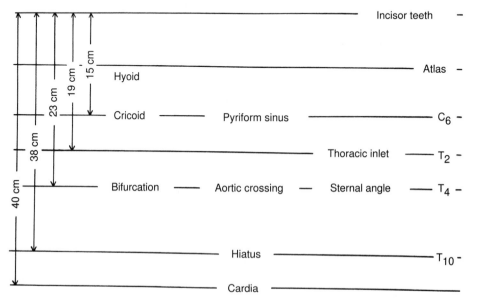

Figure 13-9.   Relative landmarks for esophagoscopy.

Left Lung: Lobes and Segments

1. Upper division of upper lobe
    a. Apical–posterior
    b. Anterior
2. Lower division of upper lobe
    a. Superior
    b. Inferior
3. Lower lobe
    a. Superior
    b. Anteromedial basal
    c. Lateral basal
    d. Posterior basal

Right Lung: Lobes and Segments

1. Upper lobe
    a. Apical
    b. Posterior
    c. Anterior
2. Middle lobe
    a. Lateral
    b. Medial
3. Lower lobe
    a. Superior
    b. Medial basal
    c. Anterior basal
    d. Lateral basal
    e. Posterior basal

Relative Contraindications for Esophagoscopy

1. Aneurysm of the aorta
2. Spinal deformities, osteophytes
3. Esophageal burns and steroid treatment

Relative Contraindications for Bronchography

1. Acute infection
2. Acute asthmatic attacks
3. Acute cardiac failure

Causes of Hemoptysis

In order of decreasing frequency:

1. Bronchiectasis
2. Adenoma
3. Tracheobronchitis
4. Tuberculosis
5. Mitral stenosis

Foreign Bodies

1. Right upper lobe bronchus: most common site
2. Left upper lobe bronchus: second most common site

3. Trachea: least likely site
4. Cervical esophagus: most common site for esophageal foreign bodies
5. Most common foreign bodies in children: peanuts, safety pins, coins
6. Most common foreign bodies in adults: meat and bone

VASCULAR ANOMALIES

See Chapter 10 and Figure 10-2. The normal great vessels are shown in Figure 13-10.

1. Double aortic arch: this anomaly is a true vascular ring. It is due to the persistence of the right fourth branchial arch vessel. The symptoms include stridor, intermittent dysphagia, and aspiration pneumonitis. The right posterior arch is usually the largest of the two arches.
2. Right aortic arch with ligamentum arteriosus: it is due to the persistence of the right fourth branchial arch vessel becoming the aorta instead of the left fourth arch vessel. This vessel crosses the trachea, causing an anterior compression.
3. Anomalous right subclavian artery: it is due to the right subclavian artery arising from the dorsal aorta, causing posterior compression of the esophagus. There is no constriction over the trachea.
4. Anomalous innominate and/or left common carotid: the innominate arises too far left from the aorta. It crosses the trachea anteriorly, causing anterior compression. The left common carotid arises from the aorta on the right or from the innominate artery. It also causes anterior compression of the trachea. In a variant of this anomaly, the innominate

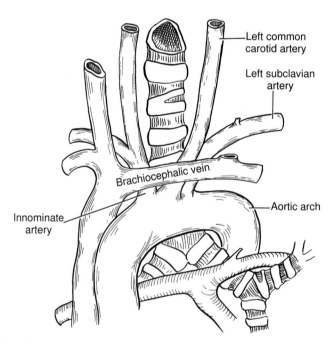

Figure 13-10.   Normal great vessels.

and the right common carotid arise from the same trunk, and when they divide they encircle the trachea and esophagus, causing airway obstruction as well as dysphagia.

5. Patent ductus arteriosus.
6. Coarctation of the aorta.
7. Enlarged heart: an enlarged heart, especially with mitral insufficiency, can compress the left bronchus.
8. Dysphagia lusoria: this term is used to include dysphagia caused by any aberrant great vessel. The common cause is an abnormal subclavian artery arising from the descending aorta.
9. Anomalous innominate arteries: they have been estimated to be the most common vascular anomaly. They cause anterior compression of the trachea. During bronchoscopy, if the pulsation is obliterated with the bronchoscope, the radial pulse on the right arm and the temporal pulse are reduced. In the case of a subclavian anomaly, the bronchoscope compressing the abnormal subclavian produces a decrease of the radial pulse, although the temporal pulse remains normal. A bronchoscope compressing a double aortic arch pulsation produces no pulse changes in either the radial or the temporal pulse.

Diseases Producing Limitation of Airflow

Pulmonary diseases that produce a reduction in the flow of air through airways more than 2 mm in diameter produce spirometric evidence for this limited airflow. Airflow limitation is reflected on the spirometer tracings as a reduction in FVC and FEV_1. In addition, the FEV_1/FVC ratio falls below the predicted normal value. Functional residual capacity is elevated, as is the RV. In more advanced cases, the total lung capacity is also increased.

An abnormal spirogram does not indicate the cause of disease, as asthma, chronic bronchitis, and emphysema all show evidence of airflow limitation. When a spirometric tracing reveals evidence of airflow limitation, the patient is normally given a bronchodilator (eg, metaproterenol) and the test is repeated.

Patients with reversible airflow limitation, such as asthma, most often demonstrate 15 to 20% improvement in dynamic lung volumes following administration of a bronchodilator. These patients are described as exhibiting "reversible airflow limitation."

Patients whose pre- and postbronchodilator tracings do not vary may have chronic bronchitis or emphysema, or may be in the throes of an asthmatic attack that is so severe the response to the bronchodilator is muted. It is, therefore, not possible to eliminate asthma as a diagnostic possibility if the postbronchodilator study does not show reversibility.

Because the incidence of postoperative pulmonary complications increases with the severity of airflow limitation, it is important to perform spirometry on all patients who, on the basis of history and physical findings, are likely to have pulmonary diseases characterized by obstruction of flow. If the spirogram is abnormal and indicative of obstruction, a bronchodilator should be given. If reversibility is demonstrated, the patient is given a bronchodilator prior to surgery to maximize his or her lung function preoperatively and reduce the incidence of postoperative complications.

Restrictive Lung Disease

The spirometric abnormality produced by patients with restrictive lung disease differs significantly from the curves produced by patients with chronic airflow limitation. Patients with restrictive lung disease exhibit a reduction in their total lung capacity. Diseases that produce restriction include diseases in which a functioning lung is replaced by granulomas or fibrosis (eg, sarcoid or interstitial fibrosis), diseases that lead to restricted expansion of the lungs as seen in primary neurologic disorders (amyotrophic lateral sclerosis) or primary muscle disorders (muscular dystrophy), diseases in which there is a reduction in the amount of functioning lung (pneumonectomy), and diseases in which there is a reduction in lung expansion (scoliosis and fibrothorax).

The spirometric tracing of a patient with restrictive lung disease demonstrates a reduction in FVC and FEV_1, but the FEV_1/FVC ratio is preserved. Whereas with chronic airflow limitation the values for functional residual capacity, RV, and total lung capacity are elevated, in restrictive lung diseases these values are reduced.

Patients with restrictive lung diseases do not demonstrate improvement after the administration of bronchodilators, as the defect in restrictive lung diseases does not lie in the airways per se.

Bibliography

Bates D. *Respiratory Function in Disease,* 3rd ed. Philadelphia: WB Saunders, 1989.

Bickerman HA. Lung volumes, capacities, and thoracic volumes. In: Chusid EL, ed. *The Selective and Comprehensive Testing of Adult Pulmonary Function.* 1983, 5.

Bone RC, Dantzker DR, George RB, et al. *Pulmonary and Critical Care Medicine.* Vols. 1 & 2. St. Louis: Mosby Year Book, 1993.

Cherniack N. *Chronic Obstructive Pulmonary Disease.* Philadelphia: WB Saunders, 1991.

Comroe JH Jr. *Physiology of Respiration,* 2nd ed. Chicago: Year Book, 1974.

Emerson P. *Thoracic Medicine.* Stoneham, MA: Butterworths, 1981.

George R, Light R, Matthay M, Matthay R, eds. *Chest Medicine: Essentials of Pulmonary and Critical Care Medicine,* 2nd ed. Baltimore: Williams & Wilkins, 1990.

Hollinshead WH. Anatomy for surgeons. *The Head and Neck,* 2nd ed. Vol. 1. New York: Harper & Row, 1968.

Kazemi H. Oxygen and carbon dioxide transport. In: *Science and Practice of Clinical Medicine.* In: *Disorders of the Respiratory System.* Vol. 2. 42.

Miller DR, Hyatt RE. Evaluation of obstructing lesions of the trachea and larynx by flow-volume loops. *Am Rev Respir Dis* 1973; 108:478.

Murray JF. *The Normal Lung—The Basis for Diagnosis and Treatment of Pulmonary Disease.* Philadelphia: WB Saunders, 1976, 82.

Murray JF, Nadel JA. *Textbook of Respiratory Medicine.* Philadelphia: WB Saunders, 1988.

Pennington J, ed. *Respiratory Infections: Diagnosis & Management,* 2nd ed. New York: Raven Press, 1989.

Related Ophthalmology 14

ANATOMY

1. The orbit forms a quadrilateral pyramid: floor, roof, medial wall, and lateral wall.
    Roof: Orbital process of the frontal bone; lesser wing of the sphenoid
    Floor: Orbital plate of maxilla; orbital surface of zygoma; orbital process of the palatine bone
    Medial wall: Frontal process of maxilla; lacrimal bone; sphenoid bone; lamina papyracea of the ethmoid bone
    Lateral wall: Lesser and greater wings of the sphenoid; zygoma

2. The trochlea, a pulley through which runs the tendon of the superior oblique muscle, is located between the roof and the medial wall. A displaced trochlea causes diplopia on downward gaze.

3. The inferior orbital fissure is in the floor of the orbit. It is bound by the greater wing of the sphenoid, orbital surface of the maxilla, and orbital process of the palatine bone. It transmits the infraorbital nerve, infraorbital vessels, zygomatic nerve, fine branches from the sphenopalatine ganglion to the lacrimal gland, and ophthalmic vein branch.

4. The anterior and posterior ethmoid foramina are situated at the junction between the frontal and ethmoid bones, in the frontal side of the suture line.

5. The superior orbital fissure lies between the roof and the lateral wall of the nose. It is a gap between the lesser and the greater wings of the sphenoid. It transmits cranial nerves III, IV, V_1, VI, the superior orbital vein, ophthalmic vein, orbital branch of the middle meningial artery, and recurrent branch of the lacrimal artery.

6. The optic canal runs from the middle cranial fossa into the apex of the orbit. It is formed by a curvilinear portion of the lesser wing of the sphenoid bone, and through it course the optic nerve and ophthalmic artery.

7. The upper lid contains:
    a. Orbicularis oculi
    b. Levator palpebrae superioris
    c. Müller's muscle
    d. Sweat glands
    e. Meibomian glands
    f. Wolfring's glands
    g. Tarsal plate

8. The lower lid contains:
    a. Tarsal plate
    b. Lower lid retractors
    c. Orbicularis oculi
    d. Sweat glands
    e. Meibomian glands
    f. Wolfring's glands

9. The lateral ends of the tarsi unite to form the lateral palpebral ligament, which fixes onto the orbital surface of the zygomatic bone. A displaced lateral canthal ligament may give rise to an inferiorly displaced canthus or slight ptosis. Also, with loss of the inferior fornix, a prosthesis will not stay in place, if such is necessary.

10. The medial ends divide into deep and superficial heads. The superficial heads unite and form the medial canthal tendon, which anchors the eyelids medially. If this support is lost, a rounding of the medial aspect of the eyelid will occur, resulting in pseudo-hypertelorism. The deep heads form the muscular diaphragm over the lacrimal fossa, envelop the punctae, and swing back to attach to the posterior lacrimal crest, establishing the "lacrimal pump" mechanism. Disruption of this muscle attachment may result in epiphora.

11. The septum orbitale is the orbital periosteum, which extends into the lid to attach to the tarsal plates. The orbital septum separates the eyelid from the orbital contents. If fat is exposed, the orbit has been entered, as there is no subcutaneous fat in the eyelids. The superior orbital septum attaches to the levator apparatus with subsequent attachment to the tarsal plate, whereas the inferior septum attaches directly into the tarsal plate. Medially, it is fused with the palpebral ligament leading toward the posterior lacrimal crest.

12. The suspensory ligament of Lockwood is a continuous band of fibrous tissue slung beneath the eyeball from side to side. The ends of the suspensory ligament blend with the cheek ligaments and with the medial and lateral horns of the aponeurosis of the levator palpebrae superioris.

13. The lower lid retractors are the capsulopalpebral heads of the inferior rectus/inferior oblique complex, and cause a slight retraction of the lower lid with forced openings. Fibers can be separated supplied by the sympathetic nerves as well as the third cranial nerve.

CONTROL OF EYE MOVEMENT

1. The upper lid is opened by the levator palpebrae superior (nerve III) and Müller's muscle (sympathetic fibers). It is closed by the orbicularis oculi (nerve VII). The ophthalmic division of nerve V is responsible for the sensory innervation to the upper lid, and the lower lid is innervated by the first two divisions of nerve V.

2. Entropion: Turning in of the lid margin. Ectropion: Turning out of the lid margin.

3. Horner syndrome: Paralysis of the sympathetic nerve, especially the superior cervical sympathetics, giving rise to ptosis, miosis, and anhidrosis. The ptosis is caused by weakness or paralysis of Müller's muscle, which can account for 3 to 6 mm of upper lid retraction.

MUSCLES

1. The six extraocular muscles and their functions are
   a. Lateral rectus, to adduct
   b. Medial rectus, to abduct
   c. Superior rectus, to elevate (and intort)
   d. Inferior rectus, to depress (and extort)
   e. Superior oblique, to intort (and depress)
   f. Inferior oblique, to extort (and elevate)

2. The lateral rectus (LR) is innervated by nerve VI. The superior oblique (SO) is innervated by nerve IV. The rest of the extraocular muscles are innervated by nerve III.

3. The inferior rectus muscle is the most commonly trapped muscle in a blowout fracture, the second being the inferior oblique. When these muscles are trapped, the patient may experience difficulty looking upward. This condition is not due to paralysis but rather to the trapping of the two muscles mentioned above. To differentiate paralysis of the elevators from trapping of the inferior rectus and the inferior oblique muscles, the "forced duction test" is performed under local or general anesthesia. The forced duction test consists of grasping the globe adjacent to the limbus with small forceps and rotating it up, down, in, and out. If the globe moves freely, there is no entrapment of these muscles. The degree of movement should be compared to that of the unaffected opposite globe.

4. There are six cardinal directions of gaze, each controlled by a set of two muscles:
    a. Eyes to right, right lateral rectus and left medial rectus
    b. Eyes to left, right medial rectus and left lateral rectus
    c. Eyes up and right, right superior rectus and left inferior oblique
    d. Eyes down and right, right inferior rectus and left superior oblique
    e. Eyes up and left, right inferior oblique and left superior rectus
    f. Eyes down and left, right superior oblique and inferior rectus

5. When diplopia occurs, it may exist in more than one direction. The muscles suspected of being involved are those controlling the direction of gaze in which the images of the diplopia are farthest apart. It is usually obvious as to which eye is involved. However, when such is not the case, each eye should be covered in turn and tested. The eye that sees the peripheral image is the one that is injured.

6. The evaluation of diplopia is very difficult and requires a detailed ophthalmologic examination. It should be ascertained whether the diplopia is vertical, horizontal, or rotational and whether it occurs in at a distance or near, up or down gaze positions.

7. Injury to the trochlea can occur during frontal sinus floor trephine or external ethmoidectomy, causing superior oblique dysfunction and subsequent diplopia.

LACRIMAL SYSTEM

1. The lacrimal gland (a serous gland predominantly) is located in a fossa within the zygomatic process of the frontal bone. The lacrimal sac lies in a fossa bound by the lacrimal bone, the frontal process of the maxilla, and the nasal process of the frontal bone.

2. The lacrimal gland secretes tears through 17 to 20 openings. Although the gland is developed, secretion of tears does not take place until 2 weeks after birth. The tears are composed of watery, oily, and mucoid components, which are present in both basic and reflex tearing.

3. When cannulating the inferior and superior canaliculi, it is important to remember that each canaliculus has a vertical portion (about 2 mm) and a longer horizontal portion (about 8 mm). The canaliculi join into a common canaliculus of variable length. A laceration of one or both canaliculi requires insertion of a silicone tube, which is looped between the inferior and superior puncti in the medial corner of the eye, brought through the nasolacrimal duct, and tied together within the nasal cavity. The laceration can be sutured over the tube, which is left in place for 6 weeks to 3 months. The lacrimal sac is about 12 mm long and the duct about 17 mm in length. The nasolacrimal duct

empties into the anterior portion of the inferior meatus. The most common site of congenital obstruction in the lacrimal system is a stricture of the valve of Hasner, of the nasolacrimal duct, at the inferior meatus. Acquired causes of the blockage, primarily in the upper collecting system, include infection (dacryocystitis)—often with the formation of dacryoliths—trauma, and idiopathic causes. The idiopathic conditions are commonly seen in postmenopausal women.

GRAVES' ORBITOPATHY

1. Malignant exophthalmos is caused by an endocrine disorder. One of the causes is an oversecretion of "exophthalmos factor" by the anterior pituitary. This factor is possibly linked to thyroid-stimulating hormone (THS). The more severe form of exophthalmos is caused by excessive orbital edema, giving rise to an increase in bulk of the extraocular muscles and adipose tissues. These adipose tissues are found at such time to contain a greater amount of mucopolysaccharides than normal. The extraocular muscles are particularly affected by this inflammatory process, which eventually leads to deposition of collagen and fibrosis. Imaging studies with computed tomography (CT) or A-scan ultrasound often demonstrate significant thickening of the middle and posterior aspects of the extraocular muscles. The globe decompresses itself through the anterior orbit, creating the observed proptosis. Upper eyelid retraction with upper scleral show may be evident. Ocular symptoms include mild burning, foreign-body sensation, and tearing from corneal exposure, progressing to severe loss of vision from compressive optic neuropathy. Management of Graves' orbitopathy is based on the severity of the disease and should be co-ordinated by a team consisting of the endocrinologist, ophthalmologist, and otorhinolaryngologist. Medical management for more severe symptoms has included the use of anti-inflammatory medications, corticosteroids, and radiation.

2. The exophthalmos is not only esthetically undesirable but can lead to
   a. Corneal exposure and desiccation due to failure to close lids over cornea.
   b. Chemosis secondary to venous stasis.
   c. Fixation of the extraocular muscles, causing ophthalmoplegia. The earliest limitation noted is in upward gaze.
   d. Retinal venous congestion leading to blindness.
   e. Conjunctivitis due to exposure, desiccation, and inflammation.

3. Because the consequences of malignant exophthalmos are grave, many surgical corrections have been devised.
   a. Kronlein's procedure removes the lateral orbital wall to allow the orbital contents to expand into the zygomatic area.
   b. Naffziger's procedure removes the roof of the orbital cavity to allow expansion of the orbital contents into the anterior cranial fossa. It does not expose any of the paranasal sinuses, and it preserves the superior orbital rim. Postoperatively, the cerebral pulsations may be noted in the orbit.
   c. Sewell's procedure consists of an ethmoidectomy and removal of the floor of the frontal sinus for expansion.
   d. Hirsch's procedure removes the orbital floor to allow decompression into the maxillary sinus. A ridge of bone around the infraorbital nerve is preserved to support the nerve.

    e. Historically, the Ogura procedure combined the floor and medial wall resections for maximal decompression.

    f. Scleral grafts to lengthen the upper lids may be required when scarring has short-ened the lids through retraction.

    g. Currently, the treatment of choice is the endoscopic decompression of the medial orbit via an ethmoidectomy with removal of the lamina papyracea and a partial resection of the floor of the orbit.

    h. Classification of thyroid ophthalmopathy has been based on Werner's detailed degree of orbital involvement (Table 14-1), with classes 5 and 6 most often requir-ing decompression surgery.

    i. Thyroid orbitopathy is primarily managed through medical control of the hyper-thyroidism. Decompression is generally indicated in euthyroid patients who con-tinue to have persistent corneal exposure, motility disturbances, and/or progressive visual loss.

EXOPHTHALMOS AND PROPTOSIS

1. Causes of exophthalmos and orbital proptosis include

    a. Pseudotumor

    b. Lymphoma

    c. Hemangioma

    d. Thyroid orbitopathy (Graves')

    e. Orbital cellulitis/abscess

    f. Metastatic tumor

    g. Paranasal sinus mass

    h. Carotid-cavernous fistula

2. Pseudotumor of the orbit is usually seen in young adults and is quite responsive to high-dose parenteral steroids. It is idiopathic in origin.

3. Lymphedema of the orbit can often be diagnosed by CT or magnetic resonance imag-ing (MRI), with a confirmatory biopsy or needle aspiration. Open biopsy may require using a medial or lateral orbitotomy approach.

4. Vascular tumors of the orbit can usually be diagnosed by orbital ultrasound with confirmation by magnetic resonance angiography (MRA) or arteriogram. Surgical approach is required to prevent impending blindness, while radiation therapy may be indicated to retard the growth of the tumor.

5. Orbital cellulitis often causes proptosis without ophthalmoplegia. When globe move-ment is reduced, presence of an orbital abscess must be suspected, and a CT or MRI

TABLE 14-1. WERNER'S DETAILED CLASSIFICATION

Class	Description
0	No physical signs or symptoms
1	Only signs (upper lid retraction, stare, and eyelid lag)
2	Symptoms (irritation, etc.) along with class 1 signs
3	Proptosis
4	Extraocular muscle involvement
5	Corneal involvement
6	Visual loss with optic neuropathy

scan obtained. Most inflammatory conditions of the orbit originate from paranasal sinus disease, with surgical drainage via an anterior orbitotomy required. Fungal orbital infection is a surgical emergency. Inflammation of the lid anterior to the orbital septum generally remains localized to the lid (preseptal cellulitis), while if posterior to the septum, it is by definition, an orbital infection.

6. Metastatic tumors of the orbit are usually of breast origin. A complete physical examination will reveal the breast tumor, although a mammogram may be indicated if not obvious. Orbital exenteration is usually not performed, in favor of chemotherapy and radiation therapy.

7. Tumors of the paranasal sinuses may encroach upon the orbit—adenocarcinoma or squamous cell carcinoma. En bloc resection of the sinus tumor with orbital exenteration is usually indicated. Polypoid disease of the sinuses, as well as a frontal sinus osteoma, may push into the orbit, causing proptosis.

8. A carotid artery–cavernous sinus fistula can occur after head or facial trauma and presents with pulsatile exophthalmos. An enhanced CT or MRA will demonstrate the fistula, and an orbital bruit can be auscultated. This condition requires intracranial closure of the fistula.

Bibliography

Char DH. *Thyroid Eye Disease.* New York: Churchill-Livingstone, 1990.

Dollinger J. Die drickentlastlung der Augenhokle durch entfurnung der aussern Orbital-wand bei hochgradigen Exophthalmos and Koneskutwer Hornhauterkronkung. *Dtsch Med Wochenschr* 1911;37:1888–1890.

Levine MR, ed. *Manual of Oculoplastic Surgery,* 2nd ed. USA: Butterworth-Heinemann, 1966.

Naffziger HC. Progressive exophthalmos following thyroidectomy: Its pathology and treatment. *Ann Surg* 1931;94:582–586.

Nesi FA, Lisman RD, Levine MR, eds. *Smith's Ophthalmic Plastic and Reconstructive Surgery.* St. Louis: Mosby, 1998.

Rootman J. *Diseases of the Orbit.* Philadelphia: JB Lippincott, 1988.

Shields JA. *Diagnosis and Management of Orbital Tumors.* Philadelphia: WB Saunders, 1989.

Sisler HA, Jakobiac FA, Trokel SL. Ocular abnormalities and orbital changes of Graves' disease. In: Duane TD, Jaeger EA, eds. *Clinical Ophthalmology.* Vol 2. Philadelphia: Harper & Row, 1986.

Steward WB, ed. *Surgery of the Eyelid, Orbit and Lacrimal System.* Vol 3.: American Academy of Ophthalmology, 1995.

Werner SC. Modification of the classification of the eye changes of Graves' disease. *Am J Ophthalmol* 1977;83:725–727.

Zide BM, Barry M, Jelks GW. *Surgical Anatomy of the Orbit.* New York: Raven Press, 1985.

Related Neurology and Neurosurgery

15

MULTIPLE SCLEROSIS

Multiple sclerosis (MS) is a central nervous system demyelinating disease of unknown cause. Multifocal plaques of demyelination are found in the optic nerves, cerebral hemispheres, brain stem, and spinal cord. The clinical syndrome is classically one of a relapsing-remitting disorder with onset in young adulthood.[1]

Epidemiology

The peak incidence is between ages 20 and 40.

Women are affected nearly twice as often as men.

The prevalence rises with increasing distance from the equator.

There is a genetic predisposition. Family members, particularly siblings, are at increased risk. Familial occurrence is in the range of 15 to 20%.

Pathogenesis

There is indirect evidence for the involvement of immunologic mechanisms. The accumulated data suggest a genetic predisposition to the disease, which may be triggered by additional factors perhaps related to environmental exposure.

The disorder displays marked clinical heterogeneity (Table 15-1).

Diagnosis

The clinical diagnosis of MS requires at least two attacks over a span of 6 months and evidence of at least two separate central nervous system lesions.

Diagnostic Studies

Magnetic resonance imaging (MRI) of the brain and spinal cord: MRI yields positive results in 85 to 90% of patients with clinically definite MS.

Examination of the cerebrospinal fluid (CSF)
Elevated immunoglobulin (Ig) G
Oligoclonal bands
Mild lymphocytosis in some cases

Evoked potential studies:
Visual evoked potentials.
Somatosensory evoked potentials are of possible value.
Brain stem auditory evoked potentials are not of value in MS.

Treatment

Immunoprophylactic therapy is widely used. Available agents include

1. Interferon β
   Interferon β-1a (Avonex, Rebif)
   Interferon β-1b (Betaseron)
2. Glatiramer acetate (Copaxone)

TABLE 15-1.   CLINICAL FINDINGS IN MULTIPLE SCLEROSIS

Common presenting symptoms*
  Focal weakness
  Numbness or tingling in a limb
  Unsteadiness
  Sudden loss or blurring of vision in one eye
  Diplopia
  Urinary urgency or hesitancy
Common signs

Hyperreflexia	Lower extremity ataxia
Babinski signs	Impaired alternating movements
Impaired vibratory sensation	Optic neuritis
Nystagmus	Impaired joint position sense
Cerebellar tremor	Spasticity
Impaired pain and temperature sense	Dysarthria
Paraparesis	Internuclear ophthalmoplegia (INO)

*Vertigo is a reported symptom in 30–50% of MS patients.

3. Mitoxantrone (Novantrone)
4. Other prophylactic therapy of possible value include
    Intravenous immunoglobulins
    Cytotoxic agents—eg, cyclophosphamide, azathioprine, or methotrexate

Therapy for Acute Exacerbations
Intravenous methylprednisolone followed by a course of oral prednisone.

Symptomatic Therapy
For the following:

>   *Fatigue:* amantadine
>   *Spasticity:* baclofen, tizanidine, diazepam; intrathecal baclofen
>   *Neurogenic bladder:* depending on symptoms
>   *Bowel dysfunction:* stool softeners, laxatives, enemas
>   *Sexual dysfunction:* counseling
>   *Pain, trigeminal neuralgia, painful tonic spasms, and other paroxysmal symptoms:* carbamazepine
>   *Tremor:* propanolol or primidone; thalamotomy
>   *Ataxia:* physical therapy

Exercise is an important component of management of the patient with MS.

HEADACHE AND FACIAL PAIN (TABLE 15-2)

Migraine
Diagnostic criteria for migraine without aura (Table 15-3):

A. At least five attacks fulfilling criteria B to D.
B. Headache lasting 4 to 72 hours (untreated or unsuccessfully treated).
C. Headache has at least two of the following characteristics:
    1. Unilateral location
    2. Pulsating quality
    3. Moderate or severe intensity (inhibits or prohibits daily activities)
    4. Aggravation by walking stairs or similar routine physical activity

TABLE 15-2. PAIN-SENSITIVE STRUCTURES OF THE CRANIUM

Intracranial	Extracranial
Venous sinuses	Cranial periosteum
Anterior and middle meningeal arteries	Skin, subcutaneous tissue, muscle, and arteries
Dura at the base of the skull	Neck muscles
Cranial nerves V, IX, and X	Second and third cervical nerve roots
Internal carotid arteries to the circle of Willis	Eyes, ears, teeth, sinuses, and oropharynx
Brain stem periaqueductal gray matter	Mucous membranes of the nasal cavity
Sensory nuclei of the thalamus	

D. During headache, at least one of the following:
1. Nausea and/or vomiting
2. Photophobia and phonophobia

E. History, physical examination, and/or investigations do not suggest an alternative cause of headache.

Migraines are frequently mistaken for sinus headaches.

Management of Migraine[2]

Identification and elimination of triggers

Lifestyle adjustments and understanding of the relative importance of diet, exercise, sleeping habits, hydration, and stress

Drug therapy

  Acute

  Specific

  5-HT$_{1b/1d}$ agonists

  Naratriptan, rizatriptan, sumatriptan, zolmitriptan

  Dihydroergotamine (IM, IV, IN)

  Nonspecific

  Acetaminophen, aspirin, caffeine combination

  Aspirin

TABLE 15-3. NEW INTERNATIONAL HEADACHE SOCIETY CLASSIFICATION OF HEADACHE (ABRIDGED)

1. Migraine
    1.1 Migraine without aura
    1.2 Migraine with aura
2. Tension-type headache
3. Cluster headache and chronic paroxysmal hemicrania
4. Miscellaneous headaches unassociated with structural lesion
5. Headache associated with head trauma
6. Headache associated with vascular disorders
7. Headache associated with nonvascular intracranial disorder
8. Headache associated with substances or their withdrawal
9. Headache associated with nonspecific infection
10. Headache associated with metabolic disorder
11. Headache or facial pain associated with disorder of cranium, neck, eyes, ears, nose, sinuses, teeth, mouth, or other facial or cranial structures
12. Cranial neuralgias, nerve trunk pain, and deafferentation pain
13. Headache not classifiable

Ibuprofen, naproxen

Perchlorphenazine (IM, IV, PR)

Butalbital, aspirin, caffeine combination

Isometheptine

Narcotics

Preventive (prophylactic)

Antidepressants

Amitriptyline, nortriptyline

Anticonvulsants

Divalproate sodium, neurontin, lamotrigine

Beta blockers

Propanolol, timolol, metoprolol

Nonsteroidal anti-inflammatory drugs (NSAIDs)

Others

Feverfew, magnesium, vitamin B_2

Headache is sometimes a symptom of a condition requiring immediate attention or emergency care. These conditions may present either acutely or subacutely (Table 15-4).

TRIGEMINAL NEURALGIA

Trigeminal neuralgia is a paroxysmal pain disturbance in which pain is felt within the distribution of one or more divisions of the trigeminal nerve. Paroxysms of pain are usually triggered by a sensory stimulus and each attack lasts only seconds. MS, cerebellopontine angle tumors, schwannomas, and other local lesions account for some cases, and vascular compression of the nerve root has been postulated as a cause in other cases. The course is commonly one of exacerbations and remissions. Carbamazepine is the most effective drug for the treatment of trigeminal neuralgia. Surgical management is appropriate for medical therapy failures. Options include alcohol block of the involved division of the trigeminal nerve, percutaneous radiofrequency thermocoagulation of the trigeminal sensory root as it exits the gasserian ganglion, and microvascular decompression of the nerve root via a posterior

TABLE 15-4. ACUTE AND SUBACUTE HEADACHE SYNDROMES

Condition	Symptoms and signs
Acute	
Subarachnoid hemorrhage	Sudden onset, "worst headache of my life"
Intracerebral hemorrhage	Diffuse or focal headache, focal CNS signs, altered mental status
Meningitis or encephalitis	Diffuse headache, neck stiffness, fever
Hypertensive encephalopathy	Diffuse headache, elevated blood pressure, signs of diffuse or focal CNS dysfunction
Angle closure glaucoma	Periorbital and frontal pain
Carotid artery dissection	Ipsilateral neck and facial pain and Horner's syndrome
Subacute	
Giant cell arteritis	>50 years of age, scalp tenderness, jaw claudication, myalgias, elevated sedimentation rate
Intracranial mass	Signs of focal CNS dysfunction, worse upon awakening and with coughing and bending over
Pseudotumor cerebri	Papilledema, blurred vision, obesity; female predominance

fossa approach. Recently, Gamma Knife stereotactic radiosurgery has been shown to obtain results (up to 75 to 80% remission/improvement) comparable to invasive techniques.

The pain of trigeminal neuralgia is excruciating, occurs spasmodically in lightning-like jabs, and is almost always confined to the area of the face innervated by the second and third divisions of the trigeminal nerve.

Trigeminal neuralgia may be a manifestation of MS; in younger individuals, this diagnosis should always be considered.

There is a high remission rate in response to carbamazepine, the dose of which is titrated to patient response. Stereotactic radiosurgery is used for cases refractory to drug therapy.

Glossopharyngeal Neuralgia

The quality of the pain of glossopharyngeal neuralgia is identical to that of trigeminal neuralgia. Pain is localized to the oropharynx, the tonsillar pillars, the base of the tongue, or the auditory meatus; it is commonly triggered by swallowing or talking.

There is frequently an excellent symptomatic response to carbamazepine.

CEREBROVASCULAR DISEASE[3]

Vertebrobasilar arterial disease enters into the differential diagnosis of vertigo of acute onset or recurrent vertigo. The posterior circulation supplies blood to the medulla, pons, cerebellum, midbrain, thalamus, occipital lobes, and mesial temporal lobes. Ischemia of the occipital lobes results in visual loss in the form of complete or partial homonymous hemianopsia, which is not uncommonly accompanied by confusion or memory loss; ischemia of the brain stem may result in symptoms of diplopia, periorbital numbness, clumsiness, weakness, ataxia, dysarthria, or drop attacks. Clinical signs may include nystagmus of the central type, internuclear ophthalmoplegia, a homonymous visual field deficit, limb or truncal ataxia, motor weakness, sensory loss, and pathologic reflexes. Cranial nerve involvement on one side with contralateral limb involvement, described as a "crossed deficit," is good evidence of brain stem dysfunction.

Sudden hearing loss with moderate dizziness may be due to infarction in the distribution of the internal auditory artery.

When nystagmus is present, as is often the case in cerebellar infarction, nystagmus is direction-changing with gaze but is more prominent to the side of the lesion, and the tendency to sway or fall is in the same direction as the nystagmus. Whereas with acute peripheral vestibulopathy, nystagmus is usually unidirectional, with the fast phase away from the side of the lesion, and swaying occurs toward the lesion or in the opposite direction as the nystagmus.

The clinical picture of acute cerebellar hemorrhage is one of sudden onset of headache, which is accompanied by symptoms of nausea, vomiting, vertigo, and ataxia evolving over a period of hours. Upon presentation, patients may be alert, confused, or comatose. Computed tomography (CT) scan confirms the diagnosis. Emergency surgical evacuation of the hematoma can be lifesaving.

MYASTHENIA GRAVIS

Myasthenia gravis (MG) is an antibody-mediated disease of the neuromuscular junction in which antibodies to the nicotinic receptor for acetylcholine at the postsynaptic endplate of the neuromuscular junction are responsible for a defect in neuromuscular transmission.

Symptoms

Early symptoms

Oculomotor weakness and ptosis

Oropharyngeal muscle weakness and difficulty chewing, swallowing, or talking

Head drop due to neck extensor muscle weakness

Limb weakness is less often the initial symptom.

Weakness is characteristically variable and is more pronounced later in the day and is manifest with sustained or repetitive activity, such as reading or chewing.

The disease is commonly progressive and progression from ocular myasthenia to generalized disease usually takes place within the first year.

Diagnosis

Pharmacologic testing with intravenous edrophonium chloride (Tensilon)

Electrodiagnostic studies:

Repetitive nerve stimulation

Single-fiber electromyography (EMG)

Immunologic studies:

Acetylcholine receptor antibodies are found in 74 to 99% of patients with MG.

Role of the Thymus Gland[4]

A tumor of the thymus occurs in 10 to 15% of patients and should be sought in all patients with MG by CT of the chest.

Thymectomy, even in the absence of tumor, should be considered as a form of treatment in patients younger than 60 years.

Treatment

Pyridostigmine bromide (Mestinon) is a cholinesterase inhibitor.

Steroids (prednisone) are used to control oculomotor symptoms if the response to Mestinon is insufficient and to control symptoms of generalized MG.

Immunosuppressant drugs: azathioprine, cyclophosphamide, and cyclosporine.

Thymectomy may be appropriate in younger patients with generalized MG.

Plasmapheresis is used in myasthenic crisis or in preparation for thymectomy.

Certain drugs may exacerbate myasthenic weakness (Table 15-5).

PITUITARY ADENOMA

The pituitary gland (hypophysis) has been described as the "master gland" of the body. It coordinates hypothalamic secretory function with organs external to the central nervous system (CNS) through its own hormonal secretions. The hypophysis has two divisions in

TABLE 15-5.   DRUGS THAT MAY EXACERBATE MYASTHENIC WEAKNESS

Succinylcholine, *d*-tubocurarine, or other neuromuscular blocking agents
Quinine, quinidine, or procainamide
Aminoglycoside antibiotics
Timolol maleate eyedrops
Beta blockers
Calcium channel blockers
D-penicillamine

humans. The anterior portion of the pituitary is called the adenohypophysis. Prolactin (PRL), growth hormone (GH), adrenocorticotropic hormone (ACTH), thyroid-stimulating hormone (TSH), follicle-stimulating hormone (FSH), and luteinizing hormone (LH) are among the hormones released by the glandular epithelial cells of the adenohypophysis. Release of all of these hormones is under the control of the hypothalamic factors, hormones, or both.

Prolactin is a 198–amino acid polypeptide. Prolactin-producing cells tend to be present in the lateral aspect of the pituitary gland and facilitate lactation. Prolactin is stimulated by thyrotropin-releasing hormone (TRH), estrogen, stress, and exercise; it is inhibited by dopamine.

Growth hormone is a 191–amino acid polypeptide hormone. Growth hormone–producing cells tend to accumulate along the lateral aspect of the adenohypophysis. Secretion occurs in episodic surges, every 3 to 4 hours. It is stimulated by growth hormone–releasing hormone (GHRH), insulin-induced hypoglycemia, arginine, L-dopa, propranolol, and exercise. It is inhibited by somatostatin (released by the hypothalamus). Growth hormone stimulates amino acid uptake and participates in glucose regulation. It opposes the effect of insulin, causes release of free fatty acids from storage sites, and mediates synthesis of insulin-like growth factors (IGFs) in the liver and other tissues. Insulin-like growth factors (also referred to as somatomedins) induce glucose oxidation in fatty tissue and protein synthesis in muscle and bone.

Adrenocorticotropic hormone is a 39–amino acid polypeptide that tends to reside in the mediolateral aspect of the pars distalis. It promotes growth of the adrenal cortex and its hormone synthesis. Adrenocorticotropic hormone is stimulated by corticotropin-releasing hormone (CRH), vasopressin, and stress. It is inhibited by the negative feedback control "loop" of cortisol. Secretion has a circadian rhythm.

Thyroid-stimulating hormone is a glycoprotein compound composed of an inactive alpha subunit and a beta subunit that is biologically active. Thyroid-stimulating hormone regulates the synthesis of triiodothyronine (T_3) and thyroxine (T_4) by the thyroid for normal metabolic function. Thyroid-stimulating hormone–producing cells tend to be located in the anteromedial aspect of the pituitary.

Gonadotropic hormone–producing cells secrete FSH and LH. They are located medially in the adenohypophysis. Both FSH and LH are glycoproteins formed by two subunits: an inactive alpha and biologically active beta subunit. They are required for normal sexual development and fertility. In the female, FSH stimulates ovarian follicular growth. In the male, testicular growth and spermatogenesis are promoted. In the female, LH stimulates ovulation and luteinization of the ovarian follicle as well as ovarian estrogen and progesterone production. In the male, LH promotes testosterone secretion of the testicle by supporting interstitial (Leydig) cell function.

The posterior portion of the pituitary gland is termed the neurohypophysis; it releases antidiuretic hormone (vasopressin) and oxytocin. Both of these hormones are actually formed in the supraoptic and paraventricular nuclei of the hypothalamus, from which they are transported via their respective axons (by the supraopticohypophyseal tract) to the neurohypophysis for storage and ultimate release. The tuberohypophyseal tract, arising from the middle and posterior portions of the hypothalamus, also sends axons to the posterior pituitary.

Vasopressin is a small, nine–amino acid peptide. It causes reabsorption of water in the kidney by increasing transepithelial permeability of the distal convoluted tubules and collecting ducts. Vasoconstriction is the other major action of the antidiuretic hormone (ADH).

Oxytocin's structure is closely related to that of ADH. It causes contraction of the smooth muscle of the uterus during labor and immediately following delivery.

The cell types of the anterior pituitary gland seen by light microscopy include chromophobe cells (comprising 50% of the total cell population), acidophils (also termed alpha cells, accounting for 40% of the pituitary cells), and basophils (also called beta cells, representing 10% of the pituitary cells). The glial cells of the neurohypophysis are termed pituicytes. The older method of classifying pituitary adenomas by light microscopy with the standard hematoxylin-eosin staining technique (chromophobe, eosinophilic, or basophilic adenoma) is no longer adequate in view of modern immunohistochemistry, electron microscopy, and serum hormone assay findings. Pituitary tumors are more appropriately classified as either functional (hormone-secreting) or nonfunctional (non-hormone-secreting). Adenomas less than 10 mm in diameter are termed microadenomas, while those greater than 10 mm in diameter are referred to as macroadenomas.

Differential Diagnosis of Sellar and Parasellar Lesions

1. Pituitary adenoma
    a. Functional tumors
        (1) PRL-secreting (most common)
        (2) GH-secreting
        (3) ACTH-secreting
        (4) Mixed secreting (PRL-GH, etc.)
        (5) Other, less common secreting tumors (thyrotropin-secreting, etc.)
    b. Nonfunctional tumors: null cell adenoma. There is no clinical evidence of increased hormone secretion. There are no recognizable hormones noted on immunohistochemical testing.
2. Pituitary carcinoma: rare
3. Meningioma: tuberculum sellae, diaphragma sellae, cavernous sinus, medial third of sphenoid wing
4. Craniopharyngioma
5. Epidermoid, dermoid, germinoma
6. Chrondro-osteal origin: chordoma, chondrosarcoma, osteochondroma, myeloma
7. Hypothalamic lesions
    a. Optic and/or hypothalamic glioma
    b. Hamartoma of the hypothalamus
8. Neurohypophyseal: infundiboma, granular cell myoblastoma
9. Metastatic neoplasms: breast, lung, prostate, etc.
10. Vascular
    a. Pituitary apoplexy
    b. Aneurysm, especially in the cavernous portion of the internal carotid artery
11. Empty sella syndrome: may be primary or secondary, with or without an enlarged third ventricle
12. Inflammatory
    a. Sellar abscess or empyema
    b. Mucocele of sphenoid sinus
    c. Granulomatous disease: sarcoidosis, tuberculosis, mycoses
    d. Lymphocytic hypophysitis

13. Cysts
    a. Rathke's cleft
    b. Arachnoidal

Signs and Symptoms

Signs and symptoms of pituitary tumors may be grouped into three categories: (1) endocrine, (2) visual, and (3) headache.

Endocrine

The endocrine functional tumors include the following:

PROLACTINOMA.   This is the most common pituitary tumor. Prolactinoma is most frequently seen in young women, presenting as amenorrhea with or without galactorrhea. Most prolactinomas (60–70%) present clinically as microadenomas. In the male, galactorrhea as a presenting symptom is unusual. Thus, males tend to present with findings of mass effect or hypopituitarism, including visual loss, impotence, and loss of fertility. As classified by light microscopy, most of these tumors are chromophobe adenomas. A majority of prolactinomas are responsive to medical therapy with dopamine receptor agonists: cabergoline or bromocriptine. These medications are tolerated by most patients. Prolactin serum levels rapidly return to normal, regular menses resume, and tumor shrinkage occurs in the vast majority of cases treated with cabergoline or bromocriptine. However, cessation of drug therapy usually results in tumor regrowth. Therefore, this medication is required permanently. The indications for surgery in prolactinomas include intolerance to medication (uncommon), patient preference, and/or failure of medication to significantly reduce hyperprolactinemia. Stereotactic radiosurgery or fractionated stereotactic radiotherapy may be used in medical and surgical failures.

GROWTH HORMONE–SECRETING ADENOMAS.   Gigantism may be seen in childhood cases before the epiphyses of the long bones have closed. Acromegaly is seen in adults. Enlargement of the jaws, hands, and/or feet is present in most adult cases. Hyperhydrosis, hypertrichosis, fatigue, decreased libido, paresthesias (including carpal tunnel syndrome), hypertension, cardiac disease, diabetes mellitus, and other findings may also be seen. Classically, these tumors were described as eosinophilic adenomas. However, most cases are chromophobe adenomas by light microscopy. Growth hormone–secreting adenomas are the second most common of the endocrine active adenomas. Most cases require surgery. The somatostatin analog octreotide has produced regression of a significant portion of acromegaly cases treated. However, its route of administration is inconvenient, requiring subcutaneous administration as often as three times a day. Bromocriptine or cabergoline do not adequately reduce GH levels in the vast majority of cases in which this has been attempted. Reoperation, stereotactic radiosurgery, or fractionated stereotactic radiotherapy may be required in recurrent/persistent tumors.

ADRENOCORTICOTROPIC HORMONE–SECRETING ADENOMAS.   These tumors present clinically as Cushing's disease. Obesity with "buffalo hump," "moon facies," abdominal stretch marks, hypertension, and hirsutism are the more common signs and symptoms seen. These tumors usually present as microadenomas. They occur much less frequently than prolactinomas and GH-secreting tumors. They are more commonly symptomatic in women. Hyperpigmentation with increasing sellar size may be seen in Cushing's syndrome after bilateral adrenalectomy. This is referred to as Nelson's syndrome. Adrenocorticotropic hormone–secreting tumors of Nelson's syndrome tend to be aggressive and large. Basophilic adenomas are usually demonstrated by light microscopy with hematoxylin-eosin staining techniques. Transsphenoidal surgery is the treatment of choice. Stereotactic radiosurgery or fractionated stereotactic radiotherapy and/or drug therapy (cyproheptadine or ketoconazole) may be used in resistant cases and/or recurrent tumors or patients who are not suitable surgical candidates.

MULTIPLE ENDOCRINE TUMORS.   Pituitary adenomas may rarely occur as part of the syndrome of multiple endocrine tumors. Most cases of Wermer's syndrome (multiple endocrine adenomatosis type 1) are associated with pituitary tumors as well as parathyroid, pancreatic, adrenal, and/or thyroid tumors.

NONFUNCTIONAL TUMORS.   These neoplasms present without endocrine deficiencies or with decreased function of one or more hormones. Panhypopituitarism with visual symptoms, signs of increased intracranial pressure, and/or extraocular muscle palsies may be seen with advanced growth. Because of their lack of secretory hormone symptomatology, these tumors tend to present as macroadenomas. Surgery, usually via a transsphenoidal approach, is indicated in most of these cases.

Visual Signs and Symptoms
1. The classic visual finding associated with enlarging suprasellar extension of pituitary adenomas is bitemporal hemianopsia associated with a progressive decrease in visual acuity.
2. If there is a significant lateral extension of tumor growth toward the cavernous sinus, extraocular muscle palsies (involving cranial nerves III, IV, and/or VI) may be noted.
3. MRI and CT scans have revealed that some bleeding into a pituitary tumor is fairly common. Fortunately, the full-blown syndrome of pituitary apoplexy is not frequent. In such cases, there is a sudden loss of vision associated with hemorrhage within a pituitary adenoma. Severe headache, decrease in level of sensorium, extraocular muscle palsies, and meningismus may also occur. Such pituitary apoplexy is a relative emergency that particularly lends itself to the transsphenoidal approach for removal of the hematoma if a patient with this syndrome is seen relatively soon after the apoplectic episode.

Headache
Headache is a common symptom associated with pituitary adenomas. Initially, the headache may be due to pressure caused by growth of the tumor along the dural covering of the cavernous sinus, stretching the dura of the diaphragma sellae, or both. With further suprasellar extension of the tumor, obstruction of the foramina of Monro may occur, with associated hydrocephalus and increased intracranial pressure. This is usually a late development. Pituitary adenomas with only headache as a symptom are not often diagnosed early because headache is such a common, nonspecific symptom.

Diagnosis and Preoperative Evaluation
Most functional pituitary adenomas are diagnosed as intrasellar lesions without signs of mass effect. Most endocrine-inactive, nonfunctional tumors are not diagnosed until signs and symptoms of hypopituitarism or mass effect evolve. An enlarged sella turcica in an asymptomatic patient is occasionally noted on skull and sinus x-rays.

Preoperative Evaluation

The team approach is essential in the evaluation of lesions in and adjacent to the pituitary gland. Evaluation and treatment include the following:

1. General medical clearance, especially in regard to cardiac, pulmonary, and renal status
2. Complete otolaryngologic evaluation, including examination of the sinuses, nasal airway, gums, and teeth
3. Complete neurologic examination
4. Neuro-ophthalmologic evaluation with emphasis on funduscopic evaluation, visual fields, and acuity
5. Endocrinologic workup: complete endocrinologic evaluation is required for pituitary adenomas preoperatively. Endocrine studies should include serum cortisol (A.M. and P.M.), GH (with concomitant serum glucose), IGF 1, PRL, thyroid function tests (including T_3 uptake and T_4, etc.), FSH, LH, and serum and urine electrolytes and osmolalities. Further tests, such as insulin tolerance test (ITT), TRH stimulation, and glucose tolerance test (GTT), may be required. The normal values of these tests vary from one laboratory to another.
6. Diagnostic imaging: MRI is the diagnostic imaging modality of choice. It does not require radiation, and adjacent vascular (carotid arteries) and neural (optic chiasm and nerves) structures are clearly seen. Multidirectional imaging is readily obtainable. Pituitary tumors are best demonstrated on sagittal and coronal views. Microadenomas usually appear as hypointense areas within the more hyperintense normal pituitary on T1-weighted images. There is enhancement of normal gland, accentuating the hypointense signal of the tumor, with the use of gadolinium, a ferromagnetic contrast agent. Macroadenomas tend to be isointense to slightly hypointense on T1-weighted images. They appear hyperintense on T2-weighted images. Blood within the pituitary usually has a high signal on T1-weighted images if methemoglobin is present. More acute apoplexy, containing deoxyhemoglobin, is hypointense on T2-weighted images. Patients with cardiac pacemakers cannot undergo an MRI scan. CT scans are performed in these cases. On contrast-enhanced CT scans, microadenomas are hypodense. Blood in the hypophysis exhibits high density on noncontrast studies.
7. Nose and throat culture sensitivity.
8. Antibiotics as indicated: usually cefazolin is used, unless the preoperative nose and throat culture indicates a resistant organism, in which case an appropriate antibiotic according to the sensitivity testing is used.
9. Pre- and intraoperative steroids with continuance into the postoperative period.
10. Informed operative consent, including detailed discussions of the indications, alternatives, possible benefits, realistic expectations, and risks of transsphenoidal surgery. All of the patient's questions should be answered.

Transseptal, Transsphenoidal Approach to the Sella Turcica

Anatomically, the important features in regard to the sella turcica include the following:

1. Inferiorly, there is a dural covering over the pituitary gland.
2. Superiorly, there is the diaphragma sellae, the hiatus of which the infundibulum of the pituitary passes through.
3. Anteriorly, the venous circular sinus is located within the dura.
4. Posteriorly, the dorsum sella may be palpated on intrasellar exploration.

5.   Located on either side laterally is the venous cavernous sinus, which contains nerves III, IV, and VI as well as the first and second divisions of cranial nerve V and the cavernous portion of the internal carotid artery.

Postoperative Endocrine Care

Many patients undergoing pituitary surgery have transient diabetes insipidus. In a few cases, it may be permanent, especially in those undergoing total or near total hypophysectomy. Hourly monitoring of urine output and specific gravity is required during the immediate postoperative period. In addition, close monitoring of serum and urine electrolytes and osmolalities is required. Acutely, one may assume that the patient has diabetes insipidus if there is prolonged urine output of more than 250 mL/h with a specific gravity of 1.005 or less and urine osmolality of less than 300 mOsm/kg H_2O. Plasma osmolality is usually greater than 290 mOsm/kg H_2O.

Initial therapy may include intravenous fluids at a rate to replace the previous hour's urinary output. However, if the volume of urinary output becomes too excessive, prolonged, or both, one may use desmopressin acetate (DDAVP), a synthetic analog of vasopressin. This may be administered intravenously or subcutaneously in acute stages. In patients with permanent diabetes insipidus, intranasal or oral DDAVP is the preferred mode of therapy.

Steroid or thyroid maintenance therapy, or both, may be required, especially in cases of preoperative panhypopituitarism. In such cases, a total of 37.5 mg of cortisone acetate and/or levothyroxine sodium 0.05 mg to 0.2 mg each day are sufficient. This dose is required in hypophysectomy cases and in instances of pituitary adenoma presenting with hypopituitary function.

Results of Surgery

The transseptal, transsphenoidal approach to pituitary tumors is, in general, a safe operation. The mortality rate for microadenomas is less than 0.5%, with a major morbidity rate of less than 2% (the most common being CSF rhinorrhea). The risks of macroadenoma surgery are greater. The mortality risk is about 1%, and the morbidity rate around 15%. The most common cause of death is hypothalamic injury.

An initial operative success rate (normalizing hypersecretory states) of 75 to 80% is obtained with microadenomas and an approximate 30 to 35% success rate is obtained for macroprolactinomas and GH-secreting macroadenomas. A greater than 50% surgical success rate may be reached with ACTH-secreting macroadenomas.

The 5-year recurrence rate appears to be about 10% with the exception of patients with Cushing's disease who present with a macroadenoma. In this latter category, the recurrence rate over 5 years appears to be significantly higher.

Increasingly, endoscopic techniques are being used for transnasal, transsphenoidal removal of pituitary adenomas, alone or in conjunction with the microscope. However, long-term results in regard to morbidity, mortality, and tumor persistence/recurrence in comparison with standard microsurgical transsphenoidal approaches are not available at this time. Early results appear encouraging.

DIFFERENTIAL DIAGNOSIS OF CEREBELLOPONTINE ANGLE TUMORS

Vestibular Schwannoma (Acoustic Neuroma)

Vestibular schwannoma is the most common primary tumor occurring in the cerebellopontine angle (CPA). Hearing loss (retrocochlear pattern) is an early symptom, usually associated with tinnitus. With a progressive increase in tumor size, involvement of the seventh cranial nerve (peripheral facial paresis) and fifth cranial nerve (decreased corneal reflex, facial hypesthesia) occurs. Further tumor growth may involve the cerebellum (gait ataxia, dysmetria, nystagmus, etc.), brain stem (hemiparesis, Babinski response, etc.), and/or jugular foramen (cranial nerves IX, X, and XI). Bilateral acoustic neuromas may be seen in von Recklinghausen's disease (neurofibromatosis type 2).

With the advancement of MRI and CT scanning techniques, angiography, conventional x-ray studies, and other diagnostic imaging studies are not usually required. The diagnostic imaging study of choice is an MRI scan. There is no ionizing radiation, subarachnoid contrast injection is avoided, bone artifacts are not present, and multiplanar imaging is accomplished. The MRI scan is particularly effective in detecting intracanalicular vestibular schwannomas. These lesions usually enhance (hyperintense signal) with the use of gadolinium. The use of thin-slice fat suppression techniques further increases the visualization of small tumors. On T1-weighted images, they are hyperintense, often with heterogenous changes due to cystic formation, tumor necrosis, or hemorrhage, or any combination of these.

A CT scan is also highly accurate in demonstrating larger tumors (5–10 mm or greater in diameter). Typically, vestibular schwannomas present as clearly demarcated masses with tissue densities close to neural tissue that significantly enhance with intravenous contrast.

Meningioma

Meningioma is the second most common primary CPA mass lesion. Hearing loss tends to occur later in the clinical course of these lesions compared to vestibular schwannomas. Multiple cranial nerve palsies and brain stem and cerebellar signs may be present with further tumor growth. Hydrocephalus may be present in larger tumors due to kinking of the aqueduct of Sylvius, blockage of CSF pathways in the posterior fossa, or both.

X-ray studies may reveal abnormal calcification, local hyperostosis involving the petrous ridge, or both, but the internal auditory meatus is normal in size. The diagnostic imaging study of choice is MRI scanning. These tumors tend to be isointense to the surrounding neural tissue on T1- and T2-weighted images. There is usually strong enhancement with gadolinium, the tumor assuming a hyperintense signal. A broad base of attachment to the petrous bone or tentorium may be present. A CT scan is also nearly always positive, with these lesions exhibiting significant contrast enhancement.

Epidermoid

Epidermoid is the third most common primary CPA mass lesion. Hearing loss, if present, tends to occur late in the patient's clinical course. Multiple cranial nerve palsies, with or without brain stem and/or cerebellar signs, may be found. A history of increasing vague, nonspecific headache or unilateral neck pain may be obtained in cases with large lesions. These tumors are slow-growing and tend to be quite large by the time they come to the attention of the clinician. Epidermoids may have a variable MRI appearance, depending on the amount of fat (including cholesterol crystals) and protein present within the tumor. Usually, they are relatively more intense in signal in comparison to surrounding neural structures on T1-weighted images. They appear more hyperintense on T2-weighted views. No significant increase in signal is seen with the use of gadolinium on T1-weighted images. A CT scan may reveal a low-density lesion in the region of the CPA that does not exhibit contrast enhancement.

The disparity between the large size of the tumor and the relative paucity of clinical findings, as well as the appearance on diagnostic imaging of finger-like interstices of tumor infiltrating the subarachnoid space, suggests the diagnosis of an epidermoid.

Metastatic Neoplasm

Metastatic tumors (lung, breast, etc.) of the CPA have a more rapid clinical course than benign lesions. Multiple, bilateral lower (and upper) cranial nerve palsies may evolve as a manifestation of meningeal carcinomatosis. Most often, a history of neoplasia is obtained. Evidence of metastatic disease elsewhere is usually present.

In these cases, MRI scans are usually more definitive than CT scans. Multiple intra-parenchymal lesions as well as meningeal carcinomatosis may be seen as areas of high signal intensity with T1-weighted contrast images. CT scans are usually positive with contrast enhancement in larger lesions. Other, multiple intracranial lesions may be diagnosed. In the initial phases of meningeal carcinomatosis, the CT scan may be negative. CSF protein may be elevated, and tumor cells may be seen on CSF cell cytologic analysis.

Glioma

Occasionally, brain stem or cerebellar gliomas (astrocytoma, subependymoma, etc.) may "escape" into the subarachnoid space and grow out toward the CPA. Such patients may present with symptoms of a lesion in this area. Examination may reveal a predominantly brain stem or cerebellar lesion.

CT scans reveal brain stem gliomas to be isodense, hypodense, or a mixture of both. About half of these tumors exhibit some contrast enhancement. Brain stem gliomas are usually hypointense on T1-weighted MRI images. They tend to be more intense on T2-weighted images. Cerebellar astrocytomas are usually hypodense on CT scans. Hypointensity is present on T1-weighted MRI images. A brighter signal is seen on T2-weighted images. In cystic lesions, nodular enhancement may be present with the use of gadolinium on T1-weighted images.

Aneurysms and Other Lesions

Aneurysms, if large enough, may be suggested on CT scanning. A large percentage of intracranial aneurysms are seen on magnetic resonance angiography (MRA) scans. They have the appearance of a signal void (black) due to blood flow. The definitive diagnosis is made by angiography. Chordoma and other bony lesions may be diagnosed by appropriate diagnostic imaging studies, including MRI and CT scans. Chordomas tend to be hyperintense on T2-weighted MRI images. Areas of bone destruction with fragments of calcification are seen within chordomas on CT scans.

Miscellaneous Disorders

Parosmia: perverted sense of smell
Hyperosmia: oversensitive sense of smell
Hyposmia: impaired sense of smell
Anosmia: total loss of smell
Cacosmia: a sense of foul smell when none is present

Carbamazepine (Tegretol) is the drug of choice for medical management of trigeminal neuralgia. Vitamin A has been used to treat anosmia (see Chapter 30). Because ammonia stimulates cranial nerve V but not cranial nerve I, it can be used as a diagnostic test when a psychogenic cause for anosmia is suspected.

Bibliography

Caplan L. Posterior circulation ischemia: Then, now, and tomorrow. *Stroke* 31:2011–2023, 2000.

Ciric I, Rosenblatt S, Kerr W, et al. Perspective in pituitary adenomas: An end of the century review of tumorigenesis, diagnosis, and treatment. In: Howard MA, ed. *Clinical Neurosurgery*. Vol 47. Philadelphia: Lippincott Williams & Wilkins, 2000.

Goodrich I, Lee KJ, eds. *The Pituitary: Clinical Aspects of Normal and Abnormal Function*. Amsterdam: Elsevier, 1987.

Gronseth GS, Barohn RJ. Practice parameter: Thymectomy for autoimmune myasthenia gravis (an evidence-based review). *Neurology* 55:7–15, 2000.

Izawa M, Hayashi M, Nakaya K, et al. Gamma knife radiosurgery for pituitary adenomas. *J Neurosurg* 93:19–22, 2000.

Jho HD, Park IS, Alfieri A. The future of pituitary surgery In: Howard MA, ed. *Clinical Neurosurgery*. Vol 47. Philadelphia: Lippincott Williams & Wilkins, 2000, 83–98.

Laske DW, Oldfield EH. Assessment of pituitary function. In: Rengachary SS, Wilkins RH, eds. *Principles of Neurosurgery*. London: Wolfe Publishing, 1994, 32.2–32.38.

Nelson PB. Antidiuretic hormone. In: *Concepts in Neurosurgery*. Vol 5. *Neuroendocrinology*. Baltimore: Williams & Wilkins, 1992, 201–207.

Noseworthy JH, Lucchinetti C, Rodriguez M, et al. Multiple sclerosis. *N Engl J Med* 343:938–952, 2000.

Physicians' Desk Reference. Oradell, NJ: Medical Economics, 1994.

Pitts LH, Jackler RK. Treatment of acoustic neuromas. *N Engl J Med* 339:1471–1473, 1998.

Pollock BE, Lunsford LD, Norén G. Vestibular schwannoma management in the next century: A radiosurgical perspective. *Neurosurgery* 43: 475–483.

Silberstein SD. Practice parameter: Evidence-based guidelines for migraine headache (an evidence based review). *Neurology* 55:754–763, 2000.

Swan IRC. Is early management of acoustic neuroma important? *J R Soc Med* 93:614–617, 2000.

Thibonnier M. Antidiuretic hormone: Regulation, disorders, and clinical evaluation. In: *Concepts in Neurosurgery*. Vol. 5. *Neuroendocrinology*. Baltimore: Williams & Wilkins, 1992, 19–30.

Fluids, Electrolytes, and Nutrition

16

Malnutrition is a common problem in patients with cancer and is present in over 20% of patients with head and neck carcinoma. Malnutrition, which may be defined as weight loss greater than 10% of ideal weight that is associated with the loss of muscle, is multifactorial in origin. The three major mechanisms in the pathogenesis of malnutrition in cancer patients include reduced dietary intake, anorexia, and cancer-induced cachexia.

Malnutrition has been associated with increased perioperative morbidity, including increased rates of postoperative sepsis and wound infection. Perioperative nutritional support, especially preoperative nutritional replacement in the severely malnourished patient, appears to be associated with a lowering of operative morbidity, mortality, and overall health care costs. It is critical that nutritional assessment be incorporated as a routine component in the workup of patients with carcinoma of the head and neck.

MALNUTRITION

The nutritional assessment begins with a complete history and physical examination as well as a diverse range of anthropometric and laboratory tests. Given that no one test or measurement can diagnose malnutrition, the clinician must incorporate a range of factors to determine the nutritional status of any given patient.

History
1. Weight loss >12 to 20% ideal body weight
2. Alcohol abuse
3. Advanced (stage III–IV) cancers of the head and neck (particularly oral cavity and oropharynx)

Physical Examination
1. Loss subcutaneous fat/muscle wasting
2. Cheilosis, stomatitis, and dry, scaling skin (various vitamin deficiencies)

Anthropometry
1. Assess body fat skinfold measurements.
2. Body mass index (BMI) = weight (kg)/height (cm) × 100 allows one to calculate/estimate lean body mass and total body fat.
3. Midarm circumference can be used to estimate skeletal muscle mass.

Laboratory Measures
1. Visceral proteins measured include albumin and transferrin. Albumin levels less than 3.0 g/dL are associated with an increased perioperative morbidity. Transferrin, an acute-phase protein with a shorter half-life (7 days), may more accurately reflect

short-term changes in nutritional status. A transferrin less than 150 mg/dL indicates a poor prognosis.

2. Transferrin may be measured directly from the serum or calculated from the total iron binding capacity (TIBC) using transferrin = $(0.68 \times TIBC) + 21$.
3. Immunologic function is closely related to nutritional status and malnutrition has been associated with decreased cellular and humoral immunity. Anergic patients have been estimated to develop septic complications one-third of the time versus only 5% in immunocompetent hosts. Cell-mediated immunity can be measured by the intradermal placement of antigens [mumps, *Candida*, purified protein derivative (PPD), tetanus, etc.].
4. A total lymphocyte count (TLC) of <1700/μL has been demonstrated to be associated with a fivefold increase in the risk of wound infection. The TLC is a gross measurement of humoral immunity.

Summary

Given that no one parameter can measure malnutrition, a formula termed the prognostic nutritional index (PNI) was developed to combine several factors.

$$PNI = 158 - 16.6 \text{ (albumin)} - 0.78 \text{ (triceps skinfold)} - 0.20 \text{ (transferrin)} - 5.8 \text{ (delayed hypersensitivity)}$$

In studies of surgical trauma, the PNI is predictive of complications and morbidity. Buzby et al. showed that in patients undergoing gastrointestinal surgery with a PNI < 40%, the complication rate was 8% and mortality 3%. In patients with a PNI > 40%, the complication rates rose to 40% with a 22% mortality. In head and neck cancer patients, Hooley et al. demonstrated a PNI > 20% to be associated with an increased risk of postsurgical complications.

NUTRITIONAL REQUIREMENTS

Once a diagnosis of malnutrition is confirmed, the clinician must accurately define the patient's nutrient and caloric requirements. The average patient will use 25 to 45 kcal/kg/day, with wide individual variation. The Harrison-Benedict formula—which incorporates age, sex, weight, height, activity, and an injury factor—can more accurately determine the patient's requirements. Once the caloric requirements are defined, a number of variables must be incorporated.

1. An average adult requires 30 to 35 kcal/kg/day. Complex cases may require assessment of nitrogen balance to determine caloric and protein status.
2. 1 g of nitrogen per 125 to 150 kcal (ie, 6.25 g of protein per 125–150 kcal). The calorie-to-nitrogen ratio is important to avoid protein-calorie malnutrition and allow restoration of protein stores.
3. Specific requirement of vitamins, minerals, and micronutrients.
4. Ongoing assessment of weight, laboratory parameters, and selective use of 24-hour urine collection to assess nitrogen balance.

NUTRITIONAL DELIVERY TECHNIQUES

All patients with malnutrition will need replacement of their deficits. Replacement can be as simple as oral supplementation with a high-calorie high-protein drink or as sophisticated as total parenteral nutrition (TPN) via central venous access. While many patients with advanced head and neck carcinoma will require perioperative nutritional support, most have a normally functioning gastrointestinal tract and will be able to utilize enteral feedings.

Enteral Feedings

There are a wide variety of enteral feeding formulations which vary in their physical and chemical composition. Depending on the medical condition of the patient one may select a formula for patients with renal failure, hepatic failure, pulmonary failure, or recent trauma. An elemental diet is residue free and contains protein in the amino acid or hydrolysate form. It provides an essentially fat free diet except for essential fatty acids and the carbohydrates are in the form of oligosaccharides. An elemental diet has particular application in patients who cannot tolerate residue in the GI tract due to low output fistula or short bowel syndrome.

The route of feeding may be nasogastric (NG), gastrostomy—either an open technique or percutaneous endoscopic gastrostomy (PEG)—or jejunostomy. Each technique has its own indications and associated advantages and disadvantages.

Nasogastric Feedings
Advantages
1. Short-term use (<2–4 weeks)
2. Ease of placement
3. Newer soft silicone catheters (8F) well tolerated

Disadvantages
1. Significant tissue reaction (nose, nasopharynx, etc.)
2. Esophageal reflux with risk of aspiration
3. Esophagitis
4. Clogging of tube

Gastrostomy Feedings
Advantages
1. Better tolerated long-term
2. Option of open technique or PEG
3. PEG allows option of local anesthesia/outpatient surgery
4. Open gastrostomy allows larger-bore tube
5. No interference with normal deglutition, airway, or voice
6. More aesthetically appealing

Disadvantages
1. Surgical procedure
2. Wound complications

Jejunostomy Indications
1. Total laryngopharyngoesophagectomy with gastric pull-up
2. Reconstruction utilizing jejunal free-flap transfer
3. Severe underlying gastric disease

Parenteral Nutrition

The use of parenteral nutrition provides the clinician with a relatively rapid nutritional replacement technique that is not dependent upon the alimentary tract. Peripheral parenteral nutrition (PPN) is given via a peripheral vein and is not adequate for complete nutritional supplementation. It may be given as a supplement composed of 5 to 10% dextrose, 3.5% amino acids, and intralipids to provide 1000 to 2000 mL per day. Total parenteral nutrition (TPN) is given via central venous access to bypass a nonfunctioning gastrointestinal tract.

Indications for TPN
1. Severe protein malnutrition with loss of a normally functioning GI system
2. Primary disease of the GI system
3. Inability to safely swallow (most cases can tolerate enteral feedings)

Advantages of TPN
1. Ability to replace calories, protein, and vitamins independent of GI function
2. Rapid replacement of nutritional deficits (1–2 weeks)
3. Maintenance of a normal growth curve
4. Restoration of nutritional and immunologic competence, thus reducing surgical morbidity and mortality

FLUID, ELECTROLYTES, AND ACID-BASE BALANCE

Trauma, operative procedures, and multiple medical diseases can produce alterations in the composition, distribution, and volume of the body fluids. Critical disturbances in the fluid, electrolyte, or acid-base balance of the body may have no outward signs or symptoms and may be diagnosed only by laboratory testing. Surgical patients are particularly prone to such disturbances due to the effects of anesthesia, parenteral feedings, underlying medical diseases, and postoperative fluid shifts.

The average 70-kg male is composed of 60% (42 L) water. Of this 42 L, approximately two-thirds (28 L) is intracellular and one-third (14 L) is extracellular. The extracellular compartment can be further divided into the interstitial fluid (10 L) and the plasma (4 L). Various electrolytes are distributed among the different fluid compartments of the body (Table 16-1).

Fluid Exchange

Routes		Average Daily Volume (mL)
Water Gains:	Oral fluids	800–1500
	Solid foods	500–700
	Water oxidation	250
Water Loss:	Urine output	800–1500
	Intestinal	250
	Insensible	500–700

TABLE 16-1. BODY FLUID ELECTROLYTE COMPOSITION

Substance	Extracellular Fluid (mEq/L)	Intracellular Fluid (mEq/L)
Sodium	140	10
Potassium	4	150
Magnesium	1.7	40
Chloride	105	10
Bicarbonate	28	10
Phosphate/sulfate	3.5	150
Protein anions	15	40

Fluid Requirements

Adults:		35 mL/kg/24 h
Children:	First 10 kg	100 mL/kg/24 h or 4 mL/kg/h
	Second 10 kg	50 mL/kg/24 h or 2 mL/kg/h
	>20 kg	25 mL/kg/24 h or 1 mL/kg/h
Fever:		500 mL/24 h above 38.3°C (101°F)

Fluid Disturbances

Overhydration (volume excess)
- Polyuria
- Urine Na >30 mEq/L
- Pulmonary edema
- Distended neck veins
- Ascites
- Peripheral edema
- Systolic hypertension
- Elevated wedge pressure

Dehydration (volume depletion)
- Oliguria
- Urine Na <10 mEq/L
- Hypotension
- Poor skin turgor
- Sunken eyeballs
- Thirst
- Tachycardia
- Hemoconcentration
- Low wedge pressure

Sodium

Normal serum Na 135–145 mEq/L
Normal intake Na 1 mEq/kg/24 h

Hypernatremia (Na >150 mEq/L)

Etiology: Loss free water: diabetes insipidus, sweating, burns, diarrhea, vomiting, osmotic diuresis, insensible losses
Solute loading: tube feeding, brain stem injury, inappropriate IV, Cushing's syndrome

Therapy: Depends on the fluid status, but basic principle is to treat underlying disorder and slowly rehydrate with hypotonic fluid. Rapid rehydration can lead to cerebral edema or congestive heart failure (CHF).

Hyponatremia (Na <130 mEq/L)

Etiology: Iatrogenic, water intoxication, sepsis, renal failure, cirrhosis, syndrome of inappropriate secretion of antidiuretic hormone (SIADH), CHF, myxedema, hyperglycemic osmotic effect (correct 2 mEq for every 100 mg of excess glucose to give a serum sodium that correctly reflects the sodium/fluid status).

Therapy: Depends upon the fluid status of the patient. If fluid overloaded (CHF, renal failure), then restrict fluid and use diuretics. If volume-depleted, then rehydrate with normal saline. If symptoms are severe [central nervous system (CNS)], then replace half the deficit over 4 to 6 hours with 3% hypertonic saline. Replace the remainder over the next 24 to 48 hours.

Potassium

Normal serum: 3.5–5.0 mEq/L
Normal intake: Adults   40–60 mEq/24 h
                  Children   2 mEq/kg/24 h

Hyperkalemia (K+ > 5.5)

Etiology: Excess intake, renal failure, rhabdomyolysis, crush injury, acidosis, angiotensin converting enzyme (ACE) inhibitors, potassium-sparing diuretics
Diagnosis: Weakness, loss of deep tendon reflexes (DTRs), confusion, irritability electroencephalographic (ECG) changes (peaked T waves, prolonged QRS, sinus arrest, asystole)
Therapy: Remove exogenous sources, Kayexalate; emergency situation with K+ > 7.5 or ECG changes combination of D_{50}/insulin/$NaHCO_3$/Ca. Consider dialysis

Hypokalemia (K+ <3.0 mEq/L)

Etiology: Decreased intake, GI loss especially NG suction, vomiting, diarrhea, laxative abuse, diuretics, steroid therapy
Diagnosis: Anorexia, nausea, vomiting, ileus, weakness, ECG changes [prolonged QT, ST-segment depression, premature ventricular contractions (PVCs)]
Therapy: Replete max rate of 40 mEq/h (monitoring)
             —*peripheral 20 mEq in 50–100 mL D_5W
             —*central 20–40 mEq in 50–100 mL D_5W

Remember serum pH will affect serum K+ (acidosis will produce an increase in serum K+ while alkalosis produces a decrease).

Calcium

Normal serum Ca^{2+} 8.5–10.6 mg/dL

Normal intake
    1–3 g/24 h
    —*total body stores 1–2 g
    —*serum Ca++ 50% ionized, 50% nonionized
    —*serum total Ca^{2+} decreases with decreasing serum protein; however, ionized Ca^{2+} remains constant. Check ionized Ca^{2+} or correct serum Ca^{2+} via decrease 0.8 mg/dL Ca^{2+} is seen with each 1.0 g/dL decrease in serum albumin below 4.0 g/dL.

Hypocalcemia (Ca^{2+} < 8 mg/dL)

Etiology: Hypoparathyroidism (iatrogenic most common), decreased albumin, pancreatitis, renal failure, hypomagnesemia, vitamin D deficiency, malabsorption, pseudohypoparathyroidism

Diagnosis: Usually symptomatic below 7.5 mg/dL, numbness, tingling, headaches, cramps, Chvostek's sign (facial nerve irritability), Trousseau's sign (carpopedal spasm)

Therapy: Emergent Ca gluconate or chloride 1 g (10 mL of 10% solution = 1 ampule) IVP over 10 to 15 minutes with cardiac monitor
—*Remember to check Mg
—*Chronic hypocalcemia replace with Os-cal 1.5 to 3.0 g/day with vitamin D (Calcitriol .50–2.0 μg/day)
—*Transient hypocalcemia (7.0–8.0) after thyroid surgery may not require therapy

Hypercalcemia (Ca^{2+} > 10.6)

Etiology: Hyperparathyroidism, ectopic parathyroid hormone production, malignancy, bony metastases, milk-alkali syndrome, vitamin D toxicity, sarcoid, tuberculosis, Paget's disease, thiazides, parathyroid malignancy

Diagnosis: Mild elevations (<11.5) often asymptomatic and may require no therapy, nocturia, polydipsia, anorexia, nausea, vomiting, abdominal pain, confusion; >14 to 16 emergency levels

Therapy: Treat underlying disorder
Hydration (normal saline 1–2 L q2h)
Diuretics
Phosphates, steroids, calcitonin, mithramycin

Magnesium

Normal serum levels: 1.6–2.5 mg/dL
Normal intake: 20 mEq/day

Hypomagnesemia Mg^{2+} < 1.5 mg/dl

Etiology: Laxative abuse, diuretics, SIADH, parathyroidectomy, burns, decreased intake (alcohol abuse, TPN, malnutrition), decreased GI absorption.

Diagnosis: Muscle weakness, cardiac arrhythmia, myoclonus

Therapy: Urgent—1 to 2 g MgSO$_4$ (8–16 mEq) over 15 to 30 minutes, then 1 g im q4-6h or Mg oxide (Uromag) 2 tabs bid

Hypermagnesemia Mg^{2+} > 3 mg/dL

Etiology: Renal failure, excess intake

Diagnosis: Hypertension, nausea, vomiting, lethargy, weakness, ECG changes (AV block, prolonged QT)

Therapy: Urgent Ca gluconate 20 mL 10% solution IVP, eliminate exogenous sources, dialysis

Acid-Base Disorders

The acid-base system is designed to maintain the pH at a level of 7.4 for optimal cellular function. A number of mechanisms including the respiratory system, renal system, extracellular buffers (primarily HCO$_3^-$), and intracellular buffers (proteins, phosphates, and hemoglobin) exist to control the pH within this narrow range (Table 16-2).

Excess hydrogen ion (acid) is eliminated by the lungs based on the reaction

$$H^+ + HCO_3^- = H_2CO_3 = CO_2 + H_2O$$

Most of the excess hydrogen is eliminated by this route, with a relatively small amount (~70 mEq) eliminated by the renal system. Both the pulmonary and renal systems make adjustments to compensate for the alterations in the acid-base balance (Table 16-2). There are four general categories of acid-base disorders; respiratory acidosis and alkalosis and metabolic acidosis and alkalosis.

Respiratory Acidosis

Primary respiratory acidosis is characterized by an increase in the partial pressure of arterial CO_2 (PCO_2) secondary to disorders that limit pulmonary function. This is most commonly seen in diseases that limit the body's ability to eliminate CO_2, such as chronic obstructive pulmonary disease, impairment of central respiration (head injuries or drugs), or chest wall trauma that prevents adequate ventilation. The diagnosis is confirmed by an arterial blood gas that demonstrates a low pH and an elevated PCO_2. The lowered pH reflects the body's attempt to compensate for the rising PCO_2, as depicted in the formula mentioned above. In chronic situations, the renal system may contribute to the compensation by retaining HCO_3^-. Treatment is centered around addressing the chronic hypoventilation and may include steroids, antibiotics, inhalers, reversal of respiratory suppression, and consideration of intubation/ mechanical ventilation.

Respiratory Alkalosis

Primary respiratory alkalosis is characterized by hyperventilation that leads to a reduction in PCO_2. The two primary etiologies are direct stimulation of the central respiratory centers [aspirin, CNS tumors/trauma/cerebrovascular accident (CVA)] or indirect stimulation through hypoxia. It may also be seen in psychogenic hyperventilation, sepsis, errors in mechanical ventilation, and fevers. The diagnosis is confirmed by an arterial blood gas that demonstrates of an elevated pH (>7.45) with a low PCO_2 (<35). Treatment is directed to the correction of the underlying disorder.

Metabolic Acidosis

Metabolic acidosis results from a variety of disorders that produce an excess acid load, decreased acid secretion, or excess bicarbonate loss. It is characterized by a low arterial pH

TABLE 16-2. ACID-BASE DISTURBANCES

Disturbance	pH	H+	Compensation	Examples
Metabolic acidosis	↓	↑	Pa_{CO_2} decreases by 1.3 mmHg for each mEq/L decrease HCO_3^-	Lactic acidosis Ketoacidosis
Metabolic alkalosis	↑	↓	Pa_{CO_2} increase by 5–7 mmHg for each mEq/L increase in HCO_3^-	Vomiting NG tube suction Cushing's syndrome
Respiratory acidosis	↓	↑	HCO_3^- increase by 1 mEq/L for each 10 mmHg increase in Pa_{CO_2}	Hypoventilation CNS lesion
Respiratory alkalosis	↓	↓	HCO_3^- decrease by 2 mEq/L for each 10 mmHg decrease Pa_{CO_2}	Hyperventilation Fever/sepsis Hypoxemia

(<7.36) and a low HCO_3 (<22). The reduction in arterial pH leads to a compensatory hyperventilation that decreases the P_{CO_2} and minimizes the change in arterial pH. Important in distinguishing among the many causes of a metabolic acidosis is the anion gap. The anion gap allows the clinician to classify the causes of metabolic acidosis into a high anion gap versus a normal anion gap (Table 16-3). The anion gap is calculated by subtracting the sum of the chloride and the bicarbonate from the sodium concentration. The usual value is 10 mEq/L.

Diagnosis is confirmed by an arterial blood gas that reflects a low pH and a lowering of the HCO_3^-. The anion gap should be calculated to help guide the determination of an etiology. Treatment is directed toward the underlying disorder. In many cases of mild metabolic acidosis (pH > 7.25), no treatment is necessary. The use of bicarbonate to treat metabolic acidosis is controversial, and in some patients with lactic acidosis and ketoacidosis it may cause more harm than benefit. In selected situations (pH < 7.20, HCO_3^- < 10 mEq/L) some clinicians would use bicarbonate while addressing the underlying cause of the acidosis.

Metabolic Alkalosis

A metabolic alkalosis is caused by a primary elevation in plasma HCO_3^- above 27 mEq/L, leading to an increased pH greater than 7.44. The increased pH stimulates a decrease in pulmonary ventilation. The drop in ventilation leads to an increase in the P_{CO_2}, thereby attempting to minimize the alterations in the blood pH. The underlying causes of metabolic alkalosis are due to a loss of acid or excess alkali intake. Table 16-4 lists the most common causes of metabolic alkalosis. By far the most common cause is related to the loss of acids (HCl). In general there is no classic clinical picture of metabolic alkalosis. Most commonly the lab values will indicate an elevated serum bicarbonate (>30 mEq/L). An arterial blood gas will then need to be obtained to assess the acid-base status and rule out a metabolic alkalosis, or the elevated bicarbonate may reflect a true respiratory acidosis with the elevated bicarbonate representing a compensatory response.

Once the metabolic workup confirms an elevated HCO_3^- with an alkalotic pH, the next step is to assess the patient's volume status. Most commonly, GI losses (vomiting, NG tube) will account for the metabolic alkalosis and treatment can be focused on restoring an adequate volume, chloride, and potassium intake, which will allow the body to self-correct the acid-base equilibrium. Obviously the underlying disorder must be addressed while at the same time providing the necessary fluids and electrolytes, which allows the renal system to excrete the excess bicarbonate. The amount of fluid and electrolytes will be guided by the patient's clinical response, but often several liters of normal saline and several hundred milliequivalents of potassium will be needed over several days.

TABLE 16-3.   ETIOLOGY OF METABOLIC ACIDOSIS

Normal anion gap
   Excess acid intake (Hcl, NH_4Cl)
   Bicarbonate loss
      GI tract (diarrhea, fistulas, NG tube)
      Proximal renal tubular acidosis
      Distal renal tubular acidosis
Increased anion gap
   Ketoacidosis (diabetes mellitus, alcohol)
   Lactic acidosis
   Poisons (aspirin, ethylene glycol)
   Renal failure

TABLE 16-4. ETIOLOGY OF METABOLIC ALKALOSIS

Acid loss (generally HCl)
  Gastrointestinal (vomiting, NG tube)
  Increased urine acidification
    Diuretics
    Aldosterone excess
    Bartter's syndrome
Excess alkali
  Alkali abuse
  Overtreatment of metabolic acidosis (ie, HCO_3^-)
Severe potassium depletion

Bibliography

Bumpous JM, Maves MD. Total lymphocyte count as a predictor of wound infections in head and neck surgery. Am J Otolaryngol (In press).

Bumpous JM, Snyderman CH. Nutritional considerations in patients with cancer of the head and neck. In Myers EN, Suen JY, eds. *Cancer of the Head and Neck.* Philadelphia: Saunders, 1996, 105–116.

Buzby GP, Mullen JL, Mathews DC, et al. Prognostic nutritional index in gastrointestinal surgery. *Am J Surg* 139:160–167, 1980.

Campos AC, Butters M, Meguid MM. Home enteral nutrition via gastrostomy in advanced head and neck cancer patients. *Head Neck* 12:137–142, 1990.

Detsky AS, Simalley PS, Chang J. Is this patient malnourished? *JAMA* 271:54–58, 1994.

Elia M. Changing concepts of nutrient requirements in disease: Implications for artificial nutritional support. *Lancet* 345:1279–1284, 1995.

Forman BH. Fluids, electrolytes, and acid-base balance. In Lee KJ, ed. *Essential Otolaryngology Head and Neck Surgery.* New Haven, CT: Medical Examination Publishing, 1991, 330–340.

Gann DS, Amaral JF. Fluid and electrolyte management. In Sabiston DC, ed. *Essentials of Surgery.* Philadelphia: Saunders, 1987, 29–61.

Hooley R, Levine H, Flores TC, et al. Predicting postoperative head and neck complications using nutritional assessment. The Prognostic Nutritional Index. *Arch Otolaryngol* 109:83–88, 1983.

Mathews TW, Johnson ML, Williams BD, et al. Nutritional status in head and neck cancer patients. *J Otolaryngol* 24:87–91, 1995.

Surgical Hemostasis 17

Hemostasis is the result of a complex interaction among blood vessels, platelets, and plasma coagulation proteins designed to prevent blood loss from the circulatory system. Following tissue injury, platelets adhere to the subendothelium of disrupted blood vessels, a process mediated by a variety of adhesive proteins including the von Willebrand factor. Platelet adhesion initiates platelet secretion, with the release of the contents of platelet intracellular storage granules. The released materials stimulate circulating platelets and cause them to acquire new adhesive properties. These stimulated platelets interact with one another during platelet aggregation to form a platelet plug to seal the injured blood vessel and prevent further blood loss.

A series of interdependent enzyme-mediated reactions initiate the formation of a chemically stable fibrin clot, which replaces the unstable platelet plug (Figure 17-1). After tissue injury (endothelial cell disruption), tissue factor (TF) expressed on cells normally separated by the endothelium from the blood binds factor VII and converts it to an active enzyme, factor VIIa.[1] The TF–factor VIIa complex subsequently activates two substrates, factors IX and X. Factor X is also activated by the factor IXa–VIIa–phospholipid–calcium ion complex. This reaction is important to supplement the direct factor VIIa–TF activation of factor X because of a naturally occurring tissue factor pathway inhibitor (TFPI) that inhibits factor Xa and the factor VIIa–TF complex. Factor Xa then complexes with factor Va, calcium ions, and anionic phospholipid (the latter derived from activated platelets and endothelial cells) to form the prothrombinase complex. This complex converts prothrombin (factor II) to thrombin (factor IIa). Thrombin acts on fibrinogen (factor I) to generate fibrin monomer and catalyzes the conversion of factor XIII to factor XIIIa. Factor XIIIa acts to cross-link fibrin monomer strands into a rigid, insoluble fibrin polymer mesh. Thrombin also catalyzes the activation of factors VIII and V.

A second pathway of blood coagulation is initiated by factor XII. Kallikrein activates factor XII to factor XIIa, a reaction facilitated by high-molecular-weight kininogen. Factor XIIa activates factor XI, and in the presence of calcium ions, factor XIa activates factor IX. Factor IXa binds to factor VIIIa in the presence of calcium ions and phospholipid.

Regulatory proteins of the coagulation system include (1) activated protein C, which, in conjunction with protein S and anionic phospholipid, inactivates factors VIIIa and Va; (2) antithrombin, which inhibits thrombin (factor IIa), factor IXa, and factor Xa; and (3) TFPI, which inhibits the factor VIIa–TF–factor Xa complex.

The fibrinolytic system plays an important role in the dissolution of blood clots and in the maintenance of a free-flowing vascular system (Figure 17-2). Two distinct types of plasminogen activators have been identified: tissue-type plasminogen activator and urokinase-type plasminogen activator. These activators convert plasminogen to its active form, plasmin, which degrades fibrin into soluble fibrin degradation products (FDPs). Plasminogen activator can also be triggered by factor XII, prekallikrein, and high-molecular-weight kininogen.

Regulatory proteins of the fibrinolytic system include two types of plasminogen activator inhibitors and alpha$_2$-antiplasmin.

352

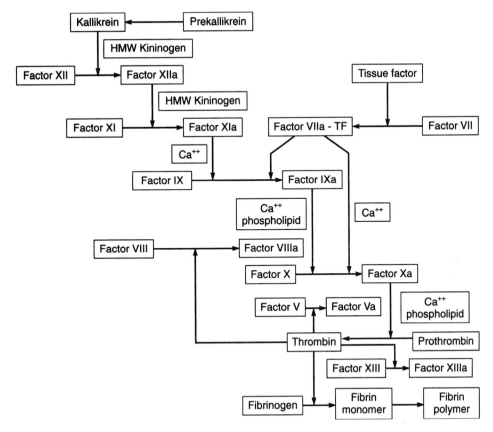

Figure 17-1. Schematic of blood coagulation.

Excessive surgical bleeding can result from vascular injury or a defect in the hemostatic mechanism. If damage to local tissue is not the apparent cause of excessive bleeding, patients should be evaluated for a defect in platelet function or plasma coagulation proteins.

CLINICAL EVALUATION

A carefully performed medical history and physical examination are paramount in assessing bleeding risk and are as important as laboratory testing. Bleeding in multiple sites and on multiple occasions suggests a systemic coagulopathy. Spontaneous bleeding or bleeding immediately after trauma suggests a platelet-vascular problem and is often characterized by bleeding from superficial surfaces, such as the skin (petechiae, ecchymoses) or mucous membranes of the nasopharyngeal, gastrointestinal, or genitourinary tracts. Bleeding that is delayed after trauma suggests clotting factor problems and is often characterized by bleeding into deep tissues, such as joints, muscles, and the retroperitoneal space. Hematomas involving the skin may also be seen.

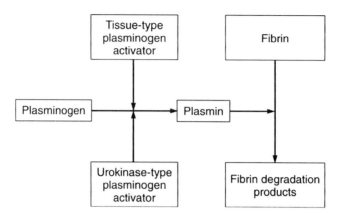

Figure 17-2. Schematic of fibrinolysis.

The history should review drug ingestion (including specific questions about over-the-counter drugs, many of which contain aspirin or a nonsteroidal anti-inflammatory agent); the family history; and the patient's response to prior stress such as dental work, tooth extractions, lacerations, formal surgical procedures, labor and delivery, and menses. A question should be asked about the need for prior transfusional therapy.

The physical examination should focus on the presence of petechiae, prominent in dependent areas and suggestive of thrombocytopenia, telangiectasias which blanch with pressure and suggest hereditary hemorrhagic telangiectasia, and ecchymoses which suggest platelet and vascular disorders. Acute hemarthroses or degenerative arthropathies suggest severe plasma coagulation disorders, such as factor VIII deficiency (hemophilia A).

LABORATORY EVALUATION

Platelet Count

The platelet count is performed to detect thrombocytopenia. Thrombocytopenia is defined as a platelet count below 150,000/µL, while thrombocytosis is defined as a platelet count above 400,000/µL. In the absence of a functional platelet defect, a platelet count greater than 100,000/µL is associated with normal hemostasis, while a platelet count less than 15,000/µL is often associated with spontaneous bleeding into skin, mucous membranes, and vital organs.

Patients with platelet counts between 50,000 and 100,000/µL are unlikely to hemorrhage except during major trauma or an operation. Patients with platelet counts between 15,000 and 50,000/µL may have spontaneous bleeding into the skin and will usually bleed excessively at the time of surgery.

The finding of thrombocytopenia should be confirmed by examination of a peripheral blood smear for several important reasons. First, large platelets observed on the peripheral blood smear suggest increased platelet turnover, as is seen in idiopathic thrombocytopenic purpura (ITP). Second, abnormal red or white cells may be observed, and this finding may provide clues indicative of a primary hematologic disorder. Third, platelet clumps provide evidence for pseudothrombocytopenia, a phenomenon not associated with any disease state. Pseudothrombocytopenia is often caused by antibodies in the patient's serum that react with platelets and blood anticoagulated with ethylenediaminetetraacetic acid (EDTA), causing agglutination and a spuriously low platelet count.[2] The agglutinated or clumped platelets are misinterpreted by the electronic counting instrument as a white cell. Pseudothrombo-cytopenia may also be caused by platelet satellitism, a phenomenon characterized by rosettes of platelets around monocytes and neutrophils.

Prothrombin Time

The prothrombin time (PT), introduced by Dr. Armand Quick in 1935, is the most common test used for monitoring oral anticoagulant therapy, as this test is responsive to reductions in the vitamin K–dependent coagulation factors II, VII, and X. Deficiencies of factors VII, V, X, II, or fibrinogen may result in prolongation of the PT. The PT is typically prolonged when factors are reduced to less than 30% of normal.

The PT is performed by adding a mixture of thromboplastin to citrate-anticoagulated plasma, recalcifying the plasma, and then measuring the clotting time. Historically, the PT has been reported as the ratio between the patient's prothrombin time and the mean control used in the laboratory. However, the actual measured PT depends on the source of the thromboplastin reagent used to initiate the "extrinsic" coagulation cascade, making it diffi-cult to compare results from different laboratories. Therefore, prothrombin times are today reported as the international normalized ratio (INR), which corrects an individual labora-tory's values to an international reference standard.[3]

The PT provides evidence about the current synthetic capacity of the liver, the adequacy of vitamin K absorption, and the inhibition of clotting factor synthesis by warfarin. The PT test is not recommended for preoperative screening of patients without evidence of a coagu-lation disorder.[4] The PT and activated partial thromboplastin time (aPTT) are recommended for patients in whom a clinical assessment cannot be made; for patients with clinical evidence to suggest a bleeding disorder, liver disease, malabsorption, or malnutrition; and for patients requiring procedures that will disrupt normal coagulation, such as a prostatectomy, proce-dures requiring extracorporeal circulation, and placement of peritoneovenous shunts.

Activated Partial Thromboplastin Time

The aPTT is dependent on factors of the "intrinsic" and "common" pathways, and it is often prolonged by deficiencies of prekallikrein; high-molecular-weight kininogen; factors XII, XI, IX, VIII, V, X, II, and fibrinogen; and von Willebrand factor. Generally speaking, pro-longation of the aPTT occurs when factors are less than 25 to 30% of normal. Circulating anticoagulants (lupus-like anticoagulants) may also prolong the aPTT.

The aPTT is performed by the addition of a surface activating agent—such as kaolin, ellagic acid, or silica—and phospholipid to citrate–anticoagulated plasma. After incubation, the plasma is recalcified and the clotting time is measured. Factor XIII deficiency and alpha$_2$-antiplasmin deficiency are not detected by the aPTT or PT assays. These two deficiencies require evaluation by specific assay techniques. Preoperative screening with the aPTT (and PT) is not recommended for patients without clinical evidence of a coagulation disorder. The aPTT is recommended as a screening test for the same cohorts of patients as outlined under the discussion of PT. A second major use of the aPTT is to monitor patients receiving the anticoagulant heparin.[5]

Bleeding Time

The bleeding-time test is based on the concept of quantifying the duration of bleeding from a standardized superficial skin wound purposely inflicted in order to test the functional integrity of the platelet-microvascular interaction. The bleeding time is difficult to standardize and is subject to variable results because of variations in operator experience, temperature of the skin, venous pressure, length and depth of the skin incision, and direction of the skin incision.

The bleeding time is not a screening test and does not predict excessive surgical bleeding.[6] This test should be reserved to evaluate abnormal bleeding. There is a linear relationship between the platelet count and the bleeding time, with the bleeding time prolonging progressively as the platelet count falls below 100,000/μL down to 10,000/μL. Below 10,000/μL, the linear relationship is lost, and the bleeding time is greater than 30 minutes. The differential diagnosis of a prolonged bleeding time with a normal platelet count is either von Willebrand disease or a qualitative platelet defect. Von Willebrand disease can be evaluated by checking factor VIII procoagulant activity, von Willebrand factor antigen, and ristocetin cofactor activity (a measurement of von Willebrand factor activity).

Functional platelet disorders can be divided into two major groups: congenital (Bernard–Soulier syndrome, Glanzmann's thrombasthenia, Scott syndrome, release defects, gray platelet syndrome, and storage pool disorders) and acquired (drugs, uremia, myeloproliferative disorders, myelodysplastic syndrome, lymphocytic or plasmacytic disorders, and antiplatelet antibodies), and appropriate tests can be pursued. The bleeding–time evaluation should be used in conjunction with the peripheral blood smear findings, platelet count, aPTT, PT, thrombin time, and a careful medical history.

Platelet Aggregation Studies

Platelet aggregation studies are the main way of studying platelet function. Platelet aggregation is monitored by the increase in light transmission through a suspension of platelet-rich plasma as aggregation occurs. Aggregating agents in the laboratory setting include collagen, adenosine diphosphate (ADP), epinephrine, arachidonic acid, and ristocetin. Studies of platelet aggregation are often complemented by studies of platelet secretion of granule contents.

Fibrinogen

Plasma fibrinogen is usually determined by adding a large excess of thrombin to a diluted plasma sample to make sure that fibrinogen is the rate-limiting step (Clauss technique). A low fibrinogen may be due to the rare disorder of congenital afibrinogenemia or to acquired hypofibrinogenemia, a finding often associated with disseminated intravascular coagulation (DIC). A low fibrinogen may also be caused by a dysfibrinogenemia, either as part of a congenital disorder (often autosomal-dominant), secondary to severe liver dysfunction or from the presence of a hepatocellular carcinoma. If a dysfibrinogenemia is present, the fibrinogen concentration may be abnormally low when measured by the Clauss technique. An immunologic assay for fibrinogen should be performed in this situation.

Fibrin Degradation Products

The enzyme plasmin degrades both fibrinogen and fibrin to form a variety of fragments named X, Y, D, and E. These fibrin degradation products or fibrin "split" products (FSPs) are not detectable in the serum of normal individuals. When FSPs are detectable, this indicates that the patient's fibrinogen, fibrin, or both have been subjected to proteolysis by the enzyme plasmin. Although elevated FSPs are most characteristically seen in DIC due to the generation of plasmin in response to the formation and deposition of fibrin, elevated FDPs are not diagnostic of DIC. Elevated FSPs may be seen in patients with severe liver disease, renal failure, deep vein thromboembolic disease, pulmonary embolism, myocardial infarction, and occasionally in low titer in postoperative patients.

Dimers of the D fragment of fibrin are one type of FSP. They are seen only when fibrin has been cross-linked by thrombin and are therefore indicative of active clotting. The combination of a D-dimer assay and a FSP assay is therefore more specific for conditions such as DIC and deep venous thrombosis (DVT). A negative D-dimer assay effectively rules out the presence of DIC or a recent DVT.[7]

Thrombin Time

The thrombin time is a clotting test done to establish that adequate levels of fibrinogen are present. The thrombin time is performed by adding a dilute solution of the enzyme thrombin to a citrated specimen of the patient's plasma and measuring the time required to convert fibrinogen to fibrin polymer. The thrombin time may be prolonged by hypofibrinogenemia (fibrinogen less than 100 mg/dL), dysfibrinogenemia, and high concentrations of fibrinogen or fibrin degradation products. Heparin, antibodies to thrombin, some monoclonal serum paraproteins, heparin-like inhibitors, and severe hypoalbuminemia are other causes of a prolonged thrombin time.

Reptilase Time

If heparin contamination is thought to be the cause of the prolonged thrombin time, a reptilase time can be performed. Reptilase is a thrombin-like enzyme that is not inactivated by heparin. In the intensive care unit setting, contamination of the blood specimen by heparin is a common problem, as blood is often drawn through arterial lines or through central venous access devices.

Specific Coagulation Factor Assays

Once it is clearly established that the PT, aPTT, or both are prolonged, further testing needs to be done to identify whether there is a factor deficiency or an acquired inhibitor is present. This is accomplished by mixing patient plasma with an equal volume of pooled plasma from normal volunteer donors. Since factor levels of 50% of normal are sufficient to produce normal PTs and aPTTs, this procedure will result in correction of the abnormality if it is caused by a deficiency of one or more factors. Specific factor assays can then be done.

If an inhibitor antibody is present, the mixing procedure will usually result in little or no correction of the abnormality. Some inhibitors can be detected only by incubating the plasma mixture for several hours, and they may not be detected immediately after mixing.

Inhibitors

Factor VIII inhibitors and circulating anticoagulants (lupus-like anticoagulants) are the most frequently encountered inhibitors. Factor IX inhibitors are rare and other inhibitors are also seen only rarely. Circulating anticoagulants are antiphospholipid immunoglobulin G or M antibodies that prolong phospholipid-dependent coagulation in vitro by binding to sites within the phospholipid component of the factor Xa–factor Va–phospholipid–calcium ion complex. The term *lupus anticoagulant* is a misnomer. It was first recognized in a patient with systemic lupus erythematosus, but it is more frequently encountered in patients without lupus. This circulating anticoagulant is associated with thrombosis rather than with bleeding. The hexagonal PTT, which uses phopholipids to neutralize the antiphospholipid antibody, is an excellent screening test for circulating lupus-like anticoagulants.[8]

Miscellaneous

Causes of bleeding not detected by the platelet count, PT, aPTT, thrombin time, fibrinogen level, or bleeding time include factor XIII deficiency (congenital and acquired), abnormal

or excessive fibinolysis (increased levels of tissue plasminogen activator, deficiency of plasminogen activator inhibitor, alpha$_2$-antiplasmin deficiency, or urokinase), and vascular pur-
puras (vasculitides, congenital tissue disorders, vitamin C deficiency, corticosteroid excess,
amyloid, senile purpura, or hereditary hemorrhagic telangiectasia).

SPECIFIC HEMOSTATIC AND COAGULATION ABNORMALITIES

Platelet Abnormalities

Thrombocytopenia

Thrombocytopenia is defined as a platelet count below 150,000/µL. Normal platelet counts
range between 150,000 and 400,000/µL. When faced with a thrombocytopenic patient, one
must ask whether true thrombocytopenia or pseudothrombocytopenia is present, what is the
cause of the thrombocytopenia, and what is the severity of the thrombocytopenia. Laboratory evaluation should include a careful examination of the peripheral blood smear and perhaps a bone marrow biopsy.

Thrombocytopenia can be divided into three categories: platelet underproduction,
increased platelet destruction, and platelet sequestration. Often more than one mechanism
may be operative.

Platelet underproduction may be caused by processes causing megakaryocytic hypoplasia (chemotherapeutic agents, bone marrow toxins, infiltrative bone marrow disorders, and
infectious agents) or by processes causing ineffective thrombopoiesis (vitamin B$_{12}$ and folic
acid deficiency, myeloproliferative disorders, and myelodysplastic syndrome).

Thrombocytopenia caused by increased platelet destruction can be arbitrarily divided
into immunologic and nonimmunologic causes. Examples of immunologic causes include
autoantibodies (idiopathic thrombocytopenic purpura), alloantibodies (neonatal alloimmune
thrombocytopenia, posttransfusion purpura, prior platelet transfusions), some cases of drug-
induced thrombocytopenia (herapin induced thrombocytopenia), malignancy-associated
thrombocytopenia, and infection (bacterial, viral). Nonimmunologically mediated platelet
destruction can occur in DIC, preeclampsia and eclampsia, thrombotic microangiopathies,
renal transplant rejection, cardiopulmonary bypass surgery, and some cardiac disorders
(valvular heart disease, severe cyanotic congenital heart disease).

Platelet sequestration disorders are characterized by hypersplenism. Under physiologic
conditions, about 30% of the total platelet mass exists as a freely exchangeable pool in the
spleen. Up to 90% of the platelets are found in the spleen of patients with hypersplenism
because of increased splenic platelet pooling. Hypersplenism is a syndrome characterized by
splenomegaly and variable cytopenias. Hypersplenism is almost always the result of an identifiable pathologic process; however, it should be noted that most patients with splenomegaly
do not have hypersplenism. Treatment is directed at the underlying pathophysiologic process.

A rare fourth category of thrombocytopenia is that of dilutional thrombocytopenia,
which may occur during massive blood loss and replacement with 4°C stored blood (which
contains no viable platelets). In this setting, the platelet count will fall from its baseline by
approximately two-thirds.

Some thrombocytopenic patients may require platelet transfusions. It is important to
remember that platelet transfusions are not innocuous! They are costly, can transmit all of
the same infections as other blood products, and can lead to the development of alloimmu-
nization. Any medications thought to be causing thrombocytopenia and all nonessential

medications should be stopped promptly. Heparin is a common culprit; even the small amounts of heparin used to flush lines may cause thrombocytopenia. Any patient who has a decrease in platelet number or function that is associated with a substantial amount of bleeding from an operative site or spontaneously from skin, mucosal surfaces, or the central nervous system is a candidate for platelet transfusions. Prophylactic platelet transfusions should be given to patients with states of platelet underproduction when the platelet count is less than 5000 to 10,000/µL.[9,10] Random donor platelet concentrates are the product of choice; they are usually ordered in a dose of four to six units of platelet concentrates per transfusion. As a general rule, each unit of a random donor platelet concentrate should increase the peripheral platelet count by at least 6000/µL and this can be checked by obtaining a platelet count 10 minutes after the transfusion. This estimate assumes normal splenic platelet pooling of about 30 to 35%.

Thrombocytosis

Thrombocytosis has been associated with a number of disorders including iron deficiency anemia, infection, inflammatory disorders, many cancers, acute hemorrhage, and the post-splenectomy state. When associated with primary myeloproliferative disorders (essential thrombocythemia, myeloid metaplasia, polycythemia vera, chronic myelocytic leukemia), there is an increased risk of both hemorrhagic and thrombotic events. Although extreme thrombocytosis (platelet count greater than 1,000,000/µL) has been associated with a much higher incidence of thrombohemorrhagic events, the degree of elevation of the platelet count does not correlate directly with the risk of hemorrhage or thrombosis.[11,12]

Platelet Qualitative Disorders

A prolonged bleeding time in the presence of a normal platelet count suggests platelet dysfunction but does not predict the risk of hemorrhage. Functional platelet disorders can be divided into congenital disorders (disorders of platelet membranes and of platelet secretion) and acquired disorders (drugs that affect platelet function, hematologic neoplasms, and systemic conditions associated with abnormal platelet function). Abnormal platelet function usually does not contribute to any bleeding problem in patients with platelet counts greater than 50,000/µL if the vascular system is intact. The one well-documented exception is open heart surgery. Bleeding times become indefinitely prolonged during the cardiopulmonary bypass procedure even at platelet counts greater than 100,000/µL.

Drugs are the most common cause of abnormal platelet function, and aspirin is probably the most commonly used drug known to affect platelet function. When a hemostatically normal patient who is taking aspirin requires an invasive procedure, aspirin should be discontinued for at least 5 days. If it is not feasible to discontinue aspirin, careful observation is required. Significant excessive bleeding attributable to aspirin is a rare occurrence. Serious bleeding, if it does occur during an operation, is usually due to a surgically correctable lesion. If severe hemorrhage due to deficient platelet function is suspected, either a random donor platelet transfusion or DDAVP (desmopressin; 1-deamino-8-D-arginine vasopressin) would be rapidly effective.[13] This should be an unusual event.

Patients with chronic renal failure have an abnormal bleeding time that may be improved with DDAVP or with packed red cells. These treatments may improve hemostasis as well. DDAVP avoids the risk of transfusion-related infection and may be associated with relatively minor side effects, such as facial swelling, mild tachycardia, water retention, and hyponatremia.

Clotting Factor Deficiencies

Fibrinogen (Factor I)

Human fibrinogen is a glycoprotein synthesized by hepatocytes and present in plasma at a concentration of approximately 300 mg/dL. Absent or very low levels of plasma fibrinogen may be associated with congenital afibrinogenemia. Acquired hypofibrinogenemia may be seen in a variety of hepatic disorders, as part of acute or chronic DIC and rarely as a manifestation of an autoantibody. Bleeding with hypofibrinogenemia usually occurs in patients with fibrinogen concentrations less than 50 mg/dL. Replacement therapy may be required to control episodes of active bleeding or in preparation for surgical procedures. Patients should receive fibrinogen replacement in the form of cryoprecipitate, which contains approximately 300 mg of fibrinogen per unit (one unit equals a 30 to 50 mL bag). The goal of replacement therapy is to raise the plasma fibrinogen to at least 100 mg/dL. The patient should receive about one-third of the starting dose daily for as long as treatment is required.

Prothrombin (Factor II)

Prothrombin is a vitamin K–dependent protein synthesized by the liver. Prothrombin deficiency may be secondary to a rare hereditary deficiency. Acquired prothrombin deficiency is seen in patients with liver disease or vitamin K deficiency and is often corrected by exogenous vitamin K administration. Circulating (lupus-like) anticoagulants have also been associated with prothrombin deficiency. Acquired prothrombin deficiency can often be corrected by exogenous vitamin K administration. Patients with a hereditary deficiency or severe liver disease may require replacement therapy. Patients are usually treated with fresh frozen plasma in loading doses of 15 to 20 mL/kg of body weight followed by 3 mL/kg of body weight every 12 to 24 hours. The half-life of prothrombin is 3 days, so once-daily dosing may be used. Plasma levels of 30% or higher are generally sufficient to treat bleeding. Factor IX concentrates, which are rich in prothrombin, can also be used, but are usually reserved to treat major hemorrhage or in anticipation of major surgery.

Factor V

Factor V is a glycoprotein synthesized by both the liver and by megakaryocytes. Factor V deficiency may be hereditary (incidence 1 in 1 million) but far more often this deficiency is associated with liver disease or disseminated intravascular coagulation. Rare factor V inhibitors have been described. Fresh frozen plasma is generally the treatment of choice for factor V deficiency, and is administered at an initial dose of 15 to 20 mL/kg of body weight followed by 3 to 6 mL/kg of body weight for 7 days following surgery. The half-life of factor V is 36 hours; hence once-daily plasma infusions are recommended, with the goal of raising the factor V level to at least 25%.

Factor VII

Factor VII is a vitamin K–dependent protein produced by the liver. Hereditary factor VII deficiency is rare (incidence 1 in 500,000). Acquired factor VII deficiency can be associated with liver disease, vitamin K deficiency, or warfarin ingestion and is recognized by deficiency of other vitamin K–dependent proteins. The half-life of factor VII is 3 to 6 hours. Factor VII deficiency is treated with fresh frozen plasma. The minimum hemostatic level of factor VII is unknown, but levels of factor VII at 15 to 25% of normal generally provide adequate hemostasis. In preparation for major surgery or to treat hemorrhage, plasma may be given at a loading dose of 20 mL/kg of body weight followed by 3 to 6 mL/kg of body weight at 6- to 8- hour intervals because of factor VII's short half-life.

Factor IX concentrates rich in factor VII have also been used in patients with factor VII deficiency, but the factor VII concentration of the product needs to be checked before use, as concentrations vary between preparations. Factor VII concentrates and recombinant factor VII preparations are in clinical trials.

Factor VIII

Hemophilia A is a bleeding disorder characterized by a genetic deficiency of the X chromosome–linked gene product, factor VIII.[14] Von Willebrand disease is a group of clinically and genetically heterogeneous inherited hemorrhagic disorders distinct from hemophilia A arising from defects in the von Willebrand factor protein. Von Willebrand factor is essential for platelet adhesion to the subendothelium and, in the laboratory, for ristocetin-induced platelet aggregation. Factor VIII and von Willebrand factor are noncovalently linked in the plasma. Von Willebrand factor stabilizes factor VIII and regulates its activity.

Factor VIII deficiency is estimated to have a worldwide incidence of about 1 in 10,000 males. In general, the degree and severity of clinical bleeding correlates well with the measurement of factor VIII procoagulant activity. Hemophilia A can be classified based on the percentage of factor VIII present:

Mild hemophilia   (5 to 50% factor VIII)
Moderate hemophilia (2 to 5% factor VIII)
Severe hemophilia   (1% factor VIII)

Patients with mild hemophilia bleed only after a severe insult. Patients with moderate hemophilia infrequently have spontaneous hemorrhage but have significant bleeding after minor trauma, while patients with severe hemophilia have frequent spontaneous hemorrhages and severe bleeding after any trauma.

The choice of treatment of factor VIII deficiency depends on the clinical severity. Patients with mild hemophilia A who have greater than 10% factor VIII procoagulant activity may be treated with DDAVP. Patients with moderate or severe disease need to receive factor VIII concentrates. Cryoprecipitate is no longer indicated for treatment of factor VIII deficiency, as factor VIII concentrates are widely available. Patients should be checked for the presence of factor VIII inhibitors prior to treatment. Aspirin and nonsteroidal anti-inflammatory drugs should be avoided entirely and intramuscular injections forbidden.

The dose of factor VIII replacement is calculated in units. Dosing has to take into account the factor VIII half-life in plasma of 8 to 12 hours. A minimum hemostatic level of factor VIII is 30% for mild hemorrhage and 50% for major hemorrhage. For life-threatening bleeding, factor VIII activity should be kept at levels of 80 to 100%. Maintenance therapy is required for a number of days after bleeding has ceased.

The amount of factor VIII concentrate that needs to be transfused initially is based on the observation that one unit of factor VIII infused per kilogram of body weight yields a 2% rise in the plasma factor VIII level. For example, 25 U/kg of factor VIII concentrate achieves a 50% factor VIII level. A 70-kg patient would, therefore, need 1750 U of factor VIII if 50% factor VIII were the goal of therapy. Subsequent treatment should consist of factor VIII concentrates administered at 8- to 12-hour intervals. For patients with severe bleeding, factor VIII should be assayed frequently to guide replacement therapy. Activated partial thromboplastin times are inappropriate for calculating and monitoring the replacement of factor VIII concentrate.

The treatment of choice for patients with mild hemophilia (factor VIII greater than 10%) who require surgery is DDAVP. DDAVP is thought to stimulate factor VIII release from storage sites. Patients who are candidates for DDAVP should receive a trial of DDAVP prior to surgery. A baseline factor VIII level is obtained. DDAVP is then administered at a dose of 0.3 μg/kg of body weight in 50 mL normal saline over 30 minutes; 30 to 45 minutes from the end of the DDAVP infusion, a factor VIII level is again checked. The factor VIII level should rise at least threefold over the baseline. Tachyphylaxis often recurs after repetitive doses of DDAVP because of depletion of factor VIII from storage sites. DDAVP can be used together with factor VIII concentrates in patients with mild hemophilia if extremely high levels of factor VIII are needed. Common side effects of DDAVP include facial warmth, flushing, and transient headaches. Rare side effects include fluid retention, abdominal cramps, diarrhea, and myalgias.

Factor VIII inhibitors are antibodies that develop in patients with hemophilia A in response to factor VIII contained in various blood products. In other patients, factor VIII antibodies develop either in the setting of an immunologic disease or spontaneously. Treatment of inhibitors is complex and requires management by an experienced hematologist.

Factor IX

Factor IX is a vitamin K–dependent protein synthesized by the liver. Hemophilia B is an X chromosome–linked recessive bleeding disorder that occurs in 1 in 30,000 live male births but rarely in females. It is a heterogeneous disorder caused by decreased or defective factor IX. The type of factor IX deficiency dictates the clinical severity of bleeding. Acquired factor IX deficiency occurs with vitamin K deficiency, severe liver disease, warfarin ingestion, and factor IX inhibitors.

Fresh frozen plasma can be used as a source of factor IX for patients with mild (factor IX: 6 to 25% of normal) or moderate (factor IX: 1 to 5% of normal) hemophilia B when small increments of factor IX levels are necessary to control bleeding. Fresh frozen plasma can at best raise plasma factor IX levels by 10 to 15%. This approach to factor IX replacement is limited by the volume of plasma that can be infused. As a rule, adult patients can be initially treated with a loading dose of 20 mL/kg of body weight of plasma followed by 3 to 6 mL/kg of body weight of plasma every 8 to 12 hours.

When higher factor IX levels are required, factor IX concentrates are administered as a loading dose followed by intermittent maintenance doses. Factor IX concentrates also contain high levels of prothrombin (factor II), factor VII, factor X, protein C, and protein S. A number of factor IX concentrates are available and each is associated with different potential risks including hepatitis, HIV, thromboembolic disease, and DIC. Newer, more purified concentrates are available that eliminate many of the risks previously associated with factor IX concentrates.

The amount of factor IX that needs to be transfused is based on the finding that one unit of factor IX infused per kilogram of body weight yields a 1% rise in the plasma IX level. For example, 25 U/kg would result in a 25% factor IX level. A 70-kg patient would, therefore, require 1750 U if a 25% factor IX was the goal of therapy.

Factor IX has a half-life of 18 to 24 hours and replacement factor IX should be administered every 12 to 24 hours using specific factor IX assays as a guideline. For mild bleeding, a factor IX level of 20 to 25% is adequate. For major bleeding, a 40 to 50% factor IX level is effective. A life-threatening bleed should be treated such that factor IX levels are maintained in the 60 to 80% range. Prior to surgery, the factor IX level should be at least 50% for several hours and should be maintained at this level for 7 to 10 days.

Factor IX inhibitors usually seen in patients with severe hemophilia B can be treated by higher than normal doses of factor IX concentrates. A hematologist should be consulted prior to ordering factor IX concentrates.

Factor X

Factor X is a vitamin K–dependent protein synthesized by the liver. The incidence of hereditary deficiency of factor X is estimated to be 1 in 500,000. Acquired factor X deficiency is associated with warfarin ingestion, vitamin K deficiency, and liver disease; it is characterized by deficiencies of other vitamin K–dependent factors. Factor X deficiency has been associated with amyloidosis and is the consequence of factor X absorption to extracellular amyloid.

The half-life of factor X is about 40 hours, and fresh frozen plasma is generally the product of choice for treating patients with hemorrhage or in preparation for surgery in those patients without vitamin K deficiency. Factor X levels of 10 to 15% generally provide adequate hemostasis; hence plasma can be administered at an initial dose of 15 to 20 mL/kg of body weight followed by 3 to 6 mL/kg of body weight every 12 to 24 hours until adequate hemostasis is achieved.

Factor IX concentrates that contain factor X have also been used successfully but are not the front-line product of choice.

Factor XI

Hereditary factor XI deficiency occurs in highest incidence in Ashkenazi Jews but rarely in non-Jewish populations. Factor XI is synthesized by the liver and acquired deficiencies are associated with inhibitor antibodies or severe liver disease. Factor XI has a long half-life of about 80 hours.

Patients with factor XI deficiency usually bleed after trauma. Prior reports have suggested that occasional patients with factor XI deficiency will not bleed after surgery. However, it is generally recommended that all patients with factor XI levels less than 20% of normal be treated with fresh frozen plasma to raise the factor XI level to 30 to 40% of normal. Plasma can be administered as a loading dose of 15 to 20 mL/kg of body weight followed by 3 to 6 mL/kg of body weight every 12 hours until hemostasis is achieved.

Factor XII, Prekallikrein, High-Molecular-Weight Kininogen

These three genetic protein deficiencies are not associated with bleeding despite prolonged activated partial thromboplastin times. Hence, no specific factor replacement is required for any of these genetic disorders.

Factor XIII

Genetic factor XIII deficiency is a rare disorder, while acquired factor XIII deficiency is secondary to the presence of inhibitor antibodies most commonly associated with isoniazid antituberculosis therapy. Severe genetic factor XIII deficiency is associated with umbilical stump bleeding in the neonatal period and with intracranial hemorrhage with little or no trauma. Bleeding associated with trauma may be of a delayed nature.

Factor XIII has a long half-life of 9 days, and prophylactic transfusions with fresh frozen plasma are often given every 4 to 6 weeks to prevent intracranial hemorrhage.

Von Willebrand Disease

Von Willebrand disease (vWD) is a group of clinically and genetically heterogeneous inherited hemorrhagic disorders arising from defects in the von Willebrand factor (vWF) protein.[15] Von Willebrand factor is a large multimeric plasma glycoprotein that plays a critical role in primary hemostasis by acting as an adhesive bridge between platelets and damaged subendothelium at the site of vascular injury. It also mediates platelet–platelet interactions for formation of platelet plugs. Additionally, vWF acts as a carrier protein for factor VIII, delivering it to sites of adherent platelets, a function essential for clot formation within damaged endothelium. Finally, vWF stabilizes factor VIII protecting it from premature activation by activated factor X or inactivation by activated protein C.

Eight-five percent of circulating vWF is synthesized in endothelial cells and stored predominantly in high-molecular-weight form in Weibel–Palade bodies before secretion into the plasma. Fifteen percent of circulating vWF is produced in megakaryocytes and stored predominantly in low-molecular-weight form in platelet alpha granules before secretion into the plasma.

It has been estimated that vWD occurs in 0.8 to 1.6% of the general population. Although more than 20 subtypes of vWD have been recognized to date, the current classification of vWD has been revised to include three types and four subtypes. Variants of vWD are classified on the basis of partial deficiencies of vWF (type 1), qualitative defects (types 2A, 2B, 2M, 2N), and complete absence of vWF (type 3).

The laboratory evaluation vWD makes use of specialized assays because the results of routine screening tests for suspected vWD (bleeding time, aPTT) are often insensitive for detecting mild or variant forms of vWD. Specific diagnostic tests include the following:[16]

1. vWF activity. Ristocetin cofactor activity (vWF:RCoF) measures vWF function and is the single most sensitive and specific assay for vWD. Measurements of vWF activity may be affected by physiologic variables that increase vWF activity (pregnancy, oral contraceptives, ABO blood group, liver disease) or decrease vWF activity (hypothyroidism).

2. vWF antigen (vWF:Ag) can be quantitated by radioimmunoassay, immunoradiometric assay, or enzyme-linked immunosorbent assay. Blood type significantly affects the normal vWF antigen level, with type AB plasma having up to twice the vWF antigen as type O plasma. vWF is an acute-phase reactant and levels will be increased during pregnancy, by oral contraceptives, by inflammatory diseases, and by chronic infections. Hypothyroidism reduces vWF antigen levels.

3. Factor VIII activity (factor VIII:C) is variably decreased in most patients with vWD but is often normal in mild disease.

4. vWF multimer analysis can detect qualitative defects of vWF very accurately and may provide some information regarding its quantity. This test is performed using sodium dodecylsulfate (SDS) agarose gel electrophoresis and measures the size distribution of plasma vWF.

5. Three highly specialized tests—the ristocetin-induced platelet agglutination (RIPA) assay, the cryoprecipitate-induced platelet agglutination assay, and gene-based diagnosis—are used to test for vWD variants with abnormal platelet function. Characteristic features of various types of vWD are shown in Table 17-1.

The goals of therapy for vWD are to prevent spontaneous bleeding, accelerate hemostasis, and prevent postoperative bleeding using one of two options:[17]

1. Administration of DDAVP to stimulate the release of endogenous vWF and factor VIII from tissue storage sites.

2. Administration of virus-inactivated, intermediate purity factor VIII concentrates rich in vWF (Humate-P, Koate-HS, Alphanate), or cryoprecipitate.

TABLE 17-1. MAJOR SUBTYPES OF VON WILLEBRAND DISEASE

	Type 1	Type 2A	Type 2B	Type 2M	Type 2N	Type 3	Platelet-Type (Pseudo-vWD)
Factor VIII:C	Decreased or normal	Decreased or normal	Decreased	Decreased or normal	Decreased	Decreased	Decreased or normal
vWF:Ag	Decreased	Decreased	Decreased	Decreased	Normal	Absent	Decreased
vWF:RCoF	Decreased	Decreased	Decreased	Decreased	Normal	Absent	Decreased
RIPA	Decreased	Decreased	Increased	Decreased	Normal	Decreased	Increased
Plasma multimeric pattern	All multimers present	Large and intermediate multimers absent	Large multimers absent	All multimers present	All multimers present	All multimers absent	Large multimers absent
Platelet count	Normal	Normal	Normal or decreased	Normal	Normal	Normal	Normal or decreased

Key: RCoF, ristocetin cofactor activity; RIPA, ristocetin-induced platelet agglutination.

Treatment strategies for patients with vWD are summarized in Table 17-2. If DDAVP is to be used as primary therapy, the patient should be given a challenge with this drug 1 to 2 weeks prior to surgery to assess responsiveness. On the day of surgery, DDAVP should be given about 45 to 60 minutes before surgery at a dose of 0.3 µg/kg body weight as a 30-minute infusion in 50 mL normal saline and once every 12 to 24 hours thereafter for three to four doses. Tachyphylaxis often occurs at this time as pre-existing stores of vWF become depleted. Factor VIII concentrates or cryoprecipitate should be available in the event that DDAVP fails to control bleeding.

Cryoprecipitate is a plasma fraction containing factor VIII, vWF, and fibrinogen. The full range of vWD multimers is present in cryoprecipitate. Humate-P, Koate-HS, and Alphanate are virus-inactivated intermediate purity factor VIII concentrates reported to contain all the vWF multimers. These are the preferred sources for factor VIII and vWF replacement, rather than cryoprecipitate, which, although richer in high-molecular-weight vWF multimers, is not routinely subjected to virucidal treatment. A typical dose of a factor VIII concentrate is factor VIII 50 U/kg body weight every 12 hours; a typical dose of cryoprecipitate is one bag per 10 kg body weight every 12 hours.

Acquired Disorders of Hemostasis
Vitamin K Deficiency

Vitamin K is an essential cofactor for the enzymatic reaction in which the glutamic acid residues on the amino terminal end of coagulation factors II (prothrombin), VII, IX, and X are converted into gamma-carboxyglutamic acid residues.[18] The gamma-carboxyglutamic acid residues confer metal binding properties on these four proteins, a property necessary for normal hemostasis to occur.

The primary source of vitamin K in humans appears to be dietary (for example, green leafy vegetables are a good source of vitamin K_1). Human intestinal bacteria synthesize vitamin K_2. Vitamin K is absorbed in the ileum in the presence of bile salts.

In the absence of dietary vitamin K, bacteria in the large intestine produce vitamin K, and passive absorption of these forms of vitamin K prevent significant vitamin K deficiency. If intestinal bacteria are destroyed by antibiotics, patients with inadequate dietary intake will become vitamin K–deficient within 1 to 3 weeks. Malabsorption syndromes from primary hepatobiliary or intestinal diseases are often associated with vitamin K deficiency.

Vitamin K in its reduced (hydroquinone) form serves as a cofactor for the enzyme that catalyzes the gamma-carboxylation reaction described earlier. In this reaction, vitamin K is

TABLE 17-2.   TREATMENT STRATEGIES IN VON WILLEBRAND DISEASE

vWD variant	Primary Therapy	Secondary Therapy
Type 1	DDAVP[a]	Factor VIII concentrate
Type 2A	DDAVP	Factor VIII concentrate
Type 2B	DDAVP in selected patients	Factor VIII concentrate cryoprecipitate
Type 2M	DDAVP	Factor VIII concentrate cryoprecipitate
Type 2N	Factor VIII concentrate	
Type 3	Factor VIII concentrate	
Platelet-type (pseudo-vWD)	Platelet transfusions	

[a]DDAVP, desmopressin; 1-deamino-8-D-arginine vasopressin.

converted to an epoxide. Warfarin and related compounds completely inhibit two enzymes (vitamin K epoxide reductase, vitamin K reductase) that are critical for conversion of vitamin K epoxide back to its hydroquinone form. This process leads to the depletion of the reduced form of vitamin K and limits the gamma-carboxylation of the vitamin K–dependent clotting factors. In addition, vitamin K antagonists limit the carboxylation of the regulatory proteins (proteins C and S) and as a result impair the function of these anticoagulant proteins.

Except in the case of life-threatening bleeding or major warfarin overdosage, reversal of vitamin K deficiency should be by the administration of vitamin K_1 (Aquamephyton).[19] The anticoagulant effect of warfarin can be overcome by low doses of vitamin K_1 because this vitamin can be reduced to its hydroquinone form through a warfarin-resistant vitamin K reductase enzyme system. Different empiric approaches have been proposed for treating patients with high INR values when rapid reversal is required. Vitamin K_1 can be given subcutaneously in a dose of 2 to 3 mg with the expectation that a demonstrable reduction of the INR will occur at 6 hours. If the INR remains high, an additional dose of vitamin, can be repeated, and the INR rechecked again in 6 hours. Some physicians prefer the use of slow intravenous infusions of vitamin K_1 because of its more predictable absorption. If the intravenous route is utilized, vitamin K_1 should be diluted and administered over 20 to 30 minutes to minimize the risk of an anaphylactic reaction.

In cases of life-threatening bleeding or serious warfarin overdosage, vitamin K_1 in a dose of 10 mg subcutaneously or intravenously should be administered and supplemented with fresh frozen plasma, a source of all the vitamin K–dependent proteins.

Heparin

Heparin is a glycosaminoglycan that, when administered parenterally, binds immediately to the plasma protein antithrombin producing a conformational change that converts the antithrombin molecule from a relatively slow inhibitor of coagulation enzymes into a very rapid inhibitor.[20] Antithrombin covalently binds to the active serine center of the coagulation enzyme, after which heparin dissociates from the ternary complex to be reutilized. The heparin-antithrombin complex inhibits factors IIa (thrombin), Xa, IXa, XIa, and XIIa. Of these coagulation enzymes, factors IIa and Xa are most responsive to inhibition by the heparin-antithrombin complex. Heparin also binds to platelets and can inhibit platelet aggregation. These properties of heparin allow it to be used for the prevention and treatment of thromboembolic disease.

Heparin can be associated with serious side effects including immune thrombocytopenia and seemingly paradoxical arterial and venous thromboemboli.[21] Thrombocytopenia without thrombosis is known as heparin-induced thrombosis type I (HIT type I), while thrombocytopenia with thrombosis is known as HIT type II. HIT type I rarely poses a threat to affected patients, but HIT type II is associated with DVT, pulmonary embolism, cerebral thrombosis, myocardial infarction, and ischemic injury to the legs and arms, producing severe morbidity and mortality. It is standard medical practice to monitor platelet counts in patients receiving heparin for any extended period.

The frequency of unfractionated heparin–induced thrombocytopenia is uncertain, but if a platelet count of 100,000/μL is used to define thrombocytopenia, bovine-derived heparin is associated with an approximate 5% incidence and porcine-derived heparin with an approximate 1% incidence of thrombocytopenia. Newer low-molecular-weight heparins (LMWHs) have been associated with thrombocytopenia, but the incidence appears to be much lower than with unfractionated heparin. Thrombocytopenia usually begins 3 to 15 days after the initiation of heparin, but it can develop within hours in patients previously exposed to the drug.

Even small doses of heparin used to maintain catheter patency may trigger thrombocytopenia. Typically, the platelet nadir in heparin-induced thrombocytopenia is between 20,000 and 150,000/μL. The finding of heparin-associated platelet antibodies confirms the diagnosis, but a negative result does not rule out the condition.

Mild thrombocytopenia alone is not a reason to discontinue heparin. However, with a fall of the platelet count to below 100,000/μL from a normal baseline, one should give strong consideration to stopping heparin as soon as is feasible. The platelet count should be monitored at least once daily, and if the platelet count drops below 50,000/μL or if arterial thrombi develop at any platelet level, heparin should be discontinued immediately. With the discontinuation of heparin, the platelet count reverts to baseline levels within 1 week.

Heparin-induced thrombosis is associated with a high morbidity and mortality and is almost always associated with a fall in the platelet count to thrombocytopenic levels. Treatment includes prompt discontinuation of heparin and avoidance of platelet transfusions. The factor Xa inhibitor danaparoid (a heparinoid) or the thrombin inhibitor lepirudin (the anticoagulant found in leeches) can be used safely to anticoagulate patients with HIT, and can prevent further damage from thrombosis in patients with HIT type 2.[22] Unproven treatments include antiplatelet agents, LMWHs, dextran, and warfarin. Clinicians should not assume that LMWHs can be used safely in patients who have heparin-induced thrombocytopenia, since LMWHs appear fully capable of promoting platelet activation by most antibodies associated with unfractionated heparin-induced thrombocytopenia.

Disseminated Intravascular Coagulation (DIC)

Disseminated intravascular coagulation is a pathophysiologic state characterized by abnormal activation of coagulation and fibrinolysis. The normal regulatory mechanisms that control physiologic coagulation and fibrinolysis break down for a variety of reasons. Multiple inciting causes of DIC have been identified, including tissue injury, cancer, infections, cardiovascular disease, obstetric disorders, immunologic phenomena, pulmonary disease, hepatic disease, neurologic disease, drugs, snake bites, and insect bites.

No single test is diagnostic of DIC. In general, DIC can be recognized in the laboratory by significantly elevated fibrin degradation products and by depletion of platelets and clotting factors. Screening tests include measurements of FSP or D-dimers, PT, aPTT, fibrinogen, and the platelet count. Serial measurements are important, as pre-existing diseases may be associated with hyperfibrinogenemia and thrombocytosis. A fall in either of these measurements early in DIC may lead to a normal laboratory value. A peripheral blood smear should be examined, but findings of thrombocytopenia or red cell fragmentation are not diagnostic of DIC.

Levels of most clotting factors drop in DIC, although factor VIII levels often increase transiently. Accelerated fibrinolysis can be recognized by measurements of antithrombin, plasminogen, and alpha$_2$-antiplasmin activity. Low levels of alpha$_2$-antiplasmin and falling levels of antithrombin and plasminogen suggest hyperfibrinolysis.

Successful treatment of DIC is highly dependent on recognizing and treating the underlying disease process triggering DIC. Additional efforts need to be made to provide for circulatory stability and adequate oxygenation. Clotting factors and inhibitors can be replaced by giving fresh frozen plasma, using the PT as a guide for adequate replacement. Cryoprecipitate is an excellent source of fibrinogen and is indicated when the fibrinogen level is less than 100 mg/dL. Random donor platelets are transfused prophylactically for platelet counts less than 15,000 to 20,000/μL and for platelet counts less than 50,000/μL in the setting of hemorrhage. Vitamin K and folic acid should be given empirically.

The use of heparin and antifibrinolytic drugs in DIC is highly controversial. The three well-defined conditions in which heparin appears to be of benefit are purpura fulminans, acute promyelocytic leukemia, and carcinomas associated with chronic DIC.

Liver Disease

The coagulopathy of advanced liver disease is complex in origin and may mimic the laboratory findings of DIC. Coagulation abnormalities may result from decreased synthesis of coagulation proteins, dietary vitamin K deficiency, malabsorption leading to vitamin K deficiency, dysfibrinogenemia, enhanced fibrinolysis due to decreased synthesis of alpha$_2$-antiplasmin (the major inhibitor of plasmin) and thrombocytopenia secondary to hypersplenism, coincident folic acid and vitamin B$_{12}$ deficiency, or concomitant alcohol-induced bone marrow suppression.

Therapy is directed at replacing deficient vitamins and using, when appropriate, fresh frozen plasma, cryoprecipitate, random donor platelet concentrates, or a mixture of these. DDAVP has no proven role in treating the coagulopathy of liver disease, and factor IX concentrates are contraindicated.

Chronic Renal Failure

The clinical significance of bleeding in chronic renal failure is difficult to assess by laboratory testing. The primary hemostatic abnormality in uremia is thought to be a defect in platelet function.[23] Laboratory testing has focused on both abnormal platelet aggregation and a prolonged bleeding time. Platelet aggregation studies are frequently abnormal in uremic patients but do not correlate well with the degree of renal failure or with the occurrence of bleeding. The bleeding time has been reported to correlate with the risk of bleeding in uremic patients, but even this has been questioned.

Anemia in chronic renal failure is an independent cause of a prolonged bleeding time. The prolonged bleeding time noted in renal failure can be corrected in part by either transfusions with packed red cells or by the administration of recombinant erythropoietin. In addition, abnormal platelet function contributes to the prolonged bleeding time of patients with chronic renal failure. Multiple functional platelet defects have been described by various laboratories.

The prolonged bleeding time and abnormal platelet aggregation studies noted commonly in uremic patients do not reliably predict an increased risk of hemorrhage and hence are not an indication for transfusional therapy or for therapeutic intervention per se. A careful medical history and physical examination are paramount in assessing the potential risk for bleeding in conjunction with appropriate clotting tests. If bleeding complicates a surgical procedure in a uremic patient, a prolonged bleeding time can be corrected with DDAVP or with packed red cells. DDAVP is administered intravenously over 30 minutes at a dose of 0.3 μg/kg of body weight. DDAVP in this setting may shorten the bleeding time for about 4 hours on average. DDAVP stimulates the release of von Willebrand factor from endothelial cells, and platelets, and this may be the mechanism of the shortened bleeding time.

The effectiveness of DDAVP in preventing bleeding at surgery in uremic patients has never been studied in a prospective randomized, double-blind clinical trial. Retrospective data suggest a low incidence of bleeding at the time of surgery in uremic patients who have not received specific treatment previously.

Packed red cells should be reserved for clinically significant problems and not for correction of laboratory abnormalities. Packed red cells can transmit viral infections and are associated with other potential serious side effects.

References

1. Rappaport SI. Blood coagulation and its alterations in hemorrhagic and thrombotic disorders. *West J Med* 158:153–161, 1993.
2. Wong VK, Robertson R, Nagaoka G, et al. Pseudothrombocytopenia in a child with the acquired immunodeficiency syndrome. *West J Med* 157:1603, 1992.
3. Nichols WL, Bowie EJW. Standardization of the prothrombin time for monitoring orally administered anticoagulant therapy with use of the international normalized ratio system. *Mayo Clin Proc* 68:897, 1993.
4. Suchman AL, Griner PF. Diagnostic uses of the activated partial thromboplastin time and prothrombin time. *Ann Intern Med* 104:810, 1986.
5. Raschke RA, Reilly BM, Guidry JR, et al. The weight based heparin dosing nomogram compared with a "standard care" nomogram. *Ann Intern Med* 119: 874, 1993.
6. Lind SE. The bleeding time does not predict surgical bleeding. *Blood* 77:2547, 1991.
7. Yu M, Nardella A, Pechet L. Screening tests of disseminated intravascular coagulation: guidelines for rapid and specific laboratory diagnosis. *Crit Care Med* 28:1777, 2000.
8. Triplett DA, Barna LK, Unger GA. A hexagonal (II) phase phospholipid neutralization assay for lupus anticoagulant identification. *Thromb Haemost* 70:787, 1993.
9. Slichter SJ. Platelet transfusion therapy. *Hematol Oncol Clin North Am* 4:291, 1990.
10. Heckman KD, Weiner GJ, Davis CS, et al. Randomized study of prophylactic platelet transfusion threshold during induction therapy for adult acute leukemia: 10,000/μL versus 20,000/μL. *J Clin Oncol* 15:1142, 1997.
11. McIntyre KJ, Hoagland HC, Silverstein MN, Petitt RM. Essential thrombocythemia in young adults. *Mayo Clin Proc* 66:149, 1991.
12. Mitus AJ, Schafer AI. Thrombocytosis and thrombocytopenia. *Hematol Oncol Clin North Am* 4:157, 1990.
13. Mannucci PM. Desmopressin: A nontransfusional form of treatment for congenital and acquired bleeding disorders. *Blood* 5:1449, 1988.
14. Furie B, Furie BC. Molecular basis of hemophilia. *Semin Hematol* 27:270, 1990.
15. Ginsburg D, Bowie EJW. Molecular genetics of von Willebrand disease. *Blood* 10:2507, 1992.
16. Triplett DM. Laboratory diagnosis of von Willebrand's disease. *Mayo Clin Proc* 66:832, 1991.
17. Aledort LM. Treatment of von Willebrand's disease. *Mayo Clin Proc* 66:841, 1991.
18. Furie B, Furie BC. Molecular basis of vitamin K-dependent carboxylation. *Blood* 9:1753, 1990.
19. Hirsh J, Dalen JE, Deykin D, et al. Oral anticoagulants. Mechanism of action, clinical effectiveness and optimal therapeutic range. *Chest* 108(4 Suppl):231S, 1995.
20. Hirsh J, Rashcke R, Warkentin TE, et al. Heparin: Mechanism of action, pharmacokinetics, dosing, considerations, monitoring, efficacy and safety. *Chest* 108 (4 Suppl):258S, 1995.
21. Aster RH. Heparin-induced thrombocytopenia and thrombosis. *N Engl J Med* 332:1374, 1995.
22. Farner B, Eichler P, Kroll H, et al. A comparison of danaparoid and lepirudin in heparin-induced thrombocytopenia. *Thromb Haemost* 85:950, 2001.
23. Carvalho AC. Acquired platelet dysfunction in patients with uremia. *Hematol Oncol Clin North Am* 4:129, 1990.

Bibliography

Colman RW, Hirsh J, Marder VJ, et al. *Hemostasis and Thrombosis. Basic Principles and Clinical Practice,* 4th ed. Philadelphia: Lippincott, 2000.

Hoffman R, Benz EJ, Shattil SJ, et al. *Hematology. Basic Principles and Practice,* 3rd ed. New York: Churchill Livingstone, 2000.

Chemotherapy of Head and Neck Cancer

18

In the United States, approximately 40,000 new cases of head and neck cancer are diagnosed each year, and 11,500 patients per year die of these lesions. Of these cancers, 60% are locally advanced (stages III and IV), and the vast majority are squamous cell carcinoma (SCC) when diagnosed. The survival rate for this group of patients, even when the cancer is resectable, is only 10 to 60%, depending on tumor site and stage. Even when cured, these patients face a 3 to 7% risk of a second primary tumor in each year of follow-up.[1]

Because of their tendency toward localized spread and progression, as well as their propensity to recur loco-regionally, squamous cell carcinomas of the head and neck (SCCHN) have traditionally been treated by the oncologic surgeon and the radiation oncologist. But as local treatment modalities have been pushed to their limits and their results remain suboptimal for patients with stage III or IV disease, a coordinated oncologic team approach has become essential for optimal patient management and the hope of improvement in the long-term outcome. While the surgical and radiation oncologist is trained to respond to the primary location and extent of the tumor as well as lymphatic metastatic pathways, the medical oncologist tends to see these tumors in their advanced state with similar epidemiology, histology, and drug sensitivity.

Failure in SCCHN almost always means loco-regional recurrence. A loco-regional cure will continue to be the objective in any treatment protocol for SCCHN. Chemotherapy must impact this objective if it is to play an essential role in the management of these tumors. As systemic treatment modalities have become more sophisticated and successful, especially in malignancies where death is related more to systemic than primary failure, local primary treatment may be de-emphasized (eg, breast cancer). In patients with SCCHN, the primary objective must be to attain loco-regional cure before the control of distant micrometastatic disease can become paramount.

The need to improve the overall outcome for patients with advanced SCCHN, as well as the desire to reduce the morbidity of ablative surgery have led to the incorporation of chemotherapy into the traditional interventions with surgery and radiation (Table 18-1).

PATHOLOGY

Basic pathologic determinants influence the stage of the tumor at presentation and its pre- and posttreatment patterns of spread and recurrence. Pathologists grade SCCHN into well-, moderately, and poorly differentiated cancers by the amount of keratinization seen microscopically. Nuclear size and percentage of mitosis coupled with host inflammatory response and pattern of border spread (infiltrating versus pushing) help to further demarcate these tumors pathologically and are predictors of clinical outcome. The grading parameters influence primary management considerations.

TABLE 18-1.   OBJECTIVES OF CHEMOTHERAPY IN HEAD AND NECK CANCER

Act as an adjunct to primary radiation and surgical treatment
Increase loco-regional control and cure
Decrease bulky tumor
Decrease morbidity of ablative surgery
Treat radiation resistant tumor cells
Increase tumor cell sensitivity to radiation
Treat distant metastatic disease
Not compromise surgical or radiation treatment
Improve overall cure rate

Molecular and oncogenetic targets and pathways of carcinogenesis are being rapidly clarified and provide powerful prognostic probes and potential therapeutic targets. Cytogenetic abnormalities are often detectable in SCCHN, more often in chromosomes 1, 9, and 11. Mutations in the p53 tumor suppression gene are present in over 50% of SCCHN. P53 protein inhibits DNA synthesis inducing apoptosis and mutations in the p53 gene predict a poorer prognosis and reduced chemotherapy sensitivity.[2] The use of "gene therapy" to introduce normal p53 genes by way of intratumoral delivery with an adenoviral vector may provide a novel treatment approach.[3] Vascular endothelial growth factor (VEGF) is a promoter of angiogenesis and thus cancer cell growth and spread. In SCCHN, VEGF expression is present in 40% of cases and predicts local recurrence and poor survival.[4] Epithelial growth factor receptor (EGFR) tyrosine kinases are involved in cell growth by signal transduction pathways, which are being targeted with novel molecules and monoclonal antibodies.[3] Ras, an intracellular growth regulator, is mutated in 25% of SCCHN. Ras functions through the enzyme farnesyl transferase (FT) inhibitors, which are being developed to target this signaling pathway.[3]

Nasopharyngeal cancers presenting with lymphoepithelial histology represent a unique clinico-pathologic entity. Epstein-Barr virus infection predisposes to the development of these tumors, which, because of their enhanced radio- and chemotherapy responsiveness have a better outcome than SCCHN, which comprise the bulk of head and neck cancers and are to be discussed in this chapter.

RATIONALE FOR CHEMOTHERAPY IN HEAD AND NECK CANCERS

It has long been known that local factors, such as the location and size of the tumor, as well as the extent of tissue invasion and lymph node spread, greatly influence the outcome of treatment for patients with SCCHN. The prognostically reliable tumor/lymph node metastasis (TNM) staging system incorporates the clinical variables. The surgical specialist of head and neck cancer understands the regional lymph node anatomy and drainage patterns that allow him or her to surgically cure a high percentage of patients with low-stage lesions. When tumors present at a more advanced stage (III or IV), are biologically more aggressive, or both, these surgical approaches are less successful.

Despite its loco-regional spread, SCCHN is known to be influenced by systemic factors. Smoking and heavy alcohol use not only predispose to the development of SCCHN but also influence the general health of the patient. Overall treatment outcome is then impacted because the patient's ability to withstand aggressive treatment is limited. Nutritional factors resulting in weight loss, vitamin deficiency, and immune incompetence have a significant impact on the outcome of therapy. Comorbid disease, such as emphysema or cirrhosis, impacts the ability to deliver definitive therapies and their outcome. Attention to the general health of the patient, nutritional repletion, and treatment of comorbid illness will all have an impact on the outcome of the treatments for SCCHN. When necessary, a tracheostomy and/or a feeding jejunostomy will need to be placed prior to the initiation of definitive treatment.

Chemotherapeutic agents that are delivered systemically are capable of acting locally to reduce tumor size, promote sensitivity to radiation, and reduce the extent of surgery. At the same time, they offer the potential of treating distant micrometastatic disease. Agents that are capable of enhancing or reconstituting the immune system may also act as adjuncts to traditional primary treatments.

With an improved understanding of head and neck carcinogenesis, systemic agents (eg, retinoids) may have the ability to impede the development of SCC, reduce the incidence of a second tumor, and perhaps reduce the propensity toward the recurrence of a cancer that has been brought into a complete remission with primary therapy.[5,6]

Systemic chemotherapy can result in impressive tumor responses in a fraction of our patients with recurrent or metastatic SCCHN. The percentage and extent of these responses is increased when chemotherapy is administered prior to other therapies. Despite impressive results, the overall impact of chemotherapy on SCCHN outcome is still limited.[7] The challenge remains of how to optimally incorporate chemotherapeutic agents into the primary treatment strategy for patients with stage III or IV cancer in order to translate objective response into improved overall cure (Table 18-2).

SINGLE-AGENT CHEMOTHERAPY

The traditional approach to define the activity and use of a chemotherapeutic agent in treating a malignant disease is to test its activity as a single agent in patients suffering from advanced stages of the cancer. Once activity has been demonstrated, patients can be treated with varying dosages of the drug and in a variety of treatment schedules to maximize response. The route and schedule of administration may also be varied. Finally, the timing of the treatment with other therapies and in combination with other drugs may be important to the response and overall effectiveness of the treatment. Chemotherapy administered concurrently with radiation as a radiosensitizer will have to be modified in dose and schedule.

Methotrexate

Methotrexate is an antimetabolite that interferes with folic acid metabolism by tightly binding the enzyme dihydrofolate reductase. It is effective by mouth, but it is usually given by intravenous weekly injection at a standard dose of 40 to 60 mg/m². Methotrexate has traditionally been the single-agent drug of choice for palliation in treating patients with recurrent or metastatic disease. Ten to 20% of patients will respond to this therapy, sometimes dramatically. For maximal response, the dose must be accelerated within the patient's tolerance. The dose-limiting toxicity is usually mucositis, especially in patients who have been previously treated with irradiation. Because methotrexate is excreted through the kidneys,

TABLE 18-2. VARIABLES IN CHEMOTHERAPY TREATMENT

Chemotherapeutic drug dosage
Treatment schedule
Route of administration
Combination with other chemotherapeutic agents
Timing with other non-chemotherapy treatments

its toxicity is markedly accentuated by alterations in renal function. Patients receiving stable weekly injections of methotrexate can develop severe toxicity if renal function changes and therefore must be closely monitored. Methotrexate plasma half-life can be prolonged by leaching from third space fluid (pleural and ascitic), thus causing unacceptable toxicity.

Methotrexate can be administered with relative safety in moderately high (500 mg/m^2) or very high (5000 mg/m^2) doses with the use of the vitamin leucovorin to rescue normal cells from the effects of the drug. There is no clear therapeutic advantage, however, to administering methotrexate in high doses to patients with SCCHN. A number of analogs of methotrexate have been used in clinical trials in an attempt to improve therapeutic efficacy or decrease toxicity, but thus far an antifol more effective than methotrexate has not been found.

5-Fluorouracil (5-FU)

5-FU is a fluoropyrimidine antimetabolite whose activated form (FdUMP) poisons cells by binding the enzyme thymidylate synthetase. It exerts a 10 to 15% single-agent activity against recurrent and metastatic head and neck cancer.[5] The relatively low single-agent activity is improved when the drug is administered by continuous intravenous infusion (eg, 600–1000 mg/m^2/day × 4 days).[8] It is generally well tolerated when given by intravenous weekly injection (400–600 mg/m^2). Its greatest toxicity is on the gastrointestinal tract, especially in causing in-field mucositis in patients previously treated or undergoing active treatment with radiation. The drug sensitizes cancer cells to the toxic effects of x-irradiation. The activity of 5-FU can be enhanced by the administration of leucovorin or interferon-alpha-2b or hydroxyurea.[9] The dose of 5-FU may have to be attenuated when it is used with leucovorin so as to avoid mucositis.

Leucovorin (Tetrahydrolic Acid)

Leucovorin is a metabolite of folic acid. It is active distal to the block in folic acid metabolism exerted by methotrexate. Leucovorin can rescue cells from the toxic effects of methotrexate even when the drug remains in the circulatory system. Leucovorin can thus be used as an antidote to methotrexate toxicity. High-dose methotrexate therapy exposes cells for 24 to 36 hours to the toxic effects of the drug in levels not attainable in conventional dosing. The addition of leucovorin (in appropriate dose and schedule) competitively overcomes the metabolic blockade and can prevent subsequent toxicity. In some tumors, this improves the therapeutic activity of methotrexate.

Leucovorin can also affect intracellular pools of deoxyuridine monophosphate (dUMP). By this mechanism it can enhance the cytotoxic effects of 5-FU.[9] 5-FU toxicity can also be enhanced (especially mucositis), which can be dose-limiting when combined with radiation.

Bleomycin

Bleomycin is an antitumor antibiotic that induces breaks in DNA. It has single-agent activity of 10 to 20% in treating SCCHN and can enhance the activity of radiation on cancer cells. It has the distinct advantage, especially when used in combination with other drugs, of causing little bone marrow toxicity. Its dose-limiting toxicity is that of mucositis, especially in patients previously irradiated or undergoing simultaneous radiation treatment. It is administered by weekly intravenous or intramuscular injection (10 U/m^2) or continuous intravenous infusion (15 U/day × 4 days). Bleomycin can cause severe lung toxicity, especially in patients with antecedent lung disease. Although related to cumulative total drug dose (250 to 450 mg/m^2), pulmonary fibrosis can be quite unpredictable even with the use of pulmonary function tests with diffusing capacity.

Mitomycin-C

Mitomycin-C is also an antitumor antibiotic that crosslinks DNA. Although it exerts little single-agent activity in SCCHN, it is a radiosensitizer and is active against hypoxic cells.[9] Hypoxic cells are two to three times less sensitive than oxygenated cells to radiation.[7] This is especially a factor in bulky tumors, and this limits their radiocurability. Mitomycin-C has been used simultaneously with radiation in an attempt to exploit these properties and improve the local response.[10]

Mitomycin-C is administered by brief intravenous infusion at a dose of 10 to 15 mg/m^2 every 4 to 6 weeks. Mitomycin-C is a strong vesicant and can cause tissue damage at intravenous infusion sites even in the hands of the most experienced practitioner. This drug has a strong, delayed, and cumulative effect on the bone marrow, especially causing prolonged thrombocytopenia. Blood counts must be closely monitored.

Hydroxyurea

Hydroxyurea is an orally effective antimetabolite that inhibits ribonucleotide reductase. Although it has low single-agent activity, it can modulate the effectiveness of 5-FU by depleting cellular pools of dUMP, potentially increasing tumor responses.[11] It also has the ability to act as a radiation enhancer and is being used in experimental treatment protocols combining 5-FU and hydroxyurea with radiation therapy.[11,12] Hydroxyurea is given by mouth at a dose of 500 to 1000 mg/m^2 one to two times daily. The drug can cause a moderate amount of nausea as well as some mucositis, but bone marrow depression is dose-limiting.

Platin Compounds

Cisplatin exhibits high single-agent activity against SCCHN (20 to 30%). The drug is a heavy metal that acts as an alkylating agent, binding both DNA and RNA. It is excreted through the kidneys, where it can cause significant toxicity. Cisplatin administration results in severe nausea and vomiting, which can be ameliorated with the use of strong antiemetics, such as steroids, serotonin antagonists, or metoclopramide and sedatives. Creatinine clearance must be monitored throughout treatment, and the drug given only to patients with clearance greater than 70 mL/min. In order to prevent nephrotoxicity, the drug must be administered following initial hydration with posttreatment diuresis of 4 to 6 hours. It is administered by standard 80 to 100 mg/m^2 infusion every 3 to 4 weeks but can be given in smaller doses (eg, 20 to 50 mg/m^2) weekly or by 24-hour infusion, where it may produce maximal radiosensitization.

Carboplatin is a cisplatin analog administered with no risk of nephrotoxicity. Because of this and its reduced tendency to cause nausea and vomiting, carboplatin can be administered in the outpatient setting. The drug, however, causes severe bone marrow suppression, which is dose-limiting. It has less single-agent activity than cisplatin.

Platin drugs act as radiation enhancers and have the distinct advantage of not significantly increasing the infield mucositis of radiation treatment. They are also associated with cumulative neurotoxicity. Platin treatment is continuing to be investigated in a variety of schedules in combination with radiation therapy.

Vinca Alkaloids

The vinca alkaloids, which damage intracellular microtubules, also have a limited single-agent activity in SCCHN. Vincristine, while not inducing bone marrow suppression, causes neurotoxicity with repeated injections. Because of its lack of bone marrow suppression, vincristine has been used in combination with other drugs that have hematologic toxicity. Vinblastine has more bone marrow and less neurotoxicity. These drugs are usually administered by weekly intravenous injection.

Taxanes

Taxoids are a family of compounds with a taxane skeleton. Taxane compounds promote microtubular assembly and stability and exert their cytotoxicity by preventing microtubular depolymerization thereby inhibiting the normal dynamic reorganization of microtubular networks.[13] The first taxoid was extracted from the bark of Pacific Yew tree and became available in 1992 as paclitaxel (Taxol). Docetaxel (Taxotere) is a semisynthetic extract of yew tree needles.

Taxoids major toxicity is dose-dependent neutropenia occurring 7 to 10 days after administration. Alopecia is almost universal. Patients experience cumulative neurotoxicity with repeated dosing, which can be exacerbated by the use of other drugs that cause neurotoxicity. Oral mucositis and myalgias as well as hypersensitivity reactions at the onset of intravenous infusions must also be watched for (pretreatment with steroids, antihistamines and H-2 blockers).

Taxoids appear to exert a high overall response rate (~40%) when used alone[13] and can be effective in patients previously refractory to cisplatin.[5] Because of their high rate of activity and differing site of cytotoxicity, taxoids (especially docetaxel) are being incorporated into regimens containing 5-FU and cisplatin.

Paclitaxel as a radiation cell sensitizer may be most effective when given by a continuous intravenous infusion.[14–16]

Biologic Response Modifiers

Although biologic response modifiers have demonstrated some but limited single-agent activity in SCCHN,[6,17] they could still prove to have some role to play in conjunction with x-irradiation. Interferons (IFNs) modulate 5-FU antimetabolite activity and have thus been integrated with infusional 5-FU and cisplatin in an attempt to increase the activity of this regimen. IFNs may play a role in decreasing field carcinogenesis.[6] Interleukin-2 has a greater toxicity profile[18] that requires intensive support throughout therapy, but it has a potential for response even in resistant tumors[18] and an ability to increase cytotoxic tumor infiltrating lymphocytes.[19] Cytokines (eg, G-CSF and GM-CSF) have demonstrated an ability to ameliorate myelosuppression and will probably play a role in reducing toxicity and enhancing results in some combination protocols.[16]

Gemcitabine

Gemcitabine is a deoxycytidine analog antimetabolite which has proven to have clinically useful antitumor activity in a variety of carcinomas, including SCCHN. Its incorporation into DNA interferes with DNA synthesis and polymerization and makes it a potent radiosensitizer. Its major toxicity is myelosuppression when given on a weekly intravenous dose schedule (1000 mg/m^2) but it does not cause mucositis. In nonmyelotoxic or noncytotoxic doses, it radiosensitizes tumor cells but appears to sensitize normal mucosa as well and cause unacceptable mucositis and deep ulcerations.[20] A better dose and schedule may permit use of this promising drug in the future.

Signal Transduction Inhibitors

These are a new class of anticancer agents which have been developed as a direct result of increased understanding of normal cellular and cancer subcellular biology. Signal transduction pathways are important targets for anticancer drugs. By interrupting signaling pathways, which are essential for normal cellular metabolism, tumor cell survival is also markedly suppressed.

Epidermal growth factor receptor (EGFR) is part of a family of transmembrane receptor tyrosine kinase (RTK) molecules which promote growth factor-induced mitogenic proliferation of cells. Anti-EGFR antibody cetuximab (C225) is a murine monoclonal antibody that binds EGFR and is being combined with radiation and chemotherapy in an effort to improve the potency and specificity of these treatments.[21] Fever and chills, skin rash, and hepatitis develop as a manifestation of protein allergic reactions.

Hypoxic Cell Sensitizers

Since many SCCHN contain necrotic centers with hypoxic cells at a distance from capillary oxygen sources, the ability of external beam radiation to kill these cells is limited. In addition to the radiosensitizing chemotherapeutic agents already mentioned, the correction of anemia as well as hyperbaric oxygenation have been used to reduce hypoxia during treatment of these patients.[22] The use of recombinant erythropoietin prior to the initiation of radiation to correct anemia or even to induce relative polycythemia may be an avenue of future investigation. Perfluorocarbon chemicals have been used in these patients to exploit their ability to alter the oxygen affinity of hemoglobin.[22] Tirapazamine (a new agent active as a hypoxic cell sensitizer) is being used alone or in combination with cisplatin concurrently with radiation and does not enhance normal tissue radiation toxicity.[23]

Radioprotective Agents

Radiation therapy toxicity in SCCHN is manifested most commonly as acute mucositis and acute and chronic xerostomia. These toxicities are generally enhanced by radiosensitizing agents and chemotherapy drugs which themselves cause mucositis. Thiol-containing compounds exhibit radioprotection by scavenging for radiation-induced free radicals. By accumulating in epithelial tissue and salivary glands and the kidneys, amifostine can protect tissues from infield radiation toxicities, especially xerostomia without protecting tumor cells or reducing treatment efficacy.[24] The drug must be given intravenously 15 to 30 minutes prior to radiation by intravenous infusion at a dose of 200 mg/m^2 and thus significantly complicates standard treatment. It can cause nausea and vomiting and allergic reactions.

Chemopreventive Agents

Retinoids are natural and synthetic analogs of vitamin A that play a role in the suppression of epithelial carcinogenesis.[5] The epidemiology of SCC of the aerodigestive system has identified alcohol and tobacco use as independent and additive risk factors. These carcinogens affect the entire epithelial lining of the aerodigestive system and place the patient previously treated for SCCHN at an annual risk of 3 to 7% for a second primary tumor.[1] Retinoids can modulate the growth and differentiation of normal and malignant epithelial cells in culture. Carotenoids are a family of compounds, one of which, beta-carotene, is a naturally occurring substance and are precursors of vitamin A. Beta-carotene and synthetic retinoids can produce objective responses in the premalignant process of leukoplakia. Beta-carotene is less toxic, but synthetic retinoids (13-cis-retinoic acid, isotretinoin) produce a greater effect.[25] Trials are ongoing to incorporate retinoids as adjuvant treatment of primary disease and chemoprevention of second primary tumors, but to date no consistent positive results or treatment recommendations have emerged.

Refer to Table 18-3 for a summary of single-agent drug therapy.

TABLE 18-3. SINGLE-AGENT DRUG THERAPY

Drug	Class	Response	Route				Dose	Combination	Sensitizer
			PO	IM SC	IV Push	Infusion			
Methotrexate	Antimetabolite	10–20%	+	–	+	–	40–60 mg/m^2 IV/wk	Yes	No
5-Fluorouracil	Antimetabolite	10–15%	–	–	+	+	600 mg/m^2 IV/wk; 800–1000 mg/m^2/d 5 d q 3 wk	Yes	Yes
Leucovorin	Vitamin	0	+	–	+	+	40–400 mg/m^2	Yes	No
Bleomycin	Antitumor antibiotic	10–20%	–	+	+	+	10 U/m^2 IV/wk; 15 U/day × 4 q 3–4 wk	Yes	Yes
Cisplatin	Heavy metal	20–30%	–	–	+	+	80–100 mg/m^2 IV q 3–4 wk	Yes	Yes
Carboplatin	Heavy metal	15–20%	–	–	+	+	300 mg/m^2 IV q 3–4 wk	Yes	Yes
Mitomycin-C	Antitumor antibiotic	5%	–	–	+	–	10–12 mg/m^2 q 4–6 wk	No	Yes
Hydroxyurea	Antimetabolite	5–10%	+	–	–	–	500–1000 mg/m^2 PO 1 d	Yes	Yes
Vincristine	Vinca-alkaloid	10%	–	–	+	–	1 mg/m^2 IV/wk	Yes	No
Vinblastine	Vinca-alkaloid	10%	–	–	+	–	4–5 mg/m^2 IV q wk	Yes	No
Paclitaxel	Antimicrotubule	40%	–	–	–	+	175–250 mg/m^2 over 4 h q 3–4 wk	?	Yes
Interferon	Biologic response modifier	5–10%	–	+	–	–	5×10^6 IM qd	Yes	No
Interleukin-2	Biologic response modifier	10–20%	–	–	–	+	3×10^6/m^2 qd × 4 d q 3–4 wk	Yes	No
β-Carotene	Retinoid	0	+	–	–	–	30–90 mg/day	Yes	Yes
Isotretinoin	Retinoid	0	+	–	–	–	1–2 mg/kg/day	Yes	No
Amifostine	Radioprotective	0	–	–	+	+	200 mg/m^2 qd with radiation	Yes	No
Gemcitabine	Antimetabolite	10%	–	–	–	+	50–300 mg/m^2 weekly	–	Yes
Cetuximab (C225)	Monoclonal antibody	0	–	–	–	+	100–400 mg/m^2 weekly × 4	Yes	Yes

Drug	Toxicity (1–4+)									
	N + V	Mucositis	Bone Marrow	Alopecia	Heart	Lung	Kidney	Nerve	Vesicant	Other
Methotrexate	1+	4+	2+	1+	–	1+	1+	–	–	Watch renal function
5-Fluorouracil	1+	3+	2+	1+	–	–	–	–	–	Rescue MTX; 5-FU toxicity
Leucovorin	–	–	–	–	–	–	–	–	–	
Bleomycin	1+	4+	–	–	–	4+	–	–	–	Fever within 24-h of injection
Cisplatin	4+	–	3+	2+	–	–	4+	3+	–	
Carboplatin	3+	–	4+	2+	–	–	–	3+	–	
Mitomycin-C	1+	–	4+	–	–	1+	2+	–	–	
Hydroxyurea in 24 h of injection	2+	1+	3+	1+	–	–	–	–	–	Jaw pain within 24 h of injection
Vincristine	–	–	–	3+	–	–	–	4+	3+	
Vinblastine	2+	–	4+	3+	–	–	–	2+	3+	
Paclitaxel	4+	–	4+	4+	1+	–	–	3+	–	Hypersensitivity nonallergic reactions
Interferon	1+	–	2+	1+	–	–	2+	–	–	Capillary leak syndrome
Interleukin-2	2+	–	2+	1+	2+	3+	2+	3+	–	Fevers, malaise, myalgias
β-Carotene	1+	–	–	–	–	–	–	1+	–	Yellowing skin
Isotretinoin	1+	–	–	–	–	–	–	1+	–	Cheilitis, conjunctivitis, dermatitis, hypertriglyceridemia
Amifostine	1+	–	–	–	–	–	–	–	–	Hypotension, allergic reactions
Gemcitabine	+	–	3+	1+	–	–	–	–	–	Enhances mucositis with radiation
Cetuximab (C225)	1+	–	–	–	–	–	–	–	–	Fever + chills, rash, transaminase

COMBINATION CHEMOTHERAPY

After single-agent activity has been demonstrated, the next logical step has been to combine the active agents to obtain additive or even synergistic results. When chemotherapeutic agents have overlapping toxicities, their doses must be lowered when used together. However, when the toxicities do not overlap, the agents may often be used in full strength in combination. Using effective agents with toxicities that do not overlap has been the strategy behind most drug combinations.

In SCCHN, significantly improved response rates are attainable with combination chemotherapy over single-agent chemotherapy.[26] These improved responses have not yet translated into improved survival of patients either with advanced recurrent or metastatic disease. Improved responses and especially improved percentages of complete responses are, however, a prerequisite for advances in the treatment of these cancers. These improved results are translating into prolonged survival in patients with locally advanced, unresectable cancers when chemotherapy is given in conjunction with radiotherapy.[5,27]

Cisplatin and 5-FU

Since cisplatin does not cause mucositis, it can be administered in combination with 5-FU given in continuous infusion without significantly altering the maximally tolerated dose of either drug. Bone marrow toxicity is additive but generally manageable; it can be countered with the use of G-CSF. Response rates of over 30% of patients with recurrent or metastatic disease and 60 to 80% in previously untreated patients are seen with this combination.[28] However, the treatment must generally be given in hospital (cisplatin 80 to 100 mg/m², 5-FU 800 to 1000 mg/m²/day × 4 days every 3 weeks), and it is expensive. In comparison with single-agent methotrexate, responses are three times higher, but response duration and median survival have not been clearly improved.

Cisplatin, 5-FU, and Leucovorin

Because leucovorin improves the therapeutic efficacy of 5-FU, it is being added to the drug combination.[9,12,29–37] This combination looks to exploit drug synergism (5-FU, leucovorin), improved pharmacokinetics of infusional cisplatin, and dose intensity to push for maximal results. Significant variables in these programs include the cisplatin infusion dose (75–125 mg/m² for 4 to 5 days), the 5-FU infusion dose (500–1000 mg/m² × 5 to 6 days) and the amount of leucovorin (100–500 mg/m² × 5 to 6 days). This combination is very toxic and requires hospitalization for a reliable, generally younger patient with minimal comorbid disease. Hospitalization for complications of therapy is high (20 to 30%), and patient deaths from toxic complications (2 to 10%) are anticipated. Approximately 40% of patients will develop grade III/IV mucositis and 60% grade III/IV neutropenia. Often second and third cycles cannot be given or are administered in attenuated doses.

But results are impressive: 30 to 50% complete responses and 80 to 90% complete and partial responses. In addition, this regimen has reduced the development of distant metastatic disease.[29–31]

Cisplatin, 5-FU, and Taxoids

Taxanes have high single-agent response rates[32,33] are logical drugs to incorporate into previously successful treatment combinations. This is especially true because of the unique mechanism of action and additive effect with cisplatin.[35] But overlapping toxicities, especially neutropenia, will present dose limitations and serious toxicity.[37,38] Docetaxel is given at a dose of 50 to 80 mg/m^2 for 1 to 4 hours infusion prior to the other drugs. Results of these regimens are encouraging, with 25 to 65% complete and 75 to 100% complete and partial responses.[33–40] Although the best way to use the taxanes in chemotherapy combination has yet to be defined, they should improve the results of prior regimens in the neoadjuvant setting as well as possibly in concomitant chemoradiotherapy and adjuvant applications.

Paclitaxel alone by weekly (30 mg/m^2), 3-weekly (75 mg/m^2), or continuous infusion (5–10 mg/m^2/day) may be more tolerable when given concurrently with radiation.[14,15]

APPLICATIONS OF CHEMOTHERAPY

Chemotherapy is the standard treatment for recurrent or metastatic SCCHN but is only of limited benefit. The integration of chemotherapy into surgical and radiation therapy treatments is being pursued with initial, concurrent, and adjunctive timing patterns. The optimal combinations, treatment sequences, and drug administration schedules have yet to be determined. Increasingly, however, concurrent chemoradiation therapy is becoming standard for patients with unresectable SCCHN and for organ preservation in laryngeal cancer.[41–43]

When analyzing reports on the use of combined modality therapy, the reader must bear in mind a number of variables which can have bearing on treatment outcome. Patient selection including age, performance status, comorbid illness and reliability as well as tumor stage, location and histology can markedly influence results. The timing of chemotherapy (including pre-, post-, or concurrent) with radiotherapy must be considered. The drug(s) selection and dose as well as administration schedule can all influence outcome, toxicity, and practicality. Finally, the total dose, dose-intensity, and administration schedule of radiation will impact outcome and tolerance. All of these variables are mixed up in the literature and make comparisons difficult. Some conclusions can be drawn from this quagmire and are reviewed below, but the overall impact of chemotherapy for SCCHN in meta-analysis remains marginal.[7]

Chemotherapy of Locally Recurrent or Metastatic Disease

Patients who have previously undergone definitive local management and have failed to respond or those who have developed locally recurrent or metastatic disease have traditionally been considered for a trial of systemic chemotherapy. This treatment is of a palliative nature only. It is capable of inducing tumor regression at the locally recurrent site or in a distant metastatic location. Overall response rates range from 20 to 40%, but the duration of these responses—when they occur—is measured in weeks, with a significant clinical advantage for only a small percentage of the patients.

When treating these patients, one must keep in mind the frequent accompaniment of hypercalcemia due to the production of a parathyroid-like hormone by these tumors. In addition, when the cancer involves the spine (usually causing pain), one must be aware of the risk of spinal cord compression, which is generally treated with radiation therapy.

Methotrexate, when administered by weekly intravenous injection at a dose of 40 mg/m^2, is generally well tolerated, but repeated injections tend to induce mucositis, and one must be aware of and monitor kidney function. Cisplatin by single-agent infusion, usually given every 3 weeks, has a higher response rate but results in a greater toxicity. The combination of 5-FU with cisplatin is as effective a regimen for recurrent or metastatic disease as is presently available, but it will only induce an overall response of about 6 months duration in about one-third of the patients. Docetaxel should also be considered in these patients and may be useful in patients who are cisplatin failures.[14]

Induction Chemotherapy

Induction chemotherapy refers to the use of systemic treatment at the outset, prior to intervention with either surgery or radiation therapy. Patients are often debilitated following initial surgical and radiation treatment. Tumor vascularity is adversely affected by antecedent radiation, thereby limiting drug penetration and concentration. It was, therefore, anticipated that responses in patients to chemotherapy at the outset would be higher than those seen in patients with recurrent disease. It had also been anticipated that patients responding to initial chemotherapy could require less and have more successful surgical treatment, as well as more effective radiation for disease rendered less bulky.

For medical oncologists who have been used to treating chronically ill patients SCCHN with recurrent disease, the responses seen to neoadjuvant chemotherapy have been dramatic and gratifying. Sixty to 90 percent of the patients show tumor regression and 20 to 40% show a complete response.[29–38,44–48] These responses have been documented in the primary site and are also seen, though less frequently, in metastatic lymph nodes at the time of surgical removal or rebiopsy.

Induction chemotherapy has been most frequently used and for which there is the most experience is the use of 5-FU by continuous infusion in conjunction with cisplatin. Those patients who achieve a complete response with upfront chemotherapy identify patients who do well with subsequent radiation therapy.[48]

The initial exciting results of these treatments, however, have been tempered because of the only small improvement in overall patient survival in patients treated with induction chemotherapy.[7] This has led to the conclusion that a response to chemotherapy is simply selecting a more favorable group of patients who would have responded to conventional therapy alone. Randomized studies in large groups of patients have, however, begun to demonstrate a survival advantage to neoadjuvant chemotherapy.[27] Longer follow-up may demonstrate survival advantages for more aggressive induction regimens. New induction protocols can and are being continuously tested and developed.

The results of these trials have demonstrated several important principles. Chemotherapeutic agents have been shown to induce responses, including complete responses, against SCCHN in a high percentage of patients when administered prior to radiation therapy. Induction chemotherapy has not adversely affected subsequent surgical or radiation therapy results nor has it increased complications. Response to chemotherapy predicts a response to radiation; complete responders have a predictably longer survival. Nonresponders may be candidates for more intensive chemoradiation therapy.[39] Finally, the frequency of distant metastases as a cause of treatment failure has been reduced in many of the neoadjuvant trials.[40] This important finding implies that the more effective the local treatment is for bulky SCCHN, the more likely treatment failure will result from metastatic disease. This in turn, will increase the role and importance of systemic therapy in any treatment protocol.

Chemoradiation Therapy

Although induction chemotherapy has not resulted in markedly improved survival of patients with locally advanced SCCHN, there have been hopeful trends seen from this approach, and meta-analysis has shown a small but definitive increase in overall survival.[7,49,50] These findings have led investigators to use chemotherapy simultaneously with radiation therapy treatments in an effort to maximize the benefits of both. The concurrent use of chemotherapy and radiation therapy offers the potential for improving the overall results of x-irradiation, the single modality capable of curing patients with advanced SCCHN. This approach aims to exploit the high response rate of previously untreated patients to chemotherapy as well as to improve the therapeutic advantage of external beam radiation by using chemotherapeutic agents that sensitize malignant cells to radiation. Systemic chemotherapy will also simultaneously reach micrometastatic disease when it is present.

Chemotherapeutic agents may be more effective against cell populations that are also relatively radioresistant.[9] Mitomycin-C has shown activity against hypoxic cells,[22] while antimetabolite drugs are most effective against cells that are actively cycling; both of these cell populations are more resistant to external beam irradiation.[9] At the same time, these drugs can increase the radiosensitivity of radiation-responsive cells. The challenge of these protocols is to incorporate effective drug treatment schedules concurrent with radiation without unacceptable degrees of toxicity that can result in potentially harmful delays in radiation treatment.

One of the major difficulties with chemoradiotherapy is infield mucositis. The problem is seen with 5-FU, methotrexate, bleomycin, taxanes, and gemcitabine. Cisplatin does not produce overlapping mucous membrane toxicity but does induce radiation enhancement against tumor cells. As the single agent with the highest activity against SCCHN, it is an ideal drug to incorporate into chemoradiotherapy protocols.[51] The addition of other drugs to cisplatin such as 5-FU, taxanes or newer signal transducer inhibitors to radiation offers the hope of higher response rates, especially in poorer- prognosis tumors.[39,52,53] The difficulty is to maintain these aggressive treatments with "acceptable" degrees of toxicity without compromising radiation dosing and treatment schedules at the same time. By paying attention to the patient's nutritional status (where necessary, providing alternate means of enteral alimentation), as well as being familiar with and aware of the toxicities and safe methods of administering the drugs, toxicity can be reduced and managed. Radiochemotherapy has emerged as the standard of care for SCCHN in the oropharynx and hypopharynx.[17,31,54–56]

Chemoradiation with the Goal of Organ Preservation

The functional, psychologic, and cosmetic deficits produced by ablative surgery on SCCHN are considerable. By using combinations of induction chemotherapy or concurrent chemotherapy and radiation (chemoradiation), better overall responses and survivals are being obtained, frequently with less debilitating or disfiguring surgery. The traditional paradigm of initial surgery followed by adjuvant radiation is being displaced by chemoradiation followed, if necessary, by surgery for stage III and IV disease. It must be stressed that the goal of these therapies is still improved overall cure and secondarily preservation of organ function.

In no site has this approach been as well studied as in the larynx and hypopharynx. Laryngeal carcinomas overall do better than other SCCHN, and the goal of speech preservation is a high priority. Trials have suggested that surgery is avoidable without compromising the chance of cure in patients treated with combination chemoradiation.[57–59] As clinical trials have matured, an evolving pattern has been towards improved results with chemoradiation over induction chemotherapy or radiotherapy alone. The Intergroup Trial R91-11 randomized patients with larynx and supraglottal larynx tumors to radiation alone, induction chemotherapy with cisplatin/5-FU or chemoradiotherapy with cisplatin.[59] Larynx preservation was achieved at 2 years in 68% of patients in the chemoradiotherapy arm and 58% with induction chemotherapy versus 53% with radiation alone. Distant metastases occurred in 15% of patients treated with radiation alone versus 7% of the patients in the two chemotherapy arms.

Other Radiation and Chemotherapy Combinations

As has already been discussed, chemotherapy can be employed prior to or concurrently with radiation. Traditional adjuvant chemotherapy may also have a role if the goal of loco-regional cure has been achieved by primary treatment and the patient, therefore, becomes at greater risk for metastatic disease. In an effort to reduce the toxicity of concurrent therapy, radiation, and chemotherapy have been administered sequentially. This approach may reduce nonmalignant tissue toxicity and enhance patient tolerance. Although the sequential approach has shown promise[46] and overall survival equivalent to concurrent therapy, relapse-free survival appears better in patients treated concurrently with radiation and chemotherapy.[47–51]

CONCLUSIONS

Despite the natural history of SCCHN for loco-regional spread and recurrence, the majority present in advanced stages and are not cured with conventional surgical and radiation therapy approaches. The addition of systemic therapy to reduce the bulk of tumor, enhance the effectiveness of radiation, modify the morbidity of surgery, attack micrometastatic disease, and improve overall cure makes logical sense. Some of these goals have been attained and much knowledge and experience gained in the last decade. Physicians caring for these patients have seen improved results with combined modality therapy and longer follow-up has confirmed these impressions. We can now say that combined modality therapy should be considered the standard for patients with unresectable SCCHN.

Although the standard use of systemic chemotherapy for locally recurrent or metastatic SCCHN has resulted in only small overall clinical improvement of these patients, it has led to the investigation and improved understanding of the actions of these drugs and their interactions with each other and with radiation. Significant improvement in tumor responses have been realized with better combinations applied earlier in the disease. Although impacting survival rates only slightly at present, the incorporation of chemical agents into the combination treatment protocol of the stage III or IV SCCHN patients remains the most rational approach.

Tolerable and reasonably effective chemotherapy programs are available to patients with SCCHN. Significant and frequent responses are seen in patients with recurrent or metastatic disease, and these are more frequent and dramatic in patients previously untreated. Why, then, is cure not achieved in a higher percentage of patients treated with chemoradiotherapy or sequential therapy, or both? Why are the results of adjuvant chemotherapy achievable in breast cancer not realized in SCCHN, or the favorable and organ-preserving results of chemoradiotherapy in SCC of the anus[60] not achievable in SCCHN? The answer must lie in the basic biology of the tumor. As more efforts and trials are directed toward the treatment of this cancer, more favorable results will be forthcoming.

As radiation therapists and radiobiologists become more knowledgeable in the dose and scheduling of radiation treatments, the simultaneous use of systemic agents (in conjunction with improved supportive care) has already resulted in a better outlook for SCCHN patients. A better understanding of the molecular biology of these cancers is also translating into more specific molecular targets for treatment as further adjuncts to their surgical, radiotherapeutic, and chemotherapeutic treatments. Better and more tolerable chemoprotective agents should also become available. Finally, better patient and population education of the causes and lifestyle alterations necessary to the prevention of these malignancies may reduce their overall incidence.

References

1. Vokes EE, Weichselbaum RR, Lippman SM, Hong WK. Head and neck cancer. *N Engl J Med* 328:184–193,1993.
2. Temam S, Flahault A, Périé S, et al. p53 gene status as a predictor of tumor response to induction chemotherapy in patients with locoregionally advanced squamous cell carcinomas of the head and neck. *J Clin Oncol* 18:385–394, 2000.
3. Khuri FR, Kim ES. Molecularly targeted strategies for the treatment of upper aerodigestive tract cancers. In Perry MC, ed. *American Society of Clinical Oncology Educational Book.* Alexandria, VA, 2001, 347–358.
4. Smith BD, Smith GL, Carter D, et al. Prognostic significance of vascular endothelial growth factor protein levels in oral and oropharyngeal squamous cell carcinoma. *J Clin Oncol* 18: 2046–2052, 2000.
5. Hong WK, Lippman SM, Itri LM, et al. Prevention of second primary tumor with isotretinoin in squamous cell carcinoma. *N Engl J Med* 323:795–801,1990.
6. Shin DM, Khuri FR, Murphy B, et al. Combined interferon-alfa, 13-*cis*-retinoic acid, and alpha-tocopherol in locally advanced head and neck squamous cell carcinoma: novel bioadjuvant phase II trial. *J Clin Oncol* 19:3010–3017, 2001.
7. Pignon JP, Bourhis J, Domenge C, *et al.* Chemotherapy added to locoregional treatment for head and neck squamous-cell carcinoma: three meta-analyses of updated individual data. MACH-NH Collaborative Group. Meta-Analysis of Chemotherapy on Head and Neck Cancer. *Lancet* 355:949–955, 2000.
8. Vokes EE, Schilsky RL, Weichselbaum RR, et al. Induction chemotherapy with cisplatin, fluorouracil and high-dose leucovorin for locally advanced head and neck cancer. *Clin Pharmacol. Anal. J Clin Oncol* 8:241–247,1990.
9. Vokes EE, Weichselbaum RR. Chemoradiotherapy for head and neck cancer. *Prin Pract Oncol* 1933;7(PPO Updates):1–12.
10. Weissberg JB, Son YH, Papac RJ, et al. Randomized clinical trial of mitomycin C as an adjunct to radiotherapy in head and neck cancer. *Int J Radiat Oncol Biol Phys* 17:3–9,1989.
11. Vokes EE, Kies MS, Haraf D, et al. Concomitant chemoradiotherapy as primary therapy for locoregionally advanced head and neck cancer. *J Clin Oncol* 18:1652–1661, 2000.
12. Vokes EE. Interactions of chemotherapy and radiation. *Semin Oncol* 20:70,1993.
13. Cortes JE, Pagdur R. Docetaxel. *J Clin Oncol.* 13:2643–2655,1995.
14. Sunwoo JB, Herscher LL, Kroog GS, *et al.* Concurrent paclitaxel and radiation in the treatment of locally advanced head and neck cancer. *J Clin Oncol* 19:800–811, 2001.
15. Rosenthal DI, Lee JH, Sinard R, et al. Phase I study of paclitaxel given by seven-week continuous infusion concurrent with radiation therapy for locally advanced squamous cell carcinoma of the head and neck. *J Clin Oncol* 19: 1363–1373, 2001.
16. Forastiere AA, Leong T, Rowinsky E, et al. Phase III comparison of high-dose paclitaxel + cisplatin + granulocyte colony-stimulating factor versus low-dose paclitaxel + cisplatin in advanced head and neck cancer: Eastern Cooperative Oncology Group Study #1393. *J Clin Oncol* 19:1088–1095, 2001.
17. Schantz SP, Dimery I, Lipman SM, et al. A phase II study of interleukin-2 and interferon-alpha in head and neck cancer. *Invest New Drugs* 10:217–223,1992.
18. Valone FH, Gandara DR, Deisseroth AB, *et al.* Interleukin-2, cisplatin, and 5-fluorouracil for patients with nonsmall cell lung and head/neck carcinomas. *J Immunother* 10:207–213,1991.
19. Vokes EE, Ratain MJ, Mick R, et al. Cisplatin, fluorouracil and leucovorin augmented by interferon alfa-2b in head and neck cancer. A clinical and pharmacologic analysis. *J Clin Oncol* 11:360–368,1993.
20. Eisbruch A, Shewach DS, Bradford CR, et al. Radiation concurrent with gemcitabine for locally advanced head and neck cancer: a phase I trial and intracellular drug incorporation study. *J Clin Oncol* 19:792–799, 2001.
21. Robert F, Ezekiel MP, Spencer SA, et al. Anti-epidermal growth factor receptor antibody Cetuximab (C255) in combination with radiation therapy in patients with advanced head and neck cancer. *Cancer Invest* 19(Suppl 1):45–47, 2001.
22. Beard CJ, Coleman CM. current therapeutic strategies toward hypoxic tumor cells. *Prin Pract Oncol Updates* ;5:1,1991.
23. Harari PM. Integration of novel biologic approaches combined with radiation in the treat-

ment of head and neck cancer. In Perry MC, ed. *American Society of Clinical Oncology Educational Book.* Alexandria, VA, 2001, 342–346.

24. Brizel DM, Wasserman TH, Henke M, et al. Phase III randomized trial of amifostine as a radioprotector in head and neck cancer. *J Clin Oncol* 18:3339–3345, 2000.

25. Lippman S, Batsakis JG, Toth BB, et al. Comparison of low dose isotretinoin with beta carotene to prevent oral carcinogenesis. *N Engl J Med* 328:15–20,1993.

26. Jacobs C, Lyman G, Velez-Garcia E, et al. Induction chemotherapy in advanced head and neck tumors: results of two randomized trials. *Int J Radiat Oncol Biol Phys* 23:483–489,1992.

27. Pfister DG, Strong E, Harrison L, et al. Larynx preservation with combined chemotherapy and radiation therapy in advanced but resectable head and neck cancer. *J Clin Oncol* 9: 850–859,1991.

28. Forastiere AA, Metch B, Schuller CE, et al. Randomized comparison of cisplatin plus fluorouracil and carboplatin plus fluorouracil versus methotrexate in advanced squamous cell carcinoma of the head and neck: A Southwest Oncology Group study. *J Clin Oncol* 10: 1245–1251,1992.

29. Laramore GE, Scott CB, Al-Sarraf M, et al. Adjuvant chemotherapy for resectable squamous cell carcinomas of the head and neck: report on intergroup study 0034. *Int J Radiat Oncol Biol Phys* 23:705–713,1992.

30. Jaulberry C, Rodrigues J, Brunin F, et al. Induction chemotherapy in advanced head and neck tumors: results of two randomized trials. *Int J Radiat Oncol Biol Phys* 23:483–489,1992.

31. Papadimitrakopoulou V, Dimery I, Lee J, et al. Cisplatin, fluorouracil, and I-leucovorin induction therapy for locally advanced head and neck cancer; the MD Anderson Cancer Center experience. *Cancer J Sci Am* 3:92–99,1997.

32. Forastiere A, Neuberg D, Taylor SIV, et al. Phase II evaluation of Taxol in advanced head and neck cancer: an Eastern Cooperative Oncology Group trial. *Monogr Natl Cancer Inst* 15:181–184,1993.

33. Dreyfuss A, Clark J, Norris C, et al. Taxotere for advanced, inoperable squamous cell carcinoma of the head and neck (abstract). *Proc ASCO* 13:931,1994.

34. Schneider M, Etienne M, Milano G, et al. Phase II trial of cisplatin, fluorouracil, and pure folinic acid for locally advanced head and neck cancer: a pharmacokinetic and clinical survey. *J Clin Oncol* 13:1656–1662,1995.

35. Schöffski P, Wanders J, Catimel G, et al for the EORTC Early Clinical Trials Group. Docetaxel and cisplatin: A highly active regimen for squamous cell carcinoma of the head and neck. *Proc Am Soc Clin Oncol* 16:402A; AB:1436,1997.

36. Clark J, Busse P, Norris C, et al. Long term results of induction chemotherapy with cisplatin, 5-FU and high dose leucovorin (PFL) for squamous cell carcinoma of the head and neck (SC-CHN) (abstract). *Proc ASCO* 15:317,1996.

37. Janinis J, Papadakou M, Panagos G, et al. A phase II study of combined chemotherapy with docetaxel, cisplatin and 5-fluorouracil (5-FU) in patients with advanced squamous cell carcinoma of the head and neck (SCCHN) and nasopharyngeal carcinoma (NC). *Proc Am Soc Clin Oncol* 15:310; AB:871,1996.

38. Posner M, Norris C, Colevas A, et al. Phase I/II trial of docetaxel, cisplatin, 5-fluorouracil and leucovorin (TPFL) for curable, locally advanced squamous cell cancer of the head and neck (SCCHN). *Proc Am Soc Clin Oncol* 16: 387A; AB:1380,1997.

39. Posner MR, Glisson B, Frenette G. Multicenter phase I–II trial of docetaxel, cisplatin, and fluorouracil induction chemotherapy for patients with locally advanced squamous cell cancer of the head and neck. *J Clin Oncol* 19: 1096–1104, 2001.

40. Tischler R, Colevas AD, Norris CM, et al. A phase I/II trial of concurrent docetaxel (T) and once daily radiation following induction chemotherapy in squamous cell cancer of the head and neck. Program and abstracts of the 37th Annual Meeting of the American Society of Clinical Oncology; May 12–15, 2001, San Francisco, California. Abstract 930.

41. Wendt TG, Grabenbauer GG, Rödel CM, et al. Simultaneous radiochemotherapy versus radiotherapy alone in advanced head and neck cancer: a randomized multicenter study. *J Clin Oncol* 16:1318–1324,1998.

42. Wanebo HJ, Chougule P, Ready N, et al. Preoperative paclitaxel, carboplatin, and radiation therapy in advanced head and neck cancer

(stage III and IV). *Semin Radiat Oncol* 9 (2 Suppl 1):77–84,1999.

43. Forastiere AA, Berkey B, Maor M, et al. Phase III trial to preserve the larynx: induction chemotherapy and radiotherapy versus concomitant chemoradiotherapy versus radiotherapy alone, Intergroup Trial R91-11. Program and abstracts of the 37th Annual Meeting of the American Society of Clinical Oncology; May 12–15, 2001; San Francisco, California, Abstract 4.

44. Merlano M, Benasso M, Corvo R, et al. Five-year update of a randomized trial of alternating radiotherapy and chemotherapy compared with radiotherapy alone in treatment of unresectable squamous cell carcinomas of the head and neck. *J Natl Cancer Inst* 88:583–589,1996.

45. Head and Neck Contracts Program. Adjuvant chemotherapy for advanced head and neck squamous carcinoma: Final report of the head and neck contracts program. *Cancer* 60: 301–311,1987.

46. Kish J, Drelichman A, Jacobs J, et al. Clinical trial of cisplatin and 5-FU infusion as initial treatment for advanced squamous cell carcinoma of the head and neck. *Cancer Treat Rep* 66: 471–474,1982.

47. Dreyfuss AI, Clark JR, Wright JE, et al. Continuous infusion high-dose leucovorin with 5-fluorouracil and cisplatin for untreated stage IV carcinoma of the head and neck. *Ann Intern Med* 112:167–172,1990.

48. Rooney M, Kish J, Jacobs, J, et al. Improved complete response rate and survival in advanced head and neck cancer after three-course induction therapy with 120-hour 5-FU infusion and cisplatin. *Cancer* 55:1123–1128,1985.

49. El-Sayed S, Nelson N. Adjuvant and adjunctive chemotherapy in the management of squamous cell carcinoma of the head and neck region: A meta-analysis of prospective and randomized trials. *J Clin Oncol* 14:838–847,1996.

50. Munro A. An overview of randomised controlled trials of adjuvant chemotherapy in head and neck cancer. *Br J Cancer* 71:83–91,1995.

51. Al-Sarraf M, Pajak TF, Marcial VA, et al. Concurrent radiotherapy and chemotherapy with cisplatin in inoperable squamous cell carcinoma of the head and neck: an RTOG study. *Cancer* 59:259–265,1987.

52. Gray J, Meluch A, Greco F, et al. Induction paclitaxel/carboplatin/5FU followed by concurrent radiotherapy and weekly paclitaxel/carboplatin for patients with locally advanced head and neck cancer (HNC): a Minnie Pearl Cancer Research Network Trial. Program and abstracts of the 37th Annual Meeting of the American Society of Clinical Oncology; May 12–15, 2001; San Francisco, California. Abstract 900.

53. Urba S., Wolf G, Eisbruch A, et al. One cycle of chemotherapy followed by concurrent chemoradiation for laryngeal preservation. Program and abstracts of the 37th Annual Meeting of the American Society of Clinical Oncology; May 12–15, 2001; San Francisco, California. Abstract 899.

54. Forastiere AA, Trotti A. Radiotherapy and concurrent chemotherapy: a strategy that improves locoregional control and survival in oropharyngeal cancer. *J Natl Cancer Inst* 91: 2065–2066,1999.

55. Brizel DM, Alberts ME, Fisher SR, et al. Hyperfractionated irradiation with or without concurrent chemotherapy for locally advanced head and neck cancer. *N Engl J Med* 338:1798–1804,1998.

56. Calais G, Alfonsi M, Bardet E, et al. Randomized trial of radiation therapy versus concomitant chemoradiotherapy and radiation therapy for advanced-stage oropharynx carcinoma. *J Natl Cancer Inst* 91:2081–2086,1999.

57. Paccagnella A, Orlando A, Marchiori C, et al. Phase III trial of initial chemotherapy in stage III or IV head and neck cancers: a study by the Gruppo di Studio sui Tumori della Testa e del collo. *J Natl Cancer Inst* 86:265–272,1994.

58. Lefebvre J, Chevalier D, Luboinski B, et al. Larynx preservation in pyriform sinus cancer: preliminary results of a European Organization for Research and Treatment of Cancer phase III trial. *J Natl Cancer Inst* 88:890–898,1996.

59. The Department of Veterans Affairs Laryngeal Cancer Study Group. Induction chemotherapy plus radiation compared with surgery plus radiation in patients with advanced laryngeal cancer. *N Engl J Med* 324:1685–1690,1991.

60. Miller EJ, Quan SH, Thaler T. Treatment of squamous cell carcinoma of the anal canal. *Cancer* 67:2038–2041,1991.

The Paranasal Sinuses: Embryology, Anatomy, Endoscopic Diagnosis, and Treatment

19

Endoscopic sinus techniques have evolved from diagnosis, through basic surgery for inflammatory disease, and into approaches for a variety of neoplastic and skull base lesions. Endoscopic approaches are now widely utilized for the management of mucoceles, benign tumors, skull base defects, orbital and optic nerve decompression, and dacryocystorhinostomy as well as adjunctively in the management of some malignancies. The surgery for inflammatory disease itself has also evolved as a result of increasing recognition of the importance of mucoperiosteal preservation and improving knowledge with regard to disease pathogenesis and management. Because of the variability of the anatomy and the critical relationships of the sinuses, endoscopic surgical techniques require a detailed knowledge of the anatomy and embryology as well as the surgical techniques.

Embryology

Traditional Teaching

1. Development heralded by the appearance of a series of ridges or folds on the lateral nasal wall at approximately the eighth week.
2. Six to seven folds emerge initially. Through regression and fusion, three to four ridges ultimately persist.
3. Ridges that persist throughout fetal development and into later life are referred to as "ethmoturbinals." These structures are all considered to be ethmoid in origin.
   a. First ethmoturbinal; rudimentary and incomplete in humans
      (1) Ascending portion forms the agger nasi
      (2) Descending portion forms the uncinate process
   b. Second ethmoturbinal; ultimately forms the middle turbinate
   c. Third ethmoturbinal; forms the superior turbinate
   d. Fourth and fifth ethmoturbinals; fuse to form the supreme turbinate

Furrows form between the ethmoturbinals and ultimately establish the primordial nasal meati and recesses.

1. First furrow (between the first and second ethmoturbinals)

388

    a.   Descending aspect forms the ethmoid infundibulum, hiatus semilunaris, and middle meatus. (The primordial maxillary sinus develops from the inferior aspect of the ethmoid infundibulum).

    b.   Ascending aspect can contribute to the frontal recess.

2.   Second furrow (between the second and third ethmoturbinals)

    a.   Forms the superior meatus.

3.   Third furrow (between the third and fourth ethmoturbinals)

    a.   Forms the supreme meatus.

The *frontal sinus* originates from the anterior pneumatization of the frontal recess into the frontal bone. A series of one to four folds and furrows arise within the ventral and caudal aspect of the middle meatus. Typically,

- The first frontal furrow forms the agger nasi cell.
- The second frontal furrow forms frontal sinus (usually).
- The third and fourth furrows form other anterior ethmoid cells.

The sphenoid sinus:

- During the third month, the nasal mucosa invaginates into the posterior portion of the cartilaginous nasal capsule to form a pouch-like cavity referred to as the cartilaginous cupolar recess of the nasal cavity.
- The wall surrounding this cartilage is ossified in the later months of fetal development and the complex is referred to as the ossiculum Bertini.
- In the second and third years the intervening cartilage is resorbed, and the ossiculum Bertini becomes attached to the body of the sphenoid.
- By the sixth or seventh year, pneumatization progresses.
- By the 12th year, the anterior clinoids and pterygoid process can become pneumatized.
- Sphenoid sinus pneumatization is typically completed between the 9th and 12th years.

Recent Contributions in Sinus Embryology

In addition to the traditional ridge-and-furrow concept of development, a cartilaginous capsule surrounds the developing nasal cavity and plays a role in sinonasal development.

- At 8 weeks, three soft tissue elevations or preturbinates are seen that correlate to the future inferior, middle, and superior turbinates.
- At 9 to 10 weeks, a soft tissue elevation and underlying cartilaginous bud emerges that corresponds to the future uncinate process.
- By 13 to 14 weeks, a space develops lateral to the uncinate anlage which corresponds to the ethmoid infundibulum.
- By 16 weeks, the future maxillary sinus begins to develop from the inferior aspect of the infundibulum. The cartilaginous structures resorb or ossify as development progresses.

All three turbinates and all the paranasal sinuses arise from the cartilaginous nasal capsule. The outpouching of the nasal mucous membranes is thought to be only a secondary phenomenon rather than the primary force in sinonasal development.

Certainly, all is not known about the complex mechanisms involved in sinus development. However, if the practicing otolaryngologist achieves a basic grasp of sinonasal embryology, this will facilitate understanding the complex and variable adult paranasal sinus anatomy encountered in his or her surgical patients.

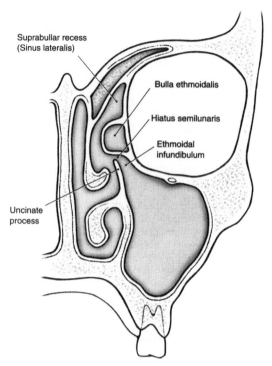

Figure 19-1.   Coronal illustration of the ethmoid sinus anatomy at the level of the maxillary sinus ostium. (*Reproduced with permission from Kennedy DW, Bolger WE, Zinreich SJ, eds.* Diseases of the Sinuses: Diagnosis and Management. *Hamilton, Ontario, Canada: Decker, 2001.*)

Anatomy

The ethmoid sinus is commonly referred to as "the labyrinth" due to its complexity and intersubject variability. In this section, paranasal sinus anatomy is discussed, with special emphasis on the ethmoid sinus and ethmoid structures important in endoscopic sinus surgery (Figure 19-1). The complex ethmoid labyrinth of the adult can be reduced into a series of lamellae based on embryologic precursors. These lamellae are obliquely oriented and lie parallel to each other. They are helpful in maintaining orientation in ethmoid procedures.

- The first lamella is the uncinate process.
- The second lamella corresponds to the ethmoid bulla.
- The third is the basal or ground lamella of the middle turbinate.
- The fourth is the lamella of the superior turbinate.

The basal lamella of the middle turbinate is especially important, as it divides the anterior and posterior ethmoids. The frontal, maxillary, and anterior ethmoids arise from the region of the anterior ethmoid and therefore drain into the middle meatus. The posterior ethmoid cells lie posterior to the basal lamella and therefore drain into the superior and supreme meati, while the sphenoid sinus drains into the sphenoethmoid recess. The lamellae are relatively constant features, which can help the surgeon maintain anatomic orientation when operating within the ethmoid "labyrinth" of the ethmoid sinus.

Agger Nasi
- Mound or prominence on the lateral wall just anterior to the middle turbinate insertion.
- Frequently pneumatized by an agger nasi cell that arises from the superior aspect of infundibulum.
- The agger nasi cell is bordered anteriorly by the frontal process of the maxilla, superiorly by the frontal recess/sinus, anterolaterally by the nasal bones, inferomedially by the uncinate process of the ethmoid bone, and inferolaterally by the lacrimal bone.

Uncinate Process
- Derived from the Latin *uncinatus,* which means hook-like or hook-shaped.
- Approximately 3 to 4 mm wide and 1.5 to 2 cm in length and nearly sagittally oriented. It is best appreciated by viewing a sagittal gross anatomic specimen after reflecting the middle turbinate superiorly.
- Through most of its course, its posterior margin is free and forms the anterior boundary of the hiatus semilunaris.
- The uncinate process forms the medial wall of the ethmoid infundibulum.
- Attaches anteriorly and superiorly to the ethmoid crest of the maxillae. Immediately below this, it fuses with the posterior aspect of the lacrimal bone. The anteroinferior aspect does not have a bony attachment.
- Posteriorly and inferiorly, the uncinate attaches to the ethmoid process of the inferior turbinate bone. At its posterior limit, it gives off a small bony projection to attach to the lamina perpendicularis of the palatine bone.

The superior, middle, and inferior parts of the *uncinate process* are related to three different sinuses:

- Superior aspect most commonly bends laterally to insert on the lamina papyracea. Inferior and lateral to this portion of the uncinate lies the blind superior pouch of the infundibular airspace, the recessus terminalis. Superior and medial to this portion of the uncinate lies, most commonly, the floor of the frontal recess. This portion of the uncinate process is therefore important in frontal recess surgery. Alternatively, the uncinate process may occasionally attach superiorly to the ethmoid roof or even bend medially to attach to the middle turbinate.
- The middle aspect parallels the ethmoid bulla. For this reason, removal of the uncinate is one of the first steps in endoscopic sinus surgery, as this allows surgical access of the ethmoid bulla and deeper ethmoid structures.
- The inferior aspect forms part of the medial wall of the maxillary sinus. The maxillary sinus ostium lies medial and superior to this part. Thus this part must be removed to widen the natural ostium.

Nasal Fontanelles
- They lie immediately anterior (anterior fontanelle) and posterior (posterior fontanelle) to the inferior aspect of the uncinate, where the lateral nasal wall consists only of mucosa.
- The posterior fontanelle is much larger and more distinct than its anterior counterpart.
- The fontanelles (especially posterior) may be perforated, creating an accessory ostium into the maxillary sinus (20–25% of patients). These accessory ostia may be indicators of prior sinus disease.

Ethmoid Bulla

The ethmoid bulla is one of the most constant and largest of the anterior ethmoid air cells, located within the middle meatus directly posterior to the uncinate process and anterior to the basal lamella of the middle turbinate.

- Based on the lamina orbitalis, it projects medially into the middle meatus and has the appearance of a "bulla," a hollow, thin-walled, rounded prominence.
- Superiorly, the anterior wall of the ethmoid bulla (or bulla lamella) can extend to the skull base and form the posterior limit of the frontal recess. If the bulla does not reach the skull base, a suprabullar recess is formed between the skull base and superior surface of the bulla.
- Posteriorly, the bulla may blend with the basal lamella or have a space between it and the basal lamella of the middle turbinate (retrobullar recess).
- The retrobullar recess may invaginate the basal lamella for a variable distance, occasionally extending the anterior ethmoid air cell system as far posteriorly as the anterior wall of the sphenoid sinus.

See Figure 19-2.

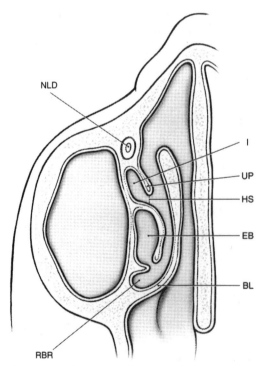

Figure 19-2.   Axial illustration of the anterior naso-sinus anatomy. NLD = nasolacrimal duct, UP = uncinate process; EB = ethmoid bulla; I = infundibulum; HS = hiatus semilunaris; RBR = retro-bullar recess. (*Reproduced with permission from Kennedy DW, Bolger WE, Zinreich SJ, eds.* Diseases of the Sinuses: Diagnosis and Management. *Hamilton, Ontario, Canada: Decker, 2001.*)

Hiatus Semilunaris

The hiatus semilunaris is a cresent-shaped gap between the posterior free margin of the uncinate process and the anterior wall of the ethmoid bulla. It is through this two-dimensional, sagittally oriented cleft or passageway that the middle meatus communicates with the ethmoid infundibulum.

Ethmoid Infundibulum

The ethmoid infundibulum is the funnel-shaped passage through which the secretions from various anterior ethmoid cells, the maxillary sinus and in some cases the frontal sinus, are transported or channeled into the middle meatus.

- It is bordered medially by the mucosa-covered uncinate process, laterally by the lamina orbitalis, anteriorly and superiorly by the frontal process of the maxilla, and superolaterally by the lacrimal bone.
- The ethmoid infundibulum communicates with the middle meatus through the hiatus semilunaris.

Ostiomeatal Unit

The term *ostiomeatal unit* does not refer to a discrete anatomic structure but rather to several middle meatal structures collectively: the uncinate process, ethmoid infundibulum, anterior ethmoid cells and ostia of the anterior ethmoid, and maxillary and frontal sinuses. *Ostiomeatal unit* is a functional rather than an anatomic designation, a term coined by Naumann (1965) in discussing the pathophysiology of sinusitis.

Frontal Recess and Sinus

The frontal recess is the most anterior and superior aspect of the anterior ethmoid sinus, forming the connection with the frontal sinus.

The boundaries of the frontal recess are

- The lamina papyracea laterally
- The middle turbinate medially
- The posterosuperior wall of the agger nasi cell (when present)
- The anterior wall of the ethmoid bulla posteriorly

The frontal recess tapers as it approaches the superiorly located internal os of the frontal sinus; above the os, it again widens as the anterior and posterior tables diverge to their respective positions. An hourglass-like appearance is evident, with the narrowest portion being the frontal ostium. There is tremendous variation with respect to the pattern of the nasofrontal connection, but most frequently the recess opens just medial to the posterior aspect of the uncinate process.

Middle Turbinate

The middle turbinate of the ethmoid bone has several important features, which, if understood well by the surgeon, are helpful in leading to safe, sophisticated surgical treatment.

- In its anterior aspect, the middle turbinate attaches laterally at the agger nasi region, specifically at the crista ethmoidalis (ethmoid eminence) of the maxilla.
- It courses superiorly and medially to attach vertically to the lateral aspect of the lamina cribrosa (cribriform plate). The anterior cranial fossa dura may invaginate into this attachment with the olfactory filae.

- The cribriform attachment is maintained for a variable distance until the insertion courses horizontally across the skull base and inferiorly to attach to the lamina orbitalis and/or the medial wall of the maxillary sinus. This segment is oriented in a near coronal plane anteriorly and an almost horizontal plane more posteriorly. It divides the ethmoid labyrinth into its anterior and posterior components (basal lamella of the middle turbinate).
- The most posterior aspect of the middle turbinate is its inferior attachment to the lateral wall at the crista ethmoidalis of the perpendicular process of the palatine bone, just anterior the sphenopalatine foramen.
- Variability in the middle portion of the basal lamellae of the middle turbinate is important to appreciate. Various posterior ethmoid cells can indent the structure anteriorly, and anterior ethmoid cells and the retrobulbar recess can indent the structure posteriorly.
- The shape of the middle turbinate is highly variable, as it can be paradoxically curved or pneumatized. If the vertical portion or lamella of the middle turbinate is pneumatized, the cell that is formed is referred to as the interlamellar cell. Pneumatization of the head of the middle turbinate is referred to as a concha bullosa.

Ethmoid Roof and Cribriform Plate

Typically, the ethmoid roof slopes inferior medially, and is thinner medially than laterally (by a factor of 10). Medially, the roof is formed by the lateral lamella of the cribriform, which is variable in its vertical height.

Keros described three types of formation of the ethmoid roof based upon the vertical height of the lateral lamella:

- Keros type I: short vertical height to the lateral lamella (1–3 mm)
- Keros type II: 4- to 7-mm depth to the olfactory fossa
- Keros type III: 8- to 16-mm depth to the olfactory fossa

Keros type III, with a long, thin lateral lamella forming a significant part of the medial part of the ethmoid sinus, is said to carry the greatest risk of inadvertent intracranial injury.

Sphenoethmoid (Onodi) Cell

Onodi stressed that when the most posterior ethmoid cell was highly pneumatized, it could extend posteriorly along the lamina papyracea into the anterior wall of the sphenoid sinus. If this occurred, the optic nerve and the carotid artery, both usually considered to border the lateral aspect of the sphenoid sinus, would actually become intimately related to the posterior ethmoid cell. Dissection in the posterior ethmoid could thus result in trauma to the optic nerve or carotid rupture if the anatomic variation were not appreciated (Figure 19-3).

Sphenoid Sinus

Located centrally within the skull, the sphenoid sinuses are separated by an intersinus septum that is highly variable in position and may attach laterally to one side in the region of the carotid artery, an important consideration if it is being surgically removed. As in the case of the other sinuses, pneumatization is highly variable. Laterally, the sinus may pneumatize for a variable distance under the middle cranial fossa (lateral recess); inferiorly, it may pneumatize to a variable extent into the pterygoid processes; and posteriorly, it may pneumatize for a variable distance inferior to the sella turcica.

The sphenoid sinus has critical anatomic relationships. Lateral to the sinus lie the carotid artery, the optic nerve, the cavernous sinus, and the third, fourth, fifth, and sixth cra-

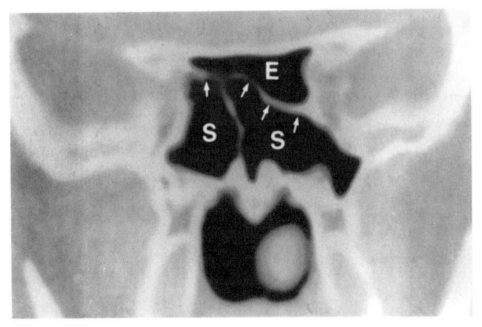

Figure 19-3. Coronal CT cut through the sphenoid sinus reveals a "horizontal septum" (*arrows*). The cell above the septum (E) represents a sphenoethmoid cell (Onodi cell) that has pneumatized above the sphenoid sinus (S), bringing the ethmoid sinus into close proximity to the optic nerve and carotid artery. (*Reproduced with permission from Kennedy DW, Bolger WE, Zinreich SJ, eds.* Diseases of the Sinuses: Diagnosis and Management. *Hamilton, Ontario, Canada: Decker, 2001.*)

nial nerves. If the sphenoid sinus is well pneumatized, the optic nerve and carotid artery can indent the sinus covered only by thin bone. The carotid canal is clinically dehiscent in 22% of specimens. The optic canal may also be dehiscent approximately 6% of the time, particularly in the presence of mucoceles, tumors, or allergic fungal sinusitis.

Concepts in Chronic Rhinosinusitis

The ostiomeatal unit plays a significant role in the pathogenesis of sinusitis. Obstruction here predisposes to inflammation, which can become chronic in the dependent sinuses. However, multiple predisposing factors are associated with the onset of chronic rhinosinusitis. These may be broadly classified into environmental, general host, and local host factors:

- Environmental factors
    Smoking, allergy, pollution, chemical and dust exposure, fungi, bacteria, and stress
- General host factors
    Reactive airways disease, genetic predisposition, specific genetic diseases (eg, cystic fibrosis, Young's syndrome), immunodeficiency, and ciliary dysfunction
- Local host factors
    Anatomic narrowing (eg, paradoxical turbinate, concha bullosa, septal deformity), persistent mucosal inflammation, osteitis, and recirculation of mucus

Since chronic sinusitis is typically a multifactorial disease, surgery is only a small part of the overall management in the majority of patients. Smoking is a relative contraindication to elective endoscopic sinus surgery. Following surgery and medical management in the postoperative period, patients require prolonged endoscopic surveillance for evidence of persistent or recurrent disease. In most cases, endoscopic evidence of disease is visible in the postoperative patient long before the return of symptoms.

Patient Selection

A decision in favor of surgical intervention is relatively easy in the presence of a large mucocele, inflammatory complication, or in the presence of diffuse nasal polyposis unresponsive to medical therapy. However, this decision is considerably more difficult when the disease is less serious or the primary complaint is recurrent sinusitis or headache. Some general *guidelines* areas follows:

- The patient should have had a trial of maximal medical therapy.
- Computed tomography (CT) should be performed at least 4 weeks following the onset of medical therapy for the most recent episode of sinusitis and at least 2 weeks following the most recent upper respiratory infection.
- There should be persistent evidence (radiographic or endoscopic) of mucosal disease.
- Nasal congestion, obstruction, decreased olfaction, and nasal/sinus fullness are generally good signs of chronic rhinosinusitis.
- Headache correlates poorly with sinus disease, and severe pain is unusual in chronic sinusitis.
- The performance of elective sinus surgery on patients who continue to smoke may result in severe scarring and worsening of symptoms.

Diagnostic Nasal Endoscopy

The development of the modern rigid nasal endoscope represents a major advance in rhinologic diagnostic capability. Nasal endoscopy is more sensitive for the diagnosis of accessible disease than CT and provides essential complementary information for diagnosis. Endoscopy permits detailed evaluation of the critical areas for sinusitis, the ostiomeatal complex and sphenoethmoid recess. The superiority of endoscopy over anterior rhinoscopy in providing a more accurate and thorough diagnostic evaluation was demonstrated in a recent evaluation of patients with sinonasal complaints. Nasal pathology was identified by nasal endoscopic examination in almost 40% of patients deemed normal by traditional rhinologic examination.

Equipment for diagnostic nasal endoscopy includes a 30-degree 4-mm endoscope, 30-degree 2.7-mm endoscope, Freer elevator, light source, fiberoptic cable, and an assortment of suction tips. The 30-degree 4-mm scope is the most useful endoscope, as it provides superb illumination, an ample viewing field, and is well tolerated by most patients. Most diagnostic endoscopy can be performed with these few basic pieces of equipment, making it easily affordable for most otolaryngologists.

Diagnostic nasal endoscopy is typically performed in an orderly fashion, with the patient sitting or supine.

- The nasal cavities are sprayed with a topical decongestant and local anesthetic.
- Topical anesthetic is applied to the inferolateral surface of the middle turbinate and to other sites where passage of the endoscope may exert pressure.

- The examiner should always take appropriate precautions when dealing with secretions and blood. Gloves, mask, and eye protection are recommended.
- A complete examination can be successfully accomplished in an organized manner with three passes of the endoscope.
- The 4-mm 30-degree telescope is usually selected first. The endoscope lens is treated with a thin film of anti-fog solution and then held lightly in the left hand by the shaft with the thumb and first two fingers and introduced slowly, under direct vision.
- The telescope is initially passed along the floor of the nose. The overall anatomy, presence of pathologic secretions or polyps, and condition of nasal mucosa may be identified. In some cases it may also be possible to identify the nasolacrimal duct within the inferior meatus. Thereafter, the scope is advanced through the nasal cavity and toward the nasopharynx. As the scope is advanced into the nasopharynx, the entire nasopharynx, including the contralateral eustachian tube orifice, can be examined by rotating the telescope.
- The second pass of the telescope is made between the middle and inferior turbinates. While the scope is being directed posteriorly, the inferior portion of the middle meatus, fontanelles, and accessory maxillary ostia can be examined. The scope is then passed medial to the middle turbinate and advanced posteriorly to examine the sphenoethmoid recess. Rotating the scope superiorly and slightly laterally allows for visualization of the superior turbinate and meatus as well as the slit-like or oval ostia of the sphenoid sinus.
- The third pass of the examination is made as the telescope is withdrawn. As the scope is brought back anteriorly, it can frequently be rotated laterally under the middle turbinate into the posterior aspect of the middle meatus. The bulla ethmoidalis, hiatus semilunaris, and infundibular entrance are inspected. Withdrawing the telescope further can provide an excellent view of the middle turbinate, uncinate process, and surrounding mucosa. In selected patients, this portion of the examination can be conducted from an anterior approach if the anatomy is favorable. Alternatively, additional topical anesthetic may be placed within the middle meatus and in the region of the anterior insertion of the middle turbinate. The middle turbinate is then gently subluxed medially, using a cotton-tipped applicator moistened with topical anesthetic, so as to allow insertion of a telescope into the middle meatus.

Diagnostic and Therapeutic Applications

In addition to the initial identification of disease, another crucial application of nasal endoscopy is to evaluate the patient's response to medical treatment, such as topical nasal steroids, antibiotics, oral steroids, and antihistamines. Through serial endoscopic examinations, resolution of polyps, pathologic secretions, mucosal edema, and inflammatory changes can be followed. These objective data, combined with the patient's subjective response, are valuable in determining the need for further treatment. Endoscopy may greatly reduce and in many cases eliminate the need for repeated radiographic examination during and after medical or surgical therapy.

An especially important diagnostic application of nasal endoscopy is to identify the causative organism in sinusitis. A small malleable culture swab or suction trap aspirator is carefully directed to the middle meatus or other site of origin of purulent drainage and submitted for culture.

Diagnostic nasal endoscopy is especially useful in the follow-up evaluation after functional endoscopic sinus surgery (FESS). Endoscopic examination provides early objective data regarding recurrence of polyps, hyperplastic mucosa, and chronic infection, often long before symptoms occur. Although diagnostic nasal endoscopy was originally used primarily for the evaluation of sinusitis, it has proved invaluable in postoperative surveillance following intranasal tumor resection and for the evaluation of cerebrospinal fluid (CSF) rhinorrhea.

One of the most common diagnostic and therapeutic uses of nasal endoscopy in the clinical setting is postoperative care after FESS. Nasal endoscopic examinations and sinus cavity debridement are essential to promote consistent ethmoid cavity healing. Under appropriate topical anesthesia, clot, mucus, and fibrin are removed from the nasal and sinus cavities and the openings to the maxillary, sphenoid, and frontal sinuses are cleared of obstructive fibrin and forming scar tissue. Removal of osteitic bone can reduce foci of inflammation and further promote healing.

Preoperative Patient Management

- Minimize infection.
- Pretreat with steroids if mucosa is hyperreactive, marked polyposis is present, or the patient has asthma (prednisone 20–40 mg/day for 2–6 days).
- Carefully and systematically reevaluate the CT scan.

CT Evaluation of the Preoperative Patient

All patients should have coronal CT scans with 3-mm cuts. Additionally, axial scans are particularly helpful in patients where a frontal sinusotomy or sphenoidotomy is likely to be performed. In these latter situations or in revision surgery, the use of computer-assisted surgical navigation is also a reasonable consideration.

The *key points in reviewing the CT* scan prior to surgery are

- Shape, slope, and thickness of skull base
- Shape and dehiscences of medial orbital wall
- Vertical height of the posterior ethmoid (in relation to the posteromedial roof of the maxillary sinus) (Figure 19-4)
- Presence of a sphenoethmoid (Onodi) cell
- Position of intrasinus sphenoid septae (in relation to carotid)
- The presence of maxillary sinus hypoplasia or infundibular atelectasis

Extent of Surgery

General guidelines for *chronic sinusitis* are as follows:

- Preserve the mucoperiosteum and try not to leave exposed bone.
- Remove bony partitions and osteitic bone in the area of disease as completely as possible.
- Extend the dissection one step beyond the extent of disease (if possible).
- Preserve the middle turbinate if possible (ie, if not markedly diseased and covered with mucoperiosteum at the end of the surgery).

General guidelines for *mucoceles* are

- Identify skull base posteriorly (for frontal mucoceles).
- Marsupialize widely, removing osteitic bone from the opening.
- Make the opening flush with the surrounding bone.

General guidelines for *inverted papillomas* are

- Obtain permission to convert to an open procedure.
- Meticulously identify the site or sites of tumor attachment.

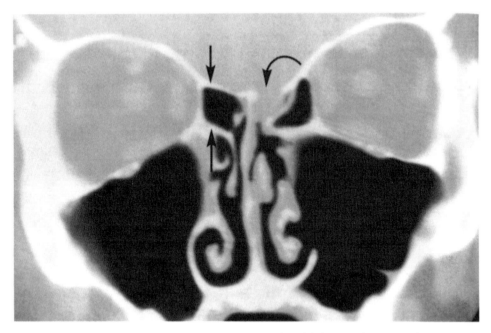

Figure 19-4. Coronal CT at the level of the posterior ethmoid sinuses demonstrating a narrow vertical height to the posterior ethmoid (*arrows*). On the left side, the skull base has been violated (*curved arrow*), apparently as a result of the limited vertical height posteriorly. (*Reproduced with permission from Kennedy DW, Bolger WE, Zinreich SJ, eds. Diseases of the Sinuses: Diagnosis and Management. Hamilton, Ontario, Canada: Decker, 2001.*)

- Remove or burr the bone at the site(s) of tumor attachment.
- Convert to an open approach if you cannot adequately access the site(s) of attachment.
- Create a widely patent cavity which allows for easy long-term endoscopic surveillance.

Anesthesia

Endoscopic sinus surgery can be performed under local anesthesia with sedation or under general anesthesia. In general, meticulous techniques have become increasingly successful in preserving mucosa. Additionally, the headsets required for computer-assisted surgical navigation are uncomfortable to wear for long periods of time. The tendency, therefore, has been to move toward general anesthesia. However, general anesthesia has the disadvantage that it does not allow monitoring of vision should an intraorbital hematoma occur or provide the same feedback of pain seen when the anterior or posterior ethmoid neurovascular bundles are approached under local anesthesia. Under general anesthesia, mild hypotension is preferable.

Under local or general anesthesia, the nose is decongested with oxymetazoline prior to surgery. Before surgery is begun on the first side, this decongestion can be supplemented with 100 to 150 mg of topical cocaine on Farrell nasal applicators. The lateral wall is then infiltrated with 1% lidocaine with 1:100,000 adrenaline, as follows:

- Anterior to the attachment of the middle turbinate

- Anterior to the inferior portion of the uncinate process
- Inferior aspect of middle turbinate
- At the midpoint of the root of the inferior turbinate

These injections may be augmented by a sphenopalatine block (transnasal or transoral) if the posterior ethmoid or sphenoid sinus requires dissection. However, this injection must be performed slowly and carefully following aspiration. Loss of vision has been reported (Figure 19-5).

SURGICAL TECHNIQUE

Uncinectomy

- Anterior attachment recognized by a semilunar depression in the lateral nasal wall.
- Incision typically begins adjacent to the anterior attachment of the middle turbinate.

If site of attachment not evident, it is preferable to make the incision posterior to its attachment and remove any residual uncinate later.

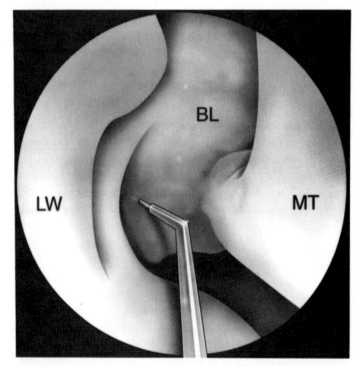

Figure 19-5. Endoscopic representation of the posterior middle meatus during transnasal injection of the sphenopalatine foramen. An angled tonsil needle is inserted in an upward and lateral direction through the inferior portion of the basal lamella (BL). The needle tip is used to feel for the foramen and the injection must be performed very slowly, after aspiration. LW = lateral wall, MT = middle turbinate. (*Reproduced with permission from Kennedy DW, Bolger WE, Zinreich SJ, eds.* Diseases of the Sinuses: Diagnosis and Management. *Hamilton, Ontario, Canada: Decker, 2001.*)

Ethmoidectomy

- Use 0° telescope until the major landmarks have been identified (to avoid disorientation)
- Identify and open bulla (forceps or microdebrider)
- Identify the medial orbital wall as early as possible during the procedure
- Work close to the medial orbital wall (skull base thin and downsloping medially)
- Identify the retrobullar and suprabullar recesses and basal lamella

If the posterior ethmoid cells are to be entered,

- Withdraw the telescope slightly to provide an overview of the basal lamella.
- Perforate the basal lamella immediately superior to its horizontal part.
- Use upbiting forceps to ensure that there is a space behind the bony lamella.
- Remove the lamella laterally and posteriorly with microdebrider or forceps (Figure 19-6).

Additional intercellular partitions are entered and removed in manner similar to that with the basal lamella. The most posterior ethmoid cell characteristically has a pyramidal shape, with the apex pointing posteriorly, laterally, and superiorly toward the optic nerve. The sphenoid sinus lies inferiorly, medially, and posterior to this cell. If a superior ethmoid or frontal recess dissection is planned, the skull base should be identified, when possible, within the

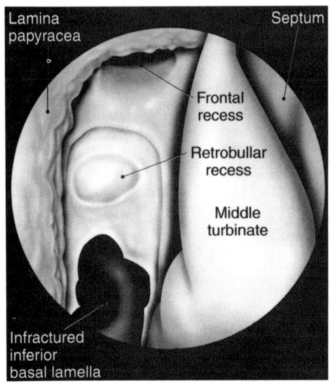

Figure 19-6. With the lamina papyracea already identified, the basal lamella may be infractured with either forceps or a microdebrider, just superior to the horizontal portion. (*Reproduced with permission from Kennedy DW, Bolger WE, Zinreich SJ, eds.* Diseases of the Sinuses: Diagnosis and Management. *Hamilton, Ontario, Canada: Decker, 2001.*)

posterior ethmoid sinus. In general, the cells here are larger and the skull base is more horizontal, making identification significantly easier and safer than in the anterior ethmoid sinus. If disease extent makes identification of the skull base difficult at this time, sphenoidotomy should be performed and the skull base identified within the sphenoid sinus (Figure 19-7).

Sphenoidotomy with Ethmoidectomy

The safest method of entering the sphenoid from within the ethmoid sinus is as follows:

- Identify the superior meatus and the superior turbinate by palpating medially between the middle and superior turbinate.
- Resect the most inferior part of the superior turbinate with a through cutting forceps or with a microdebrider.
- Palpate the sphenoid sinus ostium just medial to where the superior turbinate was resected.
- Enlarge the ostium with a Stammberger mushroom punch and Hajek rotating sphenoid punch (Figure 19-8).

Frontal Recess Surgery (Draf Type 1)

Because of the difficult anatomic relationships, it is very important to rereview the CT before working in the region of the frontal sinus. The frontal sinus may then be accessed as follows:

- Dissect from posterior to anterior along the skull base, skeletonizing the medial orbital wall.

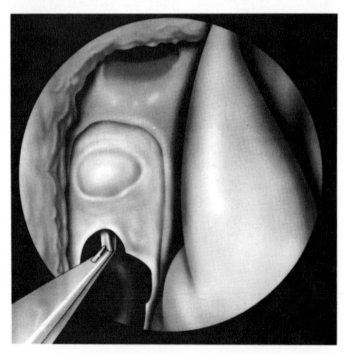

Figure 19-7. Upbiting forceps are utilized to feel for a space behind the bony partitions before they are taken down superiorly or toward the medial orbital wall. (*Reproduced with permission from Kennedy DW, Bolger WE, Zinreich SJ, eds.* Diseases of the Sinuses: Diagnosis and Management. *Hamilton, Ontario, Canada: Decker, 2001.*)

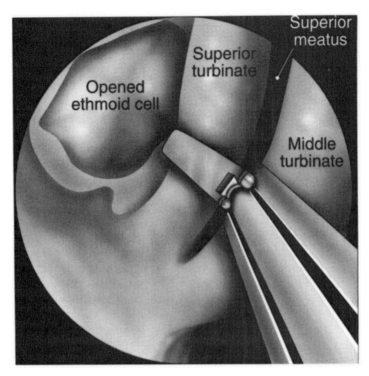

Figure 19-8. After identifying the superior meatus medially within the right ethmoid cavity, the inferior part of the superior turbinate is removed with a straight through-cutting forceps. (*Reproduced with permission from Kennedy DW, Bolger WE, Zinreich SJ, eds.* Diseases of the Sinuses: Diagnosis and Management. *Hamilton, Ontario, Canada: Decker, 2001.*)

- Remember that the anterior ethmoid vessel typically lies posterior to the supraorbital ethmoid cells and may lie up to 4 mm below the skull base.
- Remain laterally close to the medial orbital wall (thicker skull base).
- After opening the recess, carefully look for the opening to the frontal sinus; typically, it is medial, but this is variable.
- A small seeker or frontal recess curette may be used to palpate the opening, but a fine Kennedy malleable frontal sinus probe (Medtronic-Xomed, Inc., Jacksonville, Florida) is less traumatic and therefore preferable.
- A curette is then introduced, and the bony roof of the agger nasi cell is fractured anteriorly or laterally, depending on whether the opening is posterior or medial.
- The bone fragments are then painstakingly removed, taking care to avoid stripping mucosa.
- Document frontal sinus opening photographically for later comparison.

See Figure 19-9.

Draf Type 2 Frontal Sinusotomy

In a Draf 2A, the frontal sinus is opened between the lamina papyracea and the insertion of the middle turbinate. In a Draf 2B, the frontal sinus is opened medial to the middle turbinate by removal of the most anterior attachment of the middle turbinate to the skull base. These pro-

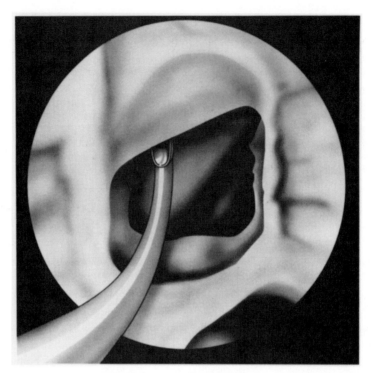

Figure 19-9.   With use of an angled telescope to view the frontal recess, a curved curette can be introduced posterior to the agger nasi cell and the roof of the cell fractured anteriorly ("uncapping the egg"). (*Reproduced with permission from Kennedy DW, Bolger WE, Zinreich SJ, eds.* Diseases of the Sinuses: Diagnosis and Management. *Hamilton, Ontario, Canada: Decker, 2001.*)

cedures are best reserved for revision procedures where (1) the anterior portion of the middle turbinate has become osteitic and tends to scar laterally and (2) the internal os of the frontal sinus is small.

Draf Type 3 Frontal Sinusotomy

Also known as a transseptal frontal sinusotomy or endoscopic Lothrop procedure, this operation removes part of the nasal septum and part of the frontal sinus septum to create one large opening accessible from both sides of the nose. Although, when the anatomy is favorable (a frontal sinus which pneumatizes extensively posteriorly superior to the nasal septum), this operation can be performed with minimal mucosal loss, in most cases use of a drill is required and extensive mucosal loss and bone exposure occurs. Thus this operation is best reserved for situations where more conservative and time-tested endoscopic procedures have failed.

Even in skilled hands, this procedure carries up to a 10% risk of CSF leak; this procedure therefore should only be undertaken by those skilled in this surgery. The basic steps of the procedure are as follows:

- Carefully evaluate the axial and coronal CT scans to determine anatomic suitability and the extent of bone that may need to be removed by drill.

- Identify the skull base posteriorly on each side and follow forward into each frontal recess.
- After injection, fenestrate and remove the most anterosuperior nasal septum.
- Using the frontal recess as a guide and preferably with image guidance, remove bone from the floor of the frontal sinus bilaterally (with punch or drill).
- Extend the opening laterally across, removing any residual anterior middle turbinate attachment. In general, it is better to look with the endoscope through one nostril and to instrument through the other, using the septal opening for visualization.
- Remove the frontal sinus intersinus septum as widely as possible. The size of the frontal opening created will depend upon the degree of bony thickening and mucosal inflammation present.
- As with openings made into other sinuses, it is important that the opening communicate with the natural ostium if good mucociliary clearance is to be achieved and subsequent closure avoided.

Maxillary Antrostomy

There is significant debate regarding the appropriate size for a maxillary antrostomy. Theoretically, a smaller ostium should be more efficient as long as removal of thick inspissated material is not required. On the other hand, the uncinate process is typically involved early in the disease process, forms a significant part of the medial maxillary sinus wall, and, if involved in the disease process, should be removed. Such removal of a diseased uncinate process will inevitably result in a wide antrostomy. The key points in maxillary antrostomy are:

- Identify the inferior cut edge of the uncinate process and pull it medially with a ball-tipped seeker.
- If the ostium is not visible lateral to uncinate remnant, press on the posterior fontanelle and look for a bubble.
- Resect the residual uncinate process with a back biting forceps and then extend the antrostomy inferiorly and posteriorly as necessary.

Management of the Nasal Septum

The nasal septum is addressed during sinus surgery if it is markedly deviated to where it significantly interferes with nasal airflow or if the deviation is such that access to the antero-superior attachment of the middle turbinate is not possible with the 0° telescope. Typically, the ethmoidectomy is performed on the wider side first. The septum is then addressed, the incision being made on the side of previously performed ethmoidectomy so as to avoid unnecessary bleeding onto the telescope during the second ethmoidectomy.

Typically, septal corrections during FESS are best achieved with an endoscopic approach. This allows the deviated nasal septum to be addressed under excellent visualization without the necessity to either change to a headlight or change instrumentation. After making the incision using overhead lighting and initiating the flap elevation, the flaps are elevated with the use of a suction elevator and bony cartilaginous resection is performed in the usual manner. We have found the 1-mm Acufex orthopedic punch particularly helpful in this regard. Septal reconstruction, if necessary, can be performed following the second ethmoidectomy by replacing crushed cartilage into the septal pocket. The septal flaps are then quilted with a running chromic suture on a small straight needle.

Packing

In general, postoperative packing is minimized following FESS. A small Merocel sinus sponge placed into the middle meatus absorbs blood and provides a gentle tamponade. Should significant bleeding be present, it is our preference not to perform a tight nasal packing but to cauterize the bleeding site with either a monopolar suction cautery or bipolar cautery, depending upon the site of origin.

Postoperative Care

MEDICAL THERAPY

- Antibiotic coverage is started in the operating room, either based upon preoperative culture or so as to provide coverage for the more frequently found organisms.
- Saline spray and topical steroids are instituted in the early postoperative period. The topical steroids are continued until the cavity is endoscopically normal.
- Oral steroids (if required) are tapered during the postoperative period based upon the endoscopic appearance of the mucosa.
- If the cavity demonstrates evidence of increasing inflammation at any point during the postoperative healing period, it is recultured under endoscopic visualization and the antibiotics are changed appropriately.

The most common site of persistent disease is the frontal recess. Therefore, when using steroid sprays, consider the use of one of the various positions that increase the dosage of steroid to that site. This includes Moffat's head-down kneeling position or a position favored by the senior author, in which the patient sprays the nose sitting in bed, then assumes a prone position with the neck hyperflexed and slightly turned to the side, alongside a large pillow. Nasal irrigations are usually reserved for patients with severe chronic hypertrophic disease and are not usually started in the immediate postoperative period so as to reduce the potential for the introduction of gram-negative organisms. During the first year or so postoperatively, patients with reactive mucosa may require both short courses of antibiotics and oral steroids in order to avoid recurrent mucosal disease and bacterial sinusitis following a viral upper respiratory infection.

Local Management of the Postoperative Cavity

- Merocel sponges are typically removed on the first postoperative day and the cavities suctioned free of blood under local anesthetic.
- Nasal endoscopy and cleaning of the cavity are repeated on a weekly basis until the cavity is healed. At each visit, crusts are removed, the cavity is examined for areas of persistent inflammation, and any residual fragments of exposed or osteitic bone are removed. Scars are divided and particular attention is paid to the all-important frontal recess region.

Symptoms—with the exception of postnasal discharge—usually resolve early following endoscopic sinus surgery. Pain and pressure in the postsurgical period are very uncommon and should be considered as signs of persistent infection or inflammation requiring additional management. Olfaction is the symptom that appears to be the most sensitive indicator of persistent or recurrent disease. Indeed, patients should be instructed to follow their sense of smell and to obtain additional medical therapy and follow-up endoscopic examination if they experience a significant decrease in their ability to smell.

Surgical Complications and Postoperative Care

Possible complications of ethmoid sinus surgery include hemorrhage, CSF leak, orbital injury, nasolacrimal duct injury, and recurrence, regardless of whether an external, intranasal, or endoscopic intranasal approach is used. In this section we summarize and review the complications of endoscopic ethmoidectomy.

Preoperative Planning to Prevent Ethmoid Sinus Complications

Reduce Intraoperative Bleeding

- Assess the patient's hemostatic system, as hemorrhage that obscures visualization appears to be a common cause of intraoperative complications. A screening history should include questions about bleeding during prior surgery, liver disease, use of antiplatelet or anticoagulant medications, or a family history of a bleeding disorder.
- Obtain screening coagulation studies or formal hematology consultation when appropriate.
- Discontinue aspirin and other nonsteroidal anti-inflammatory agents and restrict use of herbal dietary supplements for an appropriate period prior to surgery.
- For patients with sinonasal polyposis, a course of oral corticosteroid therapy can reduce polyp size and vascularity. Similarly, bleeding can be reduced in patients with reactive nasal mucosa by stabilizing the mucosa with steroids prior to surgical intervention.
- When chronic infection is present, a preoperative course of oral antibiotic therapy will help reduce tissue inflammation and vascularity.
- If the preoperative CT evaluation reveals an area of opacification adjacent to a skull base erosion, magnetic resonance imaging (MRI) should be performed to rule out a meningoencephalocele prior to surgery.
- Carefully reexamine the CT scan just prior to surgery.
- With patients who have distorted anatomy due to prior surgery, potential landmarks should be identified on the CT scan.

Intraoperative Strategies for Avoiding and Managing Complications

Prevention of Bleeding

- Provide careful topical and infiltrative vasoconstriction.
- Minimize mucosal trauma, especially to the nasal mucosa anteriorly in the nose.
- Avoid trauma to the anterior ethmoid artery. Approximately 40% of these arteries are dehiscent, as the artery can travel beneath the ethmoid roof along a bony mesentery, in some cases 1 to 3 mm from the roof [Kainz (1989)]. Care must be taken not to mistake the artery for a bony septa of an ethmoid cell and therefore to attempt resection.
- Limit dissection in the region of the sphenopalatine artery and its branches. Care should be taken to avoid dissecting the basal lamella too far inferiorly upon entering the posterior ethmoids. Bleeding can result, as the sphenopalatine artery lies just behind the inferior aspect of the basal lamellae in most patients.
- If, during surgery, bleeding persists so that it interferes with visualization, it is safer to stop the procedure and, if necessary, return at a later time.

Management of Intraoperative Bleeding
- Pack the surgical cavity with cottonoid pledgets soaked in vasoconstrictive agents.
- Persistent bleeding or bleeding from the sphenopalatine, anterior, or posterior ethmoid arteries or their branches may require a small microfibrillar collagen pack or electrocautery.
- The use of an Endoscrub (Medtronic-Xomed Inc., Jacksonville, Florida) device to clear the endoscope lens of blood is extremely helpful in maintaining good visualization and thereby reducing complications from bleeding.

Prevention of Orbital Injury
- Identify the lamina orbitalis positively and do so early in the dissection.
- Initially, limit dissection in the lateral aspect of the most posterior ethmoid cells and the sphenoid to avoid trauma to the optic nerve. This is extremely important in cases where a sphenoethmoid cell (Onodi cell) is present.
- Identify and preserve the anterior ethmoid artery. Should this artery be inadvertently divided during surgery, the lateral aspect of the vessel can retract within the orbit and bleed, with a resultant and dramatic orbital hematoma.

Management of Orbital Complications
- If the lamina papyracea is entered during intranasal ethmoidectomy and orbital fat is exposed, further dissection should be terminated in the immediate region and the fat not be removed or resected.
- Monitor for signs of an orbital hematoma, such as lid edema, ecchymosis, and proptosis. Vision is checked if the patient is under local anesthesia.
- In all cases where the lamina papyracea has been violated, tight packing of the ethmoid cavity is prohibited, as this can increase intraorbital pressure.
- When orbital hematoma is suspected and a sudden dramatic onset of progressive proptosis occurs, a "compartment syndrome" quickly results. To decrease the pressure within the orbit, initially perform a canthotomy and cantholysis and then follow with orbital decompression and ophthalmology consult.
- For smaller orbital hematomas from capillary rather than arterial bleeding, remove nasal packing, check vision, and consult ophthalmology. Medical measures such as topical timolol, intravenous acetazolamide, mannitol, and high-dose steroids as well as CT scan should be considered.

Prevention of Skull Base Injury
- Identify the ethmoid roof positively and then work anteriorly, feeling behind bony partitions before they are removed.
- Use a zero-degree telescope to reduce the possibility of disorientation associated with the deflected-angle endoscopes. After the skull base is identified, a 30-degree scope can be used more safely.
- When dissecting along the ethmoid roof, use caution clearing tissue from the medial aspect.

Management of Skull Base Injury/Cerebrospinal Fluid Rhinorrhea
- Inspect the area endoscopically to determine the site and size and whether intradural injury has occurred.
- Consider neurosurgical and infectious disease (I.D.) consultations.
- Reflect the sinus mucosa adjacent to the leak site for several millimeters.
- Place intracranial bone graft if defect is greater than 6 mm.

- Place a free overlay nasal mucosal or fascial graft over the leak site.
- Secure the graft with several layers of absorbable collagen-based packing.
- Consider a postoperative CT scan of the head to rule out the possibility of intracranial bleeding (Figure 19-10).

Postoperative Management of Complications

Immediate Postoperative Complications and Their Management

MANAGEMENT OF POSTOPERATIVE EPISTAXIS

- Application of topical hemostatic vasoconstrictive agents.
- Endoscopic localization of the bleeding site with treatment via electrocautery or direct packing of the bleeding site.
- Consider arterial ligation or embolization for refractory cases.

Management of Postoperative Cerebrospinal Fluid Rhinorrhea

Establish the diagnosis of CSF leak and determine the leak site using appropriate tests, such as endoscopy, CT scan, beta-2 transferrin test, intrathecal water-soluble contrast CT, intrathecal radioactive indium or technetium and pledget scanning, and intrathecal fluorescein (0.1 mL of 10% intravenous fluorescein diluted in 10 mL of the patient's CSF and injected over 5 minutes).

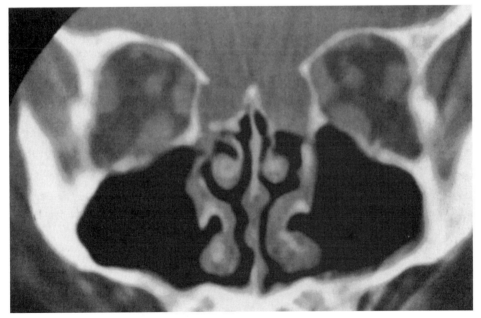

Figure 19-10. Coronal CT of a patient with complaint of anosmia, chronic nasal congestion, and discharge following prior sinus surgery at another institution. Nasal endoscopy demonstrated bilateral soft tissue masses and computed tomography shows bilateral ethmoid roof defects. Magnetic resonance imaging confirmed bilateral encephaloceles. (*Reproduced with permission from Kennedy DW, Bolger WE, Zinreich SJ, eds.* Diseases of the Sinuses: Diagnosis and Management. *Hamilton, Ontario, Canada: Decker, 2001.*)

Bibliography

Bingham B, Wang RG, Hawke M, Kwok P. The embryonic development of the lateral nasal wall from 8 to 24 weeks. *Laryngoscope* 101:912–997, 1991.

Bolger WE, Mawn C. Analysis of the sinus lateralis for endoscopic sinus surgery. *Ann Otol Rhinol Laryngol* 110 (Suppl 186):1–14, 2001.

Grunwald L. Deskriptive und topographische Anatomie der Nase und ihrer Nebenhoglen. In: Denker A, Kahler O, eds. *Handbuch der Hals-Nasen-Ohrenheilkunde.* Vol I. Berlin: Springer-Bergmann, 1925: 1–95.

Hwang PH, McLaughlin RB, Lanza DC, Kennedy DW. Endoscopic septoplasty: indications, technique, and results. *Otolaryngol Head Neck Surg* 120:678–682, 1999.

Kasper KA. Nasofrontal connections: a study based on one hundred consecutive dissections. *Arch Otolaryngol* 23:322–344, 1936.

Kennedy DW, Zinreich SJ, Hassab M. The internal carotid artery as it relates to endonasal sphenoethmoidecomy. *Am J Rhinol* 4:7–12, 1990.

Kennedy DW. Functional endoscopic sinus surgery: anesthesia, technique, and postoperative management. In: Kennedy DW, Bolger WE, Zinreich SJ, eds. *Diseases of the Sinuses: Diagnosis and Management.* Hamilton, Ontario, Canada: Decker, 2001, 211–221.

Kennedy DW. Functional endoscopic sinus surgery: concepts, surgical indications and instrumentation. In: Kennedy DW, Bolger WE, Zinreich SJ, eds. *Diseases of the Sinuses: Diagnosis and Management.* Hamilton, Ontario, Canada: Decker, 2001, 197–210.

Libersa C, Laude M, Libersa JC. The pneumatization of the accessory cavities of the fossae during growth. *Anat Clin* 2:265–273, 1981.

Naumann H. Patholische anatomic der chronischen Rhinitis und Sinusitis. In: Proceedings VIII International Congress of Oto-rhino-laryngology. Amsterdam: Excerpta Medica, 1965, 80.

Onodi A. The optic nerve and the accessory sinuses of the nose. London: Bailliere, Tindall and Cox, 1910, 1–26.

Orlandi RR, Lanza DC, Bolger WE, et al. The forgotten turbinate: the role of the superior turbinate in endoscopic sinus surgery. *Am J Rhinol* 13: 251–259, 1999.

Schaeffer JP. *The Nose, Paranasal Sinuses, Naso-lacrimal Passageways and Olfactory Organ in Man: A Genetic, Developmental, and Anatomico-Physiological Consideration.* Philadelphia: Blakiston's, 1920.

Stammberger H. *Functional Endoscopic Sinus Surgery: The Messerklinger Technique.* Philadelphia: Decker, 1991.

Stammberger HR, Bolger WE, Clement PAR, et al. Anatomic terminology and nomenclature in sinusitis. *Ann Otol Rhinol Laryngol* 104(Suppl 167):7–19, 1995.

Stedman's Medical Dictionary, 24th ed. Baltimore: Williams & Wilkins, 1982, 710.

Van Alyea OE. Ethmoid labyrinth: anatomic study, with consideration of the clinical significance of its structural characteristics. *Arch Otolaryngol* 29:881–901, 1939.

Van Alyea. Ostium maxillare: anatomic study of its surgical accessibility. *Arch Otolaryngol Head Neck Surg* 24:552–569, 1939.

Vidic B. The postnatal development of the sphenoidal sinus and its spread into the dorsum sellae and posterior clinoid processes. *AJR* 104:177–183, 1968.

Wang RG, Jiang SC, Gu R. The cartilaginous nasal capsule and embryonic development of human paranasal sinuses. *J Otolaryngol* 23:239–243.

Antimicrobial Therapy in Otolaryngology-Head and Neck Surgery

20

In the United States, more than $7 billion is spent annually on antibiotics, much of which is for treatment of infections in the ears, nose, throat, head, and neck. The otolaryngologist–head and neck surgeon, therefore, must be especially current in his knowledge of these drugs.

This chapter categorically lists the drugs that are most commonly employed in this specialty, with their major indications and drawbacks for usage. For more detailed information, the reader is referred to more comprehensive publications.[1-4]

ANTIMICROBIAL AGENTS FOR USE IN HEAD/NECK INFECTIONS

Penicillins (Beta-Lactam Antibiotics)

Beta lactams are bactericidal antibiotics. Penicillins penetrate into the cerebrospinal fluid (CSF) well in the presence of inflammation.

Penicillin-induced rashes are common, recur in only 50% of subsequent uses of the penicillins, and are not related to anaphylaxis. But anaphylaxis can be life-threatening, does not necessarily occur in patients with previous rashes, and constitutes a lifelong contraindication to future penicillin use. Fatality is most likely from parenteral use.

A. Penicillin G or V
   1. Active against:
      a. Most *Streptococcus pneumoniae*
      b. *Streptococcus pyogenes* (beta-hemolytic)
      c. Many (not all) oral anaerobes
   2. Drawbacks:
      a. Gastric acid degrades
      b. Rashes (5%)
      c. Anaphylaxis (1/10,000)
      d. Inactivated by beta lactamases (from *Moraxella catarrhalis, Haemophilus, Staphylococcus,* etc.)
      e. Relative resistance: Many *Streptococcus pneumoniae*
B. Antistaphylococcal (penicillinase-resistant) penicillins (ie, methicillin, oxacillin, dicloxacillin, nafcillin)
   1. Active against:
      a. *Staphylococcus aureus*
      b. *Streptococcus pyogenes*

        c.   Most *Streptococcus pneumoniae*

        d.   Many anaerobes (oral/respiratory)

    2.   Drawbacks:

        a.   Gastric acid degrades

        b.   Penicillin hypersensitivity

        c.   Bitter taste (suspension)

        d.   Methicillin-type resistant *Staphylococcus aureus* (up to 10%)

C.   Amino-penicillins (ie, ampicillin, amoxicillin)

    1.   Active against:

        a.   Many *Haemophilus influenzae*

        b.   *Escherichia coli* and *Proteus*

        c.   *Streptococcus pyogenes* (beta-hemolytic)

        d.   Most *Streptococcus pneumoniae*

        e.   Many anaerobes

    2.   Drawbacks:

        a.   *Staphylococcus aureus* resistance

        b.   *Haemophilus* resistance (>30%)

        c.   *Moraxella catarrhalis* resistance (>90%)

        d.   Penicillin hypersensitivity

D.   Augmented penicillins. These penicillins are combined with beta-lactamase inhibitors [ie, amoxicillin plus clavulanate (Augmentin oral), ampicillin plus sulbactam (Unasyn IV)]

    1.   Active against:

        a.   *Haemophilus influenzae*

        b.   *Moraxella catarrhalis*

        c.   *Staphylococcus aureus*

        d.   *Streptococcus pyogenes*

        e.   Most *Streptococcus pneumoniae*

        f.   Most anaerobes, etc.

    2.   Drawbacks:

        a.   Nausea, diarrhea (oral administration)

        b.   Yeast overgrowth

        c.   Penicillin hypersensitivity

        d.   *Pseudomonas* resistance—except for ticarcillin plus K^+ clavulanate (Timentin IV) and piperacillin plus tazobactam (Zosyn IV), active against *Pseudomonas aeruginosa*, etc.

E.   Anti-*Pseudomonas* penicillins are synergistic with gentamicin, tobramycin, amikacin [ie, ticarcillin (Ticar IV), mezlocillin (Mezlin IV), piperacillin (Pipracil IV)]

    1.   Active against: *Pseudomonas aeruginosa*, etc.

    2.   Drawbacks:

        a.   *Staphylococcus aureus* resistance

        b.   Penicillin hypersensitivity

        c.   Parenteral use only

Cephalosporins (Beta-Lactam Antibiotics)

The chemical relationship to penicillin probably means that patients with history of a penicillin anaphylactic reaction should avoid use of cephalosporins. However, in patients with history of penicillin rash-type reactions, cephalosporins are commonly employed.

Cephalosporins are categorized into first, second, and third generations. In general, first-generation agents are most active against gram-positive cocci, while third-generation agents are most active against gram-negative bacteria. Second-generation agents are more or less active against bacteria in each category.

A. First-generation cephalosporins
[ie, cephalexin (Keflex oral), cefadroxil (Duricef oral), cefazolin (Ancef, Kefzol, etc., IV)]
1. Active against:
   a. *Staphylococcus aureus*
   b. Streptococci and most pneumococci
   c. *Escherichia coli, Proteus, Klebsiella*
2. Drawbacks:
   a. Poor against *Haemophilus, Moraxella catarrhalis, Pseudomonas, Bacteroides*
   b. Possible penicillin anaphylaxis
   c. Many pneumococcal strains resistant

B. Second-generation cephalosporins and second-generation equivalents
[ie, cefuroxime (Ceftin oral, Zinacef IV), cefaclor (Ceclor oral), cefprozil (Cefzil oral), cefpodoxime (Vantin oral), loracarbef (Lorabid oral), cefdinir (Omnicef oral)]
1. Active against:
   a. *Haemophilus influenzae*
   b. *Moraxella catarrhalis*
   c. *Neisseria gonorrhoeae*
   d. Streptococci and most pneumococci (intermediate-level penicillin-resistant pneumococci somewhat susceptible to cefpodoxime and cefuroxime)
2. Drawbacks: Poor against *Pseudomonas, Bacteroides*
3. Many pneumococcal strains resistant
4. Poor cerebrospinal fluid (CSF) penetration (except cefuroxime)
5. Cefaclor: *Haemophilus/Moraxella* resistance, and serum sickness

C. Third-generation cephalosporins, oral
[ie, cefixime (Suprax oral), ceftibuten (Cedax oral)]
1. Active against:
   a. *Haemophilus*
   b. *Moraxella catarrhalis*
   c. *Neisseria gonorrhoeae*
2. Drawbacks:
   a. Less active against *Staphylococcus aureus*
   b. Less active against pneumococci

D. Third-generation cephalosporins, parenteral
[ie, ceftriaxone (Rocephin IV-IM), cefotaxime (Claforan IV-IM)]
1. Active against:
   a. *Haemophilus* and *Moraxella catarrhalis*
   b. *Streptococcus pneumoniae*
   c. *Neisseria meningitides*
   d. *Neisseria gonorrhoeae*
2. Advantages: High cerebrospinal fluid penetration
   [ie, ceftazidime (Fortaz, et al., IV–IM), cefepime (Maxipime IV–IM)]

3. Active against:
   a. *Pseudomonas aeruginosa,* etc.
4. High CSF penetration

Other Beta-Lactam Agents

A. Imipenem with cilastatin (Primaxin IV), meropenem (Merrem IV)
   1. Active against:
      a. *Staphylococcus aureus*
      b. *Streptococcus pyogenes* and *Streptococcus pneumoniae*
      c. *Haemophilus influenzae*
      d. *Neisseria gonorrhoeae*
      e. *Pseudomonas aeruginosa*
      f. *Escherichia coli, Klebsiella*
      g. *Bacteroides fragilis* and other anaerobes
   2. Drawbacks:
      a. Penicillin hypersensitivity
      b. Staphylococcal resistance (methicillin type)
      c. *Pseudomonas* resistance can develop (use with aminoglycoside)
B. Aztreonam (Azactam IV), suitable for penicillin-hypersensitive patients
   1. Active against:
      a. *Escherichia coli, Klebsiella, Proteus*
      b. *Pseudomonas,* etc.
      c. Gram-negative bacteria

Macrolides

A. Erythromycin (E-Mycin, ERYC, PCE, EES, etc.)
   1. Active against:
      a. *Streptococcus pyogenes* (beta hemolytic)
      b. Many *Streptococcus pneumoniae*
      c. *Staphylococcus aureus* (80%)
      d. *Haemophilus influenzae* (when combined with sulfonamides)
      e. *Mycoplasma, Legionella, Chlamydia, Corynebacterium diphtheriae, Bordetella pertussis, Clostridium tetani*
   2. Drawbacks:
      a. Many *Streptococcus pneumoniae* resistant
      b. Many *Staphylococcus aureus* resistant
      c. Nausea, cramps, vomiting
      d. Food interferes with oral use (except ethyl succinate form)
      e. Jaundice (reversible)
      f. Ototoxic (rare: ie, IV use of over 4 grams/day)
      g. Potentiates theophylline, cimetidine, digoxin, phenytoin, triazolam, warfarin, etc.
      h. Adverse interactions with terfenidine and others
B. Azithromycin (Zithromax) and clarithromycin (Biaxin)
   1. Similar activity and properties as erythromycins except:
      a. Long-acting, less nausea
      b. Azithromycin causes fewer drug interactions
      c. Clarithromycin may be taken with meals

Clindamycin (Cleocin Oral and IV)

A. Active against:
1. Anaerobic bacteria (oral, respiratory, *Bacteroides fragilis,* etc.)
2. *Staphylococcus aureus* (most strains)
3. *Streptococcus pyogenes* (beta hemolytic)
4. Most *Streptococcus pneumoniae*

B. Drawbacks:
1. Nausea, cramps, diarrhea
2. Pseudomembranous enterocolitis
3. Some *Streptococcus pneumoniae* resistant

Tetracyclines (Doxycycline Oral and Others)

A. Active against:
1. *Mycoplasma, Chlamydia, Legionella*

B. Useful against:
1. Aphthous stomatitis (as mouthwash)

C. Drawbacks:
1. Streptococci resistant (50–70%)
2. Pneumococci resistant (most)
3. *Staphylococcus aureus* resistant (most)
4. *Haemophilus* resistant (most)
5. Photosensitivity
6. Food/milk/antacid interference
7. Teeth staining and dysgenesis

(Do not administer in last half of pregnancy or to children ages 6 months to 8 years.)

Chloramphenicol (Chloromycetin)

Penetrates into cerebrospinal fluid well. Oral preparation is no longer available in the United States. Intravenous form is for treatment of life-threatening infections (ie, epiglottitis or intra-cranial spread of sinusitis/otitis media) when no alternatives are available (eg, with penicillin/cephalosporin anaphylaxis history, and when gatifloxacin or trovafloxacin is unavailable).

A. Active against:
1. *Haemophilus influenzae*
2. *Streptococcus pyogenes*
3. Many *Streptococcus pneumoniae*
4. *Neisseria meningitides*
5. Anaerobes, etc.

B. Drawbacks:
1. Many *Streptococcus pneumoniae* resistant
2. Bone marrow suppression, fatal in 1/24,000

Sulfonamides

When combined with erythromycins, penicillins, or cephalexin, can be useful treatment for acute respiratory tract infections.

A. Active against:
1. *Haemophilus influenzae*
2. *Moraxella catarrhalis*
3. Some *Streptococcus pneumoniae*

B.   Drawbacks:
   1.   Staphylococcal and streptococcal resistance
   2.   *Streptococcus pneumoniae* resistance
   3.   Rashes, hives, photosensitivity

Fluoroquinolones

A.   "Antipseudomonal" quinolones [ie, ciprofloxacin (Cipro oral, otic drops), ofloxacin (Floxin oral, otic drops)]. These are the only oral agents available for head and neck pseudomonal infections. They are potent as ototopicals and are not ototoxic.
   1.   Active against:
      a.   *Pseudomonas aeruginosa* and other gram-negative bacteria
      b.   *Haemophilus influenzae*
      c.   *Moraxella catarrhalis*
      d.   *Neisseria gonorrhoeae*
   2.   Drawbacks:
      a.   Poor against anaerobes
      b.   Poor against *Streptococcus pyogenes*
      c.   Poor against *Streptococcus pneumoniae*
      d.   Resistance develops during treatment and in communities where use is common
      e.   Potentiates theophylline (ciprofloxacin), etc., like erythromycin (see above)
      f.   Central nervous system stimulation
      g.   Antacids interfere with absorption
      h.   Not approved for children
B.   "Respiratory" quinolones [ie, levofloxacin (Levaquin oral), gatifloxacin (Tequin oral, IV), moxifloxacin (Avelox oral)]. These are active against a wide variety of respiratory pathogens, and they exhibit few drug-drug interactions.
   1.   Active against:
      a.   *Streptococcus pyogenes* (beta hemolytic)
      b.   *Streptococcus pneumoniae* (including multidrug, highly resistant strains)
      c.   *Mycoplasma, Chlamydia, Legionella*
      d.   *Staphylococcus aureus* (not methicillin-resistant)
   2.   Drawbacks: Antacids, zinc, and iron impair absorption
   3.   Not yet approved for children
   4.   Not yet approved for meningitis but probably effective (ie, trovafloxacin)

Aminoglycosides

[Ie, gentamicin (Garamycin IM/IV), tobramycin (Nebcin IM/IV), amikacin (Amikin IM/IV).] When combined with certain beta-lactam agents, these are especially effective for treatment of pseudomonal infections. Also, when combined with clindamycin, they are useful for mixed infections/prophylaxis.
   1.   Active against:
      a.   *Pseudomonas aeruginosa*
      b.   *Escherichia coli, Klebsiella, Serratia*
      c.   *Enterobacter, Proteus*
   2.   Drawbacks:
      a.   Ototoxicity
      b.   Nephrotoxicity
      c.   Not effective orally

    d.   Anaerobes resistant

    e.   Gram-positive cocci resistant

Metronidazole (Flagyl Oral and IV)

This is bactericidal against anaerobes; it may be combined with any other antibiotic for mixed infections with aerobes.

1.   Active against:

    a.   Anaerobic organisms

    b.   *Bacteroides fragilis*

    c.   *Clostridium difficile* (antibiotic-induced pseudomembranous enterocolitis)

2.   High cerebrospinal fluid penetration

3.   Drawbacks:

    a.   Inactive against aerobes such as *Staphylococcus, Streptococcus pyogenes, Streptococcus pneumoniae,* etc.

    b.   Adverse interactions with alcoholic beverages

Vancomycin (Vancocin IV)

1.   Active against:

    a.   *Staphylococcus aureus* (including methicillin-resistant)

    b.   *Streptococcus pyogenes* (beta hemolytic)

    c.   *Streptococcus pneumoniae* (multidrug, highly resistant strains)

    d.   Most other cocci

    e.   *Clostridium difficile* (antibiotic-induced enterocolitis)

2.   Drawbacks:

    a.   Ototoxic in high doses

    b.   Nephrotoxic

    c.   IV use only (except enterocolitis)

Rifampin

This is useful for prophylaxis and treatment of the carrier state of nasal/nasopharyngeal infections.

1.   Active against:

    a.   *Staphylococcus aureus*

    b.   *Streptococcus pyogenes*

    c.   *Streptococcus pneumoniae*

    d.   *Haemophilus influenzae*

    e.   *Neisseria meningitides*

    f.   *Neisseria gonorrhoeae*

    g.   *Legionella*

    h.   Anaerobes

2.   Drawbacks:

    a.   Resistance develops under therapy when used as a single agent for established infections.

Antifungal Agents

A. Amphotericin B:

    1.   Active against most systemic fungal infections (*Aspergillus, Mucor*)

    2.   Drawbacks: a. IV only; b. Nephroxicity.

B. Flucytosine: Oral against candidiasis etc.

C. Nystatin: Topical against mucosal candidiasis

    D. Miconazole: Topical against mucosal candidiasis
- a. Clotrimazole: Topical against mucosal/skin candidiasis and tenia
- b. Ketoconazole*: Oral/topical against mucosal/skin candidiasis
- c. Fluconazole*: Oral/IV against mucosal/skin candidiasis
- d. Itraconazole*: Oral against candidiasis and aspergillus
- e. Griseofulvin: Oral against dermatophytes
- f. Terbinafine: Oral against dermatophytes

Antiviral Agents (For anti-HIV agents, refer to comprehensive texts.)

    A. Acyclovir, valacyclovir, famciclovir: Oral. Active against herpes simplex and zoster infections
    B. Amantadine (Symmetrel oral): Active against influenza A
    C. Rimantadine (Flumadine oral): Active against influenza A
    D. Oseltamivir (Tamiflu oral): Active against influenza A and B
    E. Zanamivir (Relenza inhale): Active against influenza A and B

TREATMENT OPTIONS AND RECOMMENDATIONS

Acute Otitis Media

Acute otitis media may be viral, but the following bacterial pathogens should be considered and treated:

Streptococcus pneumoniae accounts for 25% of cases. It is the most virulent pathogen, is invasive, and leads to most complications of otitis media, including mastoiditis. It resolves without proper antibiotic therapy in less than 20%. Resistance to penicillin, amoxicillin, cephalosporins, macrolides (erythromycins), and clindamycin is increasing.

Haemophilus influenzae accounts for 20 to 25% of cases. Half of them will resolve without antibiotics. About 40% of strains are resistant to amoxicillin and first-generation cephalosporins. Most are resistant to the macrolides or clindamycin.

Moraxella catarrhalis accounts for 10 to 25% of cases. Over 80% of them will resolve without antibiotics. *Moraxella catarrhalis* is almost always resistant to amoxicillin, first-generation cephalosporins, erythromycin, and clindamycin.

Drug Choices

Over half of acute otitis media cases will resolve without antibiotics (or with antibiotic choices that are illogical). But well-chosen antibiotics help to relieve pain and to prevent hearing loss and mastoiditis. The following can be recommended:

1. Amoxicillin is low in cost and treats most cases, but many of the above pathogens are resistant.
2. Erythromycin (or clindamycin) for nonresistant pneumococcus—plus a sulfonamide for *Haemophilus* and *Moraxella catarrhalis*—is a low-cost alternative for penicillin-allergic patients.

The following alternatives are preferred if resistances are prevalent in the community or if amoxicillin fails to bring improvement in 5 days:

1. Augmented amoxicillin: Amoxicillin (enhanced dose) for pneumococci (intermediate-level resistance) plus clavulanate for *Haemophilus* and *Moraxella catarrhalis*

---

*Avoid concurrent use with terfenadine, phenytoin, triazolam, oral anticoagulants, etc., and many other drugs.[1]

2. Cefuroxime or cefpodoxime for pneumococci (intermediate-level resistance) and other pathogens
3. Ceftriaxone (three injections) for resistant pneumococci, *Haemophilus,* and *Moraxella catarrhalis*
4. Gatifloxacin or moxifloxacin (in adults) for multidrug highly resistant pneumococci, *Haemophilus,* and *Moraxella catarrhalis*

Chronic Suppurative Otitis Media

Chronic suppurative otitis media (with perforation) requires treatment for *Pseudomonas aeruginosa, Staphylococcus aureus,* and occasionally anaerobic bacteria. Choices include:

1. Ciprofloxacin or ofloxacin (as ear drops)
2. Ciprofloxacin (oral)
3. Clindamycin (if anaerobes or staphylococci are present)

Acute Otitis Externa

Acute otitis externa requires treatment for *Pseudomonas aeruginosa* and occasionally *Staphylococcus aureus.* Choices include:

1. Ciprofloxacin or ofloxacin (ear drops)
2. Neomycin/polymyxin (ear drops)
3. Gentamicin (eye/ear drops)
4. Oral ciprofloxacin, cephalexin, or clindamycin

Acute Rhinosinusitis

Acute rhinosinusitis (unless of dental origin) is caused by the same organisms as in acute otitis media. Likewise, many cases resolve without antibiotics. But for relief of pain and avoidance of complications, similar drug choices are recommended:

1. Amoxicillin
2. Augmented amoxicillin (high-dose amoxicillin)
3. Cefuroxime or cefpodoxime
4. Erythromycin (or clarithromycin) plus sulfonamide
5. Clindamycin plus sulfonamide
6. Ceftriaxone (IM)
7. Gatifloxacin or moxifloxacin or levofloxacin (in adults)

Acute Sinusitis with Orbital/CNS Extension

Acute sinusitis with orbital/CNS extension requires treatment for the same organisms as those named above but with intravenous agents that penetrate the blood-brain barrier:

1. Ceftriaxone
2. Trovafloxacin or gatifloxacin
3. Vancomycin plus either meropenem or aztreonam

Chronic Rhinosinusitis

Chronic rhinosinusitis is generally a mixed infection that includes a number of anaerobic organisms and often *Staphylococcus aureus.* Acute exacerbations of chronic sinusitis may be caused by the aerobic organisms of acute sinusitis. *Pseudomonas* predominates in patients with nasal/sinus polyps (eg, cystic fibrosis and asthma/aspirin-allergy patients).

Noninvasive fungal disease is also common.

Treatment options include the following:

1. Augmented amoxicillin
2. Clindamycin
3. Metronidazole plus cephalexin
4. Ciprofloxacin (if polyps)
5. Itraconazole (if fungus)

Tonsillitis

Tonsillitis in acute stages may be predominantly a *Streptococcus pyogenes* infection. But other bacteria are often present as copathogens that are resistant to penicillin, rendering it ineffective. Epstein-Barr (infectious mononucleosis) and other viruses do not respond to antibiotics, but secondary infection with mixed anaerobic/aerobic bacteria improves with antibiotic therapy. Amoxicillin given to a mononucleosis patient will likely cause a rash. The following agents are useful in both acute and chronic tonsillitis:

1. Cephalexin with metronidazole
2. Clindamycin (eg, if mononucleosis or abscess)
3. Augmented amoxicillin (if not mononucleosis)

Deep Neck Abscess

Deep neck abscess is generally a mixed anaerobic infection. Treatment decisions are made empirically or on the basis of a Gram's stain of pus, since anaerobes grow so slowly. Choices include the following:

1. Augmented ampicillin/amoxicillin
2. Clindamycin
3. Metronidazole plus either cefazolin or cephalexin

Add gentamicin, tobramycin, or amikacin to any of the above for necrotizing abscesses.

Pharyngitis

Pharyngitis may be viral, but 30% of cases in wintertime North America are from *Streptococcus pyogenes* (beta hemolytic). Other streptococcus strains also cause symptomatic sore throat, as do *Mycoplasma, Chlamydia,* and gonococcal organisms, all of which yield negative "strep" cultures. Therapeutic choices include the following:

1. Erythromycin or clarithromycin
2. Cephalexin
3. Penicillin (but copathogens give resistance)

For gonococcal infection, assume coexisting *Chlamydia* and treat with ceftriaxone (or cefixime) plus either doxycycline or erythromycin or azithromycin.

Tracheobronchitis

Tracheobronchitis is usually viral, but a long, persistent cough may be caused by *Mycoplasma, Chlamydia, Bordetella pertussis, Haemophilus,* or pneumococcal organisms. Treatment may include the following:

For viral:	Amantadine, zanamivir, oseltamivir, etc.
For bacterial:	Erythromycin (or clarithromycin) plus sulfonamide
	Doxycycline plus sulfonamide
	Levofloxacin or gatifloxacin or moxifloxacin

Laryngitis

Laryngitis is usually viral, but sometimes the same bacteria listed above for tracheobron-chitis can be involved. Treatment options are the same:

1. Symptomatic care
2. Erythromycin (or clarithromycin) plus sulfonamide
3. Doxycycline plus sulfonamide
4. Levofloxacin (or gatifloxacin or moxifloxacin)

Croup

Croup (subglottic) is generally a viral infection, but 10% of cases (especially protracted ones) are secondarily infected with *Staphylococcus aureus*. *Haemophilus* would be less likely. Choose from the following:

1. Augmented ampicillin/amoxicillin
2. Cefuroxime or ceftriaxone
3. Erythromycin (or clarithromycin) plus sulfonamide
4. Gatifloxacin or trovafloxacin (if penicillin anaphylaxis history)

Epiglottitis

Epiglottitis is almost always caused by *Haemophilus influenzae*. Treatment for it would also cover the rarer pathogens. Choices are as follows:

1. Ampicillin/sulbactam
2. Ceftriaxone or cefuroxime
3. Gatifloxacin or trovafloxacin (if penicillin anaphylaxis history)

Prophylaxis for Surgery

1. For skin incisions, treat against *Staphylococcus aureus:* cefazolin or clindamycin.
2. For mucosal incisions, treat against anaerobes: clindamycin or ampicillin/sulbactam.
3. For major head/neck surgery, treat against *Staphylococcus aureus,* anaerobes, and *Pseudomonas:* clindamycin plus gentamicin.
4. For open pharyngeal wounds, treat against anaerobes: amoxicillin suspension (eg, tonsillectomy).

References

1. *The Sanford Guide to Antimicrobial Therapy 2001.* Also, *The Sanford Guide to HIV/AIDS.* Antimicrobial Therapy, Inc., PO Box 70, Hyde Park, VT 05655.
2. *The Medical Letter Handbook of Antimicrobial Therapy.* Medical Letter, Inc., 56 Harrison Street, New Rochelle, NY 10801.
3. Johnson JT, Yu VL, eds. *Infectious Diseases and Antimicrobial Therapy of the Ears, Nose, and Throat.* Philadelphia: Saunders, 1997.
4. Fairbanks DNF. *Pocket Guide to Antimicrobial Therapy in Otolaryngology—Head and Neck Surgery,* 10th ed. American Academy of Otolaryngology–Head and Neck Surgery, One Prince Street, Alexandria, VA 22314-3357.

Neck Spaces and Fascial Planes 21

The morbidity and mortality rates of deep neck infections have improved dramatically since the appearance of classic monographs on the subject by Grodinsky and Holyoke[1] in 1938 and Beck[2] in the 1940s and 1950s. Knowledge of the neck spaces and fascial relationships is a prerequisite to understanding the etiology, symptoms, complications, and treatment of deep neck infections. The fascia invests muscles and organs, thus forming planes and spaces that direct and limit the spread of the infection. Infection of certain of the cervical spaces is considered life-threatening. These spaces include the submandibular, lateral pharyngeal, and retropharyngeal-danger-prevertebral spaces. Infections in these spaces exert fatal effect by either local airway occlusion or extension to vital areas, such as the mediastinum or carotid sheath. Infections involving other deep spaces become dangerous only as they spread into the above-mentioned spaces.

TRIANGLES OF THE NECK

See Figure 21-1.

Anterior Cervical Triangle

1. Boundaries

Superior:	mandible
Anterior:	midline
Posterior:	sternocleidomastoid

2. Subordinate triangles
    a. Submaxillary (digastric) triangle

Superior:	mandible
Anterior:	anterior belly of digastric
Posterior:	posterior belly of digastric

    b. Carotid triangle

Superior:	posterior belly of digastric
Anterior:	superior belly of omohyoid
Posterior:	sternocleidomastoid

    c. Muscular triangle

Superior:	superior belly of omohyoid
Anterior:	midline
Posterior:	sternocleidomastoid

    d. Submental (suprahyoid) triangle

Superior:	symphysis of mandible
Inferior:	hyoid bone
Lateral:	anterior belly of digastric

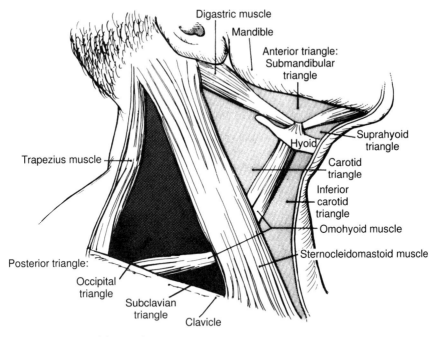

Figure 21-1.   Triangles of the neck.

Posterior Cervical Triangle

1.   Boundaries

    Anterior: sternocleidomastoid
    Posterior: trapezius
    Inferior: clavicle

2.   Subordinate triangles
    a.   Occipital triangle

    Anterior: sternocleidomastoid
    Posterior: trapezius
    Inferior: omohyoid

    b.   Subclavian triangle

    Superior: omohyoid
    Inferior: clavicle
    Anterior: sternocleidomastoid

FASCIAL PLANES OF THE NECK

    See Figure 21-2.

Superficial Cervical Fascia

1.   Envelopes
    a.   Platysma
    b.   Muscles of facial expression

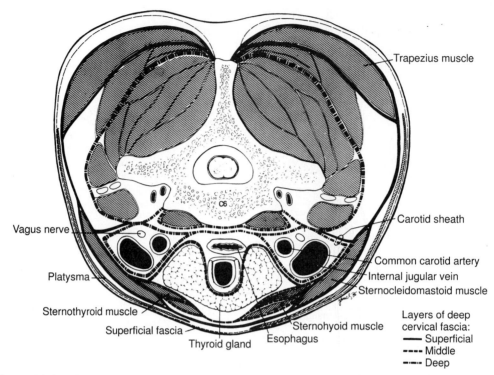

Figure 21-2.   Fascial planes of the neck. *(Adapted from Paonessa DF, Goldstein JG.* Otolaryngol Clin North Am. *1978;9:561.)*

2.   Boundaries

Superior: zygoma
Inferior: clavicle

Platysma is supplied by the cervical branch of the facial nerve and protects the mandibular branch of the facial nerve, which lies deep to it. Deep to the superficial cervical fascia and platysma lies a well-defined potential fascial space that separates the superficial fascia from deep cervical fascia. This space allows free movement of the skin and superficial fascia on deeper structures, and it also serves as an excellent cleavage plane during dissection.

Deep Cervical Fascia

1.   Superficial layer—investing fascia
    a.   Envelopes
        (1)   Trapezius, sternocleidomastoid, strap muscles
        (2)   Submandibular and parotid glands
        (3)   Muscles of mastication: masseter, pterygoids, temporalis
    b.   Boundaries

Superior: mandible and zygoma
Inferior: clavicle, acromion, spine of scapula

Anterior: hyoid bone

Posterior: mastoid process, superior nuchal line, cervical vertebrae

Superficial layer of deep cervical fascia outlines masticator space superiorly, forms stylomandibular ligament posteriorly, and splits to form suprasternal space of Burns anteroinferiorly.

2.   Middle layer—visceral fascia
    a.   Envelopes
        (1)   Pharynx, larynx, trachea, esophagus
        (2)   Thyroid and parathyroid glands
        (3)   Buccinator and constrictor muscles of the pharynx
        (4)   Strap muscles of the neck: sternohyoid, sternothyroid, thyrohyoid, and omohyoid
    b.   Boundaries

Superior: base of skull

Inferior: mediastinum

Middle layer of deep cervical fascia forms pretracheal fascia, which overlies the trachea and buccopharyngeal fascia, which lies in the pharyngeal wall. Buccopharyngeal fascia forms a midline raphe in the posterior midline, which adheres to the prevertebral fascia, and a pterygomandibular raphe in the lateral pharynx.

3.   Deep layer—prevertebral fascia
    a.   Envelopes
        (1)   Paraspinous muscles
        (2)   Cervical vertebrae
    b.   Boundaries

Superior: base of skull

Inferior: chest

Deep layer of deep cervical fascia comprises two layers: The prevertebral layer lies just anterior to the bodies of the vertebrae from the base of the skull to the coccyx and laterally attaches to transverse processes of cervical vertebrae; the alar layer lies between the prevertebral layer of deep fascia and the visceral layer of middle fascia and extends from the base of the skull to the mediastinum.

4.   Carotid sheath fascia (Figure 21-3)
    a.   Envelopes
        (1)   Common carotid artery
        (2)   Internal jugular vein
        (3)   Vagus nerve
    b.   Boundaries

Superior: base of skull

Inferior: thorax

This is a pipe-like fibrous sheath composed of all three deep fascial layers: investing, visceral, and prevertebral; it is a potential avenue for infection spread, called "The Lincoln Highway of the Neck."

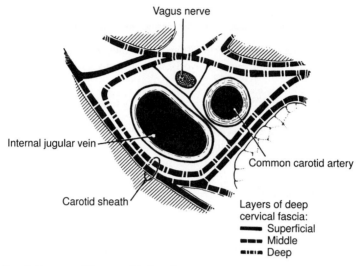

Figure 21-3. Fascial layers of the carotid sheath.

NECK SPACES

Lateral Pharyngeal Space (Pharyngomaxillary Space)

This is a cone-shaped space with its base at the base of the skull, petrous portion of temporal bone, and its apex at the hyoid bone. See Table 21-1.

1. Boundaries

Superior: base of skull
Inferior: hyoid bone
Anterior: pterygomandibular raphe
Posterior: prevertebral fascia
Medial: superior constrictor
Lateral: parotid gland, mandible, lateral pterygoid

2. Contents: styloid process divides this space into two compartments
   a. Prestyloid compartment—muscular (anterior to styloid process)
      (1) Fat
      (2) Lymph nodes

TABLE 21-1. COMPARISON OF PERITONSILLAR AND LATERAL PHARYNGEAL SPACE INFECTIONS

Parameter	Peritonsillar Infection	Lateral Pharyngeal Space Infection
Trismus	Not as pronounced	Marked
Parotid involvement	Minimal	More commonly affected (deep lobe)
Sepsis	Low-grade fever	Fever and sepsis more common
Soft palate	Edematous	Often normal
Tonsil	Acute exudate	Often normal

After Beck A. Deep neck infection. Ann Otol Rhinol Laryngol *1947;56:439.*

        (3)   Internal maxillary artery

        (4)   Inferior alveolar, lingual, auriculotemporal nerves

  b. Poststyloid compartment—neurovascular (posterior to styloid process)

        (1)   Carotid artery

        (2)   Internal jugular vein

        (3)   Sympathetic chain

        (4)   IX, X, XI, XII nerves (XI nerve courses posterolaterally after leaving the jugular foramen and is not involved to any extent in lateral pharyngeal space infections)

3. Infection

  a. Source

        (1)   Tonsils: every peritonsillar space abscess is a potential pharyngomaxillary space abscess

        (2)   Pharynx

        (3)   Teeth: most commonly from third mandibular molar; mandibular dental abscesses are notorious for their ability to spread to submandibular and lateral pharyngeal spaces

        (4)   Petrous portion of temporal bone

        (5)   Parotid gland (deep lobe)

        (6)   Lymph nodes draining nose and pharynx

  b. Pathway of spread

        (1)   Direct extension from communicating spaces: parotid, submandibular, retropharyngeal, masticator, and carotid sheath spaces

        (2)   Extension from peritonsillar abscess via direct dissection through pharyngeal wall, lymphatic spread, perivascular extension, or septic thrombosis of the peritonsillar veins

  c. Manifestations

        (1)   Medial displacement of lateral pharyngeal wall and tonsil

        (2)   Trismus: indicates infection of anterior compartment with involvement of muscles of mastication

        (3)   Parotid edema

        (4)   Retromandibular neck fullness

        (5)   Dysphagia

  d. Treatment

        (1)   External drainage through the submaxillary fossa with major vessel control; find the carotid sheath and follow it to all areas of pus in the neck, since all three layers of the deep cervical fascia enter into the formation of this sheath; lateral pharyngeal space abscess should never be approached via an intraoral route

        (2)   Tracheostomy

  e. Complications

        (1)   Septic thrombosis of the internal jugular vein: the most common complication

            (a)   Clinical features: shaking chills, spiking fever, prostration, tenderness at the mandibular angle or along the sternocleidomastoid

            (b)   Diagnosis: angiography or computed tomography (CT) scan; Tobey–Ayer test confirms jugular vein thrombosis when lumbar puncture is

done to monitor cerebrospinal fluid (CSF) pressure, occlusion of throm-
bosed vein gives no change in CSF pressure, occlusion of the contralateral vein causes marked elevation of CSF pressure

(c) Treatment: intravenous antibiotics—2 to 3 weeks; vein ligation (no
longer widely recommended); heparin therapy (controversial)

(d) Consequences: bacteremia in 50% of cases, septic pulmonary emboli,
suppurative subclavian phlebitis, lateral sinus thrombosis, cavernous
sinus thrombosis, brain abscess, metastatic abscesses

(2) Carotid artery erosion: the most common fatal complication with mortality
rate of 20 to 40% irrespective of treatment[3]

Frequency of bleed[4]

Internal carotid artery	49%
Common carotid artery	9%
External carotid artery	4%
Miscellaneous	14%

(a) Clinical features

(i) Sentinel bleeds: recurrent small hemorrhages from nose, mouth, or
ear. The extravasation of blood into tissues is most likely secondary
to arterial erosion. Venous erosion usually causes thrombosis

(ii) Protracted clinical course

(iii) Hematoma in surrounding tissues

(iv) Onset of shock

(v) Persistent peritonsillar swelling after peritonsillar abscess resolution

(vi) Ipsilateral Horner syndrome

(vii) Unexplained IX to XII cranial nerve palsies

(b) Diagnosis: angiography to localize the bleed and assess collateral flow

(c) Treatment: sentinel pharyngeal bleeding is an acute emergency, necessitating external drainage and major vessel ligation. Common carotid
artery ligation usually controls hemorrhage, but ligation of the external
carotid artery may also be required if bleeding is from the internal maxillary artery. Ligation of the common carotid artery lowers pressure in
both internal and external carotid arteries, with lower morbidity than ligation of the internal carotid artery secondary to backflow.[3]

(3) Cranial nerve involvement: Horner syndrome (cervical sympathetic chain);
hoarseness (X nerve); tongue paresis (XII nerve). The spinal accessory nerve
runs deeper and is rarely compromised.

(4) Mediastinitis: infection spread along carotid sheath

Pterygopalatine (Pterygomaxillary) Fossa

Pterygopalatine fossa is in open communication laterally via sphenomaxillary fissure with
the infratemporal fossa.

1. Boundaries

Superior:	orbital apex, sphenoid and palatine bones
Anterior:	posterior wall of maxillary antrum

Posterior: pterygoid process, greater wing of sphenoid
Medial: palatine bone, nasal mucoperiosteum
Lateral: temporalis muscle

2. Contents
   a. Maxillary nerve
   b. Sphenopalatine ganglion
   c. Internal maxillary artery
3. Infection
   a. Source
      (1) Maxillary molar teeth, especially the third molar
      (2) Osteomyelitis of the maxilla in infants
   b. Pathway of spread: cellulitis of the upper molar gingiva extends to the ptery-gopalatine, then to the infratemporal and temporal fossae
   c. Manifestations
      (1) Painful swelling of gingiva
      (2) Cellulitis of the entire side of the head: cheek, nose, auricle, upper neck, temporalis muscle
      (3) Eye: lid swelling with complete closure, globe proptosis and fixation or abducens paralysis
      (4) Severe trismus (distinguishes accompanying orbital involvement from orbital cellulitis or abscess)
      (5) Secondary maxillary sinus infection
   d. Treatment—external drainage through:
      (1) Alveobuccal sulcus above third molar with tunnel dissected posteriorly, superiorly, and medially around tuberosity of maxilla leading to pterygopalatine fossa via sphenomaxillary fissure
      (2) Caldwell–Luc with removal of posterior wall of antrum and direct exposure of pterygopalatine fossa

Masticator Space

1. Boundary: subperiosteal space between mandible and its periosteal covering
2. Contents
   a. Masseter muscle
   b. External and internal pterygoid muscles
   c. Ramus and posterior body of the mandible
   d. Tendon of insertion of temporalis muscle
   e. Inferior alveolar nerve
   f. Internal maxillary artery
3. Infection
   a. Source: molar teeth (most commonly the third molar)
   b. Manifestations
      (1) Extreme trismus
      (2) Edema and tenderness over the posterior ramus of the mandible
   c. Treatment: external drainage below the horizontal ramus of the mandible with incision carried down to the periosteum of the mandible

Parotid Space

1. Contents
   a. Parotid gland
   b. Facial nerve
   c. External carotid artery
   d. Posterior facial vein
2. Infection
   a. Source: parotid gland
   b. Manifestations: marked swelling of the angle of the jaw without associated trismus or pharyngeal swelling
   c. Treatment: external drainage via standard parotidectomy incision
3. Complications: the medial parotid space communicates directly with the pharyngomaxillary space; passage of infections into the pharyngomaxillary space and then into the mediastinum is one of the complications of parotitis

Peritonsillar Space

1. Contents: loose connective tissue lying between the capsule of the fascial tonsil medially and the superior constrictor muscle laterally (see Table 21-1).
2. Infection
   a. Source: tonsils, pharynx
   b. Manifestations:
      (1) Dysphagia, odynophagia
      (2) Drooling
      (3) Muffled voice ("hot potato" voice)
      (4) Referred otalgia
      (5) Trismus (not as pronounced as in lateral pharyngeal space infection)
      (6) Tonsil displaced toward midline, forward, and downward
      (7) Uvular deviation across midline to opposite side
   c. Treatment: peroral drainage through upper half of anterior tonsillar pillar
   d. Complications: spread into pharyngomaxillary space through posterior pharyngeal wall (following drainage of peritonsillar abscess the tonsils should be removed)

Submandibular Space

See Figure 21-4.

1. Boundaries

Superior:	mucosa of the floor of mouth
Inferior:	digastric
Anterior:	mylohyoid and anterior belly of digastric
Posterior:	posterior belly of digastric and stylomandibular ligament
Medial:	hyoglossus and mylohyoid
Lateral:	skin, platysma, mandible

2. Contents—the mylohyoid muscle divides the submandibular space into:
   a. Sublingual (supramylohyoid) space (superior)
      (1) Sublingual gland

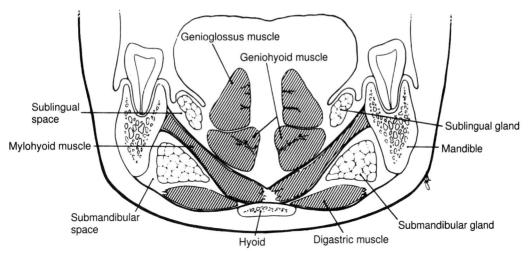

Figure 21-4. Division of the submandibular space into supramylohyoid and inframylohyoid spaces by the mylohyoid muscle. *(Adapted from Hollingshead WH. Fascia and fascial spaces of the head and neck. In: Hollingshead WH, ed. Anatomy for Surgeons, Head and Neck. Vol. I. Philadelphia: Harper & Row, 1982, 269–289.)*

  b. Submaxillary (inframylohyoid) space (inferior)
    (1) Submandibular gland
    (2) Lymph nodes
  Submaxillary space is in continuity with sublingual space along the posterior edge of the mylohyoid muscle. The submandibular gland lies within both spaces.
  3. Infection
    a. Source
      (1) Teeth (majority of infections): The relation of the apices of the teeth to the mylohyoid line determines the most likely spread of odontogenic infection. Anterior to the second molar, the sublingual space is initially involved, as the tooth apices lie superior to this line. Infections involving the second and third molars initially affect the submandibular or lateral pharyngeal space, as their roots extend to below the mylohyoid line.
      (2) Salivary glands
      (3) Pharynx and tonsils
      (4) Sinuses
    b. Pathway: direct extension and lymphatic spread
    c. Manifestations
      (1) Dysphagia
      (2) Odynophagia
    d. Treatment
      (1) Treatment of underlying pathology
      (2) External drainage if it progresses
        (a) Sublingual space: intraoral drainage if infection localizes in the floor of mouth above the mylohyoid muscle; avoid the posterior lateral region of the floor of mouth, which contains lingual artery, vein, and nerve

        (b)   Submandibular space: external drainage via transverse incision below the body of the mandible

   e.   Complications: Ludwig's angina[5] is a severe infection involving the floor of the mouth and the submental and submandibular spaces. It spreads through fascial planes and not by way of lymphatics. Typical history includes dental extraction followed by localized inflammation. Involvement of the floor of the mouth follows, with swelling and displacement of the tongue superiorly and posteriorly against the palate, causing respiratory embarrassment. Infection then spreads around the mylohyoid muscle to involve the submandibular space. Once the infection penetrates the mylohyoid muscle, symptoms progress at a rapid rate, with marked trismus, odynophagia, and hard and woody induration in the neck. Sepsis and dehydration ensue. It may progress to airway obstruction. Treatment is with intravenous antibiotics, tracheostomy, and wide external drainage. Maintenance of proper airway is of the utmost importance in the treatment of Ludwig's angina. Asphyxia is the most frequent cause of death in this disease.

Carotid Sheath Space

See Figure 21-3.

  1. Boundaries

Anterior:	sternocleidomastoid
Posterior:	prevertebral space
Medial:	visceral space
Lateral:	sternocleidomastoid

  2. Contents
    a.   Carotid artery
    b.   Internal jugular vein
    c.   X nerve
  3. Infection
    a.   Source
        (1)   Lateral pharyngeal space
        (2)   Submandibular space
        (3)   Visceral space (contamination by esophageal perforation, tracheotomy, thyroidectomy)
    b.   Pathway: local invasion from adjacent fascial spaces
    c.   Manifestations
        (1)   Pitting edema over sternocleidomastoid
        (2)   Torticollis [tortus (twisted) + collum (neck)]: neck contraction with the head turned to the normal side and chin rotated to the diseased side
    d.   Treatment
        (1)   External drainage
        (2)   Intravenous antibiotics
        (3)   Possible ligation of internal jugular vein
    e.   Complications
        (1)   Septic shock (indicates phlebitis or thrombosis of jugular vein)
        (2)   Carotid artery erosion

(3) Endocarditis

(4) Cavernous sinus thrombosis

Visceral Space

See Figure 21-5.

1. Boundaries

Superior: hyoid bone
Inferior: mediastinum
Anterior: superficial layer of deep cervical fascia
Posterior: retropharyngeal space, prevertebral space
Lateral: parapharyngeal space, carotid fascia

2. Contents
    a. Pharynx
    b. Esophagus
    c. Larynx
    d. Trachea
    e. Thyroid gland
3. Infection
    a. Source
        (1) Tonsils
        (2) Esophageal injury (foreign body, iatrogenic)
        (3) Blunt laryngeal trauma with mucosal tear
        (4) Acute thyroiditis
        (5) Chest infection

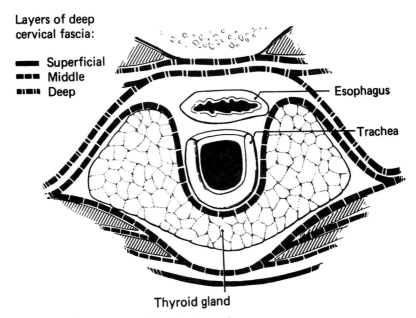

Figure 21-5. Fascial layers surrounding the visceral space.

b. Pathway of spread: direct extension from parapharyngeal or prevertebral space; from pharynx, esophagus, or larynx; from thyroid or chest
c. Manifestations
    (1) Dysphagia
    (2) Odynophagia
    (3) Hoarseness
    (4) Dyspnea
    (5) Emphysema
d. Treatment
    (1) Fasting
    (2) Intravenous hydration
    (3) Antibiotics
    (4) Tracheotomy
    (5) Surgical drainage through transverse incision along anterior border of sternocleidomastoid muscle; carotid sheath is retracted laterally; larynx, trachea, and esophagus retracted medially
e. Complications
    (1) Infections of this space are always serious because of possible extension into anterior and/or posterior mediastinum
    (2) Laryngeal edema
    (3) Mediastinal emphysema
    (4) Bronchopneumonia
    (5) Sepsis

Retropharyngeal (Retrovisceral) Space

See Figure 21-6.

1. Boundaries

    Superior: base of skull
    Inferior: superior mediastinum; tracheal bifurcation (T4); middle layer of deep cervical fascia fuses with alar layer of deep cervical fascia
    Anterior: pharynx and esophagus (middle layer of deep cervical fascia—buccopharyngeal fascia)
    Posterior: alar fascia
    Lateral: carotid sheath

    The terminology and precise division of the spaces located posterior to the viscera are controversial and confusing. The retropharyngeal space refers to the lymph node–containing space that lies anterior to the alar fascia and posterior to the pharynx and esophagus. Just posterior to this space is the potential space, which lies between the alar fascia anteriorly and the prevertebral fascia posteriorly. It was termed the danger space or space 4 by Grodinsky and Holyoke.[1] It is an area of loose connective tissue that extends from the base of the skull to the diaphragm. Although some refer to this as the prevertebral space, that name should be reserved for the space bounded anteriorly by the prevertebral fascia and posteriorly by the vertebral bodies (Table 21-2 and Figure 21-6).

2. Contents
    a. Lymph nodes
    b. Connective tissue

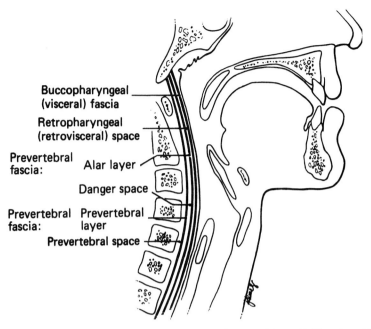

Figure 21-6. Fascial layers of the retrovisceral space. *(Adapted from Hollingshead WH. Fascia and fascial spaces of the head and neck. In: Hollingshead WH, ed.* Anatomy for Surgeons, Head and Neck. *Vol. I. Philadelphia: Harper & Row, 1982, 269–289.)*

3. Infection
   a. Source
      (1) Nose
      (2) Sinuses
      (3) Adenoids
      (4) Nasopharynx
   b. Pathway of spread
      (1) Direct spread from lateral pharyngeal space
      (2) Lymphatic spread from primary source to involve retropharyngeal lymph nodes

TABLE 21-2. COMPARISON OF THE THREE POSTVISCERAL SPACES

Space	Boundaries				Contents
	Anterior	*Posterior*	*Superior*	*Inferior*	
Retrovisceral	Buccopharyngeal fascia	Alar fascia	Skull base	Mediastinum	Lymph nodes; connective tissue
Danger	Alar fascia	Prevertebral fascia	Skull base	Diaphragm	Areolar tissue
Prevertebral	Prevertebral fascia	Vertebrae	Skull base fascia	Coccyx	Connective tissue; longus colli

The greatest number of retropharyngeal lymph nodes are found in children under age 4 and account for the relatively greater incidence of retropharyngeal abscesses in this age group. In adults, infection of this space is rare and most often is secondary to trauma.

   c. Manifestations
     (1) Seen primarily in infants and young children as a complication of acute upper respiratory infections
     (2) Odynophagia and dysphagia
     (3) Drooling and difficulty in expelling secretions
     (4) Cervical rigidity: neck is held rigid and tilted toward the uninvolved side
     (5) "Hot potato" voice
     (6) Dyspnea
     (7) Unilateral bulging of posterior pharyngeal wall: midline raphe formed by superior constrictor is attached to prevertebral fascia, therefore abscess is unilateral
     (8) Sepsis
   d. Treatment
     (1) Fasting
     (2) Intravenous antibiotics
     (3) Tracheotomy
     (4) Emergent surgical drainage:
       (a) Peroral drainage through posterior pharyngeal wall when abscess is caught early and is not complicated by respiratory obstruction.
       (b) External drainage with transverse incision along anterior or posterior border of sternocleidomastoid muscle. Abscess is opened between carotid sheath, which lies laterally, and inferior constrictor muscle, which lies medially.
   e. Complications
     (1) Rupture of abscess with aspiration and pneumonia
     (2) Mediastinitis characterized by chest pain, severe dyspnea, persistent fever, and x-ray evidence of a widened mediastinum (retropharyngeal space abscess is most likely source of mediastinitis originating in the neck)[6]
     (3) Airway obstruction

Danger Space

See Figure 21-6.

1. Boundaries

Superior:	base of skull
Inferior:	diaphragm
Anterior:	alar fascia
Posterior:	prevertebral fascia
Lateral:	transverse processes of vertebrae

2. Contents: loose areolar tissue
3. Infection
   a. Source
     (1) Retropharyngeal space
     (2) Prevertebral space
     (3) Lateral pharyngeal space

b.   Pathway of spread: direct extension from adjoining spaces
c.   Manifestations
    (1)   Same as primary space infection
    (2)   Severe sepsis should mediastinal involvement ensue
d.   Treatment: same as for primary space infection
e.   Complications—the term "danger space" refers to:
    (1)   The potential for rapid spread through the loose areolar tissue of this space
    (2)   The inferior spread to involve the posterior mediastinum to the level of the diaphragm

Prevertebral Space

See Figure 21-6.

1.   Boundaries

Superior:	base of skull
Inferior:	coccyx
Anterior:	prevertebral fascia
Posterior:	vertebral bodies
Lateral:	transverse processes of vertebrae

2.   Contents: dense areolar tissue forming a very compact space
3.   Infection: acute infections are relatively uncommon and much less frequent than those involving more anteriorly located spaces. Prior to good antitubercular therapy, abscesses in this space were common and most often due to direct extension from tuberculosis in the cervical vertebrae.
    a.   Source
        (1)   Vertebral bodies
        (2)   Penetrating injuries
    b.   Pathway of spread
        (1)   Direct extension from vertebral bodies or from adjacent neck spaces
        (2)   Tuberculosis of the spine may break through and form cold abscess (cervical Pott's abscess)
    c.   Manifestations
        (1)   Midline abscess (to differentiate from retropharyngeal abscess, which is usually unilateral)
        (2)   Cold abscess posterior to the pharynx from tuberculosis of the spine; vertebral body erosion, chronically ill patient, lymphocytosis, low-grade fever
        (3)   Suppuration in this space usually does not spread rapidly in any direction because of the compactness of this compartment
    d.   Treatment
        (1)   Needle aspiration with subsequent antituberculosis therapy
        (2)   Stabilization of spine
    e.   Complications
        (1)   Progression of vertebral process may lead to spine instability

MICROBIOLOGY OF NECK SPACE INFECTIONS

Common microorganisms in neck space infections:

1. *Staphylococcus aureus*
2. *Streptococcus pyogenes*
3. *Peptostreptococcus*
4. *Bacteroides melaninogenicus*
5. *Fusobacterium*

Bacteroides melaninogenicus may be related to a fetid odor in odontogenic infections.[7] Polymicrobial infections are the rule; Bartlett and Gorbach[8] cultured more than five microorganisms per case.

Actinomyces can cause deep neck infection that does not stay within fascial compartments but spreads indiscriminately across fascial planes. *Actinomyces* often resides in the tonsillar crypts and gingivodental sulci. Teeth can be the origin of infection. *Actinomyces* is a bacterium, although for many years it was considered a fungus; it is a Gram-positive bacillus that often branches, giving it a fungal appearance. The hallmark of actinomycosis is a chronic granuloma with sulfur granules. Diagnosis is best made by biopsy, since the bacillus is fastidious and hard to grow. Penicillin is the drug of choice and should be given for 6 to 12 months.

References

1. Grodinsky M, Holyoke E. The fascia and fascial spaces of the head and neck and adjacent regions. *Am J Anat* 1938;63:367.
2. Beck A. Deep neck infection. *Ann Otol Rhinol Laryngol* 1947;56:439.
3. Alexander D, Leonard J, Trail M. Vascular complications of deep neck abscesses. *Laryngoscope* 1968;78:361.
4. Salinger S. Hemorrhage from pharyngeal and peritonsillar abscess. *Laryngoscope* 1934;44:765.
5. Von Ludwig FW. *Medicinisches Correspondez Blait des Wurttem Bergischen Arztuchien Vereins.* 1836;6:32.
6. Pearse HE Jr. Mediastinitis following cervical suppuration. *Ann Surg* 1938;108:588.
7. Griffee MB, et al. The relationship of *Bacteroides melaninogenicus* to symptoms associated with pupal necrosis. *Oral Surg* 1980;50:457.
8. Bartlett JG, Gorbach SL. Anaerobic infections of the head and neck. *Otolaryngol Clin North Am* 1976;9:655.

Bibliography

Scully RF, Galdabini JJ, McNeely BU. Case records of the Massachusetts General Hospital: Weekly clinicopathological exercises. *N Engl J Med* 1978;298:894.

The Oral Cavity, Pharynx, and Esophagus

NORMAL ANATOMY

Oral Cavity

Boundaries: Vermilion border to junction of hard and soft palate and circumvallate papillae (linea terminalis).

Subunits: Include lip, buccal mucosa, upper and lower alveolar ridges, retromolar trigones, oral tongue (anterior to circumvallate papillae), hard palate, and floor of mouth.

Oropharynx

Boundaries: From junction of hard and soft palate and circumvallate papillae to valleculae (plane of hyoid bone).

Subunits: Include soft palate and uvula, base of tongue, pharyngoepiglottic and glossoepiglottic folds, palatine arch (including tonsillar fossae and pillars), valleculae, and lateral and posterior oropharyngeal walls.

Hypopharynx

Boundaries: From level of hyoid bone (pharyngoepiglottic folds) to level of inferior border of cricoid cartilage.

Subunits: Include pyriform (piriform) sinus (laryngopharyngeal sulcus), which is bordered by aryepiglottic folds medially and thyroid cartilage anteriorly, with its apex at the level of the cricoid cartilage, posterior and lateral pharyngeal walls (lateral merges with lateral wall of pyriform sinus), and postcricoid region, which is inferior to the arytenoids, extends to inferior margin of cricoid cartilage, and is contiguous with medial walls of pyriform sinuses.

Esophagus

Boundaries: From cricoid cartilage to cardia of stomach.

Subunits: Include upper esophageal sphincter, body (cervical–thoracic–intra-abdominal), and lower esophageal sphincter.

Dimensions: Incisors to cricopharyngeal sphincter is approximately 16 cm, to stomach, 38 to 40 cm (in adults).

Anatomy of the Oral Cavity

Salivary Ducts

1. Parotid (Stensen's): Orifice is lateral to second molars.
2. Submaxillary (Wharton's): Orifice is in midline floor of mouth adjacent to lingual frenulum.
3. Sublingual (Rivinus's): Multiple orifices draining into floor of mouth or into submaxillary duct.

Teeth

Deciduous Teeth: 20

Adult: 32, which are numbered superiorly right to left, inferiorly left to right. (Table 22-1 shows approximate time schedule for tooth eruption.)

Tongue

SURFACE ANATOMY

1. Papillae: Cover the anterior two-thirds of the tongue, including filiform (no taste function) fungiform (diffuse), and foliate (lateral tongue). The circumvallate papillae are large and lie in a V shape at the junction of the anterior and posterior portions of the tongue.
2. Sulcus terminalis: A groove at the anterior margin of the circumvallate papillae.
3. Foramen cecum: A pit at the junction of the sulcus terminalis from which the embryologic thyroid begins its descent (etiology of thyroglossal duct cyst).
4. Frenulum: Anterior fold of mucous membrane attaches the anteroinferior aspect of the tongue to the floor mouth and gingiva. Wharton's ducts open on either side of the frenulum. May be congenitally short (tongue-tied).
5. Lingual tonsil: Lymphoid tissue extending over the base of the tongue (considered to be in oropharynx). Size varies among individuals. Blood supply from lingual artery and vein.
6. Valleculae: Depressions on either side of the midline glossoepiglottic fold extending to the level of the hyoid bone. (Considered to be in oropharynx.)

MUSCLES

1. Extrinsic muscles of the tongue (cranial nerve XII): Include the geniglossus, hyoglossus, styloglossus, and palatoglossus.
2. Intrinsic muscles (cranial nerve XII): Include superior and inferior longitudinal, vertical, and transverse.
3. Fibrous septa (septum linguae): Defines midline and contains a triangular fat pad that is visualized on axial computed tomography (CT) scan.

SENSORY INNERVATION.   Anterior different from posterior.

1. Anterior two-thirds (oral tongue): Sensations of touch, pain, temperature transmitted via lingual nerve (V_3). Taste sensation is transmitted via lingual nerve to chorda tympani.

Taste:

Papillae $\longrightarrow$ afferent fibers $\longrightarrow$ lingual nerve $\longrightarrow$ chorda tympani $\longrightarrow$ geniculate ganglion $\longrightarrow$ intermediary nerve $\longrightarrow$ nucleus solitarius

TABLE 22-1. APPROXIMATE TIME SCHEDULE FOR TOOTH ERUPTION

Deciduous	Age (months)	Permanent	Age (years)
Medial incisors	7	First molar	6
Lateral incisors	9	Medial incisor	6–7
First molar	15	Lateral incisor	8–9
Canine	18	First premolar	10–11
Second molar	20–24	Canine	10.5–11.5
		Second premolar	11–12
		Second molar	12–13
		Third molar	17–25

2. Posterior third (tongue base): Touch and gag (visceral afferent) sensation is transmitted via cranial nerve IX to nucleus solitarius.

Taste: Circumvallate papillae and mucosa of epiglottis and valleculae → nucleus solitarius of the pons via cranial nerve IX

VASCULAR SUPPLY
1. Lingual artery: Second branch external carotid.
2. Lingual vein: Travels with hypoglossal nerve (ranine veins). (This places the hypoglossal nerve at risk during attempts to control bleeding.)

LYMPHATIC DRAINAGE
Anterior tongue: Central drains to ipsilateral and contralateral nodes, tip to submental nodes, and marginal (lateral) to ipsilateral nodes. Skip nodes may be encountered in level 4.

Posterior tongue: Drains to both ipsilateral and contralateral deep cervical nodes (jugulodigastric).

Hard palate: Forms the anterior two-thirds of the palate and consists of the palatine process of the maxilla and horizontal plates of the palatine bones. Covered with stratified squamous epithelium attached firmly to underlying bone.

Palate
FORAMINA OF THE PALATE
1. Greater palatine foramen: Conveys descending palatine branch of nerve V_2 to innervate palate as well as descending palatine artery (third division of maxillary artery); is 1 cm medial to second molar.
2. Accessory palatine foramen: Posterior to greater palatine foramen, conveys lesser descending palatine artery to soft palate.
3. Incisural foramen: Lies in midline of anterior palate, transmits incisural artery to anterior septum.

BLOOD SUPPLY TO PALATE

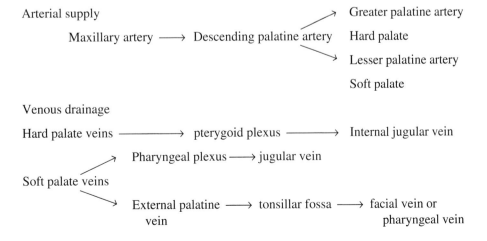

Saliva (See Also Chapter 25)

1. Total of 1500 mL/day. When unstimulated, two-thirds is secreted by submaxillary glands, when stimulated, two-thirds by parotid glands.
2. Is 99.5% water with only 0.5% organic/inorganic solids. Electrolyte composition is sodium 10 mEq/L, potassium 26 mEq/L, chlorine 10 mEq/L, and bicarbonate 30 mEq/L. pH is 6.2 to 7.4.
3. Organic component includes glycoprotein and amylase. (Circulating amylase of salivary origin can be distinguished from that of pancreatic origin.)

Muscles of Mastication

Masseter, temporalis, lateral pterygoid, medial pterygoid
Blood supply: Branches of maxillary artery
Nerve supply: V_3 (motor branch)

Anatomy of the Pharynx

Soft Palate

MUSCLES

1. Palatoglossus (anterior pillar): Approximates palate to tongue and narrows oropharyngeal opening.
2. Palatopharyngeus (posterior pillar): Raises larynx and pharynx, closing oropharyngeal aperture.
3. Musculus uvulae: Shortens uvula.
4. Levator veli palatini: Raises soft palate to contact posterior pharyngeal wall.
5. Tensor veli palatini: Pulls soft palate laterally to give rigidity and firmness to palate. Muscle originates in part on the eustachian tube cartilage, so contraction opens tube.

MOTOR INNERVATION

1. V_3 motor division $\longrightarrow$ pharyngeal plexus $\longrightarrow$ tensor veli palatini
2. X $\longrightarrow$ pharyngeal plexus $\longrightarrow$ remainder of palatal muscles

SENSORY INNERVATION

Cranial nerves V_2, IX, X.

BLOOD SUPPLY (SEE ABOVE)

MINOR SALIVARY GLANDS

Palatine Tonsils

EMBRYOLOGY.   The lateral extension of the second pharyngeal pouch is absorbed, and the dorsal remnants persist to become epithelium of palatine tonsil. The tonsillar pillars originate from the second and third branchial arches. The tonsillar crypts are first noted during the 12th week of gestation and the capsule during the 20th week.

ANATOMY.   Composed of lymphoid tissue with germinal center containing 6 to 20 epithelium-lined crypts. There is a capsule over deep surface, separated from the superior constrictor by thin areolar tissue. The palatine tonsil is contiguous with the lymphoid tissue of the tongue base (lingual tonsil).

ARTERIAL BLOOD SUPPLY TO THE TONSIL.   The plica triangularis is a variable fold consisting of lymphatic tissue and connective tissue; it lies between the tongue and palatoglossus, dorsal to the glossopalatine arch.

1. Facial ⟶ tonsillar branch ⟶ tonsil (main branch)
2. Facial ⟶ ascending palatine ⟶ tonsil
3. Lingual ⟶ dorsal lingual ⟶ tonsil
4. Ascending pharyngeal ⟶ tonsil
5. Maxillary ⟶ lesser descending palatine ⟶ tonsil

Gerlach's tonsil—lymphoid tissue within lip of fossa of Rosenmüller—involves the eustachian tube.

VENOUS BLOOD SUPPLY
1. Lingual vein
2. Pharyngeal vein

IMMUNOLOGY
1. B lymphocytes proliferate in germinal centers.
2. Immunoglobulins (IgG, A, M, D), complement components, interferon, lysozymes, and cytokines accumulate in tonsillar tissue.
3. The role of the tonsil remains controversial and to date there is no proven immunologic effect from tonsillectomy.

Microbiologic Environment of the Adult Mouth
1. Staphylococci (first oral microbe in neonate, from skin contamination)
2. Nonhemolytic streptococci
3. Lactobacilli
4. *Actinomyces*
5. *Leptothrix*
6. *Neisseria*
7. *Bacteroides*
8. Spirochetes
9. Micrococci
10. Viruses
    a. Myxovirus
    b. Adenovirus
    c. Picornavirus
    d. Coronaviruses

Oropharyngeal Walls
PASSAVANT'S RIDGE.   This is a visible constriction of the superior end of the superior constrictor, where fibers of the palatopharyngeal constrictor interdigitate. It is seen during approximation of the palate to the posterior pharyngeal wall and during elevation of the pharynx during swallowing.

LATERAL PHARYNGEAL BANDS.   These are rests of lymphoid tissue just behind posterior pillars.

MUSCLES

Pharyngeal Constrictors

1. Superior constrictor: Originates on the medial pterygoid plate, mandible, and base of tongue and inserts on median raphe.
2. Middle constrictor: Originates on the hyoid bone and stylohyoid ligament.
3. Inferior constrictor: Origin is on the oblique line of thyroid cartilage.

Pharyngeal and Laryngeal Elevators (Shorten Pharynx)

4. Salpingopharyngeus: Origin is on the temporal bone and eustachian tube.
5. Stylopharyngeus: Origin is on the styloid process.
6. Stylohyoid: Origin is on the styloid process.

Upper Esophageal Sphincter. The cricopharyngeus muscle is the most inferior portion of inferior constrictor and is separated from it by a triangular dehiscence termed Killian's dehiscence (through which a Zenker's diverticulum can form). Other dehiscences include the triangular Laimer-Haeckerman space between the posterior cricopharyngeus and the esophageal musculature and the Killian-Jamieson space, a lateral dehiscence inferior to the cricopharyngeus through which branches of the inferior thyroid artery pass. During rest, the muscle is in tonic contraction; it relaxes during swallowing. The sphincter is actively dilated by laryngeal elevation during deglutition.

PHYSIOLOGY OF NORMAL SWALLOWING

Overview

The laryngopharynx functions as a "time share" for respiration and deglutition. The most basic function of the larynx is airway protection. Some herbivores and infants are able to breathe and swallow simultaneously, whereas adults must interrupt respiration (usually during expiration) to swallow. During deglutition, the formed bolus must be moved completely through the pharynx while the glottis is closed. Defective deglutition results in either inadequate nutrition, aspiration due to failure to protect the airway, or both. The normal swallow is best understood by dividing it into three phases (Figure 22-1).

1. The oral phase prepares the food for delivery to the pharynx (some authors term this the oral preparatory phase). Components include:
    a. Mastication
    b. Addition and mixing of saliva
    c. Control of bolus—tongue, lips, buccinator, palate
    d. Selection and verification of safety of bolus (volume, taste, fish bones, etc.)
        The oral phase is under voluntary control and ends when the bolus is pressed against the faucial arches to precipitate the involuntary pharyngeal phase. Most sensitive receptors are on the anterior tonsillar pillar (IX, X)
2. The pharyngeal phase of the swallow moves the bolus quickly (in less than 1 second) past the closed glottis and through upper esophageal sphincter (UES) into the esophagus. The components of the pharyngeal phase are:
    a. Nasopharyngeal closure with palate elevation (levator, tensor veli palatini) and contraction of superior constrictor (Passavant's ridge).
    b. Cessation of respiration (during expiration).

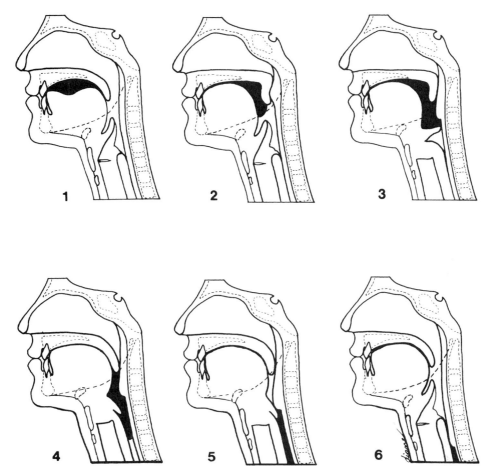

Figure 22-1. Summary of oral pharyngeal swallow. (1) Oral phase after preparation of the bolus by mastication and admixture of saliva. The bolus is positioned in the midportion of the tongue. (2) The oral phase ends when the bolus is pressed against the faucial arches by the tongue base and the pharyngeal phase of swallowing begins. (3) The pharyngeal phase begins with cessation of respiration, glottic closure, and palatal elevation. The bolus is propelled by a combination of tongue-base propulsion, contraction of pharyngeal constrictors, and laryngeal elevation. (4) Epiglottic rotation occurs due to laryngeal elevation and the pressure of the bolus. The upper esophageal sphincter is dilated through the combined action of cricopharyngeal relaxation and laryngeal elevation. (5) The bolus passes through the upper esophageal sphincter, ending the pharyngeal phase of the swallow. (6) The esophageal phase continues the transit of the bolus into the stomach. *(Prepared by Diane Robertson, AMI.)*

    c.   Glottic closure: Occurs with approximation of true vocal cords, false vocal cords, and arytenoids to epiglottis (in order).

    d.   Bolus propulsion: Requires tongue base elevation and contraction of the pharyngeal constrictor muscles.

    e.   Laryngeal elevation and pharyngeal shortening: Results in protection of laryngeal vestibule, epiglottic rotation, and active dilatation of cricopharyngeal sphincter.

    f.   Epiglottic rotation: Active due to laryngeal elevation, passive due to pressure of bolus.

    g.   Relaxation of cricopharyngeus muscle: Permits UES dilatation when combined with active dilatation by laryngeal elevation and pressure of bolus.

3.   The *esophageal phase* conveys bolus to the stomach in an average of 3 to 6 seconds with primary peristalsis and relaxation of lower esophageal sphincter.

4.   Nerves of swallowing

    a.   Sensory receptors: Found on soft palate, tongue base, tonsillar pillars, posterior pharyngeal wall.

    b.   Central ganglions: V, gasserian; IX, inferior (Andersch's), superior (petrosal); X, inferior (jugular), superior (nodose).

    c.   Efferent pathways:

        V: Teeth, jaw, masticators, buccinator

        V, X: Palate

        VII: Lips, facial musculature

        IX: Pharynx

        X: Pharynx, larynx, esophagus

        XII: Tongue

Anatomy of the Esophagus

40 cm in length in adult

Muscles

1.   No serosa; esophagus is fixed only at level of carotid.
2.   Outer longitudinal layer.
3.   Inner circular layer.
4.   Upper 5 cm skeletal muscle.
5.   Lower half smooth muscle.
6.   Upper midportion is overlap of striated and smooth muscle.
7.   Innervation: Myenteric plexus of Auerbach within muscle layers (parasympathetic ganglion cells).
8.   Vagus nerves rotate clockwise when viewed from above. Left moves to anterior surface, right moves to posterior surface.

Bolus transit: Upper one-third is striated muscle and has most rapid peristalsis—less than 1-second transit. Lower two-thirds smooth muscle, approximately 3-second transit. Gravity plays only minor role in normal swallowing, so position changes minimal. Overdistention of esophagus leads to spasm.

Peristalsis

1.   Primary: Physiologic propulsive wave of sequential constriction and shortening.
2.   Secondary: Non-physiologic retrograde peristalsis
3.   Tertiary: Non-physiologic segmental constriction without propulsion

Submucosa
Contains connective tissue, blood and lymphatic vessels, and parasympathetic ganglion cells and fibers; myenteric plexus of Meissner.

Mucosa
Contains muscularis mucosae, lamina propria, and stratified squamous epithelium with minimal secretory function and poor absorption.

Lower Esophageal Sphincter (LES)
1. Functions to prevent reflux of gastric contents into esophagus.
2. Is not a true anatomic structure but an active zone of high pressure extending 1 to 2 cm above and below diaphragm that relaxes during passage of the peristaltic wave.
3. The angle of His is the oblique angle of entry of the esophagus into the stomach. It is absent in infants, predisposing them to reflux.
4. LES function is controlled by parasympathetic tone (acetylcholine) and gastrin.
5. The diaphragmatic crurae surrounding the hiatus create a sling that assists in sphincteric function. This effect is lost with a hiatus hernia.

DISORDERS OF THE ORAL CAVITY, PHARYNX, AND ESOPHAGUS

Disorders of the Oral Cavity

Dental Developmental Abnormalities
1. Anodontia (partial or complete): The hereditary absence of teeth.
2. Dilaceration: The tooth root, as a result of trauma, fails to develop normally, resulting in an angular malformation of the root. The condition is associated with rickets and cretinism.
3. Supernumerary teeth.
4. Enamel hypoplasia.
5. Enamel discoloration: Often due to antibiotic exposure (tetracycline) prior to eruption.

Periapical Disease
1. Granuloma (asymptomatic).
2. Alveolar abscess (due to caries involving the root canal); may lead to sinusitis, osteomyelitis, Ludwig's angina, or bacteremia.
3. Radicular cyst.

Inflammation of Oral Mucosa
Stomatitis is the general term for any inflammatory disorder of the oral mucosa. It can be associated with the following diseases:

1. Gingivitis.
2. Periodontitis (pyorrhea).
3. Periodontosis is chronic degenerative destruction of the periodontal tissue. Papillon-Lefèvre syndrome comprises periodontosis, hyperkeratosis of the soles of the feet and palms of the hands, and calcification of the dura.
4. Acute necrotizing ulcerative gingivitis (ANUG, Vincent's angina, trench mouth) is due to synergistic mixed anaerobic infection including *Borrelia vincentii* (fusiform bacillus). Symptoms are a fetid odor to the breath, excessive salivation, and bleeding gingiva. Treatment is oral hygiene and penicillin.

5. Herpetic gingivostomatitis and herpes labialis are usually due to herpes simplex. Herpes labialis is the most common viral infection of the mouth. Shingles due to herpes zoster is rare.
6. Herpangina (group A coxsackievirus) is a vesicular eruption of the soft palate usually associated with fever and coryza.
7. Noma is an acute necroting gingivitis that rapidly spreads into adjacent soft tissue. It is most commonly seen in third world countries, with the highest incidence in children. *Borrelia* and other anaerobic fusiform bacilli are always present.
8. Bacterial stomatitis (due to streptococci, staphylocci, gonococci).
9. Thrush (*Candida albicans*) may present as an early manifestation of AIDS, in the elderly, or in patients who are using inhaled steroids. It also may be seen in patients who have received radiation and have decreased salivary gland output. Topical or systemic therapy may be used for treatment.
10. Actinomycosis (filiform bacillus) forms abscesses with masses of bacteria that resemble "sulfur granules."
11. Blastomycosis.
12. Histoplasmosis (*Histoplasma caspsulatum*).
13. Pyogenic granuloma. When forms on gingiva, termed *epulis*.
14. Mucositis—commonly encountered as a result of chemotherapy or radiation therapy.

Noninfectious Lesions

1. Sutton disease [recurrent aphthous ulcers (RAU)] forms multiple large, deep ulcers that can cause extensive scarring of the oral cavity.
2. Erythema multiforme produces "iris-like" lesions that may involve the oral cavity, conjunctiva, and skin. Often preceded by upper respiratory infection (URI).
3. Pemphigus vulgaris (intraepidermoid bullae).
4. Pemphigoid (subepidermoid bullae). Differentiation from pemphigus requires histologic examination with staining for basement membrane.
5. Lichen planus seen as a reticular branching pattern of leukoplakia with most common site on buccal mucosa. Advanced cases termed erosive lichen planus and have a 10 to 15% chance of developing into squamous cell carcinoma. Treatment is topical steroids.
6. Systemic lupus erythematosus.
7. Behçet's disease: Oral ulcerations, conjunctivitis, iritis, and urethretis.

Oral Mucosal Manifestations of Systemic Processes

1. Pernicious anemia: Caused by a lack of vitamin B_{12}. The tongue may show lobulations on its surface or, in advanced cases, be shiny, smooth, and red. Oral mucosa may exhibit an irregular erythema.
2. Iron deficiency anemia: Oral mucosa is ash gray (may be associated with Plummer-Vinson syndrome). Tongue is smooth and devoid of papillae.
3. Thalassemia (Mediterranean anemia): Oral mucosa has diffuse pallor and is cyanotic.
4. Polycythemia: Oral mucosa is bright blue-red with gingival bleeding.
5. Osler-Weber-Rendu disease (hereditary hemorrhagic telangiectasia): Forms spider-like blood vessels or angiomatous-appearing lesions on the oral mucosa, tongue, and nasal mucosa and is associated with recurrent epistaxis. The gastrointestinal tract may be involved and transfusion may be required.
6. Sturge-Weber syndrome: Seen as a port-wine stain of the face, oral cavity, or tongue associated with vascular malformations of the meninges and cerebral cortex.

7. Thrombocytopenic purpura: A marked decrease in platelets from a variety of causes. Initial manifestations are often oral petechiae and ecchymosis.
8. Menopausal gingivostomatitis (senile atrophy): Dry, shiny oral mucosa with a burning sensation, diffuse erythema, and occasionally fissuring in the melobuccal fold. Treatment is symptomatic.
9. Nutritional pathology (deficiency).
   a. Riboflavin: Atrophic glossitis, angular cheilosis, gingivostomatitis.
   b. Pyridoxine: Angular cheilosis.
   c. Nicotine acid: Angular cheilosis.
   d. Vitamin C: Gingivitis and "bleeding gums."
10. Kaposi's sarcoma: Often presents as violaceous macules on the oral mucosa. Uncommon except in association with AIDS, where it is considered an AIDS-defining condition.

Pigmentation Changes of the Oral Cavity
1. Melanosis: Physiologic pigmentation, often seen as dark patches of the oral mucosa.
2. Amalgam tattoo: Inadvertent tattoo of gingiva from dental amalgam introduced through a mucosal laceration.
3. Peutz-Jeghers syndrome: Melanotic macules periorally.
4. Bismuth: Black pigmentation.
5. Lead: Blue-gray line (Burton's line) that follows the gingival margin.
6. Mercury: Gray/violet pigmentation.
7. Silver: Violet/blue/gray pigmentation.
8. Addison's disease: Brown pigmentation.
9. Hemochromatosis: Bronze pigmentation.
10. Xanthomatous disease: Yellow/gray pigmentation.
11. Kaposi's sarcoma: Violaceous macules.

Common Childhood Diseases with Oral Cavity Manifestations
1. Measles (rubeola): Koplik's spots (pale round spots on erythematous base) seen on buccal and lingual mucosa
2. Chickenpox (varicella): Vesicles
3. Scarlet fever: Strawberry tongue
4. Congenital heart disease: Gingivitis, cyanotic gums
5. Kawasaki disease: Strawberry tongue

LEUKOPLAKIA (WHITE PLAQUE).   A white, hyperkeratotic lesion that may or may not be associated with dysplastic change on histologic examination. It occurs most frequently on the lip (vermilion) and then, in descending order of frequency, on the buccal mucosa, mandibular gingiva, tongue, floor of mouth, hard palate, maxillary gingiva, lip mucosa, and soft palate. Less than 10% of *isolated* (see nodular variant below) leukoplakia will demonstrate carcinoma or severe dysplasia on biopsy.

ERYTHROPLAKIA (RED PLAQUE).   A granular erythematous area often encountered in association with leukoplakia (nodular leukoplakia). Some 50% will demonstrate severe dysplasia or carcinoma in situ on biopsy.

NODULAR LEUKOPLAKIA (MIXED WHITE AND RED PLAQUES).   Greater malignant potential, similar to erythroplakia in risk of malignancy. May be seen in association with frank invasive cancer.

MEDIAN RHOMBOID GLOSSITIS.   A smooth reddish midline area of the midline of the tongue devoid of papillae. It is a developmental anomaly, and may be associated with candida overgrowth.

FORDYCE GRANULES.   Painless, pinpoint yellow nodules that occur bilaterally on the posterior buccal mucosa. These represent enlarged ectopic sebaceous glands and are a benign development anomaly.

MACROGLOSSIA.   Can be due to several causes:
1. Hemangioma
2. Lymphangioma
3. Myxedema
4. Acromegaly
5. Amyloidosis
6. Benign cysts
7. Pierre Robin (actually relative macroglossia due to micrognathia) syndrome
8. Tertiary syphilis
9. Von Gierke disease (glycogen storage disease type I)
10. Hurler's syndrome (mucopolysaccharidosis)
11. Down syndrome
12. Infection—i.e., actinomycosis

Tumors of the Mandible Excluding Carcinoma
1. Mandibular tori: Benign bony exostoses commonly seen on medial aspect of anterior mandible.
2. Odontogenic fibroma: Presents as a circumscribed radiolucency with smooth borders occurring around the crown of unerupted teeth in children, adolescents, and young adults. Radiographically, it resembles a dentigerous cyst. Treatment is excision and is nearly always curative.
3. Ameloblastoma: A neoplasm of enamel origin that presents in the third and fourth decades. The most common site is the mandible, especially the molar region. Tumors are slow-growing and painless, expanding bone. Treatment is excision.
4. Cementomas: A broad class of lesions that form cementum (bone-like connective tissue that covers the tooth root). Tumors usually arise at the tips of tooth roots in young adults. The radiographic appearance can vary from radiolucent to densely radiopaque, depending on the lesion. Treatment is simple enucleation.
5. Odonotoma: A tumor composed of ameloblasts (enamel) and odontoblasts (dentin). It appears as an irregular radiopaque mass, often between tooth roots, and is associated with unerupted teeth. Simple enucleation is sufficient treatment.
6. Adenoameloblastoma: A well-encapsulated follicular cyst occurring most commonly in the anterior maxilla of adolescent girls in association with impacted teeth. Treatment is excision. A rare malignant variant exists.
7. Ameloblastic fibroma: A slow-growing, painless lesion seen in the molar area of the mandible in adolescents and children. It contains both epithelial and mesenchymal tissue and is radiographically similar to an ameloblastoma.

8. Ameloblastic sarcoma: A malignant, fast-growing, painful, and aggressive variant of ameloblastic fibroma. Occurs most commonly in young adults. Treatment is surgical excision. Recurrence is common.
9. Ewing's sarcoma: A rapidly growing tumor causing local pain and swelling. It is most common between the ages of 10 and 25 years. The mandible is the most common site in the head and neck. Other tumors such as lymphoma, which may mimic Ewing's sarcoma, must be ruled out. Treatment is radiation and chemotherapy. Survival is about 50%.
10. Osteogenic sarcoma: A fast-growing, aggressive malignant tumor of bone. It occurs primarily in adolescents and young adults. Survival of the mandibular variant better than that of the long bone. Treatment is surgical. Combined therapy often utilized.

Odontogenic Cysts

1. Radicular cyst: The most common cyst, called a periapical cyst when it involves the tooth root. It is commonly caused by dental infection and is usually asymptomatic. It presents as a radiolucent area on x-ray. Treatment is extraction or root canal therapy.
2. Dentigerous (follicular) cyst: A developmental abnormality caused by a defect in enamel formation. It is always associated with an unerupted tooth crown and most common in the mandibular third molar or maxillary cuspid. Ameloblastoma formation occurs in the cyst wall.
3. Odontogenic keratocyst: Mimics dentigerous cysts if associated with a tooth root. If not, it is called a primordial cyst. Diagnosis is based on histology, and treatment is excision and curettage. There is a high rate of recurrence.

Other Oral Cavity Lesions

1. Hairy tongue: Due to hyperplasia of the filiform papillae. It may be black, blue, brown, or white, depending on microflora and nicotine staining, and is often associated with candidal overgrowth.
2. Epulis: A nonspecific term for a tumor or tumor-like mass of the gingiva, often a pyogenic granuloma. Common in pregnancy. Congenital epulis is rare and resembles a granular cell myoblastoma. A giant cell epulis (giant cell reparative granuloma) is more common, and histologic examination demonstrates reticular and fibrous connective tissue with numerous giant cells. Radiographs show cuffing or sclerotic margins of bone.
3. Ranula: A mucocele of the sublingual gland that presents in the floor of the mouth. If it penetrates the mylohyoid muscle and presents as a soft submental neck mass, it is termed a plunging ranula. Excision should include the entire sublingual gland in order to prevent recurrence, with care taken to protect the submandibular duct and the lingual nerve.
4. Torus palatini: A benign excessive bone growth in midline of palate that continues to enlarge beyond puberty. Occasionally it must be removed in order to prevent denture irritation.
5. Cleft palate: See Chapter 11.

Disorders of the Oropharynx
Soft Palate

1. Cleft palate: Due to failure of fusion and associated with a characteristic voice change and nasal regurgitation of liquids. A submucous cleft may be present. Eustachian tube disorder is due to failure of tensor veli palatini to open eustachian tube on swallowing (see Chapter 11).

2. Congenital elongation of the uvula.
3. Squamous papillomas.
4. Aphthous ulcers.
5. Leukoplakia, erythroplakia, squamous cell cancer.
6. Minor salivary gland tumors.
7. Quinke's disease: Swelling of the uvula, often in association with acute bacterial tonsillitis. Uvular swelling can also occur with trauma (heroic snoring, burn from hot food or beverage).
8. Angioneurotic edema: Can occur as a familial (C1 esterase deficiency) or allergic condition or due to angiotensin converting enzyme (ACE) inhibitor use. ACE inhibitor–induced angioedema is more common in those of African descent, can occur at any time following initiation of therapy, and may be a "sentinel event" for more severe involvement.

Palatine Tonsils

Differential diagnosis of tonsilar mass:

1. Acute tonsillitis
2. Tonsillith
3. Peritonsillar abscess
4. Mononucleosis
5. Parapharyngeal space mass
6. Lymphoma
7. Squamous cell cancer

Acute Tonsillitis

1. Etiology
   a. Group A beta-hemolytic streptococci (GABHS)
   b. *Haemophilus influenzae*
   c. *Streptococcus pneumoniae*
   d. Staphylococci (with dehydration, antibiotics)
   e. Tuberculosis (in immunocompromise)
2. Differential diagnosis
   a. Infectious mononucleosis
   b. Malignancy (lymphoma, leukemia, carcinoma)
   c. Diphtheria
   d. Scarlet fever
   e. Vincent's angina
   f. Leukemia
   g. Agranulocytosis
   h. Pemphigus

Acute Peritonsillar Abscess

1. Pus located deep to tonsil capsule between tonsil and superior constrictor muscle.
2. Presents with deviation of the tonsil and uvula toward the midline, swelling of soft palate, often with trismus.
3. Complications of peritonsillar abscess.
   a. Parapharyngeal abscess (due to rupture through superior constrictor).
   b. Venous thrombosis, phlebitis, bacteremia, endocarditis.

    c.   Arterial involvement to include thrombosis, hemorrhage, pseudoaneurysm.

    d.   Mediastinitis.

    e.   Brain abscess.

    f.   Airway obstruction.

    g.   Aspiration pneumonia.

    h.   Nephritis (due to streptococcal antigen).

    i.   Peritonitis.

    j.   Dehydration.

Tonsillectomy

1. Procedure referred to by Celsus in *De Medicina* (10 A.D.).
2. First documented surgery by Cague of Rheims (1757).
3. Indications:
    a. Recurrent infections—3 per year for 3 years, 5 per year for 2 years, 7 or more in 1 year, or greater than 2 weeks of school or work missed in 1 year.
    b. Hypertrophy causing upper airway obstruction (obstruction, sleep apnea).
    c. Peritonsillar abscess.
    d. Possibility of malignancy, either unilateral enlarged or search for unknown primary.
    e. Hypertrophy causing deglutition problems.
    f. Recurrent tonsillitis causing febrile seizures.
    g. Diphtheria carrier.
4. Morbidity: Post-operative hemorrhage 2 to 4%.
5. Mortality: 1 in 25,000 (hemorrhage, airway obstruction, anesthesia).

Disorders of the Tongue Base

1. Lingual tonsillar hypertrophy
2. Lingual tonsillitis
3. Lingual thyroid (failure of the descent)
4. Benign vallecular cysts
5. Neoplasms
    a. Squamous cell cancer (see Chapter 26)
    b. Lymphoma
    c. Minor salivary gland tumors (usually malignant)
    d. Lingual thyroid (due to failure of descent)

Disorders of the Oropharyngeal Walls

1. Inflammation of the lateral pharyngeal bands
2. Cobblestoning of posterior wall (inflammation of lymphoid rests)
3. Trauma (child falling with stick in mouth)
4. Squamous cell cancer
5. Eagle's syndrome (pain due to elongated styloid process)

Diseases of the Hypopharynx

1. Inflammation (associated with supraglottis)
2. Angioneurotic edema
3. Osteophyte
4. Aberrant carotid artery

5. Carotid aneurysm
6. Parapharyngeal space mass
7. Hypopharyngeal carcinoma–see Chapter 26.

DYSPHAGIA

May be oral, pharyngeal, or esophageal.

History: Note underlying disease, onset and progression, weight loss, odynophagia, dietary changes and consistencies, coughing with meals, "mucus," and pneumonia. Ask and note voice change.

Oropharyngeal symptoms: Aspiration (especially liquids) "sticking" of food in upper neck, nasal regurgitation, failure of swallowing initiation.

Esophageal symptoms: Sticking of food in suprasternal or substernal area, pain, heartburn.

Evaluation: Perform complete head and neck exam. Radiographic studies considered standard. Esophagram evaluates esophagus. Modified barium swallow (three-phase swallow, "cookie" swallow) evaluates pharyngeal function. Consider fiberoptic examination of swallowing (FEES) with or without sensory testing at same time as physical exam. May need to obtain both studies.

Radiographic findings: Pharyngeal dilatation, penetration or aspiration into trachea, into larynx, stenosis, obstruction, disorders of peristalsis, persistent cricopharyngeal bar.

Pathologic Entities

1. Anatomic defects such as cleft palate, tumor, head and neck surgery, stenosis.
2. Timing: Usually neurologic defects such as stroke or head injury, alterations in level of consciousness, injury to brain stem, cerebellum, long tracts, or peripheral cranial nerves, either sensory or motor.
3. Motor: Muscle weakness due to primary myopathy, peripheral neuropathy, injury to cranial nerve or myoneural plexus, or central injury to brain stem or cerebellum. Disorders of peristalsis.

Diseases with Dysphagia

1. Inflammatory lesions of the pharynx associated with viral infections
2. Vincent's angina
3. Thrush (*Candida*)
4. Tonsillitis (peritonsillar abscess and lingual tonsillitis)
5. Retropharyngeal abscess
6. Plummer-Vinson syndrome
7. Polio
8. Pseudobulbar palsy
9. Cerebrovascular accident
10. Acute myelogenous leukemia
11. Multiple sclerosis
12. Myasthenia gravis
13. Polyneuritis
14. Dermatomyositis
15. Myotonia congenita
16. Myotonia dystrophica

17. Muscular dystrophy
18. Primary muscular tumors
19. Primary muscular invasion due to tumor
20. Zenker's diverticulum
21. Squamous cell carcinoma
22. Adenocarcinoma
23. Laryngeal carcinoma
24. Thyroid mass
25. Achalasia
26. Chagas' disease
27. Scleroderma
28. Raynaud's phenomenon
29. Esophageal webs
30. Esophageal spasm
31. Psychologic illness
32. Schatzki's ring (lower esophageal)
33. Burns
34. Dysphagia lusoria
35. Leiomyoma (benign)

Specific Neurologic Disorders of Swallowing

1. Tongue base weakness: Associated with neuromuscular disease, stroke, brain stem disorder; manifest by poor bolus propulsion with residue in vallecula and over tongue base. Treatment is chin tuck to close vallecula, tongue base–strengthening exercises, and liquid rinse during meals.

2. Oral dysfunction: Associated with stroke (especially brain stem), articulation defect, and other neuromuscular disorders. It is manifest by poor oral control, oral residue, and failure to initiate swallow. Treatment is tongue-strengthening exercises and articulation exercises.

3. Pharyngeal sensory loss: Associated with stroke gastroesophageal reflux, aging, or surgical injury. It is manifest by retained pharyngeal secretions, decreased sensation on sensory testing, silent (without coughing) penetration of laryngeal vestibule, and aspiration, typically worse with thin liquids. Treatment is thickening of liquids to provide more time for pharyngeal response.

4. Vocal cord paralysis: Associated with brain stem stroke or peripheral nerve injury. It is manifest by a paralyzed vocal cord, typically with aspiration of thin liquids. Treatment is vocal cord medialization.

5. Vocal cord weakness: Associated with aging, general debilitation, and Parkinson's disease. It is manifest by failure of glottic closure, vocal cord bowing, and weak, breathy voice. Treatment is vocal cord adduction exercises and vocal cord augmentation.

6. Failure of laryngeal elevation: Associated with neuromuscular disorders, generalized debilitation, and stroke (especially brain stem). It is manifest by tongue base and pyriform sinus residue and failure of cricopharyngeal opening. Treatment is laryngeal elevation exercises, Mendelson maneuver (hold larynx as high as possible for as long as possible with each swallow), and electromyographic (EMG) biofeedback.

7. Generalized pharyngeal weakness: Associated with stroke and a variety of general and neuromuscular diseases. It is manifest by moderate to severe residue with failure to

clear completely on subsequent swallows, secondary penetration/aspiration, often worse with solids than with liquids. Treatment is multiple consecutive swallows, small bites, and liquid wash between bites.

8. Cricopharyngeal achalasia: Associated with failure of laryngeal elevation, gastro-esophageal reflux, neuromuscular disease, and Zenker's diverticulum. It is manifest by a cricopharyngeal "bar" or a pharyngeal diverticulum seen on radiographic examina-tion, pharyngeal residue, or regurgitation following a swallow. Treatment is laryngeal elevation exercises (EMG biofeedback), chemodenervation of the cricopharyngeus muscle with botulinum toxin (Botox), transcervical division of the cricopharyngeus muscle, or transoral diverticulotomy.

9. Disorders of peristalsis: Reduced (atony), excessive (spasm), or disordered (secondary or tertiary).

Diseases of the Esophagus
Inflammatory Disease
1. Gastroesophageal reflux with esophagitis
2. Barrett's esophagitis: Metaplasia of squamous epithelium to columnar mucosa.
3. Infections: Candidiasis; common in HIV. Treat with antifungal, including topical and systemic.

Diverticuli
1. Zenker's diverticulum: Occurs in Killian's dehiscence inferior to fibers of the inferior constrictor and superior to cricopharyngeus. Associated with failure of cricopharyn-geal dilatation due to failure of muscle relaxation, muscle fibrosis, or failure of active dilatation due to failure of laryngeal elevation. Symptoms include regurgitation of undigested food, dysphagia and weight loss, aspiration, and cough. Treatment is cricopharyngeal myotomy (with or without excision, suspension, or inversion of sac) or endoscopic diverticulotomy with either laser or stapler.
2. Epiphrenic diverticulum: Occurs just superior to cardioesophageal junction, usually on the right side. Symptoms are minimal. Constitutes 13% of all esophageal diverticula.
3. Traction diverticulum: Usually midesophageal, typically on left side, and often due to traction of adjacent inflammatory process (usually tuberculosis).

Hiatal Hernia (HH)
Defined as a portion of the stomach passing up through the esophageal hiatus of the diaphragm. HH may be either *sliding* (most common), in which the esophagogastric junction (EGJ) her-niates into the thorax, or *paraesophageal,* in which the EGJ is below the diaphragm while the fundus of the stomach bulges around it and through the diaphragm into the chest cavity. Asso-ciated conditions for sliding HH include the following:

1. Increased intra-abdominal pressure due to pregnancy, obesity, tight clothing, ascites, constipation.
2. Age: The incidence is 30% in the older population.
3. Weakness of esophageal hiatus: Results in incompetence of the LES.
4. Kyphoscoliosis.
5. Sandifer syndrome: Abnormal contortions of the neck associated with unrecognized hiatal hernia in children.
6. Saint's triad: Gallbladder disease, colonic diverticular disease, and hiatal hernia.

Motility Disorders

Diagnosis made with contrast barium study and manometry. Radiographic findings include tertiary contractions trapping barium in segments, retrograde displacement of barium, spontaneous waves not preceded by a swallow, or three to five repetitive waves following a single swallow. Some common causes of motility disorders are:

Polymyositis: Muscle weakness secondary to inflammatory and degenerative changes in *striated muscle*. Proximal muscle weakness (hip and shoulder) is the most common presenting symptom. When associated with skin rashes, this is termed dermatomyositis. It involves the striated muscle of the hypopharynx and upper esophagus. Peristalsis is diminished and poorly coordinated, and the esophagus may be dilated. Manometric evaluation demonstrates decreased UES pressure and reduced peristaltic waves. Hiatal hernia and reflux are absent.

Scleroderma (progessive systemic sclerosis): Involves smooth muscle with a marked decrease in lower esophageal sphincter pressure, associated reflux, and esophagitis. May include Raynaud's phenomenon. Some 60% of patients have significant dysphagia and up to 40% develop a stricture secondary to reflux. Normal peristalsis may be seen in the upper esophagus, with aperistalsis, dilation, and gastroesophageal reflux distally. Barium may distend the esophagus in the supine position, with free passage in the upright position.

Achalasia: A disorder of esophageal motility characterized by aperistalsis, esophageal dilatation, and failure of LES relaxation. Primary achalasia is due to idiopathic degeneration of the ganglion cells of Auerbach's plexis. Secondary achalasia can be caused by carcinoma, cerebrovascular accident, Chagas' disease, postvagotomy syndrome, or diabetes mellitus. Barium swallow demonstrates failure of peristalsis, dilatation, and an air-fluid level in the upright position.

Other Motility Disorders of the Esophagus

1. Esophageal spasm: Simultaneous, repetitive, nonperistaltic, and often powerful contractions of the esophagus.
2. Presbyesophagus: Associated with age and manifest by incoordination of sphincter function, reduced peristalsis, and frequent tertiary contractions.
3. Ganglionic degeneration: Associated with achalasia and Chagas' disease; seen in the elderly.
4. Motility disorder due to irritant such as gastroesophageal reflux or corrosive injury.
5. Neuromuscular disorder due to diabetes, alcoholism, amyotrophic lateral sclerosis, or other dysautonomia.
6. Spasm may be described as "curling," "tertiary contractions," "corkscrew esophagus," or "rosary bead esophagus."
7. Cricopharyngeal achalasia: Failure of UES dilatation (see discussion above).

Lower Esophageal Ring (Shatzki's Ring)

A concentric ring that occurs at the esophagogastric junction (EGJ). It is encountered in 6 to 14% of barium studies, but only one-third are symptomatic. Symptoms are rare unless the lumen is less than 13 mm. Dysphagia is intermittent and primarily to solid food. Heartburn is rare and manometry is normal. Is best seen in barium studies done in recumbent position or esophagogastroduodenoscopy (EGD). Often not seen on rigid esophagoscopy. A Shatzki's ring involves only mucosa, whereas peptic stricture due to reflux involves both mucosa and muscle layers.

Esophageal Webs

Dysphagia develops slowly. These are asymmetric (as opposed to rings and strictures). Usually on anterior wall, often associated with Plummer-Vinson syndrome (Patterson-Kelly, sideropenic dysphagia).

Plummer-Vinson Syndrome

Most common in females (10:1) typically of Scandinavian descent. Syndrome is associated with iron deficiency anemia, upper esophageal web, hypothyroidism, glossitis, cheilitis, and gastritis. Dysphagia may be present even in the absence of a web. Anemia may precede other features. There is an increased risk of postcricoid carcinoma (15% in one study). Diagnosis is by barium swallow (which may show abnormalities in esophageal propulsion and/or a web). Check complete blood count, serum iron, ferritin levels. Treatment is with iron replacement and dilatation of the web. Etiology is unclear; possible relationship to GERD.

Esophageal Trauma

Boerhaave syndrome—a linear tear 1 to 4 cm in length through all three layers of the esophagus due to sudden increase in esophageal pressure, usually due to vomiting. Rare, occurs on left side 90% of time, encountered in males more commonly (5:1). Presents with severe knife-like epigastric pain radiating to left shoulder, may not cause significant hematemesis. Respiratory difficulty, subcutaneous emphysema, and shock develop. Chest x-ray demonstrates initially widened mediastinum, then left pleural effusion or hydro-pneumothorax. Tear may be difficult to differentiate from myocardial infarction, pulmonary embolus, or perforated ulcer. Treatment is thoracotomy and repair of tear.

Mallory-Weiss Syndrome

Tear of cardia of stomach due to forceful vomiting. Most commonly encountered in alcoholics (usually men above age 40) and presents with massive hematemesis.

Esophageal Foreign Bodies

Most common location is at site of physiologic or pathologic narrowing, such as cricopharyngeus, scar from prior burn or surgery, or at site of peptic stricture. Use of barium studies and flexible endoscopy is controversial. Appropriate instrumentation and experience in esophagoscopy necessary to assure optimal outcome.

Iatrogenic Perforation

Most commonly occurs at sites of narrowing. Clinical picture is sore throat, neck and chest pain following procedure, often with tachycardia out of proportion to fever. Fever and subcutaneous emphysema develop later. Chest radiograph and computed tomography required if clinical suspicion present. Antibiotics, fluid resuscitation, and early surgical exploration with repair are required to assure optimal outcome.

Esophageal Compression

May be either anatomic or pathologic.

> Anatomic: Includes cricopharyngeus (UES), aorta, left mainstem bronchus, and diaphragm (LES).
>
> Pathologic: Includes enlarged thyroid or thymus, osteophyte of cervical spine, mediastinal mass, cardiac enlargement or aortic aneurysm, or massive enlargement of the liver.

Gastroesophageal Reflux Disease (GERD)

> Symptoms: May be typical (substernal chest pain, waterbrash) or atypical (laryngeal symptoms of hoarseness, voice change, sore throat, globus, or cough).

Diagnosis: Is often made by history, laryngeal examination, or response to empiric therapy. Barium swallow may demonstrate esophagitis, stricture, etc. Occasionally reflux may be seen, but absence of reflux of barium does not rule out GERD. Measurement of pH with indwelling probe (single or double) is often helpful to confirm the diagnosis. Normal values for distal esophagus have been defined; normal values for pharynx are not known. A positive Bernstein's test (reproduces symptoms by instillation of acid into esophagus) may be helpful. Esophagoscopy may be required for diagnosis and to rule out Barrett's esophagitis.

Complications: May be esophageal (ulceration, stricture, Barrett's esophagitis, carcinoma), laryngeal (chronic laryngitis, vocal process granulomata, ulceration, or subglottic edema), or pulmonary (asthma). Role in sinusitis, pediatric otitis media, and laryngeal cancer remains controversial.

Barrett's Esophagitis

Lower esophagus lined with (columnar) gastric epithelium instead of squamous epithelium, noted to have an increasing incidence and progresses to cancer of the esophagus in 10 to 15% of cases. Barrett's ulcer is a deep peptic ulceration in an area of Barrett's esophagitis.

Treatment of Gastroesophageal and Gastropharyngeal Reflux

Includes elevation of head of bed; dietary changes; and avoidance of caffeine, nicotine, and antacids. Many patients respond to H2 blockers, but proton pump inhibitors are now commonly used. Open or laparoscopic surgical procedures may be required but do not always eliminate the need for pharmacologic treatment.

Carcinoma of the Esophagus

Accounts for 4% of cancer deaths, with a male preponderance of 5 : 1. It is increasing in incidence and is associated with alcohol and tobacco usage, Barrett's esophagitis, or prior burn, scar, or stricture, but there is no gastric predisposition. Cancers arising in the upper third are usually squamous cell carcinoma, whereas those in the distal two-thirds are likely to be adenocarcinomas. In decreasing order, most common are distal one-third (40 to 50%), next is middle one-third (30 to 40%), and less than 33% arise in upper one-third. Other malignant neoplasms include sarcomas such as leiomyosarcoma or fibrosarcoma. Benign tumors of the esophagus are rare and include leiomyoma, fibroma, or lipoma.

Congenital Lesions

Congenital diaphragmatic hernias: Posterior termed pleuroperitoneal (Bochdalek's), whereas anterior is retrosternal (Morgagni's). Treatment is surgical.

Tracheoesophageal fistulae (TEF): Occur in 1 in 3000 births and are associated with polyhydramnios (16%), cardiac abnormalities, vestibular abnormalities, imperforate anus, and genitourinary abnormalities. These may be of various types; the most common (85%) is a distal TEF with upper esophageal atresia. Less common are blind upper and lower esophageal pouches without a connection to the trachea (8%) and a true H-type fistula (4%). In less than 1% does the proximal esophagus open into the trachea. Infants present with drooling and feeding difficulties, coughing, abdominal distention, vomiting, and cyanosis. Radiographs demonstrate marked air filling the stomach and proximal intestine and often right-upper-lobe pneumonia (aspiration). Passage of a nasogastric tube that meets obstruction 9 to 13 cm from the nares suggests the diagnosis. A chest radiograph with the catheter in place can demonstrate position of pouch as well as air in stomach and intestine. Some 60 to 80% of patients survive; however, if cardiac or genitourinary abnormalities are present, survival drops to 22%. Barium study is diagnostic.

Dysphagia Lusoria (Bayford Syndrome): Symptomatic compression of the esophagus by anomalous location of the right subclavian artery. Instead of arising from the innominate artery, the anomalous right subclavian originates from the descending aorta distal to the left subclavian and passes posterior to the esophagus to get to the arm. It is associated with a nonrecurrent right recurrent laryngeal nerve and aneurysms of the aorta and the aberrant right subclavian artery. Dysphagia is intermittent but can lead to weight loss. Barium swallow will show posterior compression. CT is diagnostic. Treatment is ligation and division with anastomosis of distal subclavian artery to carotid.

Chalasia (reflux in infants, thought to be normal)

Esophageal duplication

Esophageal rings

Esophageal webs

Esophageal Burns.   These have become more rare since improvements in public awareness and packaging. Bases (lye) are more likely to cause deep burns than acids. Concentrated acids, however, are associated with gastric rupture. Oral burns are not present in 8 to 20% of those with esophageal burns. Esophagoscopy is warranted within 24 hours. If no burn is found, follow up with a barium swallow in 2 weeks. If a burn is identified, do not advance beyond burn. Admit, watch for airway compromise, and treat with antibiotics and steroids (2–3 weeks). Nasogastric intubation is controversial; it can function as a lumen-finder. Pathologic sequence of burns is as follows:

1. 0 to 24 hours: dusky cyanotic edematous mucosa.
2. 2 to 5 days: gray-white coat of coagulated protein fibroblasts appears.
3. 4 to 7 days: slough with demarcation of burn depth. Esophageal wall is weakest from days 5 through 8.
4. 8 to 12 days: appearance of collagen.
5. 6 weeks: scar formation and evident stricture.

Bibliography

Armstrong RB. Cutaneous aids in the diagnosis of ulcers. *Laryngoscope* 1981;91:31–37.

Asheraft KW, Holder TM. The story of esophageal atresia and tracheoesophageal fistula. *Surgery* 1969;65:332–340.

Aviv JE, Martin JH, Kenn MS, et al. Air pulse quantification of supraglottic and pharyngeal sensation: a new technique. *Ann Otol Rhinol Laryngol* 1993;102(10):777–780.

Bailey, *Otolaryngology—Head and Neck Surgery.* Philadelphia: Lippincott, 1999.

Bastian RW. Videoendoscopic evaluation of patients with dysphagia: an adjunct to the modified barium swallow. *Otolaryngol Head Neck Surg* 1991; 104:339–350.

Bennet JR. Esophageal strictures. *Gastroenterol Clin North Am* 1978;7:555–569.

Bhaskar SN. *Synopsis of Oral Pathology,* 5th ed. St Louis: Mosby, 1977.

Bouquot JE, Gorlin RJ. Leukoplakia, lichen planus and other oral keratoses in 23,616 white Americans over the age of 35 years. *Oral Surg Oral Med Oral Pathol* 1986;61:373–381.

Boyce TM, Potter-Boyne G, Dziobek L, Solomon SL. Nosocomial pneumonia in Medicare patients: hospital cost and reimbursement. *Arch Intern Med* 1991;151:1109–1114.

Braunwald E, Isselbacker KJ, Petersdorf RG, et al. *Harrison's Principles of Internal Medicine,* 12th ed. New York: McGraw Hill, 1991.

Bredenkamp JK, Castro DJ, Mickel RA. Importance of iron repletion in the management of Plummer-Vinson syndrome. *Ann Otol Rhinol Laryngol* 1990;99:51–54.

Brown DL, Chapman WC, Edwards WH, et al. Dysphagia lusoria: aberrant right subclavian artery with a Kommerell's diverticulum. *Am Surg* 1993; 59:582–586.

Buchholz DW. What is dysphagia? *Dysphagia* 1996; 11:23–24.

Carrau RL, Murry T: *Comprehensive Management of Swallowing Disorders.* San Diego, CA: Singular Publishing Group, 1999.

Cummings CW, Fredrickson JM, Harker LA, et al. *Otolaryngology—Head and Neck Surgery.* St. Louis: Mosby, 1986.

Ekbert O, Nylander G. Cineradiography of the pharyngeal stage of deglutition in 150 individuals without dysphagia. *Br J Radiol* 1982;55: 253–257.

English GM. *Otolaryngology,* rev ed. New York: Harper & Row, 1990.

Ganong WF. *Review of Medical Physiology,* 14th ed. Norwalk, CT: Appleton & Lange, 1989.

Garibaldi RA, Brodine S, Matsumiya S. Infections among patients in nursing homes. *N Engl J Med* 1981;305:731–735.

Giordano A, Adams G, Boies L Jr, Meyerhold W. Current management of esophageal foreign bodies. *Arch Otolaryngol* 1981;107:249–251.

Gross JS, Neufeld RR, Libow LS, et al. Autopsy study of the elderly institutionalized patients—review of 234 autopsies. *Arch Intern Med* 1988; 4:173–174.

Harvey AM, Johns RJ, McKusick VA. *Principles and Practice of Medicine,* 22nd ed. Norwalk, CT: Appleton & Lange, 1988.

Hawkins DB, Demeter MJ, Barnett TE. Caustic ingestion: controversies in management: review of 214 cases. *Laryngoscope* 1980;90:98–109.

Hollingshead WH. *Textbook of Anatomy,* 3rd ed. New York: Harper & Row, 1974.

Horner J, Massey EW, Riski JE, et al. Aspiration following stroke: clinical correlates and outcome. *Neurology* 1988;38:1359–1362.

Langmore SE, Schatz K, Olsen N. Fiberoptic endoscopic examination of swallowing safety: a new procedure. *Dysphagia* 1998;2:216–219.

Lassen PE, Hegtuedt AK. Odontogenesis and odontogenic cysts and tumors. In: Cummings CW, et al, eds. *Otolaryngology Head and Neck Surgery.* St Louis: Mosby–Year Book, 1993.

Lee KJ, ed. *Essential Otolaryngology,* 7th ed. New York: Elsevier Science, 1987.

Logemann J. *Evaluation and Treatment of Swallowing Disorders.* San Diego, CA: College-Hill Press, 1983.

Miller A: Deglutition. *Physiol Rev* 1982;62:129–184.

Robbins SL. *Pathologic Basis of Disease.* Philadelphia: Saunders, 1989.

Sasaki CT, Isaacson G. Functional anatomy of the larynx. *Otolaryngol Clin North Am* 1988;21: 595–612.

Sasaki CT, Levine PA, Laitman JT, et al. Postnatal descent of the epiglottis in man: a preliminary report. *Arch Otolaryngol* 1977;103:169.

Scherr SA, Naspeca JA, McKaelian DO, Simonian SK. Chronic candidiasis of the oral cavity and esophagus. *Laryngoscope* 1980;90:769–774.

Sleisenger MN, Fordtran JS. *Gastrointestinal Disease,* 2nd ed. Philadelphia: Saunders, 1987.

Spiro HM. *Gastroenterology,* 2nd ed. New York: Macmillan, 1977.

Tucker JA, Yarington CT Jr. The treatment of caustic ingestion. *Otolaryngol Clin North Am* 1979; 12(2):343–350.

Welsh JJ, Welsh LW. Endoscopic examination of corrosive injuries of the upper gastrointestinal tract. *Laryngoscope* 1978;88:1300–1309.

Infections of the Ear 23

INFECTIONS OF THE PINNA

Skin

Bacterial infections of the auricle are often related to underlying patient comorbidities as well as trauma. Common sources of trauma include ear piercing, boxing, blunt trauma, burns, and iatrogenic insults. The common manifestations of bacterial infections are discussed below.

Bacterial

Epidemiology and Pathophysiology

Cellulitis of the ear is most commonly secondary to otitis externa[1] or due to trauma (ie, ear piercing), with the common pathogens being staphylococcal and streptococcal species.[2] There appears to be little gender difference in the incidence of cellulitis. Often, underlying comorbidities such as diabetes contribute to the development of cellulitis, as seen in a recent series by Kimura et al.[1] of hospitalized patients. There is an increased incidence in warmer climates as well. Other predisposing factors include the technique of ear piercing and "high" ear piercing (cartilaginous). Prior to piercing, ear preparation with benzalkonium chloride, a typical antiseptic, is not effective against pseudomonas; whereas 70% alcohol is effective against many skin bacteria except fungal organisms.[2] Keeping the ear clean, dry, and protected from trauma would appear prudent after piercing to decrease the incidence of perichondritis and abscess.[3]

Erysipelas or St. Anthony's fire of the pinna is an infection caused by involvement of the skin with group A beta-hemolytic streptococci, which may be similar in presentation to cellulitis of the external ear.[4] The histologic difference between these two entities lies in the depth of invasion; erysipelas is a more superficial infection than cellulitis.

Signs and Symptoms

Induration, warmth, erythema, tenderness, and fever are commonly seen. A chronic infection may develop over time that is possibly perpetuated by stasis of lymph flow.[5] Reports of toxic shock syndrome (fever, hypotension, diarrhea, strawberry tongue, erythroderma) even after a simple ear piercing are noted in the literature.[6] Clinically, erysipelas manifests itself as a raised, salmon-red, warm, and well-circumscribed area with progressing borders.[7]

Common Pathogens

Cultures often reveal *Staphylococcus aureus,* coagulase-negative *Staphylococcus, Pseudomonas aeruginosa,* and *Streptococcus* species.[1,2] Group A beta-hemolytic streptococci are especially common in erysipelas.

Diagnostic Workup

Culture is rarely necessary. If there is no resolution, consider fungal origin or biopsy for neoplasm.

462

Treatment Options

Treatment varies depending on the severity of the infection. Due to the long-term cartilaginous deformity (cauliflower ear) associated with severe perichondritis and abscess, aggressive treatment is warranted early in the course of infection. Both oral and intravenous quinolones and intravenous antipseudomonal aminopenicillins can be used for treatment, depending on the severity.[8] Oral antistaphylococcal and antistreptococcal antibiotics are adequate for simple infections; if complications are suspected, intravenous antibiotics are recommended. For treatment of perichondritis, see below.

Viral

Epidemiology and Pathophysiology

Viral infections of the external ear are relatively uncommon. The most often cited is herpes zoster oticus or the Ramsay Hunt syndrome, first cited in 1907.[9] Patients with a history of varicella zoster virus (VZV) are susceptible to this infection during times of immunosuppression. In addition, VZV reactivation may be responsible for delayed facial palsy and Ramsay Hunt syndrome after dental procedures and orofacial surgery.[10] This syndrome is responsible for 2 to 10% of all facial paralysis. The cause appears to be a recrudescence of a latent VZV infection of the geniculate ganglion and possibly throughout the facial nerve.[9] Multiple reports confirm the presence of genomic VZV DNA in the geniculate segment of the facial nerve as well as the spiral ganglion, aural vesicles, cerebrospinal fluid (CSF), middle ear mucosa, and facial canal; thus it appears to be a widespread infection.[11] It is important to note that in control temporal bones, it is common to see VZV DNA in unaffected adults.[10]

Human papillomavirus can also infect the external ear in the form of verrucae and thus represents another common viral infection of the external ear.

Signs and Symptoms

Patients with Ramsay Hunt syndrome may exhibit a combination of pathologies. It was first classified as (1) a disease affecting the sensory portion of the seventh cranial nerve, (2) a disease affecting the sensory and motor divisions of the seventh cranial nerve, (3) a disease affecting the sensory and motor divisions of the seventh cranial nerve with auditory symptoms, and (4) a disease affecting the sensory and motor divisions of the seventh cranial nerve with auditory and vestibular symptoms. In this syndrome, pain around the ear and a vesicular eruption (80–90% of patients) in the area of the conchal bowl, oral mucosa, or neck may precede, follow, or occur simultaneously with a rapidly progressive facial palsy that is House-Brackmann grade IV to VI in 50% of patients.[12] Also, sensorineural hearing loss (50%), and vertigo (30%) may occur.[13] The prognosis for recovery from facial paralysis is poorer than that of idiopathic Bell's palsy and exhibits a more severe denervation.[14] Other cranial nerves (V, IX, X, XI, and XII) can be affected as well.[15] Ramsay Hunt syndrome is also seen infrequently in children, with an improved prognosis and a less severe clinical course.[12]

Common Pathogen

Varicella zoster virus.

Diagnostic Workup

This should include a Tzanck smear, isolation of virus from the ear vesicles, and magnetic resonance imaging (MRI) of temporal bones and internal auditory canal to rule out concomitant cause of facial paralysis. Laboratory confirmation of increasing viral serum titers on complement fixation test can also be helpful.[13,15]

Treatment Options

Valacyclovir for 14 days or famciclovir for 10 days with steroids.[9] Acyclovir given intravenously appears to improve the outcome in retrospective case series, whereas it is generally considered to have poor bioavailability by the oral route.[15] Facial nerve decompression has been advocated in the past, typically in the area of the labyrinthine and geniculate segments; however, evidence of widespread inflammation along the entire course of the nerve may argue against this limited decompression.

Fungal

Epidemiology and Pathophysiology

Fungal infections of the pinna are usually secondary to extension from external otitis, which is covered in the next section. Rare causes of cellulitis of the pinna should be considered when the patient does not respond to traditional therapy, in cases of underlying immunosuppression, or based upon a characteristic patient history. A wide variety of fungal organisms have been implicated, including those involved in chromoblastomycosis.[16] A detailed patient history that includes the patient's geographical region, hobbies, and occupation will aid in diagnosis. Rarely, these uncommon pathogens, such as *Sporothrix schenckii,* may present with erythema as well as non-healing ulcers.[17]

Signs and Symptoms

Patients with fungal and unusual infections of the pinna usually will offer few distinguishing clues as to the particular pathogen. The ear often appears erythematous, tender, and edematous, as in most cellulitis. Systemic syndromes of disseminated fungal infections may also be present.

Common Pathogens

Aspergillus, Histoplasma, Mucor, Candida, Coccidiomyces, Blastomyces, Penicillium, dermatophytes (*Microsporum, Epidermophyton, Trichophyton*), and those involved in chromoblastomycosis.

Diagnostic Workup

Biopsy and fungal staining is appropriate; chest x-ray and serologic titers may also be considered.[18]

Treatment Options

Treat according to the specific etiology, with systemic therapy reserved for immunocompromised hosts or severe infections, etc. Debridement may be necessary in advanced cases.

Other Infections of the External Ear

Borrelia burgdorferi, the cause of Lyme disease, is transmitted by the tick *Ioxedes dammini.* It may be noted in the first stage by the characteristic rash, erythema chronicum migrans, and during the second stage as lymphocytoma with intensely red and violet nodules seen on the earlobe.

Treponema pallidum, the causative agent of syphilis, is rarely involved in infections of the external auditory canal, although a gumma, a lesion of tertiary syphilis, may be seen in the external canal.

Tuberculoid and lepromatous leprosy, cutaneous leishmaniasis, pediculosis, and scabies are other uncommon infections of the external ear.[19]

Perichondritis and Chondritis

Epidemiology and Pathophysiology

These infections of the auricle represent a more severe infection of the mesenchymal elements of the auricle. Typically, an inciting event such as ear piercing, a burn, surgery, or blunt or penetrating trauma (wrestling, acupuncture) may develop into a more severe infection threatening the integrity of the underlying cartilage due to vascular compromise. It is important to distinguish this entity from relapsing polychondritis, malignancy (lymphoma), and other inflammatory disorders, as the treatment differs considerably. With the advent of improved antipseudomonal antibiotics in burn patients, the incidence has decreased appreciably over the past decades.[20] The diagnosis is often based upon the clinical appearance of the ear as warm and fluctuant—it may or may not be tender—with drainage. The distinction between perichondritis and chondritis can be made only at the time of surgery, with the presence of necrotic cartilage indicating chondritis. After initial trauma, blood or serum collects in the subperichondrial potential space and may become secondarily infected with *S. aureus, P. aeruginosa,* and *Proteus* species.[21] Once this subperichondrial space is evacuated, cartilage deposition begins in 2 to 4 weeks from the remaining perichondrium, and an uneven matrix may lead to a cauliflower ear deformity.[22]

Signs and Symptoms

These infections may be acute or chronic, presenting even a few weeks after the initial inciting event.[23] After trauma, a fluctuant swelling from a hematoma or a chronically erythematous, tender, and draining ear is seen.

Common Pathogens

In order of decreasing incidence, *P. aeruginosa, S. aureus, Enterobacter, Proteus mirabilis* and other gram-negative organisms may be causative.[20]

Diagnostic Workup

Culture and sensitivity, biopsy in the clinic or operating room.

Treatment Options

The treatment goals for perichondritis and chondritis are eradiction of the infection and optimization of the final cosmetic outcome of the patient's ear. These patients are often litigious over the final cosmetic outcome; therefore it is important to caution the patient from the outset of the possibility of a significant auricular deformity. In addition, a prolonged treatment course of 1 to 2 months is not unusual.[21,22] Since the final outcome of these infections is often poor, prevention of the initial infection is the most important intervention. Careful attention to wound care, evacuation of hematoma or seroma, ear bolsters, gentle handling of the ear, and prophylactic topical (in burn patients) and systemic antibiotics are standard procedure after trauma.[20]

Management consists of antibiotic therapy, repeated surgical debridement, and meticulous local wound care. Antibiotic therapy is directed to gram-negative organisms and *S. aureus.* This may consist of an antipseudomonal aminopenicillin or a fluoroquinolone for 2 to 4 weeks.[8] Inpatient observation and intravenous antibiotics are usually recommended until clinical improvement is obtained, with outpatient use of directed antimicrobials.

The goal of surgery is to eliminate necrotic cartilage and minimize subsequent deformity. Surgical techniques vary from complete cartilage excision with a bivalve incision along the rim of the pinna to instillation of multiple catheters for irrigation of antibiotic solutions; however, only isolated case reports are available for comparison of these techniques.[20,24,25] The use of catheters may involve up to 1 month of irrigation with antibiotic solutions. Debridement is accomplished in the operating room, as these infections are severely painful. The final result of intervention is often disappointing when the disease is addressed late in its course.

INFECTIONS OF THE EXTERNAL AUDITORY CANAL

Bacterial (Acute)

Epidemiology and Pathophysiology

The skin of the external auditory canal may become infected with a variety of bacteria when host defenses are altered. Approximately 10% of all people may be affected at one point in their lives, and 90% of the time the infection is unilateral.[26,27] This disease occurs with a higher frequency in warm, humid climates and is more common in swimmers due to local maceration of the canal skin with hypothesized entry of pathogenic bacteria (eg, swimmer's ear). Infection occurs with occlusion of the apopilosebaceous units and subsequent bacterial proliferation.[28] Interestingly, the source of the problem from swimming pools appears to be an alkaline pH of the implicated pool water rather than the introduction of pathogenic bacteria. For example, the water from suspect pools often does not grow out the offending organism.[29] This change in pH appears to affect the susceptibility of the external auditory canal to bacterial overgrowth and subsequent infection. Another common predisposing factor is trauma to the canal with removal of cerumen by cotton-tipped applicators or other instrumentation. This mechanical removal of cerumen predisposes the canal skin to maceration.[28] Human cerumen is hydrophobic and acidic (pH 4–5); it contains lysozyme and immunoglobulin. A wide body of literature provides conflicting results on the bacteriostatic or bactericidal properties of human cerumen, and there is no consensus at this time.[30] Underlying skin disorders—such as atopic dermatitis, psoriasis, and seborrheic dermatitis—also predispose individuals to acute bacterial otitis externa by breaks in the skin barrier and probably by local trauma from instrumentation for itching.[28,31] Other co-morbidities, such as diabetes mellitus and human immunodeficiency virus, predispose patients to otitis externa due to immune dysfunction. Finally, hearing aids, absence of cerumen, a narrow and long external canal with poor self-cleaning ability, foreign bodies, and allergy to medications may also be causative factors.

Furuncles and carbuncles are also acute bacterial infections of the external auditory canal at the apopilosebaceous unit. The confluence of multiple infected hair follicles constitutes a carbuncle.

Signs and Symptoms

The diagnosis of otitis externa is straightforward in the adult but can be confusing in the child.[29] Severe otalgia, pruritus, erythema, edema of the external auditory canal, and discharge are all commonly seen. The canal may be completely stenosed with edema, and a conductive hearing loss may also be present. Otoscopic examination may reveal a tympanic membrane with significant debris; however, pneumotoscopy should confirm mobility and the absence of a middle ear effusion. Because of these symptoms, the patient continues to traumatize the ear and further exacerbate the infection. The diagnostic dilemma in the child is evident in younger, less cooperative patients with a possible otitis media with perforation or even a mastoiditis masquerading as a severe external otitis. The patient with otitis media will often have otalgia and fever preceding aural discharge, and the ensuing physical examination can mimic external otitis.[29] Fever is seldom seen with uncomplicated external otitis unless there is a significant cellulitis or necrotizing otitis externa. Debris from external otitis can mimic otitis media; therefore, pneumotoscopy is important during the physical examination.

Senturia has divided the stages of external otitis into preinflammatory, acute inflammatory, and chronic inflammatory stages.[32] The preinflammatory stage is characterized by loss of cerumen and mild edema of the canal. The acute inflammatory stage is marked by a progression in severity of pruritus, edema, and otalgia. The chronic stage is noted as atrophic canal skin, a paucity of cerumen, and stenosis of the canal with minimal pain. This may progress to a more complicated course of postinflammatory medial canal fibrosis characterized by a thick, fibrous plug occluding the external canal and conductive hearing loss.[33]

The symptoms of a furuncle and carbuncle consist of a painful, raised papule or pustule, usually at the meatus of the external canal.

Common Pathogens

P. aeruginosa, Staphylococcus, Proteus, and other gram-negative rods.[28,29]

Diagnostic Workup

Culture. If there is no response to traditional empiric therapy, workup for necrotizing otitis externa (malignant otitis externa) if this is suspected.

Treatment Options

The management of bacterial otitis externa consists of prevention through risk-factor modification, gentle debridement of the external auditory canal, re-establishment of an acidic pH, topical antibiotics that can be delivered in high nontoxic concentrations, and treatment of any underlying skin or medical problems.

Risk-factor modification revolves around reducing trauma to the external auditory canal by refraining from the use of cotton-tipped swabs and eliminating exposure to water through the use of earplugs or cotton balls with petrolatum jelly on the outside.[28] After water exposure, the use of a hair dryer and alcohol/vinegar (acetic acid) or commercial acetic acid preparations is also useful.

Early otitis externa can be managed with meticulous cleaning under the microscope with a suction aspirator on a daily or every-other-day basis if needed. This will provide symptomatic relief and allow topical medicine to reach the skin. Topical antibiotics usually contain boric or acetic acid to decrease the pH of the canal and the following antibiotics: neomycin, active against *S. aureus, Proteus, Klebsiella, Escherichia coli* but not against *Pseudomonas;* polymyxin B or E, active against *Pseudomonas, E. coli, Klebsiella* but not against *Proteus* or many gram-positives; gentamicin, active against *Pseudomonas.* Combination preparations of the above antimicrobials with hydrocortisone are available. It is important to note that a neomycin allergy may be present in a few percent of patients. Newer quinolone preparations of ciprofloxacin and ofloxacin appear to be equally efficacious in controlling acute otitis externa.[29] Topical benzocaine can be used for topical relief of pruritus in otitis externa.[34] The presence of anaerobic bacteria such as *Bacteroides fragilis* mandates the use of an agent such as chloramphenicol; however, this is more commonly seen in the chronic draining ear.

For mild and moderate forms of otitis externa, risk-factor avoidance, frequent cleaning of the external canal, and the aforementioned topical antibiotics with or without hydrocortisone is recommended.

Severe otitis externa is differentiated from the earlier forms by severe canal edema and stenosis with similar microbiology. The treatment principle of advanced cases remains the same with the addition of an ear wick to help expand the canal and deliver topical antibiotics deep in the canal. Topical antibiotics such as gentamicin have been tested for their duration of action in the external ear with an ear wick, and approximately 12 hours appears to be the time when effectiveness may decrease, enabling twice-a-day dosing.[35] In the absence of systemic symptoms, necrotizing otitis externa, or a significant surrounding cellulitis, topical antibiotics alone are sufficient to treat otitis externa, with adequate cleaning of the canal.[36] The wick is changed in 24 to 48 hours and replaced only if there is inadequate expansion of the canal. Frequent cleaning is often necessary in the early treatment stages. If cellulitis, fever, or canal granulation is present, systemic antibiotics should be considered, with the consideration of skull base osteomyelitis.

The treatment of furuncles and carbuncles consists of systemic antibiotics against staphylococcal organisms, topical preparations, and the placement of an ear wick if needed. The thoroughness of control of the underlying chronic staphylococcal carrier state may be a factor in reducing recidivistic disease. In cases where a small abscess is clinically evident, the area of skin pointing can be incised after injection of a local anesthetic.

Malignant Otitis Externa (Necrotizing Otitis Externa, Skull Base Osteomyelitis)

Epidemiology and Pathophysiology

This was first described as a severe, potentially life-threatening infection of the external auditory canal seen in elderly diabetic or immunocompromised patients.[37] Typically, the disease occurs in the elderly diabetic patient with an underlying microangiopathy and cellular immune dysfunction that predisposes the patient to infection.[38] Necrotizing otitis externa can also occur in other immunocompromised patients, such as those with AIDS or malignancies. *P. aeruginosa* is the usual causative agent.[39] In patients with AIDS, the disease affects a younger population and appears to follow a more lethal course.[39] The pathology consists of a severe external otitis and an osteomyelitis of the base of the skull that may lead to lower cranial neuropathies, lateral sinus thrombosis, severe headache, meningitis, and death.[37] Nadol reviewed the histopathology in two patients and noted the following: chronic osteomyelitis of the temporal bone with new bone formation, lateral sinus thrombosis, facial nerve sheath inflammation with degeneration, meningeal inflammation, destruction of otic capsule bone by osteomyelitis, and labyrinthitis. Also, cavernous sinus obliteration with soft tissue was seen in one specimen.[40] Nadol defines the somewhat orderly progression of the disease as the following: (1) external auditory canal with invasion through the fissures of Santorini or the tympanomastoid suture to the retromandibular fossa, (2) involvement of the stylomastoid and jugular foramina, (3) septic thrombosis of the lateral venous sinus, (4) spread to petrous apex through vascular and fascial planes and not air cells.[40]

Signs and Symptoms

The course of the disease may be insidious in its onset, and a high index of suspicion is paramount for diagnosis in susceptible individuals. A gradual progression is not always the rule, and occasional improvement followed by worsening of symptoms is sometimes seen. Hallmarks of the disease include external otitis with granulation tissue along the posteroinferior aspect of the external auditory canal (EAC) (tympanomastoid suture line), lower cranial neuropathies (VII, IX, X, XI), and—commonly—deep, severe pain of the affected side. Exudate from the EAC is also common. The differential diagnosis includes Paget's disease, granulomatous disorders, and carcinoma.[38] Necrotizing external otitis has been staged by Benecke as follows: stage I, infection limited to soft tissue and cartilage; stage II, soft tissue involvement and bony erosion of the temporal bone; and stage III, intracranial extension or erosion beyond the temporal bone.[41] In children, skull base osteomyelitis may be seen with an improved prognosis, more commonly involving middle ear disease and a shorter treatment course.[38] In patients with AIDS, less canal granulation is seen; consequently, a heightened suspicion is necessary for diagnosis.[39]

Common Pathogens
These include *P. aeruginosa* and *S. aureus;* others, such as *Aspergillus* and *Proteus,* may be seen rarely.[38]

Diagnostic Workup
The canal exudate is cultured using a calcium alginate swab. The serum white blood cell count may be normal or slightly elevated, and the sedimentation rate is often markedly elevated.[42] Workup for underlying comorbidities is essential if these are not already known (ie, diabetes, HIV, etc.). Imaging studies are useful to delineate the extent of the disease and follow disease progression or resolution. Computed tomography (CT) documents extent of disease and shows bony involvement, which may not change with disease resolution. Therefore only an initial scan is needed. Bone scan may document the presence of osteomyelitis (nonspecific), which may not resolve for months after resolution has occurred. Gallium-67 scan—an indicator of active inflammation—is useful for tracking the state of disease; this study is also positive in soft tissue and bone infections. Slattery and Brackmann advocate repeating the gallium scan every 4 weeks to determine length of treatment.[38] A newer method of interpreting the gallium scan involves looking at the count ratio of the affected to nonaffected sides; this may add a more objective measure in determining the degree of disease resolution.[43]

Treatment Options
The basic principles of treatment are (1) early diagnosis in high-risk populations, (2) prolonged intravenous (and possibly oral) antibiotic therapy, (3) fastidious cleaning of the external auditory canal, (4) clinical examination and serial gallium scans to assess for resolution, and (5) surgical intervention for intra- or extratemporal abscesses. Early reports from Chandler document a mortality rate of 38% with the use of combined-modality treatment comprising surgery and antimicrobials.[42] Due to the widespread pathologic process outlined above, the current role for surgery may be limited due to the improvement in antipseudomonal antibiotics. Recent reports by Martel et al., using antibiotics alone with local external canal cleaning, and Davis et al., with dual-modality therapy (antibiotics and hyperbaric oxygen therapy), show improved success rates of upward of 90 to 100%.[44,45]

Antibiotic treatment for this disease is often long-term (2–4 months); consequently there is an increased risk of developing resistance to *P. aeruginosa.* The organism's resistance to antibiotics is deterred if two drugs with alternate modes of action are used; for example, a third-generation cephalosporin (ceftazidime) plus a quinolone.[38] Other commonly used regimens include an aminoglycoside (tobramycin) and an antipseudomonal aminopenicillin. No controlled studies are available at this time comparing dual antimicrobial regimens with single-drug therapy. Oral ciprofloxacin has been used as a single agent with success.[46] Due to the severe nature of the disease, drug resistance, and the potential for multiple complications including death, it is prudent to treat aggressively with two-drug therapy until significant resolution is noted. A common management dilemma is knowing when to stop treatment, because the patient may feel better soon after starting antibiotics. A normal-appearing canal is not a sensitive indicator of resolution, and recurrences are seen 2 to 3 months after apparent cure. The gallium scan may still be positive when the clinical examination is normal.[42] The resolution of otalgia, granulation in the canal, and improved gallium scans are useful indicators of improvement.

Refractory, advanced, and recurrent cases are candidates for adjuvant hyperbaric oxygen therapy (HBO) for 30 treatments.[45] The mechanisms of action include improved phagocytic killing due to higher tissue oxygen tension levels and improved activity of aminoglycoside antibiotics.[45] The authors propose the routine use of HBO in combination with antibiotics in advanced (stages II and III) and refractory cases.

Current treatment of necrotizing otitis externa is more successful than in the past due to improved antimicrobial therapy; however, prolonged follow-up is still necessary, as mortality rates are still high, especially in patients with AIDS.

Chronic Otitis Externa

Epidemiology and Pathophysiology

Acute otitis externa may evolve into a more chronic form, with distinct histologic changes in some patients. Skin changes of acanthosis, increased size of rete pegs, inflammation around apocrine glands, and absence of sebaceous glands is seen.[19] Chronic disease may also evolve from underlying skin disorders such as seborrheic and atopic dermatitis. Prolonged treatment with antimicrobial drops and steroid creams is seen often, and topical allergies (neomycin) may contribute to the disease.

Signs and Symptoms

The skin is often thickened and the canal may be stenosed. Lichenification, excoriations, and dry adherent debris (keratosis) are often seen in affected individuals. Often the patient does not complain of pain at this stage. Conductive hearing loss may be present and may signify progression to postinflammatory medial canal fibrosis.[33] The patient may have a history of an underlying skin disorder or diabetes.

Common Pathogens

Gram-negative bacilli such as *Proteus*.[19]

Diagnostic Workup

Culture. Biopsy if there is persistent granulation, ulcer, and lack of response to therapy.

Treatment Options

The principles of treatment are similar to those for acute bacterial otitis externa, including gentle debridement of the external auditory canal, re-establishment of an acidic pH, topical antibiotics that can be delivered in high nontoxic concentrations, and treatment of any underlying skin or medical problems. In addition, direct injection of corticosteroids (Kenalog, etc.) may be useful for persistent edema of the canal skin. Finally, in the most recalcitrant cases, canalplasty, excision of canal skin, and split-thickness skin graft may be useful.[19]

Fungal

Epidemiology and Pathophysiology

The rate of fungal otitis externa (otomycosis) in the general population varies by geographic location from 9 to over 50% of all patients with otitis externa.[28] Moist and tropical environments provide the required milieu for fungal proliferation, and the increased incidence may be attributed to increased sweat and environmental humidity altering the surface epithelium of the external canal. The epithelium of the external canal is known to absorb water in these environments, possibly making it more susceptible to infection. A wide variety of organisms are seen; any of these may be the primary pathogen or may be superimposed upon a bacterial infection; in the past, the existence of primary otomycosis was questioned.[19] At this time, it is agreed that mycotic infection of the external canal represents a distinct pathologic entity. This disease also commonly occurs in postsurgical patients with mastoid bowls. Rarely, in immunocompromised patients, invasive otomycosis (*Mucor, Aspergillus*) is diagnosed.[47] The overgrowth of fungi is sometimes seen in the presence of antibacterials that alter the normal flora of the host. Although use of topical ear preparations is hypothesized to lead to an increased incidence of fungal infections, this is probably not true.[48]

Signs and Symptoms

Often the presenting symptoms of bacterial otitis externa and otomycosis are indistinguishable; however, later in the course of disease, pruritus is more frequently characteristic of mycotic infections. Also common are discomfort, hearing loss, tinnitus, and discharge.[19] There appears to be no reported difference in presentation based on the most prevalent organisms. The characteristic physical examination of fungal infections resembles that of common molds, with visible, delicate hyphae and spores (conidiophores) being seen in *Aspergillus. Candida,* a yeast, often forms mats of mycelia that are white in character; when mixed with cerumen, they appear yellowish. In the case of invasive fungal disease or unusual organisms, additional local and systemic manifestations are expected, such as cranial nerve paralysis, etc.

Common Pathogens

Prevalence depends on geographic locale: *Candida, Aspergillus niger, Aspergillus fumigatus, Penicillium,* and many others.

Diagnostic Workup

Culture is rarely needed and does not alter management. In severely immunocompromised hosts or in patients with atypical presentations, biopsy is indicated.

Treatment Options

The treatment of dermatophytosis consists of elimination of predisposing factors, the use of antifungal agents, and thorough cleaning of the canal. Antifungal preparations can be divided into nonspecific and specific types. Nonspecific antifungals include acidifying and dehydrating solutions such as boric acid, aluminum sulfate–calcium acetate, gentian violet 2%, Castellani's paint (acetone, alcohol, phenol, fuchsin, resorcinol), and Cresylate (Merthiolate, M-Cresyl acetate, propylene glycol, boric acid, and alcohol). In a nonblinded prospective study, gentian violet was 80 to 90% successful in 19 patients.[48] Also, Cresylate appears to have effective antifungal activity in vitro.[19]

Specific antifungal treatments consist of creams, solutions, and powders. In vitro studies and a prospective trial confirm clotrimazole as one of the most effective agents against *Aspergillus* and *Candida.*[19,48] Other commonly used antifungals include amphotericin B, tolnaftate, miconazole, and nystatin. In the presence of an uncomplicated otomycosis with an intact tympanic membrane, many of these agents are effective when combined with thorough cleaning of the canal.

When the patient has an open middle ear cavity such as pressure equalization tubes, radical mastoidectomy, and perforation, additional caution is necessary in the application and choice of preparations. Cresylate and gentian violet are known to be irritating to the middle ear mucosa. In addition, gentian violet appears to be vestibulotoxic and to incite middle ear inflammation in animal models; therefore, it should be used with caution in the presence of an open middle ear cleft.[49] Common nonspecific preparations such as acetic acid and propylene glycol have been shown to elevate brain stem response thresholds in animal models and can be painful on application.[50] A recent animal study showed no hair cell loss in the presence of clotrimazole, miconazole, nystatin, and tolnaftate.[49] A conservative choice for therapy with an open tympanic membrane is warranted—for example, careful cleaning and a specific antifungal medication with a minimum of additives.

Other special circumstances include otomycosis in older patients with hearing aids and immunocompromised patients. In patients with hearing aids, creams and solutions may exacerbate the moist environment, so dusting with specific antifungal therapy is recommended. It is also prudent to remove the hearing aid until the infection is resolved in order to help dry the ear. Immunocompromised patients can develop invasive fungal infections and biopsy with systemic therapy may be necessary, as these infections are often fatal.[39]

Other Organisms

As in infections of the auricle, rare organisms infect the EAC. Syphilis, Lyme disease, tuberculoid and lepromatous leprosy, cutaneous leishmaniasis, pediculosis, and scabies are some examples.[19]

INFECTIONS OF THE TYMPANIC MEMBRANE

Epidemiology and Pathophysiology

Infections limited to the tympanic membrane are less common than those previously discussed and several clinical entities are described. Bullous and granular myringitis (myringitis chronica granulosa, tympanic membrane epithelitis) are the most prevalent manifestations of infection of the tympanic membrane.[51,52] The present literature defines the differences between these diseases poorly, and the terminology is often confusing and inconsistent. This is most likely due to the fact that a disparate group of diseases are defined under the current nosology.

Bullous myringitis (myringitis bullosa) as an entity is typically described as an acute, self-limiting disease, usually unilateral, that is seen in adolescents and young adults. The pathology demonstrates inflammation of all the layers of the tympanic membrane, with bullae forming under the epithelial surface layer.[53] This disease should be divided into a primary form with no underlying otitis media and a secondary form as a sequela of middle ear disease.

Chronic granular myringitis is defined as a loss of tympanic membrane epithelium for greater than 1 month without middle ear disease.[51] It is a rare disease with an incidence of approximately 1% in a recent review from an otologist's practice and is more common in older individuals. The disorder is usually unilateral and can be associated with previous otitis media, trauma, or ventilation tubes. No associated underlying medical problems are related to the disorder, although trauma in the form of tympanomastoid surgery is a common pathogenic factor.[51]

Signs and Symptoms

Bullous myringitis typically presents with severe otalgia and bullae of the tympanic membrane that may be hemorrhagic or serous in character. The disease is typically self-limited lasting 3 or 4 days and may demonstrate a mild conductive hearing loss.[54] This may follow a viral upper respiratory infection or even be secondary to otitis media.

The symptoms and appearance of chronic granular myringitis can be confused with chronic otitis media as well as external otitis. Raised, pale granulation tissue is present on a portion (usually posterosuperior) or all of the tympanic membrane in up to 55% of the patients; recurrent perforations, thickened tympanic membrane, myringosclerosis, and external auditory canal involvement are sometimes seen. The drum typically is mobile on pneumatic examination. Otorrhea and pruritus are also common complaints.[51,52] The patients may also have a conductive hearing loss of up to 40 dB.[51] In contrast to chronic otitis media, no middle ear involvement is noted. Some authors conclude that the absence of a perforation is a prerequisite for diagnosis. Also, the involvement of the external auditory canal is usually limited to the portion near the tympanic membrane, in distinction to generalized otitis externa.

Common Pathogens

Bullous myringitis may be due to a group of different viruses, bacteria, and atypicals: *Haemophilus influenzae, S. pneumoniae, Moraxella catarrhalis,* parainfluenza virus, *Mycoplasma,* and others. Although a relationship is postulated between the *Mycoplasma* organism and bullous myringitis from studies by Rifkind et al., more recent data appear to refute this claim.[55,56] A wide variety of organisms, both viral and bacterial, are currently implicated in this disease, including the most common agents of otitis media.

Chronic granular myringitis may be due to a group of different viruses, bacteria, and atypicals including *S. aureus, S. epidermis, and P. aeruginosa.* There is again a debate in the literature regarding the pathogenic organisms. Bacterial, viral, and fungal organisms have been cultured in this disease.

Diagnostic Workup

Culture does not appear to influence management in bullous myringitis, as it is a self-limiting disease. The choice of therapy in chronic granular myringitis is also not influenced by culture results.[51] An audiogram may be helpful in documenting a conductive hearing loss.

Treatment

Primary bullous myringitis will resolve on its own in 3 to 4 days. Antibiotic drops are discouraged and do not appear to influence the resolution of disease or degree of symptoms. The use of a myringotomy knife to open the bullae is advocated to decrease pain, taking caution not to enter the middle ear space.

The basic principle of treatment for secondary bullous myringitis is to address the underlying otitis media with appropriate antibiotics.

The treatment of chronic granular myringitis is more controversial and less rewarding. Many patients are referred to the otologist after 5 or more years of symptoms and multiple courses of topical antibiotics.[51] The proposed treatment options consist of dry ear precautions, antibiotic drops, curettage, skin grafting, cauterization, and tympanoplasty for recalcitrant cases. A favorable response to treatment is common with conservative therapy when it is continued for weeks to months; however, recurrence should be expected. On the other hand, formal curettage and tympanoplasty may offer more long-lasting effects, with only occasional recurrences noted in one recent study.[52]

INFECTIONS OF THE MIDDLE EAR

Infections of the middle ear are broadly classified under the heading of otitis media. Strictly speaking, the term *otitis media* implies inflammation of the middle ear without regard to etiology or pathogenesis. Otitis media may be further subclassified in a number of ways according to the chronicity of the disease, presence of symptoms, appearance of the ear, or presumed etiology and pathogenesis. For the purposes of this chapter, the classification scheme proposed by Bluestone[57] is used.

Acute Otitis Media

Definition

Acute otitis media (AOM) involves the rapid onset of a constellation of signs and symptoms including otalgia and otoscopic evidence of middle ear effusion. Associated systemic manifestations may include anorexia, fever, vomiting, and diarrhea. The term *acute otitis media* implies a suppurative process of the middle ear space.

Epidemiology and Cost

AOM is one of the most common diseases of childhood. It has been estimated that children in the United States will experience 9.3 million episodes of AOM in the first 2 years of life.[58] In fact, Teele and colleagues found that otitis media accounted for 22.7% of visits to the pediatrician's office in the first year of life and up to 40% of visits during years 4 and 5.[59] Moreover, about one in three visits to the doctor's office for an illness were for the diagnosis of otitis media, and nearly 75% of follow-up visits were for otitis media.[59] Studies indicate that 19 to 62% of children have had at least one episode of AOM by 1 year of age, and as many as 85% of children have had at least one episode of AOM by 3 years of age.[59-65] The peak incidence of AOM is found during the second half of the first year of life. Recurrent AOM is also common, with three or more episodes occurring in 20% of children prior to 1 year of age and overall in nearly 40% of children. Risk factors for the development of AOM have been well documented and include age < 6 years, male gender, group day care, lack of breast feeding, secondhand smoke exposure, craniofacial growth abnormalities, the presence of frequent upper respiratory tract viral infections, underlying immunodeficiency, and genetic predisposition.[66]

The socioeconomic impact is also quite impressive, with billions of dollars being spent annually on the medical and surgical treatment of otitis media.[67] Gates recently estimated that AOM accounts for approximately $3.15 billion in total costs annually, of which $1.4 billion represented direct health care costs and the remaining $1.75 billion indirect costs related to family expenses.[68]

Pathogenesis

The pathogenesis of AOM is multifactorial.[69] In general, the two most clearly documented factors are bacterial infection of the middle ear space and eustachian tube dysfunction. In addition, there is growing evidence for the role of viral upper respiratory tract infections as a cause for episodes of AOM. In many cases, all three of these factors may be at work, with a viral upper respiratory tract infection (ie, the common cold) resulting in eustachian tube dysfunction and improved bacterial adherence to the upper respiratory tract mucosa, thereby allowing for altered regulation of middle ear pressure and middle ear underpressure formation. Middle ear underpressures combined with increasing numbers of microorganisms in the region of the eustachian tube orifice may predispose to bacterial and/or viral insufflation or aspiration into the tympanic cavity, with resultant suppuration and symptoms.[69-71]

Signs and Symptoms

The hallmark symptom of a child with AOM is otalgia. Best evidence suggests that otalgia is present in 50 to 75% of children with AOM.[72-74] By contrast, otalgia appears to be less frequently reported for children less than 2 years of age. In babies, symptoms such as irritability, fussiness, constant crying, lethargy, sleeplessness, or pulling at the affected ear(s)—with associated anorexia, fever, or vomiting—are frequently reported. Fever is also a common finding, being present between 21 and 45% of the time.[73,74] In older children and adults, hearing loss may also be a prominent symptom. In both adults and children, a viral upper respiratory tract infection precedes new episodes of AOM nearly 50% of the time.[75] In the early stages of infection, physical examination usually reveals a bulging, immobile, opaque tympanic membrane with some degree of erythema. In the later stages, the tympanic membrane is usually thick, with varying degrees of surface desquamation and possible perforation as well as purulent otorrhea and bleeding. During the resolution stages, the symptoms are mostly resolved except for the hearing impairment that results from residual middle ear effusion.[76]

Diagnostic Workup

For most patients with AOM, a history and physical examination are all that is needed to make a correct diagnosis. Further diagnostic studies are necessary only when the diagnosis is unclear, treatment is ineffective, or an intratemporal or intracranial complication is present or suspected. Diagnostic studies available to the physician include standard pneumatic otoscopy, otomicroscopy with a Breuning's pneumatic lens, audiologic testing (ie, tympanometry and audiometry), radiologic studies (ie, computed tomography, magnetic resonance imaging), surgical interventions (tympanocentesis, myringotomy +/− tympanostomy tube placement), and microbiologic testing. When the diagnosis is not evident, use of the operating microscope with the pneumatic lens will usually help to make the diagnosis. Tympanometry may confirm the altered mobility of the tympanic membrane; however, the lack of tympanometric immobility should not exclude the diagnosis. In numerous studies, the presence of a flat (type B) tympanogram was 94% sensitive but only 53 to 75% specific.[76–78] Diagnostic audiometry is not routinely used for children with AOM. Diagnostic tympanocentesis or myringotomy at the time of initial presentation should probably be reserved for those patients that are severely toxic, very young (neonate), in the intensive care unit setting, or have associated immunodeficiency.

For patients in whom treatment has been ineffective, the diagnosis of AOM must be reconsidered and the efficacy of the therapeutic intervention reassessed. When the diagnosis is still clear and evident, specific attention should be given to the possibility of a pathogen that is not being addressed by the particular treatment regimen (eg, resistant bacteria, virus, or fungus) or that the prescribed drug is not being delivered effectively (eg, malabsorption or poor patient compliance). Should the patient have or be suspected of having an intratemporal or intracranial complication or a resistant or atypical microorganism, tympanocentesis or myringotomy with Gram's stain, culture, and antimicrobial sensitivity testing should be undertaken immediately. Tympanocentesis should be used when organism identification is all that is needed, whereas myringotomy with aspiration should be used for middle ear drainage. Imaging studies are usually reserved for patients with suspected intratemporal or intracranial complications (see below).

In children with recurrent AOM, the history should attempt to uncover risk factors such as secondhand smoke exposure, bottle feeding, and group day care attendance. Physical examination for an occult submucous palatal cleft should be performed. Ancillary studies should attempt to evaluate for respiratory allergies, chronic sinonasal disease, immune deficiencies, primary ciliary dyskinesia, and vaccine status (ie, pneumococcal vaccine).

Common Pathogens

Numerous studies have assessed the microbiology of AOM.[69] In general, bacteria, viruses, and rarely fungi can all cause AOM.

BACTERIA   In studies that have performed diagnostic tympanocentesis, bacterial species have been isolated from the middle ear fluids in patients with AOM between 65 and 80% of the time. Although geographic regional variations occur, the three most common bacterial species responsible for AOM in children are *S. pneumoniae* (27–52%), *H. influenzae* (16–52%), and *M. catarrhalis* (2–15%). Other less common organisms include *Streptococcus pyogenes* (group A beta-hemolytic), *S. aureus* (coagulase-positive), *S. epidermidis* (coagulase negative), and gram-negative species. In neonates, there are some differences regarding the frequency of isolation of the various bacterial species, with the gram-negative organisms playing a slightly more prominent role.[79–83] Adults with AOM have microbiologic results similar to those of children.[84]

In general, bacterial resistance to antimicrobial agents has been a constant problem since the 1930s, following the introduction of the sulfonamides. In terms of AOM, resistant strains of the three most common bacterial species have frequently been identified in recent years and appear to account for numerous treatment failures and some increases in the frequency of infection-related complications. For *S. pneumoniae,* penicillin-resistant species were first identified in 1965. For this organism, susceptibility is defined by a mean inhibitory concentration (MIC) of <0.1 μg/mL, intermediate resistance as an MIC between 0.1 and 1.0 μg/mL, and resistance as MIC >1.0 μg/mL. Penicillin resistance is conferred to *S. pneumoniae* by changes in the penicillin-binding proteins in the cell wall of the bacteria, resulting in reduced affinity for beta-lactam-containing drugs. The incidence of penicillin-resistant strains of *S. pneumoniae* varies widely, with reported rates between 1 and 40% of isolates.[85,86]

H. influenzae and *M. catarrhalis* both produce beta-lactamase, thus conferring resistance to many penicillins and cephalosporins. For *H. influenzae,* the frequency of beta-lactamase production is between 20 and 40% of middle ear isolates. *M. catarrhalis* produces beta-lactamase in as high as 90 to 100% of isolates.[87] Equally worrisome is the fact that in a manner similar to *S. pneumoniae,* non-beta-lactamase-mediated resistance is occurring in strains of *H. influenzae*.[88]

VIRUSES   Respiratory viruses have been implicated as causative agents in AOM. Upper respiratory tract viral infections have been shown to precede as many as 50% of episodes of AOM.[75] Using standard culture techniques, viruses have been isolated from middle ear fluids of children with AOM 4.4 to 46% of the time.[89] Using virus-specific enzyme-linked immunoabsorbent assay (ELISA) and polymerase chain reaction (PCR) diagnostic techniques, viruses have been isolated in nearly 75% of middle ear fluids in children with AOM.[74,90,91] The most common viruses identified in cases of AOM include respiratory syncytial virus, influenza A and B viruses, rhinoviruses, mumps virus, enteroviruses, parainfluenza virus, and adenovirus.[92] Human viral challenges with various respiratory viruses have also resulted in AOM, proving a causal effect.[70,93–95] Viruses have also been implicated as a cause of treatment failure in cases of AOM.[96]

Treatment Options

Numerous studies have addressed therapies for AOM and recurrent AOM.[71,97] In general, the goals of therapy include symptomatic relief, clinical resolution, prevention of suppurative complications, clearance of residual middle ear fluid, and reduced incidence of future episodes of AOM. In this regard, only antimicrobial therapy and surgery have had a demonstrated therapeutic effect in well-controlled, randomized clinical trials. At this time, other therapies should be considered experimental. Caution should also be used when generalizing the results of randomized clinical trials to the entire population of patients with AOM. Due to the extensive selection criteria for study entry, most trials exclude children who are very young and/or have craniofacial growth abnormalities, immune deficiencies, severe infections, or other chronic illnesses. Thus, therapy must be individualized for each patient. The data below should serve only as general guidelines for therapy.

A. Acute Otitis Media

1. *Natural History:* In a summary of placebo-treated children with nonsevere AOM, resolution of fever and pain occurred in 59, 87, and 88% of children by 24 hours, 2 to 3 days, and 4 to 7 days following onset, respectively. Clinical resolution including all presenting signs and symptoms (except middle ear fluid) occurred in 73% of children by 7 to 14 days. The natural history of middle ear effusion following a single episode of AOM is that 47% of untreated children clear the fluid by 2 weeks, 60% clear the fluid by 1 month, and 75% clear the fluid by 3 months.[97]

2. *Antibiotics:* Two metanalyses of eight randomized, placebo-controlled clinical trials have demonstrated some positive effects for antibiotics on the outcome measures above.[98,99] Specifically, antimicrobial therapy has been shown to provide symptom relief significantly better than placebo by 2 to 7 days after treatment. Moreover, antibiotics were 13% more effective than placebo at achieving a complete clinical resolution. It should, however, be noted that these trials excluded children below age 2 and those who were severely ill, had associated complication, or any immunodeficiency, as placebo therapy of this high-risk group of patients would be considered unethical.

    Numerous observational studies have also demonstrated a dramatic drop in the frequency of suppurative complications. Acute mastoiditis complicating AOM has declined from an incidence of 20% in the preantibiotic era to a current rate of less than 0.1%.[100,101]

3. *Drug Choice*
    - *Initial Therapy:* The high spontaneous resolution rate of cases of AOM and the lack of bacteriology in most clinical cases makes the possibility of demonstrating efficacy of one antimicrobial agent over another impossible. Thus, initial therapy should begin with amoxicillin (40 mg/kg/day in divided doses for 10 days) because of its palatability, low cost, and low rate of adverse side effects. For children allergic to penicillin, trimethoprim-sulfamethoxazole is a suitable alternative. Second-line drugs may be necessary as initial therapy in previously treated cases, complicated cases, or in children with conjunctivitis suggesting *Haemophilus influenzae* infection. Intramuscular dosing of ceftriaxone should only be used for patients with significant compliance issues. In children at high risk for penicillin-resistant organisms (group day care, geographic high incidence, previous antibiotic therapy within 30 days), amoxicillin at 75–90 mg/kg/day is recommended.[102]
    - *Treatment Failures:* Treatment failure should be considered when symptoms and signs of AOM persist 48 to 72 hours after initial therapy. At this point, resistant organisms should be considered, although many cases will result from persistent middle ear inflammation without live bacteria. Nevertheless, second-

line drugs such as amoxicillin-clavulanate, ceftriaxone, or another beta-lactamase stable alternatives should be considered. Should the patient be severely ill, toxic, or have a complication, diagnostic tympanocentesis or myringotomy with culture is indicated.

4. *Analgesics:* All patients with AOM should receive an analgesic preparation during the initial treatment phase, as pain and fever resolution may take 2 to 7 days.

5. *Surgery:* Randomized clinical trials have shown that myringotomy alone is no better than placebo or, when used with antimicrobial therapy, is no better than antibiotics alone at achieving complete clinical resolution in patients with AOM.[103] Thus, myringotomy should be used for patients with severe AOM with associated complications or suspected complications as an adjunct to antimicrobial therapy.

6. *Follow-up:* Most children with AOM should receive follow-up examination between 1 and 3 months to ensure resolution of effusion.

B. Recurrent Acute Otitis Media

1. *Natural History:* Recurrent AOM implies multiple episodes of AOM separated by intervals of normal middle ear status (ie, no effusion). Most clinical trials use three or more episodes of AOM in a 6- to 12-month period as a liberal definition of recurrent AOM. Of untreated children meeting this criterion in clinical trials, 50% went on to have no further episodes of AOM in the following 6 months and 87% had less than three more episodes. Although these results occurred in highly selected children with nonsevere episodes of AOM, the possibility of spontaneous resolution of recurrent AOM should always be considered. Predisposing factors such as nasal allergy, group day care, secondhand smoke exposure, vaccination, and immune status should all be considered.[97]

2. *Antibiotic Prophylaxis:* Thirteen randomized, placebo-controlled trials have been performed to evaluate antimicrobial prophylaxis for recurrent AOM.[104] Of these trials, 11 demonstrated a positive effect of prophylaxis in decreasing the frequency of AOM episodes. As a whole, prophylaxis decreased AOM by 0.12 episode per patient-month (ie, 1 to 2 episodes per year for 95% of children). This result implies either that one child would need to be treated for 8 months or eight children would need to be treated for 1 month to prevent a single episode of AOM. Nevertheless, these results are highly statistically significant. Thus, the use of antimicrobial prophylaxis is effective when restricted to *highly* selected children. Patients with intercurrent or chronic otitis media with effusion are not candidates. Moreover, evidence suggests that long-term, low-dose antibiotics will select for resistant bacteria.[105] It is reasonable that prophylaxis be limited to a maximum of 6 months of therapy through the high-risk winter months. Two breakthrough episodes should be considered a prophylaxis failure, and insertion of a tympanostomy tube should then be considered.

3. *Vaccination:* Two randomized clinical trials recently studied the effect of a new seven-valent pneumococcal polysaccharide-protein conjugate vaccine (PCV7) (Prevnar; Wyeth Lederle Vaccines, Pearl River, NY) for the prevention of AOM. Generally, both studies showed a reduction in the overall AOM attack rate of 6 or 7%. Although only a modest result, this translates into a 57% reduction in AOM episodes caused by the vaccine serotypes and a 34% reduction in AOM due to all pneumococcal strains. Importantly, 98% of resistant pneumococcal strains are cov-

ered by the vaccine, hopefully resulting in a decrease in resistant AOM. Thus, children with recurrent AOM should be considered for vaccination.[106–108]

Vaccinations against the other common bacteria (*H. influenzae, M. catarrhalis*) and viruses that cause AOM are still being investigated and are not recommended for routine use at this time.

4. *Surgery:* Surgical options for the prevention of recurrent AOM include myringotomy with tubes, adenoidectomy, and tonsillectomy. It should be emphasized that these results refer to children with recurrent AOM with clearing middle ear effusions. (See below for children with *otitis media with effusion.*)

   • *Myringotomy with Tympanostomy Tube:* Three prospective, randomized trials have compared the efficacy of prophylactic antibiotics, tympanostomy tubes, and placebo for the prevention of recurrent AOM.[109–111] In each study, tubes were no better than placebo at decreasing the AOM attack rate, although the episodes were typically asymptomatic in the tube group except for otorrhea. Moreover, the time spent with otitis media or middle ear effusion was significantly less in the tube group ($p < 0.001$). Thus, tympanostomy tubes significantly decrease the morbidity (ie, otalgia, middle ear effusion, hearing loss) of AOM when compared to placebo.

   • *Adenoidectomy:* Only three studies have assessed the efficacy of adenoidectomy for recurrent AOM.[112–114] In the study with more severely affected children, adenoidectomy with tympanostomy tubes significantly decreased the AOM attack rate when compared with tubes alone. In another study by Paradise et al in children less severely affected by recurrent AOM with or without OME, adenotonsillectomy or adenoidectomy alone without tympanostomy tubes both resulted in minor reductions in the number of AOM episodes as well as time with otitis media when compared to controls.[113] These benefits appeared short-lived and the complications in the surgical group were significant in 14% of patients. Thus, adenoidectomy should probably be reserved for severely affected children with recurrent AOM or when symptomatic nasal obstruction accompanies recurrent AOM.

   • *Tonsillectomy:* The efficacy of tonsillectomy alone for recurrent AOM has not been assessed in a controlled trial. Thus, tonsillectomy alone is not indicated unless severe obstructive symptoms or recurrent adenotonsillar infections are also evident.

Otitis Media with Effusion (OME)

Definition

Otitis media with effusion is an inflammation of the middle ear space resulting in a collection of fluid behind an intact tympanic membrane. This process may be further categorized as acute, subacute, or chronic based on the duration of the disease process. In general, OME implies that severe pain and associated constitutional symptoms (ie, signs of suppuration) are lacking. Hearing loss and aural pressure may be present.

Epidemiology and Cost

The epidemiology of OME is less well known than that of AOM because the clinical manifestations of this condition in children may be subtle. Numerous short observation intervals are needed to accurately record the onset and duration of OME, as the natural history is one of resolution. With this shortcoming, studies performing screenings of asymptomatic children with tympanometry have estimated the frequency of OME. In those studies, 17 to 41% of children between 2 and 3 years of age were found to have OME during a 3-month screening period.[115–117] In another group of studies using both tympanometry and otoscopy over a 1-year period, 22 to 61% of children 2 to 6 years of age were found to have OME at some point.[118–120] In general, the frequency of OME increases with age, reaching a maximum between 1 and 2 years. Nearly all children studied have had at least one episode of OME by 3 years of age. Most episodes of OME resolve spontaneously (see "Natural History," below). By 6 to 7 years of age, eustachian tube function normalizes and the incidence of OME decreases substantially.

The socioeconomic impact of OME is quite similar to that of AOM. Gates estimated that OME accounted for approximately $1.85 to $5 billion annually in total costs, of which $1.48 to $3.9 billion were direct health care costs and the remaining $0.37 to $2.1 billion were indirect, family-related expenditures.[68] These numbers are not surprising given the fact that a relatively large number of children require surgical treatment for chronic OME.

Pathogenesis

The pathogenesis of OME is less well understood than that of AOM. It is generally accepted that OME can arise either as a result of eustachian tube obstruction or due to previous or ongoing middle ear inflammation. Eustachian tube obstruction may result from either intra- or extraluminal forces that preclude tubal opening. According to the *hydrops ex vacuo* theory, tubal obstruction alters normal middle ear pressure regulation and ultimately results in middle ear underpressures (ie, negative pressure). When underpressures are of significant magnitude and duration, effusion formation occurs through either transudation or exudation. In this way, nasal inflammation secondary to an antecedent upper respiratory tract viral infection or allergic rhinitis, adenoid hypertrophy, or a nasopharyngeal tumor mass can adversely affect normal eustachian tube function and result in OME. Alternatively, a previous episode of AOM will nearly always be associated with OME for some variable duration following treatment. In these cases, OME is usually inflammatory in nature and may have associated bacteria within the middle ear space.[69,121,122]

Signs and Symptoms

By definition, OME is not associated with the signs and symptoms of acute inflammation. Thus, fever and otalgia are absent. There are no available data describing the frequency of symptoms in children with OME. For the most part, such children appear relatively asymptomatic. They may occasionally pull at their ears or complain of a clogged sensation. Parents of children with OME may report poor hearing, speech and language developmental delay, or poor balance and clumsiness. Adults with previously normal hearing will find OME to be quite troublesome. They often present to the physician for evaluation of aural pressure, hearing loss, clicking, popping, or a sense of imbalance. In both adults and children, a previous upper respiratory tract viral infection and/or AOM are common. Patients without such a history should be carefully evaluated for other potential etiologies of eustachian tube obstruction, such as adenoid hypertrophy or a nasopharyngeal tumor.

Physical examination commonly reveals a poorly mobile tympanic membrane with either a yellow color (serous effusion), a gray color (mucoid effusion), or significant opacity. The membrane may be in either the neutral position, bulging, or retracted. In cases of serous effusion, air bubbles may also be visible, creating an air-liquid interface within the tympanic cavity. As previously stated, a thorough examination of the structures of the head and neck including the nasopharynx is indicated to evaluate for the possibility of a nasopharyngeal tumor obstructing the eustachian tube lumen.

Diagnostic Workup

Indications for diagnostic studies beyond the history and physical examination for most patients with OME are dictated by the chronicity of the disease, diagnostic uncertainty, or in unilateral cases to assess the anatomic status of the eustachian tube. For patients in whom the diagnosis is unclear, pneumatic otomicroscopy combined with tympanometry usually can clinch the diagnosis. The sensitivity and specificity of this procedure should be greater than 90% for an experienced clinician.[76] In rare cases, diagnostic myringotomy may be needed. In both adults and children with unilateral persistent OME, an etiology should be sought. Flexible fiberoptic nasopharyngoscopy in both patient groups is usually able to distinguish significant pathology. Should this be impossible, computed tomography (CT) scans of the nasopharynx, eustachian tube, and middle ear are indicated to better delineate the anatomy. Finally, patients with persistent OME should undergo an audiometric evaluation to assess the degree of hearing impairment. This is especially true in patients with associated risk factors for hearing loss, such as craniofacial anomalies, neurologic and cognitive impairment, psychomotor retardation, or known syndromes associated with sensorineural hearing loss. Chronic OME associated with significant hearing impairment may result in significant speech and language developmental delay. Should this condition exist, early intervention may be warranted.

Common Pathogens

Numerous studies have assessed the microbiology of middle ear effusions from children with long-standing OME undergoing tympanostomy tube placement.

BACTERIA   Using standard culture techniques, approximately 30 to 50% of middle ear effusions taken from children with chronic OME have bacterial species isolated.[69] Using PCR-based techniques, the bacterial identification rate is substantially higher, with as many as 75% of middle ear effusions having evidence of bacterial species.[121,122] The most commonly identified bacterial species in cases of OME are similar to those for AOM and include *S. pneumoniae, H. influenzae,* and *M. catarrhalis* (see "Acute Otitis Media," above). In children and adults with previous acute, subacute, or untreated OME, the microbiology is unknown, as most patients go untreated and the middle ear effusion resolves spontaneously.

VIRUSES   Common respiratory viruses [respiratory syncytial virus (RSV), adenovirus] have also been discovered in the effusion of children with chronic OME undergoing tympanostomy tube insertion.[123,124] The significance of these viruses in the maintenance of middle ear effusion is unknown.

Treatment Options

Numerous studies have addressed treatment options for patients with OME. In 1994, the Agency for Health Care Policy and Research (AHCPR) developed a set of clinical practice guidelines based on the best available evidence.[125] These guidelines focused on treatment of OME in otherwise healthy children aged 1 to 3 years. This section attempts to use the guidelines as well as to fill in the gaps not covered by the guidelines for the treatment of patients with OME. The book by Rosenfeld and Bluestone (1999) is an excellent review of the best available evidence for the treatment of this common condition.[126]

Generally, OME is treated to decrease symptoms, relieve conductive hearing loss, and prevent potential long-term sequelae of chronic eustachian tube obstruction (ie, retraction pockets and cholesteatomas). Thus, patients with significant symptoms, hearing loss, speech and language developmental delay, or structural abnormalities of the tympanic membrane or middle ear should be considered for active treatment. Patients with a high probability of spontaneous resolution can be observed and followed closely. Substantial controversy exists regarding the effects of mild to moderate degrees of conductive hearing loss resulting from OME on speech and language development.[127] The effects of aggressive intervention as a prevention of speech and language delay in otherwise normal children has also been disputed. By contrast, children with conditions that are associated with significant speech and language delay (sensorineural hearing loss, craniofacial developmental abnormalities, neurologic and cognitive deficits, psychomotor retardation) should be treated aggressively for OME, as this may compound communication difficulties.

1. *Natural History:* In general, OME can be categorized based on the chronology of the process. That is, acute OME represents new-onset middle ear effusion of less than 10 days duration. By contrast, chronic OME has been present for at least 3 months. Middle ear effusions present between 10 days and 3 months may be termed subacute OME. The spontaneous resolution rate of these differing clinical entities varies greatly. For instance, children with OME following a recent episode of AOM have the best prognosis, with a spontaneous resolution rate of 60% at 1 month and approximately 75% by 3 months. In children with OME detected by screening, an excellent prognosis also exists, with spontaneous resolution occurring in 50% of ears at 1 month, 75% of ears by 6 months, and nearly 90% of ears by 1 year. By contrast, children in randomized clinical trials for chronic (>3 months duration), refractory OME have a relatively poor prognosis, with only 25% spontaneous resolution at 6 months and 1 year and 31% clearing at 2 years. Thus, a relatively clear delineation exists for children with long-standing OME, as the natural history indicates a protracted course.[97] Unfortunately, similar data do not exist for adults with OME. In fact, most adult patients refuse protracted observation periods for middle ear effusion, as the constant clogged sensation, hearing loss, fullness, cracking, popping, and imbalance is intolerable. The fact that adults rarely accept prolonged observation as a treatment strategy is worth noting in considering pediatric patients with OME.

2. *Antibiotics:* Three metanalyses of 13 randomized clinical trials have shown a modest but statistically significant benefit of antimicrobial therapy for subacute and chronic OME in children.[104,125,128] Summary statistics for these trials suggest a 22% absolute increase in OME resolution attributable to antibiotic therapy. However, significant heterogeneity exists between the various studies, with some demonstrating a treatment effect and others not. Children with immune deficiencies, craniofacial growth abnormalities, and prior tubes were usually excluded from the studies. Thus, these study results should be interpreted with caution. The combination of a small clinical benefit, limited serious health consequences from nontreatment, and growing concerns of antimicrobial resistance make routine antibiotic therapy less appealing. Antibiotics are recommended in children with OME of 4 to 12 weeks duration who are considered at high risk (ie, associated sensorineural hearing loss, neurologic or cognitive deficits,

psychomotor retardation) or when OME has been present for more than 3 months but surgery is contraindicated because of anesthesia risk.

3. *Corticosteroids:* Three randomized clinical trials have shown some effect of corticosteroids on the resolution of OME.[129–131] In these trials, effusion was 20% more often resolved in the steroid group than in the placebo group at the 2-week follow-up interval. However, this effect was lost by 4 to 6 weeks. These studies suffered from relatively low power. Thus, the utility of these drugs remains in question and their routine use is discouraged at this time.

4. *Decongestant-Antihistamines:* Three randomized clinical trials have demonstrated no benefit from the use of decongestant-antihistamine preparations in the treatment of OME.[132–134]

5. *Surgery:* Surgical options for the treatment of persistent OME include myringotomy, myringotomy with tympanostomy tube, adenoidectomy, tonsillectomy, and mastoidectomy. Randomized controlled clinical trials have been performed for many of these procedures and the data, with recommendations, are summarized below.

   • *Myringotomy with or without Tympanostomy Tubes:* At least three studies have evaluated the effects of myringotomy with or without tubes for the treatment of OME refractory to antibiotics.[135–137] Two of these showed that myringotomy with tubes was significantly better than either myringotomy alone or no surgery in preventing future AOM episodes (otorrhea) as well as decreasing the percentage of time with middle ear effusion.[135,136] Specifically, myringotomy with tubes resulted in 0.41 less AOM episodes per person-year than no surgery and 0.47 less episodes per person-year than myringotomy alone. In terms of time with middle ear effusion, tubes resulted in 26% less time with effusion than no surgery and 19% less time with effusion than myringotomy alone. These studies confirm that myringotomy with tubes is highly effective in treating children with chronic OME. Clear indications for myringotomy and tympanostomy tube placement in children with chronic OME include (1) significant hearing loss (>20 dB); (2) high risk for speech and language developmental delay (sensorineural hearing loss, craniofacial abnormalities, neurologic or cognitive impairment); (3) ongoing speech and language delay; (4) recurrent AOM in conjunction with OME; (5) structural changes to the tympanic membrane, including severe retraction pocket formation with or without adhesion. Other potential indications for tympanostomy tube placement in children with chronic OME include (1) bilateral involvement for 3 months or (2) unilateral OME for 6 months.

   • *Adenoidectomy:* Three randomized clinical trials have shown that adenoidectomy is effective for chronic OME.[112,137,138] In the study by Gates, 4- to 8-year-old children with OME refractory to medical therapy were randomized to myringotomy alone, myringotomy with tubes, adenoidectomy with myringotomy, or adenoidectomy with tubes. In both groups undergoing adenoidectomy, children had significantly less time with middle ear effusion, better hearing, longer time to first recurrence, and fewer surgical retreatments than children not receiving adenoidectomy. The effect of adenoidectomy in this study was irrespective of adenoid size.[137] In a study by Paradise et al., children with previous tympanostomy tubes were randomly assigned to receive either adenoidectomy with tubes or tubes alone.[137] The adenoidectomy group had 28% less time with AOM (otorrhea) and spent 47% fewer days with otitis media of any type than the tube-only group. Unfortunately, neither of these studies included a significant number of children under 4 years of age; thus, the AHCPR guidelines issued a statement that adenoidectomy was not indicated for this group of children. In general, adenoidectomy should be reserved for children with chronic OME refractory to medical therapy after a previous set of tympanostomy tubes.

- *Tonsillectomy:* Tonsillectomy has not been shown to be effective for chronic OME.[113,138]

Chronic Suppurative Otitis Media (CSOM) with or without Cholesteatoma

Definition

Chronic suppurative otitis media (CSOM) involves a long-standing discharge through a non-intact tympanic membrane from either a perforation or a tympanostomy tube. It is important to recognize that not all cases of CSOM are associated with cholesteatomas. Conversely, not all cases of cholesteatoma are associated with CSOM. However, the two processes frequently coexist. Throughout the literature, the terminology is often intermixed, and the term *chronic otitis media,* without distinction, is applied. Unfortunately, this term is intrinsically not descriptive and may refer to chronic otitis media with effusion, CSOM without cholesteatoma, and CSOM with cholesteatoma. These distinctions in terminology are important, since they refer to different conditions with varying treatment needs and prognoses.

Epidemiology

The true incidence of CSOM (with or without cholesteatoma) is unknown. This is partly because of the problems in terminology discussed above. In general, CSOM is more common in certain racial groups. Specifically, Native Americans, Alaskan natives (Eskimos), Greenland natives (Inuits), Australian aborigines, and New Zealand natives all have a higher incidence of CSOM than American whites. These children have chronic otorrhea through a tympanic perforation in most cases. Interestingly, cholesteatoma is not frequently associated with CSOM in these populations, such an association being reported in only 1 to 3% of children with CSOM.[139] In children with tubes, the rate of CSOM is quite low, occurring in less than 1–3% of children.

Pathogenesis

The pathogenesis of CSOM without cholesteatoma is somewhat speculative. Since the disorder requires a communication between the middle ear and external auditory canal, a perforation or tympanostomy tube must be present. Many cases of tympanic membrane perforation result from episodes of AOM. In some instances, the perforation remains dry, and in others the ear drains. In the former situation and in cases of dry tympanostomy tubes, chronic suppurative otitis media results from superinfection of the middle ear mucosa, from organisms in either the external auditory canal or nasopharynx. Investigators have shown that the eustachian tubes in some Eskimos, Native Americans, and blacks may be abnormally patent, thereby predisposing to recurrent or chronic nasopharyngeal–middle ear reflux of secretions. The presence of a chronic tympanic membrane opening (tympanostomy tube or perforation) also obviates the normal middle ear "air cushion," thus perpetuating the problem. Another plausible theory is that CSOM develops as a result of chronic exposure of the middle ear to flora or contamination from the external auditory canal. Chronic middle ear infection through either of these two mechanisms may then allow mastoid contamination and chronic otomastoiditis. In cases of cholesteatoma, similar mechanisms may also be at work. As squamous debris in the cholesteatoma is inherently avascular, this provides the nidus for bacterial superinfection.[139]

Signs and Symptoms

The typical signs of CSOM are long-standing otorrhea through a nonintact tympanic membrane. The ear is usually painless except when eczematoid otitis externa intervenes, significant intratemporal or intracranial complications occur, or malignancy is present. Patients usually report a hearing loss as well. Examination frequently reveals a tympanic membrane perforation with moderately edematous middle ear mucosa. There may be associated granulation tissue in and around the perforation. When a cholesteatoma is present, a retraction pocket or squamous debris may be present. In these cases, there may also be evidence of bony external auditory canal erosion. Tuning fork examination will confirm an associated conductive hearing loss in most cases unless a complication is present. Long-standing cholesteatomas may result in erosion into the otic capsule, with resulting vertigo and sensorineural hearing loss. Erosion of the fallopian canal may also result in facial paralysis. Rarely, cholesteatomas can involve the central nervous system.

Diagnostic Workup

The diagnostic evaluation rarely requires more than a thorough clinical examination. Specific attention should be paid to the presence or absence of a cholesteatoma. Cholesteatoma is generally a surgical disease, whereas many cases of CSOM without cholesteatoma can be managed medically. This should include otomicroscopy with suctioning of secretions. Gram's stain and culture is useful in cases of medical therapy failure. Diagnostic audiometry should be performed in most cases to assess the degree and type of hearing loss. CT scanning should be performed when intratemporal or intracranial complications are suspected or when surgical intervention is being planned. These studies should include both axial and coronal fine cuts (1–1.5 mm) through the temporal bones using bone algorithms. When there is no response to medical therapy, biopsy of persistent granulation tissue in the ear canal should be considered to rule out malignancy, a granulomatous process, or other pathologies. Tissue cultures should be obtained as well. Caution should be exercised in these cases and general anesthesia considered to prevent biopsy-related complications.

Common Pathogens

The most common pathogens isolated from the ears of patients with CSOM (with or without cholesteatoma) are *P. aeruginosa* and *S. aureus*. Anaerobic bacteria have also been frequently isolated in some studies. Fungi may rarely be present when superinfection of the external auditory canal is present.[139]

Treatment Options

Initial treatment of patients with CSOM (with or without cholesteatoma) should be directed at clearing the infection. Long-term management frequently requires addressing issues such as recurrent otorrhea, hearing loss, and the management of cholesteatomas.

1. *Antibiotics:* Antimicrobial therapy is the standard for treating CSOM. Usually, suctioning the ear (ie, aural toilet) and placement of ototopic medication is all that is needed to stop the chronic otorrhea. Numerous topical preparations are available for the treatment of ear infections; however, only ofloxacin otic drops (Floxin Otic, Daichi Corp.) are approved by the Food and Drug Administration (FDA) for application when the tympanic membrane is not intact. This quinolone-class drug has a broad spectrum of action

and is useful against most bacterial species that cause CSOM. Other topical preparations frequently used in cases of CSOM combine antibiotics (neomycin, polymixin B, ciprofloxacin) with steroids (hydrocortisone). With all otic formulations, concentrations well above the mean inhibitory concentrations (MIC) for most pathogens can be obtained. The addition of corticosteroids aids in resolution of the inflammatory reaction. Caution must be used in applying aminoglycoside- (neomycin, gentamicin, tobramycin) containing preparations to the open middle ear, as this class of antibiotics may rarely cause sensorineural hearing loss. In most cases, these medications do not penetrate the inner ear (round window), presumably because of decreased permeability of the round window secondary to inflammation. Topical antimicrobial therapy frequently results in rapid resolution of the otorrhea in 1 to 2 weeks. Oral antimicrobial agents are frequently ineffective in treating CSOM. This is because most oral agents except the quinolone class of drugs have limited activity against *Pseudomonas aeruginosa.* The quinolones have had limited use in children because of their potential for affecting bone growth adversely.

In patients with refractory otorrhea, consideration must be given to a resistant organism, poor drug delivery, the presence of chronic otomastoid osteitis, or cholesteatomas. When cholesteatoma is not readily evident, CT imaging and culture-directed intravenous antibiotics are a reasonable approach. Usually, an antipseudomonal penicillin or a second-generation cephalosporin will cover the offending organisms. Daily suctioning and instillation of ototopic agents is also useful. In these cases, 7 to 10 days of treatment will usually dry the ear without the need for further therapy.[140] Should this therapy fail, surgery should be considered.

2. *Surgery:* Surgical therapy for CSOM is directed at revealing and treating previously unrecognized cholesteatomas, removing infected granulations, identifying rare underlying pathologies, and providing middle ear–mastoid communication and drainage. This usually requires mastoidectomy and tympanoplasty through an intact canal wall approach. Added communication between the middle ear and mastoid can be obtained by opening the facial recess (ie, posterior tympanotomy). Should a cholesteatoma be evident, complete removal (ie, intact canal wall mastoidectomy with tympanoplasty) or exteriorization (ie, canal wall down mastoidectomy) is indicated. The details of these surgical procedures are beyond the scope of this chapter and can be found elsewhere.[141]

3. *Prevention:* Patients with recurrent otorrhea that readily clears with otic preparations may suffer from recurrent middle ear contamination from repeated water exposure, recurrent nasopharyngeal–middle ear contamination, a tympanostomy tube chronically colonized by bacteria, a foreign-body reaction, immunocompromise, or an unrecognized cholesteatoma. Repeated water exposures may require only judicious use of ear plugs during swimming or bathing. When this is ineffective, tympanostomy tube removal or tympanic membrane closure (ie, tympanoplasty) may be indicated. Should recurrent nasopharyngeal–middle ear reflux be suspected, tympanic membrane closure may also restore the normal middle ear "air cushion," thus obviating the problem. In children with recurrent upper respiratory tract infections and recurrent otorrhea, antimicrobial prophylaxis should be considered, as well as vaccination (see "Recurrent Acute Otitis Media," above). A complete immune evaluation should also be entertained. Finally, cholesteatoma is generally considered a surgical disease and complete removal or exteriorization is advocated to control infection, progressive bone erosion, and complications.

Complications of Otitis Media

Definition

Intratemporal/intracranial complication of otitis media refers to the development of an infectious or inflammatory process within either the temporal bone or intracranial cavity that occurs either concurrently with or immediately following otitis media and as a direct result of it.

Extracranial/Intratemporal

Complications of otitis media are fortunately quite rare since the institution of routine antimicrobial therapy. For instance, in the preantibiotic era, acute mastoiditis complicated AOM in up to 20% of cases, as compared to <0.1% of cases in the post-antibiotic era.[100,101] Few data exist regarding the relative frequency of the various intratemporal complications. Most likely, hearing loss is the most common complication, occurring to some degree in nearly every ear infection, and labyrinthitis and petrous apicitis are the least common.

1. *Tympanic Membrane Perforation:* Tympanic membrane perforation as a result of AOM is relatively uncommon, although the true incidence of this complication is unknown. The clinical signs and symptoms of AOM with perforation are typically seen in a child with AOM who subsequently develops purulent otorrhea accompanied by a substantial decrease in pain. The organisms responsible for perforated AOM are the same as those mentioned for AOM without perforation. A very small percentage of children with AOM and tympanic membrane perforation go on to develop a chronic perforation with or without CSOM (see below). Most tympanic membrane perforations following episodes of AOM heal spontaneously in a few days. Occasionally, tympanoplasty is needed to close a chronic tympanic membrane perforation.

2. *Tympanosclerosis:* Tympanosclerosis is a common sequela of otitis media, although there are few data to indicate its true incidence. Usually, there is an asymptomatic white patch on the tympanic membrane that moves with pneumatic otoscopy. In some cases, tympanosclerosis can involve the middle ear. In rare instances, tympanosclerosis is so extensive that an associated conductive hearing loss is present. Histologically, Sorenson and True described a fibroblastic invasion of the submucosal layer of the tympanic membrane followed by thickening and fusion of the collagen fibers into a mass and finally scattered calcifications within the intracellular and extracellular spaces.[142] The cause of tympanosclerosis remains unknown. In most cases, tympanosclerosis requires no further treatment.

3. *Hearing Loss:* In regard to otitis media, hearing loss may occur during or following episodes of AOM, as a result of middle ear effusion, tympanic membrane perforation, ossicular erosion, serous labyrinthitis, or suppurative labyrinthitis. Since routine audiometry is not performed in children with uncomplicated AOM, the incidence of this complication is unknown. In children with chronic middle ear effusion (OME) or tympanic membrane perforation, relatively minor degrees (10–30 dB) of conductive hearing loss are common.[143,144] When more serious complications such as ossicular erosion or labyrinthitis occur, significant hearing loss is the norm. In an adult, the diagnosis is usually readily evident and confirmed by conventional audiometry. In contrast, a high degree of suspicion is needed to discover a unilateral hearing loss in a child. Thus, children with a unilateral hearing loss are usually discovered at the time of screening audiometry in elementary school. Treatment of the hearing loss is based on etiology

(see discussions of otitis media with effusion, tympanic membrane perforation, ossicular erosion, and labyrinthitis).

4. *Ossicular Erosion:* Ossicular erosion is uncommon following episodes of AOM. One exception to this is the case of necrotizing AOM resulting from group A beta-hemolytic streptococcal infection. This disease usually occurs in severely immunocompromised patients and results in complete tympanic membrane perforation, ossicular erosion, and often suppurative labyrinthitis. CSOM (with or without cholesteatoma) more frequently results in ossicular erosion and associated hearing loss. Ossicular erosion with or without discontinuity is most commonly seen to involve the long process of the incus near the incudostapedial joint. The predilection for this particular portion of the incus is unknown, although numerous investigators speculate that the blood supply of this ossicle is most tenuous in this region, thereby predisposing to osteitis and necrosis with resultant discontinuity. The treatment for ossicular discontinuity is either surgical ossicular reconstruction or hearing amplification.

5. *Facial Paralysis:* Facial paralysis may accompany episodes of either AOM or CSOM (with or without cholesteatoma). In the preantibiotic era, between 1906 and 1938, 105 (0.8%) out of 13,125 patients treated for acute or chronic otitis media had peripheral facial weakness. It was estimated that 0.5% of patients with AOM and 1.7% of patients with chronic OM (with or without cholesteatoma) developed facial palsy. These authors concluded that cholesteatoma was a major cause of facial palsy related to otitis media.[145] In the post-antibiotic era, facial paralysis is less common than in the preantibiotic era.[146] In a recent review of the intratemporal complications related to AOM over a 15-year period at a major U.S. medical center, 22 cases of facial paralysis were treated in association with AOM. Compared to the total number of patients with AOM, the incidence of this complication is quite small.[147] In another study from Denmark, it was estimated that facial paralysis complicated cases of AOM in approximately 2.3 cases per million inhabitants.[148] Of 1024 surgically treated cases of CSOM with cholesteatoma, 11 (1%) presented with preoperative facial paralysis.[149] Most investigators believe that inflammation in the middle ear space extends to the confines of the fallopian canal through either congenital dehiscences (in AOM) or osteitic erosion (in CSOM) in the tympanic segment of the facial nerve. Neural inflammation or compression results in edema and varying degrees of entrapment within the bony canal, with consequent neural dysfunction. Most patients with AOM present with partial facial paralysis, although 5 of the 22 (22.7%) patients in the Pittsburgh study had House-Brackmann (HB) grade VI dysfunction at the time of presentation.[147] Diagnostic evaluation should include CT scanning as well as audiometry to evaluate for associated intratemporal or intracranial complications as well as the possibility of an unrecognized erosive process (cholesteatoma, malignancy, etc.). In patients with complete facial paralysis, electrical diagnostic testing (ie, electroneuronography) should be performed to assess the degree of neural degeneration. The microbiology of AOM associated with facial paralysis is similar to that of uncomplicated AOM. In patients with partial paralysis and associated AOM, myringotomy is indicated for culture and sensitivity testing and for middle ear drainage. Culture-directed intravenous antibiotics are appropriate in this setting. Routine mastoidectomy is not indicated unless acute coalescent mastoiditis or an erosive process is evident on radiographic imaging. Complete neural degeneration on electroneuronography (ENOG) may be an indication for nerve decompression, although this remains contro-

versial. For patients with CSOM with cholesteatoma, surgical therapy to either eradicate or exteriorize the disease is indicated. Outcomes for patients with AOM and associated facial paralysis are generally good. In the Pittsburgh study, all but one patient (HB grade V) had normal (HB grade I) or near normal (grade II) facial function at resolution.[147] For patients with CSOM with cholesteatoma, the data suggest a somewhat worse outcome.

6. *Acute Mastoiditis:* Acute mastoiditis most commonly occurs from contiguous spread of AOM to the mastoid portion of the temporal bone. When mucosal edema and infection are all that occurs, the mastoid infection is mostly subclinical and manifest as clouding of the mastoid air cells on CT scanning. The incidence of this condition in patients with AOM is unknown but probably approaches 100% in children with uncomplicated AOM.

A more important distinction is the presence of clinical mastoiditis. In these cases, mastoid infection may present in a number of stages based on the degree of involvement of the bone, periosteum, overlying skin, upper neck, and lymphatic system. From the mastoid air cells, infection can extend through (a) the mastoid cortex, resulting in a subperiosteal abscess; (b) the aditus ad antrum into the middle ear; (c) the zygomatic root cells to form a supra-auricular or temporal abscess; (d) the inferior and lateral regions of the mastoid into the soft tissues of the neck as a Bezold's abscess; (e) the posterior air cells into the occipital bone and result in osteomyelitis of the calvarium (ie, Citelli abscess); (f) the retrofacial, infralabyrinthine, or supralabyrinthine air cells into the petrous apex (ie, petrositis); and (g) the bony covering of the posterior or middle fossa plates, to result in intracranial complications (see below).

Although the frequency of these various conditions is unknown, most reports suggest that the frequency of mastoiditis has decreased markedly since the institution of antibiotic therapy for AOM. Most series report 40 to 70 patients collected over a 10-year period.[150–152]

Acute mastoiditis most frequently occurs as a sequela of partially or untreated cases of AOM in children. In recent studies, investigators have shown that a previous history of recurrent AOM or OME is usually not present in patients with acute mastoiditis. The mean age is usually 3 years at presentation.[150–152]

Diagnosis is based on the clinical features and CT scanning. Patients will usually have significant signs of toxicity, with fever and significant otalgia. Mastoiditis will be manifest as significant retroauricular pain, ear protrusion, and sagging of the skin of the posterosuperior external auditory canal, with postauricular tenderness to palpation and edema. A peripheral blood smear will frequently reveal a leukocytosis. The tympanic membrane will frequently have characteristics of AOM (see "Acute Otitis Media," above). Weber and Rinne testing will usually be consistent with a conductive hearing loss. CT scanning is needed to delineate the extent of the infection and the degree of mastoid osteitis and abscess formation. CT scanning may or may not reveal rarefying osteitis of the mastoid with destruction of the bony trabeculae, resulting in coalescence. This is an important distinction in that coalescence (or mastoid abscess formation) is considered to be an absolute indication for surgical intervention, whereas noncoalescence is initially treated medically.

The microbiology of acute mastoiditis is somewhat different from that of uncomplicated AOM. *S. pyogenes* (group A beta-hemolytic) is the leading cause of acute mastoiditis, followed by *S. pneumoniae* and *H. influenzae*.[150–152] Interestingly, *P. aeruginosa* (8.5%) and anaerobes (5%) account for a significant number of cases.

Most children or adults presenting with noncoalescent mastoiditis can be treated with myringotomy and drainage of the middle ear and culture-directed intravenous antibiotics. Prior to organism identification, empiric therapy using a second-generation cephalosporin or an antipseudomonal aminopenicillin is usually adequate. After symptom resolution, oral antimicrobial therapy should continue for 10 to 14 days. Should this therapy fail over 24 to 48 hours, further surgical intervention should be considered in the form of simple mastoidectomy.

Surgical intervention is indicated when (a) CT scanning reveals coalescence, (b) the symptoms and clinical signs (fever, leukocytosis, otorrhea) fail to respond to intravenous antibiotics, (c) a significant abscess (subperiosteal, cervical, occipital, temporal) exists, or (d) intracranial complications are associated. For coalescent mastoiditis, simple mastoidectomy to the level of the mastoid antrum with wound drainage is adequate. When extratemporal abscess formation is present, incision and drainage is indicated. Mastoidectomy in these cases is indicated when coalescent mastoiditis accompanies the abscess or the abscess fails to respond to incision, drainage, and antibiotics.[53]

7. *Labyrinthitis:* Labyrinthitis can occur as a complication of both AOM and CSOM (with or without cholesteatoma). This is discussed in detail under infections of the inner ear.

8. *Petrous Apicitis:* The petrous apex is divided into anterior and posterior compartments by the internal auditory canal.[153] The anterior compartment may be further subdivided into the peritubal and apical regions.[154] Petrous apicitis has been categorized as acute, chronic, and complicated.[155] Acute petrositis develops rapidly as an extension of AOM and mastoiditis occurring typically in a well-pneumatized temporal bone. By contrast, chronic petrositis evolves as a complication of CSOM (with or without cholesteatoma) and develops as an extension along fascial planes, vascular channels, or direct erosion. Complicated petrositis can occur in both acute and chronic forms and is frequently associated with intracranial complications.

Petrositis is rather frequently noted in asymptomatic patients on radiographic imaging. In these cases, careful observation and follow-up is all that is needed. Clinical signs and symptoms of petrositis are most notably deep pain and persistent aural discharge following simple mastoidectomy. Posterior petrositis usually results in suboccipital headache, and anterior petrositis results in retro-orbital pain. When petrositis is accompanied by retro-orbital pain, a sixth nerve palsy (diplopia), and persistent otorrhea, Grandenigo's syndrome is present. In these cases, pain occurs as a result of trigeminal nerve involvement and the sixth nerve is involved as it enter Dorello's canal in the petroclinoid ligament. Further symptoms of apicitis are dictated by the degree of involvement of the other intratemporal and intracranial structures.

CT scanning is the initial imaging modality of choice for patients with suspected petrositis. Usually, clouding of the petrous apex region with varying degrees of erosion is obvious. When intracranial complications are also suspected, MRI is also useful to delineate soft tissue involvement.

Treatment of acute petrositis is similar to that of acute mastoiditis (see above). In general, acute, noncoalescent petrositis is best managed with culture-directed intravenous antibiotics obtained at the time of myringotomy or mastoidectomy. Further surgical intervention is indicated when (1) CT scanning reveals coalescence and the symptoms and clinical signs (fever, leukocytosis, otorrhea) fail to respond to intravenous antibiotics or when (2) a significant abscess (intracranial) exists. Surgical approaches to the petrous apex are predominantly along drainage pathways and the otic capsule, carotid artery, jugular foramen, and the intracranial structures limit wide exposure. The typical approaches include transcanal-infracochlear, transmastoid-retrofacial-infralabyrinthine, transmastoid-supracochlear, transmastoid-retrolabyrinthine, transmastoid-translabyrinthine, transmastoid-transcochlear, and finally the middle fossa–subtemporal. Choice of surgical approach is dictated by the location of the lesion, degree of pneumatization, and status of the hearing.[156] Consultation with a neurosurgeon is frequently useful to help in the management of the associated intracranial complications in these patients.

9. *Chronic suppurative otitis media (with or without cholesteatoma):* See above.

Intracranial

Intracranial complications are generally considered to be less common than the intratemporal complications previously described.[157] Prior to the antibiotic era, death from intracranial complications of otitis media was common. In the 1920s and 1930s it was estimated that 6% of patients with AOM or CSOM went on to develop an intracranial complication.[158] In fact, during this era, 1 out of every 40 deaths at the Los Angeles County Medical Center was related to an intracranial complication of otitis media. The mortality rate for otitic meningitis was ~90%[159]; for brain abscess, it was ~80%.[160] Following the institution of the sulfonamides and penicillin, the frequency of these complications and the related mortality rate decreased dramatically.[161,162] In terms of the relative frequency of occurrence of the various intracranial complications, most studies find that meningitis is most common and otitic hydrocephalus and subdural empyema the least common. Prior to the institution of routine antibiotic therapy for AOM, acute infection accounted for most intracranial complications. Subsequently, it has been estimated that 75% of intracranial complications occur as a result of CSOM with or without cholesteatoma.[162] Finally, CSOM with cholesteatoma seems to result in intracranial complications more frequently than CSOM without cholesteatoma.[163] Presumably, the erosive nature of cholesteatoma can break down the natural barriers to infection, ultimately resulting in intracranial penetration.

1. *Meningitis:* Despite antibiotic therapy, meningitis may still complicate episodes of otitis media. Overall, approximately 80% of otitic meningitis occurs in patients with AOM, while 20% follows CSOM.[164] In children, Friedman et al. found that 36% of cases of central nervous system infection were associated with otitis media, and 91% of these were otitic meningitis.[165] In adults, CSOM is twice as common as AOM as a precursor to meningitis. In patients with AOM, best evidence suggests that meningitis most frequently results from hematogenous dissemination to the dura, while direct, transtemporal penetration is less common. One exception to this is in children with known inner ear malformations such as Mondini's deformity. Cases of recurrent meningitis in these children presumably result from spread along preformed pathways between the middle ear, labyrinth, and subarachnoid space.

    Clinical symptoms of meningitis include headache, restlessness, irritability, fever, chills, vomiting, and photophobia. Examination will usually reveal an ill patient with significant lethargy and diminished mental status. Signs of meningeal irritation include nuchal rigidity and positive Kernig's and Brudzinski's signs. Further progression will lead to seizures, coma, and death. Diagnostic studies should include a CT scan of the brain and temporal bones to evaluate for an associated intratemporal or intracranial complication and for the presence of increased intracranial pressure. From an otologic perspective, a myringotomy with culture or a culture of otorrheal fluid should be performed to drain the middle ear and to determine the offending organism. Lumbar puncture should be undertaken immediately if increased intracranial pressure (ICP) is not suspected on CT imaging. Cerebrospinal fluid (CSF) analysis should include Gram's stain, culture and sensitivity testing, and glucose and protein determination. Rapid identification of the offending organism(s) may now be possible in some institutions using PCR-based diagnostic techniques. Should ICP be elevated, appropriate pressure-lowering measures (mannitol, acetazolamide, hyperventilation) should be undertaken prior to CSF determination, or a ventriculostomy may be needed. The most common offending organism today is probably *S. pneumoniae.* In years prior to the routine use of the *H. influenzae* type B vaccine, this organism accounted for many cases. In patients with CSOM, gram-negative organisms such as *P. aeruginosa, Proteus, Klebsiella,* and anaerobic species are more common. Empiric antibiotics should have substantial central nervous system penetration and cover the presumed bacterial pathogens. Culture-directed intravenous antibiotics should be begun as soon as possible. In children with meningitis, the addition of intravenous dexamethasone to antibiotics has been shown to decrease the neurologic and audiologic sequelae.[166] Mastoidectomy should be performed in neurologically stable patients when coalescent mastoiditis, CSOM with cholesteatoma, epidural abscess, or sigmoid sinus thrombosis is evident.[157] In children with AOM and associated meningitis, modern-day mortality rates are less than 3%. In patients with CSOM, the mortality rates are somewhat higher, presumably as a result of the gram-negative organisms and the invasive disease.

2. *Epidural Abscess:* Epidural abscess involves a collection of pus or purulent granulation tissue between the temporal bone and dura. This complication is the second most common intracranial complication of otitis media[167] and is more frequently associated with CSOM. According to Snow (1980), epidural abscess more frequently involves the posterior fossa dura in acute coalescent mastoiditis, while either the middle or posterior fossa dura can be associated with CSOM with cholesteatoma.[168] Most patients with epidural abscess that is uncomplicated by meningitis, sigmoid sinus thrombosis, hydrocephalus, or meningitis are asymptomatic. In fact, this complication is frequently recognized only at the time of mastoidectomy for CSOM with cholesteatoma. Occasionally, patients will complain of deep ear pain. Examination will be similar to that in patients with AOM or CSOM without complications. CT imaging of a patient with an epidural abscess will demonstrate a contrast-enhancing lesion adjacent to the temporal bone. MRI studies will show a lesion that is hyperintense to CSF on both T1- and T2-weighted algorithms. Treatment of epidural abscess associated with otitis media is usually surgical. That is, the epidural space should be opened and allowed to communicate freely with the pneumatized spaces of the temporal bone. Thick granulation tissue should be removed to identify relatively normal dura. Associated intracranial complications should be treated as described in the other sections.

3. *Sigmoid Sinus Thrombosis:* In cases of otitis media, sigmoid sinus thrombosis comprises infectious thrombophlebitis of the sigmoid dural venous sinus. Prior to antibiotic therapy, sigmoid sinus thrombosis was found in nearly 20% of autopsies performed for

otogenic intracranial complications.[169] Currently, sigmoid sinus thrombosis is quite rare. In older series, there are conflicting reports regarding whether this condition more frequently arises from complicated AOM or CSOM. Two theories exist regarding the presumed pathogenesis of infectious sigmoid sinus thrombosis. The first involves direct extension from perisinus bone erosion with transmural sinus wall inflammation, mural thrombus formation, and subsequent propagation with obstruction. The second hypothesis is that small vessels within the temporal bone become inflamed and obstructed with infected thrombus, subsequently propagating to involve the larger dural venous sinus.[157]

The most common finding in patients with sigmoid sinus thrombosis is fever, which is usually sustained or occurs in a spiking ("picket fence") pattern. Unfortunately, other symptoms are uncommon except when there is associated meningitis, hydrocephalus, or significant thrombus propagation. When the petrosal sinuses are involved to result in septic cavernous sinus thrombosis, chemosis, proptosis, and ophthalmoplegia will occur. When posterior clot propagation involves the confluence of sinuses (torcula), significant hydrocephalus and cerebral edema will ensue. Distal propagation to the neck can result in a palpable cord in the neck and, rarely, septic pulmonary emboli. Involvement of the mastoid emissary vein will result in edema, erythema, and tenderness over the mastoid (Griesinger's sign). In modern times, CT and MRI will usually make the diagnosis, with angiography reserved for nondiagnostic studies. Studies such as lumbar puncture with ipsilateral (Queckenstedt's test) or contralateral (Tobey-Ayer test) jugular venous compression are of historic interest only. Contrast-enhanced CT imaging may show a delta sign—a central nonenhanced clot surrounded by enhancing dural sinus wall. MRI has more recently proven superior to CT for diagnosing infectious thrombosis of dural venous sinuses because of its ability to demonstrate low or absent flow, clot formation, and the presence of enhancing regions consistent with inflammation. Early clot formation, rich in deoxyhemoglobin, appears of intermediate intensity on T1-weighted images and hypointense on T2-weighted images. As the clot matures, methemoglobin accumulates, giving the thrombus high intensity on both T1- and T2-weighted images. MR angiography allows assessment of blood flow and velocity.

Management of infectious sigmoid sinus thrombosis should initially be directed at controlling severe neurologic sequelae such as meningitis, hydrocephalus, and abscess formation. Culture-directed intravenous antibiotics should be instituted early on. The usage of anticoagulation therapy is controversial. For cases where sigmoid sinus thrombosis is not complicated by cavernous sinus thrombosis, thrombolysis is probably not justified, as this may increase the risk of venous infarction.[170] In cases of cavernous sinus involvement, anticoagulation may be justified. Surgical intervention should include at least wide decompression of the sigmoid sinus with excision of perisinus granulation tissue. The sinus should be opened in cases where an intrasinus abscess is present. Needle aspiration of the sinus may help to determine the presence of sinus abscess. Complete evacuation of the sinus thrombus is probably not justified. In cases of severe septic pulmonary emboli complicating sigmoid sinus thrombosis, jugular venous ligation may be useful.[157]

4. *Brain Abscess:* Otogenic brain abscess is an uncommon complication of otitis media. Although the incidence of this complication is unknown, it is estimated that less than 20% of all brain abscesses are otitic in origin.[171] They are more common in adults than in chil-

dren[172]; occur more commonly in CSOM than in AOM patients[173]; and more frequently involve the cerebrum than the cerebellum.[167] In most cases, otogenic brain abscess arises as a complication of venous thrombophlebitis rather than direct dural extension. Local cerebritis (encephalitis) results in necrosis and liquefaction, which is then walled off by fibrosis and granulation tissue. As the abscess expands, it may rupture into the ventricles or subarachnoid space, resulting in overwhelming meningitis and death. The bacteriology of otogenic brain abscess is similar to that of either CSOM or AOM, depending on the etiologic process. In general, most abscesses are polymicrobial. Common organisms isolated include streptococcal and staphylococcal species; the gram-negative species such as *Pseudomonas, Proteus,* and *Escherichia coli;* and anaerobes.[157]

There are four clinical stages of brain abscess, including (1) invasion (cerebritis), (2) localization (quiescent abscess), (3) enlargement (manifest abscess), and (4) termination (abscess rupture).[174] Early symptoms are fever, headache, and drowsiness, followed by a clinically silent stage that can last days to weeks. Later, the fever, headache, and lethargy return, with associated focal neurologic symptoms. Finally, if rupture occurs, the patient dies rapidly.

Diagnostic studies are similar to those for other suspected intracranial complications. Usually both CT and MRI scanning are obtained. The CT scan will often show the abscess with peripheral rim enhancement. MRI is better at detecting subtle cerebritis without abscess formation and allowing for the assessment of dural venous sinus flow.

Management of brain abscess requires intravenous antibiotics. Other important issues include determining the risk of increased intracranial pressure and abscess rupture as well as controlling the source of infection. Surgical intervention is indicated in large or expanding abscesses, especially when they are refractory to medical therapy.

5. *Subdural Empyema:* Subdural empyema is a severe, purulent bacterial infection of the space between the dura mater and the arachnoid membrane. Otogenic subdural empyema is the least common of all of the intracranial complications of otitis media; it is most common in cases of complicated CSOM with cholesteatoma and can involve either the supratentorial or posterior fossa regions. The three proposed mechanisms of subdural empyema involve direct spread through the dura, retrograde venous thrombophlebitis, or brain abscess rupture into the subdural space.[169] In most cases, subdural empyema presents with signs and symptoms of severe meningitis and possibly seizures. Diagnosis is readily apparent on MRI scanning. Usually, immediate neurosurgical intervention is indicated and wide opening of the infected space is needed. Despite early diagnosis and treatment, this condition is often fatal.

6. *Otitic Hydrocephalus:* Otitic hydrocephalus is a condition characterized by signs of increased intracranial pressure (headache, vomiting, papilledema) without abscess formation, clear CSF, and associated otitis media.[175] Interestingly, enlargement of the ventricles is not characteristic, making the term *hydrocephalus* a misnomer. Otitic hydrocephalus is second only to subdural empyema as the least common intracranial complication of otitis media. It may be associated with either AOM or CSOM. Symonds proposed the theory that this condition arises as a result of arachnoid villus obstruction secondary to retrograde thrombophlebitis extension from the lateral sinus to the sagittal sinus.[176] The diagnosis is made by demonstrating increased intracranial pressure, clear CSF, and lateral and possibly sagittal sinus thrombosis on MRI. Management of the increased intracranial pressure and otitis media are the primary goals. The intracranial

pressure can usually be lowered medically with steroids, acetazolamide, furosemide, and mannitol. Should this prove unsuccessful, CSF drainage procedures such as serial lumbar puncture, lumbar drainage, or ventriculo- or lumbar-peritoneal shunting may be needed. Failure to control increased pressure can result in focal neurologic deterioration with blindness and ultimately death.[157]

INFECTIONS OF THE INNER EAR

Bacterial

Epidemiology and Pathophysiology

Acute bacterial infection of the inner ear or labyrinthitis is divided into serous or toxic labyrinthitis and suppurative labyrinthitis. These diseases occur in the presence of an acute or chronic bacterial otitis media, spreading from the middle ear and round window membrane or a horizontal canal fistula, respectively.[53] In addition, suppurative labyrinthitis is divided into otogenic (tympanogenic) and meningogenic labyrinthitis. The presumed route of spread for otogenic labyrinthitis is through the round window membrane, oval window, a labyrinthine fistula, or congenital abnormalities of the temporal bone. The route of inoculation for meningogenic labyrinthitis is through the internal auditory canal or the cochlear aqueduct to the membranous labyrinth.[177]

Serous labyrinthitis is a complication of otitis media and is thought to occur when toxic mediators from otitis media reach the membranous labyrinth with an absence of bacteria in the inner ear.[178] The incidence of this complication of otitis media is unknown, but it is uncommon and represented 3% of all intratemporal complications in a recent study.[147] Another large study from Thailand demonstrated a complication rate of less than 1% in otitis media; however, 34% of the patients with complications had labyrinthitis. It was not specified whether these were serous or suppurative in nature.[179] The pathogenesis of the disease is based on extrapolation from animal data and findings of sensorineural hearing loss in humans with otitis media. In animal models with otitis media, permeability studies of the round window membrane demonstrate the passage of macromolecules in the presence of toxic mediators such as streptolysin O.[180] Although animal data exist to prove the hypothesis that acute otitis media can affect the membranous labyrinth to cause labyrinthitis and hearing loss, human data are still less conclusive.[181,182]

In suppurative labyrinthitis, whether otogenic or meningogenic, there is a more severe infection of the labyrinth. The etiology of acute suppurative labyrinthitis involves direct access of the infecting organism to the bony and membranous labyrinth. The incidence of this infection is rare and currently represents only a few percent of all intratemporal complications of otitis media.[179] In the preantibiotic era, there were reports of an incidence between 1.5 and 16% of all patients with otitis media.[181] The incidence of meningogenic suppurative labyrinthitis is related to the severity of meningitis; however, there does not appear to be a relationship to the duration of meningitis or causative organism.[177] The pathology of suppurative labyrinthitis is well documented in the literature and shows a wide variety of findings. Although it is commonly assumed that suppurative labyrinthitis results in irreversible damage to the cochlea and vestibular end organs, histopathologic evidence often demonstrates intact neurosensory epithelium and the organ of Corti. A large study of the temporal bone in meningogenic suppurative labyrinthitis produced the following findings: (1) inflammation confined to the perilymphatic spaces of the cochlea and vestibular organs; (2) eosinophilic staining of inner ear fluids (a finding of unresolved significance); (3) loss of spiral ganglion cells in 12% of patients; (4) the modiolus and cochlear aqueduct as the presumed routes of inoculation.[177] Other temporal bone studies demonstrate contrasting pathology, with lymphocytes in the endolymph spaces and labyrinthitis ossificans.[178] In some patients, there appear to be several stages after acute suppurative labyrinthitis, leading to the development of fibrous tissue and ossification of the membranous labyrinth over a period of up to 1 year.[181] These changes usually occur at the region of the scala tympani in the basal turn of the cochlea and have clinical implications for patients undergoing cochlear implantation.

Signs and Symptoms

The differentiation between serous labyrinthitis and suppurative labyrinthitis is based upon a continuum of clinical findings. A clear division between the two diseases is difficult to make based upon clinical grounds alone; the two can probably be definitively separated only by temporal bone histopathology.[177]

Classically, serous labyrinthitis is seen in the patient with AOM, CSOM, or cholesteatoma and is characterized by the sudden onset of mild to moderate hearing loss and occasionally vertigo. In most cases, the symptoms resolve with time, pointing to reversible damage thought to be due to changes in cochleovestibular ionic potential and inflammatory toxic mediators.

Suppurative labyrinthitis is distinguished in the child by profound sensorineural hearing loss, otalgia, nausea, fever, emesis, and vertigo or clumsiness.[147,178] It often coexists with AOM, CSOM, cholesteatoma, or meningitis. Another acute finding may be the presence of nystagmus either toward or away from the involved ear when there is vestibular dysfunction. The classical description of the disease states that the otologic changes are irreversible; however, Merchant's temporal bone histopathology argues against this because many of the neurosensory elements are intact even in the presence of lymphocytes. The disease may progress to facial paralysis, meningitis, and other intracranial complications.[139]

Hearing loss in meningogenic suppurative labyrinthitis is most common following infection with *S. pneumoniae* (30%), followed by *H. influenzae* (11%) and *N. meningitides* (7%); it occurs very early in the illness.[183,184]

Common Pathogens

SEROUS LABYRINTHITIS   The common pathogens of acute otitis media—*S. pneumoniae, H. influenzae,* and *M. catarrhalis*—are commonly thought to cause serous labyrinthitis.[180]

SUPPURATIVE LABYRINTHITIS   Otogenic pathogens are similar—*S. pneumoniae, H. influenzae,* and *M. catarrhalis*—and include the pathogens associated with chronic otitis media, such as *Proteus, Klebsiella, and P. aeruginosa,* etc. Also, the anaerobes *Bacteroides* and *Peptococcus* species have been implicated in suppurative labyrinthitis.[180]

Meningogenic pathogens are typically *H. influenzae, S. pneumoniae,* and *N. meningitides* and are changing due to the use of vaccines.

Diagnostic Workup

The studies needed for the diagnosis of serous labyrinthitis are limited to an audiogram and a CT scan. Culture of middle ear fluid from otorrhea, a myringotomy, or typanocentesis is essential as well.

The increased severity of suppurative labyrinthitis mandates an audiogram, culture of the otogenic or meningogenic source, and CT scan of the temporal bones and brain to rule out other complications.

Treatment Options

The treatment goals for serous labyrinthitis are (1) prevention of further progession of the disease into suppurative labyrinthitis and (2) resolution of the underlying infectious disease. This is accomplished by treatment of the underlying AOM, CSOM, or cholesteatoma with appropriate culture-directed antibiotics. If the middle ear is not draining, a myringotomy is advised, with or without placement of a tympanostomy tube.[139]

Similarly, the treatment goals for suppurative labyrinthitis are (1) prevention of further cochleovestibular damage and (2) resolution of the underlying infectious disease. Due to the severity of this disease, the potential for hearing impairment, and otitic meningitis, aggressive medical and surgical therapy is indicated. The mainstays of therapy are culture-directed intravenous antibiotics and myringotomy with or without tube placement.

Controversy exists in the literature with respect to the addition of steroid therapy to prevent hearing loss and labyrinthitis ossificans. In a large, multi-institutional randomized prospective placebo-controlled study, there was no difference in neurologic sequelae or hearing loss between patients treated with antibiotics alone or antibiotics in combination with steroids.[184] Another prospective placebo-controlled trial by Lebel et al. was able to demonstrate a significant improvement in hearing outcome with the addition of steroid therapy in patients with *H. influenzae* meningitis.[185] More recently, a retrospective study examining the effect of steroids on the progression of suppurative labyrithitis to labyrinthitis ossificans demonstrated a possible benefit to the administration of steroids in a small number of patients with *S. pneumoniae* meningitis.[186] This is also supported by a recent animal model for pneumococcal meningitis that showed improved hearing outcome with early steroid administration.[187] At present, the decision to administer steroid therapy is still controversial and should be individualized to each patient.

Viral

Viral Labyrinthitis

Viral labyrinthitis is characterized by a variety of different diseases with different clinical presentations. Although the membranous labyrinth is one continuous structure, viral infections do not affect all of the neurosensory epithelium universally and a particular virus will not always infect the same structures when comparative temporal bone anatomy is studied. In addition, due to the inaccessibility of the otic capsule structures, definitive culture and pathology study can be done only on postmortem examination. Various techniques such as acute and convalescent serologies have been used to suggest the diagnosis of viral labyrinthitis; however, more definitive diagnostic tests remain elusive at this time. The route of inoculation offers another diagnostic dilemma, as many of these diseases appear to affect the inner ear with no other systemic effects. The clinical diagnoses of sudden sensorineural hearing loss and acute viral labyrinthitis are also postulated by many to be vascular-occlusive in nature.

The terminology of labyrinthitis is also confusing, as the diseases represented by this single term cannot be categorized into a distinct nosology. A wide variety of terms are currently used to describe these diseases, such as *vestibular neuronitis, cochlear neuronitis, viral labyrinthitis, cochleitis, vestibulitis,* and *cochleovestibulitis.* It is important to recognize that different viruses and different sites of pathology often represent one clinical syndrome. Sudden sensorineural hearing loss is addressed in another chapter. Therefore, the following discussion addresses specific etiologic agents rather than clinical syndromes in order to avoid further confusion. The following viruses are described: cytomegalovirus, rubella, measles, and mumps virus. Although many other viruses have been implicated, these are mentioned only briefly.

Cytomegalovirus

Epidemiology and Pathophysiology

The cytomegalovirus (CMV), a DNA virus, is a member of the herpesvirus group and has widespread prevalence throughout the population, with excretion rates of up to 70% of children in day care centers.[188] The disease is expressed in both primary and latent forms and is spread by horizontal and vertical transmission. In addition, there is a high rate of asymptomatic excretion, confounding the diagnosis unless a targeted organ demonstrates recovered virus. The classified forms of this disease include congenital, asymptomatic, and reactivated (in immunocompromised hosts). This disease is the most common nongenetic cause of congenitally deafened infants each year in the United States.[189] This is one of the few diseases listed that continues to be commonly seen by the otolaryngologist, as vaccine use is not currently widespread (the Towne strain).[190]

The temporal bone anatomy demonstrates the following pathology: viral inclusion–bearing cells in the scala media, Reissner's membrane, stria vascularis, semicircular canals, utricle, and saccule.[189] Also CMV has been isolated by culture of aspirated perilymph and endolymph.[191] Although this continues to be a common cause of hearing loss in infants, treatment protocols are currently inconclusive as to their effect on the course of neonatal disease.[192]

Signs and Symptoms

Approximately 1 to 2% of all infants are infected with CMV.[54] Although CMV infection can be severe at birth (cytomegalic inclusion disease), these cases represent only about 5% of infected patients.[188,189] Cytomegalic inclusion disease is characterized by intrauterine growth retardation, neonatal jaundice, purpura, hepatosplenomegaly, microcephaly, retinitis, and intracerebral calcifications. Deafness occurs in 20 to 65% of infants with cytomegalic inclusion disease and is typically bilateral. In affected patients, the hearing loss follows no consistent pattern and may progress over a period of years. For asymptomatic patients, the rate of hearing loss varies from 7 to 13% of children and thus should be considered in infants and children with nonsyndromic and nongenetic hearing loss.[189] Vestibular abnormalities are less consistently demonstrated in these patients on electronystagmography, although pathologic specimens will demonstrate involvement of the vestibular system.[189]

Common Pathogens

Cytomegalovirus—a herpesvirus, DNA virus.

Diagnostic Workup

Currently there is no universal screening recommendation for congenital CMV infection and the "gold standard" for diagnosis is isolation of the virus from the urine of the affected infant. Because of the significant number of asymptomatic patients and the confounding variable of reactivation of disease, the diagnosis of infection can be difficult. Serum IgM and IgG are diagnostic early in disease; however, later in infancy the differentiation between reactivation, primary infection, and a causal relationship for hearing loss is difficult to ascertain, as no specimen from the inner ear fluid can be obtained. For example, the case of a 2-year-old with deteriorating sensorineural hearing loss and a positive IgG serology for CMV is suggestive of a causal relationship but difficult to prove. Rising IgG titers in the patient with a history of seropositivity in the past must be interpreted with caution and can indicate a reinfection with another strain rather than a reactivation.[190]

Treatment Options

Currently the therapy for cytomegalovirus inclusion disease is supportive in the infant, although a recent phase II trial shows stabilization of the hearing loss in treated infants with ganciclovir.[192] Older individuals such as the immunocompromised population will benefit from the administration of ganciclovir for other indications.[188] There is no current preventive strategy for transmission as well.

Rubella (German Measles)
Epidemiology and Pathophysiology

The diseases of measles, mumps, and rubella (MMR) are less commonly seen at this time, secondary to the widespread use of the MMR vaccine. There has been an approximately 99.7% decrease in incidence.[192,193] The most current reports on this disease and its effect on hearing come from international sources such as second and third world countries.

Congenital rubella syndrome is most commonly seen in infants whose mothers acquire maternal infection in the first trimester.[192,193] This virus has not yet been isolated from perilymph or endolymph.

The histopathology of the disease demonstrates cochlear and saccular degeneration and atrophy of the stria vascularis. The utricle, semicircular canals, and vestibular sensory epithelium are typically not involved.[54]

There are scattered reports in the literature of hearing loss after the measles, mumps, and rubella vaccine.[194]

Signs and Symptoms

Rubella causes the following symptoms: retroauricular, posterior cervical, and postoccipital lymphadenopathy; a viral enanthem (Forschheimer spots) on the soft palate; a maculopapular rash beginning on the face and spreading to the entire body; and low-grade fever. Hearing loss is not present in the acquired form.[54,193]

Congenital rubella syndrome (Gregg's syndrome) affects most organ systems: cataracts, microphthalmia, cardiac defects, "blueberry muffin" skin lesions, growth retardation, and hearing loss are all characteristics of the disease. The hearing loss is usually present in approximately 50% of affected individuals and is often severe to profound.[54,195] It is important to note that in patients with congenital rubella, hearing changes may occur months to years after initial infection.[195]

Common Pathogens

Rubella virus, a togavirus, RNA virus.

Diagnostic Workup

Specific IgG and IgM tests. ELISA and hemagglutination tests are also used. Also, culture of rubella from the nasopharynx, urine, etc. may be done.[193]

Treatment Options

A specific treatment does not exist for this disease. Interferon gamma and other nonspecific antiviral therapies have been tried in the past.

Measles (Rubeola)
Epidemiology and Pathophysiology

The measles virus is now infrequent in the United States and the incidence has dropped by 99.7% in the last 60 years.[193] This disease is still encountered in countries without widespread vaccine programs and therefore is occasionally seen in the United States. The transmission is by respiratory droplets, and it is highly contagious.

The hearing loss in measles accounted for up to 5 to 10% of all cases of profound bilateral deafness prior to the widespread use of the vaccine.[196]

The temporal bone pathology of this disease consists of the following: severe degeneration of the organ of Corti, striae, cochlear neurons, and vestibular damage. Inflammation, fibrous deposition, and ossification have been noted in the basal turns of the cochlea in some specimens.[196]

The measles virus is also linked to otosclerosis by studies using electron microscopy and immunochemistry.[197]

Signs and Symptoms

Measles can be divided into three stages: (1) incubation stage (7–10 days with minimal symptoms); (2) prodromal stage (cough, coryza, conjunctivitis, Koplik's spots—white spots on the buccal mucosa), and (3) a maculopapular rash with high fever for 2 to 3 days.[193]

The hearing loss in measles occurs in the presence or absence of encephalitis and is often asymmetric, bilateral, and severe.[13] Vestibular abnormalities are not uncommon.

Common Pathogens

Measles virus—a paramyxovirus, RNA virus.

Diagnostic Workup

The diagnosis is straightforward in the face of an epidemic or in isolated cases; therefore, serology is rarely needed. An audiogram should be obtained only if there is clinical suspicion of hearing loss.

Treatment

The treatment for measles virus is supportive. Vitamin A has been used in the past.

Mumps

Epidemiology and Pathophysiology

Mumps, like measles and rubella, is now infrequent in the United States due to the use of the MMR vaccine. Mumps infection in many instances is subclinical, and positive serology is frequent in the general population—up to 80 to 90%.[198] Approximately 10% of patients with mumps will have a meningitis, usually after the onset of parotitis. A greater number of patients, 60 to 70%, will have increased lymphocytes in the CSF.[196,198] The disease is spread by infected salivary secretions. A viremia occurs as well, which is thought to be the route of spread in the body.

The temporal bone pathology of mumps infection shows atrophy of the organ of Corti and striae, with minimal effect on the vestibular system. Also, endolymphatic hydrops and obliteration of the endolymphatic duct is also seen.[13,196] The route of infection to the inner ear is thought to be due to a viremia or through the cochlear aqueduct.[13]

Mumps infection is also associated with various other otologic syndromes. There is evidence for mumps as an etiologic agent of sudden sensorineural hearing loss, delayed endolymphatic hydrops, and Ménière's disease.[199,200]

Signs and Symptoms

The clinical features of mumps are typically salivary adenitis, epididymoorchitis, pancreatitis, meningitis, and hearing loss.[13,54] Hearing loss occurs in 5 per 10,000 cases of mumps, is typically sudden in onset, and may occur a few days or weeks after the onset of parotitis.[13,201] The patients may complain of tinnitus, dizziness, and hearing loss, which is unilateral in 80% of patients.[13,201] The hearing loss is typically in the higher frequencies, and reduced caloric responses may be noted on vestibular testing.

Common Pathogens
Mumps virus—a paramyxovirus, RNA virus.

Diagnostic Workup
This includes an audiogram and vestibular testing in those with specific complaints. Mumps virus can be isolated from throat culture or CSF. The presentation is usually typical.

Treatment Options
There is no specific antiviral therapy for mumps. Treatment is supportive. For sudden hearing loss, carbogen, steroids, vasodilator, adenosine triphosphate (ATP), and vitamin B_{12} have been tried with varying success.[201]

Other Viral Infections

A variety of other viruses are implicated in the literature as agents of inner ear infection. Herpesvirus and influenza virus are also implicated in the pathogenesis of sudden sensorineural hearing loss, with a variety of clinical, pathologic, and experimental evidence.[202] Parainfluenza virus, adenovirus, and HIV virus are also suspected of causing damage to the inner ear.

The HIV virus is suspected to cause vertigo and hearing impairment, and otologic complaints are common in patients with this disease.[203] A temporal bone study of patients who died of AIDS reveals changes in the vestibular end organs of the maculae and cristae ampullarae as well as what appears to be a viral cytopathic effect.[204] There are a number of confounding variables, including other viruses in these patients, that make it difficult to draw definitive conclusions as to cause and effect.

Other

A variety of other organisms are documented to infect the inner ear structures, such as *T. pallidum* and *M. tuberculosis*. These are discussed because they are seen in the immunocompromised host.

Otosyphilis

Epidemiology and Pathophysiology
Luetic inner ear disease can be classified as congenital or acquired. Further breakdown exists but is not addressed here. In recent years, the number of new cases of syphilis approximates 8500 in 1997, with 1000 cases of congenital syphilis.[205,206] The demographics of the disease have shifted to a greater proportion of African Americans and females and away from male homosexuals.[207]

In congenital syphilis, hearing loss occurs in approximately one-third of patients studied.[207] For symptomatic neurosyphilis, up to 80% of patients will have hearing loss.[200]

The histopathology of otosyphilis is divided into two predominant pathologies. In early congenital syphilis and the meningitis of secondary and tertiary syphilis, a meningo-neuro-labyrinthitis is seen. For late congenital, latent, and tertiary syphilis, there is an osteitis of the temporal bone. Affected temporal bones will demonstrate an obliterative endarteritis, microgummata, endolymphatic hydrops, ossicular involvement, degeneration of the organ of Corti, and cochlear neuron loss.[200]

Signs and Symptoms

The symptoms of otosyphilis may present as sudden sensorineural hearing loss, fluctuating hearing loss, episodic vertigo, unilateral or bilateral progressive hearing loss, and tinnitus.[207,208] The various presentations are seen in both congenital and acquired disease, the manifestations of which are reviewed elsewhere.[206,207] The sensorineural hearing loss is flat or greater in the lower frequencies and often shows no typical pattern.[209] Otologic symptoms are seen in all three stages of syphilis, and because of the clinical diversity, syphilis should be included in the workup of sudden sensorineural hearing loss, Ménière's disease, autoimmune inner ear disease, and vestibular neuritis.

Hennebert's sign is a positive fistula test in the absence of middle ear disease and is postulated to be secondary to fibrous bands between the stapes footplate and the oval window.[200]

Tullio's sign is the presence of vertigo and nystagmus in response to a loud sound. Again, the pathophysiology is thought to be due to fibrous bands between the stapes footplate and the oval window. This test is not specific for otosyphilis.

Vestibular testing reveals abnormalities in up to 50% of patients.[209]

Pathogen

T. pallidum.

Diagnostic Workup

The most challenging aspect of otosyphilis is making a positive diagnosis. The current literature advocates the specific treponemal test FTA-ABS (fluorescent treponemal antibody absorption) because of the low prevalence of the disease in the general population. Also, many otologic symptoms occur in late stages of syphilis when the venereal disease research laboratory (VDRL) and rapid plasma reagin (RPR) tests may be negative. The positive predictive value of this test is reviewed by Hughes and Rutherford and because of the low prevalence, only 22% of positive tests will be true positives even with a specificity of 98%.[210]

An audiogram and typically an examination for retrocochlear pathology (MRI or ABR) is also indicated. If the presence of neurosyphilis is suspected, a lumbar puncture is performed. These patients should also have testing for HIV and tuberculosis.[206,211]

Therapeutic Options

The treatment of otosyphilis has met with varied success in the past. Traditionally, the patients are treated with penicillin G and steroids.[205,209] It has recently been advised that patients with neurosyphilis be treated with high-dose intravenous procaine penicillin for 10 to 14 days, as adequate CSF levels are not obtained in patients treated with intramuscular pencillin; however, other intramuscular regimens are also advocated.[206] In view of many of these patients' socioeconomic status, compliance may be an issue and hospitalization advised. Treatment of syphilis, even in its late stages, can prevent further sequelae.[206]

The expected outcome from treatment with antibiotics and steroids for 2 weeks is the following: (1) hearing, approximately 20 to 30% will improve; (2) discrimination, approximately 30% will improve; (3) tinnitus and vertigo, up to 75% will improve.[211] Unfortunately, many of the treatment responses do not appear to have lasting effects once the steroids are tapered; therefore prolonged steroid therapy may be required.

Aural Tuberculosis

Epidemiology and Pathophysiology

Aural *Mycobacterium tuberculosis* represents one of the infrequent types of head and neck tuberculosis; in a recent review, only one case had been seen in the previous 10 years at a major university hospital.[212] The incidence of tuberculosis in developed countries is low, approximately 5 to 20 cases per 100,000 population; however, it can be seen in the immuno-compromised host. The more recent publications on this topic are from second and third world nations. This is often a disease of childhood in developing countries.

The presumed route of spread is hematogenous in origin, whereas in the past spread was thought to be from the eustachian tube.[200] The bacilli affect the middle ear mucosa and temporal bone with the typical pathology of caseating granulomas, causing otitis media, mastoiditis, and tympanic membrane perforations.[200]

Signs and Symptoms

Tuberculosis of the ear follows an insidious course and should be suspected when aural discharge is profuse and painless. A review of 43 patients from South Africa highlights the following features: painless, profuse otorrhea; multiple perforations; pale granulation tissue; hearing loss; and facial palsy.[213] The patient may also present with painful, acute mastoiditis and a central perforation.[214] At surgery, the findings of pale granulation tissue, bone necrosis, and sequestrum formation are common. Also, the finding of active tuberculosis at other sites is suggestive of otologic tuberculosis.

Complications such as facial paralysis, postauricular fistula, and intracranial extension have been described.[215]

Pathogen

M. tuberculosis.

Diagnostic Workup

The diagnosis of tuberculous otomastoiditis is often delayed, and a high index of suspicion is needed based on the above-mentioned signs and symptoms. Histology from granulation tissue, AFB staining of discharge, PCR for *M. tuberculosis,* and culture of discharge are commonly the methods of choice for diagnosis. Histology is the most useful and demonstration of the organism can be difficult.[213,214] An audiogram and a CT scan are ordered if complications are noted. A purified protein derivative (PPD) test, chest x-ray, and search for other extrapulmonary tuberculosis are standard. Culture may commonly reveal gram-negative organisms in addition to the tuberculous bacilli.[214]

Treatment Options

The treatment of tuberculous otitis is typically medical to begin with, using multidrug therapy because of changing resistance patterns. Cure rates are high with medical therapy; however, in patients with acute mastoiditis, surgery has also proved useful.[214] Even in the presence of facial palsy, the rapid institution of antituberculous chemotherapy can reverse the facial weakness.[213] The duration of medical treatment depends on underlying host immune function, multidrug-resistant tuberculosis, and primary or reactivation state, etc.; in general, a dry ear is expected within 2 to 4 months of treatment.

References

1. Kimura AC, Pien FD. Head and neck cellulitis in hospitalized adults. *Am J Otolaryngol* 1993; 14(5):343–349.
2. More DR, Seidel JS, Bryan PA. Ear-piercing techniques as a cause of auricular chondritis. *Pediatr Emerg Care* 1999;15(3):189–192.
3. Hanif J, et al. "High" ear piercing and the rising incidence of perichondritis of the pinna. *BMJ* 1991;322:906–907.
4. Bisno AL, Stevens DL. Streptococcal infection of skin and soft tissues. *N Engl J Med* 1996; 334(4):240–245.

5. Indianer, L. Chronic cellulitis—Left ear. *Arch Dermatol* 1969;100:505–506.

6. McCarthy VP, Peoples WM. Toxic shock syndrome after ear piercing. *Pediatr Infect Dis J* 1988;7(10):741–742.

7. Sardick NS. Current aspects of bacterial infections of the skin. *Dermatol Clin* 1997;15(20):341–349.

8. Noel SB, et al. Treatment of *Pseudomonas aeruginosa:* Auricular perichondritis with oral ciprofloxacin. *J Dermatol Surg Oncol* 1989; 15(6):633–637.

9. Wackym PA. Molecular temporal bone pathology: II. Ramsey Hunt syndrome (herpes zoster oticus). *Laryngoscope* 1997;107:1165–1175.

10. Furuta Y, Ohtani F, Fukuda S, et al. Reactivation of varicella-zoster virus in delayed facial palsy after dental treatment and oro-facial surgery. *J Med Virol* 62(1):42–45, 2000.

11. Murakami S, et al. Varicella zoster virus distribution in Ramsay Hunt syndrome revealed by Polymerase Chain Reaction. *Acta Otolaryngol (Stockh)* 1998;118:145–149.

12. Hato N, et al. Ramsay Hunt syndrome in children. *Ann Neurol* 2000;48:254–256.

13. Davis LE, Johnsson LG. Viral infections of the inner ear: Clinical, virologic, and pathologic studies in humans and animals. *Am J Otolaryngol* 1983;4(5):347–362.

14. Robillard RB, Hilsinger RL Jr, Adour KK. Ramsay Hunt facial paralysis: Clinical analysis of 185 patients. *Otolaryngol Head Neck Surg* 1986;95:292–297.

15. Uri N, Greenberg E, Meyer W, et al. Herpes zoster oticus: Treatment with acyclovir. *Ann Otol Rhinol Laryngol* 1992;101:161–162.

16. Iwatsu T, Takano M, Okamoto S. Auricular chromomycosis. *Arch Dermatol* 1983;119:88–89.

17. Cox RL, Reller LB. Auricular sporotrichosis in a brick mason. *Arch Dermatol* 1979;115:1229–1230.

18. Busch RF. Coccidioidomycosis of the external ear. *Otolaryngol Head Neck Surg* 1992;107(3):491–492.

19. Lucente FE, Lawson W, Novick NL. *The External Ear.* Philadelphia: Saunders, 1995.

20. Mills DC II, Roberts LW, Mason AD Jr, et al. Suppurative chondritis: Its incidence, prevention, and treatment in burn patients. *Plast Reconstr Surg* 1988;82(2):267–276.

21. Martin R, Yonkers AJ, Yarington CT Jr. Perichondritis of the ear. *Laryngoscope* 1976; 86:664–673.

22. Bassiouny A. Perichondritis of the auricle. *Laryngoscope* 1981;91:422–431.

23. Fisher JK. Chronic cellulitis, left ear. *Arch Dermatol* 1969;100:505–506.

24. Dowling JA, Foley FD, Moncrief JA. Chondritis in the burned ear. *Plast Reconstr Surg* 1968;42:115.

25. Wannamaker HH: Suppurative perichondritis of the auricle. *Trans Am Acad Ophthalmol Otolaryngol* 1972;76:1289.

26. Raza SA, Denholm SW, Wong JC. An audit of the management of acute otitis externa in an ENT casualty clinic. *J Laryngol Otol* 1995; 109:130.

27. Yelland M. Otitis externa in general practice. *Med J Aust* 1992;156:325.

28. Selesnick SH. Otitis externa: Management of the recalcitrant case. *Am J Otol* 1994;15(3):408–412.

29. Guthrie et al. Diagnosis and treatment of acute otitis externa—an interdisciplinary update. *Ann Otol Rhinol Laryngol* 1999(Suppl)176:1–23.

30. Campos A, et al. Influence of human wet cerumen on the growth of common and pathogenic bacteria of the ear. *J Laryngol Otol* 2000;114:925–929.

31. Shea CR. Dermatologic diseases of the external auditory canal. *Otolaryngol Clin North Am* 1996;29(5):783–794.

32. Senturia BH, Marcus MD, Lucente FE. *Diseases of the External Ear: An Otologic-Dermatologic Manual.* New York: Grune & Stratton, 1980.

33. Slattery WH, Saadat P. Postinflammatory medial canal fibrosis. *Am J Otol* 1997;18:294–297.

34. Fairbanks DNF. *Pocket Guide to Antimicrobial Therapy in Otolaryngology—Head and Neck Surgery,* 8th ed. Alexandria, VA: The American Academy of Otolaryngology—Head and Neck Surgery Foundation, 1996, 36–42.

35. Rakover Y, et al. Duration of antibacterial effectiveness of gentamicin ear drops in external otitis. *J Laryngol Otol* 2000;114:827–829.

36. Hannley MT, Denneny JC III, Holzer SS. Use of ototopical antibiotics in treating 3 common ear diseases. *Otolaryngol Head Neck Surg* 2000;122(6):934–940.

37. Chandler JR. Malignant external otitis. *Laryngoscope* 78;1257:1968.

38. Slattery WH, Brackman DE. Skull base osteomyelitis—malignant external otitis. *Otolaryngol Clin North Am* 1996;29(5):795–806.

39. Ress BD et al. Necrotizing external otitis in patients with AIDS. *Larygoscope* 1997;107: 456–460.

40. Nadol JB. Histopathology of *Pseudomonas* osteomyelitis of the temporal bone starting as malignant external otitis. *Am J Otolaryngol* 1980;1(5):359–371.

41. Benecke JE Jr. Management of osteomyelitis of the skull base. *Laryngoscope* 1989;99:1220.

42. Chandler JR. Malignant external otitis and osteomyelitis of the base of the skull. *Am J Otol* 1989;10(2):108–110.

43. Stokkel MPM, et al. The value of quantitative gallium-67 single-photon emission tomography in the clinical management of malignant external otitis. *Eur J Nucl Med* 1997;24(11): 1429–1432.

44. Martel J, et al. Malignant or necrotizing otitis externa: Experience in 22 cases. *Ann Otolaryngol Chir Cervicofac* 2000;117(5):291.

45. Davis JC, et al. Adjuvant hyperbaric oxygen in malignant external otitis. *Arch Otolaryngol Head Neck Surg* 1992;118:89–93.

46. Lang R, et al. Successful treatment of malignant external otitis with oral ciprofloxacin: A report of experience with 23 patients. *J Infect Dis* 1990;161:537–540.

47. Haruna S, et al. Histopathology update: Otomycosis. *Am J Otolaryngol* 1994;15(1): 74–78.

48. Paulose KO, et al. Mycotic infection of the ear (otomycosis): A prospective study. *J Laryngol Otol* 1989;(103):30–35.

49. Tom LW. Ototoxicity of common topical antimycotic preparations. *Laryngoscope* 2000; 110(4):509–516.

50. Marsh RR, Tom LW: Ototoxicity of antimycotics. *Otolaryngol Head Neck Surg* 1989; 100(2):134–136.

51. Blevins NH, Karmody CS. Chronic myringitis: Prevalence presentation, and natural history. *Otol Neurotol* 2001;22:3–10.

52. El-Seifi A, Fouad B. Granular myringitis: Is it a surgical problem? *Am J Otol* 2000;21: 462–467.

53. Canalis RF, Lambert PR. Acute suppurative otitis media and mastoiditis. In: Canalis RF, Lambert PR, eds. *The Ear. Comprehensive Otology.* Philadelphia: Lippincott Williams & Wilkins, 2000, 397–408.

54. Nager GT. *Pathology of the Ear and Temporal Bone.* Baltimore: Williams & Wilkins, 1993.

55. Rifkind A, Chanock RM, Kravetz HM, et al. Ear involvement (myringitis) and primary atypical pneumonia following inoculation of volunteers with Eton agent. *Am Rev Respir Dis* 1962;85:479–489.

56. Roberts DB. The etiology of bullous myringitis and the role of mycoplasmas in ear disease: A review. *Pediatrics* 1980;65(4):761–766.

57. Bluestone CD. Definitions, terminology, and classification. In: Rosenfeld RM, Bluestone CD, eds. *Evidence-Based Otitis Media.* Hamilton, Ontario, Canada: Decker, 1999, 85–104.

58. Berman S. Otitis media in children. *N Engl J Med* 1995;332:1560–1565.

59. Teele DW, Klein JO, Rosner B. Greater Boston Otitis Media Study Group. Epidemiology of otitis media during the first seven years of life in children in the greater Boston: A prospective cohort study. *J Infect Dis* 1989;160:83–94.

60. Pukander J, Sipila M, Karma P. Occurrence of and risk factors in acute otitis media. In: Lim DJ, Bluestone CD, Klein JO, Nelson JD, eds. *Recent Advances in Otitis Media with Effusion. Proceeding of the Third International Symposium.* Philadelphia: Decker, 1984, 9–12.

61. Stangerup SE, Tos M. Epidemiology of acute suppurative otitis media. *Am J Otolaryngol* 1986;7:47–54.

62. Sipila M, Pukander J, Karma P. Incidence of acute otitis media up to the age of 1½ years in urban infants. *Acta Otolaryngol (Stockh)* 1987; 104:138–145.

63. Ingvarrson L, Lundgren K, Stenstrom C. Occurrence of otitis media in children: Cohort studies in an urban population. In: Bluestone CD, Casselbrant ML, eds. Workshop on epidemiology of otitis media. *Ann Otol Rhinol Laryngol* 1990;99(Suppl 149):17–18.

64. Alho O, Koivu M, Sorri M, Rantakallio P. The occurrence of otitis media in infants. *Int J Pediatr Otorhinolaryngol* 1991;21:7–14.

65. Casselbrant ML, Mandel EM, Rockett HE, Bluestone CD. Incidence of otitis media and

bacteriology of acute otitis media during the first two years of life. In: Lim DJ, Bluestone CD, Klein JO, Nelson JD, eds. *Recent Advances in Otitis Media with Effusion. Proceedings of the Fifth International Symposium.* Philadelphia: Decker, 1993, 1–3.

66. Casselbrant ML, Mandel EM. Epidemiology. In: Rosenfeld RM, Bluestone CD, eds. *Evidence-Based Otitis Media.* Hamilton, Ontario, Canada: Decker, 1999, 117–136.

67. Stool SE, Field MJ. The impact of otitis media. *Pediatr Infect Dis J* 1989;8:S11–S14.

68. Gates GA. Cost-effectiveness considerations in otitis media treatment. *Otolaryngol Head Neck Surg* 1996;114:525–530.

69. Bluestone CD, Klein JO. Otitis media, atelectasis, and eustachian tube dysfunction. In: Bluestone CD, Stool SE, eds. *Pediatric Otolaryngology.* Philadelphia: Saunders, 1990, 320–486.

70. Buchman CA, Doyle WJ, Skoner DP, et al. Influenza A virus-induced acute otitis media. *J Infect Dis* 1995;172:1348–1351.

71. Bluestone CD, Lee D. What to expect from surgical therapy. In: Rosenfeld RM, Bluestone CD, eds. *Evidence-Based Otitis Media.* Hamilton, Ontario, Canada: Decker, 1999, 207–221.

72. Niemela M, Uhari M, Jounio-Ervasti K, et al. Lack of specific symptomatology in children with acute otitis media. *Pediatr Infect Dis J* 1994;13:765–768.

73. Hayden GF, Schwartz RH. Characteristics of earache among children with acute otitis media. *Am J Dis Child* 1985;139:721–723.

74. Pitkaranta A, Virolainen A, Jero J, et al. Detection of rhinovirus, respiratory syncytial virus, and coronavirus infection in acute otitis media by reverse transcriptase polymerase chain reaction. *Pediatrics* 1998;102:291–295.

75. Arola M, Ziegler T, Ruuskanen O, et al. Rhinovirus in acute otitis media. *J Pediatr* 1988; 113:693–695.

76. Carlson LH, Stool SE. Diagnosis. In: Rosenfeld RM, Bluestone CD, eds. *Evidence-Based Otitis Media* Hamilton, Ontario, Canada: Decker, 1999, 105–115.

77. Fields MJ, Allison RS, Corwin P, et al. Microtympanometry, microscopy, and tympanometry in evaluating middle-ear effusion prior to myringotomy. *N Z Med J* 1993;106: 386–387.

78. Ovesen T, Paaske PB, Elbrond O. Accuracy of an automatic impedance apparatus in a population of secretory otitis media: Principles in the evaluation of tympanometrical findings. *Am J Otolaryngol* 1993;14:100–104.

79. Berman SA, Balkany TJ, Simmons MA. Otitis media in the neonatal intensive care unit. *Pediatrics* 1978;62:198.

80. Bland RD. Otitis media in the first six weeks of life. Diagnosis, bacteriology, management. *Pediatrics* 1972;49:187.

81. Shurin PA, Howie VM, Pelton SI, et al. Bacterial etiology of otitis media in the first six weeks of life. *J Pediatr* 1978;92:893.

82. Tetzlaff TR, Ashworth C, Nelson JD. Otitis media in children less than 12 weeks of age. *Pediatrics* 1977;59:827.

83. Karma P, Pukander J, Sipila M, et al. Middle ear fluid bacteriology in neonates and very young infants. *Int J Pediatr Otorhinolaryngol* 1987;14:141.

84. Celin SE, Bluestone CD, Stephenson J, et al. Bacteriology of acute otitis media in adults. *JAMA* 1991;266(16):2249–2252.

85. De Neeling AJ, Van Leeuwen WJ, Van Klingeren B, et al. Epidemiology of resistance of *Streptococcus pneumoniae* in the Netherlands. *Abstracts of the 36th Interscience Conference on Antimicrobial Agents and Chemotherapy,* New Orleans, LA, 1996, 44, abstract No C57.

86. Committee on Infectious Disease, American Academy of Pediatrics. Therapy for children with invasive pneumococcal infections. *Pediatrics* 1997;99:289–299.

87. Bluestone CD, Stephenson JS, Martin LM. Ten year review of otitis media pathogens. *Pediatr Infect Dis J* 1992;11:75–115.

88. Doern GV, Jorgenson JH, Thronsberry C, et al. National collaborative study of the prevalence of antimicrobial resistance among clinical isolates of *Haemophilus influenzae. Antimicrob Agents Chemother* 1988;32:180–185.

89. Ruuskanen O, Arola M, Putto-Laurila A, et al. Acute otitis media and respiratory virus infections. *Pediatr Infect Dis J* 1989;8:94–99.

90. Heikkenen T, Thint M, Chonmaitree T. Prevalence of various respiratory viruses in the middle ear during acute otitis media. *N Engl J Med* 1999;340:260–264.

91. Okamoto Y, Kudo K, Ishikawa K, et al. Presence of respiratory syncytial virus genomic sequences in middle ear fluid and its relationship to expression of cytokines and cell adhesion molecules. *J Infect Dis* 1993;168(5):1277–1281.

92. Henderson FW, Collier AM, Sanyal MA, et al. Longitudinal study of respiratory viruses and bacteria in the etiology of acute otitis media with effusion. *N Engl J Med* 1982;306:1377–1383.

93. Buchman CA, Doyle WJ, Skoner D, et al. Otologic manifestations of experimental rhinovirus infection. *Laryngoscope* 1994;104:1295–1299.

94. Buchman CA, Doyle WJ, Alper CM, et al. Comparison of nasal and otologic responses following intranasal challenge with influenza A virus or rhinovirus-39. *Proceedings of the Sixth International Symposium on Recent Advances in Otitis Media*, June 1995, 137:235.

95. Buchman CA, Doyle WJ, Pilcher O, et al. Nasal and otological effects of experimental respiratory syncytial virus infection in adults. *Am J Otolaryngol.* 2002;23:70-75.

96. Chonmaitree T, Owen MJ, Patel JA, et al. Effect of viral respiratory tract infection on outcome of acute otitis media. *J Pediatr* 1992;120(6):856–862.

97. Rosenfeld RM. Natural history of untreated otitis media. In: Rosenfeld RM, Bluestone CD, eds. *Evidence-Based Otitis Media.* Hamilton, Ontario, Canada: Decker, 1999, 157–177.

98. Rosenfeld RM, Vertrees JE, Carr J, et al. Clinical efficacy of antimicrobial drugs for acute otitis media: Meta-analysis of 5400 children from 33 randomized trials. *J Pediatr* 1994;124:355–357.

99. Del Mar C, Glasziou P, Hayem M. Are antibiotics indicated as initial treatment for children with acute otitis media? *BMJ* 1997;314:1526–1529.

100. Rudberg RD. Acute otitis media: Comparative therapeutic results of sulphonamide and penicillin administered in various forms. *Acta Otolaryngol* 1954;113(Suppl)1–79.

101. Nadal D, Herrman P. Bauman A, Fanconi A. Acute mastoiditis: Clinical, microbiological, and therapeutic aspects. *Eur J Pediatr* 1990;149:560–564.

102. Dowell SF, Butler JC, Giebink GS, et al. Acute otitis media: Management and surveillance in an era of pneumococcal resistance—a report from the Drug-resistant *Streptococcus pneumoniae* Therapeutic Working Group. *Pediatr Infect Dis J* 1999;18(1):1–9.

103. Kaleida PH, Casselbrant ML, Rockette HE, et al. Amoxicillin or myringotomy or both for acute otitis media: Results of a randomized clinical trial. *Pediatrics* 1991;87:466–474.

104. Williams RL, Chalmers TC, Stange KC, et al. Use of antibiotics in preventing recurrent acute otitis media and in treating otitis media with effusion: A meta-analysis attempt to resolve the brouhaha. *JAMA* 1993;270:1344–1351.

105. Guillemot D, Courvalin P. Better control of antibiotic resistance. *Clin Infect Dis* 2001;15;33(4):542–547.

106. Black S, Shinefield H, Fireman B, et al. Efficacy, safety, and immunogenicity of heptavalent pneumococcal conjugate vaccine in children. *Pediatr Infect Dis J* 2000;19:187–195.

107. Eskola J, Kilpi T, Palmu A, et al for the Finnish Otitis Media Study Group. Efficacy of pneumococcal conjugate vaccine against acute otitis media. *N Engl J Med* 2001;344:403–409.

108. Bluestone CD. Pneumococcal conjugate vaccine: Impact on otitis media and otolaryngology. *Arch Otolaryngol Head Neck Surg* 2001;127(4):464–467.

109. Gebhart DE. Tympanostomy tubes in otitis media-prone children. *Laryngoscope* 1981;91:849–866.

110. Gonzalez C, Arnold JE, Woody EA, et al. Prevention of recurrent acute otitis media: Chemoprophylaxis versus tympanostomy tubes. *Laryngoscope* 1986;96:1330–1334.

111. Casselbrant ML, Kaleida PH, Rockette HE, et al. Efficacy of antimicrobial prophylaxis and of tympanostomy tube insertion for prevention of recurrent acute otitis media: Results of a randomized clinical trial. *Pediatr Infect Dis J* 1992;11:278–286.

112. Paradise JL, Bluestone CD, Rogers KD, et al. Efficacy of adenoidectomy for recurrent otitis media in children previously treated with tympanostomy-tube placement. Results of parallel randomized and nonrandomized trials. *JAMA* 1990;18:263(15):2066–2073.

113. Paradise JL, Bluestone CD, Colborn DK, et al. Adenoidectomy and adenotonsillectomy for recurrent acute otitis media: Parallel random-

ized clinical trials in children not previously treated with tympanostomy tubes. *JAMA* 1999; 8:282(10):945–953.

114. van Cauwenberge PB, Bellussi L, Maw AR, et al. The adenoid as a key factor in upper airway infections. *Int J Pediatr Otorhinolaryngol* 1995;32(Suppl):S71–S80.

115. Poulsen G, Tos M. Repetitive tympanometric screenings of two years old children. *Scand Audiol* 1980;9:21–28.

116. Tos M, Holm-Jensen S, Sorensen CH, Mogensen C. Spontaneous course and frequency of secretory otitis media in four-year-old children. *Arch Otolaryngol* 1982;108:4–10.

117. Fiellau-Nikolajsen M. Epidemiology of secretory otitis media: A descriptive cohort study. *Ann Otol Rhinol Laryngol* 1983;92:172–177.

118. Louis J, Fiellau-Nikolajsen M. Epidemiology of middle ear effusion and tubal dysfunction: A one-year prospective study comprising monthly tympanometry in 387 non-selected seven-year-old children. *Int J Pediatr Otorhinolaryngol* 1981;3:303–307.

119. Casselbrant ML, Brostoff LM, Cantekin EI, et al. Otitis media with effusion in preschool children. *Laryngoscope* 1985;95:428–436.

120. Casselbrant ML, Brostoff LM, Cantekin EI, et al. Otitis media in children in the United States. Acute and secretory otitis media. *Proceedings of the International Conference on Acute and Secretory Otitis Media,* Part I. Amsterdam: Kugler, 1996, 161–164.

121. Post JC, Preston RA, Aul JJ, et al. Molecular analysis of bacterial pathogens in otitis media with effusion. *JAMA* 1995;24–31:273(20): 1598–1604.

122. Rayner MG, Zhang Y, Gorry MC, et al. Evidence of bacterial metabolic activity in culture-negative otitis media with effusion. *JAMA* 1998;28;279(4):296–299.

123. Shaw CB, Obermyer N, Wetmore SJ, et al. Incidence of adenovirus and respiratory syncytial virus in chronic otitis media with effusion using the polymerase chain reaction. *Otolaryngol Head Neck Surg* 1995;113(3):234–241.

124. Moyse E, Lyon M, Cordier G, et al. Viral RNA in middle ear mucosa and exudates in patients with chronic otitis media with effusion. *Arch Otolaryngol Head Neck Surg* 2000;126(9): 1105–1110.

125. Stool SE, Berg AO, Berman S, et al. *Otitis Media with Effusion Young Children.* Clinical practice guideline number 12. AHCPR Publication No. 94-0622. Rockville, MD: Agency for Health Care Policy and Research, Public Health Service, US Department of Health and Human Services; July 1994.

126. Rosenfeld RM. What to expect from medical therapy. In: Rosenfeld RM, Bluestone CD, eds. *Evidence-Based Otitis Media.* Hamilton, Ontario, Canada: Decker, 1999, 179–205.

127. Vernon-Feagans L. Impact of otitis media on speech, language, cognitive, and behavior. In: Rosenfeld RM, Bluestone CD, eds. *Evidence-Based Otitis Media.* Hamilton, Ontario, Canada: Decker, 1999, 353–373.

128. Rosenfeld RM, Post JC. Meta-analysis of antibiotics for the treatment of chronic otitis media with effusion. *Otolaryngol Head Neck Surg* 1992;106:378–386.

129. Giebink GS, Batalden PB, Le CT, et al. A controlled trial comparing three treatments for chronic otitis media with effusion. *Pediatr Infect Dis J* 1990;9:33–40.

130. Macknin ML, Jones PK. Oral dexamethasone for treatment of persistent middle ear effusion. *Pediatrics* 1985;75:329–335.

131. Niederman LG, Walter-Bucholtz V, Jabalay T. A comparative trial of steroids versus placebo for treatment of chronic otitis media with effusion. In: Lim DJ, Bluestone CD, Klein JO, Nelson JD, eds. *Recent Advances in Otitis Media with Effusion. Proceeding of the Fourth International Symposium.* Burlington, Ontario, Canada: Decker, 1988, 273–275.

132. Cantekin EI, Mandel EM, Bluestone CD, et al. Lack of efficacy of decongestant-antihistamine combination for otitis media with effusion ("secretory" otitis media) in children: Results of a double-blind randomized trial. *N Engl J Med* 1983;308:297–301.

133. Dusdieker LB, Smith G, Booth BM, et al. The long-term outcome of chronic otitis media with effusion. *Clin Pediatr* 1985;24:181–186.

134. Haugeto OK, Schroder KE, Mair IWS. Secretory otitis media, oral decongestant, and antihistamine. *J Otolaryngol* 1981;10:359–362.

135. Mandel EM, Rockette HE, Bluestone CD, et al. Myringotomy with and without tympanostomy tubes for chronic otitis media with effusion.

Arch Otolaryngol Head Neck Surg 1989;115: 1217–1224.

136. Mandel EM, Rockette HE, Bluestone CD, et al. Efficacy of myringotomy with and without tympanostomy tubes for chronic otitis media with effusion. *Pediatr Infect Dis J* 1992;11: 270–277.

137. Gates GA, Avery CS, Prihoda TJ, Cooper JC. Effectiveness of adenoidectomy and tympanostomy tubes in the treatment of chronic otitis media with effusion. *N Engl J Med* 1987; 317:1444–1451.

138. Maw AR, Bawden R. Spontaneous resolution of severe chronic glue ear in children and the effect of adenoidectomy, tonsillectomy, and insertion of ventilation tubes (grommets). *BMJ* 1993;306:756–760.

139. Bluestone CD, Klein JO: Intratemporal complications and sequelae of otitis media. In: Bluestone CD, Stool SE, Kenna MA, eds. *Pediatric Otolaryngology,* 3rd ed. Philadelphia; Saunders, 1996.

140. Kenna MA. Treatment of chronic suppurative otitis media. *Otolaryngol Clin North Am* 1994; 27(3):457–472.

141. Brackmann DE, Shelton C, Arriaga M. *Otologic Surgery*. Philadelphia: Saunders, 2001.

142. Sorenson H, True O. Histology of tympanosclerosis. *Acta Otolaryngol* 1972;73(1):186–26.

143. Fria TJ, Cantekin EI, Eichler JA. Hearing acuity in children with effusion. *Arch Otolaryngol* 1985;11:10–16.

144. Karma PH, Laitila PME, Sipila M, et al. Sensorineural hearing and childhood acute otitis media in adolescence. In: Lim DJ, Bluestone CD, Casselbrant ML, et al., eds. *Proceeding of the Sixth International Symposium on Recent Advances in Otitis Media*. Hamilton, Ontario, Canada: Decker, 1995, 387.

145. Kettel K. Facial palsy of otitis origin. *Arch Otolaryngol* 1943;37:303–348.

146. Juselius H, Kaltiokallio K. Complications of acute and chronic otitis media in the antibiotic era. *Acta Otolaryngol* 1972;74:445–450.

147. Goldstein NA, Casselbrant ML, Bluestone CD, Kurs-Lasky M. Intratemporal complications of acute otitis media in infants and children. *Otolaryngol Head Neck Surg* 1998;119(5): 444–454.

148. Ellefsen B, Bonding P. Facial palsy in acute otitis media. *Clin Otolaryngol* 1996;21:393–395.

149. Sheehy JL, Brackmann DE, Graham MD. Cholesteatoma surgery: Residual and recurrent disease. A review of 1024 cases. *Ann Otol Rhinol Laryngol* 1977;86:451–454.

150. Rubin JS, Wei WL. Acute mastoiditis: Review of 34 patients. *Laryngoscope* 1985;95:963–965.

151. Hawkins DB, Dru D, House JW, Clark RW. Acute mastoiditis in children: A review of 54 cases. *Laryngoscope* 1983;93:568–572.

152. Rosen A, Ophir A, Marchak G. Acute mastoiditis: A review of 69 patients. *Ann Otol Rhinol Laryngol* 1986;95:222–224.

153. Chole RA. Petrous apicitis surgical anatomy. *Ann Otol Rhinol Laryngol* 1985;94:251–257.

154. Schuknecht HF, Gulya AJ. *Anatomy of the Temporal Bone with Surgical Implications*. Philadelphia: Lea & Febiger, 1986.

155. Allam AF, Schuknecht HF. Pathology of petrositis. *Laryngoscope* 1968;78:1813.

156. Thedinger BA, Jackler RK. Lesions of the petrous apex. In: Jackler RK, Brackmann DE, eds. *Neurotology*. St Louis: Mosby, 1994, 1169–1188.

157. Neely JG, Doyle KJ. Facial nerve and intracranial complications of otitis media. In: Jackler RK, Brackmann DE, eds. *Neurotology*. St Louis: Mosby, 1994, 905–918.

158. Kafka MM. Mortality of mastoiditis and cerebral complications with review of 3225 cases of mastoiditis and complications. *Laryngoscope* 1935;45:790–822.

159. House HP. Otitis media: Comparative study of results obtained in therapy before and after introduction of sulfonamide compounds. *Arch Otolaryngol* 1946;43:371–378.

160. Ballantine HT, White JC. Brain abscess: Influence of the antibiotics on therapy and mortality. *N Engl J Med* 1953;248:14–19.

161. Dawes JD. Discussion of intracranial complications of otogenic origin. *Proc R Soc Med* 1961;54:315–319.

162. Proctor CA. Intracranial complications of otitic origin. *Laryngoscope* 1966;76:288–308.

163. Matthews TJ, Marus G. Otogenic intradural complications: A review of 37 patients. *J Laryngol Otol* 1988;102:121–124.

164. Gower D, McGuirt WF. Intracranial complications of acute and chronic ear disease: A problem still with us. *Laryngoscope* 1983; 93:1028–1033.

165. Friedman EM, McGill TJ, Healy GB. Central nervous system complications associated with acute otitis media in children. *Laryngoscope* 1990;100:149–151.

166. Odio CM et al. The beneficial effects of early dexamethasone administration in infants and children with bacterial meningitis. *N Engl J Med* 1991;324:1525–1531.

167. Samuel J, Fernandez CM, Steinberg JL. Intracranial otogenic complications: A persisting problem. *Laryngoscope* 1986;96:272–277.

168. Snow JB. Cranial and intracranial complications of otitis media. In: English GM (ed). *Otolaryngology.* Philadelphia: JB Lippincott, 1980(1), 1–32.

169. Courville CB, Nielson JM. Fatal complications of otitis media and mastoiditis in the antibiotic era. *Laryngoscope* 1955;19:451–501.

170. Doyle KJ, Jackler RK. Otogenic cavernous sinus thrombosis. *Otolaryngol Head Neck Surg* 1991;104:873–877.

171. LeBeau J, et al. Surgical treatment of brain abscesses and subdural empyema. *J Neurosurg* 1973;38:198–203.

172. Spires JR, Smith RJ, Catlin FI. Brain abscesses in the young. *Otolaryngol Head Neck Surg* 1985;93:468–473.

173. Myers EN, Ballantine HT. The management of otogenic brain abscess. *Laryngoscope* 1965; 75:273–288.

174. Bluestone CD, Klein. Intracranial complications of otitis media and mastoiditis. In: Bluestone CD, Stool SE (eds). *Pediatric Otolaryngology.* Philadelphia: Saunders, 1990, 537–546.

175. Foley J. Benign forms of intracranial hypertension—"toxic" and "otitic" hydrocephalus. *Brain* 1955;78:1–41.

176. Symonds CP. Hydrocephalus and focal cerebral symptoms in relation to thrombophlebitis of the dural sinuses and cerebral veins. *Brain* 1937;60:531–550.

177. Merchant SN, Gopen Q. A human temporal bone study of acute bacterial meningogenic labyrinthitis. *Am J Otol* 1996;17:375–385.

178. Slattery WH, House JW. Complications of otitis media. In: Lalwani AK, Grundfast KM, eds. *Pediatric Otology and Neurotology.* New York: Lippincott-Raven, 1998.

179. Kangsanarak J, et al. Extracranial and intracranial complications of suppurative otitis media, report of 102 cases. *J Laryngol Otol* 1993; 107:999–1004.

180. Engel F, Blatz R, Schliebs R, et al. Bacterial cytolysin perturbs round window membrane permeability barrier in vivo: Possible cause of sensorineural hearing loss in acute otitis media. *Infect Immun* 1998;66(1):343–346.

181. Paparella MM, Sugiura S. The pathology of suppurative labyrinthitis. *Ann Laryngol Otol* 1967;76:554–586.

182. Paparella MM, Goycoolea MV, Meyerhoff WL. Inner ear pathology and otitis media. *Ann Otol Rhinol Laryngol* 1980;89:249.

183. Fortnum HM. Hearing impairment after bacterial meningitis: A review. *Arch Dis Child* 1992;67:1128–1133.

184. Wald ER, et al. Dexamethasone therapy for children with bacterial meningitis. *Pediatrics* 1995;95(1):21–28.

185. Lebel MH, Freij BJ, Syrogiannopoulos GA, et al. Dexamethasone therapy for bacterial meningitis. Results of two double-blind, placebo-controlled trials. *N Engl J Med* 1988; 319(15):964–971.

186. Hartnick CJ, Kim HY, Chute PM, et al. Preventing labyrinthitis ossificans—the role of steroids. *Arch Otolaryngol Head Neck Surg* 2001;127:180–183.

187. Rappaport JM, Bhatt SM, Burkard RF, et al. Prevention of hearing loss in experimental pneumococcal meningitis by administration of dexamethasone and ketorolac. *J Infect Dis* 1999;179(1):264–268.

188. Red Book: *Report of the Committee on Infectious Diseases.* Elk Grove Village, IL: American Academy of Pediatrics, 2000, 25.

189. Strauss M. Human cytomegalovirus labyrinthitis. *Am J Otolaryngol* 1990;11:292–298.

190. Stagno S. Cytomegalovirus. In: Behrman RE, Kliegman RM, Jenson HB, eds. *Nelson's Textbook of Pediatrics,* 16th ed. Philadelphia: Saunders, 2000.

191. Davis LE, Rarey KE, Stewart JA, et al. Recovery and probable persistence of cytomegalovirus in human inner ear fluid without cochlear damage. *Ann Otol Rhinol Laryngol* 1987;96: 380–383.

192. Whitley RJ, Cloud G, Gruber W, et al. Ganciclovir treatment of symptomatic congenital cytomegalovirus infection: Results of a phase

II study. National Institute of Allergy and Infectious Diseases Collaborative Antiviral Study Group. *J Infect Dis* 1997;175(5):1080–1086.

193. Maldonado Y. Rubeola. In: Behrman RE, Kliegman RM, Jenson HB, eds. *Nelson's Textbook of Pediatrics,* 16th ed. Philadelphia: Saunders, 2000.

194. Stewart BJ, Prabhu PU. Reports of sensorineural deafness after measles, mumps, and rubella immunisation. *Arch Dis Child* 1993;69(1):153–154.

195. Niedzielska G, Katska E, Szymula D. Hearing defects in children born of mothers suffering from rubella in the first trimester of pregnancy. *Int J Pediatr Otolaryngol* 2000;54:1–5.

196. McKenna MJ. Measles, mumps, and sensorineural hearing loss. *Ann N Y Acad Sci* 1997;830:291–298.

197. Chole RA, McKenna MM. Pathophysiology of otosclerosis. *Otol Neurotol* 2001;22:249–257.

198. Ray G. Mumps. In: Isselbacher KJ et al, eds. *Harrison's Principles of Internal Medicine,* 13th ed. New York: McGraw-Hill, 1994.

199. Koga K, Kawashiro N, Nakayama T, et al. Immunologic study on association between mumps and infantile unilateral deafness. *Acta Otolaryngol (Stockh)* 1988;456(Suppl):55–60.

200. Schuknecht HF. *Pathology of the Ear,* 2nd ed. Baltimore: Lea & Febiger, 1993.

201. Yamamoto M, Watanabe Y, Mizukoshi K. Neurotological findings in patients with acute mumps deafness. *Acta Otolaryngol (Stockh)* 1993;504(Suppl):94–97.

202. Wilson WR. The relationship of the herpesvirus family to sudden hearing loss: A prospective clinical study and literature review. *Laryngoscope* 1986;96:870–877.

203. Chandrasekhar SS, Connelly PE, Brahmbhatt SS, et al. Otologic and audiologic evaluation of human immunodeficiency virus–infected patients. *Am J Otolaryngol* 2000;21(1):1–9.

204. Pappas DG Jr, et al. Ultrastructural findings in the vestibular end-organs of AIDS cases. *Am J Otol* 1995;16(2):140–145.

205. Gleich LL, Linstrom CJ, Kimmelman CP. Otosyphilis: A diagnostic and therapeutic dilemma. *Laryngoscope* 1992;102:1255–1259.

206. Lukehart SA. Chapter 172. In: Braunwald E, Fauci AS, Kasper DL, et al, eds. *Harrison's Principles of Internal Medicine,* 15th ed. New York: McGraw-Hill, 2001.

207. Smith ME, Canalis RF. Otosyphilis. In: Canalis RF, Lambert PR, eds. *The Ear: Comprehensive Otology.* Philadelphia: Lippincott Williams & Wilkins, 2000.

208. Balkany TJ, Dans PE. Reversible sudden deafness in early acquired syphilis. *Arch Otolaryngol Head Neck Surg* 1978;104:66–68.

209. Zoller M, Wilson WR, Nadol JB. Treatment of syphilitic hearing loss. *Ann Otol* 1979;88:160–165.

210. Hughes GB, Rutherford I. Predictive value of serologic tests for syphilis in otology. *Ann Otol Rhinol Laryngol* 1986;95:250–259.

211. Linstrom CJ, Gleich LL. Otosyphilis: Diagnostic and therapeutic update. *J Otolaryngol* 1993;22(6):401–408.

212. Konishi K, Yamane H, Iguchi H, et al. Study of tuberculosis in the field of otolaryngology in the past 10 years. *Acta Otolaryngol (Stockh)* 1998;538(Suppl):244–249.

213. Singh B. Role of surgery in tuberculous mastoiditis. *J Laryngol Otol* 1991;105:905–915.

214. Yaniv E. Tuberculous otitis—An underdiagnosed disease. *Am J Otolaryngol* 1987;8:356–360.

215. Greenfield BJ, Selesnick SH, Fisher L, et al. Aural tuberculosis. *Am J Otol* 1995;16(2):175–182.

Noninfectious Disorders of the Ear

24

EXTERNAL EAR

Pinna, external auditory canal

Trauma

Lacerations

Simple laceration—skin +/– cartilage
Stellate—blunt trauma or crush injury
Avulsion—tear or separation

TREATMENT   Deep cleaning, debridement, surgical repair. May require stage or flap reconstruction. Dressing-stint, systemic antibiotics.

COMPLICATIONS   Perichondritis, cartilage necrosis

Hematoma

Blunt trauma

TREATMENT   Incision and drainage with through-and-through sutures and bolster dressing.

ANTIBIOTICS   Systemic antibiotics

LATE TREATMENT   Repeated aspiration, mild pressure dressing

COMPLICATIONS   Fibrosis, cauliflower ear, perichondritis

Acute Burns

Thermal, electrical, chemical. 25% of facial burns lead to infected auricle.

TREATMENT   Dependent on degree: first, second, or third; tissue loss, second- and third-degree burns. Topical and systemic antibiotics, local injection of gentamicin, surgical debridement

Radiation Burns

Acute first-degree burns. Late changes, skin dryness, telangiectasia, atrophy, cartilage necrosis

TREATMENT   Prolonged wound care; hyperbaric oxygen for poor healing controversial.

Frostbite

Exposure to subfreezing temperature and wind leading to disruption of endothelial layer with extravasation of erythrocytes, platelet aggregation, and sludging

SYMPTOMS   Pain, burning, discoloration; reduced pliability; loss of sensation

TREATMENT   Slow warming; antibiotics; anticoagulants; debridement of necrotic tissue after demarcation. No pressure or pressure dressing to the ear.

Bites

Human or animal; most common site: lobe of the ear

TREATMENT   Meticulous cleaning; systemic antibiotics; surgical repair and/or debridement

Keloids, Hypertrophic Scars

Occur in up to 30% of blacks and Hispanics

TREATMENT   Steroid injection, surgical excision

External Ear—Systemic Diseases

Contact Dermatitis

SIGNS AND SYMPTOMS   Erythema; pruritus; blisters; weeping; crusting extending to face and neck, associated with systemic allergies

OFFENDING AGENTS   Topical antibiotics [neomycin, quinolones (ciprofloxacin)]; nickel and chromium found in stainless steel, jewelry; plastic and latex; hair coloring agents; shampoos

TREATMENT   Removal of offending agent or agents, topical steroids +/− systemic steroids (severe reactions), Benadryl (diphenhydramine HCl).

Differential diagnosis is cellulitis or herpes zoster oticus, may require treatment with antibiotics or antiviral agents.

Gout

Nodular tophi, deposits of uric acid crystals in helix or antihelix, which may ulcerate

Diabetes Mellitus

Small vessel disease, tissue necrosis following trauma or surgery

Hypothyroidism

Dry, thick skin, pinna, and external canal; acromegaly; enlarged pinna

Hyperlipidemia

Xanthoma, yellowing plaques over helix.

Relapsing Perichondritis

Recurring erythema; pain and swelling regressing to cartilage loss

Wegener's Granulomatosis

Three percent of patients with symptoms similar to perichondritis

Carcinoma of the External Ear

General

Six percent of skin cancers involve the pinna.

Lymphatic drainage: Anterior auricular nodes, lateral pinna and anterior canal wall; postauricular nodes, superior and upper posterior pinna, posterior canal wall; superficial and deep cervical nodes, lobule and floor of external ear canal.

Metastasis more common with perichondrial and cartilage invasion.

Basal Cell Carcinoma

Erythematous lesion with raised margins; silvery scales most common, occurring on the pinna and external canal

TREATMENT   Biopsy, wide local excision; may require cartilage excision, skin graft, or local flaps

Squamous Cell Carcinoma

Most common malignancy of pinna and external ear canal

SIGNS   Pain, bloody discharge, granular appearance

TREATMENT   Biopsy, wide surgical excision, may require parotidectomy, block resection of ear canal or temporal bone resection, possible postoperative radiation

Malignant Melanoma

Seven percent of head and neck sites involve the ear.

Other Tumors of the Ear

Adenoid cystic carcinoma, adenocarcinoma, adenoma, pleomorphic adenoma

TREATMENT   Depending on tissue type

External Ear Canal

Seborrheic Dermatitis

Eczematoid external otitis, the most common dermatologic condition of the external canal, may be associated with dandruff.

SIGNS AND SYMPTOMS   Itching; weeping; recurrent external otitis; canal stenosis; dry, scaly, fissured skin

TREATMENT   Good cleaning with irrigation and drying (hair dryer), 1% hydrocortisone solution or lotion, 3% salicylic acid solutions

Psoriasis

Affects 2 to 5% of the population. In 18% with systemic psoriasis, the ear is affected. It also affects the scalp and postauricular sulcus.

TREATMENT   Local control, 1% hydrocortisone lotion or solution

Keratosis Obturans

Rapid accumulation of keratin debris; casts; plugged external auditory canal; painless erosion and expansion of external canal; may be associated with drainage, foul odor, and secondary external otitis

PATHOLOGY   Chronic inflammation and poor epithelial migration

TREATMENT   Frequent cleaning, irrigation; topical 1% hydrocortisone; 3% salicylic acid

Cholesteatoma

Keratin accumulation in the external canal associated with osteitis and bone necrosis; usually occurs on the floor of the external canal; commonly associated with pain and keratin invasion of bone

TREATMENT   Frequent cleaning of the external auditory canal; topical steroids; may require surgical debridement of osteitic bone

Radiation Necrosis

Late complication of radiation therapy: atrophic epithelium; exposed necrotic bone; accumulation of squamous debris and cholesteatoma formation

TREATMENT   Frequent cleaning and irrigation; lubrication with mineral oil; local debridement of bone; may involve ear canal, mastoid, and glenoid fossa. Surgery usually complicated by delayed and poor healing.

Osteoma

Pedunculated bone mass developing along suture lines, tympanosquamous, tympanomastoid occluding osteoma may require surgical removal. In surgery, care should be taken to protect tympanic membrane.

Exostosis

Lamellar thickening of bone of external ear canal, less commonly anterior and posterior canal wall associated with exposure to cold water. May cause canal stenosis, cerumen impaction, or limited exposure of the tympanic membrane.

TREATMENT   Canaloplasty, skin graft, and meatoplasty

Hemangioma

Soft, reddish or purple mass of external ear canal pulsating on microscopic examination.

Capillary hemangioma usually involutes in childhood. Cavernous does not involute and may extend to surrounding structures.

Cholesterol Granuloma

Blue-domed cyst; fluid "motor oil" color, often thought to be blood

TREATMENT   Aspiration; surgery rarely needed

Other Benign Lesions

Adenoma, lipoma, fibroma, chondroma, keratoacanthoma, monosalivary gland tumors; diagnosis and treatment dependent on biopsy

Secondary Stenosis or Atresia

CAUSES   Recurrent or chronic external otitis often associated with acute anterior tympano-medial angle, trauma, repeated instrumentation, or previous surgery

SIGNS AND SYMPTOMS   Recurrent external otitis, conductive hearing loss, narrowing of external auditory canal, blunting and loss of normal drum landmarks, 30- to 40-dB conductive hearing loss

TREATMENT   Early—expandable wick and packs, topical antibiotics and steroids.
Late—excision of fibrosis and epithelium, canaloplasty, thin split-thickness skin graft, and meatoplasty. Prolonged postoperative packing reduces recurrent stenosis.

Foreign Body

Insects, nuts, beans, gum, putty, beads, toys, etc. Avoid irrigation—vegetable matter will expand; blind instrumentation may cause bleeding or swelling of the ear canal and may impale the foreign material through the eardrum.

TREATMENT   Local anesthetic block, microscopic examination and instrumentation for removal of foreign body, mineral oil or antibiotic solution may facilitate removal, antibiotic pack

MIDDLE EAR AND MASTOID

Trauma

Temporal Bone Fractures, Basilar Skull Fractures

LONGITUDINAL FRACTURES   70 to 90% of temporal bone fractures; parietal bone fracture.
Extending to external ear canal, middle ear, eustachian tube, and foramen lacerum. Frequent disruption on tympanic membrane, ossicular chain, and may involve the geniculate ganglion.

Presentation   Bleeding from external canal; conductive hearing loss; cerebrospinal fluid (CSF) otorrhea; facial paralysis

TRANSVERSE FRACTURES   20 to 30% of temporal bone fractures; usually, more severe occipital bone injury

Presentation   Hemotympanum; CSF rhinorrhea; sensorineural hearing loss; facial paralysis in 50% of cases

Evaluation   Examination for multisystem, neurologic, cervical, and cranial nerve VII and VIII injuries; computed tomography (CT); audiogram; electroneurography (ENOG); facial paralysis

Treatment   Stabilize for other neurologic and life-threatening injuries; observation; antibiotic coverage; surgery: for persistent tympanic membrane perforation; conductive hearing loss; facial paralysis (greater than 90% weakness on ENOG); persistent CSF leak

Tympanic Membrane Injuries

PERFORATIONS

Penetrating injuries—cotton applicators, sticks, and bobby pins tend to involve the posterior drum and may involve the ossicular chain

Burns—welder's slag burn, acid, lightning—usually involve the anterior drum and annulus; poorer chance of spontaneous healing

Blast and barotrauma—weakened central drum, water exposure and diving, fall, slap

EVALUATION   Microscopic examination; audiogram; clinical evaluation for vertigo; CT if foreign body or ossicular discontinuity suspected

TREATMENT

Acute   Prevention of secondary infection—antibiotic pack and drops with water exposure; oral antibiotics; keep the ear dry; infection adversely affects spontaneous healing.

Observation—spontaneous healing usually more successful in 78 to 94% than early surgical intervention; drum skin margins may be microscopically realigned in the first 24 hours.

Emergency Surgery   Penetrating injury with sensorineural hearing loss and vertigo, suggest fracture and impaction of the stapes footplate into the vestibule or perilymph fistula.

Emergency Treatment   Seal the oval window and repair the tympanic membrane. Reconstruct the ossicular chain as a secondary procedure depending on residual hearing and bone conduction audiogram.

Late Treatment   Tympanoplasty—indications: Persistent perforation after 4 months; conductive hearing loss >20 dB.

Potential Problem at Surgery   Squamous epithelium (cholesteatoma) in growth onto the medial surface of drum may extend farther than anticipated on clinical examination to involve the anterior annulus and eustachian tube as well as the ossicular chain.

Tympanoplasty   78 to 94% of traumatic perforation will heal spontaneously within 4 months.

MIDDLE EAR AND MASTOID—SYSTEMIC DISEASES

Wegener's Granulomatosis

19% ear involvement

Signs and Symptoms

Conductive hearing loss, serous otitis media

Pathology

Chronic inflammation and granulation tissue formation

Tuberculosis

Hematogenous or lymphatic spread to temporal bone

Signs and Symptoms

Thickened tympanic membrane with loss of landmarks, conductive hearing loss, multiple or total perforation with serous drainage

Polyarteritis Nodosa

Sensorineural hearing loss, sudden hearing loss, facial paralysis

Sarcoidosis

Facial paralysis

Osteogenesis Imperfecta

Van der Hove's syndrome: inherited autosomal dominant; conductive hearing loss; blue sclerae; stapes footplate thickening

Treatment

Stapedectomy, generally good results

Paget's Disease

Osteitis deformans: male : female ratio 4 : 1; inherited autosomal dominant; thickening of the skull; mixed conductive hearing loss; thickening of the ossicles with fixation

CT Scan

Shows thickening of cortical bone

TREATMENT   Stapedectomy

CONDUCTIVE HEARING LOSS

Otosclerosis

Incidence

White population 8 to 12%, clinical disease 0.5 to 2%; black population 1%, clinical disease 0.1%. Female : male ratio 2 : 1.

Genetics

Family history: 49 to 58%, selective population 70%, autosomal-dominant penetrance 25 to 40%, osteogenesis imperfecta, 6% have otosclerosis.

Pathology

Enchondrial bone—early phase: vascular, spongy bone progressing to fibrosis; late phase: new bone replaced with sclerotic bone.
Foci: 67%, one; 27%, two; three or more, 6%.
Anterior oval window, fistulae, antefenestrum, 70 to 90%.
Round window, 30 to 70%; cochlear, 14%; extensive involvement, 10 to 12%.
Measles virus associated with otosclerotic foci.

Clinical Presentation

Progressive conductive or mixed hearing loss; most common presentation ages 30 to 50; hearing loss also seen at ages 20 to 30 in 42%; at less than age 20, in 31%; associated with pregnancy in 30 to 63%; paracusis willisiana (hearing better in noise), 36 to 85%; tinnitus, 75 to 100%; imbalance, 22%; vertigo, 26%; Schwartze's sign (promontory hyperemia), 10%

Audiometry

Progressive, low-frequency, conductive or mixed hearing loss; maximum conductive component, 60 dB; Carhart notch, depressed bone thresholds, 1,000 to 2,000 Hz (over closure—air–bone gap); word discrimination good, 70% or better

Acoustic Reflex

No reflex: fixed stapes

Diphasic reflex (on-off): occurs in 94% with symptoms of less than 5 years and in 9% greater than 10 years. (40% of normals have diphasic acoustic reflexes.)

Tuning Forks

Webber, lateralizes to affected ear; Rinne, negative—bone greater than air, masking the opposite ear with unilateral hearing loss. Applying the tuning forks to the teeth rather than the mastoid will increase the sensitivity 5 to 10 dB.

Tuning Fork	Air–Bone Gap
Negative 256 Hz Rinne	15 dB or more
Negative 512 Hz Rinne	25 dB or more
Negative 1024 Hz Rinne	35 dB or more

Vestibular Testing

Vestibular testing only when indicated

Reduced caloric response, 40 to 57%

Directional preponderance, 37 to 53%

Positional vertigo, 33%

Computed Tomography (CT)

Thin section (0.5–1.5 mm) of labyrinth, axial and coronal views; areas of reduced bone density, cochlear deformity. Indications—rapid loss of bone threshold, cochlear otosclerosis.

Surgical Indications

Conductive hearing loss 20 dB or greater

Negative Rinne test, 256 and 512 Hz (good candidate)

Negative 1024 Hz (excellent candidate)

Good bone conduction threshold

Speech discrimination 70% or better

Stable middle and inner ear

Poorer-hearing ear done first

Other Considerations

Hearing disability; occupation; hobbies (scuba diving); inability to use a hearing aid at air conduction thresholds but aidable bone thresholds

Surgical Contraindications

Only or better-hearing ear; ear with better speech discrimination; perforated tympanic membrane; active middle ear disease; active Ménière's disease

Relative Contraindications

Age: child less than 18 years of age

Poor eustachian tube function

Air conduction threshold < 30 dB

Air–bone gap < 15 dB

Aidable hearing with bone conduction > 40 dB

Occupation: roofer, acrobat, scuba diver

ALTERNATIVE TREATMENTS   None. Good hearing in one ear; hearing aid

MEDICAL TREATMENT   Sodium fluoride, calcium, vitamin D (widely accepted but not FDA approved)

Indications   Cochlear otosclerosis; bone conduction loss > 5 dB in less than 12 months

Surgical Results
Dependent on surgeon's experience more than prosthesis; prosthesis—personal preference, Teflon wire and stainless steel bucket comparable results
Experienced surgeon: Closure of air–bone gap, < 10 dB, 90 to 95%
Revision surgery, 2%
Significant sensorineural hearing loss, < 0.5%
Mild transient vertigo, 5%
Severe persistent vertigo, < 0.5%
Preservation of chorda tympani nerve, 95%
Dysgeusia, 5% to 10%
Facial paralysis, rare
Resident: Closure of air–bone gap, < 10 dB, 65% to 90%

Intraoperative Complications
Torn tympanomeatal flap
Dislocation of incus
Fractured long process of incus
Perilymph gusher (1/300)
Bleeding
Vertigo
Sensorineural hearing loss
Floating footplate
Depressed footplate

Postoperative Complications
Acute otitis media
Suppurative labyrinthitis and meningitis
Vertigo
Reparative granuloma
Perilymph fistula (0.3–2.5%)

Revision Stapes Surgery
2% of cases

Displaced prosthesis, 44%
Incus necrosis, 28%
Perilymph fistula, 8%
Tympanic membrane perforation, 6%
Cholesteatoma, 7%

HEARING RESULTS—REVISION SURGERY
Closure of air–bone gap < 10 dB 46 to 80%; results dependent on cause of failure
Sensorineural hearing loss (bone conduction) 0.8 to 7.7%; use of the laser has improved the results of revision stapes surgery

Causes of vertigo and hearing loss in stapes surgery: suction in the oval window; excessive manipulation of stapes or prosthesis; long prosthesis; failure to seal oval window, perilymph fistula; disruption of membranous labyrinth; removal of prosthesis; heat from laser

Fixed Malleus or Incus

Onset
Usually after age 50; 3% of stapes revisions; congenital

Examination
Reduced mobility of malleus handle on pneumatic otoscopy or palpation

Audiogram
Flat conductive hearing loss; 15- to 20-dB air–bone gap; congenital, 35- to 50-dB air–bone gap

CT Scan
Attic fixation of ossicle; congenital deformed and fixed ossicular mass

Pathology
Ossification of anterior malleolar ligament

Treatment
Tympanoplasty III; transection of malleus neck and anterior malleolar ligament; incus interposition or partial ossicular prosthesis between stapes and malleus handle and drum

Ossicular Discontinuity

Etiology
Trauma, basilar skull fracture; chronic otitis media; eustachian tube dysfunction; previous surgery

Examination
Hypermobile drum and malleus handle on pneumatic otoscopy or palpation

Audiometry
Conductive hearing loss 25 to 60 dB; tympanogram hypermobile eardrum

Treatment
Tympanoplasty with ossicle interposition or partial ossicular prosthesis (PORP) or total ossicular prosthesis (TORP)

Congenital Atresia
(See Chapter 10: "Clefts and Pouches," "Embryology of the Ear," "Congenital Deformities")

Facial Nerve Prolapse
Dehiscent facial nerve impinging on stapes superstructure; occurs in children (congenital) and adults; flat conductive hearing loss 15 to 25 dB; may cause a 10- to 20-dB conductive loss after successful stapes surgery

Congenital Cholesteatoma
Cholesteatoma developing behind an intact tympanic membrane; no significant history of otitis media

Etiology

Epithelial rest cells; sites—anterosuperior quadrant mesotympanum and tympanic membrane adjacent to malleus and posterior mesotympanum

Presentation

Tympanic membrane—2 to 6 years of age—white mass beneath drum, usually adjacent to malleus

Middle ear—6 to 12 years of age—white middle ear mass, white drum

Mastoid—12 to 30 years of age—white middle ear mass, hearing loss, vertigo

Petrous apex, geniculate ganglion—20 to 45 years of age—facial paralysis or paresis, sensorineural hearing loss, vision changes, facial hypesthesia

Posterior fossa—40 to 60 years of age—sensorineural hearing loss, vertigo, headache, visual changes

Evaluation

Audiogram; facial paralysis electroneurography (ENOG), vestibular testing (ENG) if indicated

CT of temporal bone

Magnetic resonance imaging (MRI) posterior fossa and petrous apex lesions

Treatment

Dependent on location and associated complications

Cholesterol Granuloma

Blue-domed cyst, blue eardrum

Presentation

Mastoid—conductive hearing loss, drainage fluid "motor oil" color, often thought to be blood; blue eardrum

Petrous apex, posterior fossa—pain, headache, visual changes, sensorineural hearing loss

Pathology

Cyst or fluid within mastoid or petrous apex; may expand into posterior fossa; contains hemosiderin, cholesterol crystals, chronic inflammation; thought to be caused by bleeding or negative pressure; usually develops in previously pneumatized temporal bones

Evaluation

Audiogram; CT scan—diffuse soft tissue density (fluid), cystic lesion in the petrous apex; MRI scan—(increased signal T1 and T2), nonenhancing lesion with contrast

Management

Mastoid/middle ear—large-diameter ventilation tubes, mastoidectomy with expanding lesions, may ultimately lead to radical mastoidectomy and maximum conductive hearing loss

Petrous apex—expanding cyst; drainage through the hypotympanum, or infralabyrinthine approach for hearing preservation; translabyrinthine or transcochlear with profound hearing loss

Intracranial—depending on location, posterior or middle fossa approach

INNER EAR DISORDERS

Ménière's Disease (Endolymphatic Hydrops)

SYMPTOMS   Aural fullness, roaring tinnitus, fluctuating hearing loss, severe episodic whirling vertigo

ASSOCIATED SYMPTOMS   Nausea, vomiting, diplacusis, recruitment, and anxiety

Atypical Ménière's Disease
Incomplete symptom complex, vestibular hydrops—episodic vertigo, cochlear hydrops—fluctuating hearing loss

Lermoyez Syndrome
Increasing oral fullness and tinnitus, hearing loss relieved with vertigo attack

Crisis of Tumarkin
Otolithic crisis, drop attacks

HISTOLOGY   Endolymphatic hydrops, distention of Reisner's membrane, ruptures of Reisner's membrane with attacks and fluctuation in hearing, endolymphatic sac, fibrosis, reduced vascularity and reduced lumen size

OTHER ETIOLOGIES   Autoimmune sensorineural inner ear disease, 15 to 20%; syphilis, 6%

INCIDENCE   46 to 128 per 100,000; bilateral disease 3 to 8% after 5 years, 8 to 42.5% after 20 years; male = female

ONSET   45 to 50 years

NATURAL HISTORY   Episodic vertigo and fluctuating hearing loss; progressive loss of hearing usually to 50 dB and 50% speech discrimination; reduced attacks of vertigo over several years; may occur as a single attack with profound hearing loss

DIAGNOSTIC STUDIES
   Audiogram, low-frequency sensorineural hearing loss; repeat audiograms, fluctuating or progressive hearing loss; glycerol test, threshold improved 10% or speech discrimination improved 12%
   ECOG, elevated summating potential, summating potential > 40% of action potential
   Electronystagmography (ENG), caloric testing, vestibular weakness in affected ear
   Rotational testing, reduced response, prolonged latency, vestibular recruitment
   Laboratory studies, rule out autoimmune inner ear disease or syphillis, RPR, FTA; inner ear antibodies when indicated

STAGING: AMERICAN ACADEMY OTOLARYNGOLOGY HEAD AND NECK SURGERY   Stages 0–VI; stage 0, no disability; IV, frequent recurrent vertigo > 4 weeks per year; VI, chronic or incapacitating vertigo

MEDICAL TREATMENT
   Diet: Low salt (< 2000 mg/day); dietary log to identify sources of salt
   Diuretics: Hydrochlorothiazide; carbonic anhydrase inhibitors, acetazolamide

Labyrinthine suppressants: Dimenhydrate; meclizine; diazepam (Valium); promethazine HCl (Phenergan)

CHEMICAL LABYRINTHECTOMY AND SURGICAL INDICATIONS   Medical failure; intractable and frequent disabling vertigo

Chemical Labyrinthectomy   Gentamicin profusion of round window, 80 to 90% control; 30 to 68% profound sensorineural hearing loss (depending on technique and dosage); IM streptomycin bilateral Ménière's.

SURGICAL PROCEDURES

Endolymphatic sac procedures—vertigo control 60 to 80%; hearing preservation
Labyrinthectomy—vertigo control 90 to 95%; complete hearing loss
Vestibular nerve section—vertigo control 90 to 95%; hearing preservation

Autoimmune Sensorineural Hearing Loss, Autoimmune Inner Ear Disease
General
Inner ear and central nervous system (CNS) capable of immune response; normal cochlea, contains no immune immunocompetent cells; endolymphatic sac, helper and suppressor T cells, lymphocytes, macrophages; B cells lymphocytes; immunoglobins IgM, IgA, IgG

Systemic Autoimmune Disorders Associated with Autoimmune Inner Ear Disease
Polyarteritis nodosa; Wegener's granulomatosis; systemic lupus erythematosus; rheumatoid arthritis; ulcerative colitis.

Cogan's Syndrome
Interstitial keratitis
Vertigo, bilateral progressive sensorineural hearing loss
Hypersensitivity with vasculitis
Bilateral symptoms of Ménière's disease, 15 to 20%

Syphilis
TREATMENT

High-dose steroids, prednisone, 40 to 60 mg per day for 30 days; slowly tapered dosage, reinstitute higher dose if hearing deteriorates with tapering steroids; cytotoxic medication with prolonged high dose of steroids or failure to respond to steroids
Methotrexate: 7.5 to 15 mg per week with folic acid
Cyclophosphamide (cytoxin), 1 to 2 mg per week
Monitor for toxicity: CBC platelets, BUN, creatinine, liver function, urinalysis
Plasmapheresis when patient does not respond to medical treatment

Idiopathic Sudden Sensorineural Hearing Loss (SSNHL)
Abrupt or rapidly progressing hearing loss over minutes or days

Incidence
5 to 20 per 100,000 per year, median age 40 to 54 years, of distribution, male = female

Pathology

Viral: Loss of hair cells and supporting cells; tectorial membrane disruption; stria vascularis atrophy; neuronal loss; seen in mumps and measles

Vascular: Small vessel thrombosis, inner ear fibrosis

Etiology

Bacterial: Bacterial meningitis; bacterial labyrinthitis; syphilis; mycoplasmal bacteria

Viral: Mumps, cytomegalovirus, influenza virus, herpes simplex, and human immuno-deficiency virus (HIV)

Vascular: Thromboembolic disorders; vasculitis; coronary artery bypass surgery; macroglobulinemia; sickle cell disease; radiation therapy

Autoimmune inner ear disease

Trauma

Barotrauma, perilymph fistula

Post–stapes surgery, perilymph fistula

Acoustic blast injury

Temporal bone fracture

Tumors: Cerebellopontine angle tumors, 1 to 3%; cranial nerves VIII, VII, schwanno-mas, meningiomas, leptomeningeal carcinomatosis, metastatic disease

Ototoxic medications

Congenital inner ear deformities

Intracochlear membrane rupture

Diagnostic Studies

Audiometry: air–bone and speech; tympanometry; stapedial reflex; otoacoustic emis-sions (OAE), auditory brain stem response (BSRA)

Vestibular testing: when indicated

Radiographic: MRI with gadolinium-DPTA—internal auditory canal and cerebello-pontine angle (CPA); CT of temporal bone with congenital deformity, hearing loss, or trauma

Laboratory: CBC and differential, sedimentation rate, coagulation studies, FTA, ABS-RPR, thyroid function, inner ear antibodies, lipid profile

Recovery

Spontaneous recovery: to 10 dB of opposite ear 47 to 63%

Treatment

Considerations based on possible etiologies:

No treatment

Vasodilators—reverse hypoxia

Carbogen (95% O_2 + 5% CO_2), increased oxygen tension in cochlea

Medication: Histamine; nicotinic acid; procaine

Anticoagulant: Heparin; warfarin; low-molecular-weight dextran

Steroids: Prednisone, 40 to 60 mg, systemic (middle ear perfusion)

Antiviral: Acyclovir, famciclovir antibodies

Antibiotics: Erythromycin (macrolide antibiotic family)

Diuretics: Possible hydrops

Perilymph Fistulas

Sudden or progressive hearing loss associated with roaring tinnitus, dysacusis, dysequilibrium

History

Stapes surgery, trauma; exertion, barotrauma, spontaneous in children or congenital hearing loss

Examination

Normal; Hennebert's sign (fistula test—vertigo with pneumatic otoscopy)

Diagnostic Studies

Serial audiograms, monitoring hearing, MRI with contrast to rule out CPA lesion

Treatment

Observation 7 to 10 days; bed rest; head elevation; stool softener

Surgical Indications

Progressive hearing loss with persistent symptoms

Surgical Findings

Perilymph leak around annular ligament of stapes; leak around stapes prosthesis; round window leak

Ototoxicity

Aminoglycosides

AUDIOGRAM   High frequency progressing to all frequencies

PATHOLOGY   Outer hair cell loss; progression basal turn to apex

VESTIBULAR TO COCHLEAR TOXICITY (INCREASING COCHLEAR TOXICITY)   Streptomycin, gentamicin, netilmicin, tobramycin, amikacin, neomycin

PREVENTION   Therapeutic drug monitoring (peak and trough drug levels) twice weekly; periodic audiograms; BUN and creatinine levels twice weekly; drug dosage adjusted to remain in therapeutic range

Macrolide Antibiotics

Erythromycin, clarithromycin, azithromycin

AUDIOGRAM   Bilateral flat sensorineural hearing loss

PATHOLOGY   Stria vascularis

TOXICITY   Dose-dependent and usually reversible

Diuretics

Loop diuretics, ethacrynic acid, furosemide; affects 0.7 to 6.4% of patients

PATHOLOGY   Stria vascularis

Salicylates

AUDIOGRAM   Bilateral flat sensorineural hearing loss

TOXICITY   Dose-dependent and usually reversible

Antineoplastic Drugs
AUDIOGRAM   High- and mid-frequency loss

TOXICITY   Cisplatin; dose-dependent

PATHOLOGY   Outer hair cell loss; high- to mid-frequency

Radiation
AUDIOGRAM   High- and mid-frequency loss, poor discrimination, progression to complete hearing loss

PATHOLOGY   Late—atrophy of membranous labyrinth, degeneration of spiral and annular ligament, organ of Corti. Early—serous labyrinthitis

TUMORS OF THE MIDDLE EAR AND MASTOID

Multiple Myeloma
Slight male predominance; onset, 60 years old, round lytic lesions on CT scan; bone marrow, myeloma cells

Leukemia
Submucosal infiltrate of pneumatized spaces, conductive hearing loss, chronic middle ear effusion

Neurofibroma Facial Nerve
Pale middle ear mass, involvement of facial nerve, conductive or sensorineural hearing loss, facial weakness

CT Scan
Middle ear soft tissue mass; enlarged fallopian canal and geniculate ganglion

MRI Scan
Enhancing mass—middle ear, geniculate ganglion

ENOG
Reduced wave amplitude to no wave formation

Fibrous Dysplasia
Types: Polyostotic or monostotic

Findings
Enlargement and thickening of temporal bone, occlusion of external auditory canal with loss of mastoid air space, skull deformities and conductive hearing loss

CT Scan
Characteristic ground-glass appearance

Treatment
Conservative, long-term follow-up

Complications
Cholesteatoma formation, conductive hearing loss

Eosinophilic Granuloma
Common in children: histiocyte proliferation

Presentation
Most common in children; conductive hearing loss; bleeding, polyp, or pain; more severe forms and Hand-Schüller-Christian disease or Letterer-Siwe disease

Metastatic Carcinoma to the Temporal Bone
Primary tumor site: breast cancer, prostate cancer, renal cell carcinoma, bronchogenic squamous cell carcinoma, lymphoma

Glomus Tumors: Chemodectoma, Paraganglioma

Definition
Vascular tumor arising from neuroectodermal tissue, glomus bodies

GLOMUS TYMPANICUM   Develops on the promontory of the middle ear along the course of Arnold's nerve and Jacobson's nerve; may extend to mastoid or petrous apex via air cell tracts; jugular bulb not involved

GLOMUS JUGULARE   Arising within the jugular bulb; may involve middle ear, mastoid, petrous apex, neck, and intracranial space of the posterior fossa

GLOMUS VAGALE   Originates along vagus nerve; involves neck, jugular bulb, temporal bone, and posterior cranial fossa

Pathology
Nest of round or cuboidal cells—"Zellballen"—supported by reticular tissue and vascular channels; electron microscopy and immunohistochemical stains demonstrate neurosecretory granules containing catecholamines and serotonin.

Presentation
Fifth decade most common; female 1.5 : 1 male; larger, more aggressive tumors third decade with male predominance; multiple tumors, 10%; malignancy, 3%; catecholamine-secreting, 1%

Signs and Symptoms
Pulsating tinnitus; conductive hearing loss; large tumors—sensorineural hearing loss; cranial nerve palsy—involving cranial nerves VII, IX, X, XI, XII; bleeding

Examination
Red, pulsating mass—high-power magnification; Brown's sign—blanching and pulsation seen with pneumatic otoscopy; cranial nerve paralysis

Evaluation
AUDIOGRAM   Air, bone, speech

RADIOLOGY   CT of temporal bone with and without contrast; MRI of skull base with and without gadolinium contrast, MR arteriogram with venous phase; arteriogram preoperative, may be combined with embolization

LABORATORY   Vanillylmandelic acid (VMA), metanephrine, serotonin when indicated; history of hypertension, headache, diarrhea

CLASSIFICATION

Location	Fisch	Glasscock-Jackson
Middle ear	A	Tympanicum type I, II
Middle ear, mastoid, hypotympanum	B	Tympanicum III, IV Jugulare I
Infralabyrinthine, jugular bulb, petrous apex, neck	C	Jugulare I, II, III
Infralabyrinthine, jugular bulb, petrous apex, neck, intracranial extending beyond temporal bone	D	Jugulare II, III Jugulare IV

Management
SURGICAL APPROACH
Tympanicum: margins seen—transcanal; transcanal hypotympanotomy
Tympanicum: margins not seen—transcanal hypotympanotomy; extended facial recess
Jugulare: Dependent on tumor extension—infratemporal fossa approach; extended hypotympanotomy

COMPLICATIONS   Primarily with larger tumors; cranial nerve paralysis worse than preop: cranial nerve VII, 13%; IX and X, 33%; XI, 17%; XII, 11%
CSF leak; hearing loss; bleeding; wound infection; wound breakdown; death

RADIATION   Tumor control; recurrence; unresectable lesion; poor surgical candidate

POSTERIOR FOSSA, CEREBELLOPONTINE ANGLE TUMORS
Acoustic Neuroma, Schwannoma
General
Cerebellopontine angle (CPA) tumors—10% of intracranial tumors
Vestibular schwannoma (acoustic neuroma)—78% of CPA tumors
Meningiomas—3% of CPA tumors

Occurrence
0.8 to 2.7% of population; 0.7 to 1 per 100,000

Pathology
Vestibular division of cranial nerve VIII; Schwann cells; originate in Scarpa's ganglion (vestibular ganglion)

Type 2 Neurofibromatosis
Bilateral tumors; chromosome 22 abnormality; transmission autosomal dominant

Symptoms
Unilateral progressive sensorineural hearing loss, 85%; sudden hearing loss, 15 to 20%; 1 to 2% of patients with sudden hearing loss have acoustic schwannoma; tinnitus, 56%; vestibular dysfunction: vague disequilibrium, 50%; vertigo, 19%

Midface hypesthesia, cranial nerve V; facial paresis; diplopia; dysphagia; hoarseness; aspiration; cerebellar ataxia

Hydrocephalus: headache, vomiting

Signs

Hitzelberger's sign—reduced sensation of the posterior external meatus; reduced corneal reflex; facial weakness; reduced cerebellar function

Audiometry

Usually high-frequency sensorineural hearing loss with reduced word recognition

INDEX OF SUSPICION   Asymmetric high-frequency hearing loss 15 dB, 12% difference in word recognition; hearing complaints disproportional to audiologic findings; rollover—loss of word recognition with increased volume; acoustic reflex decay

BRAIN STEM EVOKED RESPONSE AUDIOMETRY (BERA)   Sensitivity, 85 to 90% of tumors; may not detect smaller tumors; intra-aural difference wave V > 0.4 msec, significant; wave V > 0.2 msec, 40 to 60% of tumors; no wave formation, 20 to 30% of tumors

Vestibular Testing

Unilateral weakness 70 to 90%; spontaneous nystagmus, larger tumors

MRI

Internal auditory canal and cerebellopontine angle with and without gadolinium DPTA (diethylenetriamine pentaacetic acid) contrast enhancement; detects tumors < 5 mm; T2 fast spin echo MRI, enhances fluid resolution, which contrasts contents of internal auditory canal (IAC); screen for acoustic schwannoma; acoustic schwannoma = "light bulb" centered at IAC; meningioma, broad-based, dural tail

Treatment

OBSERVATION   50 to 55% show little or no growth in 1 to 3 years; growth < 0.2 mm per year

Repeat MRI in 6 months and then annually with solid tumors; repeat MRI every 4 to 6 months with tumors > 1 cm, cystic tumors, enlarging tumors

SURGICAL RESECTION

Translabyrinthine Approach   Tumors of all sizes; discrimination, < 70%; pure-tone > 30 dB intra-aural difference

Advantages—early facial nerve identification, less cerebellar retraction

Disadvantages—complete hearing loss; facial nerve preservation 90 to 98.5% (experienced surgeons); facial paralysis dependent on tumor size: small tumors (< 2 cm) 75% House-Brackman grade I to II; large tumors, 42% grade I to II and 75% grade I to IV; CSF leak, 4 to 14%

Middle Fossa Approach   Intracanalicular tumor or < 1 cm extension into the posterior fossa; hearing preservation, < 30 dB pure-tone intra-aural difference; word recognition, > 70%; complete tumor removal, 98%; hearing preservation, 71%; facial nerve function grade I to II, 92%

Suboccipital Retrosigmoid Approach   Popular neurosurgical approach; can be used for all size tumors; most commonly done in "park bench" or supine position to reduce air embolization; commonly used for hearing preservation

Surgical Results   Complete tumor removal, 95%, depending on tumor size; facial nerve near normal, 58 to 93%; Hearing preservation, 17 to 65%; postoperative headache, 23 to 64%; CSF leak, 11 to 15%; meningitis, 1 to 7%; death, < 1%

STEREOTATIC RADIOSURGERY   Multisource cobalt-60 gamma (gamma knife), linear accelerator

Indications   Usually reserved for patients who are poor surgical risk; elderly, who refuse surgical removal of tumor

Results   Tumor growth at 1 year, 4 to 15%; hearing preservation, 22 to 50%; facial weakness, 17 to 66.5%

Potential Concerns   Removal of residual or recurrent tumor more complex with greater risk of complications

Meningioma

3% of CPA tumors; MRI shows less involvement of internal auditory canal, characteristic dural tail

Facial Nerve Schwannoma

Gradual facial paresis, hearing loss; may present like acoustic schwannoma; MRI with gadolinium DPTA—enhancement in fallopian canal, geniculate ganglion, parotid gland

Treatment

Surgical resection with cable graft from greater auricular nerve or sural nerve

References

1. Bardach J. Surgery for congenital and acquired malformations of the auricle. In: CW Cummings, JM Fredrickson, LA Harker, et al, eds. *Otolaryngology Head and Neck Surgery.* Vol 4. *Ear and Skull Base.* St Louis: Mosby, 1986, 2861–2898.
2. Lucente FE, Smith PG, Thomas JR. Diseases of the external ear. In: Alberti PW, Reuben RJ, eds. *Otologic Medicine and Surgery.* Vol 2. New York: Churchill Livingstone, 1988, 1073–1092.
3. Graham MD, Lee KJ, Goldsmith MM III. Noninfectious disorders of the ear. In: Lee KJ. *Essential Otolaryngology Head and Neck Surgery,* 7th ed. Stamford, CT: Appleton & Lange, 1999, 721–746.
4. Shea CR. Dermatologic disorders, diseases of the external ear canal. *Otolaryngol Clin North Am* 1996;29:783–794.
5. Tran LP, Grundfast KM, Selesnick SH. Benign lesions of the external auditory canal. *Otolaryngol Clin North Am* 1996;29:807–826.
6. Kuhel WI, Hume CR, Selesnick SH. Cancer of the external auditory canal and temporal bone. *Otolaryngol Clin North Am* 1996;29:827–852.
7. Backous DD, Minor LB, Niparko JK. Trauma to the external auditory canal and temporal bone. *Otolaryngol Clin North Am* 1996;29: 853–866.
8. Parisier SC, Levenson MJ, Hanson MB. Canaloplasty. *Otolaryngol Clin North Am* 1996;29: 867–886.
9. Kinney SE. Trauma. In: Cummings CW, Fredrickson JM, Harker LA, et al, eds. *Otolaryngology Head and Neck Surgery.* Vol 4. *Ear and Skull Base.* St Louis: Mosby, 1986, 3033–3045.

10. Schucknecht HF. *Trauma.* In: Schucknecht HF, ed. *Pathology of the Ear.* Cambridge, MA: Harvard University Press, 1974, 291–316.

11. Griffin WL. A retrospective study of traumatic tympanic membrane perforations in a clinical practice. *Laryngoscope* 1979;89:261–282.

12. Lindeman P, Edstrom S, Grandstrom G, et al. Acute traumatic tympanic membrane perforations: Cover or observe? *Arch Otolaryngol Head Neck Surg* 1987;113:1285–1287.

13. Morrison AW, Booth JB. Systemic disease and otology. In: Alberti PW, Ruben RJ, eds. *Otologic Medicine and Surgery.* Vol 1. New York: Churchill Livingstone, 1988, 855–883.

14. Nager GT. *Pathology of the Ear and Temporal Bone.* Baltimore: Williams & Wilkins, 1993.

15. Nadol B. Manifestations of systemic disease. In Cumming CW, Fredrickson JM, Harker LA, et al, eds. *Otolaryngology Head and Neck Surgery.* Vol 4. St Louis: Mosby, 1986, 3017–3032.

16. Gristwood RE. Otosclerosis (otospongiosis: treatment). In: Alberti PW, Ruben RJ, eds. *Otologic Medicine and Surgery.* Vol. 2. New York: Churchill Livingstone, 1988, 1241–1260.

17. Evitar A. Stapes surgery. In: Alberti PW, Ruben RJ, eds. *Otologic Medicine and Surgery.* Vol 2. New York: Churchill Livingstone, 1988, 1261–1276.

18. Houck JR, Harker LA, McCabe BF. Otosclerosis. In: Cummings CW, Fredrickson JM, Harker LA, et al, eds. *Otolaryngology Head Neck Surgery.* Vol 4. *Ear and Skull Base.* St Louis: Mosby, 1986, 3095–3112.

19. McKenna MJ, Mills BG. Ultrastructural and immunohistochemical evidence of measles virus in active otosclerosis. *Acta Otolaryngol* 1990;470 (Suppl):130–139, discussion 139–140.

20. Niedermeyer HP, Arnold W. Otosclerosis and measles virus associated inflammatory disease. *Acta Otolaryngol* 1995;115:300–303.

21. Shambaugh GE. *Diagnosis of Ear Disease, Surgery of the Ear,* 2nd ed. Philadelphia: Saunders, 1967, 71–98.

22. Shea JJ Jr. Forty years of stapes surgery. *Am J Otol* 1998;19:52–55.

23. Moon CN, Hahn MJ. Partial or total footplate removal and stapedectomy a comparative study. *Laryngoscope* 1984;94:912–915.

24. Wiet RJ, Causse JB, Shambaugh GE. *Otosclerosis, Otospongiosis.* Alexandria, VA: American Academy Otolaryngology Head and Neck Surgery, 1991.

25. Farrior JB. Small fenestra stapedotomy for management of progressive conductive deafness. *South Med J* 1994;87:17–22.

26. De La Cruz A, Fayad JN. Revision stapedectomy. *Otolaryngol Head Neck Surg* 2000;123:728–732.

27. Farrior JB, Temple AE. Teflon wire piston or stainless steel bucket stapes prosthesis, does it make a difference? *Ear Nose Throat J* 1999;78:252–253, 257–260.

28. De La Cruz A, Angeli S, Slattery WH. Stapedotomy in children. *Otolaryngol Head Neck Surg* 1999;120:487–492.

29. Farrior J, Sutherland A. Revision stapes surgery. *Laryngoscope* 1991;101:1155–1161.

30. Haberkamp TJ, Harvey SA, Khafagy Y. Revision stapedectomy with and without the CO_2 laser: An analysis of results. *Am J Otol* 1996;17:225–229.

31. Silverstein H, Bendet E, Rosenberg S, Nichols M. Revision of stapedectomy with and without the laser, a comparison. *Laryngoscope* 1994;104:1431–1438.

32. Prasad S, Kramer DB. Results of revision stapedotomy for conductive hearing loss. *Otolaryngol Head Neck Surg* 1993;109:742–747.

33. Pedersen CB. Revision surgery in otosclerosis, operative findings in 186 patients. *Clin Otolaryngol* 1994;19:446–450.

34. Hammerschlag PE, Fishman A, Scheer AA. A review of 308 cases of revision stapedectomy. *Laryngoscope* 1998;108:1794–1800.

35. Han WW, Incesulu A, McKenna MJ, et al. Revision stapedectomy: Intraoperative findings, results and review of the literature. *Laryngoscope* 1997;107:1185–1192.

36. Coker NJ, Duncan NO III, Wright GL, et al. Stapedectomy trends for the resident. *Ann Otol Rhinol Laryngol* 1988;97:109–113.

37. Burns JA, Lambert R. Stapedectomy in residency training. *Am J Otol* 1996:17:210–213.

38. Hendley GH, Hicks JN. Stapedectomy in residency, the UAB experience. *Am J Otol* 1990;11:128–130.

39. Zappia JJ, Weit RJ. Congenital cholesteatoma. *Arch Otolaryngol Head Neck Surg* 1995;121:19–22.

40. Robert Y, Carcasset S, Rocourt N, et al. Congenital cholesteatoma of the temporal bone, MR

findings and comparison with CT. *AJNR* 1995;
16:755–761.

41. Karmody CS, Byahatti SV, Belvins N, et al. Origin of congenital cholesteatoma. *Am J Otol* 1998;19:292–297.

42. Weber PC, et al. Meniere's disease. *Otolaryngol Clin North Am* 1997;30:1166.

43. Schucknecht HF. *Meniere's Disease, Pathology of the Ear.* Cambridge, MA: Harvard University Press, 1974, 453–464.

44. Gantz BJ, Gidley PW. Meniere's disease: Medical therapy. In: Gates G, ed. *Current Therapy in Otolaryngology Head and Neck Surgery,* 6th ed. St Louis: Mosby, 1998, 79–80.

45. Kartush JM, Larouere MJ. Meniere's disease: Surgical therapy. In: Gates G, ed. *Current Therapy in Otolaryngology Head and Neck Surgery,* 6th ed. St Louis: Mosby, 1998, 81–86.

46. Nedzelski JM, Chiong CM, Fradet G, et al. Intratympanic gentamicin installation as treatment of unilateral Meniere's disease: Update of an ongoing study. *Am J Otol* 1993;14:278–282.

47. Hirsch BE, Kramer DB. Intratympanic gentamicin therapy for Meniere's disease. *Am J Otol* 1997;18:44–71.

48. Garcia-Ibanez E, Garcia-Ibanez JL. Middle fossa vestibular neurectomy: A report of 373 cases. *Otolarygol Head Neck Surg* 1980;88: 846–890.

49. Glasscock ME, Johnson GD, Poe TS. Long term hearing results following middle fossa vestibular nerve section. *Otolaryngol Head Neck Surg* 1989; 97:135–140.

50. Graham MD, Sataloff RT, Kemink JL. Titration streptomycin therapy for bilateral Meniere's disease, a preliminary report. *Otolaryngol Head Neck Surg* 1984;92:440–447.

51. Singleton GF, Schuknecht HF. Streptomycin sulfate in the management of Meniere's disease. *Otolaryngol Clin North Am* 1968;1:531–539.

52. Thomsen J et al. Placebo effect in surgery for Meniere's disease, a double-blind, placebo-controlled study on endolymphatic sac shunt surgery. *Arch Otolaryngol* 1981;107–127.

53. Pillsbury HD, Arenberg I, Ferraro J, Ackley R. Endolymphatic sac surgery: The Danish sham study: An alternative analysis. *Otolaryngol Clin North Am* 1983;16:123–127.

54. Poliquin JF. Immunology of the ear. In: Alberti PW, Ruben RJ, eds. *Otologic Medicine and Sur-*
gery. Vol 1. New York: Churchill Livingstone, 1988, 813–829.

55. McCabe BF. Autoimmune sensorineural hearing loss. *Ann Otol Rhinol Laryngol* 1979;88: 585–589.

56. McCabe BF. Autoimmune inner ear disease: Therapy. *Am J Otol* 1989;10:196–197.

57. Harris JP, Sharp PA. Inner ear autoantibodies in patients with rapidly progressive SNHL. *Laryngoscope* 1990:100:516–524.

58. Wilson WR. Sudden sensorineural hearing loss. In: Cummings CW, Fredrickson JW, Harker LA, et al, eds. *Otolaryngology Head and Neck Surgery.* Vol 4. *Ear and Skull Base.* St Louis: Mosby, 1986, 3219–3224.

59. Hughes GB, Freedman MA, Haberkamp TJ, Guay ME. Sudden sensorineural hearing loss. *Otolaryngol Clin North Am* 1996;29:393–405.

60. Harris JP. Autoimmune inner ear disease. In: Bailey BY, ed. *Head Neck Surgery Otolaryngology,* 2nd ed, Vol 2. Philadelphia: Lippincott-Raven, 1998, 2207–2218.

61. Hashisaki GT. Sudden sensorineural hearing loss. In: Bailey BY, ed. *Head Neck Surgery Otolaryngology,* 2nd ed, Vol 2. Philadelphia: Lippincott-Raven, 1998, 2193–2198.

62. Riggs LC, Matz GH, Rybak LP. Ototoxicity. In: Bailey BY, ed. *Head Neck Surgery Otolaryngology,* 2nd ed, Vol 2. Philadelphia: Lippincott-Raven, 1998, 2165–2170.

63. May JS, Fisch U. Neoplasm of the ear and lateral skull base. In: Bailey BY, ed. *Head Neck Surgery Otolaryngology,* 2nd ed, Vol 2. Philadelphia: Lippincott-Raven, 1998, 1981–1996.

64. Farrior JB, Packer JT. Glomus tumors of the temporal bone: Electron microscopic and immunohistochemical evaluation. *Otolaryngol Head Neck Surg* 1991;4:24–28.

65. Farrior J. Infratemporal approach to the skull base for glomus tumors: Anatomic considerations. *Ann Otol Rhinol Laryngol* 1984;93: 616–622.

66. Farrior JB. Anterior hypotympanic approach for glomus tumors of the inferotemporal fossa. *Laryngoscope* 1984;94:1016–1021.

67. Pensak ML. Skull base surgery. In: Glasscock ME, Shambaugh GE, eds. *Surgery of the Ear,* 4th ed. Philadelphia: Saunders, 1990, 503–533.

68. Schwaber MK. Acoustic neuroma and tumors of the cerebellopontine angle; In: Glasscock ME,

Shambaugh GE, eds. *Surgery of the Ear,* 4th ed. Philadelphia: Saunders, 1990, 535–570.

69. Brackmann DE, Green JD Jr. Cerebellopontine angle tumors. In: Bailey BY, ed. *Head Neck Surgery Otolaryngology,* 2nd ed, Vol 2. Philadelphia: Lippincott-Raven, 1998, 2171–2192.

70. Tos M, Thomsen J, Charabi S. Incidence of acoustic neuromas. *Ear Nose Throat J* 1992;72: 391–393.

71. Saunders JE, Luxford WM, Devgan KK, Fetterman BL. Sudden hearing loss in acoustic neu-

roma patients. *Otolaryngol Head Neck Surg* 1995;133:23–31.

72. Rosenberg SI. Natural history of acoustic neuromas. *Laryngoscope* 2000;110:497–505.

73. Warrick P, Blance M, Routka J: The risk of hearing loss in non-growing conservatively managed acoustic neuromas. *Am J Otol* 1999;20: 758–762.

74. Kondziolka D, Lunsford LD, Flickeri JC. Gamma knife radiosurgery for vestibular schwannomas. *Neurosurg Clin North Am* 2000;11:651–658.

Salivary Glands: Benign and Malignant Diseases

25

This chapter highlights the anatomy and physiology of the salivary glands and outlines the diseases that affect them. An extensive bibliography is provided for further study.

The salivary glands are of the exocrine type. Saliva functions as a

Lubricant
Debriding agent
Buffer
Contributor to the digestion of food

ANATOMY

Parotid Gland

Largest of the major glands (approximately 20 g).
Deep portion of the gland is in contact with the parapharyngeal space.
> Contains the styloid process and its three muscles (stylopharyngeus, styloglossus, and stylohyoid).
> Prestyloid portion contains only muscles and fat.
> Poststyloid portion (also referred to as the neurovascular space) contains the internal jugular vein, internal carotid artery, and cranial nerves IX through XII.

Deep cervical fascia splits to enclose the parotid gland.
Anteroinferior portion is the stylomandibular ligament, which separates the parotid from the submandibular gland.
Deep portion may extend between this ligament and the posterior border of the ramus of the mandible into the prestyloid compartment of the parapharyngeal space, forming a parapharyngeal tumor (Figure 25-1).
Stensen's duct parallels the zygoma (about 1 cm inferior to it) and enters the oral cavity opposite the second upper molar tooth.
Facial nerve is the most superficial structure passing through the parotid gland.
Facial nerve divides at the pes anserinus into five main branches: temporal, zygomatic, buccal, mandibular, and cervical.
Zygomatic branch crosses the zygoma directly over the periosteum.
Mandibular and cervical branches lie directly under the platysma in the plane of the deep cervical fascia.
Superficial temporal and maxillary veins unite to form the retromandibular vein, which passes just deep to the facial nerve.
Retromandibular vein divides into an anterior and a posterior branch; the former joins facial vein to form the common facial vein, which is a major superior tributary to the internal

535

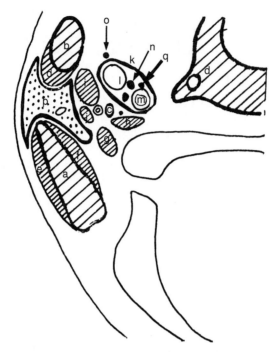

Figure 25-1.   Axial sectional anatomy of the parotid gland. a, mandible; b, mastoid; c, styloid; d, vertebra; e, masseter; f, medial pterygoid; g, styloglossus; h, stylopharyngeus; i, stylohyoid; j, digastric; k, carotid sheath; l, internal jugular vein; m, internal carotid artery; n, vagus nerve; o, accessory nerve; p, parotid; q, sympathetic nerve.

jugular vein, whereas the lateral joins the postauricular vein over the sternocleidomastoid muscle to form the external jugular vein.

Parasympathetic supply originates in the inferior salivatory nucleus (medulla) and travels with the glossopharyngeal nerve and then Jacobson's nerve to the otic ganglion, where it synapses.

Postganglionic fibers are carried by the auriculotemporal branch of V_3 to the parotid gland.

Sympathetic fibers travel in the spinal cord, exit with the superior thoracic nerves, and finally synapse in the superior cervical ganglion.

Postganglionic fibers travel via arterial plexuses and sensory nerves to innervate the salivary and sweat glands as well as cutaneous blood vessels.

Both the postganglionic sympathetic and parasympathetic nerves have acetylcholine as their neurotransmitter.

Submandibular Gland

Second largest salivary gland in size (10 g), wraps around the posterior edge of the mylohyoid muscle.

Deep cervical fascia splits to enclose the gland.

Ramus mandibularis nerve passes through the superficial layer of the deep cervical fascia and is directly superficial to the gland.

Ramus mandibularis nerve may course inferiorly as low as the hyoid bone (also a derivative of the second branchial arch).

Hypoglossal nerve courses deep to the tendon of the digastric and then lies medial to the deep leaf of the deep cervical fascia.

Hypoglossal nerve then runs anteriorly along the hyoglossus deep to the mylohyoid muscle (Figure 25-2).

Facial artery courses medial to the posterior belly of the digastric muscle and then hooks over that structure to enter the submandibular gland, exiting it at the inferior border of the mandible at a point marked by the facial notch.

Lingual artery courses along the lateral surface of the middle constrictor, deep to the digastric muscle, and then runs anteriorly medial to the hyoglossus muscle.

Lingual nerve passes between the medial pterygoid muscle and ramus of the mandible, entering the mouth just below the lower third molar, and courses in a submucosal plane along the hyoglossus.

Midway along that muscle it sends two branches to the submandibular ganglion.

Parasympathetic supply to the submandibular gland originates in the superior salivatory nucleus (pons) and travels via the nervus intermedius and chorda tympani (which is carried by the lingual nerve in its distal portion) to the submandibular ganglion.

Some fibers synapse in the ganglion and others synapse in the gland itself.

Sympathetic supply to the submandibular gland is the same as for the parotid gland.

Wharton's duct courses between the sublingual gland and the hyoglossus and opens through a small punctum just lateral to the frenulum in the floor of the mouth, behind the lower incisor tooth.

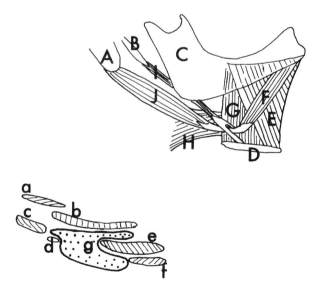

Figure 25-2. (*Top*) Anatomy of the submandibular triangle. A, mastoid; B, styloid; C, mandible; D, hyoid; E, mylohyoid; F, anterior belly of digastric; G, hyoglossus; H, middle constrictor; I, stylohyoid; J, posterior belly of digastric. (*Bottom*) Axial sectional anatomy of the submandibular gland. a, middle constrictor; b, hyoglossus; c, posterior belly of digastric; d, stylohyoid; e, mylohyoid; f, anterior belly of digastric; g, submandibular gland.

Sublingual Gland

Smallest of the major salivary glands, the sublingual gland lies in a submucosal plane in the anterior floor of the mouth and opens through numerous ducts (of Rivinus) into the oral cavity just posterior to orifice of Wharton's duct (Figure 25-3).

Minor Salivary Glands

Some 600 to 1000 minor salivary glands are distributed throughout the oral cavity and oropharynx, with the greatest density in the hard and soft palates (the hard palate has 250 glands and the soft palate, 150).[1-3]

EMBRYOLOGY

Oral cavity develops from the ectodermal stomodeum and endodermal foregut.

Ectodermal-endodermal junction lies approximately at the junction of the oral cavity and oropharynx.

Portions of the floor of the mouth are of endodermal origin.[4,5]

Parotid gland is the first to make its appearance, at the sixth gestational week.

Originates from buds in the posterior stomodeum that elongate, forming solid cords (it is therefore of ectodermal origin).

Cords extend laterally through the mesenchyme across the developing masseter muscle toward the ear.

Cords canalize and form ducts, and their distal portions form acini.

Surrounding mesenchyme forms the capsule of the gland at a relatively late developmental stage.

Lymph nodes are therefore incorporated within the gland.

Submandibular glands first appear at the end of the sixth gestational week as small buds in the floor of the mouth lateral to the tongue.

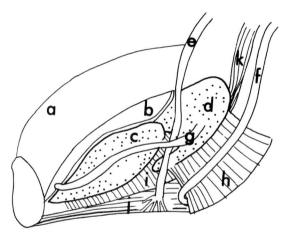

Figure 25-3.   Sagittal section through the tongue demonstrating the anatomy of the sublingual gland. a, mandible; b, floor of mouth mucosa; c, sublingual gland; d, submandibular gland; e, lingual nerve; f, hypoglossal nerve; g, Wharton's duct; h, hyoglossus; i, mylohyoid; j, genioglossus; k, stylohyoid.

Buds then grow posteriorly, curve around the mylohyoid muscle, and appear in the sub-mandibular triangle.

Sublingual glands develop from multiple buds in the floor of the mouth at the eighth gestational week. (The latter glands are consequently of endodermal origin.)

Capsule of these glands is formed at an early stage from the surrounding mesenchyme; therefore, associated lymph nodes are located outside the gland.[6]

HISTOLOGY

Secretory unit consists of the acinus at one end and the ductal elements at the other.

Ducts are arranged sequentially away from the acinus as the intercalated duct, striated duct, and excretory duct.

Myoepithelial cell is situated around the acinus and extends to the intercalated duct region (Figure 25-4).

Acinar cells, characterized by a dense concentration of secretory cellular organelles (rough endoplasmic reticulum, Golgi apparatus, and secretory granules), produce the saliva.

Striated duct cells contain abundant mitochondria necessary for the metabolic demands of transport of both water and electrolytes.

Myoepithelial cells, which are characterized by cytoplasmic filaments on the basal side, can contract about the acinus (forcing secretions through the duct), aid in transport, and contribute to the basement membrane.

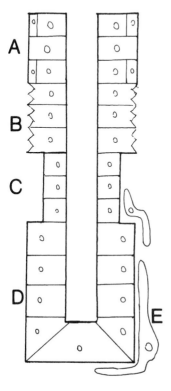

Figure 25-4. Salivary gland unit. A, excretory duct; B, striated duct; C, intercalated duct; D, acinus; E, myoepithelial cell.

Cells of the intercalated and excretory ducts are less differentiated.[7]

Sebaceous glands are closely juxtaposed to the ducts.

Lymphoid tissue is either arranged diffusely or organized into specific lymph nodes within the parotid.[8]

PHYSIOLOGY

Saliva contains both inorganic and organic compounds.

Inorganic compounds include all the electrolytes found within normal human fluids.

The sodium concentration is low and the potassium level is high (as in intracellular fluid).

Sodium concentration is directly proportional to the salivary flow rate.

Sodium is actively transported, whereas chloride and water are passively transported into the lumen.

Salivary glands also have the ability to trap iodide and technetium from plasma and can excrete it in saliva.

Organic compounds within saliva include such proteins as mucin and amylase, many other enzymes, carbohydrates, and blood clotting factors.

Approximately 80% of the population are "secretors"; that is, their saliva contains the isohemagglutinogens corresponding to their individual ABO grouping.

Another constituent is "secretory piece," which is necessary to form secretory immuno-globulin A (IgA); the latter has antimicrobial activity.[9]

Saliva is actually produced in the acinus by active transport and is stored there, with modifications made by the ductal cells.

Alterations in the tonicity of saliva are made as it passes down the duct.

Parotid gland consists almost entirely of serous cells; its secretion is watery, low in mucin, but high in enzymes.

Sublingual gland is mainly of the mucous type; its secretion is therefore high in mucin content and thus quite viscid.

Between 500 and 1500 mL of saliva is produced daily.

Basal secretion rate is minimal but can be augmented by numerous factors acting locally as well as through the autonomic nervous system.

Salivary flow is higher in perimenopausal women than in those who are postmenopausal; quantity and quality can be improved by hormone replacement therapy.[10]

With aging, the number of acini is reduced, fatty and fibrous tissue increases, and there is a decreased synthesis of proteins (by 60%), including sIgA.

This leads to xerostomia, an increased susceptibility to environmental factors, and the development of caries.[11]

There is a diurnal rhythm, with the ebb taking place during sleep.

Parasympathetic effect is to increase ionic and organic secretion from all the major salivary glands; sympathetic effect is less consistent.

Several reflexes are initiated to augment the secretion rate during eating.

Sight and smell of food, the actual chewing and taste of the food, and finally esophageal and gastric reflexes induced by the bolus cause an increased rate of secretion.

Saliva is crucial for maintaining the moistness of the oral and pharyngeal linings and protects these surfaces from chemical, mechanical, and thermal trauma.

Important as a lubricator and a vehicle for the transmission of taste information.

Buffer against acidic fluids and aids in the dissolution and digestion of carbohydrates (amylase).

Saliva also has a specific antibacterial activity related to leukotaxins, opsonins, lysozymes, and antibodies (IgA).

Particularly important in preventing dental caries by cleaning the teeth and gums of foreign material and reducing the friction of chewing; it promotes the calcification of teeth as well.[12,13]

Opposite reaction is manifest by the rapid dental decay following ablation of salivary glands by radiation therapy.[14]

TESTS OF FUNCTION

Salivary flow rate determined by cannulating the salivary duct and measuring volume over time with and without stimulation.

Citric acid 1% provides minimal stimulation, while 10% citric acid results in maximal stimulation of the salivary glands.

Chemical analysis of the produced saliva can then also be performed.

DIAGNOSTIC STUDIES

Sialography

Contrast study of a particular salivary gland.

Low-viscosity, water-soluble contrast medium is injected into the cannulated ducts, after which the gland is studied by conventional or computed radiology.

Can determine the size, functional characteristics, and morphology of the salivary gland.

Conventional sialography has a limited role in the diagnosis of sialectasia; it may itself trigger an episode of acute sialoadenitis.[15,16]

Computed Tomography (CT)

Used alone, with intracanalicular or intravenous contrast, to study the structure and dimension of a given salivary gland.

CT sialography is unnecessary, as CT with contrast alone can yield sufficient detail.

CT is useful for assessing deep lobe parotid tumors or parapharyngeal tumors, adjacent tissue invasion/extension, or cervical node metastasis (Figure 25-5).

Magnetic Resonance Imaging (MRI)

Useful in assessing parapharyngeal space lesions.[17–19]

Current MRI may be more advantageous than CT in differentiating neoplastic from inflammatory conditions.

Radiosialography

Useful for studying the dynamic activity of a given salivary gland as well as for specific histology.

During flow phase, the vascularity of the gland is demonstrated.

During concentration phase, the radioisotope is concentrated in the gland.

During "washout" phase, after citric juice is given, the gland excretes the isotope into the oral cavity.

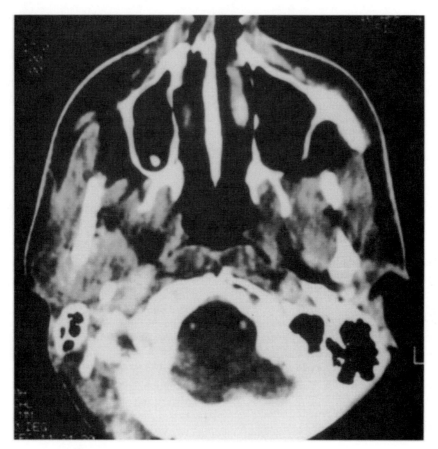

Figure 25-5. Transaxial CT demonstrates a right parotid deep lobe tumor extending into the parapharyngeal space. CT scan shows an inhomogeneous uptake within the mass. The speckled calcium deposits are often seen in pleomorphic adenomas. (*Courtesy of Morton Jacobs, MD.*)

Diffuse dysfunction of the salivary glands (as in Sjögren's syndrome, radiation sialoadenitis, diabetes, cirrhosis, malnutrition, or drug effect) is characterized by diffusely decreased activity within the glands.

Focally increased activity within a tumor mass is characteristic of Warthin's tumor and the much rarer oncocytoma.

Warthin's tumors concentrate the isotope but do not have a patent duct system and therefore collect the isotope.

Oncocytomas have a high concentration of mitochondria and consequently increased activity on scans.

Inflammatory lesions are characterized by an increased washout phase (Figure 25-6).[20]

Diagnostic Ultrasound

Limited applicability to the evaluation of salivary gland diseases.

Tumors are usually echogenic; inflammatory lesions are less echogenic.

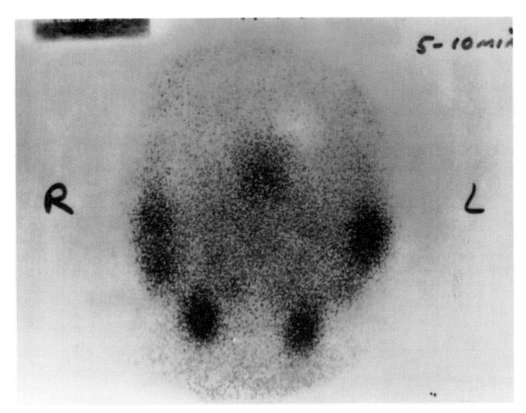

Figure 25-6. Salivary nuclear scan shows elevated uptake in both parotid glands, strongly suggesting bilateral Warthin's tumors. (*Courtesy of Martin Barandes, MD.*)

Benign tumors usually have distinct margins, whereas malignant tumors are irregular and infiltrative.

Main advantage of ultrasound is that it can study all planes of extension within a short period of time.

Salivary Gland Endoscopy

First introduced in 1991.

Useful for diagnosing and extracting posteriorly situated sialoliths.[21,22]

Fine Needle Aspiration Biopsy (FNAb)

Useful in differentiating benign from malignant tumors and inflammatory lesions from lymphoproliferative disorders.

Most successful for the diagnosis of squamous cell carcinoma.[23]

Sensitivity of FNA has been reported as 91%, with a specificity of 98%.[24]

Immunocytochemical markers [cytokeratin, vimentin, S-100, glial fibrillary acid protein (GFAP)] may further enhance the ability of FNAb to distinguish between monomorphic adenoma and adenoid cystic carcinoma.[25]

Core needle biopsies have the advantage of providing tissue for histologic examinations, with the small risk of spreading the tumor.

Labial Biopsy

Useful in the diagnosis of Sjögren's syndrome, as it can demonstrate lymphoid and plasma cell infiltration and acinar atrophy.

Can discriminate between Sjögren's and sarcoidosis.[26,27]

A patient presenting with a mass in one of the salivary glands should first undergo a careful, complete history and physical examination. The particular gland is carefully palpated (bimanually if possible) and the duct inspected. Saliva is expressed and its character noted. If a stone is suspected, plain or occlusal views of the floor of the mouth and mandible views are helpful for demonstrating a radiopaque stone (which is present in only 40% of cases). If a tumor is suspected, no additional salivary studies need be done unless the tumor arises in the deep lobe of the parotid gland. In such cases CT or MRI is useful. A parotid tumor presenting in the parapharyngeal space should not be punch- or open-biopsied per os, as these methods contaminate the oral lining with tumor and necessitate its resection along with the tumor mass. A careful evaluation for cervical metastases is performed and a chest x-ray film obtained. Needle aspiration biopsy may yield a diagnosis of cancer, which can then prepare both the patient and surgeon and influence the surgical approach. Minor salivary gland tumors should be punch-biopsied preoperatively when possible. Unless superficial, they should all undergo evaluation with a CT scan.

SALIVARY GLAND DISEASES

Classification

1. Nonneoplastic
   a. Infectious
   b. Noninfectious
2. Neoplastic
   a. Benign
   b. Malignant
      (1) Primary
      (2) Secondary

NONNEOPLASTIC DISEASES

Infectious Diseases

Acute Sialoadenitis

Acute inflammation of the gland.

Causes erythema, pain, tenderness, swelling, and a purulent discharge from the affected duct.

Found in debilitated and dehydrated patients, especially with major surgery, trauma, radiation therapy, immunosuppression, chemotherapy, or Sjögren's syndrome.

Typically due to *Staphylococcus aureus.*

Treatment includes rehydration, warm compresses, antistaphylococcal antibiotics, and oral irrigations.

Chronic Recurrent Sialoadenitis

Recurrent, slightly painful enlargement of the gland, especially noted on eating.

Caused by decreased salivary flow (stones), stasis, and alteration in composition.

Treatment: sialogogues, massage, hydration, salivary duct dilation, with sialoadenectomy reserved for refractory cases.

Parotid Abscess

Progression of the acute parotitis into a stage of suppuration with multiloculated areas and pitting edema.

Treatment: antibiotics, incision (parallel to the nerve) and drainage.

Viral Parotitis or Mumps

Common viral (paramyxovirus) infection of children between the ages of 4 and 10 years. The infection period is 14 to 21 days; the duration is 7 to 10 days.

Symptoms: bilateral painful swelling of the parotid glands, malaise, and trismus.

Other target organs may be affected, causing orchitis, pancreatitis, nephritis, encephalitis, meningitis, and cochleitis.

Diagnosis: measuring titers, specifically antibodies to the S&V antigen (titers of more than 1 : 192).

The condition is usually self-limited.

Adults who have frequent exposure to children but did not have mumps during childhood are advised to have the mumps vaccine.

Adults with mumps orchitis should be treated with interferon alpha 2B to prevent testicular atrophy.[28]

Granulomatous Sialoadenitis

Seen in sarcoidosis, tuberculosis, and syphilis, especially in association with HIV infection.[29]

Actinomycosis

Acute infection characterized by inflammation and trismus.

Chronic variant characterized by a firm, progressively enlarging, painless facial swelling with progressively increasing trismus.

Often confused with a parotid tumor.

Prior history usually includes previous dental trauma.

Diagnosis can be made with anaerobic cultures.

Treatment is long-term penicillin therapy.[30]

Noninfectious Diseases

Recurrent Parotitis

Result of congenital or acquired sialectasis.

Calculi or strictures produce the sialectasis.

Characterized by hypertrophy, stenosis, and duct dilatation resulting in pain and swelling while eating.

Treatment is usually conservative, with tympanic neurectomy[31] or parotidectomy reserved for patients who are symptomatic.

Sialolithiasis

Usually affects the submandibular glands (80% of cases).

Calculi are often composed of hydroxyapatite and are multiple in 25%.

65% of parotid calculi are radiolucent, while 65% of submandibular ones are radiopaque.[32,33]

More common in men of middle age; characterized by pain and swelling of the affected gland, which worsens at mealtime.

Stones within Wharton's duct can be removed transorally by sialodochoplasty, sialolithectomy using the CO_2 laser,[34] sialolithotripsy using the pulsed dye laser,[35] or extracorporeal electromagnetic shock-wave lithotripsy.[36,37]

If the stone(s) is/are situated toward the hilum, sialoendoscopy or submandibular gland resection is advocated (if the patient is symptomatic).

Branchial Apparatus Anomalies

Anomalies of the first branchial cleft: two subtypes.

Type I is a duplication anomaly of the external auditory canal (ectoderm); cyst is antero-inferior to the lobule.

Type II defect is derived from the first cleft and arch (ectoderm and mesoderm) and may open onto the sternocleidomastoid muscle or external auditory canal.

Type II sinus tract is commonly interdigitated with the facial nerve at its exit from the stylomastoid foramen.

Treatment for type I or II defects is surgical excision.[38,39]

Sjögren's Syndrome

Autoimmune disorder, characterized by keratoconjunctivitis sicca, xerostomia, abnormal taste, intermittent unilateral or bilateral salivary gland enlargement, and dry tongue with atrophy of the papillae.

Associated with connective tissue diseases: eg, rheumatoid arthritis, systemic lupus erythematosus, and polyarteritis nodosa.

Most commonly occurs in menopausal women.

May progress to pseudolymphoma and rarely Waldenström's macroglobulinemia.

Absolute concentrations of albumin, cystatin C, cystatin S, total IgA, and total protein are increased; the output per minute of total protein, albumin, amylase, and IgA is decreased.[40]

Diagnosis is made by performing a minor salivary gland biopsy (lip, septum, or hard palate) in conjunction with laboratory tests (rheumatoid factor, antinuclear factor, protein electrophoresis, autoantibodies as SS-A and SS-B, etc.).[41]

Pathologic findings in these cases are a lymphocytic infiltrate, acinar atrophy, and ductal epithelial hyperplasia and metaplasia.

Treatment for the xerostomia and xerophthalmia in these cases is symptomatic.[42,43]

Benign Lymphoepithelial Lesion (of Godwin)

Inflammatory condition affecting the salivary glands, characterized by a mass of lymphoid tissue, either of the diffuse type or organized with germinal centers, containing scattered foci of epithelial cells of ductal origin.[44]

May present as bilateral salivary cysts, which can be diagnosed and symptomatically treated by needle aspiration.

Condition has been increasingly seen in association with HIV infection.

Incidence of lymphoma in such cases is 10%; rarely, Kaposi's sarcoma is found.[45,46]

Xerostomia—Dry Mouth

Several local and systemic diseases can cause this condition (Table 25-1).

Makes deglutition difficult, decreases taste sensation, and promotes dental decay.

TABLE 25-1. DIFFERENTIAL DIAGNOSIS OF XEROSTOMIA

Local
   Irradiation
   Chronic sialoadenitis
   Interruption of chorda tympani
   Surgery
Systemic
   Sjögren's syndrome
   Diabetes
   Dehydration
   Debilitation
   Mental stress
   Infection
   Anemia
   Drugs
      Analgesics, anticonvulsants, antiemetics, antihistamines, antihypertensives, antinauseants, anti-Parkinson agents, antipruritics, antispasmodics, appetite suppressants, cold medications, diuretics, expectorants, muscle relaxants, psychotropic drugs, sedatives

Both teletherapy and endogenous radiotherapy, such as iodine[131] for thyroid cancer, can affect salivary gland function.[47]

Treatment involves managing the underlying condition and symptomatically treating the patient with artificial saliva and mouthwashes.[48,49]

Amifostine coadministered with radiation therapy (given IV 15 minutes prior to RT) prevents the development or reduces the severity of postradiation xerostomia.

Incidence of acute and late xerostomia was reduced by 20% in those taking the drug.

Acupuncture has been used in the treatment of radiation-induced xerostomia.[50]

Ptyalism

Hypersalivation, caused by a number of conditions (Table 25-2).

Treatment usually requires surgery: transection of the chorda tympani, sialoadenectomy, and ligation or transposition of the ducts.[51]

Intraparotid injection of botulinum toxin A or Nd:YAG intraductal.

Photocoagulation of both Wharton's ducts is among newer treatment techniques.

TABLE 25-2. CAUSES OF HYPERSALIVATION (PTYALISM)

Inflammatory
   Stomatitis
   Rabies
Endocrine
   Pregnancy
   Graves' disease
Neuropsychiatric
   Epilepsy
   Cerebral palsy (oral incompetence)
   Hysteria
Drugs
   Mercury
   Iodine
   Pilocarpine

Sialosis

Bilateral recurrent salivary gland swelling characterized histologically by acinar cell hypertrophy, striated duct atrophy, and interstitial edema; several causes have been identified (Table 25-3).

Mucoceles

Pseudocysts arising from minor salivary glands.

Sites of predilection: lower lip (70%), floor of mouth (15%).

Ranula = mucocele in floor of mouth.

Plunging ranula originates from sublingual gland and extends below the mylohyoid into the submandibular space.

May result from trauma,[52] obstruction, or congenital anomalies.[53]

Can be treated with aspiration, injection of a sclerosing agent, marsupialization with or without laser, incision and drainage, or complete excision with/without resection of the major salivary gland.

NEOPLASTIC DISEASES

Etiologic Factors

Previous radiation therapy associated with the development of pleomorphic adenoma and mucoepidermoid tumors, with a latency of 7 to 30 years after the initial radiation dose.[54–57]

Increased percentage of smokers among patients with Warthin's tumor.[58]

Alcohol consumption among women has been determined to cause a 5.5-fold elevated risk for the development of a salivary cancer.[59]

Patients with mucoepidermoid carcinoma have been shown to have a high risk for the development of breast cancer.[60,61]

Eskimos appear to be particularly prone to develop malignant oncocytomas[62] and malignant lymphoepithelial lesions (as a group, they have the highest incidence of salivary gland cancers).

Familial traits for salivary gland.

TABLE 25-3. DIFFERENTIAL DIAGNOSIS OF BILATERAL SALIVARY GLAND ENLARGEMENT (SIALOSIS)

Nutritional
  Vitamin deficiency
  Malnutrition
  Bulimia
Endocrine
  Diabetes
  Hypothyroidism
Metabolic
  Obesity
  Malabsorption
  Cirrhosis
  Anemia
Inflammatory
  Sjögren's syndrome
Drugs
  Thiourea

Occupational agents have been associated with minor gland adenocarcinoma in the sinonasal region (furniture and woodworking, boot and shoe manufacturing, asbestos,
rubber).[63,64]

Correlation with prior skin cancer among men has been proposed.[65]

See Tables 25-5 to 25-9.

Epidemiology

Five percent of all head and neck tumors (excluding skin tumors), with an incidence of
1 to 3 per 100,000.

Incidence of salivary cancer in the United States is 0.9 per 100,000.

The distribution of salivary gland cancers is 1.2 per 100,000 among men and 0.7 per
100,000 among women.

Warthin's tumor affects men more than women.

Peak incidence is in the oldest age group.

Histologic distribution of salivary gland tumors among the pediatric age group is listed
in Table 25-4.[66,67]

Pediatric mucoepidermoid carcinomas are of low or intermediate grade.[68]

Parotid is the most common site of all salivary neoplasms (73%), followed by minor
glands (14%) and submandibular gland (11%)[69] (Figure 25-7).

Benign Tumors (Table 25-5)

Pleomorphic Adenoma

PLEOMORPHIC ADENOMA

Most common benign salivary tumor.

Slightly more common in women, with a peak incidence during the fifth decade.

Slow-growing, well demarcated, and usually encountered in the parotid gland, in the
posterior region.

There is morphologic diversity, including mucoid, chondroid, osseous, and myxoid
elements.

Myoepithelial cell is thought to be the cell of origin.

Visible excrescences and microscopic prolongations account for the high recurrence
rate if enucleation alone is performed.[70]

MONOMORPHIC ADENOMA

Clinical features similar to those of pleomorphic adenoma except that only one morphologic type is present.

TABLE 25-4. PEDIATRIC SALIVARY TUMORS

Benign (68%)		Malignant (32%)	
Type	**%**	**Type**	**%**
Mixed tumor	48	Mucoepidermoid	37
Hemangioma	31	Acinic cell	22
Neurofibroma	6	Rhabdomyosarcoma	9
Miscellaneous	15	Lymphomas	9
		Miscellaneous	23

Modified from Krolls[66]

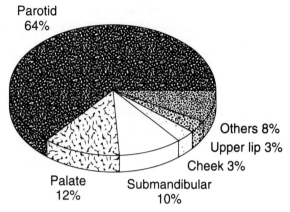

Figure 25-7. Salivary gland tumors: site distribution.

Subclassified as basal cell adenoma, trabecular adenoma, canalicular adenoma, or tubular adenoma.

Occurs more commonly in the parotid gland, is slow-growing, and is solitary.[71–73]

WARTHIN'S TUMOR

Papillary cystadenoma lymphomatosum.

Occurs far more commonly in men than women (5 : 1), is more common in whites, has a peak incidence during the fifth and sixth decades, and accounts for 5 to 10% of all parotid tumors.

Painless masses are slow-growing, nontender, cystic, and compressible.

On needle aspiration, a thick, turbid fluid is sometimes found.

Some 2 to 6% are bilateral and 12% are multicentric.

Classically demonstrate increased activity on radiosialography.

Histologic appearance is classic on light microscopy (Figure 25-8).

TABLE 25-5. HISTOLOGIC CLASSIFICATION OF SALIVARY TUMORS

Tumor	Incidence (%)
Benign	
Pleomorphic adenoma	52
Warthin's tumor	5
Monomorphic adenoma	3.4
Oncocytoma	1.4
Malignant	
Mucoepidermoid	12.4
Acinic cell	6.4
Adenocarcinoma	6.2
Adenoid cystic	4.3
Malignant mixed	2.3
Squamous cell	1.6
Others	5
Total	100

AFIP Registry (13,749 cases).[98]

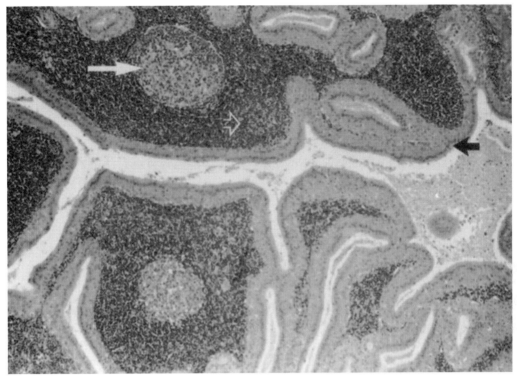

Figure 25-8. Warthin's tumor. Note the characteristic biphasic composition: (1) abundant lymphoid sheets (open white arrow) with conspicuous follicles and germinal centers (*white arrow*); and (2) lining of epithelium consisting of a bilayer of oncocytic cells (*black arrow*).

On electron microscopy, the cells are characterized by a high density of mitochondria. Tumor is thought either to arise in heterotopic salivary duct tissue or to represent a hypersensitivity disease triggered by metaplasia of the strained duct.[74,75]

ONCOCYTOMA

Oncocytoma accounts for less than 1% of salivary gland tumors.

Usually occurs in the parotid with a peak incidence during the sixth decade of life.

Circumscribed but unencapsulated and characterized by a slow growth rate.

Can be bilateral and multinodular and is typically "hot" on radiosialography.

The oncocyte (an epithelial cell mutant rarely present before the age of 50) is seen on light microscopy and derived from the intercalated duct reserve cell.

On electron microscopy, this cell is characterized by a high concentration of mitochondria.[76]

Malignant Tumors (See Tables 25-5, 25-6, 25-7)

Mucoepidermoid Carcinoma (Figure 25-9)

Most common malignant salivary tumor.

Arises most often in the parotid gland (70% of all mucoepidermoid cancers), although it accounts for only 10% of all parotid tumors.

TABLE 25-6. STAGING OF SALIVARY GLAND TUMORS: AMERICAN JOINT COMMITTEE ON CANCER, 1988

All categories are subdivided
  a. No local extension
  b. Local extension (clinical or macroscopic evidence of invasion of skin, soft tissues, bone, or nerve)
T_1: < 2 cm
T_2: 2.1–4.0 cm
T_3: 4.1–6.0 cm
T_4: > 6 cm

N_1: single ipsilateral lymph node < 3 cm
N_{2a}: single ipsilateral lymph node 3.1–6 cm
N_{2b}: multiple ipsilateral lymph nodes < 6 cm
N_{2c}: bilateral/contralateral lymph nodes < 6 cm
N_3: > 6 cm

Stage I:	$T_{1a}/T_{2a}N_0M_0$
Stage II:	$T_{1b}/T_{2b}/T_{3a}N_0M_0$
Stage III:	T_1/T_2 with N_1M_0
	$T_{4a}/T_{3b}N_0M_0$
Stage IV:	T_{4b} any N_1M_0
	any T with N_2/N_3M_0
	any T, any N with M_1

The most common type of salivary malignancy induced by radiation.

Peak age incidence is during the third to fifth decades.

More than 75% of the patients present with an asymptomatic swelling, 13% present with pain, and a smaller number present with facial nerve paralysis.

Tumor is derived from the epithelial cells of the interlobar and intralobar salivary ducts.

The tumor is unencapsulated, and lymph node metastases are found in 30 to 40%.

Low-, intermediate-, and high-grade variants are described pathologically.

Low-grade tumors resemble pleomorphic adenoma (oval, well circumscribed, and mucoid material present); the intermediate- and high-grade subtypes are characterized by an infiltrative process.

Young patient usually presents with a low-grade tumor.[77,78]

Malignant Mixed Tumors

Accounts for 6% of all parotid tumors.

Histologically resembles the pleomorphic adenoma, although metastases to cervical nodes are found.

Characterized by an explosive growth rate and most commonly occurs in older patients (sixth to seventh decades).[79]

TABLE 25-7. SALIVARY GLAND TUMORS: MALIGNANCIES ARISING IN THE GLANDS

Gland	Percent of Malignancies
Parotid	32
Submandibular	41
Minor	60

Source: Armed Forces Institute of Pathology.

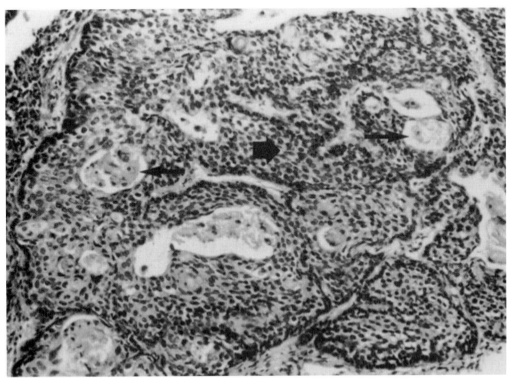

Figure 25-9. Mucoepidermoid carcinoma. Note the disorganized clusters of epithelium displaying both epidermoid (*wide black arrow*) and glandular areas (*thin black arrows*).

Carcinoma Ex Pleomorphic Adenoma

Patients with this tumor have frequently undergone previous salivary gland resection. Pathologically, remnants of the benign mixed tumor are identified, although metastases from this tumor contain only the carcinoma element.

Adenocarcinoma

Accounts for 4% of all parotid tumors and 20% of minor salivary gland tumors.

Most patients (80%) are asymptomatic, 40% of the tumors are found to have fixation to underlying or overlying structures, 30% of the patients develop cervical node metastases, 20% have facial nerve paralysis, and 15% have facial pain.

Arises from the terminal tubules and intercalated or strained duct cells.

Many varieties of adenocarcinoma have been described (conventional adenocarcinoma, mucinous adenocarcinoma, papillary adenocarcinoma), and they are graded as of low, intermediate, or high grade.[80]

Adenoid Cystic Carcinoma (Figure 25-10)

Accounts for 3% of parotid tumors, 15% of submandibular tumors, and 30% of minor salivary gland tumors.

Most common malignant tumor of the submandibular or minor salivary glands.

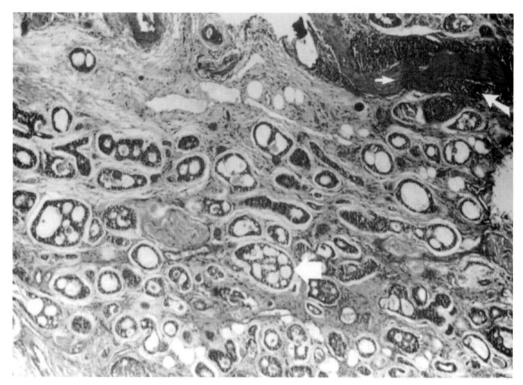

Figure 25-10.   Adenoid cystic carcinoma. It is composed of infiltrating clusters of epithelial cells with a prominent cribriform ("Swiss cheese") pattern (wide white arrow). Note the characteristic perineural invasion by tumor (nerve, *small white arrow;* tumor cells, *angled white arrow*).

Women with the tumor slightly outnumber men.

Half of the patients are asymptomatic on presentation, although a large percentage of the tumors are fixed to overlying or underlying structures.

Bone involvement is present in one-half, 25% have facial pain, 20% have facial nerve involvement, and lymphatic metastases occur in 15%.

Tumor is characterized by early perineural spread and an indolent course.

Origin is thought to be the myoepithelial cell.[81–83]

Three growth patterns have been described: cribriform, solid, and tubular.

Acinic Cell Carcinoma

Occurs almost exclusively in the parotid gland, although it accounts for only 3% of parotid tumors.

Affected women slightly outnumber men.

Rarely multifocal, but 3% are bilateral.

Peak age incidence is between the fifth and sixth decades.

Cervical node metastasis is present in 15%.

Pathologic hallmark is the presence of amyloid.

Cell of origin is thought to be the serous acinar components and the intercalated duct cell.[84]

Squamous Cell Carcinoma

Occurs more commonly in men of older age and is characterized by rapid growth. Incidence of lymph node metastasis is 47%.

The tumor usually arises in the parotid gland.

Primary squamous cell carcinoma of salivary origin must be differentiated from metastatic disease, which initially involves the lymph nodes and then spreads to the gland proper.

Thought to arise from the excretory duct cells.[85,86]

Malignant Oncocytoma

Similar to the benign variety except that it is characterized by distant metastases, cervical node metastases, and blood vessel, nerve, or lymphatic invasion as well as malignant cytologic features.

Salivary Duct Carcinoma

Rare tumor resembles mammary ductal cancer.

Stensen's duct is more frequently involved than Wharton's duct.

Tend to recur locally (35%) and develop distant metastases (62%), with only 23% of patients alive at 3 years.[87]

Malignant Lymphoepithelial Lesion

Rare entity characterized by both benign and malignant areas within a given tumor.

The malignant portion represents anaplastic cancer of ductal origin.

Nodal metastases have been frequently noted.[88–90]

Myoepithelial Carcinoma

Rare tumor.

Myoepithelial differentiation with unique immunohistochemical and ultrastructural properties.

Biologic behavior is unpredictable.

Treat with postoperative radiation therapy and chemotherapy when indicated.[91]

Malignant Lymphoma

Primary malignant lymphomas of the salivary glands are rare, with about 150 cases reported in the world literature and only 8 originating in the submandibular gland.

Optimal treatment is biopsy with radiation therapy to the region.

Prognosis is better for salivary gland lymphoma than for nodal lymphoma of similar histology.[92]

Metastases

Metastases to the parotid gland may travel to the intraparotid lymph nodes, extend directly into the parotid, or involve paraglandular lymph nodes.

Most common primaries are melanoma and squamous cell carcinoma.

Tumors in the region of the temporal, scalp, and external auditory canal usually metastasize to the paraglandular nodes, whereas those originating in the mucosal lining of the oral cavity, sinus tissues, or pharynx spread to the intraglandular nodes.[93,94]

MINOR SALIVARY GLAND TUMORS (SEE TABLE 25-8)

Despite the abundance of minor salivary glands, they serve as the origin for only 15% of all salivary gland tumors.

Benign tumors (55%) slightly outnumber malignant ones, with pleomorphic adenoma accounting for the bulk of cases.

Oral pathologists[95] have found that the commonest type is mucoepidermoid cancer, followed by adenocarcinoma, adenoid cystic, acinic, and malignant mixed.

General pathologists,[96] looking at all sites of minor salivary gland malignancies (ie, including paranasal sinuses), have found that the commonest is adenoid cystic, followed by adenocarcinoma, mucoepidermoid carcinoma, malignant mixed, and acinic carcinoma.

TREATMENT

The minimal diagnostic and therapeutic procedure for parotid tumors is a superficial parotidectomy (also referred to as lateral parotidectomy or supraneural parotidectomy) unless a lipoma or isolated Warthin's tumor is found under the skin flap. This procedure is advocated so as to avoid facial nerve injury and incomplete tumor removal (even the benign tumors are characterized by excrescences and pseudopod formation). However, if the tumor is confined to the tail, an inferior superficial parotidectomy may suffice once the facial nerve is identified and preserved provided that the tumor is benign.[97] Similarly, if the tumor is benign and confined to the deep lobe, the superficial lobe may be reflected forward, allowing for complete resection of the deep lobe, following which the superficial lobe can be returned to the original position. It should be noted, however, that not all physicians share this opinion; in fact, several English authors have advocated enucleation combined with postoperative radiotherapy. They have demonstrated low rates of complications and recurrence.[98,99]

Short-duration paralytics (mivacurium, 10–15 minutes; atacurium, 30 minutes) may be employed so that the sternocleidomastoid muscle and digastric muscles do not twitch excessively during dissection. The anesthesiologist should ensure that the paralysis is reversed once the facial nerve dissection commences.

Parotidectomy may be accomplished through the modified Blair incision, or a facelift approach may be employed. The latter is more time-consuming but the cosmesis is excellent.[100,101] The great auricular nerve may be preserved, but the ultimate sensory deficit is sim-

TABLE 25-8. DISTRIBUTION OF MINOR SALIVARY GLAND CANCERS ACCORDING TO SITE (MSKCC)

Site	Percent of Total
Palate	40
Antrum	14
Tongue	11
Cheek/lips	10
Nasal fossa	10
Gingiva	6
Floor of mouth	3.5
Other	5.5
Best prognosis with cheek/lips	
Worst prognosis with sinonasal tumors	

Key: MSKCC = Memorial Sloan Kettering Care Center.

ilar to that after sacrifice of the great auricular nerve.[102] Other authors have determined that there is a higher rate of sensory deficit if the nerve is cut.[103]

Total parotidectomy is favored by most when there is involvement of the superficial and deep lobes of the parotid gland by either a benign or a malignant tumor. Some advocate total parotidectomy for any malignant tumor (even if it is confined to the lateral portion of the gland) or when combined with resection of adjacent or metastatic skin cancers.[104] Facial nerve sacrifice is recommended by most authors only if a malignant tumor involves the nerve. When such is the case, one may occasionally need to extend the resection into the mastoid and remove an additional proximal portion of the nerve. Most authors agree that facial nerve grafting should be performed at the initial surgery if a proximal stump is available, acknowledging that postoperative radiotherapy does not interfere with nerve regrowth.[105] Otherwise, a nerve XII or VII crossover graft with or without a digastric or masseter sling may be performed.

Minor salivary gland tumors are primarily treated surgically. The site of origin determines the particular type of resection. Malignant minor salivary gland tumors should be resected with an adequate margin of normal tissue (>1 cm). With adenoid cystic carcinoma, surgery may involve resecting associated nerves proximally until clear margins are obtained, as this tumor has a high propensity for perineural spread.

Deep lobe parotid tumors with parapharyngeal extension or parapharyngeal space salivary tumors may be resected through a lateral approach (under the nerve, or the nerve may be transected), a paramandibular approach (after removing the submandibular gland), median mandibulotomy, paralingual extension, or transparotid cervical approach. The clinical evaluation and radiographic analysis help determine the proper method. Higher cranial nerve neuropathy may lead to postoperative morbidity in resections of these larger lesions.

Benign tumors of the submandibular gland are treated with complete transcervical resection of the gland. Some authors have recently described an intraoral surgical approach.[106]

The indications for concomitant radical neck dissection include obvious cervical metastases, cancers arising in the submandibular gland, primary squamous cell carcinoma, undifferentiated carcinoma, larger tumors (>4 cm), or high-grade mucoepidermoid carcinoma of advanced stage.[107] When dealing with extensive cancers, surrounding structures such as the adjacent nerves and muscles may need to be sacrificed in order to secure clear margins. Selective neck dissection may be employed in an N_0 neck to remove those nodes at risk when the histology or tumor characteristics favor nodal spread.[108]

Radiation therapy is no longer used as primary therapy for salivary gland tumors. As mentioned above, some English authors advocated radiotherapy following enucleation for pleomorphic adenoma.[109] It may be employed for microscopically positive margins after resection of a salivary neoplasm or in conjunction with revision surgery for recurrences.[110] Most authors use postoperative radiotherapy for intermediate- and high-grade mucoepidermoid carcinoma, malignant mixed tumor, adenocarcinoma, adenoid cystic carcinoma, high-grade acinic cell carcinoma, all squamous cell carcinomas, insecure margins, and any malignant tumor of stage 2 or greater.[111–113] A clear survival advantage for combined surgery and radiation therapy at 5 and 10 years was shown for large cancers where the removal was incomplete or in doubt.[114–119] While survival may not be improved for adenoid cystic carcinoma, the local recurrence rate is reduced with adjunctive teletherapy.[120,121] Combined therapy (surgery followed by radiation therapy) has superior local control and rates of freedom from relapse as compared with single-modality therapy for the treatment of malignant minor salivary gland tumors.[122] Radiation therapy may be complicated by xerostomia,[123] trismus, and serous otitis media.

Several authors have used chemotherapy for recurrent or residual carcinomas. The partial responders have had an average response duration of 3 months. The anthracyclines are most effective.[124] Others have used cisplatin, doxorubicin, and cyclophosphamide with a similar duration of response.[125]

PROGNOSIS

The single most important factor in the prognosis of salivary gland tumors with a given histology is the stage of the disease on initial presentation[126] (Figures 25-11 and 25-12). The grade of the tumor is the second most important determinant, especially with mucoepidermoid carcinoma. The site of the primary tumor is most important with adenocarcinoma and adenoid cystic carcinoma, with the outlook worse in the sinonasal and laryngeal regions. Overall, parotid malignancies had a better survival than minor salivary gland cancers, which themselves have better survival than submandibular ones.[127] Facial nerve paresis or paralysis is an ominous finding (Table 25-9).[128,129] The prognosis for each tumor is presented in Table 29–10.

Although local failure is most common among all the malignant tumors, a high proportion of the adenoid cystic carcinomas and adenocarcinomas fail distally. The most common site of distant metastasis for both these tumors is the lung. The other sites are disseminated: bone or brain. The sites of failure for the malignant tumors are outlined in Table 25-11.

COMPLICATIONS AFTER PAROTIDECTOMY

Frey's Syndrome

Gustatory sweating following parotidectomy is acknowledged by 50% of patients, although it can be demonstrated with the Minor starch-iodine test in virtually 100% of patients.

Cross-reinnervation of the autonomic supply to the parotid gland occurs after parotidectomy; the parasympathetic fibers, stimulated by the smell and taste of food, now innervate sweat glands and blood vessels through acetylcholine, thereby causing sweating and erythema of the skin overlying the region.

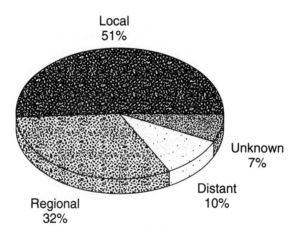

Figure 25-11.   Historical stage distribution of salivary gland cancer.

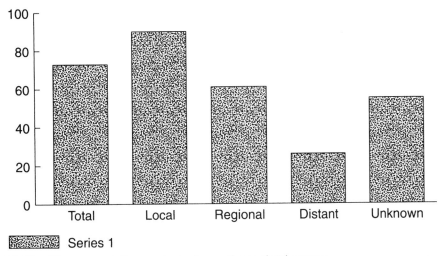

Figure 25-12.   Five-year relative survival rate—salivary gland cancer.

Can be demonstrated by painting the patient's face with iodine, spraying starch over the
    area, and then giving the patient a lemon to chew.
Most patients are not troubled by this phenomenon.
Treatment:
1.   Apply 3% scopolamine cream over the area.
2.   Apply antiperspirant.
3.   Section Jacobson's nerve through a tympanotomy approach.
4.   Create sternocleidomastoid muscle flap.
5.   Interpose a sheet of fascia lata, dermis, expanded Polytef, or allograft between the skin
    and parotid bed.[130]
Extensive defects may be reconstructed with pectoralis major myocutaneous flaps, pedicled
    or free latissimus dorsi flaps with/without skin grafts.[131]

Facial Nerve Paresis/Paralysis

Facial nerve paresis/paralysis after surgery for benign salivary tumors should be mini-
    mal (<5%).
If all patients are carefully examined, even after the most meticulous dissection and
    preservation of the nerve, some facial weakness can usually be found, represent-
    ing a neuropraxia of the terminal branches, or it may relate to sectioning of the
    platysma muscle.
If the main trunk or a branch is severed accidentally during surgery, it should be imme-
    diately repaired with a fine monofilament nonabsorbable suture.

TABLE 25-9. SALIVARY GLAND CANCERS PRESENTING WITH FACIAL NERVE ABNORMALITY

Malignant mixed
High-grade mucoepidermoid
Squamous cell
Adenoid cystic

TABLE 25-10. DETERMINATE SURVIVAL FOR SALIVARY GLAND CANCERS (MSKCC)

Tumor Type	Determinate Survival (percent)		
	5 years	10 years	15 years
Mucoepidermoid, low grade	92	90	82
Mucoepidermoid, high grade	49	42	33
Acinic cell	76	63	55
Adenocarcinoma	41	34	28
Malignant mixed	40	24	19
Adenoid cystic	30	20	10
Squamous cell cancer	26	19	NA

Following deliberate division after resection of a malignant tumor, either a graft (great auricular or sural) is interposed or a hypoglossal-facial nerve anastomosis is performed (if distal branches are intact).

Postoperative radiation therapy will not interfere with return of facial nerve function.[132]

Sialoceles and Salivary Fistulas

After superficial parotidectomy, a small amount of saliva occasionally collects in the wound or drains through the incision.

Usually resolves within 2 or 3 weeks after an adequate parotidectomy with ligation of Stensen's duct.

If necessary, an anticholinergic agent (topical scopolamine discs) may be applied to decrease the drainage and encourage closure of the fistula.

Botulinum toxin type A may be injected subcutaneously once the salivary fluid is aspirated.

Wound exploration is seldom required.

ACKNOWLEDGMENT

The photomicrographs in this chapter were kindly provided by Winston Harrison, M.D. Gratitude is expressed to Rita Maier for librarian assistance.

TABLE 25-11. SITES OF FAILURE FOR SALIVARY GLAND CANCERS (MSKCC)

Tumor Type	Failure (%)	
	Local Site	Distant Site
Mucoepidermoid	26	15
Acinic cell	33	12
Adenocarcinoma	51	26
Adenoid cystic	67	42
Squamous cell	57	23

From Ellis GL, Auclair PL, Gnepp DR. *Surgical Pathology of the Salivary Glands.* Philadelphia: Saunders, 1991. With permission.

References

1. Grant JCB. *An Atlas of Anatomy,* 6th ed. Baltimore: Williams & Wilkins, 1972.
2. Basmajian JU. *Grant's Method of Anatomy,* 10th ed. Baltimore: Williams & Wilkins, 1980.
3. Hollinshead WH. *Anatomy for Surgeons: The Head and Neck,* 2nd ed. New York: Harper & Row, 1968.
4. Wilson DB. Embryonic development of the head and neck. The face. *Head Neck Surg* 1979; 2:145.
5. Moore KC. *The Developing Human,* 3rd ed. Philadelphia: Saunders, 1982.
6. Johns ME. The salivary glands: anatomy & embryology. *Otolaryngol Clin North Am* 1977; 10: 261.
7. Batsakis JG. *Tumors of the Head and Neck.* Baltimore: Williams & Wilkins, 1979.
8. Martinez-Madrigal F, Micheau C. Histology of the major salivary glands. *Am J Surg Pathol* 1989;13:879.
9. Rice DH. Salivary gland physiology. *Otolaryngol Clin North Am* 1977;10:273.
10. Laine M, Leimola-Virtanen R. Effect of hormone replacement therapy on salivary flow rate, buffer effect and pH on perimenopausal and postmenopausal women. *Arch Oral Biol* 1996;41:91–96.
11. Vissink A, Spijkervet FK, Van Nieuw Amerongen A. Aging and saliva. *Spec Care Dentist* 1996;16:95–103.
12. Ganong WF. *Review of Medical Physiology.* Los Altos, CA: Lange, 1985.
13. West JB. *Physiological Basis of Medical Practice.* Baltimore: Williams & Wilkins, 1985.
14. Beumer J, Curtis T, Harrison R. Radiation therapy of the oral cavity: sequelae and management. *Head Neck Surg* 1979;1:301.
15. Kushner DC, Weber AL. Sialography of salivary gland tumors with fluoroscopy and tomography. *Am J Radiol* 1978;130:941.
16. Rabinov K, Weber AL. *Radiology of the Salivary Glands.* Boston: GK Hall, 1985.
17. Schaefer SD. Evaluation of NMR vs CT for parotid masses. *Laryngoscope* 1985;95:945.
18. Casselman JW, Mancuso AA. Major salivary gland masses: comparison of MRI and CT. *Radiology* 1987;165:183.
19. Tabor EK, Curtin HD. MR of the salivary glands. *Radiol Clin North Am* 1989;27:379.
20. Greyson ND, Noyek AM. Radionuclide salivary scanning. *J Otolaryngol* 1982;10 (Suppl): 1, 1982.
21. Nahlieli O, Baruchin A. Endoscopic technique for the diagnosis and treatment of obstructive salivary gland diseases. *J Oral Maxillofac Surg* 1999;57:1394.
22. Marchal F, Dulguerov P, Lehmann W. Interventional sialendoscopy. *N Engl J Med* 1999; 341:1242.
23. Sismanis A, Strong MS, Merrian S. Fine needle aspiration biopsy of neck masses. *Otolaryngol Clin North Am* 1980;13:421.
24. Layfield LJ, Tan P, Glasgow BJ. Fine needle aspiration of salivary gland lesions. *Arch Pathol Lab Med* 1987;111:346.
25. Gupta RK, Naran S, Dowle C, Simpson JS. Coexpression of vimentin, cytokeratin and S-100 in monomorphic adenoma of salivary gland: value of marker studies in the differential diagnosis of salivary gland tumors. *Cytopathology* 1992;3:303–309.
26. Giotaki H, Constantopoulos SH, et al. Labial minor salivary gland biopsy. *Respiration* 1986; 50:102.
27. Lindvall AM, Jonsson R. The salivary gland component of Sjögren's syndrome: an evaluation of diagnostic methods. *Oral Surg Oral Med Oral Pathol* 1986;62:32.
28. Yeniyol CO, Sorguc S, Minareci S, et al. Role of interferon-alpha-2B in prevention of testicular atrophy with unilateral mumps orchitis. *Urology* 2000;55:931.
29. van der Walt JD, et al. Granulomatous sialadenitis of the major salivary glands. *Histopathology* 1987;11:131.
30. Fenton RS, Rotenberg D. Actinomycosis of the parotid. *J Otolaryngol* 1977;6:233.
31. Long term results of tympanic neurectomy for chronic parotid sialectasis. *Rev Laryngol Otol Rhinol* 2000;121:95.
32. Langlais RP, Kasle MJ. Sialolithiasis: the radiolucent ones. *Oral Surg* 1975;40:686.
33. Langlais RP, Benson BW, Barnett DA. Salivary gland dysfunction. *Ear Nose Throat J* 1989; 68:758.
34. Azaz B, Regev E, Casap N, Chicin R. Sialolithectomy done with a CO_2 laser. *J Oral Maxillofac Surg* 1996;54:685–688.

35. Ito H, Baba S. Pulsed dye laser lithotripsy of submandibular gland salivary calculus. *J Laryngol Otol* 1996;110:942–946.

36. Ottaviani F, Capaccio P, Campi M, Ottaviani A. Extracorporeal electromagnetic shock-wave lithotripsy for salivary gland stones. *Laryngoscope* 1996;106:761–764.

37. Yoshizaki T, Maruyama Y, Motoi I, et al. Clinical evaluation of extracorporeal shock wave lithotripsy for salivary stones. *Ann Otol Rhinol Laryngol* 1996;105:63–67.

38. Work WP. Newer concepts of first branchial cleft defects. *Laryngoscope* 1972;82:1581.

39. Aransohn RS. Anomalies of the first branchial cleft. *Arch Otolaryngol* 1976;102:737.

40. van der Reijden WA, van der Kwaak JS, Veerman EC, Nieuw Amerongen AV. Analysis of the concentration and output of whole salivary constituents in patients with Sjögren's syndrome. *Eur J Oral Sci* 1996;104:335–340.

41. Fox RI. Sjögren's syndrome: immunobiology of exocrine gland dysfunction. *Adv Dent Res* 1996;10:35–40.

42. Moutsopoulos HM. Sjögren's syndrome. *Ann Intern Med* 1980;92:212.

43. Lyons GD. Sicca syndrome. *Laryngoscope* 1983;93:880.

44. Godwin JT. Benign lymphoepithelial lesion of the parotid gland. *Cancer* 1952;5:1089.

45. Finfer MD, Schinella RA, et al. Cystic parotid lesions in patients at risk for AIDS. *Arch Otolaryngol* 1988;114:1290.

46. Sperling NM, Lin PT. Parotid disease associated with HIV infection. *Ear Nose Throat J* 1990;69:475.

47. Malpani BL, Samuel AM, Ray S. Quantification of salivary gland function in thyroid cancer patients treated with radio iodine. *Int J Radiat Oncol Biol Phys* 1996;35:535–540.

48. Glass BJ. Drug-induced xerostomia as a cause of glossodynia. *Ear Nose Throat J* 1989;68:776.

49. Rhodus NL. Xerostomia and glossodynia in patients with autoimmune disorders. *Ear Nose Throat J* 1989;68:791.

50. Blom M, Dawidson I, Fernberg JO, et al. Acupuncture treatment of patients with radiation-induced xerostomia. *Eur J Cancer B Oral Oncol* 1996;32B:182–190.

51. Eilkie TF, Brody GS. The surgical treatment of drooling. *Plast Reconstr Surg* 1977;59:791.

52. Canosa A, Cohen M, Dent M. Post-traumatic parotid mucocele. *J Oral Maxillofac Surg* 1999; 57:745.

53. Anastassov GE, Halavy J, Solodnik P, et al. Submandibular gland mucocele. *Oral Surg Oral Med Oral Pathol* 2000;89:159.

54. Schneider AB. Salivary gland neoplasms as a late consequence of head and neck irradiation. *Ann Intern Med* 1977;87:160.

55. Sener SF, Scanlon EF. Irradiation-induced salivary gland neoplasms. *Ann Surg* 1980;138:46.

56. Land CE, Saku T, Hayashi Y, et al. Incidence of salivary gland tumors among atomic bomb survivors, 1950–1987. *Radiat Res* 1996;146:28–36.

57. Schneider AB, Favus MJ, Stachura ME, et al. Salivary neoplasms as a late consequence of head and neck irradiation. *Ann Intern Med* 1977;87:160–164.

58. Monk JS, Church JS. Warthin's tumor: a high incidence and no sex predominance in central Pennsylvania. *Arch Otolaryngol* 1992;118: 477–478.

59. Spitz MR, Fueger JJ, et al. Salivary gland cancer. A case-control investigation of risk factors. *Arch Otolaryngol* 1990;116:1163.

60. Abbey LM, Schwab BH, Landau GC, Perkins ER: Incidence of second primary breast cancer among patients with a first primary salivary gland tumor. *Cancer* 1984;54:1439.

61. Berg JW, Hutter RV, Foote FW. The unique association between salivary gland cancer and breast cancer. *JAMA* 1968;204:771.

62. Arthaud JB. Anaplastic parotid carcinoma in seven Alaskan natives. *Am J Clin Pathol* 1972; 57:275.

63. Roush GO. Epidemiology of cancer of the nose and paranasal sinuses. Current concepts. *Head Neck Surg* 1979;2:3.

64. Keller AZ. Residence, age, race and related factors in the survival and associations with salivary tumors. *Am J Epidemiol* 1969;90: 269.

65. Spitz MR, Tilley BC, Batsakis JG, et al. Risk factors for major salivary gland carcinoma. *Cancer* 1984;54:1854.

66. Krolls SO. Salivary gland lesions in children. *Cancer* 1972;30:459.

67. Schuller DE, McCabe BF. The firm salivary mass in children. *Laryngoscope* 1977;87:1891.

68. Callender DL, Frankenthaler RA, Luna MA, et al. Salivary gland neoplasms in children.

Arch Otolaryngol Head Neck Surg 1992;118: 472–476.

69. Eveson JW, Cawson RA. Salivary gland tumors. A review of 2410 cases with particular reference to histological types, site, age and sex distribution. *J Pathol* 1985;146:51.

70. Conley J, Clairmont A. Facial nerve in recurrent benign pleomorphic adenoma. *Arch Otolaryngol* 1979;105:247.

71. Dardick I, Kahn HJ, Van Nostrand AW, Baumal R. Salivary gland monomorphic adenoma. *Am J Pathol* 1984;115:334.

72. Mintz GA, Abrams AM, Melrose RJ. Monomorphic adenomas of the major and minor salivary glands. *Oral Surg Oral Med Oral Pathol* 1982; 53:375.

73. Batsakis JG, Brannon RB, Sciubba JJ. Monomorphic adenomas of major salivary glands. *Clin Otolaryngol* 1981;6:129.

74. Chapnik JS. The controversy of Warthin's tumor. *Laryngoscope* 1983;93:695.

75. Batsakis JG, Regezi JA. The pathology of head and neck tumors: salivary glands, Part 1. *Head Neck Surg* 1978;1:59.

76. Hastrup N, Bretlau P, Krogdahl A, Melchiors H. Oncocytomas of the salivary glands. *J Laryngol Otol* 1982;96:1027.

77. Batsakis JG, Regezi JA, Repola DA. The pathology of head and neck tumors: salivary glands, Part 2. *Head Neck Surg* 1978;1:167.

78. Spiro RH, Huvos AG, Berk R, Strong EW. Mucoepidermoid carcinoma of salivary gland origin. *Am J Surg* 1978;136:461.

79. Foote FW, Frazell EL. Tumors of the major salivary glands. *Cancer* 1953;6:1065.

80. Spiro RH, Huvos AG, Strong EW. Adenocarcinoma of salivary origin. *Am J Surg* 1982; 144:423.

81. Batsakis JG, Regezi JA. The pathology of head and neck tumors: salivary glands, Part 4. *Head Neck Surg* 1979;1:340.

82. Spiro RH, Huvos AG, Strong EW. Adenoid cystic carcinoma of salivary origin. *Am J Surg* 1974;128:512.

83. Spiro RH, Huvos AG, Strong EW. Adenoid cystic carcinoma: factors influencing survival. *Am J Surg* 1979;138:579.

84. Spiro RH, Huvos AG, Strong EW. Acinic cell carcinoma of salivary origin. *Cancer* 1978;41: 924.

85. Shemen LJ, Huvos AG, Spiro RH. Squamous cell carcinoma of salivary gland origin. *Head Neck Surg* 1987;9:235.

86. Marks MW, Ryan RF, et al. Squamous cell carcinoma of the parotid gland. *Plast Reconstr Surg* 1987;79:550.

87. Lewis JE, McKinney BC, Weiland LH, et al. Salivary duct carcinoma. *Cancer* 1996;77: 223–230.

88. Amaral AL, Nascimento AG. Malignant lymphoepithelial lesion of the submandibular gland. *Oral Surg* 1984;58:184.

89. Bosch JD. Malignant lymphoepithelial lesion of the salivary glands. *J Otolaryngol* 1988;17: 187.

90. Shemen LJ, Saw D. Malignant lymphoepithelial lesion. Wu D, Shemen L, Brady T, Saw D: Malignant lymphoepithelial lesion of the parotid gland. *ENT Journal.* 2001;80:803.

91. Savera A, Sloman A, Huvos A, et al. Myoepithelial carcinoma of salivary glands. *Am J Pathol* 2000;24:761.

92. Hyman GA, Wolff M. Malignant lymphomas of the salivary glands. *Am J Clin Pathol* 1976; 65:421–438.

93. Conley J, Arena S. Parotid gland as a focus of metastasis. *Arch Surg* 1963;87:69.

94. Nichols RD. Metastases to parotid nodes. *Laryngoscope* 1980;90:1324.

95. Waldron CA, El-Mofty SK, Gnepp DR. Tumors of the intraoral minor salivary glands: a demographic and histologic study of 426 cases. *Oral Surg Oral Med Oral Pathol* 1988; 66:323.

96. Spiro RH. Salivary neoplasms. *Head Neck Surg* 1986;8:177.

97. Shemen LJ. Conservative vs. superficial parotidectomy. *Arch Otolaryngol* 1999;125:1166.

98. McEvedy B, Ross WM. The treatment of mixed parotid tumors by enucleation and radiotherapy. *Br J Surg* 1976;63:341.

99. Armitstead PR, Smiddy FG, Frank HG. Simple enucleation and radiotherapy in the treatment of the pleomorphic salivary adenoma of the parotid gland. *Br J Surg* 1979;66:716.

100. Hagan WE, Anderson JR. Rhytidectomy techniques utilized for benign parotid surgery. *Laryngoscope* 1980;90:711.

101. Teres DJ, Tuffo KM, Fee WE. Modified facelift incision for parotidectomy. *J Laryngol Otol* 1994;108:574.

102. Porter ME. Great auricular nerve during parotidectomy. *Clin Otolaryngol* 1997;22: 251.

103. Christensen NR, Jacobsen SD. Parotidectomy. Preserving the posterior branch of the great auricular nerve. *J Laryngol Otol* 1997; 111:556.

104. Martins AS, Souza ALG, Souza LS, et al. Surgical procedures for primary, metastatic or adjacent parotid tumors. *Int Surg* 1999;84: 318.

105. Gullane PJ, Havas TJ. Facial nerve grafts: effects of postoperative irradiation. *J Otolaryngol* 1987;16:112.

106. Hong KH, Kim YK. Intraoral removal of the submandibular gland. *Otolaryngol Head Neck Surg* 2000;122:798.

107. Armstrong JG, Harrison LB, Thaler HT, et al. The indications for elective treatment of the neck in cancer of the major salivary glands. *Cancer* 1992;69:615–619.

108. Spiro RH. Management of the neck in parotid cancer. *Am J Surg* 1996;172:695.

109. Renehan A, Gleave EN, Hancock BD, et al. Long-term follow-up of over 1000 patients with salivary gland tumors treated in a single centre. *Br J Surg* 1996;83:1750–1754.

110. Buchman C, Stringer SP, Mendenhall WM, et al. Pleomorphic adenoma: effect of tumor spill and inadequate resection on tumor recurrence. *Laryngoscope* 1994;104:1231–1234.

111. Elkon D, Colman M, Hendrickson FR. Radiation therapy in the treatment of malignant salivary gland tumors. *Cancer* 1978;41:502.

112. Reinfuss M, Korzeniowski S. The role of radiotherapy in the treatment of malignant tumors of the salivary glands. *Tumor* 1980;66:467.

113. Sadeghi A, Tran LM, Mark R, et al. Minor salivary gland tumors of the head and neck: treatment strategies and prognosis. *Am J Clin Oncol* 1993;16:3–8.

114. Fitzpatrick PJ, Theriault O. Malignant salivary gland tumors. *Int J Radiat Oncol Biol Phys* 1986;12:1743.

115. Tran L, Sidrys J, Sadeghi A, et al. Salivary gland tumors of the oral cavity. *Int J Radiat Oncol Biol Phys* 1990;18:413.

116. van der Wal JE, Snow GB, et al. Intraoral adenoid cystic carcinoma: the role of postoperative radiotherapy in local control. *Head Neck* 1989;11:497.

117. Spiro RH, Armstrong J, et al. Carcinoma of major salivary glands. Recent trends. *Arch Otolaryngol* 1989;115:316.

118. Bissett RJ, Fitzpatrick PJ. Malignant submandibular tumors. *Am J Clin Oncol* 1988; 11:46.

119. Armstrong JG, Harrison LB, Spiro RH, et al. Malignant tumors of salivary gland origin: a matched pair analysis of the role of combined surgery and post-operative radiation therapy. *Arch Otolaryngol* 1990;116:290–293.

120. Migilianico L, Eschwege F, Marandas P, Webault P. Cervicofacial adenoid cystic carcinoma: study of 102 cases. *Int J Radiat Oncol Biol Phys* 1987;13:673–678.

121. Fitzpatrick PJ, Theriault C. Malignant salivary gland tumors. *Int J Radiat Oncol Biol Phys* 1986;12:1743–1748.

122. Parsons JT, Mendenhall WM, Stringer SP, et al. Management of minor salivary gland carcinomas. *Int J Radiat Oncol Biol Phys* 1996; 35:443–454.

123. Liem IH, Olmos RAV, Balm AJM, et al. Evidence for early and persistent impairment of salivary gland excretion after irradiation of head and neck tumors. *Eur J Nucl Med* 1996; 23:1485–1490.

124. Rentschler R, Burgess MA, Byers R. Chemotherapy of malignant major salivary gland neoplasms. *Cancer* 1977;40:619.

125. Licitra L, Cavina R, Grandi C, et al. Cisplatin, doxorubicin and cyclophosphamide in advanced salivary gland carcinoma. *Ann Oncol* 1996;7: 640–642.

126. Spiro RH, Huvos AG. Stage means more than grade in adenoid cystic carcinoma. *Am J Surg* 1992;164:623–628.

127. Spiro RH. Salivary neoplasms: overview of a 35-year experience with 2807 patients. *Head Neck Surg* 1986;8:177.

128. Conley J, Hamaker PC. Prognosis of malignant tumors of the parotid gland with facial paralysis. *Arch Otolaryngol* 1975;110:39.

129. Vrielinck LJG, Ostyn F, et al. The significance of perineural spread in adenoid cystic carcinoma of the major and minor salivary glands. *Int J Oral Maxillofac Surg* 1988;17:190.

130. Shemen LJ. Expanded polytetrafluoroethylene for reconstructing postparotidectomy defects and preventing Frey's syndrome. *Arch Otolaryngol Head Neck Surg* 1995;121:1307–1309.

131. Ioannides C, Fossion E. Reconstruction of extensive defects of the parotid region. *J Craniomaxillofac Surg* 1997;25:57.

132. Reddy PG, Reden RL, Mathog RH. Facial nerve rehabilitation after radical parotidectomy. *Laryngoscope* 1999;109:894.

Carcinoma of the Oral Cavity and Pharynx

26

Cancers of the oral cavity and pharynx annually account for 363,000 new cases worldwide and almost 200,000 deaths.[1] In 2001, these tumors accounted for 30,100 new cancer cases or 3% of all cancers in the United States.[2] They are at least 2.5 times more common in men than in women.

Greater than 90% of malignant neoplasms arising within the oral cavity and pharynx are squamous cell carcinomas (SCCs). Tumors of a variety of histologic types, which arise from minor salivary glands distributed throughout the oral cavity, are the second most common. Tobacco and alcohol use, advanced age, and male gender are the risk factors most commonly associated with oral and pharyngeal epidermoid cancer.[3] Excessive combined use of tobacco and ethanol results in a 15-fold increased risk to develop these cancers.[4]

ANATOMY

Traditionally, the oral cavity and pharynx have been grouped together for epidemiologic study and ease of categorization. However, the carcinomas of the oral cavity and pharynx differ greatly in anatomic, biologic, and pathologic features. Furthermore, the pharynx is subdivided into three distinct regions: the oropharynx, hypopharynx, and nasopharynx (see Figure 26-1)[5].

Oral Cavity

The oral cavity extends from the cutaneous-vermilion junction of the lips to the oropharynx. The posterior border of the oral cavity includes the circumvallate papillae, anterior tonsillar pillars, and junction of the hard and soft palate. Subsites within the oral cavity include

- Lips
- Oral tongue, anterior two-thirds
- Floor of mouth
- Buccal mucosa
- Gingival mucosa (alveolar ridge), upper and lower
- Retromolar trigone
- Hard palate

Oropharynx

The oropharynx begins anteriorly at the circumvallate papillae, tonsillar pillars, and the junction between the hard and soft palate. The oropharynx extends vertically from the inferior surface of the soft palate superiorly to the plane of the superior surface of the hyoid bone. The oropharynx is divided into six subsites:

- Base of tongue
- Soft palate and uvula
- Tonsillar pillars

566

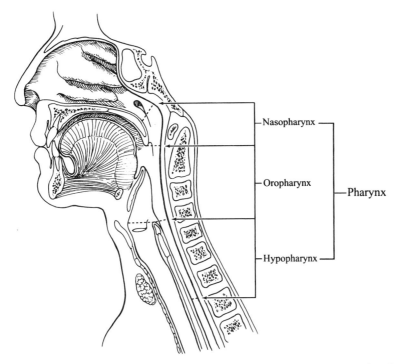

Figure 26-1.   The pharynx is divided into three distinct anatomic subsites. The soft palate, hyoid bone, and cricoid cartilage serve to demarcate each region.

- Pharyngeal tonsils
- Glossotonsillar sulci
- Oropharyngeal walls, lateral and posterior

Hypopharynx

The vertical limits of the hypopharynx are the superior border of the hyoid and the lower border of the cricoid cartilage. It includes three subsites:

- Pyriform sinus (or fossa), left and right
- Hypopharyngeal walls, lateral and posterior
- Postcricoid region (area of the pharyngoesophageal junction)

The postcricoid area extends from the arytenoid cartilages to the inferior aspect of the cricoid. This watershed area connects the two pyriform sinuses, thus forming the anterior wall of the hypopharynx. Each pyriform sinus extends from the pharyngoepiglottic folds to the upper end of the cervical esophagus and is bounded laterally by the thyroid cartilage and medially by the surface of the aryepiglottic fold and the arytenoid and cricoid cartilages.

Nasopharynx

The posterior choanae* form the anterior limit of the nasopharynx. The nasopharynx is divided into three subsites:

---

*The posterior nasal septum and choanae are considered part of the nasal cavity.

- Lateral walls (including the fossa of Rosenmüller and torus tubarius)
- Vault (including the superior surface of the soft palate)
- Posterosuperior wall (extending laterally from the vault to the base of skull, including the adenoid)

TNM STAGING

The *tumor,* lymph *node,* systemic *metastasis* (TNM) system is a clinical staging schema based on the extent of disease as determined by physical examination and imaging prior to initial treatment.[5] TNM staging provides a useful estimation of prognosis, aids in treatment selection, and permits the assessment of treatment outcomes. The American Joint Committee for Cancer (AJCC) coordinates and periodically updates the criteria for assessment and staging. While these schemas are useful to clinicians and their patients, they are imperfect in precisely assessing a tumor's biologic potential and its response to treatment. Additional predictive factors include aspects of the primary tumor, such as depth of invasion, growth pattern (exophytic versus infiltrative), and the degree of adjacent soft tissue and/or osseous spread. The presence of and characteristics of lymph node metastasis, such as immobility or ulceration through the skin, are also important. Finally, important adverse pathologic criteria of the primary tumor—such as perineural invasion, thickness, depth of invasion, and degree of differentiation—are not yet included in any staging system but correlate with poor treatment outcomes. Extracapsular spread of metastatic tumor outside a lymph node is the most reliable predictor of poor treatment outcomes.

TNM Staging for Oral Cavity, Oropharynx, Hypopharynx

T Stage, Primary Tumor

ORAL CAVITY

T_X: Primary tumor cannot be assessed

T_0: No evidence of primary tumor

Tis: Carcinoma in situ

T_1: Tumor <2 cm in greatest dimension

T_2: Tumor >2 cm but not >4 cm in greatest dimension

T_3: Tumor >4 cm in greatest dimension

T_4 (lip): Tumor invades adjacent structures (eg, through cortical bone, inferior alveolar nerve, floor of mouth, skin of face)

T_4 (oral cavity): Tumor invades adjacent structures [eg, through cortical bone, into deep (extrinsic) muscles of tongue, maxillary sinus, skin. Superficial erosion alone of bone/tooth socket by gingival primary is not sufficient to classify as T_4]

OROPHARYNX

T_X: Primary tumor cannot be assessed

T_0: No evidence of primary tumor

Tis: Carcinoma in situ

T_1: Tumor <2 cm in greatest dimension

T_2: Tumor >2 cm but not >4 cm in greatest dimension

T_3: Tumor >4 cm in greatest dimension

T_4: Tumor invades adjacent structures [eg, pterygoid muscle(s), mandible, hard palate, deep muscle of tongue, larynx]

HYPOPHARYNX

T_X: Primary tumor cannot be assessed

T_0: No evidence of primary tumor

Tis: Carcinoma in situ

T_1: Tumor limited to one subsite and <2 cm in greatest dimension

T_2: Tumor involves more than one subsite or an adjacent site, or measures >2 cm but not >4 cm in greatest diameter without fixation of hemilarynx

T_3: Tumor measures >4 cm in greatest dimension or with fixation of hemilarynx

T_4: Tumor invades adjacent structures (eg, thyroid/cricoid cartilage, carotid artery, soft tissues of neck, prevertebral fascia/muscles, thyroid and/or esophagus)

Regional Lymph Nodes (N) for Oral Cavity, Oropharynx, and Hypopharynx

N_X: Regional lymph nodes cannot be assessed

N_0: No regional lymph node metastasis

N_1: Metastasis in a single ipsilateral lymph node, <3 cm in greatest dimension

N_2: Metastasis in a single ipsilateral lymph node, >3 cm but not >6 cm in greatest dimension, or in multiple ipsilateral lymph nodes, none >6 cm in greatest dimension, or in bilateral or contralateral lymph nodes, none >6 cm in greatest dimension

N_{2a}: Metastasis in a single ipsilateral lymph node >3 cm but not >6 cm in greatest dimension

N_{2b}: Metastasis in multiple ipsilateral lymph nodes, none >6 cm in greatest dimension

N_{2c}: Metastasis in bilateral or contralateral lymph nodes, none >6 cm in greatest dimension

N_3: Metastasis in a lymph node >6 cm in greatest dimension

Distant Metastasis (M) for Oral Cavity, Oropharynx, Hypopharynx, Nasopharynx

M_X: Distant metastasis cannot be assessed

M_0: No distant metastasis

M_1: Distant metastasis

Stage Grouping for Oral Cavity, Oropharynx, Hypopharynx (Figure 26-2)

Stage 0:	$TisN_0M_0$
Stage I:	$T_1N_0M_0$
Stage II:	$T_2N_0M_0$
Stage III:	$T_3N_0M_0$; $T_{1-3} N_1M_0$
Stage IV:	$T_4N_{0-1}M_0$; $T_{1-4}N_{2-3}M_0$; $T_{1-4}N_{0-4}M_1$

TNM Staging for the Nasopharynx

This staging system contains several important differences as compared to the TNM staging for the oral cavity and the other pharyngeal sites. The AJCC distinguished T and N staging to account for the distinct difference in clinical behavior of nasopharyngeal carcinoma. Note the addition of T_{2a} and T_{2b}. The supraclavicular fossa is defined by three points: (1) the superior margin of the sternal end of the clavicle; (2) the superior margin of the lateral end of the clavicle; (3) the point where the neck meets the shoulder. This includes the caudal portion of levels IV and V. All cases with lymph node metastasis in this fossa are considered N_{3b}.

Primary Tumor (T)

T_X: Primary tumor cannot be assessed

T_0: No evidence of primary tumor

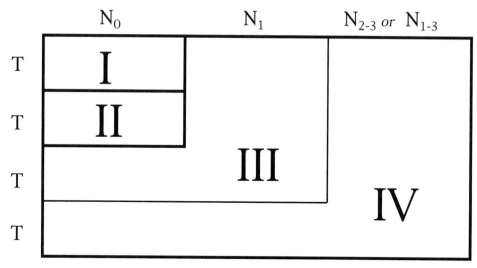

Figure 26-2. TNM staging for the oral cavity, oropharynx, and nasopharynx. Roman numerals indicate stage.

Tis: Carcinoma in situ

T_1: Tumor confined to the nasopharynx

T_2: Tumor extends to soft tissues of oropharynx and/or nasal fossa

    T_{2a}: without parapharyngeal extension

    T_{2b}: with parapharyngeal extension

T_3: Tumor invades bony structures and/or paranasal sinuses

T_4: Tumor with intracranial extension and/or involvement of cranial nerves, infratemporal fossa, hypopharynx, or orbit

Regional Lymph Nodes (N)

N_X: Regional lymph nodes cannot be assessed

N_0: No regional lymph node metastasis

N_1: Unilateral metastasis in lymph node(s), <6 cm in greatest dimension, above the supraclavicular fossa

N_2: Bilateral metastasis in lymph node(s), <6 cm in greatest dimension, above the supraclavicular fossa

N_3: Metastasis in a lymph node(s)

    N_{3a}: >6 cm in dimension

    N_{3b}: extension to the supraclavicular fossa

Distant Metastasis (M) for Nasopharynx

    M_X: Distant metastasis cannot be assessed

    M_0: No distant metastasis

    M_1: Distant metastasis

Stage Grouping for Nasopharynx

| Stage I | $T_1N_0M_0$ |
| Stage IIA | $T_{2a}N_0M_0$ |

Stage IIB $T_{1-2}N_1M_0$
                   $T_{2a}N_1M_0$
                   $T_{2b}N_{0-1}M_0$
Stage III $T_{1-2b}N_2M_0$
                   $T_{2a}N_2M_0$
                   $T_{2b}N_2M_0$
                   $T_3N_{0-2}M_0$
Stage IVA $T_4N_{0-2}M_0$
Stage IVB   Any T, N_3M_0
Stage IVC   Any T, any N, M_1

TREATMENT OF PATIENTS WITH ORAL AND PHARYNGEAL CARCINOMA

A Multidisciplinary Approach Is Crucial for Optimal Treatment

Successful oncologic management of oral and pharyngeal cancer requires the close, multi-disciplinary collaboration among head and neck radiologists, pathologists, head and neck surgical oncologists, radiation oncologists, and medical oncologists. Optimal aesthetic and functional outcomes require close coordination of reconstructive surgeons, speech pathologists, dentists, physical therapists, and maxillofacial prosthodontists.

Assessment and Evaluation

Comprehensive history and physical examination are critical for appropriate diagnosis and treatment selection. All mucosal surfaces of the upper aerodigestive tract must be carefully examined to assess for the extent of the primary lesion, regional metastasis, and second synchronous primary malignancy. Chest roentgenograms and routine serologic tests (electrolyte panel and complete blood count) are important screening tests, both for the overall health status of the patient and for the presence of distant metastasis. Panorex or dental x-rays should be considered if the patient might require radiation therapy. Computed tomography (CT) scans of the chest and abdomen are indicated when serologic tests or the screening chest roentgenogram identifies an abnormality. Bone scans are rarely needed.

Comorbid disease, such as chronic obstructive pulmonary disease, cardiovascular disease, or diabetes, is associated with increased mortality in head and neck squamous cell carcinoma (HNSCC) patients.[6,7] Piccirillo has advocated that comorbidity be included into the TNM staging for HNSCC.[8] In addition to comorbidity and past medical history, careful attention should be paid to the nutritional status of every patient. An assessment of recent weight loss should be made. Patients with >10% of weight loss during the 6 months prior to surgery are at greater risk for major perioperative complications.[9]

Treatment Selection

In general, early-stage (I–II) carcinoma of the oral cavity and pharynx (excluding nasopharynx) can be treated with radiation therapy or surgery. For advanced-stage tumors, combination modality treatment (surgery with preoperative or postoperative radiation therapy) results in improved rates of locoregional control and overall survival. The role of chemotherapy in HNSCC remains unclear.[10] However, concurrent chemotherapy with radiation therapy may improve outcome for selected patients with pharyngeal carcinoma. Chemotherapy may also improve survival in patients with extracapsular spread (ECS).[11]

Management of the N_0 Neck

The incidence of occult cervical metastasis is significant for patients with oral and pharyngeal squamous carcinoma. While the rate depends on the primary site and its size, there is little debate that most patients are at high risk for regional failure. Several treatment options are advocated for managing N_0 neck disease: (1) expectant management, (2) elective cervical lymphadenectomy, or (3) elective radiotherapy to the neck. With expectant management, the "wait and watch" policy may result in diminished regional control and overall survival.[12,13] Salvage rates for delayed regional metastasis may be lower.

Many advocate elective neck dissection over radiation therapy in patients if the incidence of occult metastasis is great than 25 to 30%. While occult metastasis can be managed with similar results, histopathologic examination of the neck dissection specimen provides important prognostic data, such as the presence of extracapsular spread.[14,15] Further adjuvant therapy can then be given to these high-risk patients. If no metastasis is present, if micrometastasis is present, or if a single node without ECS is present, the patient can be spared radiation therapy. However, the morbidity of even selective neck dissection must be considered.

Second Primary Malignancy in Head and Neck Squamous Cell Carcinoma (HNSCC)

The incidence of second primary tumors is approximately 5 to 10%.[16] A synchronous second primary tumor is found simultaneously with the initial head and neck cancer, while a metachronous tumor develops after treatment. Approximately 50% of second primaries arise within the head and neck, while the lung is the next most common site (20%). Retinoic acid compounds can diminish the rate of second metachronous primary tumors of the head and neck[17] and prevent the development of cancer from premalignant lesions of the oral cavity.[18]

Molecular Biology of HNSCC

Slaughter first elucidated the hypothesis of "field cancerization" in 1953.[18a] He speculated that carcinogen exposure is not limited to the primary tumor but is distributed throughout the mucosa of the upper aerodigestive tract. The frequency and distribution of second primary cancers in HNSCC provide strong evidence for field cancerization.

Recent advances in the molecular biology of HNSCC have provided additional support for Slaughter's hypothesis. Genetic alterations in p53, the tumor suppressor gene, are commonly present in HNSCC.[19] Brennan and colleagues demonstrated that premalignant genetic abnormalities are already present in mucosa adjacent to the primary tumor. Further research has correlated the alterations in specific loci (p16, cyclin D1, EGF-R) with the progression from normal mucosa to dysplasia, and finally to carcinoma.[20]

Distant Metastasis

Distant metastasis (DM) develops in 15% of patients with head and neck cancer.[21] While few studies have examined the incidence of DM at presentation, it is estimated to be 5 to 7%. There is a clear correlation between distant metastasis and these clinical pretreatment factors: higher nodal stage, the number of lymphatic metastases, and advanced T stage. Patients undergoing extensive surgery should also be carefully screened for the presence of DM. For an isolated pulmonary metastasis, resection may be indicated. Patients with ECS and with local and regional recurrence have a significantly higher risk for developing DM.

Follow-up

Most patients with head and neck cancer die as a result of local or regional failure. Therefore, after definitive treatment, regular follow-up examinations are important. When recurrence is identified early, salvage therapy may be effective.

Recurrences usually present in the first 2 years after treatment; thus, clinic visits should be more frequent during this time. After the first 2 years, follow-up should be at least annually, because the incidence of developing a second primary cancer remains constant at about 4 to 5% per year. If the patient should become symptomatic at any time between visits, the surgeon should perform a thorough examination and order any ancillary tests and procedures that might be necessary. Pain is a sensitive indicator for tumor recurrence and should serve as a "warning sign" for the head and neck oncologist.[22]

CARCINOMA OF THE ORAL CAVITY

Early-stage oral cavity cancer is most commonly treated with surgery, while advanced-stage disease is treated with combined-modality therapy. Since successful treatment of oral cavity cancer relies on effective management of the regional lymphatics as well as the primary tumor, elective neck dissection is recommended for most patients with adverse clinical features, including advanced T stage and depth of invasion > 4 mm. Therapeutic neck dissections are performed for patients with clinically apparent nodal disease. Postoperative radiotherapy is administered to those patients with pathologic evidence of perineural spread, extensive nodal disease, or ECS.

Carcinoma of the Lip

1. Facts and figures
   a. Histopathology: >95% of lesions are SCCs
      (1) Basal cell carcinoma, minor salivary gland also seen
   b. Location: 95% lower lip, 5% upper lip
   c. Although BCC is seen occasionally in the upper lip and rarely in the lower lip, SCC is still the most common cancer of the upper lip
   d. Age at time of diagnosis: 50% patients between 50 and 69 years
   e. Incidence: 1.8 per 100,000[23]
   f. Male predilection: 20:1 to 35:1 for lower lip, but 5:1 for upper lip
2. Diagnosis, evaluation
   a. Diagnosed early because of prominent location.
   b. Regional metastasis:
      (1) Relatively uncommon; seen in an estimated 10% of patients.
      (2) Lymphatic drainage primarily to submental, submandibular nodes.
      (3) Bilateral metastasis is always a concern because of the lymphatic drainage pattern but is rarely seen (<10%).
3. Treatment
   a. Resection and reconstruction:
      (1) Extent of resection determines reconstruction.
      (2) Proper alignment of vermilion border is critical.
      (3) Closure in four layers.
      (4) Reconstruction (lower lip) is based on the size of the defect[24]:
         (a) <¼–⅓: primary closure, facilitated by V-shaped excision
         (b) ¼–½: bilateral advancement flaps or "lip-switch" flaps: Abbe, when close to oral commissure; Estlander, when involving the oral commissure.
         (c) ½–⅔: Karapandzic flap.
         (d) ⅔–total: local flap reconstruction (Bernard-Burow or Gillies fan flap) or free tissue transfer.

    b.   Adjuvant therapy:
        (1)   Postoperative radiation therapy is indicated in high-risk patients:
            (a)   Locally advanced disease (T_3–T_4)
            (b)   Perineural invasion at the primary site[25]
            (c)   Positive margins
            (d)   Multiple lymphatic metastases or extracapsular spread
        (2)   Primary radiation for those rare patients unsuitable for or unwilling to undergo resection
4. Treatment outcomes
    a.   Local and regional control: >90%
    b.   Five-year rates of survival:
        (1)   Overall: 91%[26]
        (2)   Stage I–II: >90%
        (3)   Stage III–IV: 30–70%[27,28]

Carcinoma of the Tongue

Treatment for tongue cancer depends on the stage of the primary tumor and extent of regional metastasis. Although radiation is a potential option for the primary treatment of tongue cancers, most tongue cancers are treated surgically in this country because of treatment-related morbidity associated with radiation. In the case of more advanced disease, multi-modality therapy, consisting of surgery and postoperative radiation, is the standard of care. Since treatment may result in considerable impairment of speech and swallowing function, rehabilitation by a qualified speech pathologist should be planned before treatment and initiated early in the treatment course.

1. Facts and figures
    a.   Second most common tumor of the oral cavity (30%)
    b.   Most often arises along the lateral borders of the tongue[29]
    c.   Histopathologic criteria of the primary tumor:
        (1)   Depth of invasion >2–4 mm correlated with higher rates of regional metastasis, recurrence, and mortality.[30–32]
        (2)   Perineural invasion at the primary site is another indicator of recurrence and increased mortality.[33,34]
    d.   The incidence of SCC of the tongue in young patients has been increasing in the United States, from 4% in 1971 to 18% in 1993.[35]
    e.   No clinical features or risk factors (age, substance abuse) have been clearly identified.
        (1)   An increased genetic susceptibility to carcinogenesis has been postulated and preliminary studies using molecular epidemiology techniques support this hypothesis.[36,37]
2. Diagnosis, evaluation
    a.   Regional metastasis: common
        (1)   Incidence: depends on T stage, tumor factors
            (a)   Clinically apparent: 25–33%
            (b)   Occult: 25–33%
        (2)   Primary nodal drainage to levels I to III (see Figure 26-3). However, in one study, 16% of patients had either isolated level IV metastasis or level III node

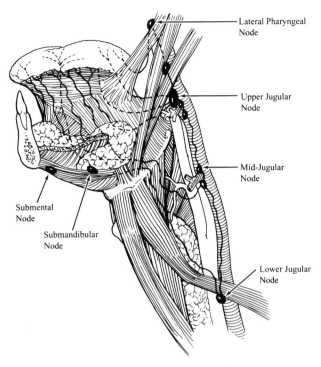

Figure 26-3. Lymphatic drainage of the oral tongue and oropharynx.

as the only pathologically positive node, without disease in levels I or II.[38] For this reason, selective cervical lymphadenopathy is recommended to include at least levels I to IV.

3. Treatment
    a. Management of the primary
        (1) Initial wide, negative margins are important. Tumor retraction into the intrinsic tongue musculature during resection is a near-catastrophic event, making complete tumor extirpation difficult.
        (2) Partial glossectomy: indicated for early T1–T2 lesions; healing by secondary intention or skin graft for reconstruction.
        (3) Total glossectomy: for advanced disease. Even with reconstruction, can result in difficulty with deglutition and maintenance of an adequate airway. Aspiration may be a chronic problem; thus laryngectomy may be necessary. In selected patients, total glossectomy may be possible without total laryngectomy.[39]
    b. Management of the mandible
        (1) Tumors involving gingiva should be resected with periosteum as the deep margin.
        (2) Tumors involving periosteum should be resected with an additional deep margin of bone—ie, a marginal mandibulectomy.
        (3) Depending on the extent of tumor involvement, *rim mandibulectomy,* removing a bicortical "rim" of bone at the upper aspect of the alveolus, or *sagittal*

mandibulectomy, taking the inner cortex using a vertical or oblique resection, is used. Standard segmental mandibulectomy is indicated for lesions directly invading bone.

   c. Management of the neck

      (1) Anatomic studies have demonstrated that the anterior portion of the tongue drains to the submental nodes and the lateral portion into the submandibular and deep jugular nodes. Bilateral nodal drainage also occurs, particularly from primaries that are located close to the midline of the tongue.

      (2) Upper jugular nodes (73%), submandibular nodes (18%), the middle jugular nodes (18%), and the submental nodes (9%) are the most frequent sites of metastasis for SCC of the oral tongue.[40]

      (3) Elective neck dissection results in better outcomes than observation.[41–44] Survival following salvage treatment for regional metastasis is approximately 35–40%.

4. Treatment outcomes

   a. Five-year locoregional control rates of 91%.[42,45]

   b. Five-year survival rates[42,46]:

      (1) 60–75% for stage I, II

      (2) 25–40% for stage III, IV

   c. Impact of extracapsular spread (ECS) on survival[15]:

      (1) Five-year disease-specific and overall survival rates for patients with pathologically negative necks (pN–) were 88% and 75%; for pN+/ECS– patients, 65% and 50%; and for pN+/ECS+ patients, 48% and 30%.

Carcinoma of the Floor of the Mouth (FOM)

1. Facts and figures

   a. Third most common oral cavity tumor.

   b. Tumors ≤ 2 cm are often asymptomatic and may appear as an erythematous discoloration of mucosa. As the lesions grow and ulcerate, extension into the root of the tongue or lingual or mental nerves may occur, resulting in decreased tongue mobility and decreased sensation in the teeth, lip, and chin. More advanced cancers arising from this site can abut or invade the mandible.

2. Diagnosis, evaluation

   a. High rate of occult metastatic nodal disease: 23–50%

   b. Cervical metastasis is most frequently seen in the submandibular (64%), upper jugular (43%), and the submental nodes (7%).[40] Bilateral metastasis is not uncommon given the midline location of the FOM.

   c. Tumor may obstruct or track along the sublingual and submandibular glands. In addition, perineural and lymphovascular invasion is often seen with FOM lesions.

3. Treatment

   a. Management of the primary

      (1) Although early-stage cancers can be treated with nearly equivalent outcomes by radiation or surgery, surgery is preferred. XRT (radiation therapy) near the mandible tends to cause greater morbidity than does surgery.

      (2) Superficial or small lesions can be resected transorally and reconstructed with split-thickness skin grafts or left to heal by secondary intention.

    (3) Larger lesions require formal resection of the FOM, including aspects of the ventral tongue and the sublingual gland. These lesions are sometimes best approached via the transcervical approach in order to achieve en bloc resection with adequate margins. Tracheotomy is often necessary due to postoperative edema.
    (4) Cancers involving the periosteum or with superficial mandibular invasion can be removed via marginal mandibulectomy.
    (5) For edentulous patients or those with limited mandibular height, segmental mandibulectomy may be necessary because of the high risk for radionecrosis and/or pathologic fracture.
    (6) A segmental resection may be necessary if there is more extensive invasion of bone. Defects of the anterior segment of the mandible require bone reconstruction, usually with a free fibular or iliac crest graft.
  b. Management of the neck
    (1) Elective treatment of the neck for FOM primary cancers is recommended because of the high rate of occult nodal disease (25–50%) and the poor salvage rate following development of cervical recurrence.
    (2) Therapeutic neck dissections are most commonly accomplished by comprehensive cervical lymphadenectomy, with postoperative radiation therapy for patients at greatest risk for recurrence.
4. Treatment outcomes
  a. Locoregional control:
    (1) Recurrence at the primary site (41%) is twice as common as failure in the neck (18.5%).[47]
    (2) The major source of treatment failure.
  b. Five-year survival rates for patients with cancer of the FOM range from 64–80% in the case of stage I disease, 61–84% in stage II, 28–68% in stage III, and 6–36% in stage IV disease.[48]

Carcinoma of the Retromolar Trigone (RMT)

1. Facts and figures
  a. *Anatomy.* The retromolar trigone is a triangulated region of gingiva overlying the ascending ramus of the mandible.
  b. The true incidence of RMT carcinoma is difficult to determine since tumors often involve both the retromolar trigone and adjacent sites, sometimes making it difficult to ascertain the tumor's epicenter.
2. Diagnosis, evaluation
  a. The RMT represents a watershed area, near the buccal mucosa, tonsillar fossa, glossopharyngeal sulcus, lateral floor of mouth, tongue base, soft palate, and, deeply, the masticator space.
  b. A thin layer of mucosa and underlying soft tissue overlies the mandible; therefore bony involvement may develop early.
    (1) For these reasons, tumors of the retromolar trigone often present at an advanced stage.
    (2) At presentation, regional metastases are common: 10–20%.[49]

3. Treatment
    a. Management of the primary
        (1) For stage I or II tumors, surgery and radiation are equally effective.[50,51]
        (2) For more extensive superficial lesions that involve the soft palate but do not invade bone, radiotherapy may be a better treatment option, since palatal resection can result in poor speech and swallowing outcomes.
        (3) Stage III and IV lesions often require combined surgery and radiation. A "composite resection" (ie, requiring extensive soft tissue and adjacent bone) is often necessary.
            (a) A visor flap or a lip-splitting incision is needed for exposure.
            (b) Osseous resection from the subcondylar region to the mental foramen.
            (c) Soft tissue resection often includes the RMT, tonsillar fossa, lateral floor of mouth, soft palate, buccal mucosa, and pterygoid musculature.
    b. Reconstruction following surgery
        (1) Reconstruction of the RMT must address the recovery of speech and swallowing functions. When oncologically safe, sparing the condyle and posterior ramus of the mandible greatly facilitates the success of bony reconstruction. Often, however, these lateral defects create little functional morbidity.
        (2) Reconstruction methods include split-thickness skin graft, a regional flap, or a free tissue transfer flap, depending on the size of the defect and the need for osseous reconstruction and/or soft tissue coverage.
        (3) Obturators may be necessary if the resection involves a significant portion of the palate. Defects that have insufficient soft tissue bulk or involve osseous reconstruction require regional flaps or free tissue transfer.
    c. Management of the neck
        (1) Patients with clinically evident cervical disease should be managed with a therapeutic neck dissection. Elective management of the neck should be considered in patients with advanced-stage primaries.
4. Treatment outcomes
    a. Locoregional recurrence:
        (1) Common without combined-modality therapy
    b. Five-year actuarial survival rates:
        (1) 80% (T_1), 57.8% (T_2), 46.5% (T_3), and 65.2% (T_4)[51]
    c. The 5-year overall survival rate:
        (1) 26–55%[50, 51]

Carcinoma of the Alveolar ridge, Gingival Mucosa, or Gums

1. Facts and figures
    a. 10% of all malignancies in the oral cavity.
    b. Most commonly arise in edentulous areas or at the free margin of the gingiva of the lower alveolar ridge.
2. Diagnosis and evaluation
    a. 40% of these patients will have invasion of the mandible or maxilla at the time of diagnosis.[52] Open tooth sockets or small defects in the edentulous mandibular ridge provide ready access for tumor invasion into bone.

     b.   Regional metastasis is clinically evident in 25–30% of these patients and the occult cervical metastatic rate is 15%. Lymphatic drainage for alveolar ridge cancers is most often to the upper deep jugular nodes.[53]

3.   Treatment
    a.   Management of the primary cancer
       (1) Small cancers of the alveolar ridge can be resected transorally.
       (2) Partial maxillectomy for lesions of the upper alveolar ridge or mandibulectomy for those of the lower alveolar ridge is often required, since invasion of mandible or maxilla is not uncommon.
       (3) Resection of lateral segments of the mandible may not require reconstruction. Major resections involving the anterior arch of the mandible do require osteomyocutaneous flaps and reconstructive plates.
    b.   Management of the neck
       (1) Therapeutic, comprehensive treatment of the neck is indicated in all patients who have clinically positive neck disease.
       (2) Early-stage primary cancers with clinically N_0 necks may be observed; however, in patients with advanced T stage, radiologic or histologic evidence of mandibular invasion, and/or decreased tumor differentiation, elective treatment of the neck is recommended.[53]
    c.   Adjuvant therapy
       (1) Adjuvant radiotherapy is recommended for patients with extensive nodal disease, histopathologic criteria (perineural invasion, lymphovascular invasion), or inadequate margins of resection.[54]
       (2) XRT as primary modality is not recommended unless the patient is an unsuitable operative candidate.

4.   Treatment outcomes
    a.   Local and regional control: 70–80%
    b.   Five-year survival rates: 50–65%[52–55]
    c.   The presence of mandibular cortical invasion decreased 5-year survival from 85 to 68%. Cervical metastases also decreased 5-year survival (86 vs. 59%).[54]

Carcinoma of the Palate

1.   Facts and figures
    a.   Only half of all tumors are SCCs.
    b.   Minor salivary gland tumors are also common.[56]
    c.   Necrotizing sialometaplasia is a benign mucosal inflammatory lesion that can be mistaken for malignancy in the hard palate.

2.   Diagnosis and evaluation
    a.   Most carcinomas manifest as a granular superficial ulceration of the hard palate. Initial growth tends to be superficial, although these tumors can extend through the periosteum of bone into adjacent regions of the oral cavity, such as the paranasal sinuses and floor of the nose.
    b.   10–25% of patients present with cervical nodal metastases. Nonetheless, preoperative imaging should be performed to assess the lateral pharyngeal nodes, since these are difficult to evaluate on clinical examination.
    c.   Careful assessment of the trigeminal nerve is crucial. Perineural invasion to the gasserian ganglion should be evaluated with magnetic resonance imaging (MRI).[57,58]

3. Treatment
    a. Although radiation can be used to treat carcinomas of this site, surgery is preferred. Radiation is more commonly reserved for adjuvant or salvage therapy.
    b. Management of the primary
        (1) Wide local excision may be adequate to obtain surgical margins. However, infrastructure maxillectomy may be necessary. For extensive involvement of the adjacent bony and soft tissue structures, a total maxillectomy, with or without orbital exenteration, may be required.
    c. Management of the neck
        (1) Elective treatment of the neck is generally not recommended for patients with primary cancer of the palate because of the low rate of occult metastases.[59]
    d. Reconstruction issues
        (1) A maxillary defect requires reconstruction. An obturator with or without a skin graft is the most common method of reconstruction. The obturator is fabricated from a synthetic polymer and provides oronasal separation, which can yield normal speech and swallowing function.
        (2) Extensive soft tissue reconstruction with either regional flap or free tissue transfer remains controversial. Concern has been raised that a bulky flap might delay the diagnosis of recurrence.
    e. Role of radiation
        (1) Radiotherapy can be selected for primary or adjuvant management of palate cancer. Postoperative radiotherapy is often recommended to decrease local and regional recurrence. Absolute indications for postoperative radiotherapy include positive surgical margins, presence of perineural invasion, neck node metastasis, and recurrent tumors.
4. Treatment outcomes
    a. Local recurrence rate: 53%
    b. Regional recurrence rate: 30%[56]
    c. Five-year survival: 44–75%[59]

Carcinoma of the Buccal Mucosa

1. Facts and figures
    a. Although tumors arising from the buccal mucosa are rare in the United States (constituting <10% of all oral cavity cancer), they are the most common oral cavity cancers in India.
    b. The high incidence of cancers at this site in India is attributed at least in part to the prevalent practice of chewing "pan," a combination of betel nut, lime, and tobacco.[60]
2. Diagnosis and evaluation
    a. Verrucous carcinoma
        (1) Verrucous carcinoma accounts for <5% of all oral cavity carcinomas, but has a predilection for the buccal mucosa.
        (2) Characterized by its whitish, warty, bulky, cauliflower-like growth, with a broad base.
        (3) Often difficult to distinguish from verrucous hyperplasia.
        (4) Carcinoma is characterized by extension of the lesion into the underlying connective tissue deep to the adjacent normal epithelium.[61]

(5) Verrucous carcinoma has a more favorable prognosis and is considered a low-grade malignancy.[62] Surgical resection remains the preferred mode of treatment for the primary lesion.[63] Adjuvant radiation treatment is usually not indicated. Since verrucous carcinomas rarely metastasize, elective neck dissection is often not indicated for patients with this disease.

b. Squamous carcinoma of the buccal mucosa
    (1) More often arises from preexisting leukoplakia than do other oral cavity cancers.[64]
    (2) Typically develops as an exophytic or verrucous process but can also be ulcerative.
    (3) As with lesions of the retromolar trigone, epidermoid cancer of buccal mucosa can quickly invade into adjacent bony structures and, as a result, often presents at an advanced stage. Posteriorly, it can extend to involve the pterygoid muscles; superiorly, it can grow to involve the alveolar ridge, palate, or maxillary sinus.
    (4) Tumor thickness (>6 mm) correlates with increased morbidity and mortality.[65]
    (5) Regional metastases are most commonly seen in the submandibular nodes.

c. Mixed verrucous-squamous carcinoma of the buccal mucosa
    (1) A hybrid of squamous carcinoma and verrucous carcinoma has been described, as 20% of verrucous lesions will have a focus of squamous carcinoma.[63]
    (2) These lesions behave more aggressively than lesions that are purely verrucous. While many have speculated that radiation therapy may induce "anaplastic transformation," there is no evidence for this correlation.[62]

3. Treatment
a. Management of the primary
    (1) Stage I and II disease: equal efficacy with surgery or radiation.[66] Transoral resection is preferred and is most convenient for small lesions.
    (2) If gingiva is involved, margin should include gingiva and periosteum.
    (3) If periosteum is involved, at least a marginal mandibulectomy is required.
    (4) For more extensive involvement, segmental mandibulectomy is needed.

b. Management of the neck
    (1) Elective management of the neck is recommended, However, no consensus has been reached as to whether elective treatment of the neck is best accomplished by radiation or surgery.[67,68]

c. Reconstruction
    (1) Early-stage lesions: skin grafts or mucosal advancement flaps.
    (2) More extensive defects may require regional or free tissue transfer.

d. Adjuvant therapy
Postoperative radiotherapy is often recommended[69,70]:
    (1) For advanced-stage buccal carcinoma (T_{3-4}).
    (2) Close surgical margins
    (3) Perineural or lymphovascular invasion
    (4) Tumor thickness >10 mm
    (5) Poor differentiation
    (6) Bone invasion

4. Treatment outcomes
   a. Locoregional recurrence is significant and ranges from 43[71] to 80%.[67]
   b. Five-year survival[72]:

Stage I	78%
Stage II	66%
Stage III	62%
Stage IV	50%

MANAGEMENT OF OROPHARYNGEAL CARCINOMAS

1. Facts and figures
   a. Most malignancies of the oropharynx (90%) are squamous cell carcinoma (SCC).
      (1) Histologic subtypes: nonkeratinizing vs. keratinizing.
      (2) Nonkeratinizing carcinomas may be well or poorly differentiated, often seen with submucosal spread and "pushing" margin.
   b. Lymphocytic malignancy
      (1) Lymphoid tissue is abundantly present in the oropharynx. As such, the next most common malignancy encountered is lymphoma, primarily of the palatine tonsils and base of the tongue.
      (2) Lymphoma of the tonsil and the base of the tongue may be the first symptom of systemic lymphoma or, more rarely, the only primary site.
   c. Salivary gland carcinoma
      (1) Malignant transformation of the minor salivary glands may result in adenoid cystic carcinomas and other histologic subtypes within the oropharyngeal area.

Diagnosis and Evaluation

1. Physical examination: careful assessment of larynx and nasopharynx is needed to assess for local tumor extension.
   a. **Bimanual palpation** often reveals important clinical details, especially in the base of the tongue.
   b. The incidence of second primary tumors is significant.[73]
2. For the soft palate, tumor thickness (>3 mm) has correlated with regional metastasis and survival.[74] Cervical metastasis is present in at least 50% of patients.
   a. For even small midline lesions of the soft palate, the propensity for regional metastasis is great (>40%).[75]
3. Often, it is difficult to distinguish between direct spread into the neck from the primary tumor and extracapsular spread outside a large nearby lymph node with metastatic tumor.
4. The jugulodigastric or subdigastric nodal groups (level II) are most commonly affected. However, posterior and retropharyngeal nodes are also often involved and must be considered during treatment planning.
5. Metastatic cervical lymph nodes from oropharyngeal sites may present as cystic in nature. As such, these metastases can easily be mistaken for branchial anomalies.[76,77]
6. Recent studies have shown a relationship between human papillomavirus, especially subtype 16 (HPV-16), and a certain subtype of oropharyngeal carcinoma arising in patients without other risk factors.[78,79]

Treatment

1. Radiation therapy
    a. Treatment philosophy for oropharyngeal carcinoma has changed much over the past 25 years. Initially, surgery was favored. As technical improvements were made, radiation therapy (external beam and/or brachytherapy) came into favor because it usually results in less morbidity and functional disturbance than surgery. Often, a combined-modality approach using surgery and radiation is selected. Combination chemotherapy and radiation therapy has been evaluated for treatment of oropharyngeal squamous cell carcinoma. Hyperfractionation delivery of XRT and concurrent "boost" radiotherapy may improve local and regional control.[80] Several studies have demonstrated outcomes comparable to those of the standard approach using surgery and postoperative radiation.[81–85]
    b. Special considerations:
        (1) *Tonsil and soft palate:* Surgeons generally agree that combining surgery and irradiation is best for treatment of lesions that extend beyond the confines of the tonsillar fossa. Tonsil SCC is treated with radiation through parallel opposed portals. Only the ipsilateral neck is treated unless (a) invasion of the soft palate is significant, especially close to the midline; (b) clinically positive nodes appear in the contralateral neck; or (c) the tongue has been invaded.
        (2) *Base of tongue (BOT):* XRT is delivered by parallel, opposed external beam portals to the primary site, including bilateral regional lymph nodes. If this is used as a primary therapeutic modality, surgery may be recommended if significant improvement does not occur with 5000 rad.
2. Radiation therapy with chemotherapy
    a. According to several preliminary studies, primary radiation therapy with concurrent chemotherapy improves local and regional control and disease-specific survival.
        (1) In a 1997 retrospective study, concomitant boost chemotherapy with hyperfractionation radiation therapy resulted in 5-year local control rates of 96, 96, and 82% in T_1, T_2, and T_3 tumors. With neck dissection as indicated, 5-year regional control rates were 92, 76, 89, and 89% for N_0, N_1, N_2, N_3.[86]
        (2) Prospective studies are under way to confirm these initial results.[87,88]
3. Surgery
    a. Approaches to the oropharynx include:
        (1) Transoral excision
        (2) Anterior mandibulotomy (mandibular swing)
        (3) Lateral mandibular osteotomy
        (4) Composite resection
        (5) Midline translingual pharyngotomy
        (6) Extended lateral pharyngotomy
        (7) Transhyoid pharyngotomy
    b. Special considerations:
        (1) Total glossectomy may be required for advanced-stage BOT lesions.
        (2) Invasion of the larynx is often seen and a laryngectomy may be needed to achieve complete tumor resection or prevent aspiration.
        (3) Neck dissection is needed for oropharyngeal carcinoma with regional metastases that does not respond or only partially responds to radiation therapy.[88,89]

Treatment Outcomes

1. Local and regional control:
   a. *Tonsil:* 75–90%, stage I–II; 50%, stage III; 20–50%, stage IV
   b. *Base of tongue:* 75–90%, stage I–II; 50%, stage III; 20%, stage IV
   c. *Soft palate:* 75–90%, stage I–II; 75%, stage III; 35%, stage IV[90]
2. Five-year survival:
   a. *Tonsil:* 80%, stage I–II; 50%, stage III; 20–50%, stage IV
   b. *Base of tongue:* 85%, stage I–II; 20–50%, stage III–IV[91]
   c. *Soft palate:* 70–80%, stage I–II; 64%, stage III; 20–40%, stage IV
3. Distant metastasis:
   a. Patients with oropharyngeal SCC may have an increased risk of developing distant metastasis. Large tumors with bulky nodal disease should be followed carefully for local and regional recurrence but also for signs of distant failure.

MANAGEMENT OF HYPOPHARYNGEAL CARCINOMAS

1. Facts and figures
   a. SCC: Most malignancies of the hypopharynx (90%) are epidermoid carcinoma. Rarely, salivary gland malignancies or sarcomas are seen.
   b. Risk factors: tobacco, ethanol,[3] possibly gastroesophageal reflux disease[92]
   c. Plummer-Vinson[93] syndrome: dysphagia, hypopharyngeal and esophageal webs, weight loss, and iron-deficiency anemia affecting women aged 30 to 50 years.
      (1) The association with postcricoid carcinoma was made because of the reverse in the usual 4:1 ratio of male:female prevalence of cancer in other areas of the head and neck.
   d. In the United States, pyriform sinus carcinoma predominates (accounting for 60–70% of cases), while in Europe postcricoid carcinomas predominate.[94]

Diagnosis and Evaluation

1. Symptoms—often present late in the disease—chronic sore throat, referred otalgia, dysphagia, neck mass.
2. 70% of patients with SCC of the hypopharynx present with stage III disease, while most laryngeal cancers are detected at an earlier stage.
3. The rich lymphatic network in the submucosal tissue surrounding the hypopharynx allows early spread to regional lymph nodes and direct extension into adjacent soft tissues.
4. 60–75% of patients with hypopharyngeal carcinoma have palpable cervical metastases at presentation.[95–97]
5. Carcinoma of the medial wall of the hypopharynx may behave differently and have a greater propensity for contralateral metastasis than lesions of the lateral wall.[98] Furthermore, lesions that involve more than one subsite within the hypopharynx have significant increase in mortality.[97]
6. There is a strong propensity for submucosal spread and "skip metastases," which should be considered during surgical resection.[99,100]

Treatment

Management of hypopharyngeal carcinoma remains both challenging and controversial. Treatment selection depends on stage, subsite, and institutional preference. While a few clear-cut recommendations can now be made, there is little consensus about the optimal therapy for hypopharyngeal tumors.

1. Radiation therapy:
   a. XRT is advocated as a primary modality of treatment for T_1 and selected T_2 lesions[101,102] with early-stage disease:
      (1) Twice-daily hyperfractionation XRT dosimetry is critical.
      (2) Local control rates: 89% for T_1 and 77% for T_2 tumors
      (3) Preradiation neck dissection may be considered in certain patients with extensive but resectable cervical metastasis.
      (4) Five-year survival rates were 68% for T_1 and 46% for T_2 lesions.
      (5) XRT may provide a better functional (organ-preserving) approach.
      (6) XRT treats bilateral cervical nodal basins as well as the retropharyngeal nodes with diminished morbidity.
   b. Postoperative adjuvant radiation therapy plays a crucial role following surgery for advanced-stage carcinomas of the hypopharynx.
      (1) Improved local and regional control, increased survival.[103,104]
      (2) *Indications:* multiple levels of or bulky nodal disease, cartilage invasion, extracapsular spread, positive surgical margins.
   c. The role of concurrent chemotherapy and radiation therapy in the treatment of hypopharyngeal SCC remains unclear.
      (1) The European Organization for Research and Treatment of Cancer (EORTC) Head and Neck Cooperative Group showed results comparable to surgery and post-operative XRT, but the 5-year survival rate was only 35%.
2. Surgery
   a. Pharyngeal wall
      (1) Selected tumors can be resected with laryngeal preservation if there is no fixation to the prevertebral fascia.[105]
      (2) Approach via transhyoid or median labiomandibular glossotomy.
   b. Postcricoid mucosa
      (1) These tumors usually present at an advanced stage and therefore require total laryngopharyngectomy.[106]
      (2) These lesions can involve the cervical esophagus, requiring laryngopharyngoesophagectomy.
   c. Pyriform sinus
      (1) Extended partial laryngopharyngectomy was first described by Ogura and may be indicated for selected T_1 and T_2 carcinomas.[107]
      (2) Supracricoid hemilaryngopharyngectomy[108] preserves cricoid integrity and the contralateral arytenoid and vocal cord. Oncologic results were comparable when adjuvant radiation therapy was used.
      (3) Total laryngopharyngectomy, however, is often required for complete oncologic resection.
3. Reconstruction
   a. Primary closure:
      (1) Possible in selected patients with adequate mucosa—ie, patients undergoing partial laryngopharyngectomy or total laryngectomy with partial pharyngectomy.

    b. Regional flap reconstruction:
       (1) Pectoralis major myocutaneous flap: useful for partial largyngopharyngectomy defects.
    c. Microvascular free-tissue transfer:
       (1) Radial forearm and rectus abdominis flaps have been used for partial pharyngectomy defects. Tubed radial forearm, rectus, or other fasciocutaneous flaps have also been described for closure of total laryngopharyngectomy defects.
       (2) Free jejunal autograft is often used for reconstruction following total laryngopharyngectomy.[109,110]
       (3) Gastric pull-up is indicated when total laryngopharyngectomy with esophagectomy is performed. Price et al. noted a high incidence (20%) of occult, synchronous esophageal carcinoma.[111]

Treatment Outcomes for Combined-Modality Therapy

1. Local and regional control:
    a. Pyriform sinus: 58–71%[97]
    b. Pharyngeal wall: 91% for T_1, 73% for T_2, 61% for T_3 lesions, and 37% for T_4 carcinomas[112]
    c. Postcricoid carcinoma: <60%[106]
2. Five-year survival rates:
    a. Pyriform sinus: 20–50%[97,103,104]
    b. Pharyngeal wall: 21%[112]
    c. Postcricoid carcinoma: 35%[106]
3. Distant metastasis and death from disease:
    a. Numerous studies have documented a high rate of systemic metastasis from hypopharyngeal SCC.[113,114]
    b. These patients may be at higher risk for hematogenous dissemination as compared to patients with SCC at other primary sites.

CARCINOMA OF THE NASOPHARYNX (NPC)

1. Facts and figures
    a. Histopathology: World Health Organization (WHO) Classification.
    b. WHO type I: keratinizing SCC, similar to other epidermoid carcinoma of the head and neck.
    c. WHO type II: non-keratinizing epidermoid carcinoma, also known as transitional cell carcinoma. Papillary features are often seen.
    d. WHO type III: undifferentiated carcinomas, historically known as lymphoepithelioma or Schmincke tumors. These poorly differentiated tumors are infiltrated by nonmalignant T-cell lymphocytes. This is the most common form of NPC.
2. Epidemiology and pathogenesis:
    a. Endemic NPC, usually WHO type II or III; 75% of cases
       (1) Found predominantly in the southern provinces of China, Southeast Asia, certain Mediterranean populations, and among the Aleut Native Americans.
       (2) Risk factors include[115] Epstein-Barr virus (EBV), genetic predisposition (HLA class I and II haplotypes),[116,117] environmental factors (food-preserving nitrosamines frequently used in Cantonese salted fish).[118]

(a) The incidence of NPC among North America–born Chinese is significantly lower than among native-born Chinese but still greater than the risk for Caucasians, emphasizing a synergistic role of environmental factors.[119]

(3) Sporadic NPC, WHO type I; 25% cases.

(a) Related to tobacco and alcohol exposure.

3. The role of EBV in NPC:

a. EBV is a double-stranded DNA virus, part of the human herpesvirus family. It establishes persistent, chronic infection, usually in B lymphocytes. Six nuclear proteins (EBNAs)[120] and three membrane proteins (LMPs)[121] are believed to mediate EBV-related carcinogenesis.

b. Prevalence of NPC: EBV-antibodies are acquired earlier in life in tropical rather than in industrialized countries, but by adulthood 90–95% of populations have demonstrable EBV antibodies.[122]

c. Serologic tests may be useful in regions where NPC is prevalent.

(1) May identify occult disease and lead to earlier diagnosis.

(2) IgA antibodies to viral capsid or to the early antigen complex are present in high titers compared to those in matched controls.[123]

(3) Prospective screening detected occult NPC and anticipated recurrences after therapy.[123]

(4) Molecular cytogenetic studies have confirmed that EBV infection is an early, possibly initiating event in the development of nasopharyngeal carcinoma. Clonal EBV DNA was present in premalignant lesions, suggesting that NPC arises from a single EBV-infected cell.[124]

(5) B-cell lymphocytes should serve as the only reservoir of EBV and persistent infection within epithelial cells strongly suggests premalignancy or NPC.[125]

(6) Nasopharyngeal brush biopsy[126] or swab[127] has been advocated for screening and early diagnosis by using polymerase chain reaction (PCR) to detect the EBV genome within nasopharyngeal epithelia. Further studies will be needed to confirm the accuracy and efficacy of this approach.[128]

Diagnosis and Evaluation

1. Peak incidence: fifth and sixth decades of life. However, (20%) of NPC develops in patients under the age of 30. These younger patients tend to have undifferentiated (WHO III) tumors.

2. Few early symptoms develop in NPC. The development of a neck mass (usually level II or V) most often leads to diagnosis and treatment[129] (see Table 26-1).

3. Initially, NPC may grow unnoticed and spread locally to the oropharynx and skull base.

4. Associated cranial neuropathies (especially cranial nerves III–VI) are common. Further extension may involve cranial nerve XII at the hypoglossal foramen or the cervical sympathetic chain, resulting in Horner's syndrome.

5. Jugulodigastric, posterior cervical, and/or retropharyngeal lymphadenopathy is frequently present at the time of diagnosis.

6. Spread to the parotid nodes can occur through the lymphatics of the eustachian tube.

7. Low cervical metastasis (to the lower jugular or supraclavicular chains) was uniformly associated with poor prognosis.[119,130]

TABLE 26-1. PRESENTING SYMPTOMS AND SIGNS OF NASOPHARYNGEAL CARCINOMA, LISTED IN ORDER OF FREQUENCY

1. Neck mass	60%
2. Aural fullness	41%
3. Hearing loss	37%
4. Epistaxis	30%
5. Nasal obstruction	29%
6. Headache, pain	16%
7. Otalgia	14%
8. Neck pain	10%
9. Weight loss	10%
10. Diplopia	8%

From Neel.[129] With permission.

8. Some 87% of patients present with palpable nodal disease and 20% have bilateral metastases.[131]
9. Computed tomography (CT) scan is critical for appropriate staging.
10. Magnetic resonance imaging (MRI) is often needed to assess for intracranial and perineural involvement.
11. For patients with a neck mass and an occult but suspected nasopharyngeal primary tumor, the presence of EBV by DNA amplification is predictive of the development of overt nasopharyngeal carcinoma.[132]
12. Distant metastasis (DM):
    a. Present or develops in 25–30% of patients.
    b. Nasopharynx is the subsite within the head and neck that has the highest rate of DM.[21]
13. Whereas local and regional failure previously accounted for most morbidity and mortality, distant metastasis now is a frequent mode of failure and death.[133,134]

Treatment

1. Radiation therapy
   a. X-ray therapy is the primary treatment modality for nasopharyngeal carcinoma. When properly delivered, external beam therapy can spare adjacent tissues and limit morbidity to the pituitary, eyes, ears, and frontal and temporal lobes. Improved imaging with CT and MRI has permitted better dosimetry and treatment outcomes.
   b. Concurrent administration of chemotherapy has been shown to improve overall survival rates in a recent phase III study performed in the United States.[135] This approach in an Asian population has shown encouraging preliminary results that are comparable to the U.S. data.[136]
   c. Reirradiation (with external beam and interstitial x-ray therapy) may play a role in the treatment of certain recurrent NPCs, especially using conformal intensity-modulated therapy.[137,138]
   d. When delivered through a traditional intracavitary approach, brachytherapy offered little advantage over external beam therapy. A transnasal interstitial implant was developed to deliver a more effective tumoricidal dose.[139]
   e. Wei and colleagues have advocated a transpalatal approach for the placement of gold grain (^{198}Au), the preferred radiation source.[140] The five-year local control rate 80%[141] was achieved when recurrent disease was localized to the nasopharynx without bony invasion.

2. Surgery
   a. Surgical resection of NPC and its metastases is technically difficult if not infeasible due to the architecture and inaccessibility of the anterosuperior skull base and the retropharyngeal lymphatics.[142]
   b. Therefore surgery is reserved for highly selected patients in cases of radiation failure or tumor recurrence.[143,144] Several approaches have been advocated:
      (1) An infratemporal fossa approach, described by Fisch.[145]
      (2) A combined transpalatal, transmaxillary, transcervical approach.[143,146]
      (3) An extended osteoplastic maxillotomy or "maxillary swing."[147,148]
   c. Salvage neck dissection for persistent postradiation lymphadenopathy is well established[149] but may be treacherous. Lateral retropharyngeal nodes may invade the base of the skull and extend medially along the tranverse process of the cervical vertebra. Tumoral involvement of the vertebral or internal carotid artery is not infrequent.

Treatment Outcomes

1. Local and regional control:
   a. Radiation: 60%[150,151]
   b. Radiation with concurrent chemotherapy: 70–80%[135,136]
2. Five-year survival:
   a. Radiation: 36–58%[150,151]
   b. Radiation with concurrent chemotherapy: 70–80%[135,136]
3. Ten-year survival:
   a. The risk of recurrence continues after 5 years.
   b. 10–40%.[133,152,153]

References

1. Parkin DM, Pisani P, Ferlay J. Global cancer statistics. *CA Cancer J Clin* 1999; 49:(1)33–64.
2. Greenlee RT, Hill-Harmon MB, Murray T, Thun M. Cancer statistics, 2001. *CA Cancer J Clin* 2001; 51:15–36.
3. Decker J, Goldstein JC. Risk factors in head and neck cancer. *N Engl J Med* 1982; 306: 1151–1155.
4. Rothman K, Keller A. The effect of joint exposure to alcohol and tobacco on risk of cancer of the mouth and pharynx. *J Chronic Dis* 1972; 25:711–716.
5. Fleming ID, Cooper JS, Henson DE, et al. *AJCC Cancer Staging Manual*. Philadelphia: Lippincott Williams & Wilkins, 1997, 28–43.
6. Piccirillo JF. Importance of comorbidity in head and neck cancer. *Laryngoscope* 2000; 110:593–602.
7. Chen AY, Matson LK, Roberts D, Goepfert H. The significance of comorbidity in advanced laryngeal cancer. *Head Neck* 2001; 23:566–572.
8. Piccirillo JF. Inclusion of comorbidity in a staging system for head and neck cancer. *Oncology (Huntingt)* 1995; 9:831–836; discussion 841, 845–848.
9. van Bokhorst-de van der Schueren MA, van Leeuwen PA, Sauerwein HP, et al. Assessment of malnutrition parameters in head and neck cancer and their relation to postoperative complications. *Head Neck* 1997; 19:419–425.
10. Adjuvant chemotherapy for advanced head and neck squamous carcinoma. Final report of the Head and Neck Contracts Program. *Cancer* 1987; 60:301–311.
11. Johnson JT, Wagner RL, Myers EN. A long-term assessment of adjuvant chemotherapy on outcome of patients with extracapsular spread of cervical metastases from squamous carcinoma of the head and neck. *Cancer* 1996; 77:181–185.
12. Haddadin KJ, Soutar DS, Oliver RJ, et al. Improved survival for patients with clinically

T1/T2, N0 tongue tumors undergoing a prophylactic neck dissection. *Head Neck* 1999; 21:517–525.

13. Yuen AP, Wei WI, Wong YM, Tang KC. Elective neck dissection versus observation in the treatment of early oral tongue carcinoma. *Head Neck* 1997; 19:583–588.

14. Alvi A, Johnson JT. Extracapsular spread in the clinically negative neck (N0): implications and outcome. *Otolaryngol Head Neck Surg* 1996; 114:65–70.

15. Myers JN, Greenberg JS, Mo V, Roberts D. Extracapsular spread. A significant predictor of treatment failure in patients with squamous cell carcinoma of the tongue. *Cancer* 2001; 92(12):3030–6.

16. Jones AS, Morar P, Phillips DE, et al. Second primary tumors in patients with head and neck squamous cell carcinoma. *Cancer* 1995; 75:1343–1453.

17. Hong WK, Lippman SM, Itri LM, et al. Prevention of second primary tumors with isotretinoin in squamous-cell carcinoma of the head and neck. *N Engl J Med* 1990; 323: 795–801.

18. Lippman SM, Batsakis JG, Toth BB, et al. Comparison of low-dose isotretinoin with beta carotene to prevent oral carcinogenesis. *N Engl J Med* 1993; 328:15–20.

18a. Slaughter DP, Southwick HW, Smejkal W. "Field Cancerization" in Oral Stratified Squamous Epithelium: Clinical Implications of Multicentric Origins. *Cancer* 1953; 6:963-968.

19. Brennan JA, Sidransky D. Molecular staging of head and neck squamous carcinoma. *Cancer Metastasis Rev* 1996; 15:3–10.

20. Califano J, van der Riet P, Westra W, et al. Genetic progression model for head and neck cancer: implications for field cancerization. *Cancer Res* 1996; 56:2488–2492.

21. Merino OR, Lindberg RD, Fletcher GH. An analysis of distant metastases from squamous cell carcinoma of the upper respiratory and digestive tracts. *Cancer* 1977; 40:145–151.

22. Smit M, Balm AJ, Hilgers FJ, Tan IB. Pain as sign of recurrent disease in head and neck squamous cell carcinoma. *Head Neck* 2001; 23:372–375.

23. Douglass CW, Gammon MD. Reassessing the epidemiology of lip cancer. *Oral Surg Oral Med Oral Pathol* 1984; 57:631–642.

24. Larrabee WF. *Principles of Facial* Reconstruction. Philadelphia: Lippincott-Raven,1995, 172–173.

25. Byers RM, O'Brien J, Waxler J. The therapeutic and prognostic implications of nerve invasion in cancer of the lower lip. *Int J Radiat Oncol Biol Phys* 1978; 4:215–217.

26. Hoffman HT, Karnell LH, Funk GF, Robinson RA, Menck HR. The National Cancer Data Base report on cancer of the head and neck. *Arch Otolaryngol Head Neck Surg* 1998; 124:951–962.

27. Heller KS, Shah JP. Carcinoma of the lip. *Am J Surg* 1979; 138:600–603.

28. Baker SR, Krause CJ. Carcinoma of the lip. *Laryngoscope* 1980; 90:19–27.

29. Frazell EL, Lucas JC. Cancer of the tongue: report of the management of 1,554 patients. *Cancer* 1962; 15:1085–1099.

30. Mohit-Tabatabai MA, Sobel HJ, Rush BF, Mashberg A. Relation of thickness of floor of mouth stage I and II cancers to regional metastasis. *Am J Surg* 1986; 152:351–353.

31. Scholl P, Byers RM, Batsakis JG, et al. Microscopic cut-through of cancer in the surgical treatment of squamous carcinoma of the tongue. Prognostic and therapeutic implications. *Am J Surg* 1986; 152:354–360.

32. Spiro RH, Huvos AG, Wong GY, et al. Predictive value of tumor thickness in squamous carcinoma confined to the tongue and floor of the mouth. *Am J Surg* 1986; 152:345–350.

33. Ballantyne AJ, McCarten AB, Ibanez ML. The extension of cancer of the head and neck through peripheral nerves. *Am J Surg* 1963; 106:651–667.

34. Fagan JJ, Collins B, Barnes L, et al. Perineural invasion in squamous cell carcinoma of the head and neck. *Arch Otolaryngol Head Neck Surg* 1998; 124:637–640.

35. Myers JN, Elkins T, Roberts D, Byers RM. Squamous cell carcinoma of the tongue in young adults: increasing incidence and factors that predict treatment outcomes. *Otolaryngol Head Neck Surg* 2000; 122:44–51.

36. Sturgis EM, Castillo EJ, Li L, et al. Polymorphisms of DNA repair gene XRCC1 in squamous cell carcinoma of the head and neck. *Carcinogenesis* 1999; 20:2125–2129.

37. Lingen M, Sturgis EM, Kies MS. Squamous cell carcinoma of the head and neck in non-

smokers: clinical and biologic characteristics and implications for management. *Curr Opin Oncol* 2001; 13:176–182.

38. Byers RM, Weber RS, Andrews T, et al. Frequency and therapeutic implications of "skip metastases" in the neck from squamous carcinoma of the oral tongue [see comments]. *Head Neck* 1997; 19:14–19.

39. Weber RS, Ohlms L, Bowman J, et al. Functional results after total or near total glossectomy with laryngeal preservation. *Arch Otolaryngol Head Neck Surg* 1991; 117:512–515.

40. Byers RM. Modified neck dissection. A study of 967 cases from 1970 to 1980. *Am J Surg* 1985; 150:414–421.

41. Johnson JT, Leipzig B, Cummings CW. Management of T1 carcinoma of the anterior aspect of the tongue. *Arch Otolaryngol* 1980; 106:249–251.

42. Lydiatt DD, Robbins KT, Byers RM, Wolf PF. Treatment of stage I and II oral tongue cancer. *Head Neck* 1993; 15:308–312.

43. Spiro JD, Spiro RH, Shah JP, et al. Critical assessment of supraomohyoid neck dissection. *Am J Surg* 1988; 156:286–289.

44. Byers RM, Wolf PF, Ballantyne AJ. Rationale for elective modified neck dissection. *Head Neck Surg* 1988; 10:160–167.

45. Spiro RH, Strong EW. Epidermoid carcinoma of the mobile tongue. Treatment by partial glossectomy alone. *Am J Surg* 1971; 122:707–710.

46. Franceschi D, Gupta R, Spiro RH, Shah JP. Improved survival in the treatment of squamous carcinoma of the oral tongue. *Am J Surg* 1993; 166:360–365.

47. Sessions DG, Spector GJ, Lenox J, et al. Analysis of treatment results for floor-of-mouth cancer. *Laryngoscope* 2000; 110:1764–1772.

48. Rodgers L Jr, Stringer S, Mendenhall W, et al. Management of squamous cell carcinoma of the floor of mouth. *Head Neck* 1993; 15:16–19.

49. Shumrick DA, Quenelle DJ. Malignant disease of the tonsillar region, retromolar trigone and buccal mucosa. *Otolaryngol Clin North Am* 1979; 12:115–120.

50. Byers RM, Anderson B, Schwarz EA, et al. Treatment of squamous carcinoma of the retromolar trigone. *Am J Clin Oncol* 1984; 7:647–652.

51. Kowalski LP, Hashimoto I, Magrin J. End results of 114 extended "commando" operations for retromolar trigone carcinoma. *Am J Surg* 1993; 166:374–379.

52. Byers RM, Newman R, Russell N, Yue A. Results of treatment for squamous carcinoma of the lower gum. *Cancer* 1981; 47:2236–2238.

53. Eicher SA, Overholt SM, el-Naggar AK, et al. Lower gingival carcinoma. Clinical and pathologic determinants of regional metastases. *Arch Otolaryngol Head Neck Surg* 1996; 122:634–638.

54. Overholt SM, Eicher SA, Wolf P, Weber RS. Prognostic factors affecting outcome in lower gingival carcinoma. *Laryngoscope* 1996; 106: 1335–1339.

55. Soo KC, Spiro RH, King W, et al. Squamous carcinoma of the gums. *Am J Surg* 1988; 156:281–285.

56. Evans JF, Shah JP. Epidermoid carcinoma of the hard palate. *Am J Surg* 1981; 142:451–455.

57. Ginsberg LE. Imaging of perineural tumor spread in head and neck cancer. *Semin Ultrasound CT MR* 1999; 20:175–186.

58. Ginsberg LE, DeMonte F. Imaging of perineural tumor spread from palatal carcinoma. *AJNR Am J Neuroradiol* 1998; 19:1417–1422.

59. Chung CK, Johns ME, Cantrell RW, Constable WC. Radiotherapy in the management of primary malignancies of the hard palate. *Laryngoscope* 1980; 90:576–584.

60. Sankaranarayanan R. Oral cancer in India: an epidemiologic and clinical review. *Oral Surg Oral Med Oral Pathol* 1990; 69:325–330.

61. Shear M, Pindborg JJ. Verrucous hyperplasia of the oral mucosa. *Cancer* 1980; 46:1855–1862.

62. Batsakis JG, Hybels R, Crissman JD, Rice DH. The pathology of head and neck tumors: verrucous carcinoma, Part 15. *Head Neck Surg* 1982; 5:29–38.

63. Spiro RH. Verrucous carcinoma, then and now. *Am J Surg* 1998; 176:393–397.

64. Vegers JWM, Snow GB, Van der Waal I. Squamous cell carcinoma of the buccal mucosa. *Arch Otolaryngol Head Neck Surg* 1979; 105:192–195.

65. Mishra RC, Parida G, Mishra TK, Mohanty S. Tumour thickness and relationship to locoregional failure in cancer of the buccal mucosa. *Eur J Surg Oncol* 1999; 25:186–189.

66. Nair MK, Sankaranarayanan R, Padmanabhan TK. Evaluation of the role of radiotherapy in

the management of carcinoma of the buccal mucosa. *Cancer* 1988; 61:1326–1331.

67. Close LG, Brown PM, Vuitch MF, et al. Microvascular invasion and survival in cancer of the oral cavity and oropharynx. *Arch Otolaryngol Head Neck Surg* 1989; 115:1304–1309.

68. Dhawan IK, Verma K, Khazanchi RK. Carcinoma of the buccal mucosa: incidence of regional lymph node involvement. *Indian J Cancer* 1993; 30.

69. Dixit S, Vyas RK, Toparani RB, et al. Surgery versus surgery and postoperative radiotherapy in squamous cell carcinoma of the buccal mucosa: a comparative study. *Ann Surg Oncol* 1998; 5:502–510.

70. Fang FM, Leung SW, Huang CC, et al. Combined-modality therapy for squamous carcinoma of the buccal mucosa: treatment results and prognostic factors. *Head Neck* 1997; 19:506–512.

71. Kroll SS, Evans GR, Goldberg D, et al. A comparison of resource costs for head and neck reconstruction with free and pectoralis major flaps. *Plast Reconstr Surg* 1997; 99: 1282–1286.

72. Diaz EM, Jr, Holsinger FC, Zuniga ER, et al. Squamous Cell Carcinoma of the Buccal Mucosa: One Institution's Experience with 119 Previously Untreated Patients. *Head Neck* 2002. In Press

73. McGuirt WF. Panendoscopy as a screening examination for simultaneous primary tumors in head and neck cancer: a prospective sequential study and review of the literature. *Laryngoscope* 1982; 92:569–5676.

74. Baredes S, Leeman DJ, Chen TS, Mohit-Tabatabai MA. Significance of tumor thickness in soft palate carcinoma. *Laryngoscope* 1993; 103:389–393.

75. Har-El G, Shaha A, Chaudry R, et al. Carcinoma of the uvula and midline soft palate: indication for neck treatment. *Head Neck* 1992; 14:99–101.

76. Thompson LD, Heffner DK. The clinical importance of cystic squamous cell carcinomas in the neck: a study of 136 cases. *Cancer* 1998; 82:944–956.

77. Gourin CG, Johnson JT. Incidence of unsuspected metastases in lateral cervical cysts. *Laryngoscope* 2000; 110:1637–1641.

78. Gillison ML, Koch WM, Capone RB, et al. Evidence for a causal association between human papillomavirus and a subset of head and neck cancers. *J Natl Cancer Inst* 2000; 92:709–720.

79. Mork J, Lie AK, Glattre E, et al. Human papillomavirus infection as a risk factor for squamous-cell carcinoma of the head and neck. *N Engl J Med* 2001; 344:1125–1131.

80. Ang KK, Peters LJ, Weber RS, et al. Concomitant boost radiotherapy schedules in the treatment of carcinoma of the oropharynx and nasopharynx. *Int J Radiat Oncol Biol Phys* 1990; 19:1339–1345.

81. Urban SG, Forastiere AA, Wolf GT, et al. Intensive induction chemotherapy and radiation for organ preservation in patients with advanced resectable head and neck carcinoma. *J Clin Oncol* 1994; 12:946–953.

82. Koch WM, Lee DJ, Eisele DW, et al. Chemoradiotherapy for organ preservation in oral and pharyngeal carcinoma. *Arch Otolaryngol Head Neck Surg* 1995; 121:974–980.

83. Calais G, Alfonsi M, Bardet E, et al. Randomized trial of radiation therapy versus concomitant chemotherapy and radiation therapy for advanced-stage oropharynx carcinoma. *J Natl Cancer Inst* 1999; 91:2081–2086.

84. Vokes EE, Kies MS, Haraf DJ, et al. Concomitant chemoradiotherapy as primary therapy for locoregionally advanced head and neck cancer. *J Clin Oncol* 2000; 18:1652–1661.

85. Kies MS, Haraf DJ, Rosen F, et al. Concomitant infusional paclitaxel and fluorouracil, oral hydroxyurea, and hyperfractionated radiation for locally advanced squamous head and neck cancer. *J Clin Oncol* 2001; 19: 1961–1969.

86. Gwozdz JT, Morrison WH, Garden AS, et al. Concomitant boost radiotherapy for squamous carcinoma of the tonsillar fossa. *Int J Radiat Oncol Biol Phys* 1997; 39:127–135.

87. Brizel DM, Albers ME, Fisher SR, et al. Hyperfractionated irradiation with or without concurrent chemotherapy for locally advanced head and neck cancer. *N Engl J Med* 1998; 338:1798–1804.

88. Clayman GL, Johnson CJ II, Morrison W, Set al. The role of neck dissection after chemoradiotherapy for oropharyngeal cancer with

advanced nodal disease. *Arch Otolaryngol Head Neck Surg* 2001; 127:135–139.

89. Peters LJ, Weber RS, Morrison WH, et al. Neck surgery in patients with primary oropharyngeal cancer treated by radiotherapy. *Head Neck* 1996; 18:552–559.

90. Weber RS, Peters LJ, Wolf P, Guillamondegui O. Squamous cell carcinoma of the soft palate, uvula, and anterior faucial pillar. *Otolaryngol Head Neck Surg* 1988; 99:16–23.

91. Lee HJ, Zelefsky MJ, Kraus DH, et al. Long-term regional control after radiation therapy and neck dissection for base of tongue carcinoma. *Int J Radiat Oncol Biol Phys* 1997; 38:995–1000.

92. Biacabe B, Gleich LL, Laccourreye O, et al. Silent gastroesophageal reflux disease in patients with pharyngolaryngeal cancer: further results. *Head Neck* 1998; 20:510–514.

93. Larsson LG, Sandstrom A, Westling P. Relationship of Plummer-Vinson disease to cancer of the upper alimentary tract in Sweden. *Cancer Res* 1975; 35:3308–3316.

94. Thawley SE, Panje WR, Batsakis JG, Lindberg RD. *Comprehensive Management of Head and Neck Tumors*. Vol. 1. Philadelphia: Saunders, 1999, 944–945.

95. Ogura JH, Biller HF, Wette R. Elective neck dissection for pharyngeal and laryngeal cancers. An evaluation. *Ann Otol Rhinol Laryngol* 1971; 80:646–650.

96. Razack MS, Sako K, Kalnins I. Squamous cell carcinoma of the pyriform sinus. Head Neck Surg 1978; 1:31–4.

97. Spector JG, Sessions DG, Emami B, et al. Squamous cell carcinoma of the pyriform sinus: a nonrandomized comparison of therapeutic modalities and long-term results. *Laryngoscope* 1995; 105:397–406.

98. Johnson JT, Bacon GW, Myers EN, Wagner RL. Medial vs lateral wall pyriform sinus carcinoma: implications for management of regional lymphatics. *Head Neck* 1994; 16:401–405.

99. Harrison DF. Surgical management of hypopharyngeal cancer. Particular reference to the gastric "pull-up" operation. *Arch Otolaryngol* 1979; 105:149–152.

100. Ho CM, Ng WF, Lam KH, et al. Submucosal tumor extension in hypopharyngeal cancer. *Arch Otolaryngol* 1997; 123:959–965.

101. Fein DA, Mendenhall WM, Parsons JT, et al. Pharyngeal wall carcinoma treated with radiotherapy: impact of treatment technique and fractionation. *Int J Radiat Oncol Biol Phys* 1993; 26:751–757.

102. Garden AS, Morrison WH, Clayman GL, et al. Early squamous cell carcinoma of the hypopharynx: outcomes of treatment with radiation alone to the primary disease. *Head Neck* 1996; 18:317–322.

103. Vandenbrouck C, Eschwege F, De la Rochefordiere A, et al. Squamous cell carcinoma of the pyriform sinus: retrospective study of 351 cases treated at the Institut Gustave-Roussy. *Head Neck Surg* 1987; 10:4–13.

104. El Badawi SA, Goepfert H, Fletcher GH, et al. Squamous cell carcinoma of the pyriform sinus. *Laryngoscope* 1982; 92:357–364.

105. Spiro RH, Kelly J, Vega AL, et al. Squamous carcinoma of the posterior pharyngeal wall. *Am J Surg* 1990; 160:420–423.

106. Stell PM, Ramadan MF, Dalby JE, et al. Management of post-cricoid carcinoma. *Clin Otolaryngol* 1982; 7:145–152.

107. Ogura JH, Jurema AA, Watson RK. Partial laryngopharyngectomy and neck dissection for pyriform sinus cancer. *Laryngoscope* 1960; 70:1399–1417.

108. Laccourreye H, Lacau St Guily J, Brasnu D, et al. Supracricoid hemilaryngopharyngectomy. Analysis of 240 cases. *Ann Otol Rhinol Laryngol* 1987; 96:217–221.

109. McKee DM, Peters CR. Reconstruction of the hypopharynx and cervical esophagus with microvascular jejunal transplant. *Clin Plast Surg* 1978; 5:305–312.

110. Bradford CR, Esclamado RM, Carroll WR, Sullivan MJ. Analysis of recurrence, complications, and functional results with free jejunal flaps. *Head Neck* 1994; 16:149–154.

111. Price JC, Jansen CJ, Johns ME. Esophageal reflux and secondary malignant neoplasia at laryngoesophagectomy. *Arch Otolaryngol Head Neck Surg* 1990; 116:163–164.

112. Meoz-Mendez RT, Fletcher GH, Guillamondegui OM, Peters LJ. Analysis of the results of irradiation in the treatment of squamous cell carcinomas of the pharyngeal walls. *Int J Radiat Oncol Biol Phys* 1978; 4:579–585.

113. Spector JG, Sessions DG, Haughey BH, et al. Delayed regional metastases, distant metastases,

and second primary malignancies in squamous cell carcinomas of the larynx and hypopharynx. *Laryngoscope* 2001; 111:1079–1087.

114. Martin SA, Marks JE, Lee JY, et al. Carcinoma of the pyriform sinus: predictors of TNM relapse and survival. *Cancer* 1980; 46: 1974–1981.

115. Henderson BE, Louie E, SooHoo Jing J, et al. Risk factors associated with nasopharyngeal carcinoma. *N Engl J Med* 1976; 295:1101–1106.

116. Simons MJ, Wee GB, Goh EH, et al. Immunogenetic aspects of nasopharyngeal carcinoma. IV. Increased risk in Chinese of nasopharyngeal carcinoma associated with a Chinese-related HLA profile (A2, Singapore 2). *J Natl Cancer Inst* 1976; 57:977–980.

117. Chan SH, Day NE, Kunaratnam N, et al. HLA and nasopharyngeal carcinoma in Chinese—a further study. *Int J Cancer* 1983; 32:171–176.

118. Ho JH, Huang DP, Fong YY. Salted fish and nasopharyngeal carcinoma in southern Chinese. *Lancet* 1978; 2:626.

119. Dickson RI. Nasopharyngeal carcinoma: an evaluation of 209 patients. *Laryngoscope* 1981; 91:333–354.

120. Huang DP, Ho HC, Henle W, et al. Presence of EBNA in nasopharyngeal carcinoma and control patient tissues related to EBV serology. *Int J Cancer* 1978; 22:266–274.

121. Fahraeus R, Rymo L, Rhim JS, Klein G. Morphological transformation of human keratinocytes expressing the LMP gene of Epstein-Barr virus. *Nature* 1990; 345:447–449.

122. Porter DD, Wimberly I, Benyesh-Melnick M. Prevalence of antibodies to EB virus and other herpesviruses. *JAMA* 1969; 208:1675–1679.

123. Zeng Y, Zhang LG, Wu YC, et al. Prospective studies on nasopharyngeal carcinoma in Epstein-Barr virus IgA/VCA antibody-positive persons in Wuzhou City, China. *Int J Cancer* 1985; 36:545–547.

124. Pathmanathan R, Prasad U, Sadler R, et al. Clonal proliferations of cells infected with Epstein-Barr virus in preinvasive lesions related to nasopharyngeal carcinoma. *N Engl J Med* 1995; 333:693–698.

125. Niedobitek G, Young LS. Epstein-Barr virus persistence and virus-associated tumours. *Lancet* 1994; 343:333–335.

126. Tune CE, Liavaag PG, Freeman JL, et al. Nasopharyngeal brush biopsies and detection of nasopharyngeal cancer in a high-risk population. *J Natl Cancer Inst* 1999; 91:796–800.

127. Sheen TS, Ko JY, Chang YL, et al. Nasopharyngeal swab and PCR for the screening of nasopharyngeal carcinoma in the endemic area: a good supplement to the serologic screening. *Head Neck* 1998; 20:732–738.

128. Chang AR, Liang XM, Chan AT, et al. The use of brush cytology and directed biopsies for the detection of nasopharyngeal carcinoma and precursor lesions. *Head Neck* 2001; 23:637–645.

129. Neel HB III. Nasopharyngeal carcinoma. Clinical presentation, diagnosis, treatment, and prognosis. *Otolaryngol Clin North Am* 1985; 18:479–490.

130. Scanlon PW, Rhodes RE Jr, Woolner LB, et al. Cancer of the nasopharynx: 142 patients treated in the 11 year period 1950–1960. *Am J Roentgenol Radium Ther Nucl Med* 1967; 99:313–325.

131. Lindberg R. Distribution of cervical lymph node metastases from squamous cell carcinoma of the upper respiratory and digestive tracts. *Cancer* 1972; 29:1446–1449.

132. Feinmesser R, Miyazaki I, Cheung R, et al. Diagnosis of nasopharyngeal carcinoma by DNA amplification of tissue obtained by fine-needle aspiration. *N Engl J Med* 1992; 326: 17–21.

133. Lee AW, Poon YF, Foo W, et al. Retrospective analysis of 5037 patients with nasopharyngeal carcinoma treated during 1976–1985: overall survival and patterns of failure. *Int J Radiat Oncol Biol Phys* 1992; 23:261–270.

134. Cheng SH, Yen KL, Jian JJ, et al. Examining prognostic factors and patterns of failure in nasopharyngeal carcinoma following concomitant radiotherapy and chemotherapy: impact on future clinical trials. *Int J Radiat Oncol Biol Phys* 2001; 50:717–726.

135. Al-Sarraf M, LeBlanc M, Giri PG, et al. Chemoradiotherapy versus radiotherapy in patients with advanced nasopharyngeal cancer: phase III randomized Intergroup study 0099. *J Clin Oncol* 1998; 16:1310–1317.

136. Cheng SH, Jian JJ, Tsai SY, et al. Long-term survival of nasopharyngeal carcinoma following concomitant radiotherapy and chemotherapy. *Int J Radiat Oncol Biol Phys* 2000; 48:1323–3130.

137. Wang CC. Re-irradiation of recurrent nasopharyngeal carcinoma—treatment techniques and results. *Int J Radiat Oncol Biol Phys* 1987; 13:953–956.

138. Dawson LA, Myers LL, Bradford CR, et al. Conformal re-irradiation of recurrent and new primary head-and-neck cancer. *Int J Radiat Oncol Biol Phys* 2001; 50:377–385.

139. Vikram B, Hilaris B. Transnasal permanent interstitial implantation for carcinoma of the nasopharynx. *Int J Radiat Oncol Biol Phys* 1984; 10:153–155.

140. Wei WI, Sham JS, Choy D, et al. Split-palate approach for gold grain implantation in nasopharyngeal carcinoma. *Arch Otolaryngol Head Neck Surg* 1990; 116:578–582.

141. Choy D, Sham JS, Wei WI, et al. Transpalatal insertion of radioactive gold grain for the treatment of persistent and recurrent nasopharyngeal carcinoma. *Int J Radiat Oncol Biol Phys* 1993; 25:505–512.

142. Lederman M. *Cancer of the Nasopharynx: Its Natural History and Treatment.* Springfield, IL: Charles C Thomas, 1961.

143. Fee WE, Jr. Surgical resection for recurrent nasopharynx cancer. *Cancer Treat Res* 1990; 52:55–59.

144. Hsu MM, Ko JY, Sheen TS, Chang YL. Salvage surgery for recurrent nasopharyngeal carcinoma. *Arch Otolaryngol Head Neck Surg* 1997; 123:305–309.

145. Fisch U. The infratemporal fossa approach for nasopharyngeal tumors. *Laryngoscope* 1983; 93:36–44.

146. Fee WE Jr, Gilmer PA, Goffinet DR. Surgical management of recurrent nasopharyngeal carcinoma after radiation failure at the primary site. *Laryngoscope* 1988; 98: 1220–1226.

147. Wei WI, Lam KH, Sham JS. New approach to the nasopharynx: the maxillary swing approach. *Head Neck* 1991; 13:200–207.

148. Catalano PJ, Biller HF. Extended osteoplastic maxillotomy. A versatile new procedure for wide access to the central skull base and infratemporal fossa. *Arch Otolaryngol Head Neck Surg* 1993; 119:394–400.

149. Yen KL, Hsu LP, Sheen TS, et al. Salvage neck dissection for cervical recurrence of nasopharyngeal carcinoma. *Arch Otolaryngol Head Neck Surg* 1997; 123:725–729.

150. Chu AM, Flynn MB, Achino E, et al. Irradiation of nasopharyngeal carcinoma: correlations with treatment factors and stage. *Int J Radiat Oncol Biol Phys* 1984;10: 2241–2249.

151. Bailet JW, Mark RJ, Abemayor E, et al. Nasopharyngeal carcinoma: treatment results with primary radiation therapy. *Laryngoscope* 1992; 102:965–972.

152. Perez CA, Devineni VR, Marcial-Vega V, et al. Carcinoma of the nasopharynx: factors affecting prognosis. *Int J Radiat Oncol Biol Phys* 1992; 23:271–280.

153. Fandi A, Bachouchi M, Azli N, et al. Long-term disease-free survivors in metastatic undifferentiated carcinoma of nasopharyngeal type. *J Clin Oncol* 2000; 18:1324–1330.

Cancer of the Larynx, Paranasal Sinuses, and Temporal Bone

27

CANCER OF THE LARYNX

Epidemiology and Pathology

Laryngeal cancer accounts for about 1% of all new cancers diagnosed in the United States and approximately 0.75% of all cancer deaths.[1] Over 90% are squamous cell carcinoma (SCC), and these account for about 30% of all head and neck cancers. The highest incidence occurs in the seventh decade and an estimated 10,000 new cases are diagnosed in the United States per year. Predominantly a disease of men, with a male:female ratio of 5:1, there has been a small but significant fall in the incidence recently, particularly in men.[1] While SCC is the most common cancer, all cell types in the larynx can give rise to malignancy, including adenocarcinoma, minor salivary gland tumors, carcinoid, oat cell carcinoma, and undifferentiated carcinoma.

Etiology

The mutagenic effects of tobacco, especially in cigarette smoke, are the most important etiologic agents. There is a linear relationship between the number of cigarettes smoked and the risk of developing laryngeal SCC.[2] All types of alcohol consumption are associated with an increased relative risk (2.2-fold) compared to that of nondrinkers, with a particular predilection to the development of supraglottic cancers.[3,4] Combined smoking and alcohol abuse increases the laryngeal cancer risk by 50% over the expected additive rate. Carcinogenic influences from a number of environmental factors—including radiation, asbestos, wood dust, mustard gas, and refinery products—have been identified.[5]

Anatomy

The larynx can be divided into supraglottic, glottic, and subglottic sites, and within each site are a number of subsites as stipulated by the International Union Against Cancer (UICC)[6] (Table 27-1). The supraglottis is separated from the glottis by a horizontal line drawn through the ventricles and the glottis from the subglottis by a line 1 cm below the free edge of the vocal cords. The subglottis extends inferiorly from this line to the lower border of the cricoid cartilage. The junction between the glottis and subglottis is ill defined; other authors have suggested it should be marked by the histologic junction of the squamous epithelium with the respiratory epithelium located about 5 mm below the free edge of the vocal cords.

A number of potential spaces or compartments surround the larynx and are vital to an understanding of the pattern of tumor spread. The pre-epiglottic space is bounded superiorly

596

TABLE 27-1. ANATOMIC SITES AND SUBSITES OF THE LARYNX (UICC)[6]

1. Supraglottis
   a. Suprahyoid epiglottis [including tip, lingual (anterior) and laryngeal surfaces]
   b. Aryepiglottic fold, laryngeal aspect
   c. Arytenoid
   d. Infrahyoid epiglottis
   e. Ventricular bands (false cords)
2. Glottis
   a. Vocal cords
   b. Anterior commisure
   c. Posterior commisure
3. Subglottis

by the hyoepiglottic ligament and the vallecula mucosa, anteriorly by the thyrohyoid ligaments, and posteriorly by the epiglottis and thyroepiglottic ligament (Figure 27-1). The epiglottic cartilage contains numerous perforations through which tumor can spread easily from its posterior surface to the space. The paraglottic space, or potential space, lies outside of the laryngeal inlet deep to the mucosa. Its lateral relation is the thyroid cartilage anteriorly and the mucosa over the medial wall of the piriform sinus posteriorly (Figure 27-2). The quadrangular membrane lies medially above and the conus elasticus lies inferiorly. This space is contiguous with the pre-epiglottic space superiorly and anteriorly, and tumor can readily spread outside the larynx from the paraglottic space inferolaterally between the

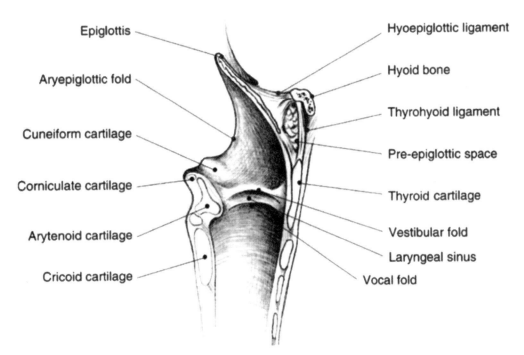

Figure 27-1. Sagittal section of the larynx demonstrating anatomic divisions of the larynx.

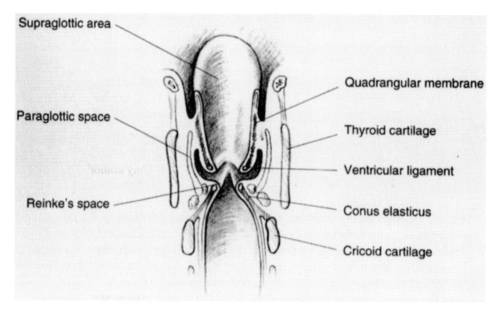

Figure 27-2.   Coronal section of the larynx illustrating barriers to the spread of carcinoma.

thyroid cartilage and cricoid cartilages. Reinke's space lies immediately below the epithelium of the vocal cord, superficial to the thyroarytenoid muscle, and is bounded superiorly and inferiorly by the junction of columnar and squamous epithelium.

Spread of Tumor

Supraglottic carcinomas most frequently arise in the central infrahyoid epiglottis and typically spread anteriorly through the fenestra of the epiglottis to reach the pre-epiglottic space, vallecula, and tongue base. Lateral extension will involve the piriform fossa and later the postcricoid region with resulting dyspnea. Deep invasion involves the paraglottic space allowing spread superiorly and inferiorly. Less commonly, inferior mucosal extension will involve the ventricle or the vocal cords. The term *transglottic* is given to a tumor from one laryngeal region that crosses the glottis in continuity with another region. The lesion, by definition, must have invaded the paraglottic space and is associated with a high incidence of cartilage invasion and cervical node metastases. Supraglottic cancers have a propensity to spread bilaterally to cervical zones II and III due to the rich lymphatic supply draining through the thyrohyoid membrane and along the superior thyroid vessels. Generally the risk of occult or actual metastases from supraglottic cancer with T_1, T_2, T_3, and T_4 tumors is 20, 40, 60, and 80% respectively.

Glottic SCC has a predilection for the anterior half of the true vocal cord and can spread to Reinke's space, where it extends anteriorly and posteriorly along the vocal cord. Deep invasion results in involvement of the vocalis muscle and the paraglottic space, causing decreased glottic mobility. Posterior extension to the arytenoid and cricoarytenoid joint will further limit cord mobility. The glottic larynx is virtually devoid of lymphatics, and consequently less than 8% of patients with T_1 and T_2 carcinoma will have nodal involvement, compared to 20 to 40% with more advanced glottic tumors. The insertion of the vocalis tendon into the thyroid cartilage, an area known as Broyle's ligament, permits tumor invasion of cartilage at this site. The Delphian node is a primary route of regional spread from the glottis and drains to paratracheal nodes and then to the superior mediastinum.

Subglottic carcinomas spread superiorly to involve the glottis and laterally to involve surrounding structures such as the thyroid. They tend to spread to paratracheal lymphatics and then to superior mediastinal nodes.

Symptoms and Signs

The history should record the duration and progression of symptoms with details of smoking and alcohol intake plus exposure to other carcinogens. Any comorbidity, particularly pulmonary or cardiovascular, and associated medications should be documented. A detailed head and neck examination, including either indirect or fiberoptic laryngoscopy, will reveal the site and extent of the lesion and document impairment of cord mobility. The examination should assess the dental status and evaluate the airway. Careful palpation of the neck will detect direct extension of the tumor through the laryngeal framework, fixation of the larynx, and splaying of the thyroid cartilage. The size, mobility, and relationship of any enlarged lymph nodes in the neck are recorded. The clinical presentation and patterns of spread of carcinoma are dictated by the anatomic location of the lesion.

In North America, approximately 30% of laryngeal carcinomas arise in the supraglottis. The signs and symptoms of supraglottic carcinoma in the early stages of the disease are nonspecific and two-thirds are not diagnosed until an advanced stage. Initially, pharyngeal discomfort or pain and varying degrees of dysphagia are the presenting features. Later bulky, exophytic tumor growth or transglottic spread may cause hoarseness, dyspnea, and stridor. A neck mass may be the presenting complaint due to metastases or direct tumor extension. Odynophagia and unilateral otalgia are acknowledged as more advanced symptoms; aspiration is not uncommon at this stage due to an incompetent supraglottic valve mechanism.

Glottic carcinomas, which constitute 50 to 70% of laryngeal cancers, are frequently associated with hoarseness in the early stages of the disease due to an alteration in the mass, shape, and mobility of the involved cord. Airway obstruction and dyspnea represent late features.

Early subglottic carcinoma may cause vague throat discomfort or be asymptomatic. Hoarseness is due to superior extension to the vocal cord or recurrent laryngeal nerve involvement. Often, dyspnea or hemoptysis are the first symptoms that bring the patient to seek medical attention.

Investigation

All patients must undergo endoscopy to confirm the diagnosis by biopsy, determine the extent of the primary carcinoma, and exclude a synchronous primary carcinoma. A representative nonnecrotic area of the lesion should be submitted for pathologic analysis. When attempting to confirm recurrent disease after radiotherapy, it is important to realize that the tumor may be entirely submucosal. The value of formal panendoscopy under general anesthesia has been questioned recently, as many lesions can be biopsied in the office under direct vision or with flexible endoscopes, and the number of second primaries and metastases not picked up on general examination, flexible endoscopy, and radiology is very low.[7] In a selected group of patients with laryngeal carcinoma formal panendoscopy may be justified, as palpation of the cricoarytenoid joint will allow a distinction to be made between direct involvement of the cricoarytenoid joint, impairment due to recurrent laryngeal nerve invasion, or extensive tumor infiltration of the vocalis muscle and paraglottic space. Sites such as the ventricles, subglottis, postcricoid region, vallecula, and piriform fossa can also be inspected, since they may harbor occult disease.

All patients must have a chest x-ray to exclude metastases, intercurrent pulmonary disease, or a synchronous lung primary. Computed tomography (CT) scanning of the chest in patients with advanced disease may help in the detection of smaller lesions.[8] If partial laryngeal surgery is considered, pulmonary function tests are required preoperatively. Imaging of the larynx with CT scans or magnetic resonance imaging (MRI) will reveal the extent of the tumor, airway patency, cartilage involvement, subglottic extension, pre-epiglottic and paraglottic space involvement, and extension to the hypopharynx. Tongue base invasion, retrocricoid invasion, extralaryngeal spread, and nodal involvement can be demonstrated effectively with CT or MRI, but MRI may be more sensitive than CT to cartilage invasion. Fine needle aspiration cytology will aid in the assessment of suspected regional metastases.

Once the clinical and radiologic information is complete, the tumor is staged according to the UICC or American Joint Committee on Cancer (AJCC) criteria[6] (Table 27-2).

Management

The approach to the management of any patient with laryngeal cancer must consider the patient's age, general condition, personal preferences, the institutional facilities available for treatment, and the location and stage of the tumor. A decision is best made following a multidisciplinary assessment with radiation oncology, speech pathology, radiology, pathology, social services, nursing, medical oncology, and anesthesiology where appropriate.

Early Laryngeal Carcinoma ($T_{1/2}$)

Early laryngeal carcinoma (T_1/T_2) is usually managed with a single modality of treatment and responds well to radiation, transoral laser resection, or partial laryngeal surgery. Primary cure rates of 80 to 85% are expected, and with the addition of second-line treatment, over 90% of patients are cured[9,10] (Tables 27-3 and 27-4). The choice between the modalities depends upon the facilities and skills available at the institution in which the patient is being treated and on patient preference.

Radiation for early glottic or supraglottic laryngeal carcinoma is usually a dose of 50 to 70Gy over 5 to 8 weeks, although the final dose and configuration vary with the extent of the tumor and cord mobility. Its advantages include the lack of surgical morbidity, absence of hospitalization, and good voice quality after completion of treatment, although the voice never completely returns to normal.[11] All patients suffer the acute mucositis and pharyngitis that accompany this treatment, both of which restrict activity during the latter part of treatment. Possible complications include chondronecrosis and laryngeal edema in the long-term laryngeal stenosis and occasionally induction of new tumors. The detection of recurrence after radiation can be difficult. Once recurrence is established, however, it is usually managed by partial or total laryngectomy, although endoscopic transoral resection has recently been described.[12]

Transoral laser resection using suspension microlaryngoscopy is rapidly gaining popularity for early laryngeal cancer, particularly in Europe, where it has been used for some time. The tumor is carefully dissected from the larynx under frozen section control. Local control rates are reported to be about 85% for T_1/T_2 glottic and supraglottic lesions,[13,14] and

TABLE 27-2. UICC TNM STAGING AND STAGE GROUPINGS FOR LARYNGEAL CARCINOMA[6]

Supraglottis

T_1	Tumor limited to one subsite of supraglottis with normal vocal cord mobility
T_2	Tumor invades mucosa of more than one adjacent region outside the supraglottis (eg, mucosa of base of tongue, vallecula, medial wall of piriform sinus) without fixation of the larynx
T_3	Tumor limited to larynx with vocal cord fixation and/or invades any of the following: postcricoid area, pre-epiglottic tissue, deep base of tongue
T_4	Tumor invades through thyroid cartilage and/or extends into soft tissue of the neck, thyroid and/or esophagus

Glottis

T_1	Tumor limited to vocal cord(s) (may involve anterior or posterior commisure) with normal mobility
T_{1a}	Tumor limited to one vocal cord
T_{1b}	Tumor involves both vocal cords
T_2	Tumor extends to supraglottis and/or subglottis and/or with impaired vocal cord mobility
T_3	Tumor limited to larynx with vocal cord fixation
T_4	Tumor invades through thyroid cartilage and/or extends to other tissue beyond the larynx—eg, trachea, soft tissue of the neck, thyroid, pharynx

Subglottis

T_1	Tumor limited to subglottis
T_2	Tumor extends to vocal cord(s) with normal or impaired mobility
T_3	Tumor limited to larynx with vocal cord fixation
T_4	Tumor invades through cricoid or thyroid cartilage and/or extends into other tissue beyond the larynx—eg, trachea, soft tissue of the neck, thyroid, esophagus

N stage

N_x	Regional lymph nodes cannot be assessed
N_0	No regional metastases
N_1	Metastases in a single ipsilateral lymph node, 3 cm or less in greatest dimension
N_{2a}	Metastases in a single ipsilateral lymph node, more than 3 cm but not more than 6 cm in greatest dimension
N_{2b}	Metastases in multiple ipsilateral lymph nodes, none more than 6 cm in greatest dimension
N_{2c}	Metastases in bilateral or contralateral lymph nodes, none more than 6 cm in greatest dimension
N_3	Metastases in a lymph node more than 6 cm in greatest dimension

M stage

M_x	Distant metastases cannot be assessed
M_0	No distant metastases
M_1	Distant metastases

Stage groupings

Stage 0	Tis	N_0	M_0
Stage I	T_1	N_0	M_0
Stage II	T_2	N_0	M_0
Stage III	T_1, T_2	N_1	M_0
	T_3	N_0, N_1	M_0
Stage IVA	T_4	N_0, N_1	M_0
	Any T	N_2	M_0
Stage IVB	Any T	N_3	M_0
Stage IVC	Any T	Any N	M_1

with salvage surgery or radiation, overall control is much higher. Its advantages include a single visit for treatment, a short hospital stay, and a rapid return to work. As radiation is not used in most of the early cases, this can be reserved for salvage should local control not be achieved. Disadvantages include the need for technical expertise in the operative technique and a relatively long operative time for each case. There is some operative morbidity, although this has been reported to be minimal.

TABLE 27-3. FIVE-YEAR SURVIVAL OF LARYNGEAL CARCINOMA IN RELATION TO TREATMENT MODALITY

Tumor	5-Year Survival %	
	Radiation and Surgical Salvage	Surgery
Glottic		
T_1	93	90
T_2	85	75
T_3	66	55
T_4	50	34
Supraglottic		
T_1	90	71
T_2	81	62
T_3	64	55
T_4	50	25
Subglottic		
T_1–T_4	36	42

Partial laryngeal surgery has been used as a primary modality for early laryngeal carcinoma for many years with excellent results,[15] but its failure to be widely adopted reflects the degree of patient selection and technical expertise that is required to obtain these results. Patient must be selected carefully for partial laryngeal surgery and must have good pulmonary and cardiac function (Table 27-5).

For glottic carcinoma, vertical partial laryngectomy is the operation of choice. Options include laryngofissure with cordectomy, hemilaryngectomy, extended or frontolateral vertical partial laryngectomy, and near-total laryngectomy.[16] As techniques for reconstruction of the larynx improve, the amount of tissue that can be resected while preserving the function of the larynx has increased.[17] Advances in surgical technique and reconstruction combined with an improved understanding of the routes of laryngeal cancer spread have facilitated this progress.[18]

Supraglottic laryngectomy can be considered when the tumor is limited to the supraglottis and not involving the anterior commisure. Some larger T_3 lesions and those extending to the piriform sinus or pre-epiglottic space can be resected with this technique as long as vocal cord mobility remains normal. Involvement of the arytenoid will necessitate its removal, with the increased risk of aspiration. Contraindications to this supraglottic laryngectomy include vocal cord fixation, interarytenoid involvement, and thyroid cartilage invasion.

TABLE 27-4. FIVE-YEAR SURVIVAL BY 1972 TNM CLASSIFICATION

Tumor	5-Year Survival %							
					N_3		N_4	
	N_0 Glottic	N_{1a} Supra	N_{1b} Glottic	N_{2b} Supra	Glottic	Supraglottic	Glottic	Supraglottic
T_{1a}	94	86	61	65	100 (1 case)	45		—
T_{1b}	93	94	—	—	—	—	—	—
T_2	85	82	62	45	—	20	—	0 (1 case)
T_3	65	76	53	36	0 (4 cases)	20	—	—
T_4	40	55	37	40	10	8	0 (2 cases)	—

TABLE 27-5. EXTERNAL LARYNGEAL SURGERY: INDICATION AND CONTRAINDICATION FOR GLOTTIC CANCER

Indications
T_1, T_2, and small T_3 lesions
    Limited to one vocal cord or not more than 5 mm of the contralateral cord
    Inferior extension not exceeding 12–15 mm at the anterior commisure (10 mm in radiation salvage cases)
        and/or 5 mm at the vocal process of the arytenoid
    Superior extension not exceeding the free edge of the false cord (lateral wall of ventricle in radiation salvage cases)

Contraindications
Large T_3 or any T_4 lesions
    Interarytenoid or cricoarytenoid joint involvement
    Bilateral arytenoid involvement or diminished mobility of both vocal cords
    Thyroid cartilage invasion
    Supraglottic or subglottic extensions exceeding those listed above
    Poor pulmonary reserve or medical contraindications

When the anterior commisure is involved in supraglottic or glottic carcinoma, supracricoid laryngectomy can be considered. This involves resection of the larynx above the cricoid with preservation of one of the arytenoids. Recent studies describe a 5-year survival of 87% and 98 to 100% local control, with laryngeal preservation for selected lesions.[19] The risk of significant complications such as aspiration or permanent tracheotomies is low.

Partial laryngeal surgery has many of the advantages of transoral laser resection, including precise tumor margin control, but the hospital stay is longer and operative morbidity and potential complications are higher (eg, aspiration, tracheostomy dependence, fistula, stenosis). Vocal function is good in successful cases and radiation can be reserved for salvage should local control not be achieved. When surgery is the first line of management, postoperative radiation is recommended for microscopically positive margins, intralymphatic or perineural invasion, multiple positive nodes, or extracapsular nodal spread of tumor.

There is no indication for neck dissection in patients with T_1N_0 or T_2N_0 glottic carcinoma, but with supraglottic carcinoma bilateral anterolateral selective neck dissections are indicated (levels II, III, IV) for the N_0 neck and modified radical or radical neck dissection performed for N+ disease. When the patient is treated with primary radiation, the neck is included in fields for supraglottic carcinoma or limited N+ disease. For larger N+ disease, planned neck dissection before or after radiation can be performed.

Advanced Laryngeal Carcinoma ($T_{3/4}$)
The optimum management of advanced laryngeal carcinoma is more controversial. The aim is to optimize disease-free and overall survival while preserving quality of life. Practices vary widely between countries and even centers in the same country. Generally, combined therapy is widely used, as it shows better survival rates than single-modality treatment in patients with advanced neck disease and advanced primary cancers (Table 27-3). The options include radiotherapy and conservative or radical surgery for salvage, chemoradiation and surgical salvage, radical surgery preceded or followed by radiotherapy. Currently the trend is toward laryngeal preservation, as studies have indicated that patients wish to preserve some laryngeal function and therefore improve quality of life, even though survival may be slightly compromised.

RADIATION WITH SURGICAL SALVAGE The main advantage of nonsurgical management of advanced laryngeal cancer is preservation of the voice provided that sufficient functional larynx is present after completion of therapy, as large tumors may destroy the laryngeal framework, leaving the patient with a nonfunctioning larynx despite a complete response to treatment. About 50% of patients will achieve local control of their disease with primary radiation of the larynx for T_3/T_4 disease. About half of those failing will be salvaged with total laryngectomy, and overall survival including those dying of other causes is about 55% at 5 years.[20-22] The need for a tracheostomy prior to treatment for advanced laryngeal carcinoma is a poor prognostic sign, but laryngeal preservation is possible in over 40% using a policy of primary radiation.[23] Epidemiologic studies of regions within North America confirm that radiotherapy with surgical salvage results in much the same overall survival when compared to primary surgery, and radiation has the significant advantage of laryngeal preservation.[24] Changes in standard radiation protocols may improve the possibility of preserving the larynx. Accelerated hyperfractionated regimens for supraglottic carcinoma show excellent primary locoregional control (64% for T_3, 40% for T_4) and overall locoregional control after salvage (88% for T_3, 51% for T_4).[25] Other advances include the use of tumor radiosensitizers[26] and hypoxia-activated cytotoxic drugs.[27]

Detection of residual or recurrent disease after radiation remains a major problem in patients with advanced laryngeal carcinoma. Sloughing of the mucosa is common and may be difficult to differentiate from disease even with the help of CT or MRI. Biopsies of the area may be difficult to interpret due to the radiation changes induced in the tissue. Positron emission tomography (PET) scanning has recently been shown to hold some promise for the future with this difficult problem.[28] Failed radiation cases are usually managed by total laryngectomy or near-total laryngectomy. One of the significant disadvantages of salvage surgery after primary radiation is the higher rate of complications, particularly pharyngocutaneous fistula.[22,29,30]

Prediction of radiation response is the key to selection of patients for primary radiation. Various molecular markers have been used, but all remain experimental and none are in wide use today. The best predictors appear to be T stage, N stage, pretreatment anemia,[31] and CT findings, particularly tumor size,[21,32,33] preepiglottic space involvement, and subglottic extension.[34] Measurement of intratumoral hypoxia with an Eppendorf probe is highly predictive of radiation response but remains experimental at this time.[35]

CONCURRENT CHEMORADIATION WITH SURGICAL SALVAGE In an attempt to improve laryngeal preservation rates, chemotherapy given before, during, or after radiotherapy for advanced laryngeal cancer has been widely used and evaluated in clinical trials over the last two decades. The advantage to patients of laryngeal preservation has been clearly demonstrated in the improved quality of life shown in the laryngeal preservation arm of the Veterans Affairs study.[36] In a large meta-analysis of all published chemoradiation trials in laryngeal carcinoma, the only significant benefit was seen with concurrent chemoradiation. The benefit was small and only seen in a heterogeneous group of trials. When a smaller number of more homogenous trials were combined, the significance was lost. The conclusion reached was that the routine use of chemotherapy was debatable and should remain in the realm of clinical trials before it can be recommended.[37]

TOTAL LARYNGECTOMY WITH POSTOPERATIVE RADIATION This approach has been widely used in the past and continues to be the mainstay of treatment in many units for larger, more invasive tumors. Due to the radical nature of the therapy and the use of two modalities at the outset of treatment, it is most likely to result in locoregional control. Its most significant disadvantage is loss of the larynx and the implications of voice rehabilitation for the patient. Recent trials have not shown any obvious survival benefit over primary radiation or chemoradiation with surgery for salvage.[37] Complications after surgery are significantly reduced without prior radiation,[29] although weight loss of more than 10% preoperatively, indicating a poor nutritional status, is still a significant risk factor.[38] The risk of recurrence is significantly increased if tumor is found in the subglottis or is found to involve the postcricoid region after laryngectomy.[39]

Voice rehabilitation after total laryngectomy is one of the areas in which significant changes have taken place over the last two decades. The introduction of indwelling prostheses to facilitate the production of tracheoesophageal speech has improved the quality of speech available to many laryngectomy patients.[11] Poor vision, poor manual dexterity, and lack of personal motivation are relative contraindications to the use of tracheoesophageal methods of rehabilitation. The main problems associated with the valves are leakage, granuloma formation, and candidiasis. Prior to the development of these valves, swallowing and controlled regurgitation of air was used to produce vibration in the pharygoesophageal segment, so-called esophageal speech. This technique was difficult to learn and required considerable effort to establish an acceptable voice. The electrolarynx is the simplest way to restore speech after laryngectomy, but the voice is quiet and monotonous. It is now reserved for patients in whom other methods of voice rehabilitation are not possible.

NOVEL STRATEGIES   Transoral resection of large supraglottic tumors has been described, with a recurrence-free survival for stage 3 disease of 74% and for stage 4 disease of 45%.[14] A number of patients in the series received postoperative radiation, making these results difficult to interpret, as the effect of debulking the tumor in those patients receiving radiation is unclear. Reconstruction of large hemicricolaryngectomy defects with a prefabricated flap of vascularized trachea has recently been described. A reasonable voice and good airway with minimal aspiration in selected patients can be achieved.[17] Advanced ($T_{3/4}$) endolaryngeal carcinomas have been treated with neoadjuvant chemotherapy and supracricoid laryngectomy with cricohyoidopexy, with an actuarial survival of 73% at 5 years and a 92% laryngeal preservation rate. The value of the chemotherapy is questioned, but it probably acts as a good indicator of suitability for surgery.[40]

NECK DISSECTION   In patients with advanced supraglottic carcinoma and a clinically negative neck, treatment in the form of bilateral neck radiation or a selective neck dissection is recommended due to the high incidence of occult nodal metastases.[41] When pathologically positive nodes are found, the use of postoperative radiation is advisable, as it significantly reduces recurrence in the neck.[42] For patients with advanced glottic carcinoma, ipsilateral neck radiation or selective dissection is recommended. Clinically positive neck nodes indicate that a modified radical or radical neck dissection should be performed at the time of surgery or before or after completion of radiation to the primary tumor.

Later development of second primary tumors in the head, neck, or lung and distant metastases represent a problem in head and neck cancer despite good locoregional control. About 15% develop a second primary[43] and 5% of patients die due to distant metastases after treatment. Risk factors for distant metastases include advanced stage and supraglottic site of primary tumor.[44]

Subglottic Carcinoma

While subglottic cancers are rare, <2% of laryngeal cancers, tend to present late with cartilage and nodal involvement, thus necessitating laryngectomy, bilateral neck dissection, and postoperative radiotherapy to the neck and upper mediastinum.[45] Radiation can be used alone with a 36% local control rate in patients with T_4 tumors,[46] but detection of residual or recurrent disease is a particular problem in this site. Peristomal recurrence after surgery and radiation is a feature of this disease.

Carcinoma in Situ

Carcinoma in situ of the vocal cord may be managed by vocal cord stripping or laser ablation using suspension microlaryngoscopy. Close follow-up of these patients with repeat laryngoscopy is necessary to exclude invasive disease, as up to 20% of dysplastic lesions progress to carcinoma.[47] When recurrence is noted, repeat stripping, laser, partial laryngeal surgery, or radiation are treatment options. Our institution recently reported excellent results with 51Gy in 20 fractions given over 4 weeks for persistent carcinoma in situ, with only 1 patient going on to develop invasive disease and with no serious acute or late complications.[48]

Verrucous Carcinoma

Verrucous carcinoma is a variant of SCC accounting for 1 to 2% of all laryngeal neoplasms. Clinically it tends to invade locally, with an exophytic appearance, and does not metastasize. Histologically it is characterized by the appearance of well-differentiated squamous cells invading the laryngeal stroma in a pushing manner, forming papillary fronds with keratosis and acanthosis. Small lesions can be excised endoscopically; larger lesions may require partial or total laryngectomy. The role of radiation therapy in the management of verrucous carcinoma remains controversial due to the possible transformation to anaplastic carcinoma.

CANCER OF THE PARANASAL SINUSES

Epidemiology and Pathology

The incidence of paranasal sinus carcinoma is less than 1 per 100,000 per year in the United States. It is twice as common in men as in women and it most commonly develops during the fifth to seventh decades. These rare malignancies account for 0.2% of all malignant tumors and 3% of upper aerodigestive tract cancers. Presenting symptoms are often nonspecific, resulting in a delay in diagnosis. About 55% start in the maxillary sinus, 35% the nasal cavity, 9% the ethmoid sinus, and 1% in the frontal and sphenoid sinuses, although many present late, making it difficult to determine the primary site.[49]

SCCs are the most common type histologically, followed by adenocarcinoma and minor salivary gland tumors particularly adenoid cystic carcinoma. Other types include melanoma, esthesioneuroblastoma, sarcoma, lymphoma, plasmacytoma, sinonasal undifferentiated carcinoma, and sinonasal neuroendocrine carcinomas. All except SCCs have a poor long-term prognosis.

Etiology

The development of sinonasal cancers has been linked to exposure to industrial environmental factors.[50] Several occupational groups including nickel refiners, woodworkers, leather workers, textile workers, petroleum refiners, and chrome pigment manufacturers have been found to be at increased risk. Nickel refiners appear to be particularly at risk of developing SCC and anaplastic carcinoma and have been shown to have an incidence of sinonasal malignancy at least 100 times that of the general population with a long latent period. Hardwood workers appear to be predisposed to the development of adenocarcinoma of the ethmoid sinus as well as SCC and anaplastic carcinoma of the maxillary sinus. Smoking is an additional independent risk factor.

Presentation

The most common presenting symptoms of paranasal sinus cancer include unilateral nasal obstruction, facial or dental pain, nasal discharge, and epistaxis. Hypoesthesia in the distribution of the infraorbital nerve suggests a superoposteriorly located lesion, whereas opthalmoplegia or visual loss imply orbital or cavernous sinus involvement. Epiphora, trismus, and facial or palatal swelling are late signs implying advanced disease.

A mass may be visible in the nose, and careful examination of the upper cranial nerves may reveal sensory changes. Proptosis and loosening of teeth indicate extensive disease. An ophthalmology consult is recommended and may reveal subtle changes in the eye, such as superior retinal vein occlusion not otherwise seen. Direct fiberoptic endoscopy or rigid endoscopy of the nose allows guided biopsy of suspicious tissue. A thorough head and neck examination should be carried out with careful assessment of the neck.

Primary malignancies arising from the sphenoid sinus are very rare. Patients often present with headaches and visual disturbance. Cranial nerve palsies are a poor prognostic sign.[51]

Investigation and Staging

CT and MRI give different and important information in the management of the patient with sinonasal cancer. CT provides detail of bone destruction and the accurate information on the status of the neck, while MRI best differentiates adjacent soft tissue involvement, intracranial extension, and perineural spread. MRI will also differentiate an obstructed sinus with fluid collection from a space-occupying lesion. A chest x-ray should be performed to exclude chest metastases.

The latest UICC staging system (1997) separates maxillary from ethmoid sinus tumors, which facilitates analysis of treatment for this disease[6] (Table 27-6). Advanced stage, orbital and dural invasion, and nodal metastases are particularly poor prognostic factors.

Management

Due to the rarity of malignant paranasal sinus neoplasms, their varied histologic type and, until recently, the lack of a uniform staging system, it is difficult to interpret the literature as to the best form of treatment for this disease. Unfortunately, the majority of patients present with late-stage disease. This poses considerable management challenges due to the proximity of these tumors to vital structures, such as the eye and brain, so that radical en bloc resection with a clear surgical margin is often not possible.

Surgery alone is indicated only for early stage disease where the tumor can be completely resected with clear margins. For more advanced disease, surgery with pre- or postoperative radiation is generally recommended, but primary radiation with surgical salvage is reported to give comparable results. With regard to the timing of radiation, primary surgery with postoperative radiation allows accurate resection of the tumor under frozen section control, but radiation of the surgical bed postoperatively will likely involve a significant dose to the eye. Preoperative radiation allows a significant dose to be given close to

TABLE 27-6. UICC TNM STAGING FOR PARANASAL SINUS NEOPLASMS[6]

Maxillary sinus	
T_1	Tumor limited to the antral mucosa with no erosion or destruction of bone
T_2	Tumor causing bone erosion or destruction except for the posterior antral wall, including extension into hard palate and/or middle nasal meatus
T_3	Tumor invades any of the following: bone of the posterior wall of the maxillary sinus, sub-cutaneous tissues, skin of the cheek, floor or medial wall of the orbit, infratemporal fossa, pterygoid plates, ethmoid sinuses
T_4	Tumor invades orbital contents beyond the floor or medial wall including the apex and/or any of the following: cribriform plate, base of skull, nasopharynx, sphenoid sinus, frontal sinus
Ethmoid sinus	
T_1	Tumor confined to ethmoid with or without bone erosion
T_2	Tumor extends into the nasal cavity
T_3	Tumor extends to anterior orbit and/or maxillary sinus
T_4	Tumor with intracranial extension, orbital extension including apex, involving sphenoid and/or frontal sinus and/or skin of nose
N stage	
N_x	Regional lymph nodes cannot be assessed
N_0	No regional metastases
N_1	Metastases in a single ipsilateral lymph node, 3 cm or less in greatest dimension
N_{2a}	Metastases in a single ipsilateral lymph node, more than 3 cm but not more than 6 cm in greatest dimension
N_{2b}	Metastases in multiple ipsilateral lymph nodes, none more than 6 cm in greatest dimension
N_{2c}	Metastases in bilateral or contralateral lymph nodes, none more than 6 cm in greatest dimension
N_3	Metastases in a lymph node more than 6 cm in greatest dimension
M stage	
M_x	Distant metastases cannot be assessed
M_0	No distant metastases
M_1	Distant metastases

but not involving the eye, clearing microscopic disease from this area prior to surgery. However, this approach is associated with a higher incidence of wound complications and renders assessment of surgical margins more difficult intraoperatively. Orbital exenteration is probably not necessary in most cases, as recent studies have indicated that survival is little changed.[52]

Primary radiation with surgical salvage has shown comparable results to planned combined treatment, and—with the increasing use of conformal radiotherapy and newer techniques such as intensity modulated radiation therapy (IMRT)—an increased dose to a more targeted volume may give better results with a further reduced dose to the eye (Table 27-7). It has been particularly successful in early T_1 and T_2 tumors, which appear to respond equally well to radiation or en bloc resection. Recent reports of aggressive management regimens involving chemotherapy followed by surgery and postoperative chemoradiation have reported excellent results—73% overall survival and 66% disease free survival at 5 years—but this is toxic therapy and only selected patients with a good performance status will be suitable.[53]

At the time of diagnosis, metastatic nodal disease from SCC of the paranasal sinuses is present in 5 to 10% of patients and is indicative of a very poor prognosis (Table 27-8). The sinus lymphatics drain into the retropharyngeal parapharyngeal, and upper cervical nodes bilaterally, and a routine elective neck dissection is probably of little benefit. Due to the

TABLE 27-7. FIVE-YEAR SURVIVAL OF MAXILLARY SINUS CARCINOMA

Study	No. of Patients	Overall (%)	Surgery and Radiation (%)	Radiation Alone (%)
Lewis and Castro[70]	191	28	33	20
Cheng and Wang[71]	17	34	48	22
Lee and Ogura.[72]	44	49	69	14
Tiwari et al.[55]	43	—	64	—
Waldron et al.[56]	110	43	—	31

aggressive behavior of these tumors, the following should be considered contraindications to radical treatment in paranasal sinus carcinoma: (1) extension of the cancer into the nasopharynx with clival destruction and gross involvement of the brain parenchyma, (2) unresectable cervical adenopathy, and (3) distant metastases.

Maxillary Sinus Carcinoma

Surgical approaches to the tumor depend on its location and the extent of disease. Inferiorly placed tumors may be accessible via a lateral rhinotomy or midfacial degloving, but more extensive disease will require an infraorbital extension of the incision to give sufficient access for a radical maxillectomy. Tumors extending up to involve the ethmoid sinus or the cribriform plate will require access from above and below in the form of a craniofacial resection to allow en bloc resection of tumor. Restoration of palatal function after maxillectomy can be achieved with a dental prosthesis for smaller defects or osseocutaneous free flap repair for larger defects.[54] Recently reported results for this approach have given overall survival figures in the region of 65%, although some patients also received induction chemotherapy.[55] A series of patients treated at our institution with primary radiation and surgical salvage has recently reported a local control rate of 40% and cause-specific survival of 43% at 5 years.[56]

Ethmoid Sinus Carcinoma

Unless the tumor is very small, most patients require craniofacial resection to allow en bloc resection of the tumor, including the cribriform plate. This is usually followed with postoperative radiation to control residual microscopic disease. As discussed previously, radiation of the surgical bed is likely to involve significant damage to the eye in the long term. Recent series report a local control rate of 75% and overall survival of 55% with this approach.[57] Primary radiation with surgical salvage for ethmoid carcinoma has been reported to give a local control rate of 50 to 65%, but salvage of recurrent disease is rarely successful.[57,58]

Sphenoid sinus neoplasms are usually treated with either primary radiation or surgery plus radiation, but the outcome is poor.[51]

TABLE 27-8. SURVIVAL OF PATIENTS WITH PARANASAL SINUS AND NASAL CAVITY MALIGNANCY

Parameter	Antrum	Frontosphenoethmoidal	Antroethmoid	Nose
No. of cases	193	105	69	130
5-year survival %	23	33	30	52
10-year survival %	10	14	9	22
With metastases				
5-year survival %	13	0	0	39
10-year survival %	0	0	0	23

Other Malignancies of the Paranasal Sinuses

Adenocarcinomas are more commonly found in the upper nasal cavity and ethmoid sinus, with a great propensity for aggressive local progression. In general they have a relatively low incidence of metastases and a poor prognosis due to local recurrent disease with a poor survival rate. Adenoid cystic carcinomas occur with the same frequency as adenocarcinomas but most commonly involve the maxillary antrum. Patients tend to present with distant rather than regional metastases, although relentless progression of the tumor at the skull base is the most likely cause of death. They usually have an acceptable 5-year survival rate of about 75%, but the 15-year control rate drops to 25%. Both types are usually managed with a combination of primary surgery and postoperative radiation. Some reported benefits have been demonstrated with the use of neutron beam radiation in locally advanced and unresectable lesions.

Osteogenic sarcomas and chondrosarcomas are seen more commonly in the mandible than in the maxilla. Due to relentless progression, these lesions are usually lethal. With induction chemotherapy, preoperative radiation, and wide-field ablative surgery, a 30% five-year survival rate has been reported. The paranasal sinuses are an unusual site of presentation for lymphoma, although within this region any of the subtypes can occur. Melanomas of the paranasal sinuses are usually advanced at the time of presentation. the patient may present with black nasal discharge accompanying the other usual symptoms of paranasal sinus malignancy. The prognosis is usually very poor, with a mean survival of about 2 years. Esthesioneuroblastomas are rare tumors of the anterior skull base; wide local resection and postoperative radiotherapy probably give the best long-term survival.[59] Plasmacytomas are again rare but, due to their radiosensitivity, are usually managed with primary radiation.

CANCER OF THE EAR CANAL AND TEMPORAL BONE

Cutaneous malignancies affecting the pinna are common, while neoplasms of the ear canal and temporal bone are rare and account for less than 0.05% of all head and neck malignancies. Typically carcinomas of the pinna occur in older men with a history of sun exposure. SCC and basal cell carcinoma are the most common histologic types, usually presenting with a history of a painless ulcerative lesion on the rim of the pinna with surrounding erythema and induration. Treatment depends on the location and extent of the lesion; small ones may be locally resected with high cure rates and satisfactory cosmetic results. Larger lesions may require complete resection of the pinna, temporal bone resection, and/or parotidectomy. Alternatively, radiotherapy may be used as the primary mode of treatment with surgery reserved for salvage. When radiotherapy is properly fractionated, the risk of osteoradionecrosis or chondronecrosis is minimal. For basal cell carcinomas, adequate cure rates have been obtained by using curettage, radiation, or Mohs chemosurgery, but, in general, radiation is reserved for recurrent lesions or those that have failed other forms of therapy. The remainder of this section focuses on malignancies of the ear canal and temporal bone.

Etiology and Pathology

Patients often have a long history of a chronically discharging ear on the side of the tumor. Although this is one of the most common presenting symptoms of carcinoma of the external ear and temporal bone, it is thought that exposure to chronic inflammation may play a role in the etiology of this condition. Exposure to aflatoxin B, produced by certain fungi, and a history of head and neck radiation also predispose to this condition.[60]

A variety of tumor types may involve the external ear and temporal bone, but the most common is SCC. Other pathologies include adenoid cystic carcinoma, adenocarcinoma, basal cell carcinoma, melanoma, and metastases. Embryonal rhabdomyosarcoma may be found in children. Tumors usually arise in the external auditory meatus and invade the middle ear, although it is frequently not possible to determine the exact site of origin.

Symptoms and Signs

Diagnosis is often delayed, as the symptoms and signs of malignancy are initially similar to those of chronic otitis externa or chronic suppurative otitis media (CSOM), with a sero-sanguineous discharge. They are usually accompanied by deep, intense pain and a sensation of fullness in the ear, with a conductive hearing loss. A fleshy mass or polyp may be visible in the ear canal. When the tumor extends more deeply, sensorineural deafness and facial nerve paralysis or other cranial nerve palsies may develop. Extension into the parotid gland may be evident. At the time of presentation, up to 20% of patients will have developed regional or distant metastatic disease.

Investigation

After audiologic investigations to establish the level of hearing, suspicious lesions within the external ear canal or middle ear should be biopsied under local or general anesthesia, taking care not to disrupt the ossicles. A contrast-enhanced CT with fine cuts through the temporal bone helps in the evaluation of bone destruction and cervical lymphadenopathy. MRI has better soft tissue discrimination and is more sensitive in the assessment of vascular involvement if there is suspicion of internal carotid artery or internal jugular vein disease, and it better defines intracranial extension.

Staging

There is no accepted staging protocol from the AJCC or UICC for malignancies of the temporal bone and ear. This may be due to the heterogeneity of histopathologic types as well as the difficulties associated with the identification of the site of origin of these tumors. One of the most widely used staging systems in the literature is from the University of Pittsburgh, which includes both clinical and radiological evaluation[61] (Table 27-9).

Management

Primary surgery with postoperative radiation in selected cases form the mainstay of treatment for this disease. The aim of surgery is to achieve a complete en bloc resection of the tumor with, where possible, preservation of hearing and facial nerve function.

Small T_1 lesions of the external ear with no evidence of bone invasion may be excised with a sleeve resection of the ear canal skin. For T_2 lesions still confined to the ear canal

TABLE 27-9. UNIVERSITY OF PITTSBURGH STAGING SYSTEM FOR CARCINOMA OF THE EXTERNAL AUDITORY MEATUS[61]

T_1	Tumor limited to the EAM without bony erosion or evidence of soft tissue extension
T_2	Tumor with limited EAM erosion (not full thickness) or radiographic findings consistent with limited (<0.5 cm) soft tissue involvement
T_3	Tumor eroding the osseous EAM (full thickness) with limited (<0.5 cm) soft tissue involvement, or tumor involving middle ear and/or mastoid, or patients presenting with paralysis
T_4	Tumor eroding the cochlea, petrous apex, medial wall of the middle ear, carotid canal, jugular foramen, or dura or with extensive soft tissue involvement (>0.5 cm)

but involving the bony canal wall, a lateral temporal bone resection is required. This involves a systematic dissection of the temporal bone around the ear canal lateral to the middle ear to remove the entire canal and tympanic membrane intact. T_3 lesions with extension to the mastoid or middle ear require a more extensive subtotal temporal bone resection with removal of the ear canal, middle ear, petrous bone, and temporomandibular joint with a partial or total parotidectomy. The facial nerve is sacrificed when invaded by malignancy; grafting with the sural or greater auricular nerve is possible provided that the proximal and distal margins are clear of disease. T_4 lesions with extension of disease to the medial aspect of the temporal bone (petrous apex) necessitate a total temporal bone resection with carotid artery sacrifice. SCC involving the petrous apex is considered incurable, although adenoid cystic carcinoma and sarcomas can be treated with this approach. After the more major resections, regional or free flap reconstruction can be used to cover exposed dura, prevent cerebrospinal fluid (CSF) leakage, and replace surgical dead space.[62] It is our practice to perform upper neck dissection (levels II and III) routinely with this resection in patients with an N_0 neck. For more extensive neck disease, a modified radical or radical neck dissection is required.

Planned postoperative radiation appears to confer a survival benefit on patients with more extensive disease[63–69] (Table 27-10). Overall control of T_1 and T_2 tumors appears to be in the range of 80 to 100%; T_3 tumors, 50 to 70%; and T_4 tumors, 10 to 40%.[66,68,69] One series has reported improved results (65% survival for T_4 disease at 3 years) with more formalized encompassing surgery and increased radiation dosage.[67] A retrospective review of cases in many series appears to indicate that primary radiation does not have a role to play in the management of this disease other than in selected T_1 tumors.[64,68]

Melanoma of the Ear

Melanomas of the ear are rare and have a poor prognosis. They comprise 7% of all head and neck melanomas and 4% of cutaneous ear malignancies. They are seen in a younger patient population than those with squamous or basal cell carcinomas. The majority of lesions are located on the periphery of the ear.

Melanomas of the ear present as superficial lesions that tend to spread toward the periphery. They tend to metastasize regionally to the preauricular parotid or jugulodigastric nodes. Histologic diagnosis should be confirmed by excision or incision biopsy where appropriate. A CT scan of the brain is performed routinely, as these lesions tend to metastasize widely. Further studies should include liver, spleen, and bone scans as well as chest x-ray. Small lesions can be excised locally with good results. Larger lesions may require a more radical excision of the ear and temporal bone in conjunction with a neck dissection and

TABLE 27-10. SURVIVAL OF CARCINOMA OF THE TEMPORAL BONE AND EAR WITH RESECTION AND RADIOTHERAPY

Study	No. of Cases	5-Year Survival %
Wang[73]	20	45
Sinha and Aziz[74]	15	40
Liu et al.[65]	15	54
Pfreunder et al.[66]	27	61
Zhang et al.[68]	33	52
Hashi et al.[64]	20	59

parotidectomy. Chemotherapy must be considered in the treatment plan and the medical oncologist should be involved early in the care of these patients. Survival is related to Breslow's levels of thickness. The metastatic rate with lesions less than 3 mm is 21% and with lesions in excess of 3 mm is approximately 60%.

Other Malignancies of the Ear and Temporal Bone

Although rare, adenoid cystic carcinoma is the most common tumor of glandular origin. It tends to spread perineurally and erodes the bone of the ear canal through the fissure of Santorini to invade the parotid gland. Pain is the presenting symptom in up to 85% of patients. It appears that the prognosis is related to the histologic type, with the tubular pattern having the best outcome. Patients with the solid histologic pattern have the worst prognosis. Primary tumors that metastasize to the temporal bone are uncommon. In most cases they originate from primary sites in the breast, lung, or kidney.

References

1. Eisner MP, Kosary CL, Hankey BF, et al, eds. *SEER Cancer Statistics Review, 1973–1998.* Bethesda, MD: National Cancer Institute, 2001.

2. Rothman KJ, Cann CI, Flanders D, Fried MP. Epidemiology of laryngeal cancer. *Epidemiol Rev* 2:195–209,1980.

3. Williams RR, Horm JW. Association of cancer sites with tobacco and alcohol consumption and socioeconomic status of patients: interview study from the Third National Cancer Survey. *J Natl Cancer Inst* 58(3):525–547,1977.

4. Silvestri F, Bussani R, Stanta G, et al. Supraglottic versus glottic laryngeal cancer: epidemiological and pathological aspects. *ORL J Otorhinolaryngol Rel Spec* 54(1):43–48,1992.

5. Wortley P, Vaughan TL, Davis S, et al. A case-control study of occupational risk factors for laryngeal cancer. *Br J Ind Med* 49(12): 837–844,1992.

6. Sobin LH, Wittekind C, eds. *TNM Classification of Malignant Tumours,* 5th ed. New York: John Wiley & Sons, 1997.

7. Davidson J, Gilbert R, Irish J, et al. The role of panendoscopy in the management of mucosal head and neck malignancy—a prospective evaluation. *Head Neck* 2000;22(5):449–454; discussion 454–455.

8. Houghton DJ, Hughes ML, Garvey C, et al. Role of chest CT scanning in the management of patients presenting with head and neck cancer. *Head Neck* 20(7):614–618,1998.

9. Spector JG, Sessions DG, Chao KS, et al. Stage I (T1 N0 M0) squamous cell carcinoma of the laryngeal glottis: therapeutic results and voice preservation. *Head Neck* 21(8):707–717,1999.

10. Orus C, Leon X, Vega M, Quer M. Initial treatment of the early stages (I, II) of supraglottic squamous cell carcinoma: partial laryngectomy versus radiotherapy. *Eur Arch Otorhinolaryngol* 257(9):516, 2000.

11. Simpson CB, Postma GN, Stone RE, Ossoff RH. Speech outcomes after laryngeal cancer management. *Otolaryngol Clin North Am* 30(2): 189–205,1997.

12. Quer M, Leon X, Orus C. Endoscopic laser surgery in the treatment of radiation failure of early laryngeal carcinoma. *Head Neck* 22(5): 520–523, 2000.

13. Eckel HE, Thumfart W, Jungehulsing M, et al. Transoral laser surgery for early glottic carcinoma. *Eur Arch Otorhinolaryngol* 257(4): 221–226, 2000.

14. Iro H, Waldfahrer F, Altendorf-Hofmann A, Weidenbecher M, et al. Transoral laser surgery of supraglottic cancer: follow-up of 141 patients. *Arch Otolaryngol Head Neck Surg* 124(11):1245–1250,1998.

15. Ferlito A, Silver CE, Howard DJ, et al. The role of partial laryngeal resection in current management of laryngeal cancer: a collective review. *Acta Otolaryngol* 120(4):456–465, 2000.

16. Lima RA, Freitas EQ, Kligerman J, et al. Near-total laryngectomy for treatment of advanced laryngeal cancer. *Am J Surg* 174(5): 490–491, 1997.

17. Delaere PR, Poorten VV, Goeleven A, et al. Tracheal autotransplantation: a reliable reconstruc-

tive technique for extended hemilaryngectomy defects. *Laryngoscope* 108(6):929–934,1998.

18. Buckley JG, MacLennan K. Cancer spread in the larynx: a pathologic basis for conservation surgery. *Head Neck* 22(3):265–274, 2000.

19. Laccourreye O, Muscatello L, Laccourreye L, et al. Supracricoid partial laryngectomy with cricohyoidoepiglottopexy for "early" glottic carcinoma classified as T1–T2N0 invading the anterior commissure. *Am J Otolaryngol* 18(6): 385–390,1997.

20. MacKenzie RG, Franssen E, Balogh JM, et al. Comparing treatment outcomes of radiotherapy and surgery in locally advanced carcinoma of the larynx: a comparison limited to patients eligible for surgery. *Int J Radiat Oncol Biol Phys* 47(1):65–71, 2000.

21. Parsons JT, Mendenhall WM, Stringer SP, Cassisi NJ. T4 laryngeal carcinoma: radiotherapy alone with surgery reserved for salvage. *Int J Radiat Oncol Biol Phys* 40(3):549–552, 1998.

22. Davidson J, Keane T, Brown D, et al. Surgical salvage after radiotherapy for advanced laryngopharyngeal carcinoma. *Arch Otolaryngol Head Neck Surg* 123(4):420–424,1997.

23. MacKenzie R, Franssen E, Balogh J, et al. The prognostic significance of tracheostomy in carcinoma of the larynx treated with radiotherapy and surgery for salvage. *Int J Radiat Oncol Biol Phys* 41(1):43–51,1998.

24. Groome PA, O'Sullivan B, Irish JC, et al. Glottic cancer in Ontario, Canada and the SEER areas of the United States. Do different management philosophies produce different outcome profiles? *J Clin Epidemiol* 54(3):301–315, 2001.

25. Nakfoor BM, Spiro IJ, Wang CC, et al. Results of accelerated radiotherapy for supraglottic carcinoma: a Massachusetts General Hospital and Massachusetts Eye and Ear Infirmary experience. *Head Neck* 20(5):379–384,1998.

26. Overgaard J, Hansen HS, Overgaard M, et al. A randomized double-blind phase III study of nimorazole as a hypoxic radiosensitizer of primary radiotherapy in supraglottic larynx and pharynx carcinoma. Results of the Danish Head and Neck Cancer Study (DAHANCA) Protocol 5-85. *Radiother Oncol* 46(2):135–146,1998.

27. Rischin D, Peters L, Hicks R, et al. Phase I trial of concurrent tirapazamine, cisplatin, and radio-

therapy in patients with advanced head and neck cancer. *J Clin Oncol* 19(2):535–542, 2001.

28. Lonneux M, Lawson G, Ide C, et al. Positron emission tomography with fluorodeoxyglucose for suspected head and neck tumor recurrence in the symptomatic patient. *Laryngoscope* 110(9):1493–1497, 2000.

29. Virtaniemi JA, Kumpulainen EJ, Hirvikoski PP, et al. The incidence and etiology of postlaryngectomy pharyngocutaneous fistulae. *Head Neck* 23(1):29–33, 2001.

30. Parikh SR, Irish JC, Curran AJ, et al. Pharyngocutaneous fistulae in laryngectomy patients: the Toronto Hospital experience. *J Otolaryngol* 27(3):136–140,1998.

31. Warde P, O'Sullivan B, Bristow RG, et al. T1/T2 glottic cancer managed by external beam radiotherapy: the influence of pretreatment hemoglobin on local control. *Int J Radiat Oncol Biol Phys* 41(2):347–353,1998.

32. Daugaard BJ, Sand HH. Primary radiotherapy of carcinoma of the supraglottic larynx—a multivariate analysis of prognostic factors. *Int J Radiat Oncol Biol Phys* 41(2):355–360,1998.

33. Mendenhall WM, Parsons JT, Mancuso AA, et al. Definitive radiotherapy for T3 squamous cell carcinoma of the glottic larynx. *J Clin Oncol* 15(6):2394–2402,1997.

34. Hermans R, Van den Bogaert W, Rijnders A, Baert AL. Value of computed tomography as outcome predictor of supraglottic squamous cell carcinoma treated by definitive radiation therapy. *Int J Radiat Oncol Biol Phys* 44(4):755–765,1999.

35. Brizel DM, Dodge RK, Clough RW, Dewhirst MW. Oxygenation of head and neck cancer: changes during radiotherapy and impact on treatment outcome. *Radiother Oncol* 53(2): 113–117,1999.

36. Terrell JE, Fisher SG, Wolf GT. Long-term quality of life after treatment of laryngeal cancer. The Veterans Affairs Laryngeal Cancer Study Group. *Arch Otolaryngol Head Neck Surg* 124(9):964–971,1998.

37. Pignon JP, Bourhis J, Domenge C, Designe L. Chemotherapy added to locoregional treatment for head and neck squamous-cell carcinoma: three meta-analyses of updated individual data. MACH-NC Collaborative Group. Meta-Analysis of Chemotherapy on Head and Neck Cancer. *Lancet* 355(9208):949–955, 2000.

38. van Bokhorst-de van der Schueren MA, van Leeuwen PA, Sauerwein HP, et al. Assessment of malnutrition parameters in head and neck cancer and their relation to postoperative complications. *Head Neck* 19(5):419–425,1997.

39. Yuen AP, Wei WI, Ho WK, Hui Y. Risk factors of tracheostomal recurrence after laryngectomy for laryngeal carcinoma. *Am J Surg* 172(3):263–266,1996.

40. Laccourreye O, Brasnu D, Biacabe B, et al. Neo-adjuvant chemotherapy and supracricoid partial laryngectomy with cricohyoidopexy for advanced endolaryngeal carcinoma classified as T3–T4: 5-year oncologic results. *Head Neck* 20(7):595–599,1998.

41. Hicks WL Jr, Kollmorgen DR, Kuriakose MA, et al. Patterns of nodal metastasis and surgical management of the neck in supraglottic laryngeal carcinoma. *Otolaryngol Head Neck Surg* 121(1):57–61,1999.

42. Byers RM, Clayman GL, McGill D, et al. Selective neck dissections for squamous carcinoma of the upper aerodigestive tract: patterns of regional failure. *Head Neck* 21(6):499–505, 1999.

43. Narayana A, Vaughan AT, Fisher SG, Reddy SP. Second primary tumors in laryngeal cancer: results of long-term follow-up. *Int J Radiat Oncol Biol Phys* 42(3):557–562,1998.

44. Leon X, Quer M, Orus C, et al. Distant metastases in head and neck cancer patients who achieved loco-regional control. *Head Neck* 22(7):680–686, 2000.

45. Dahm JD, Sessions DG, Paniello RC, Harvey J. Primary subglottic cancer. *Laryngoscope* 108(5): 741–746,1998.

46. Warde P, Harwood A, Keane T. Carcinoma of the subglottis. Results of initial radical radiation. *Arch Otolaryngol Head Neck Surg* 113(11): 1228–1229,1987.

47. Gallo A, de Vincentiis M, Della Rocca C, et al. Evolution of precancerous laryngeal lesions: a clinicopathologic study with long-term follow-up on 259 patients. *Head Neck* 23(1):42–47, 2001.

48. Spayne JA, Warde P, O'Sullivan B, et al. Carcinoma-in-situ of the glottic larynx: results of treatment with radiation therapy. *Int J Radiat Oncol Biol Phys* 49(5):1235–1238, 2001.

49. Cody DT, DeSanto LW. Neoplasms of the nasal cavity. In Schuller DE, ed. *Otolaryngology:* *Head and Neck Surgery,* 3rd ed. Vol 2. St. Louis: Mosby, 1998.

50. Rousch GC. Epidemiology of cancer of the nose and paranasal sinuses—current concepts. *Head Neck* 2:3,1979.

51. DeMonte F, Ginsberg LE, Clayman GL. Primary malignant tumors of the sphenoidal sinus. *Neurosurgery* 2000;46(5):1084–1091; discussion 1091–1092.

52. Carrau RL, Segas J, Nuss DW, et al. Squamous cell carcinoma of the sinonasal tract invading the orbit. *Laryngoscope* 109(2 Pt 1):230–235,1999.

53. Lee MM, Vokes EE, Rosen A, et al. Multimodality therapy in advanced paranasal sinus carcinoma: superior long-term results. *Cancer J Sci Am* 5(4):219–223,1999.

54. Brown JS. Deep circumflex iliac artery free flap with internal oblique muscle as a new method of immediate reconstruction of maxillectomy defect. *Head Neck* 18(5):412–421,1996.

55. Tiwari R, Hardillo JA, Mehta D, et al. Squamous cell carcinoma of maxillary sinus. *Head Neck* 22(2):164–169, 2000.

56. Waldron JN, O'Sullivan B, Gullane P, et al. Carcinoma of the maxillary antrum: a retrospective analysis of 110 cases. *Radiother Oncol* 57(2):167–173, 2000.

57. Jiang GL, Morrison WH, Garden AS, et al. Ethmoid sinus carcinomas: natural history and treatment results. *Radiother Oncol* 49(1):21–27, 1998.

58. Waldron JN, O'Sullivan B, Warde P, et al. Ethmoid sinus cancer: twenty-nine cases managed with primary radiation therapy. *Int J Radiat Oncol Biol Phys* 41(2):361–369,1998.

59. Irish J, Dasgupta R, Freeman J, et al. Outcome and analysis of the surgical management of esthesioneuroblastoma. *J Otolaryngol* 26(1): 1–7,1997.

60. Goh YH, Chong VF, Low WK. Temporal bone tumours in patients irradiated for nasopharyngeal neoplasm. *J Laryngol Otol* 113(3):222–228,1999.

61. Arriaga M, Curtin H, Takahashi H, et al. Staging proposal for external auditory meatus carcinoma based on preoperative clinical examination and computed tomography findings. *Ann Otol Rhinol Laryngol* 99(9 Pt 1):714–721,1990.

62. Gal TJ, Kerschner JE, Futran ND, et al. Reconstruction after temporal bone resection. *Laryngoscope* 108(4 Pt 1):476–481,1998.

63. Austin JR, Stewart KL, Fawzi N. Squamous cell carcinoma of the external auditory canal. Therapeutic prognosis based on a proposed staging system. *Arch Otolaryngol Head Neck Surg* 120(11):1228–1232,1994.

64. Hashi N, Shirato H, Omatsu T, et al. The role of radiotherapy in treating squamous cell carcinoma of the external auditory canal, especially in early stages of disease. *Radiother Oncol* 56(2):221–225, 2000.

65. Liu FF, Keane TJ, Davidson J. Primary carcinoma involving the petrous temporal bone. *Head Neck* 15(1):39–43,1993.

66. Pfreundner L, Schwager K, Willner J, et al. Carcinoma of the external auditory canal and middle ear. *Int J Radiat Oncol Biol Phys* 44(4):777–788, 1999.

67. Spector JG. Management of temporal bone carcinomas: a therapeutic analysis of two groups of patients and long-term followup. *Otolaryngol Head Neck Surg* 104(1):58–66,1991.

68. Zhang B, Tu G, Xu G, et al. Squamous cell carcinoma of temporal bone: reported on 33 patients. *Head Neck* 21(5):461–466,1999.

69. Moody SA, Hirsch BE, Myers EN. Squamous cell carcinoma of the external auditory canal: an evaluation of a staging system. *Am J Otol* 21(4):582–588, 2000.

70. Lewis JS, Castro EB. Cancer of the nasal cavity and paranasal sinuses. *J Laryngol Otol* 86(3):255–262,1972.

71. Cheng VS, Wang CC. Carcinomas of the paranasal sinuses: a study of sixty-six cases. *Cancer* 40(6):3038–3041,1977.

72. Lee F, Ogura JH. Maxillary sinus carcinoma. *Laryngoscope* 91(1):133–139,1981.

73. Wang CC. Radiation therapy in the management of carcinoma of the external auditory canal, middle ear, or mastoid. *Radiology* 116(3): 713–715,1975.

74. Sinha PP, Aziz HI. Treatment of carcinoma of the middle ear. *Radiology* 126(2):485–487,1978.

Thyroid and Parathyroid Glands

28

ANATOMY AND EMBRYOLOGY

> "The extirpation of the thyroid gland for goiter typifies perhaps better than any operation the supreme triumph of the surgeon's art."
>
> —Halsted, 1920[1]

The thyroid is composed of two lateral lobes connected by an isthmus, which rests at the level of the second to fourth tracheal cartilages. Each thyroid lobe measures approximately 4 cm high, 1.5 cm wide, and 2 cm deep. The ventral surface of the thyroid gland is covered by the infrahyoid strap muscle musculature. The pyramidal lobe, present in about 40% of patients, can arise from the superior aspect of the midline isthmus or from the right or left thyroid lobes.

The thyroid's medial anlage arises as a ventral diverticulum from the endoderm of the first and second pharyngeal pouches at the foramen cecum, the junction of the copula, and tuberculum impar. The diverticulum forms at 4 weeks gestation and descends from the base of tongue to its adult pretracheal position in the route of the neck through a midline anterior path, assuming its final adult position by 7 weeks gestation. As the medial anlage descends, it is joined by the lateral thyroid primordia, arising from the fourth pharyngeal pouch. Parafollicular C cells arising from the neural crest of the fourth pharyngeal pouch as ultimobranchial bodies migrate and infiltrate the forming lateral thyroid lobes.[2]

If thyroid migration is completely arrested, a lingual thyroid results without normal tissue in the orthotopic site. If the inferiormost portion of the thyroglossal duct tract is maintained, a pyramidal lobe is formed. If a remnant of thyroid tissue is left along the thyroglossal duct tract, it can cystify, enlarge, and present in the adult as a midline neck mass, frequently in close association with the hyoid bone. Surgery for thyroglossal duct cyst therefore requires resection of the midportion of the hyoid bone and identification and resection of any cranially extending track leading toward the base of the tongue.

An extensive regional intra- and periglandular lymphatic network exists in the neck base. The isthmus and medial thyroid lobes drain initially to delphian, pretracheal, and superior mediastinal nodes, while the lateral thyroid drains initially to the internal jugular chain. The inferior pole drains initially to paratracheal perirecurrent laryngeal nerve (RLN) nodes. The extensive pericapsular and intraglandular thyroid lymphatic network mediates the early intraglandular lymphatic spread of papillary carcinoma, which has in the past been viewed as multifocal carcinoma.

The cervical viscera—including trachea, larynx, and thyroid—are ensheathed in the middle or visceral layer of the deep cervical fascia. It is important to distinguish between the true thyroid capsule and the areolar tissue present in the interval between the true thyroid capsule and the undersurface of the strap muscles (ie, the perithyroid sheath). The true thyroid capsule is tightly adherent to the thyroid parenchyma and continuous with fibrous septa that divide the gland's parenchyma into lobules. As the strap muscles are elevated off the ventral surface of the thyroid, the thin areolar tissue of the perithyroid sheath is encountered as thin cob-web-like tissue that is typically easily lysed and occasionally associated with small bridging vessels extending from the undersurface of the strap muscles to the true thyroid capsule. As dissection extends around the posterolateral lobe of the thyroid during thyroidectomy, separation of the layers of the perithyroid sheath allows recognition of the superior parathyroid, which is usually closely associated with the posterolateral thyroid capsule.

Ligament of Berry

The thyroid elevates with the larynx and trachea with deglutition. It is this that allows the examiner to distinguish between a thyroid nodule, which elevates, and a perithyroid lymph node, which does not. The thyroid is attached to the laryngotracheal complex through anterior and posterior suspensory ligaments. The anterior suspensory ligament arises from the anterior aspect of the first several tracheal rings to insert on the corresponding undersurface of the thyroid isthmus. The posterior suspensory ligament of the thyroid (also known as the ligament of Berry) can be regarded as a condensation of the thyroid capsule, which extends from the lateral aspect of the upper tracheal rings to form a dense connection between the trachea and the corresponding undersurface of the bilateral thyroid lobes. This fibrous formation has been termed the ligament of Berry or Berlin's adherent zone.[3] The ligament of Berry is both dense and well vascularized, deriving a branch along its inferior edge from the inferior thyroid artery. The ligament of Berry can be closely associated with adjacent thyroid tissue, which can, to a varying degree, infuse into the substance of the ligament and in doing so approximate the RLN. Berlin and, more recently, Wafae, found that in a significant percentage of patients the RLN can actually penetrate the thyroid gland within the ligament of Berry.[3,4] It is this set of anatomic concerns that prohibits capsular dissection as a method to prevent injury to the RLN. The thyroid tissue that infuses the ligament of Berry can occasionally be seen after lobectomy in the thyroid bed as a small round profile of thyroid tissue, approximating the transected edge of the ligament of Berry. Remnants of this tissue can result in thyroid bed uptake after "total thyroidectomy."

Recurrent and Superior Laryngeal Nerves

The cervical branches of the vagus of concern during thyroid surgery include the superior laryngeal nerve (SLN), both internal and external branches, as well as the RLN (Figure 28-1). The SLN's internal branch brings general visceral afferents to the lower pharynx, supraglottic larynx, and base of tongue as well as special visceral afferents to epiglottic taste buds. The SLN's external branch brings branchial efferents to the cricothyroid muscle and inferior constrictor. The RLN contains branchial efferents to the inferior constrictor and all laryngeal intrinsics except the cricothyroid muscle as well as general visceral afferents from the larynx (vocal cords and below), upper esophagus, and trachea. These branches also convey parasympathetic innervation to the lower pharynx, larynx, trachea, and upper esophagus. The vagus exits the pars nervosa of the jugular foramen and descends the neck in the carotid sheath. As the heart descends during embryologic life, the RLN is carried caudally by the lowest persisting aortic arch. The right vagus runs from the posterior aspect of the internal jugular vein at the base of the neck to cross anterior to the first part of the right subclavian artery. The right RLN branches from the vagus and courses up and behind the right subclavian into the right thoracic inlet into the base of the neck. The left vagus courses from the carotid sheath in the left neck base anteriorly around the aortic arch. The left RLN branches from the vagus, curv-

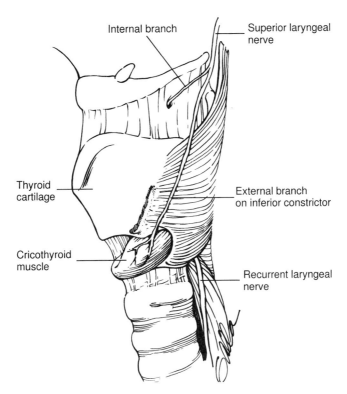

Figure 28-1.   Recurrent and superior laryngeal nerves.

ing up under the aortic arch just lateral to the obliterated ductus arteriosus. On the right, the fifth aortic arch normally degrades. This places the right RLN under the fourth arch (ie, the right subclavian artery) (see Figure 28-2). If the development of the right fourth arch fails, the right subclavian artery arises from the aorta and passes to the right with a retroesophageal course. This implies that the right RLN simply branches from the vagus in the neck and runs from the carotid sheath to its laryngeal entry point. Such a nonrecurrent RLN occurs in approximately 0.5 to 1% of cases.[5] On the left, the fifth arch forms the ductus arteriosus and the fourth arch the aorta. The left RLN comes to lie under the aorta, just lateral to the obliterated ductus arteriosus. Nonrecurrence of the left RLN has been identified in the context of transposition of the great vessels.

The right RLN enters the neck base at the thoracic inlet more laterally than does the left recurrent. The right RLN ascends the neck, traveling from lateral to medial, crossing the inferior thyroid artery. Superiorly, it travels under the inferiormost fibers of the inferior constrictor, extending up behind the cricothyroid articulation to enter the larynx. The laryngeal entry point of the RLN is marked anteriorly by the thyroid cartilage's inferior cornu. The left RLN emerges from underneath the aortic arch and enters the thoracic inlet on the left in a more paratracheal position and extends upward in or near the tracheoesophageal groove, ultimately crossing the distal branches of the inferior thyroid artery. Typically, for the last centimeter or so, the RLN, prior to laryngeal entry, travels close to the lateral border of the trachea. The RLN can be identified laterally at midpolar level near the ligament of Berry (lateral approach), infe-

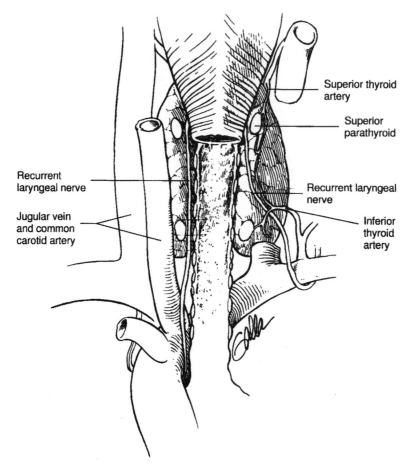

Figure 28-2.   Posterior view of thyroid showing superior and inferior thyroid arteries and their relationship to the recurrent laryngeal nerves.

riorly in the neck base at the thoracic inlet (inferior approach), or through a superior approach after dissection of the superior pole at the RLN's laryngeal entry point (superior approach). In approximately one-third of cases, the RLN branches prior to its laryngeal entry point.[6] Ninety percent of branching occurs above the level of the intersection of the RLN with the inferior thyroid artery.[7] RLN nerve branching can vary from side to side within the same patient.

The inferior thyroid artery derives as an upwardly directed branch of the thyrocervical trunk, extending under the carotid artery medially to cross the RLN. The RLN may be deep or superficial to the artery or may ramify branches of the artery. The basic relationship is, however, that the artery and nerve intersect.

RLN position may be significantly abnormal in the setting of goitrous change and substernal extension. Retrotracheal goiter may place the nerve ventral to thyroid tissue by excavating the region deep to the nerve. We have found that in about 15% of cases of large cervical or substernal goiters, the nerve is fixed or splayed over the surface of the goiter. In such cases of large goiter or substernal goiter, routine identification of the RLN in the thoracic inlet may be prohibited because of the size of the goiter. Some recommend blunt finger dissection to deliver a goiter from the wound or a substernal goiter into the neck without RLN identification. Because of the possibility of nerve fixation or nerve splaying associated with the undersurface of such a goiter, blunt dissection without nerve identification risks stretch injury. Identification of the RLN through a superior approach in these circumstances is recommended.

The SLN arises from the upper vagus just below the nodose ganglion and descends medial to the carotid sheath. It divides into internal and external branches about 2 to 3 cm above the superior pole of the thyroid. The internal branch travels medially to the carotid system, entering the posterior aspect of the thyrohyoid membrane, providing sensation to the ipsilateral supraglottis. The external branch descends to the region of the superior pole and extends medially along the inferior constrictor muscle to enter the cricothyroid muscle. As the external branch slopes downward on the inferior constrictor musculature, it has a close association with the superior pole pedicle. Typically, the external branch diverges from the superior pole vascular pedicle 1 cm or more above the superior aspect of the thyroid superior pole. However, several studies have documented that, in about 20% of cases, the external branch is closely associated with the superior thyroid vascular pedicle at the level of the capsule of the superior pole, placing it at risk during ligation of the superior pole vessels.[8,9] Depending upon the degree of superior pole development, sternothyroid muscle division may help in exposure of the superior pole region. With external branch injury there is a loss of vocal tensing, manifest by increased vocal tiredness and a loss of higher registers. Postoperative examination after unilateral external branch injury shows a bowed and somewhat lowered cord with a larynx that is slightly rotated to the affected side. Such an injury brought to an end the operatic career of Amelita Galli-Curci after thyroid surgery.

The thyroid ima artery is a separate unpaired inferior vessel which may rise from the innominate artery, carotid artery, or aortic arch directly and is present in 1.5 to 12% of cases.[10] The potential for a high-riding innominate artery or thyroid ima artery requires wide exposure and careful dissection along the anterior trachea during isthmus dissection at thyroidectomy.

The thyroid veins include the superior, middle, and inferior thyroid veins (Figure 28-3). The superior thyroid vein derives as a branch of the internal jugular vein and travels with the superior thyroid artery in the superior pole vascular pedicle. The middle thyroid vein travels without arterial complement and drains into the internal jugular vein. The inferior thyroid vein also travels without arterial complement, extending from the inferior pole to the internal jugular or brancheocephalic vein. The right and left thyroid veins can form a plexus of vessels at the lower margin of the thyroid called the plexus thyroideus impar.

THYROID FUNCTION TESTS

Thyroid hormone (TH) production and secretion is regulated by the pituitary's thyroid-stimulating hormone (TSH). The two thyroid hormones are thyroxine (T_4) and triiodothyronine (T_3). As TH decreases, TSH increases in an effort to stimulate the thyroid to maintain the pre-existing set point. Increased TSH levels stimulate gland size and vascularity. As TH increases, TSH release is suppressed. Although T_3 is more physiologically potent than T_4, it is T_4 that strongly correlates with TSH level and is believed to play a predominant role in TSH negative feedback. T_4 represents 90% and T_3 10% of the thyroid gland's production of TH. The half life of T_4 is 6 to 7 days; therefore, with change in exogenous T_4 dose, thyroid function tests are reassessed after 5 to 6 weeks. The half-life of T_3 is only 1 day, so reassessment of thyroid function tests after dose change of exogenous T_3 is performed after 1 to 2 weeks.

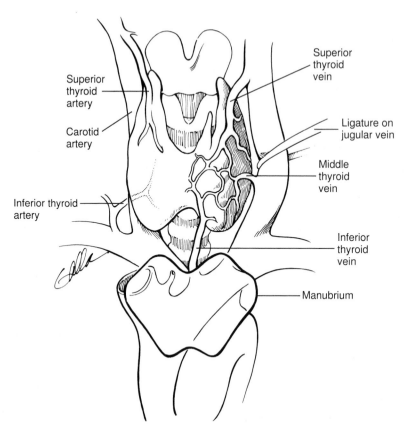

Figure 28-3.   Superior thyroid and inferior thyroid arteries (left figure) and superior, middle, and inferior thyroid veins (right figure).

Eighty percent of circulating T_3 is created from conversion of T_4 in the periphery. T_3 is physiologically several times more potent than T_4. Both T_4 and T_3 stimulate calorigenesis, potentiate epinephrine, lower cholesterol levels, and have roles in normal growth and development. Iodine is actively transported into the thyroid follicular cell and is oxidized to thyroglobulin-bound tyrosine residues. Four such iodinizations result in the formation of T_4; removal of one residue results in the formation of T_3. Both T_3 and T_4 are formed in this way within the thyrocyte and are subsequently stored bound to thyroglobulin in colloid. The stored hormone is, upon release, taken up from colloid, cleaved off thyroglobulin, and released into the circulation.

T_4 and T_3 are predominately protein-bound (mainly to thyroid-binding globulin), with less than 1% representing free (that is, unbound) hormone. Total T_4 and total T_3 laboratory tests measure total amount of protein-bound and free hormone. There can be significant fluctuation in these total measures depending upon changes in thyroid-binding globulin level. It is the T_3 resin uptake test that allows for correction of total T_4 level for fluctuation in thyroid-binding globulin. T_3 resin uptake measures the binding capacity of existing thyroid-binding globulin. The more available binding sites on native thyroid-binding globulin, the less resin uptake of radiotagged T_3. Thus, in states of thyroid-binding globulin excess, T_3 resin uptake is low. Such resin uptake is now often expressed as an index of the patient's T_3 resin uptake over normal uptake as the TH–binding ratio (THBR). High levels of thyroid-binding globulin occur in pregnancy or with use of birth control pills. Low thyroid-binding globulin levels can occur in hypoproteinemic states (example: nephrotic syndrome), in acromegaly, and with androgen and anabolic steroids. Of note, in true thyroid functional disease, total T_4 and T_3 resin uptake fluctuates in the same direction; whereas in protein-binding abnormalities, total T_4 and T_3 resin uptakes move in opposite directions (Table 28-1).

Assays of TSH (third-generation ultrasensitive assays capable of detecting 0.01 mU/L) currently available make this measure the sole test necessary to sensitively diagnose hypo- or hyperthyroidism. Measurements of TSH are now used not only to monitor replacement therapy but also to measure suppressive therapy both for thyroid nodules and postoperatively for thyroid carcinoma. Exogenous T_4 is available as levothyroxine and exogenous T_3 as lyothyronine. If TSH is high and T_4 is normal, subclinical hypothyroidism is diagnosed. Such a pattern is typically seen in early Hashimoto's thyroiditis, is believed to represent an early stage of pituitary–thyroid axis impairment, and is typically treated with T_4. If TSH is low and T_4 and T_3 are normal, subclinical hyperthyroidism is diagnosed. Such a pattern is often seen in multinodular goiter, as the patient develops progressive hyperfunctional regions within the thyroid and grades toward frank hyperthyroidism. Avoidance of iodine loads, such as seaweed-containing health foods, amiodarone, and computed tomography (CT) iodine contrast agents and intermittent monitoring of thyroid function tests are typically recommended.

BENIGN THYROID DISEASE

Hypothyroidism

Hypothyroidism is the functional state characterized by increased TSH and decreased TH. Hypothyroidism has a variety of causes and can present with a multitude of symptoms (Table 28-2). *Myxedema* refers to nonpitting edema secondary to increased glycosaminoglycans in tissue in severe hypothyroidism. Treatment for hypothyroidism is typically started at a low dose to avoid abrupt correction, especially in elderly patients or in patients with coronary artery disease. Typically, T_4 is started at 0.05 mg PO per day and is slowly increased, titrated to thyroid function levels.

Hyperthyroidism

Hyperthyroidism refers to the physiologic state of increased TH biosynthesis and secretion. *Thyrotoxicosis* refers to the clinical syndrome of TH excess. Hyperthyroidism can occur as a result of several pathologic entities and presents with characteristic symptoms (Table 28-3).

TABLE 28-1. PATTERNS OF THYROID FUNCTION TESTS

	Euthyroid	Hyperthyroid	Hypothyroid	States of High TBG	States of Low TBG
TSH	Normal	↓	↑	Normal	Normal
Total T_4	Normal	↑	↓	↑	↓
T_3 resin uptake (or THBR)	Normal	↑	↓	↓	↑
Free T_4 index	Normal	↑	↓	Normal	Normal

TBG, thyroid-binding globulin; TSH, thyroid-stimulating hormone; T_4, thyroxine; T_3, triiodothyronine.

TABLE 28-2. HYPOTHYROIDISM

Differential Diagnosis	Clinical Manifestations

1. Primary gland failure (common)
  a. Hashimoto's thyroiditis
  b. Iodine deficiency
  c. Associated with thyroiditis (lymphocytic/postpartum, subacute)
  d. Radiation-induced (I^{131} or external beam)
  e. Postsurgical
  f. Drugs (lithium, iodine)
  g. Hereditary metabolic defects in hormonogenesis
2. Central hypothyroidism (rare)
	Fatigue, slowed mentation, change in memory, depression, cold intolerance, hoarseness, brittle hair, dry skin, thick tongue, weight gain, constipation/ileus, menstrual disturbance, bradycardia, non-pitting edema, hyporeflexia, psychosis, hyponatremia, hypoglycemia, coma. In infants, mental retardation/cretinism.

By far, Graves' disease and toxic nodular goiter account for most hyperthyroidism. Hyperthyroidism referable to thyroiditis is self-limiting.

Graves' disease accounts for 60% of clinical hyperthyroidism. Graves' disease is an autoimmune disease resulting from immunoglobulin, autoantibody binding the TSH receptor, which results in TSH-like activity. Graves' disease is more common in females than in males and typically presents in the third to fourth decades. The physical examination shows a diffusely enlarged anodular thyroid. Increased metabolic activity is reflected by increased blood flow; thus a thyroid bruit can often be heard. Graves' disease is characterized histologically by scattered lymphocytic infiltration. Patients may have an infiltrative ophthalmopathy with exophthalmos. Although considered a part of Graves' disease, the ophthalmopathy typically follows an independent course. Graves' disease may also be characterized by an infiltrative dermopathy, resulting in localized myxedema (example: pretibial) and, rarely, thyroid acropachy, characterized by digital clubbing and edema of the hands and feet. Iodine-123 (I^{123}) scanning shows a diffuse increased gland uptake. Graves' disease can be treated with radioactive iodine ablation, antithyroid drugs, or surgery. Treatment of Graves' disease in the United States, except in children and young adults, usually involves radioactive iodine initially.

Hyperthyroidism can also arise from either uninodular or multinodular toxic goiter. In these cases, unlike Graves' disease, the hyperfunctional tissue is restricted to one or more regions within the thyroid gland, which is enlarged in a nodular pattern. Toxic multinodular goiter develops from pre-existing nontoxic nodular goiter. Toxic goiter occurs more frequently in endemic goiter, occurring in iodine-deficient regions, and presents more commonly in females than in males. It presents without the eye or skin findings that characterize Graves' disease. As toxic multinodular goiter evolves from pre-existing nontoxic nodular goiter over time, there is a progressive nodule formation and evolution of hyperfunctional regions, which

TABLE 28-3. HYPERTHYROIDISM

Differential Diagnosis	Clinical Manifestations
1. Graves' disease 2. Toxic nodule/multinodular goiter 3. Thyroiditis 4. Exogenous hyperthyroidism/struma ovarii/functional thyroid cancer 5. Thyrotropin, thyrotropin-like secreting tumor (pituitary, trophoblastic, other)	Weight loss, fatigue, nervousness, tremor, palpitations, increased appetite, heat intolerance, muscle weakness, diarrhea, sweating, menstrual disturbance

elaborate excess TH, resulting in suppression of TSH. This TSH suppression results in the adjacent normal gland becoming less active on I^{123} scans, with hyperfunctional areas being hot. At this stage the hyperfunctional region is not autonomous and a suppression I^{123} shows no uptake. This prehyperthyroid pattern of suppressed TSH but normal T_4 and T_3 is referred to as subclinical hyperthyroidism. The development of overt hyperthyroidism in such patients with exogenous iodine administration (example: iodine CT contrast) is referred to as the Jod-Basedow phenomenon. With time, the hyperfunctional regions become truly autonomous, continuing to secrete TH despite significant TSH suppression. When true autonomy occurs, I^{123} scanning shows focal hot regions with complete absence of adjacent normal gland. Suppression scanning at this time shows ongoing focal uptake, demonstrating autonomy despite TSH suppression. For uninodular toxic goiter, hyperthyroidism typically does not occur until the nodule is 3 cm or larger. Such nodules are usually characterized by enhanced T_3 production relative to T_4. The treatment of such toxic nodules is either surgery or radioactive iodine. Antithyroid medications are considered only as a pretreatment prior to more definitive surgical or radioablative treatment. Unlike Graves' disease, there is a low rate of spontaneous remission after antithyroid drug therapy is withdrawn in toxic nodular goiter. Surgery for toxic nodules has the advantage of quickly and definitively correcting hyperthyroidism and is associated with low morbidity. Rates of cure and subsequent development of hypothyroidism vary with the radioactive iodine ablation regimen.

Treatment of Hyperthyroidism

When medical treatment is initially offered for hyperthyroidism, treatment is usually initiated with antithyroid drugs in order to render the patient euthyroid. Radioiodine ablation represents a more definitive modality. Radioiodine ablation involves the oral administration of I^{131}. Areas of increased uptake are preferentially injured through beta-radiation. There is no evidence of genetic change or induction of malignancy with such treatment. It is, however, contraindicated in women who are pregnant or lactating. Despite its safety, it is used infrequently in children and adolescents.

The thionamides or antithyroid drugs introduced in the 1940s include propylthiouracil (PTU) and methimazole. They block iodine organification and TH synthesis. In addition, PTU blocks peripheral conversion of T_4 to T_3. Propylthiouracil is given three times a day and methimazole once a day. Both typically require administration over 6 to 8 weeks before rendering a patient euthyroid. This lag represents time necessary to exhaust preformed TH existing in colloid. Side effects include rash, fever, lupus-like reaction, and bone marrow suppression, which is reversible if detected early (bone marrow suppression occurs in 0.3–0.4% of cases). These agents are contraindicated in pregnancy and lactation.

The administration of iodides (potassium iodide, Lugol's solution) inhibits organification and prevents TH release. Iodides have been given preoperatively to decrease thyroid gland vascularity. The antithyroid effect of iodine is transient, with escape within 2 weeks, and is termed the Wolff-Chaikoff effect. If high-dose iodides are given for prolonged periods of time, especially in the setting of toxic nodular goiter, hyperthyroidism can result.

Beta-adrenergic blockers such as propranolol or nadolol do not change TH production but block peripheral TH effects. They are useful in symptomatic control while other treatments are initiated and also in transient forms of hyperthyroidism associated with thyroiditis (see below). Beta-adrenergic blockers are contraindicated in patients with asthma, chronic obstructive pulmonary disease, cardiac failure, insulin-dependent diabetes, bradyarrhythmias, and those taking monoamine oxidase inhibitors and tricyclics.

Antithyroid drugs have certain advantages in the treatment of hyperthyroidism. They have a quick onset of action and their use may allow remission with ongoing euthyroid status after discontinuation of the medicine. Such remission is more likely in patients with small goiters, mild hyperthyroidism, and those who have thyrotoxicosis characterized by elevated levels of T_3 (T_3 toxicosis).[11,12] As noted above, the rate of remission after discontinuation of antithyroid medications is quite low in toxic nodular goiter. Disadvantages of antithyroid medications include the risk of agranulocytosis, which requires ongoing concern and evaluation each time symptoms of infection arise. Also, even if a remission occurs after discontinuation of antithyroid drugs, there is a high rate of hyperthyroid relapse. One study showed that 74% of patients relapsed if followed over a period of 5 years.[13]

Radioactive iodine ablation has advantages and disadvantages. It is often definitive treatment and has no significant long-term side effects in terms of risk of developing malignancy or teratogenic effects if conception is delayed more than 6 months after radioactive iodine treatment. Some question its application to the treatment of nodules, which may be malignant, but most feel the incidence of malignancy within hot nodules is quite small. Disadvantages of radioiodine ablation include the rate of hypothyroidism after its use. Up to 80% of patients with Graves' disease and up to 50% of those with toxic nodules treated with radioactive iodine ultimately become hyperthyroid.[14,15] The incidence of hypothyroidism varies with the dosing regimen. Iodine ablation results in a less rapid normalization of TH levels than does surgery, typically requiring 6 to 8 weeks. Although radioactive iodine treatment at doses used for Graves' disease and toxic nodules has not been associated with the development of genetic mutation or malignancy, there is still reluctance to treat young patients with radioablation.[16,17]

Surgery for Hyperthyroidism

Surgery results in correction of the hyperthyroid state faster than administration of radioactive iodine and without the risks of antithyroid drugs. It is especially suited for toxic nodules, where one discrete region of the thyroid may be resected with preservation of adjacent normal tissue. Many studies show that when properly done, surgery poses a lower risk of hypothyroidism than radioactive iodine ablation.[18] Presently in the United States, surgery for Graves' disease is typically recommended if antithyroid drugs or radioactive iodine ablation fail, but it was formerly the primary treatment of Graves' disease in this country and remains such in Japan.[18] Surgery for Graves' is considered when there is: (1) failure or significant side effects after medical treatment, (2) need for rapid return to euthyroidism, (3) massive goiter, or (4) a wish to avoid radioactive iodine. For uninodular or multinodular toxic goiter, surgery and radioablation are typically considered primary treatments.

Endocrinologic management is essential in order to return the patient preoperatively to the euthyroid state so as to avoid perioperative thyroid storm. Euthyroidism is obtained typically by antithyroid drugs used for 6 weeks prior to surgery with or without beta-adrenergic blockers. When the patient is euthyroid, some consider a 2-week course of preoperative iodide (SSKI or Lugol's solution), which is believed to decrease vascularity and gland friability, although the efficacy of such treatment is controversial.[19,20]

The goal of surgery for hyperthyroidism is to remove the hyperfunctional tissue and preserve sufficient thyroid tissue to render the patient euthyroid. Implicit in the surgical philosophy is that it is preferable to render the patient hypothyroid rather than to provide inadequate resection with recurrent hyperthyroidism. The standard offering for Graves' disease is bilateral subtotal thyroidectomy with resection of any existing pyramidal lobe. Some suggest that, as an alternative to bilateral subtotal thyroidectomy, a total lobectomy on one side and contralateral subtotal resection is best. Others recommend total thyroidectomy, accepting the resulting postoperative need for TH replacement.[21] When remnants are left during surgery for Graves' disease, they generally range from 4 to 8 g.[22]

The surgery for toxic nodule involves resection of the involved portion of the gland, usually through lobectomy. With this technique there is a very low incidence of recurrent hyperthyroidism.[21] In toxic multinodular goiter, the gross or sonographically identified nodule does not always correspond to the hyperfunctional region identified on scintillography. It is then best to consider both scintillographic and sonographic information in constructing a rational surgical plan for toxic multinodular goiter.

Complication rates of bilateral subtotal thyroidectomy for Graves' disease in expert hands show an average of 0.4% permanent hypoparathyroidism and 1.2% permanent vocal cord paralysis.[23] The risk of postoperative hypothyroidism is approximately 24%. This is generally considered lower than the incidence of hypothyroidism after radioablation. The rate of postoperative recurrent hyperthyroidism after bilateral subtotal thyroidectomy for Graves' disease in expert hands is about 6% and is proportional to the size of the remnant left, the iodine content of the diet, and the degree of lymphocytic infiltration of the gland.[23]

Thyroiditis

Hashimoto's Thyroiditis

Hashimoto's thyroiditis is not only the most common form of thyroiditis but also the most common cause of goiter and the most common single thyroid disease.[24] It has an autoimmune etiology and is associated with increased thyroid peroxidase antibodies in 70 to 90% of patients.[24] Hashimoto's presents as a painless, firm, symmetric goiter, typically in a female in the third to fifth decade of life. Usually patients are euthyroid at presentation, but hypothyroid symptoms may occur at presentation in up to 20%. Hypothyroidism may develop with time, so ongoing follow-up is warranted.[25] Iodine[123] scanning typically contributes little information to the workup but, when obtained, shows patchy uptake varying with the degree of thyroid involvement. Patients usually have no regional symptoms, although pain has been reported.[26] Histologically, there is lymphocytic infiltration with germinal center formation, follicular acinar atrophy, Hürthle cell metaplasia, and fibrosis. Hypothyroidism results from progressive loss of follicular cells. Patients who are hypothyroid are simply treated with TH, which usually decreases the size of the goiter. Surgery is considered if the goiter is large, symptomatic, or refractive to TH.

Typically, both thyroid lobes are enlarged and firm. Because the lobes can be firm and discrete during the examination, the lobe may be mistaken for a focal nodule. In such cases, I[123] scanning shows that the entire lobar uptake corresponds to the "palpable nodule." It is best to avoid fine needle aspiration in patients with Hashimoto's thyroiditis, as these aspirates will confusingly show Hürthle cells and lymphocytes and may lead to a recommendation of surgery. Fibrous variants of Hashimoto's thyroiditis have been described and can form a massive, firm goiter. Although thyroid lymphoma usually arises out of a Hashimoto's gland, most patients with Hashimoto's thyroiditis do not develop lymphoma. The development of a rapidly enlarging mass within a Hashimoto's gland should raise concern regarding lymphoma and warrants fine needle aspiration or biopsy. Any discrete palpable abnormality that is not part of the diffuse goiter process despite a pre-existing diagnosis of thyroiditis should be evaluated with fine needle aspiration.

Subacute Granulomatous Thyroiditis

Subacute granulomatous thyroiditis (SGT) has also been termed deQuervain's thyroiditis. It is believed to be viral in etiology. SGT is the most common cause of painful thyroid.[27] It typically presents with an enlarged, painful thyroid, often after upper respiratory tract infection. Patients may also have malaise and fever. Pain in the perithyroid region typically radiates up the neck to the angle of the jaw. The pain and enlargement may only involve a portion of the gland (example: one lobe) and later migrate to the opposite lobe. Although pain is characteristic of SGT, it may also occur with hemorrhage into a benign nodule and with thyroid cancer. Fifty percent of patients with SGT present with hyperthyroidism with an elevated TH and sedimentation rate. I[123] scanning typically shows less than 2% uptake. It is believed that there is a virally induced follicular cell disruption with a resultant TH spill and secondary development of hyperthyroidism. The pain in hyperthyroid phase typically resolves in 3 to 6 weeks. As the acute injury improves, about 50% of patients will enter a hypothyroid phase, which typically lasts several months. Most patients ultimately revert to euthyroidism; only 5% will develop permanent hypothyroidism.[25] The low I[123] uptake in SGT distinguishes the transient hyperthyroidism of SGT from that of Graves' disease or toxic multinodular goiter. Subacute granulomatous thyroiditis is typically a self-limiting entity, treated as needed with nonsteroidal anti-inflammatory drugs such as aspirin, and, rarely, steroids.

Lymphocytic Thyroiditis

Lymphocytic thyroiditis is also termed silent, painless, or postpartum thyroiditis. Its etiology is unknown, but it is believed to be an autoimmune disease. It follows a course similar to that of subacute thyroiditis, although it is not associated with pain. Lymphocytic thyroiditis may occur sporadically but is common in postpartum females; it may occur in up to 5% of such women.[24] Patients typically present with painless, symmetric thyroid enlargement and reversible hyperthyroidism. Usually no treatment is offered, given that the thyrotoxicosis is self-limiting.

Acute Suppurative Thyroiditis

Acute suppurative thyroiditis is an exceedingly rare thyroid infection with abscess formation. It is usually bacterial (commonly due to *Staphylococcus, Streptococcus,* or *Enterobacter*) but can be fungal or even parasitic. It typically presents in the setting of an upper respiratory tract infection. Children may demonstrate left pyriform sinus fistulae.[27] Treatment is with incision and drainage and parenteral antibiotics. In children, after acute treatment, evaluation for possible pyriform sinus fistula is reasonable, including barium swallow, CT, or endoscopy.

Riedel's Struma

Riedel's struma is an unusual, rare inflammatory process of unknown etiology. It is the thyroid equivalent to sclerosing cholangitis or retroperitoneal fibrosis. Presentation is with a large, nontender goiter with a woody consistency fixed to surrounding structures with progressive regional symptoms, including dysphagia, tracheal compression, and possibly RLN paralysis. Patients present euthyroid but can progress to hypothyroidism. The clinical course is characterized by progressive regional aerodigestive track symptoms. Histologically, Riedel's struma represents an extensive fibrotic process, the hallmark of which is extrathyroidal extension of fibrosis into surrounding neck structures.[28] Treatment may require a biopsy, often in the form of isthmectomy, which may be sufficient to relieve symptoms of tracheal and esophageal pressure. Aggressive surgery is usually avoided because of the loss of surgical planes due to extensive extrathryoidal fibrosis.

Euthyroid Goiter (Nontoxic Diffuse and Multinodular Goiter)

Thyroid enlargement without significant functional derangement may occur with diffuse anodular enlargement (nontoxic diffuse goiter) or through multinodular formation (multinodular goiter). Goiter development can be sporadic or associated with iodine deficiency, inherited metabolic defects, or exposure to goitrogenic agents. In multinodular goiter, nodules may vary in size and the gland may have asymmetric involvement, with one lobe being larger than the other. Thyroid function tests are normal for nontoxic diffuse goiter. For multinodular goiter, thyroid function tests may show a normal T_4 and T_3, with TSH low normal (subclinical hyperthyroidism) as mentioned above. Over a period of years, subclinical hyperthyroidism can grade into overt hyperthyroidism, especially with increased iodine exposure. Iodine scanning typically shows heterogeneity, with some regions that are cold and some that are hot.

Goiter may be stable over a period of years or can slowly grow. Nodules within multinodular goiter may also undergo rapid, painful enlargement secondary to hemorrhage. Such a rapid increase in size may be associated with pain and an increase in regional symptoms, including airway distress.

Several studies suggest that from 15 to 45% of patients with large cervical goiters or substernal goiters may be asymptomatic.[29,30] It is of note, however, that patients may be asymptomatic and yet have radiographic evidence of tracheal obstruction and evidence of airway obstruction on flow volume studies.[31] When patients with goiter are symptomatic, they may present with chronic cough, nocturnal dyspnea, choking, and difficulty breathing in different neck positions or in recumbency. Such patients may have been erroneously diagnosed with asthma or obstructive sleep apnea. Several surgical series show that approximately 20% of patients with cervical and retrosternal goiters present with acute airway distress, with up to 10% requiring intubation.[29,30] We feel that all patients who are symptomatic, all patients with significant radiographic evidence of airway obstruction, and all patients with substernal goiter should be offered surgery.

The physical examination of such patients should include evaluation of respiratory status, tracheal deviation, and substernal extension. The development of venous engorgement or subjective respiratory discomfort with the arms extended over the head (Pemburton's sign) can suggest obstruction of the thoracic inlet from a large or substernal goiter. All patients should have vocal cord mobility assessed. Similarly, all patients should have a TSH test to rule out subclinical hyperthyroidism. Fine needle aspiration should be considered only if there is a dominant discrete mass. Sonogram and scintillography are usually not necessary. Chest x-ray can be helpful in assessing the tracheal air column. However, if there is significant concern regarding tracheal deviation or compression, axial CT scanning is the ideal study. This can assess the impact of the goiter on all adjacent cervical viscera and is also helpful in assessing the degree of substernal extension and the relationship of any substernal component with the great vessels. It is important, when ordering CT scanning, to order it without contrast until the patient's thyroid functional status is clearly understood.

Thyroxin suppression can reduce goiter size and has been found to be more helpful in diffuse than in multinodular goiter. The reduction in goiter size is, however, unpredictable.[32] Suppression is generally not recommended if TSH is less than 1 mU/L. Goiter growth typically resumes after T_4 discontinuation.[33] Radioiodine ablation has been used with multinodular goiter, but since uptake is usually low and patchy, the efficiency of this modality is limited. Also, acutely, radioiodine ablation can increase the size of goiter. Again, surgery is considered for all patients with large cervical goiters with airway or esophageal evidence of compression on x-rays or with active symptomatology. Surgery is also considered when the goiter is a significant cosmetic issue. Surgery is considered for all substernal goiters, as the substernal tissue represents abnormal tissue, which is unavailable for routine physical examination, monitoring, or fine needle aspiration. If acute enlargement of the substernal components of the goiter occur, the airway is impacted at a mediastinal level.

During the surgery for goiter, nerve identification is recommended. It may be necessary to use a superior approach with identification of the nerve at the laryngeal entry point after superior pole dissection and then retrograde dissection of the nerve away from the goiter. In our studies, we have found approximately a 15% incidence of nerve fixation or nerve splaying on the undersurface of the goiter in large cervical and substernal goiters. Multiple surgical series suggest that sternotomy for large cervical and substernal goiters is rarely needed. In our series, we have not found evidence of tracheomalacia despite significant preoperative tracheal compression. Those patients—diagnosed with tracheomalacia after cervical and substernal goiter surgery in the past—may in fact have had bilateral vocal cord paralysis. The surgery necessary for cervical and substernal goiter ranges from lobectomy to bilateral subtotal thyroidectomy. Total thyroidectomy is rarely needed.[30] The incidence of carcinoma (usually small intrathyroidal papillary carcinomas) in such multinodular goiters is approximately 7.5%.[34]

MANAGEMENT OF THYROID NODULES

1. Thyroid nodules are common. They occur in 4 to 7% of the adult population.[35] Approximately 1 in 20 new nodules can be expected to harbor carcinoma. Approximately 10,600 cases of new thyroid carcinoma are diagnosed in the United States per year. Approximately 1100 deaths from thyroid carcinoma occur in the United States per year.[36,37]

2. Ninety five percent of thyroid nodules are colloid nodules, adenomas, thyroid cysts, focal thyroiditis, or cancer. Less likely entities are also possible (Table 28-4). A colloid or adenomatous nodule is a nodule within a gland affected by multinodular goiter. It represents a focal hyperplastic disturbance in thyroid architecture and is generally not a true clonal neoplasm. True follicular adenomas are monoclonal tumors arising from follicular epithelium and can be autonomous or nonautonomous. It is unknown whether some follicular adenomas have the capability of evolving to follicular carcinoma.

3. Despite the importance of the history and physical examination, alone they are unreliable in the prediction of carcinoma. Most blatant signs of malignancy detected on physical examination occur quite late in the course of well-differentiated thyroid carcinoma or with anaplastic carcinoma. Unfortunately, many of these same findings on examination can be caused by changes associated with benign disease, such as hemorrhage into a benign cyst. The history and physical examination should provide us with a clinical setting within which we interpret the fine needle aspiration (Table 28-5). Certainly patients with chronic, stable examinations, evidence of a functional disorder, and those with a multinodular gland without a dominant nodule are of less concern in terms of malignancy. However,

TABLE 28-4. DIFFERENTIAL DIAGNOSIS OF THE THYROID NODULE

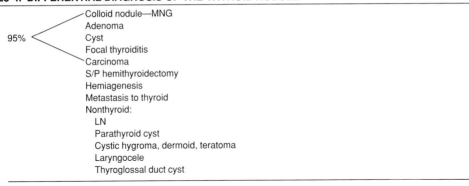

MNG, multinodular goiter; LN, lymph node; S/P, status post.

papillary carcinomas can be stable over several years. Patients with Hashimoto's thyroiditis can have papillary carcinoma or lymphoma, and patients without a dominant nodule can have thyroid malignancy. Patients who are less than 20 years of age have a higher risk of carcinoma. In patients who are above 60 years of age, nodular disease is more common and malignant disease, if ultimately found, has a considerably worse prognosis. A history of exposure to ionizing radiation is a risk factor for the development of benign and malignant thyroid nodularity, with palpable nodularity being present in up to 17 to 30% of patients exposed.[38] Approximately 1.8 to 10% of those exposed to low-dose radiation will eventually develop thyroid carcinoma.[37] Some studies suggest that patients with palpable thyroid lesions with a history of x-ray therapy may have a 30 to 50% risk of malignancy, though other studies suggest a lower incidence of malignancy.[39,40] The risk of follicular malignancy is higher in larger nodules.[41] Also, lesions greater than 4 cm are at increased risk for false-negative results during fine needle aspiration. Generally the firmer the nodule, the more one should be concerned for carcinoma. Lymphadenopathy and vocal cord paralysis are strong correlates of malignancy.[39] Family history of medullary carcinoma is certainly important to elicit but is infrequently present. Symptoms of rapid growth, pain, or aerodigestive tract compromise may occur with advanced malignancy but more commonly are associated with benign disease. Low-dose radiation therapy (example:

TABLE 28-5. DEGREE OF CLINICAL CONCERN FOR CARCINOMA IN A THYROID NODULE BASED ON HISTORY AND PHYSICAL EXAMINATION

Less Concern	More Concern
Chronic stable examination	Age < 20 > 60 years
Evidence of a functional disorder	Males
(eg, Hashimoto's toxic nodule)	Rapid growth, pain
Multinodular gland without dominant nodule	History of radiation therapy
	Family history of thyroid carcinoma
	Hard, fixed lesion
	Lymphadenopathy
	Vocal cord paralysis
	Size > 4 cm
	Aerodigestive tract compromise (eg, stridor, dysphagia)

200–500 rads), has been given in the past for adenoidal and tonsillar hypertrophy, thymic enlargement, facial acne, and tinea of the head and neck. Such treatment ended in approximately 1955 in the United States. Nodules may develop with a latency of up to 20 to 30 years, requiring ongoing vigilance. Exposure to nuclear fallout, high-dose therapeutic radiation as for Hodgkin's disease, or scatter exposure from breast radiation also seems to increase the risk of thyroid nodular disease.

4. It is best to orient toward the thyroid through adjacent cartilaginous laryngeal reference points. Once the thyroid cartilage notch (ie, Adam's apple) is identified, the anterior ring of the cricoid can be easily found. One thumb-breadth below the cricoid, the isthmus can be palpated on the underlying upper cervical trachea. When identifying the isthmus in the midline or the bilateral thyroid lobes laterally, it is useful to have the patient swallow in order to have the thyroid roll upward underneath the thumb. With such an examination, nodules of 1 cm or greater can be routinely detected. It is important, as mentioned above, to determine the firmness of the thyroid nodule and its mobility or fixation to the adjacent laryngotracheal complex. All patients with thyroid lesions should have a vocal cord examination to assess vocal cord motion. It should be strongly emphasized that voice and swallowing can be normal in the setting of complete unilateral vocal cord paralysis.

Workup: Laboratory Evaluation

1. Sensitive TSH assay represents an excellent screening test to definitively diagnose euthyroidism, hyperthyroidism, or hypothyroidism. In general, the finding of hyper- or hypothyroidism to some degree diverts attention from the workup directed toward ruling out neoplasia with fine needle aspiration and toward diagnosis of the thyroid functional disorder, such as Hashimoto's or toxic nodule, which usually does not involve fine needle aspiration. Thyroid peroxidase (TPO) antibodies are helpful if the diagnosis of Hashimoto's thyroiditis is suspected. Thyroglobulin is secreted by both normal and to some degree by malignant thyroid tissue. The assay is interfered with by antithyroglobulin antibodies. Since there is extensive overlap in thyroglobulin levels between benign thyroid conditions and thyroid carcinoma, thyroglobulin measures are not useful in the workup of the thyroid nodule. Because of the rarity of medullary carcinoma of the thyroid, calcitonin is not thought to be a reasonable screening test in patients with a solitary nodule.

2. Radionuclide scanning (with technetium 99m or I^{123}) has been used in the past for the workup of thyroid nodularity. However, 95% of all nodules are typically found to be cold. Only 10 to 15% of cold nodules are malignant.[42,43] It is generally accepted that thyroid scanning does not make it possible to separate nodules into benign and malignant categories.[35]

Ultrasonography

While ultrasonography does not distinguish benign from malignant lesions, it can provide an accurate baseline, giving baseline information as to nodule size, identifying other nodules including contralateral nodularity, and identifying cervical adenopathy. Although cystic lesions are less likely than solid lesions to be malignant, either type can be malignant. A sonogram can identify the number, size, and shape of cervical nodes surrounding and distant from the thyroid. The size and shape of such nodes has been correlated with the presence of nodal metastatic disease. Sonography may also be useful in screening the thyroid for small lesions in patients presenting with metastatic thyroid cancer and for the evaluation of the thyroid in patients with a history of head and neck radiation.[44]

Fine Needle Aspiration

Fine needle aspiration (FNA) has emerged as the central diagnostic test in thyroid nodular disease. Effectiveness of FNA is, in turn, related to the skill of both aspirator and cytopathologist. FNA has significantly decreased the number of patients being sent to surgery by 20 to 50%, and has significantly increased the yield of carcinoma found in surgical specimens by 10 to 15%.[37]

Thyroid FNA cytopathologic categories include (1) malignant, (2) suspicious, (3) benign, and (4) nondiagnostic. When FNA is read as malignant, the chance of malignancy is very high, with a false-positive rate of only 1%.[45] False-positives are usually due to the confusing cytologic picture in Hashimoto's thyroiditis, Graves' disease, or toxic nodules. Toxic nodules will often be read as microfollicular/follicular neoplasm. Hashimoto's can show high numbers of lymphocytes suggestive of lymphoma, as well as Hürthle cells and microfollicular arrays. Medullary carcinoma of the thyroid can have a variety of histologic and cytologic forms. Once medullary carcinoma is suspected, calcitonin immunohistochemistry can confirm the FNA diagnosis. Anaplastic carcinoma is often easily identified based on the degree of anaplasia. Lymphoma can be suggested by FNA, but additional tissue with open biopsy is often required to confirm the diagnosis. The main difficulty with FNA in the identification of malignancy is the differentiation of follicular adenoma from follicular carcinoma. This diagnosis hinges on a histologic finding of pericapsular vascular invasion. In order to definitively differentiate follicular adenoma from follicular carcinoma, histologic evaluation of the entire capsule is necessary. This goal cannot be obtained with FNA. The FNA of such follicular adenomas is therefore graded as to several cytopathologic features ranging from macrofollicular to microfollicular. This involves a spectrum of increasing hypercellularity, decreasing amounts of colloid, and increasing amounts of nuclear atypia. The least worrisome finding on FNA of a follicular lesion is described as a macrofollicular lesion, or as a colloid adenomatous nodule. Here, large follicular arrays with plentiful colloid and some follicular sheets can be seen. The follicles are not microfollicular and the smear is not hypercellular. In such lesions, there is believed to be little if any malignant potential. With a lesion that is read as microfollicular with little colloid and little follicular sheeting, the risk of carcinoma ranges from 5 to 15% and increases with the nodule's size.[41,45] Hürthle cells are large polygonal follicular cells with granular cytoplasm. A Hürthle cell–predominant aspirate may indicate an underlying Hürthle cell adenoma or Hürthle cell carcinoma. Hürthle cells can also be present as metaplastic cells in a variety of thyroid disorders, including multinodular goiter and Hashimoto's thyroiditis. Because of the risk of an underlying Hürthle cell carcinoma, patients with FNAs described as Hürthle cell–predominant are recommended to have surgery. Nondiagnostic aspirates occur in about 15% of cases, with about 3% of these ultimately showing malignancy. Such aspirates should be repeated, perhaps with sonographic guidance.[45]

How often will we be wrong when we tell the patient the FNA is benign?

Fine needle aspiration false-negative rate ranges from 1 to 6%.[45] False-negatives occur with greater frequency with small lesions less than 1 cm or large lesions greater than 3 cm as well as in cystic lesions.

Significant emphasis is placed during FNA on palpation and stabilization of the nodule, usually by tenting the nodule relative to the skin or by stabilizing the nodule on adjacent structures.

Options for management of patients with FNAs reported as benign include (1) following the patient with repetitive examinations and sonograms; (2) administering suppressive therapy; and, rarely (3) surgery. Lesions founds to be malignant and suspicious lesions (microfollicular, Hürthle cell–predominant) are resected.

Cysts account for about 20% of all thyroid nodules.[38] The identification of a thyroid nodule as a cyst is not necessarily equivalent to a benign diagnosis. The cyst may be a simple cyst or may hemorrhage into a colloid nodule. Papillary carcinomas can present with cystic metastasis with or without hemorrhage. In general, the color of cyst fluid is not helpful in diagnosis (except that parathyroid tumors may have clear fluid), but hemorrhagic fluid and a quick recurrence of the cyst are potentially suggestive of cystic papillary carcinoma. The technique of repetitive FNA cyst drainage plus or minus suppressive therapy is generally ineffective when cysts are greater than 3 to 4 cm in diameter.[40] Surgery is recommended in these cases. The risk of carcinoma in a cyst that has persisted after aspiration attempts ranges from 10 to 30%.[38,46]

Algorithm for the Evaluation of Thyroid Nodules

Cysts less than 4 cm can be aspirated and potentially suppressed, with surgery reserved for recurrent cyst formation. Cysts larger than 4 cm should be resected. Patients with lesions found to be malignant or suspicious on FNA should be sent for surgery. Nondiagnostic lesions should have a second FNA, perhaps sonogram-guided. Patients with benign lesions on FNA should have the option of being followed, suppressed, or operated on. Benign lesions followed or suppressed can be rebiopsied in 1 year.

Thyroid Hormone Suppression

TH has been used to shrink or stabilize thyroid nodularity. This has been proposed because of the known effect of TH treatment on goitrous enlargement of the thyroid.[17] Reduction in size of a solitary thyroid nodule in response to T_4 therapy has been thought to imply a benign hormone-dependent quality. It is, however, known that TSH receptors are present on normal as well as malignant thyroid tissue. It is also known that malignant lesions can shrink on T_4, so the response to T_4 is not specific for benign disease. Emerick showed that 11% of patients with follicular carcinoma had a decrease in size of lesion on suppressive therapy.[47] Conversely, a lack of response to T_4 suppression is not specific for malignancy; Rojeski notes surgery on nodules failing T_4 suppression found carcinoma in only 20 to 40% of cases.[38] As Mazzaferri notes, there are no randomized controlled trials clearly suggesting that T_4 is better than placebo in the treatment of solitary colloid nodules. Suppressive doses of T_4 can increase nocturnal heart rate, decrease serum cholesterol, and increase the risk of atrial fibrillation in the elderly.[48] Suppressive therapy is obviously not recommended in patients with subclinical hyperthyroidism from a nodule or multinodular goiter and is usually avoided if TSH is less than 1 mU/L. Suppressive therapy also induces loss of bone density.

Well-Differentiated Thyroid Carcinoma

Papillary Carcinoma of the Thyroid

1. Papillary carcinoma is characterized histologically by the formation of papillae and unique nuclear features. The nuclei of the neoplastic epithelium are large, with nuclear margins folded or grooved and with prominent nucleoli giving a "Orphan Annie eye" appearance. Lesions with any papillary component, even if follicular features predominate, are believed to follow a course consistent with papillary carcinoma. Papillary carcinoma primaries and nodal metastases can often cystify. Unfavorable histologic forms

of papillary carcinoma include diffuse sclerosing and tall-cell variants.[49–51] Of note, there is no benign neoplastic counterpart for papillary carcinoma of the thyroid.

2. Papillary carcinoma is strongly lymphotropic, with early spread through intrathyroidal lymphatics as well as to regional cervical lymphatic beds. It is believed that the multiple foci of papillary carcinoma often seen within the thyroid gland represent intraglandular lymphatic spread rather than true multifocality.[49]

3. When presenting in children, regional and distant metastasis is more common than in adults. Despite presentation with more advanced disease, prognosis in children is generally quite favorable.

4. The majority of papillary carcinomas arise spontaneously. Low-dose radiation exposure is thought to have an inductive role in some patients with papillary carcinoma. A RET oncogene rearrangement has been identified in 10 to 30% of patients with papillary carcinoma.[52,53]

5. At presentation, approximately 30% of patients harbor clinically evident cervical nodal disease (up to 60% of pediatric patients) with a rate of distant metastasis at presentation of approximately 3%.[54]

6. The high prevalence of microscopic disease in regional neck nodal basins and in the contralateral thyroid lobe is in stark contrast to the low clinical recurrence in the neck (<9%) and in the contralateral lobe (<5%).[55,56]

7. Most studies suggest that the presence of cervical lymph node metastasis has no significant prognostic implications. There is some evidence to suggest that the presence of cervical lymph node metastasis may increase the subsequent rate of nodal recurrence.[54,57]

Follicular Carcinoma

1. Follicular carcinoma is the well-differentiated thyroid malignancy, with follicular differentiation lacking features typical of papillary carcinoma. Follicular carcinoma, typically seen as small follicular arrays or solid sheets of cells, has significant morphologic overlap with the benign follicular adenoma. Pericapsular vascular invasion is the most reliable indication of malignancy.[58]

2. The degree of invasiveness, a strong prognostic correlate, varies. Lesions may be widely invasive or "minimally" invasive.[58,59]

3. Treatment for follicular carcinoma has been enveloped by controversy regarding the multifocal nature of papillary carcinoma. However, the vast majority of the literature supports follicular carcinoma as a unifocal thyroid lesion. Spread is not through lymphatic channels but through direct extension and hematogenously. A recent review of bilateral thyroid resections for follicular carcinoma showed that the incidence of contralateral disease for follicular carcinoma approaches zero.[60]

4. Follicular carcinoma occurs more commonly in females than in males and in an older age group than papillary carcinoma, with the median age in the sixth decade. Little is known regarding the etiology of follicular carcinoma, although there is an increased incidence in regions of iodine-deficient endemic goiter.[49]

5. True follicular carcinoma is less likely than papillary carcinoma to present with nodal metastasis (approximately 9%), but it has a higher rate of distant metastasis at presentation. Reports of distant metastasis vary, but a reasonable estimate is a rate of 16%. This makes sense intuitively, since the initial diagnosis of follicular carcinoma is made through identification of capsule-level vascular invasion.

6. Prognosis for follicular carcinoma relates to a number of patient and tumor characteristics—mainly the degree of invasiveness, the presence of metastatic disease, and age at presentation.[62] Insular and poorly differentiated forms of follicular carcinoma have a poorer prognosis than follicular carcinoma overall.

7. Hürthle cell carcinoma is considered a subtype of follicular carcinoma. It is believed to follow a more aggressive course than follicular carcinoma overall, especially with respect to distant metastasis. Radioactive iodine uptake is typically poor, with greater reliance being placed on surgery.

Prognostic Risk Grouping for WDTC

1. Starting with Woolner in the 1960s, age and degree of invasiveness were used to separate patients with well-differentiated thyroid carcinoma into diverse prognostic groups.[50] The identification of key prognostic variables makes it possible to segregate patients with well-differentiated thyroid carcinoma into a large low-risk group and a small high-risk group. Mortality in the low-risk group is approximately 1 to 2%, while in the high-risk group it is approximately 40 to 50%.[63,64] Segregation of patients into high- and low-risk groups permits appropriately aggressive treatment in the high-risk group with avoidance of excess treatment and its complications in patients in low-risk category.

2. The key elements of existing prognostic schema for well-differentiated thyroid carcinoma include:

    a. Age: Typically, for females below age 50 and for males below age 40 prognosis is improved.

    b. Degree of invasiveness/extrathyroidal extension: Increased invasiveness increases the risk of local, regional, and distant recurrence and decreases survival.

    c. Metastasis: The presence of distant metastases increases mortality.

    d. Sex: Males generally have a poorer prognosis than females,

    e. Size: Lesions larger than 5 cm have a worse prognosis and lesions smaller than 1.5 cm have a better prognosis. There is controversy as to the exact cutoff, some describing decreased prognosis with lesions greater than 4 cm.

3. The two best-known prognostic schema are those devised by Ian Hay and Blake Cady.[63,64] Hay's scheme for papillary carcinoma is summarized by the mnemonic AGES—for age, gender, extent, and size. Cady's prognostic schema is for papillary carcinoma and follicular carcinoma and is summarized by the mnemonic AMES—for age, metastasis, extent, and size.

4. Other risk factors that affect prognosis have been studied. If gross disease is left at the completion of initial surgery, prognosis is worse. If radioactive iodine and T_4 suppression are given postoperatively, prognosis generally improves.

Extent of Thyroidectomy

1. Although well-differentiated thyroid cancer certainly can represent a lethal disease, it is associated with a prolonged survival in the vast majority of patients. Surgical treatment must blend an aggressive oncologic approach with a commitment not to harm the patient with excessive treatment. Mazzaferri's recent retrospective study with long-term follow-up on 1358 patients suggests that initial treatment seems important in terms of survival. This study suggests that bilateral thyroid surgery improves survival and decreases recurrence. They recommended near-total thyroidectomy followed by radioactive iodine and T_4 suppression for lesions greater than 1.5 cm.[57] Samaan also found that survival was best

in patients treated with total thyroidectomy followed by postoperative radioactive iodine.[59] However, there are many studies showing no difference in survival between patients with well-differentiated thyroid carcinoma treated with hemithyroidectomy versus total thyroidectomy, including Shah's and Cady's.[65–67]

2. Recurrence has been shown to be favorably affected by aggressive surgery in some studies, including those of Mazzaferri, Rose, and Grant.[51,68,69] Many studies, however, question the significance of extent of thyroidectomy on recurrence rate, including those of Cady, Vickery, and Tollefsen.[56,67,70] Pasieka reviewed the literature and described a contralateral lobe recurrence rate after conservative thyroid surgery as 7%.[71]

3. Occult papillary microscopic disease in the contralateral lobe is present with much greater frequency than is clinically manifest. This is analogous to microscopic disease in the cervical and mediastinal nodal beds. In the past, elective neck dissection has been performed for papillary carcinoma, given the 68 to 80% rate of positive microscopic disease in these beds. Such neck dissections have been abandoned, since only 7 to 8% of patients develop clinically significant nodal disease.[72–75] Thus, both the contralateral lobe of the thyroid and the regional cervical lymphatics usually contain microscopic disease. It seems to make sense intuitively that the microscopic disease contained within the contralateral lobe should be as clinically silent as that in the neck.

4. One argument for total thyroidectomy is that through production of hypothyroidism (TSH >25 mU/L), it allows for whole-body scanning and use of thyroglobulin as a marker postoperatively. These goals, however, can be obtained with conservative surgery and remnant ablation.[76] Further, total thyroidectomy, even in expert hands, has a significant failure rate in terms of the postoperative need for ablation. Studies show that thyroid bed uptakes of greater than 1 to 2% occur in about 15% of patients after total thyroidectomy.[77,78]

5. The bulk of the literature supports increased complication rates, mainly RLN paralysis and permanent hypoparathyroidism, with bilateral thyroid surgery.[79,80] Anaplastic transformation of microscopic contralateral disease has been estimated as so rare an event that it should not be considered in routine surgical planning.[79]

6. In 1987, Hay provided excellent data suggesting that the extent of thyroidectomy should be tailored to the patient's prognostic risk grouping.[63] He found that survival was equivalent for low-risk-group patients with unilateral or bilateral surgery. Survival in the high-risk group was improved with the offering of bilateral thyroid surgery over unilateral thyroid surgery. However, total thyroidectomy offered no survival benefit above near-total thyroidectomy.[63]

7. A rational surgical plan for patients with well-differentiated thyroid carcinoma can be constructed despite the divergent information in the literature. Surgery should be undertaken in an attempt to encompass all gross disease in both thyroid and neck, understanding that microscopic disease, while present, generally has little clinical significance and infrequently becomes clinically manifest. Intrathyroidal contralateral disease and nodal disease should be evaluated at surgery by careful palpation and can also be detected by preoperative sonography. Most agree that bilateral thyroid surgery will optimize survival in patients in high-risk groups, with near-total thyroidectomy being equivalent to total. In patients in low-risk groups with small intrathyroidal lesions, if the contralateral lobe is negative on preoperative sonography and is negative to intraoperative palpation, unilateral surgery is appropriate. An isthmus margin frozen section should be obtained intraoperatively. It is important to note that in addition to a patient's risk grouping, extent of

thyroidectomy must be tailored to how the specific surgery has proceeded. If the first side has revealed two parathyroids of good color with good vascular pedicles and with a RLN that has been identified and stimulates well electrically, contralateral thyroid surgery can be contemplated. If the first side has not gone well, contralateral surgery should be deferred or at least postponed.

Surgical Treatment of the Neck for Well-Differentiated Thyroid Cancer

In all cases, systematic evaluation of the central neck nodal beds should be performed (including Delphian, perithyroid, pretracheal, RLN, upper mediastinal and perithymic regions), with resection of grossly enlarged lymph nodes. If nodal disease is evident in the lateral neck, a modified radical neck dissection rather than "berry picking" is recommended. Such a systematic neck dissection seems to decrease subsequent nodal recurrence but has an unclear impact on survival.[51,81]

Invasive Disease

Extracapsular disease involving the strap muscles or sternocleidomastoid muscle (SCM) is usually easily managed with resection of the involved musculature. When disease is focally adherent to a functioning RLN, it should be dissected off, removing gross disease and preserving the functioning nerve. An infiltrated RLN is resected if preoperative paralysis is present. Disease invasive to the larynx and trachea is managed with resection of gross disease, with preservation of vital structures when possible. Near-total excision with postoperative adjuvant treatment is equivalent with respect to survival to more radical resection.[82] If such a conservative approach does not allow complete removal of gross disease, then complete through-and-through resection with airway reconstruction is advocated.[83]

Postoperative Follow-up for Well-Differentiated Thyroid Cancer

1. TH, usually T_4, is given to suppress TSH to 0.1 to 0.3 mU/L or lower in high-risk patients. I^{131} can be given postthyroidectomy based on the patient's risk grouping and likelihood of harboring metastatic disease. Typically, high-risk patients with papillary carcinoma and most patients with follicular carcinoma are considered for treatment.[84]

2. I^{131} is given in ablative doses ranging from 30 to 50 mCi if patients have undergone less than total thyroidectomy and greater than 1% uptake on regional neck scanning. Such treatment completes thyroid ablation, rendering the patient hypothyroid. Thereafter, with a TSH greater than 25 mU/L, whole-body scanning can be performed. Metastatic well-differentiated thyroid carcinoma cells require increased TSH levels to drive them to take up sufficient I^{131} scanning doses to reveal their presence on whole-body scanning. If disease is identified on such whole-body scans, therapeutic doses of I^{131} (100–150 mCi) are given.

3. External beam radiation (typically using from 50 to 60 Gy) has been employed to palliate extensive central neck disease, prolong local control, and improve quality of life in inoperable cases or where gross disease persists postoperatively. It has also been used to palliate bony and CNS metastasis.[38]

4. Thyroglobulin is produced by normal and, to some degree, malignant thyroid tissue and can serve as a marker of well-differentiated thyroid cancer. Since normal thyroid cells elaborate thyroglobulin, it is of no use as a marker unless total thyroid ablation has been achieved through either surgery or surgery plus postoperative radioablation. Thyroglobulin is usually elevated after total thyroid ablation in patients with known metastatic dis-

ease and, along with whole-body scanning, can be used to assess the status of metastatic disease. If thyroglobulin is less than 2 ng/mL (on T_4 suppression) after total thyroid ablation and whole-body scanning is negative, patients rarely harbor metastatic disease.[85,86]

Medullary Carcinoma of the Thyroid

1. Medullary carcinoma of the thyroid (MTC) represents approximately 5 to 10% of all thyroid cancers, with a clinical behavior that is intermediate between well-differentiated thyroid cancer and anaplastic carcinoma.[89] This lesion arises not from thyroid follicular cells but rather from parafollicular C cells.

2. Approximately 75% of medullary carcinoma occurs as a sporadic neoplasm, typically presenting in the fourth decade as a unifocal lesion without associated endocrinopathy. Hereditary MTC accounts for the remaining 25%, occurring in a younger age group with multifocal thyroid lesions. Three distinct forms of hereditary MTC exist (Table 28-6).

3. All three forms of hereditary MTC are inherited as autosomal dominant traits and are associated with multifocal MTC. All are preceded by multifocal C-cell hyperplasia. Lack of certainty in MTC subtype diagnosis preoperatively has resulted in the surgical recommendation of total thyroidectomy for all cases of medullary carcinoma.

4. Calcitonin is secreted by normal parafollicular C cells, and calcitonin elevation occurs in C-cell hyperplasia and all forms of MTC. This tumor marker has proven extremely useful in establishing a diagnosis in asymptomatic relatives of hereditary cases and in postoperative screening for recurrent disease.

5. RET oncogene point missense germ-line mutations have been identified in patients with inherited MTC.[87,88] These mutations can be detected through a single blood test by analysis of peripheral lymphocyte DNA and are not present in patients with sporadic disease.

6. Medullary carcinoma of the thyroid has a strong tendency toward paratracheal and lateral neck nodal involvement. In fact, medullary carcinoma of the thyroid of any type that is palpable implies nodal involvement. There is no significant effective therapy available for medullary carcinoma of the thyroid other than surgery. Therefore all patients with medullary carcinoma of the thyroid should have, at time of surgery, thorough central neck dissection emphasizing the paratracheal regions. Given the high incidence of microscopic lateral neck disease, all patients with palpable medullary carcinoma of the thyroid should have ipsilateral modified radical neck dissections with a consideration for bilateral modified radical neck dissections.[90]

7. Preoperatively, for all patients suspected of having medullary carcinoma of the thyroid, a 24-hour urine collection should be obtained for urinary catecholamines, vanillylmandelic acid, and metanephrine to rule out pheochromocytoma.

8. MTC tends to metastasize early to cervical and mediastinal nodal groups and to recur locally. Eventually, MTC may metastasize hematogenously to lung, liver, or bone. For all types of MTC, the 5-year survival rate is between 78 and 91%; the 10-year survival is between 61 and 75%.[89,91]

9. During thyroidectomy, the parathyroid glands should be explored. Most recommend their excision only if they are grossly enlarged.

Lymphoma

1. Thyroid lymphoma usually occurs in the sixth decade of life, presenting typically as a rapidly enlarging firm, painless mass. If extrathyroidal spread has occurred, patients may

TABLE 28-6. SUBTYPES OF MEDULLARY THYROID CARCINOMA (MTC)

	Mode of Transmission	Family History	Age at Presentation (Decade)	Likelihood of Regional LN* Involvement	Subtypes of MTC			
					Pheochromocytoma	Hyperparathyroidism	Mucosal Neuromata Marfanoid Habitus	
Sporadic	—	Negative	4th	High	No	No	No	
MEN* IIa	Autosomal dominant	Positive or negative	3rd	High if Dx with mass Low if Dx with screen	Yes	Yes	No	
MEN IIb	Autosomal dominant	Usually negative	1st or 2nd	High	Yes	No	Yes	
FMTC*	Autosomal dominant	Positive or negative	4th	Low	No	No	No	

*LN, lymph node; MEN, multiple endocrine neoplasia; FMTC, familial nonmultiple endocrine neoplasia medullary carcinoma of the thyroid.

present with evidence of RLN paralysis, dysphagia, and regional adenopathy. Often, there is a history of pre-existing hypothyroidism. Lymphoma is associated with pre-existing Hashimoto's thyroiditis in 80% of cases.

2. Treatment is through radiation therapy and sometimes chemotherapy. Surgery is mainly restricted to biopsy.

Anaplastic Carcinoma

1. Anaplastic carcinoma represents less than 5% of thyroid cancers and occurs almost exclusively in an older age group. Anaplastic carcinoma is believed to be one of the most aggressive known human malignancies and generally is considered uniformly fatal, with an average survival of about 6 months.

2. Patients with anaplastic carcinoma typically present in the seventh decade with large, widely invasive primaries often fixed to the laryngotracheal complex, vocal cord paralysis, cervical adenopathy, and, frequently, distant metastasis. There is often a history of pre-existing goiter that has been stable for years. Surgical treatment is generally limited to isthmusectomy for biopsy, often combined with tracheotomy. It is important to obtain sufficient biopsy material to rule out lymphoma. Aggressive surgery directed toward the thyroid or laryngotracheal complex is, in general, not recommended.[92,93] Treatment recommendations generally include hyperfractionated external beam radiation combined with doxorubicin-based chemotherapy.

THYROIDECTOMY: SURGICAL ANATOMY

1. A collar-type thyroid incision is made, typically 1 or 2 finger breadths above the sternal notch in a curvilinear fashion, within a normal skin crease. Crosshatches are unnecessary. A subplatysmal skin flap is raised superiorly up to the level of the thyroid notch.

2. Strap muscles are identified in the midline, and the sternohyoid (more medial) and sternohyoid (more lateral) are elevated in one layer off the ventral surface of the thyroid lobe while controlling any small bridging veins. Assessment of frank invasion should be made as the strap muscles are elevated.

3. Through primarily blunt dissection, the lobe is dissected and mobilized. As this is done, the thyroid gland is retracted medially onto the laryngotracheal complex, and the strap muscles are retracted laterally. This typically allows identification of the middle thyroid vein, which, when taken, provides for greater lateral exposure (Figure 28-4).

4. Once the thyroid gland is mobilized, it is important to identify the cricoid and trachea in the midline just above and below the thyroid isthmus. This identification of the midline provides an anchoring landmark for further work and is of critical importance.

5. At this point the inferior pole is preliminarily dissected with an eye toward identifying the inferior parathyroid, which is typically located within 1 cm inferior or posterior to the thyroid's inferior pole. The inferior parathyroid is often within the uppermost thyrothymic horn (upper thymus). Once this inferior parathyroid is dissected off the inferior pole of the thyroid, the RLN can be identified.

6. The RLN can be identified through the lateral approach at the midpolar level just below the ligament of Berry and its laryngeal entry point. The RLN is identified as a white, wave-like structure with characteristic vascular strip. Extra laryngeal branching can occur in about one-third of patients above the crossing point of the RLN and inferior thyroid artery. The nerve should be followed through the ligament of Berry. A capsular plane of

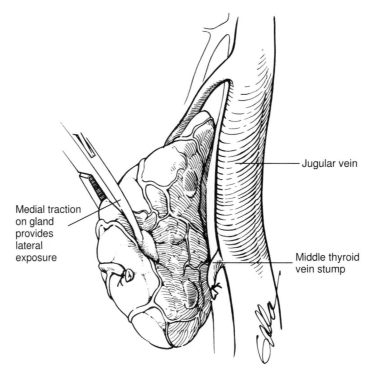

Figure 28-4.   Middle thyroid vein division provides for greater lateral exposure.

dissection on the thyroid does not prevent nerve injury in all cases. On the right, the RLN occurs somewhat more laterally than on the left. Nerve stimulation can be used to facilitate nerve identification. The laryngeal entry point is indicated by the inferior cornu of the thyroid cartilage. The possibility of a nonrecurrent RLN on the right should be kept in mind. Goitrous enlargement of the thyroid gland can significantly distort RLN position, as can peri-RLN nodal paratracheal disease. If, through goitrous enlargement or substernal extension, the nerve cannot be found laterally or as described above or inferiorly at the thoracic inlet, it should be searched for through the superior approach. In this circumstance, the superior pole is taken down proceeding from superiorly down to identify the nerve at its laryngeal entry point adjacent to the ligament of Berry.

7. Dissection of the nerve through the ligament of Berry must be slow and meticulous. Bleeding should not be met with indiscriminate clamping. In general, the bands of tissue can be bipolar, but minor bleeding is best controlled with pressure with a neurosurgical pledget. The nerve should be followed through the ligament to its laryngeal entry point, dipping underneath the lowermost fibers of the inferior constrictor.

8. The RLN should be identified in all cases both visually and electrically through neural monitoring. The electrical identification of the RLN is analogous to electrical stimulation of the facial nerve during parotid or mastoid surgery. The electrical identification reinforces its visual identification and provides the surgeon with a new functional dimension to surgical anatomy. RLN monitoring speeds nerve identification, aids in dissection

(similar to facial nerve stimulation during parotidectomy), and helps to assess RLN integrity at the completion of surgery.

9. The distal branches of the inferior and superior thyroid arteries should always be taken as close to the thyroid as possible in order to optimize parathyroid preservation (Figure 28-5). If the parathyroid has turned black as a result of its dissection or has a questionable vascular pedicle, it can be biopsied, confirmed as parathyroid, and then minced and placed into several muscular pockets in the SCM.

10. Downward and lateral retraction of the superior pole allows dissection in the interval between the thyroid cartilage medially and the superior pole laterally. The superior polar vessels are then ligated at the level of the thyroid capsule individually. If the superior pole region is hooded by the sternothyroid, this muscle can be selectively divided to improve exposure of the superior pole region. The external branch of the SLN can be, in approximately 20% of cases, closely related to the superior pole vessels at the level of the thyroid capsule and is, therefore, vulnerable to injury.[96,97]

11. In those cases where a portion of the lobe is left in place in order to preserve parathyroid tissue, it is the posterolateral portion of the thyroid lobe that should be left in situ. It is prudent, prior to making the decision about the line of resection within the thyroid lobe, to identify the RLN inferiorly so that its distal course can be judged prior to transecting the lobe.

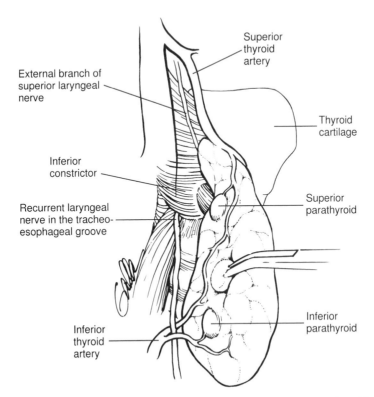

Figure 28-5. Laterally, the inferior thyroid artery and superiorly, the superior thyroid artery are followed to identify inferior and superior parathyroid glands.

Surgical Complications

1. RLN paralysis rates vary. All studies do not involve postoperative laryngeal examination, which is essential for determination of accurate postoperative paralysis rates. Many reports reveal rates of 6 to 7%, with some reports as high as 23%.[98,99] The incidence of RLN paralysis increases with bilateral surgery, revision surgery, surgery for malignancy, surgery for substernal goiter, and in patients brought back to surgery for bleeding.[99,100] The author believes that the RLN should be clearly identified and dissected along its entire course at thyroidectomy and that identification should be made both visually and through neural electric stimulation. Such stimulation is safe and allows the surgeon to identify a neurapraxic nerve injury and potentially postpone contralateral thyroid surgery.[94] Temporary RLN paralysis generally resolves within 6 months. Bilateral RLN paralysis may result in a nearly normal voice but also respiratory insufficiency with postoperative stridor. Such complications should be extremely rare if contralateral lobe surgery is deferred or staged in cases with possible ipsilateral nerve injury based on electrical intraoperative stimulation. SLN external branch paralysis occurs in 0.4 to 3% of cases and results in reduction of cricothyroid vocal cord tensing with loss of high vocal registers. The affected cord will be lower and bowed, with laryngeal rotation.[101]

2. Hypoparathyroidism can result in perioral and digital paresthesias. Progressive neuromuscular irritability results in spontaneous carpopedal spasm, abdominal cramps, laryngeal stridor, mental status changes, QT prolongation on the electrocardiogram, and ultimately tetanic contractions. Chvostek's sign is the development of facial twitching with light tapping over the facial nerve. This sign must be assessed preoperatively, as approximately 5% of the normal population has a positive Chvostek's sign in the setting of eucalcemia. Trousseau's sign is induced carpal spasm through tourniquet-induced ischemia. Treatment for hypocalcemia is usually begun when the calcium level falls below 7.5 mg/dL or in the symptomatic patient. Temporary hypothyroidism, defined as being of less than 6 months duration, occurs in from 17 to 40% of patients after total thyroidectomy.[102] Permanent hypothyroidism after total thyroidectomy in the community occurs in approximately 10% of patients.[103,104]

Parathyroid Glands

1. The parathyroid glands' hormonal product, parathyroid hormone (PTH), maintains calcium levels through increased calcium absorption in the gut, mobilization of calcium in bone, inhibition of renal calcium excretion, and stimulation of renal hydroxylase to maintain vitamin D levels.

2. Total calcium levels vary with protein fluctuation, but ionized calcium is maintained within strict ranges. In patients with normal albumin, total serum calcium can be followed. If the albumin level is abnormal, total serum calcium levels can be corrected (total serum calcium levels fall by 0.8 mg/dL for every 1 g/dL fall in albumin) or the ionized calcium can be followed.

3. Adenomatous or hyperplastic change to the parathyroid glands can increase PTH levels and produce hypercalcemia. The term *adenoma* implies a single enlarged gland, typically in the context of three other normal glands. Adenomas have been found to be benign clonal neoplasms. Such glands are hypercellular, consisting of chief and oncocytic cells, with decreased intra- and intercellular fat.[105,106] The term *hyperplasia* implies that all four glands are involved in the neoplastic change, though the gross enlargement of the glands may be quite asymmetric. Histologically, in hyperplasia there is an increased number of

chief and oncocytic cells in multiple parathyroid glands. The diagnosis of adenoma versus hyperplasia incorporates both gross surgical and histologic information. Most feel that if one gland shows gross enlargement and histologically is hypercellular with decreased fat and a second gland biopsy shows normal-appearing parathyroid, the enlarged gland should be considered an adenoma.

4. Primary hyperparathyroidism, which occurs in approximately 1 out of 500 females and 1 out of every 2000 males, can be spontaneous, familial, or associated with multiple endocrine neoplasia (MEN) syndromes; it may occur with increased frequency in patients with a past history of low-dose external beam radiation therapy. HPT is usually mediated by a single gland's adenomatous change (approximately 85%), but it can be caused by four-gland hyperplasia in approximately 5 to 15% of cases. Four-gland hyperplasia can be sporadic or can occur in familial HPT or in MEN I (Werner's) and MEN IIa (Sipple's) syndromes. Double adenomas account for 2 to 3% of cases and are more common in elderly patients. Carcinomatous degeneration of parathyroid tissue occurs rarely and accounts for approximately 1% of cases of HPT.[106] One should suspect parathyroid carcinoma if calcium and PTH levels are significantly elevated. In cases of parathyroid carcinoma, preoperative exam may be notable for a perithyroid mass. Such findings do not occur in benign HPT.

5. Secondary HPT represents a hyperplastic response of parathyroid tissue, typically to renal failure. When this parathyroid response becomes autonomous, persisting after correction of the primary metabolic derangement (typically renal transplant) with increased PTH levels despite normalization of calcium, it is termed tertiary HPT.

6. Elevated calcium and decreased phosphorus with elevated PTH help establish the diagnosis of HPT, but elevated calcium levels can be caused by many other entities (Table 28-7).

7. While the finding of high calcium and high PTH virtually diagnoses HPT, benign familial hypocalciuric hypercalcemia (BFHH) is worth considering. Like HPT, BFHH is associated with high calcium and PTH levels. It is an autosomal-dominant inherited disease characterized by excess renal calcium reabsorption, leading to high serum calcium and low urine calcium levels which are stable throughout life.

TABLE 28-7. DIFFERENTIAL DIAGNOSIS OF HYPERCALCEMIA

Primary hyperparathyroidism
Secondary hyperparathyroidism
Tertiary hyperparathyroidism
Pseudohyperparathyroidism
Sarcoid
Granulomatous disease (tuberculosis, berylliosis, eosinophilic granuloma)
Milk-alkali syndrome
Benign familial hypocalciuric hypercalcemia
Malignancy (breast, lung, multiple myeloma)
Pheochromocytoma
Vitamin D intoxication
Excess calcium intake
Lithium and thiazide diuretics
Hyperthyroidism
Adrenal insufficiency
Immobilization
Paget disease
Factitious hypercalcemia (tourniquet effect)

8. While chronically elevated calcium levels in the past have been detected through "painful bones, kidney stones, abdominal groans, psychic moans, and fatigue overtones," the majority of primary HPT today is detected in asymptomatic patients on routine laboratory screening panels.[107] Hypercalcemia, when severe and chronic, may, however, present with an impressive array of symptoms and disease (Table 28-8).

9. Most surgeons and endocrinologists agree that patients who are symptomatic from hypercalcemia warrant surgical exploration. In addition, typically all patients with significantly elevated calcium levels greater than 11.5 mg/dL are also offered surgery. Surgery is also offered for young patients under 50 years of age because of the potential for development of symptoms if followed nonsurgically. Also, surgery is offered to all patients who desire it or who have had a previous episode of life-threatening hypercalcemia. Controversy exists for patients over 50 years of age who are asymptomatic. In such patients, if there is evidence of significant bone or renal dysfunction, surgery is recommended. If creatinine clearance in this patient group is decreased by 30% for age without other obvious cause, urinary calcium is greater than 400 mg/dL, or bone density is less than two standard deviations below the mean corrected for age, gender, and race, surgery is recommended.[108]

Localization Studies

1. The use of preoperative localization studies in first-time uncomplicated cases of HPT has been controversial. Given the high success rate (95%) of such parathyroid exploration in experienced hands, the use of localization studies relates to the philosophy of unilateral versus bilateral parathyroid exploration. Most agree that localization studies are warranted in revision cases. If unilateral or minimal-access exploration is planned, localization studies should be considered (Figure 28-6).

2. Sonography is relatively inexpensive, with sensitivities in the literature ranging from 22 to 82%.[109] Sonography is, however, extremely operator-dependent, and is poor in evaluating lesions behind the larynx and trachea or in the mediastinum. CT scanning is relatively expensive and overall has been found to be less sensitive than magnetic resonance imaging (MRI). MRI is expensive, with sensitivities ranging from 50 to 80%.[109] Sestamibi scanning, initially introduced as a cardiac scan, has been found to be an excellent study for preoperative localization in HPT. Sestamibi is initially taken up by both thyroid and

TABLE 28-8. MANIFESTATIONS OF CHRONIC HYPERCALCEMIA

Weight loss
Polyuria–polydipsia
Malaise
Fatigue
Confusion
Depression
Memory changes
Hypertension
Renal dysfunction (ranging from nephrolithiasis to nephrocalcinosis)
Duodenal and peptic ulcers
Constipation
Pruritus
Pancreatitis
Arthritis
Gout
Bone pain, cysts, demineralization, fracture
Band keratitis, palpebral fissure calcium deposition

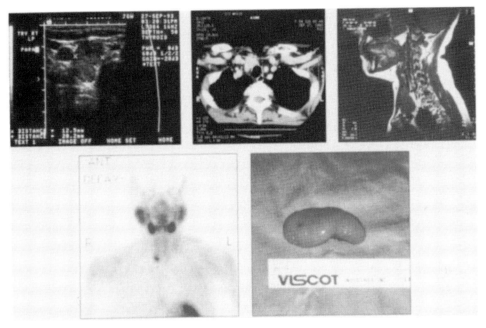

Figure 28-6. Parathyroid localization tests: parathyroid adenoma seen on sonogram, CT, MRI, (top), and sestamibi scanning (below).

parathyroids. The thyroid uptake is, over time, washed out, yet sestamibi is retained by adenomatous parathyroid glands. The uptake and retention of sestamibi is thought to be related to cellular mitochondrial content. Three-hour washout scans reveal the enlarged parathyroids. This scan seems to be one of the most sensitive tests available for HPT, with sensitivity in the literature ranging from 70 to 100%.[109,110] Such scanning is unable to detect adenomas smaller than about 200 mg or less than 5 mm and may also miss patients who have previously undergone surgery, who have multigland disease including double adenomas, or who have mediastinal disease.[111–113] Coexistent thyroid pathology also may interfere with sestamibi washout, especially Hürthle cell lesions.

Surgical Theory for Hypoparathyroidism

1. Although a single adenoma is more likely, hyperplasia must always be kept in mind when creating the surgical plan. The finding of one enlarged gland does not make the diagnosis of an adenoma. It is the histologic comparison of the presumptive adenoma with a presumptive normal parathyroid gland that makes the diagnosis of adenoma and rules out four-gland hyperplasia. Advocates of unilateral exploration suggest that adenoma resection and identification and biopsy of an ipsilateral normal gland are sufficient to rule out four-gland disease. Advocates of bilateral exploration suggest that the adenoma must be resected and all three of the remaining normal glands visualized or biopsied. Theoretically, unilateral exploration augmented by preoperative localization studies should allow shorter operative times, a decrease in postsurgical complications, and resultant cost savings.[114,115]

2. A survey of 53 surgical departments suggests that no one approach is strongly favored.[116] However, there seems to be a general trend toward unilateral surgery and minimally invasive approaches with increased reliance on preoperative localization testing and intraoperative frozen section. One of the newest trends in parathyroid surgery is intraoperative PTH assays. Given the short half-life of PTH, approximately 10 minutes after resection of an adenoma, the PTH falls to within normal limits. If strict intraoperative PTH criteria are observed once sufficient PTH fall occurs, the surgery can be successfully halted.

3. There has been controversy as to the degree of operation believed necessary for four-gland hyperplasia. Surgical strategies have ranged from resection of only the enlarged glands to 3½-gland subtotal resection to 4-gland resection with autotransplantation to the forearm. In general, the aggressiveness of the surgical approach should relate to the clinical severity of the subtype of four-gland hyperplasia. In milder forms—a four-gland hyperplasia such as nonfamilial, sporadic four-gland hyperplasia and MEN IIa—it is recommended that all four glands and supernumerary glands be identified but that only enlarged glands be resected. Such an approach has resulted in a low rate of hypercalcemic recurrence in these patients.[117] For patients with more severe forms of four-gland hyperplasia—as in familial HPT, secondary HPT, and MEN I—a more aggressive surgical approach is generally recommended.[118] For these forms, most recommend at least 3½-gland subtotal resection with clipping of the remaining remnant or total parathyroidectomy with transplantation of the remnant to the forearm.

Parathyroid: Surgical Anatomy

1. Parathyroid glands have been described as yellow-tan, caramel, or mahogany in color and are in this way distinguished from the brighter, less distinct yellow fat with which the parathyroids are typically closely associated. It is essential that the dissection be meticulous and proceed in a strictly bloodless field in order to appreciate these subtle characteristics. Parathyroids have a varying shape, which has been described elegantly by Wang as flat-bean or leaf-like, often with a vascular strip down the midline.[119] Fat is bright yellow, nonencapsulated, and less discrete. Thyroid is firmer and redder. Lymph nodes are harder, more spherical, and gray to red. Despite their characteristic size, shape, and color, one of the most typical features of the parathyroid glands is that they appear in the surgical field as discrete encapsulated structures with sharp margins. They can be observed as discrete bodies gliding within the more amorphous fat surrounding them as this fat is gently manipulated (the gliding sign).

2. The vast majority of humans have four parathyroid glands, but approximately 5% of patients will have more than four glands.

Superior Parathyroid: Surgical Anatomy

The superior parathyroid derives from the fourth branchial pouch and is associated with the lateral thyroid anlage/C-cell complex. As such, the superior parathyroid tracks closely with the posterolateral aspect of the bilateral thyroid lobes. The final adult position of the superior parathyroid is less variable than that of the inferior parathyroid because of its shorter embryologic migratory path. The superior parathyroid typically occurs at the level of the cricothyroid articulation of the larynx, approximately 1 cm above the intersection of the RLN and inferior thyroid artery. In this location, the superior parathyroid is closely related to the posterolateral aspect of the superior thyroid pole, often resting on the thyroid capsule in this location. The superior parathyroid is revealed as layers of the perithyroid sheath are serially taken dissected at this location. The superior parathyroid is located at a plane deep (dorsal) to the plane of the RLN in the neck. The superior parathyroid can lie quite deep in the neck and tends toward a retrolaryngeal and retroesophageal location. When the superior gland migrates—through either gravity, negative intrathoracic pressure, or the repetitive muscular activity of deglutition—it migrates into the posterior mediastinum.

Inferior Parathyroid: Surgical Anatomy

The inferior parathyroid enjoys a more varying adult position. This is thought to be a consequence of its longer embryologic migratory path when compared to that of the superior parathyroid. The inferior parathyroids derive from the third branchial pouch and migrate with the thymus anlage. The inferior parathyroid is found in close association with the inferior pole of the thyroid, often on the posterolateral aspect of the capsule of the inferior pole or within 1 to 2 cm. In such locations, the inferior parathyroid is often closely associated with the thickened fat of the thyrothymic horn (ie, thyrothymic ligament), a tongue of thymus which has undergone fatty degeneration and arises from the anterior mediastinum and extends up through the thoracic inlet and attaches to the undersurface of inferior thyroid pole. Failure of descent of the inferior parathyroid can result in a gland being found much higher up in the neck. The inferior parathyroid is generally located superficial (ventral) to the RLN.[120]

Parathyroid Exploration

1. The overriding technical principle in parathyroid exploration is meticulous dissection in a bloodless field to avoid blood staining of tissues. Loupe magnification is helpful. One should not rely much on preoperative localization tests and should assume multigland disease. One should have a low threshold to identify the RLN, depending on the depth of needed dissection. Mirror-image symmetry occurs for the upper parathyroids as well as for the lower parathyroids. Finding a left gland can then assist in finding the corresponding right gland. When one initially identifies a normal-appearing gland, it is appropriate to cautiously and reasonably dissect this gland so as to rule out an attached adenoma. With intraoperative PTH analysis, an area of presumptive adenoma can be palpated to generate an intraoperative PTH spike, helping to confirm parathyroid tissue in this location. During parathyroid exploration, one should never remove a normal parathyroid gland and should avoid empiric thyroidectomy. The inferior thyroid artery can be used and traced to find the parathyroid glands. However, this dissection must be done cautiously along the distalmost branches of the inferior thyroid artery to avoid parathyroid devascularization. Normal parathyroid gland biopsy can be helpful with frozen section but should not be done excessively and should be done only after all the glands are visualized. Intraoperative density tests have been used in the past but should be replaced by frozen section analysis. Intraoperative PTH drop can be extremely helpful in determining when exploration can be successfully halted as long as strict criteria for its use are met.

2. The first step in parathyroid exploration involves a full exploration of all normal parathyroid gland locations. Step 2 involves identification of the "missing gland." If the inferior gland is missing, then the thyrothymic horn is exposed/resected and the region greater than 1 cm lateral to the inferior pole and medial to the inferior pole adjacent to the trachea are dissected. If this search is unrewarding, then frank ectopic inferior gland locations are explored, including the lower thymus. An undescended ectopic gland is then considered; therefore the carotid sheath is opened and explored from hyoid to thoracic inlet. Hot spots for undescended ectopic inferior parathyroids include the carotid bifurcation and superior

thyroid artery takeoff. Consideration should also be given to a subcapsular or intrathyroidal inferior parathyroid. Should the superior parathyroid be missing, the extended normal locations for the superior gland should be explored, including the posterolateral aspect of the upper half of the thyroid lobe and retrolaryngeal, retroesophageal regions. If this search is unrewarding, then the superior gland can be searched for more inferiorly in the para- and retroesophageal region, extending from the hyoid down to the posterior mediastinum.

3.   If the above search is unrewarding and has revealed only four normal-appearing glands, one should consider a fifth gland. Such a fifth-gland adenoma is typically found in the thymus; therefore more aggressive thymic exploration and resection are warranted.

4.   The final step in parathyroid exploration would involve considerations prior to closure. First the surgeon should consider studies that have identified missed adenomas after operation. These sites include the thymus, para- and retroesophageal regions, intrathyroidal, the carotid sheath and the anterior mediastinum. Once these areas are considered, bilateral inferior jugular PTH sampling can be looked into. One should avoid empiric thyroidectomy and never remove normal thyroid gland. At this point the incision is closed and the diagnosis reconsidered with additional blood, urine, and localization testing. Such testing should include sestamibi scanning with single photon emission computed tomography (SPECT), chest imaging, and possibly selective venous catheterization. Reoperation plus or minus mediastinal dissection, is contemplated after re-evaluation of calcium, PTH, urine studies, and localization studies.

Complications of Parathyroid Surgery

In experienced surgical hands, persistent hypercalcemia occurs postoperatively in less than 5% of patients with primary HPT caused by adenoma. A higher failure rate of approximately 10 to 50% exists when HPT is caused by hyperplasia, some forms of inherited HPT (eg, familial HPT, MEN I), or secondary HPT. Reasons for failure (ie, persistent or recurrent hypercalcemia) in surgery for HPT include failure to find the adenomatous gland in a normal cervical location, failure to find a second adenoma, failure to recognize four-gland hyperplasia, failure to identify a supernumerary gland (ie, fifth gland), regrowth of adenoma from the unresected stump of a resected adenoma, unrecognized parathyroid carcinoma, or incorrect diagnosis (eg, BFHH). The most common ectopic locations for parathyroid adenomas include retroesophageal, retrotracheal, anterior mediastinal, intrathyroidal, carotid sheath, and hyoid/angle of mandible. Hypoparathyroidism can occur after surgery for HPT. Permanent hypoparathyroidism occurs after surgery for adenoma in approximately 5% of cases overall. Permanent hypoparathyroidism occurs after surgery for hyperplasia or secondary HPT in about 10 to 30% of cases.[121] In patients with severe or long-standing HPT, especially if preoperative alkaline phosphatase is elevated, bone calcium stores may be severely depleted, and bone calcium uptake after successful surgery can lead to prolonged and severe hypocalcemia, which must be aggressively repleted.

References

1. Halsted WS. The operative story of goiter, the author's operation. *Johns Hopkins Hosp Rep* 1920;19:71–257.

2. Livolsi V. *Surgical Pathology of the Thyroid.* Philadelphia: Saunders, 1990.

3. Berlin D. The recurrent laryngeal nerve in total ablation of the normal thyroid gland. *Surg Gynecol Obstet* 1935;60:19–25.

4. Wafae N, Cesar-Vieira N, Vorobieff A. The recurrent laryngeal nerve in relation to the infe-

rior constrictor muscle of the pharynx. *Laryngoscope* 1991;101:1091–1093.

5. Eisele DW. Complications of thyroid surgery. In: Eisele DW, ed. *Complications in Head and Neck Surgery.* St. Louis: Mosby, 1993, 423.

6. Rustad WH. Revised anatomy of recurrent laryngeal nerves: Surgical importance based on the dissection of 100 cadavers. *J Clin Endocrinol Metab* 1954;14:87–96.

7. Nemiroff PM, Katz AD. Extralaryngeal divisions of the recurrent laryngeal nerve: Surgical and clinical significance. *Am J Surg* 1982;144: 466–469.

8. Lennquist S, Kahlin C, Smeds S. The superior laryngeal nerve in thyroid surgery. *Surgery* 1987;102(6):1000–1008.

9. Cernea C, et al. Surgical anatomy of the external branch of the superior laryngeal nerve. *Head Neck* 1992;14:380–383.

10. Hollingshead WH. Anatomy of the endocrine glands. *Surg Clin North Am* 1958;39: 1115–1140.

11. Cooper D. Antithyroid drugs. *N Engl J Med* 1984;311(21):1353.

12. Totten MA, Wool MS. Medical treatment of hyperthyroidism. *Med Clin North Am* 1979; 63:321.

13. Reed DJ. Hyperthyroidism and hypothyroidism complicating the treatment of thyrotoxicosis. *Br J Surg* 1987;74:1060.

14. Toft AD, Irvine WJ, Seth J. Thyroid function in the long-term follow-up of patients treated with I[131]. *Lancet* 1975;2:576.

15. Wise PH, Ahmad A, Burnet R, et al. Intentional radioiodine ablation in Graves' disease. *Lancet* 1975;20:1231.

16. Holm LE, Dahlquist I, Israelsson A, et al. Malignant thyroid tumors after I[131] treatment. *N Engl J Med* 1980;303:188.

17. Freitas JE, Swanson DP, Gross MD, et al. I[131] optimal treatment for hyperthyroidism in children and adolescents. *J Nucl Med* 1979;20: 847.

18. Harada T, Catugiri M, Ito K. Hyperthyroidism: Graves' disease and toxic nodular goiter. In: Clark O, Duh Q, eds. *Textbook of Endocrine Surgery.* Philadelphia: Saunders, 1997, 47.

19. Falk S. Surgical treatment of hyperthyroidism. In: Falk S, ed. *Thyroid Disease.* New York: Raven Press, 1990, 241.

20. Coyle PJ, Mitchell JE. Thyroidectomy: Is Lugol's solution necessary? *Ann R Coll Surg Edinb* 1982;64:334.

21. Melliere D, Etienne G, Becquemin JP. Operations for hyperthyroidism. *Am J Surg* 1988; 155:395–399.

22. Hedley AG, Michie W, Duncan T, et al. The effect of remnant size on the outcome of subtotal thyroidectomy for thyrotoxicosis. *Br J Surg* 1972;59:559.

23. Silver C, Wendy S. Thyroid disease and surgery. In: Bailey B, ed. *Otolaryngology Head and Neck Surgery.* Philadelphia: Lippincott, 1993, 1229.

24. Hamburger JI. The various presentations of thyroiditis. *Ann Intern Med* 1986;104:219.

25. Hay ID. Thyroiditis: A clinical update. *Mayo Clin Proc* 1985;60:836–843.

26. Singer PA. Thyroiditis. *Med Clin North Am* 1991;75(1):61–77.

27. Farwell AP, Braverman LE. Inflammatory thyroid disorders. *Otolaryngol Clin North Am* 1996;29(4):541–556.

28. Woolner CB, McConahey WM, Beahrs OH. Invasive fibrous thyroiditis (Riedel's struma). *J Clin Endocrinol Metab* 1956;17:201.

29. Alfonso A, Christoudias G, Amaruddin Q, et al. Tracheal or esophageal compression due to benign thyroid disease. *Am J Surg* 1981; 142:350–354.

30. Katlic M, Grillo H, Wang CA. Substernal goiter: Analysis of 80 patients from MGH. *Am J Surg* 1985;149:283–287.

31. Jauregui R, Lilker E, Bayley A. Upper airway obstruction in euthyroid goiter. *JAMA* 1977; 238(20):2163–2166.

32. Zorrilla L, Tsai J, Freedman M. Airway obstruction due to goiter in older patients. *J Am Geriatr Soc* 1989;37:1153–1156.

33. Hurley D, Gharib H. Evaluation and management of multinodular goiter. *Otolaryngol Clin North Am* 1996;29(4):527–540.

34. Koh KB, Chang KW. Carcinoma in multinodular goiter. *Br J Surg* 1992;79:266–267.

35. Mazzaferri EL. Thyroid cancer in thyroid nodules: Finding a needle in a haystack. *Am J Med* 1992;93:359.

36. Leeper R. Thyroid carcinoma. *Med Clin North Am* 1985;69(5):1079–1096.

37. Hathaway H. Diagnosis and management of the thyroid nodule. *Otolaryngol Clin North Am* 1990;23(2):303–337.

38. Rojeski M, Gharib H. Nodular thyroid disease. *N Engl J Med* 1985;313(7):418–436.

39. Hamming J, et al. The value of fine needle aspiration biopsy in patients with nodular thyroid disease divided into groups of suspicion of malignant neoplasm on clinical grounds. *Arch Intern Med* 1990;150:113.

40. Daniels GH. Thyroid nodules and nodular thyroids: A clinical overview. *Compr Ther* 1996; 22(4):239–250.

41. Miller J, et al. Diagnosis of malignant follicular neoplasm of the thyroid by needle biopsy. *Cancer* 1985;55:2812–2817.

42. Ashcraft M, vanHerle A. Management of thyroid nodules I. *Head Neck Surg* 1981;Jan/Feb:216–227.

43. Ashcraft M, vanHerle A. Management of thyroid nodules II. *Head Neck Surg* 1981;Mar/Apr:297–322.

44. Simeone JS, Daniel GH, Mueller PR, et al. High resolution real-time sonography of the thyroid. *Radiology* 1982;145:431–435.

49. Rosai J, Carcangiu ML, DeLellis RA. *Atlas of Thyroid Pathology. Tumors of the Thyroid Gland.* Washington DC: Armed Forces Institute of Pathology, 1992.

50. Woolner L, Beahrs OH, Black M, et al. Classification and prognosis of thyroid carcinoma. *Am J Surg* 1961;102:354–387.

51. Mazzaferri EL, Young RL. Papillary thyroid carcinoma: A ten-year follow-up report on the impact of treatment in 576 patients. *Am J Med* 1981;70:511–518.

52. Lloyd RV. RET proto-oncogene mutation and rearrangements in endocrine disease. *Am J Pathol* 1995;147:1539–1544.

53. Takahashi M. Oncogenic activity of the RET proto-oncogene in thyroid cancer. *Crit Rev Oncogene* 1995;6(1):35–46.

54. McConahey WM, Hay I, Woolner C, et al. Papillary thyroid carcinoma treatment at Mayo Clinic 1946 through 1970: Initial manifestations, pathologic findings, treatment and outcome. *Mayo Clin Proc* 1986;61:978.

55. Maxon HR, Smith HS. Radioactive I^{131} in the diagnosis and treatment of metastatic well-differentiated thyroid carcinoma. *Endocrinol Metab Clin North Am* 1990;19(3):685–717.

56. Tollefsen HR, Shah JP, Huvos AG. Papillary carcinoma of the thyroid: Recurrence in the thyroid gland after initial surgical treatment. *Am J Surg* 1972;124:468–472.

57. Mazzaferri EL, Jhiang SM. Long-term impact of initial surgical and medical treatment for papillary and follicular thyroid cancer. *Am J Med* 1994;97(5):418–428.

58. Lange W, Georgii A, Stauch G, et al. The differentiation of atypical adenomas and encapsulated follicular carcinoma in the thyroid gland. *Virchows Arch (A)* 1980;385:125–141.

59. Samaan NA. The results of various modalities of treatment of well-differentiated thyroid cancer: A retrospective review of 1,599 patients. *J Clin Endocrinol Metab* 1992;75:7114–7120.

60. Randolph GW, Daniels GH. The incidence of follicular carcinoma in the contralateral thyroid lobe: Radioactive iodine ablation versus completion thyroidectomy. *Abstracts of the Fourth International Conference on Head and Neck Cancer—Program 7/28–8/96.* Abstract #147:95.

61. Young RL, Mazzaferri EL, Rahe AJ, et al. Pure follicular carcinoma: Impact of treatment in 214 patients. *J Nucl Med* 1980;21:733–737.

62. Lange W, Choritz H, Hundeshagen H. Risk factors in follicular thyroid carcinoma: A retrospective follow-up study covering a fourteen year period with emphasis on morphologic findings. *Am J Surg Pathol* 1986;10(4):246–255.

63. Hay ID, Grant CS, Taylor WP, et al. Ipsilateral lobectomy versus bilateral lobar resection of papillary carcinoma of the thyroid: A retrospective analysis of surgical outcome using a novel prognostic scoring system. *Surgery* 1987; 102:1088–1095.

64. Cady B, Rossi R. An expanded view of risk group definition in differentiated thyroid carcinoma. *J Surg* 1988;104:947–953.

65. Shah JP, Loree TR, Dharker D, et al. Lobectomy versus total thyroidectomy for differentiated carcinoma of the thyroid: A matched pair analysis. *Am J Surg* 1993;166:331–335.

66. Schroder DM, Chambors A, France CT. Operative strategy for thyroid cancer. Is total thyroidectomy worth the price? *Cancer* 1986;58: 2320–2328.

67. Cady B, Rossi R, Silverman M, et al. Further evidence of the validity of risk group definition in differentiated thyroid carcinoma. *Surgery* 1985;98:1171.

68. Rose RG, Kelsey MP, Russell WO. Follow-up study of thyroid cancer treated by unilateral lobectomy. *Am J Surg* 1963;106:494–500.

69. Grant CS, Hay I, Gough IR, et al. Local recurrence in papillary thyroid carcinoma: Is extent of surgical resection important? *J Surg* 1988; 104:954.

70. Vickery AL, Wang CA, Walker AM. Treatment of intrathyroidal papillary carcinoma of the thyroid. *Cancer* 1987;60:2587–2591.

71. Pasieka JL, Thompson NW, McLeod MK, et al. The incidence of bilateral well-differentiated thyroid cancer found at completion thyroidectomy. *World J Surg* 1992;16:711–717.

72. Attie JH, Khatif RA, Steckler RM. Elective neck dissection in papillary carcinoma of the thyroid. *Am J Surg* 1971;122:464–471.

73. Noguchi S, Noguchi A, Murakami M. Papillary carcinoma of the thyroid I: Developing patterns of metastasis. *Cancer* 1970;26:1053.

74. Noguchi S, Noguchi A, Murakami M. Papillary carcinoma of the thyroid II: Value of prophylactic lymph node excision. *Cancer* 1970;26:1061.

75. Harwood J, Clark OH, Dunphy JE. Significance of lymph node metastasis in differentiated thyroid carcinoma. *Am J Surg* 1978;136:107–112.

76. Randolph GW, Daniels GH. Functional efficacy of 30 mCi ablation of post-surgical thyroid remnants in patients with well-differentiated thyroid carcinoma. In press.

77. Auguste LJ, Attie JN. Completion thyroidectomy for initially misdiagnosed thyroid cancer. *Otolaryngol Clin North Am* 1990;23(3): 429–439.

78. Marchetta FC, Krause L, Sako K. Interpretation of scintigrams obtained after thyroidectomy. *Surg Gynecol Obstet* 1963;116:647–649.

79. Cohn K, Backdahl M, Forsslund G. Biologic considerations and operative strategy in papillary carcinoma of the thyroid: Arguments against the routine performance of total thyroidectomy. *Surgery* 1984;96(6):957–970.

80. Farrar WB, Cooperman M, James AG. Surgical management of papillary and follicular carcinoma of the thyroid. *Ann Surg* 1980;192(6): 701–704.

81. Randolph GW. Papillary cancer of the thyroid in low risk patients: Extent of thyroidectomy. *Arch Otolaryngol Head Neck Surg* 2001;127: 462–466.

82. Lipton RL, McCaffery TV, vanHeerden JA. Surgical treatment of invasion of the upper aerodigestive tract by well-differentiated thyroid carcinoma. *Am J Surg* 1987;154:363–367.

83. Grillo HC, Zannini P. Resectional management of airway invasion by thyroid carcinoma. *Ann Thorac Surg* 1986;42:287–298.

84. Harness J, et al. Follicular carcinoma of the thyroid gland: Trends and treatment. *Surgery* 1984;96(6):972–980.

85. Ross D. Long-term management of differentiated thyroid carcinoma. *Endocrinol Metab Clin North Am* 1990;19(3):719–739.

86. Ronga G. Can I^{131} whole body scanning be replaced by thyroglobulin measurement in postsurgical follow-up of differentiated thyroid carcinoma? *J Nucl Med* 1990;31:1766–1771.

87. Grauer A, Raue F, Gagel R. Changing concepts in the management of hereditary and sporadic medullary thyroid carcinoma. *Endocrinol Metab Clin North Am* 1990;19:613–635.

88. Eng C, Mulligan L, Smith D, et al. Mutation of RET proto-oncogene in sporadic medullary thyroid carcinoma. *Genes Chromosome Cancer* 1995;12:209–212.

89. Saad MF, Ordonez NG, Rashid RK, et al. Medullary thyroid carcinoma: A study of the clinical features and prognostic factors in 161 patients. *Medicine* 1984;63:319–342.

90. Randolph GW, Maniar D. Medullary carcinoma of the thyroid. *Cancer Control* 2000;7(3): 253–261.

91. Kakudo K, Carney JR, Sizemore GW. Medullary carcinoma of the thyroid: Biologic behavior of the sporadic and familial neoplasm. *Cancer* 1985;55:2818–2821.

92. Venkatesh YS, Ordonez NG, Shultz PN, et al. Anaplastic carcinoma of the thyroid. *Cancer* 1990;66:321–330.

93. Nel CJ, vanHeerden JA, Goellner J, et al. Anaplastic carcinoma of the thyroid: A clinicopathologic study of 82 cases. *Mayo Clin Proc* 1985;60:51–58.

94. Randolph GW, Kobler J, Montgomery W, Hillman R. Comparison of intraoperative recurrent laryngeal nerve monitoring techniques during thyroid surgery (abstract). *Otolaryngol Head Neck Surg* 1996;115:102.

95. Eisele DW. Intraoperative electrophysiologic monitoring of the RLN. *Laryngoscope* 1996; 106(4):443–449.

96. Lennquist S, Cahlin C, Smeds S. The superior laryngeal nerve in thyroid surgery. *Surgery* 1987;102(6):1000–1008.

97. Cernea C, et al. Surgical anatomy of the external branch of the superior laryngeal nerve. *Head Neck* 1992;14:380–383.

98. Eisele DW. Complications of thyroid surgery. In: Eisele DW, ed. *Complications of Head and Neck Surgery.* St. Louis: Mosby, 1993, 423.

99. Martensson H, Terins J. Recurrent laryngeal nerve palsy in thyroid gland surgery related to operations and nerves at risk. *Arch Surg* 1985;120:475–477.

100. Sinclair ISR. The risk to the recurrent laryngeal nerves in thyroid and parathyroid surgery. *J R Coll Surg Edinb* 1994;39:253–257.

101. Lore JM. Complications in the management of thyroid carcinoma. *Semin Surg Oncol* 1991;7:120–125.

102. vanHeerden JA, Groh MA, Grant CS. Early post-operative morbidity after surgical treatment of thyroid cancer. *Surgery* 1987;161:724–727.

103. Foster RS. Morbidity and mortality after thyroidectomy. *Surg Gynecol & Obstet* 1978:146:423–429.

104. Mazzaferri E, Young RL. Papillary carcinoma: A 10 year follow-up report of the impact of treatment in 576 patients. *Am J Med* 1981;70:511–518.

105. Arnold A, Staunton CE, Kim HG, et al. Monoclonality and abnormal parathyroid hormone genes in parathyroid adenomas. *N Engl J Med* 1988;318:658.

106. Delellis RA. *Tumors of the Parathyroid Glands: Atlas of Tumor Pathology.* Third Series. Fascicle 6. Washington, DC: Armed Forces Institute of Pathology, 1993.

107. Heath H, Hodgson S, Kennedy MA. Primary hyperparathyroidism: Incidence, morbidity, and potential economic impact in a community. *N Engl J Med* 1980;302:186.

108. National Institutes of Health Conference. Diagnosis and management of asymptomatic primary hyperparathyroidism. Consensus development conference statement. *Ann Intern Med* 1991; 114:593.

109. Rodriguez-Gonzalez J, Pancio PD. Localization studies in patients with persistent or recurrent hyperparathyroidism. In: Clark O, Duh Q, eds. *Textbook of Endocrine Surgery.* Philadelphia: WB Saunders, 1997, 42–341.

110. Casas AT, Burke GT, Sathyanarayan A, et al. Perspective comparison of technetium 99m sestamibi–iodine 123 scan versus high-resolution ultrasonography for pre-operative localization of abnormal parathyroid glands in patients with previously unoperated primary hyperparathyroidism. *Am J Surg* 1993;166:369.

111. Thule P, Tharoke K, Vasant J, et al. Pre-op localization of parathyroid tissue with technetium 99m sestamibi I^{123} subtraction scanning. *J Clin Endocrinol Metab* 1994;78:77.

112. Voorman S, Petti G, Chonkick G, et al. The pitfalls of technetium-thallium parathyroid scanning. *Arch Otolaryngol Head Neck Surg* 1988; 114:993.

113. Randolph GW, Gaz R, Johns R, Caradonna D, Siddiqui S. Pre-op sestamibi scanning: Where does it fail? In press.

114. Wei JP, Burke G. Analysis of savings in operative time for primary hyperparathyroidism using localization with technetium 99m sestamibi scan. *Am J Surg* 1995;170:488.

115. Russell CF, Laird JD, et al. Scan directed unilateral cervical exploration for parathyroid adenoma. A legitimate approach? *World J Surg* 1990;14:406.

116. Tibblins S, Bizard JP, Bondeson AG, et al. Primary hyperparathyroidism due to solitary adenoma: A comparative multicenter study of early and long-term results of different surgical regimens. *Eur J Surg* 1991;157:511.

117. Bonger HT, Bruining HA. Technique of parathyroidectomy. In: Clark O, Duh Q, eds. *Textbook of Endocrine Surgery.* Philadelphia: WB Saunders, 1997, 43–347.

118. Kraimts JL, Duh Q, Demeure M, et al. Hyperparathyroidism in MEN syndromes. *Surgery* 1992;112:1080.

119. Wang CA. Anatomic basis of parathyroid surgery. *Ann Surg* 1976;183:271.

120. Pyrtek LJ, Painter RL. An anatomic study of the relationship of the parathyroid glands to the recurrent laryngeal nerve. *Surg Gynecol Obstet* 1964;119:509.

121. Diagnosis of primary hyperparathyroidism. In: Clark O, Duh Q, eds. *Textbook of Endocrine Surgery.* Philadelphia: WB Saunders, 1997:297.

Carotid Body Tumors, Vascular Anomalies, Melanoma, and Cysts and Tumors of the Jaws

29

CAROTID BODY TUMORS

The normal carotid body is a chemoreceptor located at the carotid bifurcation, occasionally visualized as a pink adventitial mass measuring about 5 mm. The body is responsive to decreased arterial Po_2, increased Pco_2, pH, and temperature via catecholamines, causing increased respiratory rate and volume with concomitant elevation of pulse rate and blood pressure. It is distinct from the carotid sinus, which is a pressoreceptor. The carotid body receives innervation from a branch of the glossopharyngeal nerve and blood supply from the external carotid system, although supply via the occipital, vertebral, and thyrocervical trunk ascending cervical branches has been described. Carotid body tumors comprise about 65% of head and neck paragangliomata.

The carotid body is derived from neural crest cells of the branchiomeric group of paraganglia, which are distributed in jugulotympanic, orbital, intercarotid, laryngeal (cricotracheal membrane along the course of the superior laryngeal nerve, false vocal fold), and subclavian regions of the head and neck. Additionally, nasal and nasopharyngeal paragangliomas have been reported. Although associated with the autonomic nervous system and capable of producing and storing vasoactive and neurotransmitter substances, most carotid body tumors are nonfunctioning. The terms *nonchromaffin tumor, glomus tumor,* and *chemodectoma* are no longer recommended when referring to these paraganglionic tumors. A characteristic histologic appearance includes chief cells arranged in clusters or "zellballen," with neurosecretory granules, reticulin-staining vascular septa, and sustentacular cells.

The typical patient will present in the fourth or fifth decade with a slow-growing, painless neck mass. A history of labile hypertension or associated headache should prompt laboratory evaluation of a possible functional tumor via urine catecholamines and metabolic breakdown products. Large tumors may cause dysphagia, hoarseness, and vocal cord paralysis, with many patients relating many years of symptoms. Incidence is probably equal in male and female patients.

The critical finding on physical examination is a poorly defined neck mass at the anterior border of the sternocleidomastoid muscle, at the level of the hyoid bone, that is mobile

655

from side to side but not vertically. Arterial pulsation will be transmitted and a bruit may be auscultated. Average tumor size at presentation is about 4 cm. Associated vocal cord paralysis may be noted. Syncopal episodes may accompany larger tumors that occlude internal carotid blood flow. Bilateral tumors are present in 2 to 10% of patients, with this group typically presenting at an earlier age. Despite characteristic clinical presentation, these tumors are frequently misdiagnosed.

Preoperative fine needle aspiration (FNA) or open biopsy of a mass with the above characteristics has been described, although diagnosis should be definitive by clinicoradiographic findings, obviating the need for potentially dangerous procedures. Diagnostic radiographic evaluation may include carotid angiography with preoperative selective embolization or angiogram. The characteristic "lyre" sign is produced by splaying apart of the internal and external carotid arteries.

Differential diagnosis includes branchial cleft cyst, vagal and hypoglossal neurogenic tumors, nodal metastasis, lymphoma, aneurysm, and acquired vascular malformation.

Treatment of these tumors is surgical and should be individualized. Subadventitial dissection, after proximal and distal control of the carotid system and specific identification of the cranial nerves aided by surgical loupe magnification, is most easily begun posterolaterally. Interpositional arterial grafting may be necessary for reconstruction in unusual cases. Maintenance of normotension throughout the case is critical in the avoidance of central neurologic sequelae and is facilitated by preoperative placement of central and arterial cannulas as well as large-bore intravenous catheters. Asymptomatic tumors in the elderly with significant comorbidity may be best observed. Recurrence is about 10%, usually after an apparent long disease-free interval. Incomplete excision has also been reported. Residual tumor is not considered a contraindication to salvage surgery, as secondary treatment can be as effective as in the primary setting. External beam radiotherapy is reserved for a palliative or salvage adjuvant role. Arrest of disease progression and alleviation of symptoms is considered successful in this setting.

A familial variant (autosomal dominant with incomplete penetrance) represents about 8% of cases and is associated with pheochromocytoma, neurofibromatosis, and medullary carcinoma of the thyroid. About one-third of these cases are bilateral and have synchronous multicentric paragangliomata. Malignant carotid body tumors are more rare (3%) in the familial association than in sporadic cases (about 12%). The malignant variety is uniformly fatal, with distant metastases to nodes, lung, and bone (less frequently reported to heart, liver, kidney, pancreas, pleura, dura, and skin).

VASCULAR ANOMALIES

The lack of a rational nomenclature acknowledging clinical, histologic, and vascular dynamics of the various vascular anomalies has long been an obstacle to their understanding. This improper terminology has not uncommonly been responsible for incorrect diagnosis, illogical treatment, and misdirected therapeutic research. The standard classification system of Mulliken and Glowacki, circa 1982, provided a schema based on the *clinical* and *histologic* characteristics of vascular lesions but remained unwieldy and did not include *vascular dynamics*, which have direct relevance to their rational treatment. An updated classification system proposed by Jackson et al. has accomplished this goal and has simplified the diagnostic and therapeutic approach to these lesions:

I. Hemangioma
II. Vascular malformation
   Low-flow (venous)
   High-flow (arteriovenous)
III. Lymphatic (lymphovenous) malformation

Hemangiomas

Hemangiomas are hamartomatous neoplasms, representing mesodermal rests of vasoformative tissue (endothelial hyperplasia). Neovascularization enlargement occurs by canalization of hyperplastic solid masses of endothelial cells. Hemangiomas are the most common congenital anomalies in humans, occurring in 10 to 12% of Caucasians and in up to 22% of preterm infants weighing less than 1000 g. About one-third are present at birth as a macule, pale spot, or telangiectasia. Seventy to 90% become apparent between the first and fourth weeks of life. Overall, 85% are manifest by the close of the first year. A 3:1 female:male ratio is characteristic excepting subglottic lesions, where incidence is equal. A family history is present in about 3% of cases. About 63% of lesions are cutaneous, 15% subcutaneous, and 22% mixed. The most common site for deep hemangiomas in the head and neck region is within the masseter muscle. The lesion is typically solitary (80%), although generalized hemangiomatosis and syndromic associations exist.

A characteristic natural history distinguishes this anomaly. A rapid postnatal proliferative growth phase (8 to 18 months) is histologically accompanied by endothelial hyperplasia, increased endothelial turnover, mast cell infiltration, and upregulation of basic fibroblast growth factor (b-FGF) and vascular endothelial growth factor (VEGF). Enzymes involved in the remodeling of extracellular matrix are also increased (type IV collagenase, proteases, urokinase).

After a stable plateau, all lesions enter a slow but inevitable involutional phase occurring over the next 5 to 8 years. Spontaneous involution of even the most aggressive, complicated lesions does occur. Involution is characterized by endothelial apoptosis and the downregulation of angiogenesis with increased metalloproteinases and mast cells. Fibrosis, fatty infiltration, diminished cellularity, and normalization of mast cell count characterize this phase. Growth and involutional phases may overlap, however. Regression is complete in 50% by 5 years and in 70% by 7 years. Rate of regression is unrelated to sex, age, size, appearance, and duration of the proliferative phase. Continuing improvement is noted in the remaining children until 10 to 12 years of age. Graying of the cutaneous portion of the lesion yields the "herald spot," which signifies impending involution. Clinical history and physical examination alone should allow accurate diagnosis in 95% or more of cases.

As a rule, the treatment of uncomplicated hemangiomas should be delayed until involution is complete. Excision or suction-assisted lipectomy (SAL) of residual fibrofatty deposits and excision of redundant crepey atrophic skin or telangiectasias may then be performed. One should not, in general, yield to parents, who typically seek treatment for their children very early, largely due to the early appearance, rapid growth, and capacity of hemangiomas to produce significant deformity. *Primum non nocere* remains the dictum here. The potential for psychosocial damage during the waiting period should, however, be considered. Lesions of the nasal tip and lip are notoriously slow to regress and should probably be resected early (no evidence of change over a 6-month period), to avoid deformities that will be more difficult to manage later (eg, "Cyrano de Bergerac" nasal deformity).

Active, early treatment must be employed in complicated cases and for lesions in vital locations. Massive deforming lesions; high-output congestive heart failure; localized consumptive coagulopathy with thrombocytopenia and intravascular coagulation (Kasabach-Merritt syndrome); and ulcerating, infected, and hemorrhaging lesions are potentially lethal complicated forms and may mandate early, aggressive treatment. Overall mortality for giant lesions related to hemorrhage, airway obstruction, or infection is about 20% and is much greater than for unselected cases. Laryngeal, eyelid, periorbital, perioral, periauricular, and nasal lesions may cause severe and possibly permanent functional problems (airway obstruction, amblyopia, strabismus, orbital enlargement, and interference with hygiene and alimentation).

Pharmacologic therapy is initiated for complicated and "alarming" hemangiomas not amenable to palliative surgical resection. Corticosteroids (prednisone), 2 to 3 mg/kg per day for 2 to 3 weeks, will elicit a response in sensitive lesions within 7 to 10 days. A 30 to 60% response is typical but is variable to excellent in about 30%, doubtful in about 40%, and absent in about 30% of cases. Mortality, despite the introduction of steroids, is as high as 54% for visceral lesions and 30 to 40% in Kasabach-Merritt syndrome. The dose is lowered to 1 mg/kg per day, or an alternate-day schedule (30 to 40 mg) may be elected for a 4- to 6-week cycle. Intralesional triamcinolone may be applicable to some small, uncomplicated lesions. Multiple courses are usually effective in cases of rebound growth. Proposed mechanisms of action include increased vascular sensitivity to circulating physiologic vasoconstricting substances. Steroids appear to favorably influence the natural course of sensitive lesions, hastening an earlier involution than would otherwise occur. High-dose steroid treatment has a place in the therapy of many diseases of children, although steroids must be administered with caution. Active infection and seizure disorders must be controlled. Weekly weight and blood pressure measurements and stool occult blood tests are taken, and a balanced, nutritious diet is followed. Growth suppression (antianabolic effect) and withdrawal insufficiency phenomena are more theoretic risks and are not typically encountered or anticipated.

Interferon 2-alpha (rIFN-2a, INTRON, Hoffman-LaRoche) has been observed to inhibit endothelial proliferation and angiogenesis and is now used in recombinant form in complicated lesions refractory to steroid treatment, as such lesions are often fatal prior to involution. A dose of 1 to 3 million U/m^2 body surface area is administered as a single daily subcutaneous injection. Local and systemic complications are decreased and length of time to involution is shortened in about 90% of patients. Therapy is sustained for about 9 to 14 months to avoid regrowth (reversible by reintroduction of treatment). Fever has been the only consistent toxic side effect and is responsive to acetaminophen therapy. Monthly CBC, PT/PTT, liver enzymes, electrolytes, BUN, and creatinine test results are followed during the first year of treatment. The drug should be considered in off-protocol centers for compassionate use in selected cases. Antiangiogenesis factors hold promise for the future.

Windows for surgical intervention include the following:

Infancy: Rare, complicated, unresponsive lesions (eg, upper eyelid)
Preschool: Nasal tip lesions
Grade school: Serial excision of soft tissue residua

Compression therapy via specially fitted Jobst-type garments has limited application in the head and neck region. External beam radiotherapy has no place in the management of these lesions in the head and neck region. With the exception of subglottic (CO_2) and intralesional (Nd:YAG) treatment of obstructing hemangiomas, laser therapy is inappropriate to these tumors due to inadequate depth of penetration and potential for depigmentation.

In contrast to hemangiomas (hyperplastic), vascular malformations and lymphatic malformations (dysmorphogenetic), with normal endothelial kinetics, would *not* be expected to respond to these specific pharmacotherapeutics.

Lesions of Special Importance

SUBGLOTTIC HEMANGIOMA OF INFANCY   A subglottic hemangioma of infancy presents with a persistent croup-like syndrome with stridor, cyanosis, and weight loss but with absence of hoarseness when crying. Cyanosis is typically worsened by crying due to vascular congestion within the hemangioma. Ninety percent of these infants are symptomatic by 3 months of age. Fifty percent have associated cutaneous hemangiomas. The lesion is typically anterior. Biopsy is contraindicated because of the possibility of aspiration and exsanguination. Involution will spontaneously occur in 12 to 18 months and may be hastened by steroid treatment. Tracheotomy is the temporizing treatment of choice. CO_2 laser treatment may also be applied in specific cases.

ADULT LARYNGEAL HEMANGIOMA   Usually supraglottic or glottic, adult laryngeal hemangiomas are often polypoid or pedunculated. They rarely present with respiratory distress and can usually be observed. CO_2 laser treatment is the method of choice for symptomatic lesions.

PAROTID HEMANGIOMA   Parotid hemangioma is the commonest parotid tumor of infancy. Excision, postinvolution, sparing cranial nerve VII, is the recommended management for these tumors.

HEMANGIOMAS OF BONE.   Reported in vertebral bodies as well as frontal, parietal, and gnathic (mandible, maxilla) sites, hemangiomas of bone usually present in the second to fourth decades of life in female patients. Slow, progressive expansion with a multilocular radiographic appearance is characteristic. Surgical excision is the treatment of choice.

Vascular Malformations

Vascular malformations present at lower incidence than hemangiomas but are responsible for more significant clinical problems and are more often a source of severe cosmetic deformity. In contrast to hemangiomas, they are always present at birth, grow in proportion to body growth or in response to hemodynamic changes, never spontaneously regress, and appear with equal incidence in male and female patients. They are localized or diffuse errors of embryonic development and are most commonly sporadic. A normal flat endothelium with normal turnover and normal mast cell count with thin basement membranes and normal urinary basic fibroblast growth factor (b-FGF) are characteristic. Characterization of the molecular basis of these dysmorphogenetic lesions is just beginning to be clarified. These collections of vessels may be arterial, venous, or any combination thereof. Spontaneous enlargement may be due to thrombosis, ectasia, or the development of new arteriovenous communications in response to surgical manipulation, trauma, or the hormonal changes of puberty or pregnancy.

Vascular dynamics allow subclassification of these lesions based on speed of flow through the lesion and rate of shunting between arterial and venous components. This allows the rational selection of treatment and its timing, as these tumors exhibit very different behavior and prognosis and therefore require different approaches to treatment.

As with hemangiomas, history and physical examination are sufficient to establish a clinical diagnosis in most cases. Plain radiographs may demonstrate a soft tissue mass with calcification or phleboliths, characteristic of low-flow lesions. High-flow lesions may exhibit destructive skeletal changes, and changes in density on computed tomography (CT) may demonstrate the extent of disease and bony involvement. Magnetic resonance imaging (MRI) may characterize flow dynamics of the lesion. Selective angiography serves both a diagnostic and a therapeutic role in defining the extent of disease, supplying and runoff vessels, degree of shunting, and in catheter-directed embolic occlusion.

Low-Flow Vascular Malformations (Venous Malformations)

Low-flow vascular malformations include port-wine stain (nevus flammeus). These lesions tend to become nodular and thickened with age. Small tumors may be treated with sclerosing agents—3% sodium tetradecyl sulfate (Sotradecol) is most commonly used in this country. Intralesional injection of up to 30 mL may be repeated at intervals of several months. A combined approach with pre-embolization and excision within 48 hours may be required for large, complicated lesions. Cosmetic camouflage or pulsed dye laser photocoagulation therapy may also be used for smaller, less dynamic lesions.

High-flow Vascular Malformations (Arteriovenous Malformations)

High-flow vascular malformations exhibit more dynamic vascular behavior and seem more likely to expand rapidly in response to inadequate therapy. Clinically, a palpable thrill, auscultable bruit, and bony overgrowth are characteristic. The pain, localized temperature elevation, and a buzzing sound may be particularly bothersome to the patient. Hemorrhage may be lethal. Angiographic characteristics include high shunt and high flow with large ectatic vessels, multiple feeders, absence of parenchymal staining, and arterial and venous phases visualized on the same film. Microshunts not visualized become apparent after inadequate treatment as prompt recurrence of tumor that has been only temporarily reduced in size. This is due to a reorientation of vascular supply and hemodynamics.

An aggressive combined approach is necessary for successful control of these lesions and includes selective angioembolization, control of feeding vessels, and total resection of the lesion within 48 hours. Any single component alone constitutes inadequate treatment and will be met with prompt failure and often the development of a lesion worse than the index lesion. Significant hemorrhage should be prepared for and hypotensive anesthesia techniques should be routine. Intraoperative embolization and extracorporeal cardiac bypass with profound hypothermia and total circulatory arrest have all been described as adjunctive techniques and should be appropriately considered. Here, a team approach is as necessary as adequate preoperative planning.

Lymphatic Malformations (Lymphovenous Malformations)

The lymphatic vascular system develops concurrently with the venous system and is therefore often associated with (venous) low-flow vascular malformations. About 65% of lesions are present at birth and 90% are manifest by 2 years. Some 80% of head and neck lesions involve the neck. The parotid gland is also a common location. Respiratory decompensation and/or dysphagia due to inflammation of large cervical lesions may follow upper respiratory infection and may require urgent intervention. Surgical excision, sparing vital structures, is the mainstay of therapy. Although spontaneous resolution has been reported, it is distinctly rare. Skeletal distortion and overgrowth are common sequelae of large lesions. These are treated after completion of soft tissue procedures according to the principles of craniofacial and orthognathic surgery. Early surgery is advocated to avoid the development of lesions that might require heroic surgery.

Other Lesions

Acquired Vascular Malformations

"Spider" angiomas appear spontaneously at puberty and disappear thereafter. Similar lesions appear in about two-thirds of pregnancies, resolving spontaneously in the puerperium. "Senile" angiomas present on sun-exposed areas and may mandate excision for cosmetic reasons or to rule out malignancy.

Hemangiopericytoma

Presenting as a slowly expanding asymptomatic mass, hemangiopericytoma originates from the capillary pericyte of Zimmermann and occurs equally in both sexes. It is considered a malignant lesion with metastatic rates varying from 33 to 57%. Wide local excision (WLE) is the treatment of choice for this tumor.

Malformation Syndromes

Osler-Weber-Rendu Syndrome/Hereditary Hemorrhagic Telangiectasia (HHT)

Osler-Weber-Rendu syndrome or hereditary hemorrhagic telangiectasia (HHT) is an autosomal-dominant disorder characterized by malformed ectatic vessels (high-flow vascular malformation) in skin, mucous membranes, and viscera. Lesions often appear at puberty and increase in severity with age. Hemorrhage may present as epistaxis, hematemesis, or neurologic symptoms due to intracranial or intracordal hemorrhage.

Sturge-Weber Syndrome

Sturge-Weber syndrome is a low-flow vascular malformation (port-wine stain) of V_1/V_2 trigeminal distribution with ipsilateral malformations of the choroid and leptomeninges and possible calcifications of the posterior parietal or occipital lobes. Facial skeletal and soft tissue overgrowth are also associated. Ophthalmologic findings include glaucoma, buphthalmos, hemianopia, and optic atrophy.

MELANOMA AND PIGMENTED CUTANEOUS LESIONS

The integumentary system is the organ most commonly afflicted with malignancy. Cutaneous carcinomas represent about one-third of all new cases of carcinoma, with 25% appearing in the head and neck region. The incidence of malignant melanoma is rising more rapidly than that of any other malignancy, with a projected lifetime risk of 1 in 90 for persons born in the year 2000. Ten percent annual increases in incidence have been reported in recent years, with a 10-fold increase over the past 50 years. It is currently the leading cause of death from diseases of the skin. An estimated 7300 Americans died of metastatic melanoma in 1999. Overall mortality has decreased, however, due to early detection and treatment.

About 25% of melanomas occur in the head and neck region, with the cheek (46%) the most frequent site, followed by the neck (20%), scalp (18%) external ear (12%), nose (2%), and eyelids (1%). Fewer than 1% of melanomas of the head and neck present mucosally.

Melanocytes are derived from neural crest cells, which migrate peripherally to the integument by the 12th week of gestation. Melanin is produced by melanocytes in the basal epidermis and packaged in organelles (melanosomes). Melanosomes are distributed to keratinocytes in the malpighian layer of the epidermis and hair cortex cells via phagocytosis. All racial groups have the same number of melanocytes per unit area of skin. Racial variations in skin color are due to differences in melanosome distribution, degradation, size, and melanin content (hemoglobin redox state and dietary carotenoid intake are also influences).

Epidemiology and Risk Factors

Melanoma is primarily a disease of Caucasians, with the fair-skinned, sandy-haired phenotype at greatest risk, although it has been described in all races and climates. Estimated relative risk is increased at a rate of 1.6 for blondes, 3 for redheads, 2 for fair skin, 3 for more than 20 nevi on the body, and 7 for more than 100 nevi. The direct relationship to actinic exposure is well documented, and unlike other cutaneous malignancies, melanoma is more related to brief, intense exposures (versus chronic exposure). Studies that document the fact that about 80% of one's lifetime exposure to actinic irradiation occurs in the first 18 years underline the importance of photoprotection, which should begin in childhood (those less than 6 months of age should be protected *entirely* from exposure). Self-examination campaigns have resulted in earlier diagnosis and may be responsible for much of the apparent rise in incidence. The lifetime risk for Caucasians is about 0.6%. Once melanoma is diagnosed, the likelihood of a metachronous second primary is about 3.5%. Primary relatives have about a 1.7-times increased risk.

Benign and Premalignant Lesions

The most common pigmented lesions in Caucasians are benign nevi: junctional, intradermal, or compound. About 25% of melanomas arise from pre-existing benign nevi, usually junctional, rarely before puberty. These lesions are perhaps best diagnosed, and surveillance best performed, by the dermatologist.

Junctional Nevus

Junctional nevi occur at the dermoepidermal junction and are flat and uniform in color. They are typically smooth, macular, well defined, nonhairy, and round.

Intradermal Nevus

The common adult "mole" or intradermal nevus typically has melanocytes in the dermis. These distort normal skin topography and are raised, hairy, and pale.

Compound Nevus

Compound nevi have melanocytes in the dermis and epidermis with combined features of the other nevi and are usually darker and palpable. When surrounded by a depigmented circle, a compound nevus is known as a "halo" nevus.

Other Lesions

SPITZ NEVUS   Also known as a compound melanocytoma or juvenile melanoma, the spitz nevus is characterized by rapid growth; it is pink to red in color, appearing in children from 5 to 10 years of age.

BLUE NEVUS   Dark, smooth, round, and dome-like, the blue nevus appears in childhood. It is a lentigo-pigmented macular lesion with a reticulated pattern. The simple blue nevus is indistinguishable from a junctional nevus. Solar blue nevi are called "liver spots."

SEBORRHEIC KERATOSIS   Seborrheic keratoses are multiple raised, verrucous, variegated, stuck-on–appearing papules.

PIGMENTED BASAL CELL CARCINOMA   Pigmented basal cell carcinoma is a rare subtype to be considered in differential diagnosis.

Melanoma Subtypes

Unlike the benign pigmented lesions, melanoma subtypes are malignancies that typically present irregular borders, surface irregularity, ulceration, and multiple variegated colors. Signs of malignant degeneration include deepening pigmentation, areas of focal depigmentation, inflammation, satellite nodules, bleeding, itching, modularity, and rapid growth.

Superficial Spreading Melanoma (SSM)

Superficial spreading melanoma (SSM), the most common subtype (about 70%) of melanoma, often arises in a pre-existing junctional nevus. It initially expands (horizontal growth phase), with changes in coloration, areas of amelanosis, and surface irregularity. Development of nodules within the substance of the lesion heralds the vertical growth phase. The prognosis is intermediate between the two types of melanoma described below.

Nodular Melanoma (NM)

Comprising 15 to 30% of melanomas in reported series, the nodular melanoma (NM) typically begins in uninvolved skin and lacks a radial growth phase. About 5 to 8% are amelanotic. Overall, the NM has the worst prognosis of the various subtypes.

Lentigo Malignant Melanoma (LMM)

Representing about 4 to 10% in most series, the lentigo malignant melanoma (LMM) appears like a skin stain and is large and flat. The lesion's perimeter is highly convoluted. Cheek involvement is common (an area of high melanocyte density). Patients are usually elderly. These tumors exhibit an indolent course (5 to 15 years), with fewer than 30% metastasizing.

Clinical/Pathologic Staging

Classic Clark levels (Figure 29-1) and Breslow thickness (ocular micrometer measurement of lesion, from granular cell layer to deepest tumor involvement) have been historically important in prognosticating this malignancy, although within certain Clark levels there are gradations of thickness associated with significantly different survival rates.

Clark Levels

Level I: Tumor confined to the epidermis
Level II: Tumor invading the papillary dermis (80 to 90% 5-year survival)
Level III: Tumor filling the papillary dermis (50% 5-year survival)
Level IV: Tumor invading the reticular dermis (30% 5-year survival)
Level V: Tumor invading subcutaneous tissue (less than 20% 5-year survival)

American Joint Committee on Cancer Revised TNM Staging System for Melanoma (2002)

A completely revised staging system for cutaneous melanoma will become official with the sixth edition of the *AJCC Cancer Staging Manual* in 2002 (Tables 29-1 and 29-2). *Ulceration,* an underreported and highly significant feature, has emerged as the single most important prognostic factor influencing mortality in both localized and regional disease. This is now included with thickness in the T category. The *number* of metastatic lymph nodes and whether they are *occult* (microscopic) versus *clinically apparent* are characteristics now included in the N category. The *site* of distant metastasis and elevation of serum lactate dehydrogenase (LDH) are recognized in the updated M classification.

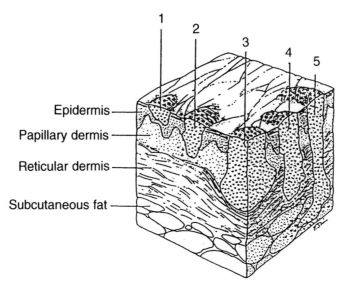

Figure 29-1. Levels of tumor invasion by the Clark microstaging criteria. *(Adapted with permission from McGovern VJ, et al. The classification of malignant melanoma and its histologic reporting.* Cancer *1973;32:1446.)*

Sentinel lymph node (SLN) status is the single most important predictor of survival in patients with melanoma, and it overpowers *both* Clark and Breslow staging systems as a prognostic factor when metastases are present.

Thirteen cancer centers and cancer cooperative groups have contributed complete staging and survival data for 17,600 melanoma patients in validating this new system, which serves as the primary stratification and end results reporting criterion for this disease.

Mucosal Melanomas

Melanomas of the mucous membranes comprise approximately 10% of head and neck melanomas. The oral cavity is the site of approximately 50% of cases, the nasal and sinus cavities 35%, and the pharynx and larynx 15%. The most common sites in the oral cavity are the palate and the inferior alveolus. Interestingly, mucosal melanomas usually do not occur in the olfactory area of the superior nasal recess, where pigmentation is a prominent feature. This subtype is extremely rare in African Americans, who have a high prevalence of melanosis, and there is no apparent relation to local irritation, chronic infection, or allergy. Nasal or paranasal sinus melanomas typically present with unilateral epistaxis or nasal obstruction in about 88% of patients. Here the nasal septum and maxillary sinus are the most common sites of origin. The highest incidence occurs between ages 50 and 70. Grossly, the lesion often appears brownish gray with a smooth, flat, lacy pattern that looks deceptively benign. Nasal melanomas usually present as dark, fleshy tumors that bleed easily. The total removal of all pigmented lesions of the mucosa in Caucasian patients for diagnostic as well as prophylactic purposes is strongly advocated. The differential diagnosis of oral pigmentation includes the following:

- *Endogenous causes:* Racial, Addison's disease, Peutz-Jeghers syndrome (intestinal polyposis), polyostotic fibrous dysplasia, jaundice, Cooley's anemia (beta thalassemia or thal-

TABLE 29-1. TNM STAGING SYSTEM FOR MELANOMA

T Classification	Thickness	Ulceration Status
T_1	</=1.0 mm	A: Without ulceration and level II/III
		B: With ulceration or level IV/V
T_2	1.01–2.0 mm	A: Without ulceration
		B: With ulceration
T_3	2.01–4.0 mm	A: Without ulceration
		B: With ulceration
T_4	>4.0 mm	A: Without ulceration
		B: With ulceration
N Classification	**No. of Metastatic Nodes**	**Nodal Metastatic Mass**
N_1	1 node	A: Micrometastasis*
		B: Macrometastasis†
N_2	2–3 nodes	A: Micrometastasis
		B: Macrometastasis
		C: In-transit metastasis(es)/satellite(s)
		without metastatic nodes
N_3	4 or more nodes or matted nodes or	
	in-transit metastasis(es)/satellite(s)	
	with metastatic nodes	
M Classification	**Site**	**Serum LDH**
M_{1a}	Distant skin, subcutaneous, or nodal	Normal
M_{1b}	Lung	Normal
M_{1c}	All other visceral	Normal
	Any distant	Elevated

*Micrometastases diagnosed after sentinel lymph node biopsy or elective lymph node dissection.
†Macrometastases: clinically detectable nodes confirmed by therapeutic lymphadenectomy or nodes with gross extracapsular extension.

assemia major), sickle cell anemia, thrombocytopenic purpura, hemochromatosis, antimalarial therapy, pregnancy, chlorpromazine (Thorazine) therapy, oral contraceptives, neurofibromatosis, hyperpituitarism, hyperthyroidism, infectious mononucleosis, benign nevi, oral melanosis, and malignant melanomas

- *Exogenous causes:* Heavy metals (bismuth, lead, mercury, silver, gold, arsenic, copper, chrome, cadmium, zinc, brass); amalgam tattoo; charcoal; intraoral trauma
- *Endocrine and metabolic causes:* Nicotinic acid deficiency (pellagra), folic acid deficiency secondary to malabsorption syndrome (sprue), vitamin A or C deficiency, hyperthyroidism, and cutaneous inflammatory diseases.

Metastasis to regional lymph nodes from mucosal melanoma has a much lower incidence than melanomas of the skin. Local recurrence after excision varies from 25% in the pharynx to 40% in the nasal cavity and sinuses.

Treatment
Wide local resection (eg, maxillectomy) is favored because of the relatively low incidence of regional metastasis due to discontinuity in the regional lymphatic system. Composite resection of the primary melanoma and the regional lymphatics is applied in continuity when surgical anatomy permits. For melanomas of the inferior alveolus, lateral pharynx, or floor of the mouth, it is the treatment of choice. Irradiation is used with palliative intent. Alter-

TABLE 29-2. STAGE GROUPINGS FOR CUTANEOUS MELANOMA

	Clinical Staging*			Pathologic Staging†		
	T	N	M	T	N	N
0	Tis	N_0	M_0	Tis	N_0	M_0
IA	T_{1a}	N_0	M_0	T_{1a}	N_0	M_0
IB	T_{1b}	N_0	M_0	T_{1b}	N_0	M_0
	T_{2a}	N_0	M_0	T_{2a}	N_0	M_0
IIA	T_{2b}	N_0	M_0	T_{2b}	N_0	M_0
	T_{3a}	N_0	M_0	T_{3a}	N_0	M_0
IIB	T_{3b}	N_0	M_0	T_{3b}	N_0	M_0
	T_{4a}	N_0	M_0	T_{4a}	N_0	M_0
IIC	T_{4b}	N_0	M_0	T_{4b}	N_0	M_0
III	Any T	**Any N**	M_0			
IIIA				T_{1-4a}	N_{1a}	M_0
				T_{1-4a}	N_{2a}	M_0
IIIB				T_{1-4b}	N_{1a}	M_0
				T_{1-4b}	N_{2a}	M_0
				T_{1-4a}	N_{1b}	M_0
				T_{1-4a}	N_{2b}	M_0
				T_{1-4a}	N_{2c}	M_0
IIIC				T_{1-4b}	N_{1b}	M_0
				T_{1-4b}	N_{2b}	M_0
				T_{1-4b}	N_{2c}	M_0
				Any T	N_3	M_0
IV	Any T	Any N	**Any M**	Any T	Any N	Any M

*Includes microstaging of primary and clinical/radiographic evaluation for metastases.
†Includes microstaging of primary and regional lymph nodes after partial or complete lymphadenectomy. Exception: Pathologic stage 0 or 1a does not require pathologic evaluation of lymph nodes.

native fractionation protocols with a high dose per fraction (400–600 rads) are of proven benefit but often limited effectiveness.

Prognosis

An overall 15% 5-year determinate cure rate, with 11% of patients living beyond 5 years and 74% dead within 5 years, has been reported. Melanoma of the nasal septum has a better prognosis than melanoma of the turbinates or sinuses.

Tumor thickness is the single most important factor determining survival for clinical stage I melanomas (greater than 3 mm, 53% 5-year survival; less than 0.76 mm, 98% 5-year survival). Thickness correlates directly with mortality and also with risk of local recurrence; satellitosis; and regional, in-transit, and distant metastasis. For stage II tumors, number of involved lymph nodes and ulceration of the primary are the most important factors. Increasing age, male sex, head and neck sites, scalp primaries, amelanotic tumors, and nodular subtype (probably) also portend a poorer prognosis. Here overall survival is 35% at 5 years; with wide local excision (WLE), 62%; with WLE with elective lymph node dissection (ELND), 76% when pathologic stage N_0, and 25% when pathologically involved.

Principles of Diagnosis

All biopsies should be performed with definitive treatment and reconstruction in mind. Destructive (electrodesiccation, cryotherapy) and shave techniques have no place in the treatment of pigmented lesions, as they prevent the assessment of tumor thickness—a critically important factor in prognosticating local disease.

Elliptical excisional biopsy is recommended for small lesions located where resection will not be disfiguring. Excision need not include underlying muscle fascia and should include a 2-cm margin in most head and neck lesions. Formal re-excision of the wound with margins adjusted for tumor thickness may follow. Definitive treatment may be delayed for up to 3 weeks without adverse effect on final outcome.

Technetium lymphoscintigraphy may be used to map cutaneous lymphatics, identifying first-echelon nodal basins that might not otherwise be predicted by traditional anatomic studies and providing information that will often modify planned surgical treatment of certain lesions in discordant cases. It is complemented by chromatic identification techniques (isosulfan blue). This in vivo mapping technique does not actually identify metastases but is highly effective in identifying first-echelon nodal basins, allowing superselective sampling of such "sentinel" lymph nodes for frozen section analysis for micrometastatic disease. Such immediate analysis has a 5% false-negative rate in routine hematoxylin and eosin (H&E) staining, which may be improved though permanent immunohistochemical staining for S-100, NK1/C3, and HMB 45 and by polymerase chain reaction (PCR) techniques. This approach has provided a low-morbidity, minimally invasive procedure on which to base a rational approach to the clinically N_0 neck. The validity of this technique has been confirmed in analysis of nodal recurrences in lymphatic fields *not* identified by radiolymphoscintigraphy. The World Health Organization (WHO) has recognized these techniques as a standard of care.

Principles of Treatment

Further understanding of tumor biology and data from mature prospective trials have provided a more rational approach to excision margins, minimizing local recurrence and maximizing cosmetic result. Surgical margins should be based on tumor thickness excepting LMM, which, because of low recurrence, justifies a 1-cm margin regardless of primary size. Margins are proportional to local recurrence though unrelated to overall survival. Recommendations include:

> *Melanoma in situ:* 0.5- to 1.0-cm excision margin
> *Tumor less than 0.76 mm:* 1.0- to 2.0-cm excision margin
> *Tumor more than 0.76 mm:* 3.0-cm excision margin

Auricular lesions may be wedge-excised, reserving more radical amputations for large, basally placed, or recurrent disease.

About 8% of patients will present with locoregional nodal metastases, and another 10% will develop them during the course of their disease. Therapeutic lymphadenectomy clearly has a place in the management of metastatic melanomas inasmuch as a significant minority of patients will be cured by the lymphadenectomy alone. Selective neck dissection techniques have not been shown to have a negative influence on survival or on local recurrence in comparison to traditional radical techniques. Extended procedures should be reserved for macroscopic extension. Regional lymph node metastases appear to be indicators of systemic disease, as a majority of patients will develop systemic disease within a few years independent of, or before, locoregional recurrence. A high incidence of asymptomatic central nervous system (CNS) metastases (11%) has been documented in CT studies, with the head and neck patient at particular risk. Findings of brain involvement should mandate local tumor control only and should modify radical traditional approaches.

ELND in patients at risk for occult metastasis has been historically controversial, although mature prospective clinical trials of SLN biopsy have clarified management of the clinically N_0 neck over the last several years. SLN superselective biopsy has improved the accuracy of staging, providing prognostic information on which to base subsequent treatment decisions. It facilitates early therapeutic lymph node dissection in patients with nodal metastases. Candidates for adjuvant therapy with interferon alpha-2b are identified through SLN biopsy. All $T_2N_0M_0$, $T_3N_0M_0$, and $T_4N_0M_0$ melanomas should have pathologic nodal staging with sentinel lymphadenectomy prior to entry onto clinical trials. Homogeneous patient populations may now be entered onto clinical trials of novel adjuvant therapy agents and regimens. SLN biopsy is appropriate for patients at significant risk for nodal metastasis, including those with Breslow thickness of 1.0 mm or greater. Thin melanomas (<1.0 mm) with poor prognostic features (eg, ulceration, Clark's levels III and IV) are at increased risk for late recurrence and metastasis and are also appropriate for SLN techniques. Multiple and multilevel SLNs are common in the head and neck region.

The recently reported ECOG trial EST 1684 demonstrated the ability of interferon 2-alpha to alter the natural history of melanoma in prolonging disease-free and overall survival by approximately 1 year for T_4 and N_1 disease. Survival advantage was restricted to patients with micrometastatic disease only (ie, no benefit for pN_0 patients). An intensive daily intravenous bolus over 1 month is followed by thrice-weekly subcutaneous daily maintenance injections for the next 48 weeks. This protocol has an acceptable toxicity profile but requires dose modification in about one-third of patients, with about three-quarters completing the prescribed year-long course. Issues of time and dose dependency and applicability to other patient groups await the results of ongoing clinical trials.

Parotidectomy

Superficial parotidectomy encompasses all paraglandular and most (about two-thirds) intraglandular parotid lymph nodes and is advocated with cranial nerve VII preservation for primary sites where the gland is in the lymphatic drainage field and for clinically metastatic disease to *either* the parotid or neck. The latter is due to the poor sensitivity of clinical examination to metastatic disease at each site. This approach is adequate in 75% of cases. There is a predilection for distant metastatic failure in patients so treated. The role of intraparotid dissection for SLN sampling as guided by chromo- (isosulfan blue) and radio-lymphoscintigraphy *in lieu of* superficial parotidectomy awaits the results of long-term follow-up of this site for late failure. This is controversial and should be undertaken by only the most experienced surgeon, inasmuch as the unidentified cranial nerve VII is placed at additional risk for temporary and permanent damage.

Local Recurrence

Local recurrence (any recurrence within 5 cm) is considered a harbinger of systemic disease. Long-term survival in this context is 20 to 30%.

Metastatic Melanomas of Unknown Primary

Metastatic melanomas of unknown primary have a better prognosis than nodal metastases from known sites and of known character. With a single node smaller than 3 cm, likelihood of control above the clavicle is 82%, with 66% survival. If nodes are multiple or larger than 3 cm, survival is 33%.

Treatment of Metastatic Disease

Although the incidence of metastatic disease has dramatically increased over the last decade, mortality has risen far less rapidly, largely due to earlier diagnosis. Regional and distant metastases are also decreasing. Within the first 3 to 4 years following primary treatment, in-transit metastasis is 2.3%. Most distant metastases are also diagnosed within this period. Isolated late metastasis, 5% at 10 or more years, is characteristic of thinner lesions. Treatment goals should be the prolongation of life, with palliation an objective worthy of intense effort. Therefore, even in disseminated disease, there may be a role for resection. Unlike the case with other histologies, direct surgical resection of distant metastases has been less effective (eg, lung, brain), with a median survival of 3 to 20 months (30% at 1 year, less than 5% at 5 years). Brain and liver metastases have been less sensitive than nodal disease to adjuvant therapies. Regimens including bacille Calmette-Guérin (BCG), dacarbazine (DTIC), nitrosoureas, and melphalan have been used. Most recently, promising results of trials of high-dose bolus interleukin-2 (IL-2) have been published. This recombinant therapy immunomodulates the host response via a unique mechanism, with 7% complete response (CR) and an additional 10 to 30% partial response (PR) and a durable response to therapy. A 3-year survival rate of 22% multiplies most series. Spontaneous regression is observed in fewer than 1% of melanomas. The most common cause of death from malignant melanoma is pulmonary failure due to pulmonary metastasis. The second commonest is elevated intracranial pressure (ICP) and hemorrhage due to brain metastasis. Multiple organ metastases are noted in 95% of patients dying from malignant melanoma.

Other Lesions

Giant Hairy Nevus

Giant hairy nevi are difficult management problems in the head and neck region. The incidence of melanoma is about 15%, most often (60%) within the first 10 years of life (peak, 3 to 5 years). Mandated fractional excision should be initiated early in life. Expectant management and dermabrasion techniques are condemned, as many who subsequently develop malignant melanoma will die of the disease.

Congenital Melanoma/Pregnancy Effect (Childhood Melanoma)

Children born to mothers with widespread malignant melanoma will die within days to months. Pregnancy after the diagnosis of malignant melanoma has no adverse effect on 5- or 10-year survival. Malignant melanoma initiated during pregnancy is hormonally sensitive and adversely affected by the pregnancy.

Childhood melanomas arise de novo in about two-thirds of cases and are clinically and biologically analogous to adult melanomas.

Familial Melanoma

About 6% of patients with melanoma have a familial tendency. Familial melanoma typically presents between ages 10 and 20. Treatment is analogous to that of the adult form. Dysplastic nevus syndrome mandates serial photographic mapping of affected families. Immunodeficiency states have been associated in familial cases.

Xeroderma Pigmentosum

There is an increased incidence of xeroderma pigmentosum due to actinic damage in the absence of a normal mechanism of DNA repair.

CYSTS AND TUMORS OF THE JAWS

Tooth development is a complex process involving interactions between ectoderm, neuroectoderm, and mesoderm. It is an ongoing process from 6 to 7 weeks in utero through early adulthood and involves multiple stages and sites. The stages of development are dependent on normal relationships, morphogenesis, and mineralization. Pathologic processes can develop in different embryonic tissues at different stages, resulting in a wide variety of cysts and tumors unique to the jaws. The accurate diagnosis and treatment of these lesions require the combination of clinical history and physical examination in addition to diagnostic imaging studies and pathologic and/or laboratory studies. Many of these lesions may appear similar to each other, without pathognomonic findings on more limited evaluation. Malignant features may be nonspecific and may be mimicked by benign disease.

Cysts of the Jaws and Oral Tissues

With rare exceptions, epithelium-lined cysts in bone are seen only in the jaws. Based on the embryonic tissue of origin, they are divided into two main groups (Table 29-3).

- *Odontogenic cysts:* The epithelial lining is derived from the epithelial remnants of the tooth-forming organ. Based on their etiology, these cysts can be subdivided into inflammatory and developmental types.
- *Nonodontogenic cysts:* The sources of the epithelium of these cysts are from tissue *other than* tooth-forming organs. Epithelial inclusions at the areas of union of embryonic facial processes are speculated to be the tissues of origin.

Odontogenic Cysts

Developmental

DENTIGEROUS CYSTS   These cysts develop from the follicular tissue covering the fully formed unerupted tooth crown. Dentigerous cysts are the second most common (18%) cysts of the jaws. The mandibular third molar and maxillary canine teeth are common sites. Radiographically, the cyst typically shows a well-defined unilocular radiolucent area with a sclerotic border encircling the crown of an unerupted tooth. In about 50% of the cases there will be evidence of resorption of adjacent roots. Neoplastic transformation of the cyst lining to ameloblastoma and rarely to squamous cell carcinoma has been reported. Treatment consists of enucleation of the cyst together with extraction of the associated tooth. A tooth in a favorable direction of eruption may be salvaged by marsupialization of the cystic wall. Recurrence after treatment is rare.

TABLE 29-3. CLASSIFICATION OF CYSTS OF THE JAWS AND ORAL TISSUES

A. Odontogenic cysts
Developmental
　Dentigerous cyst
　Eruption cyst
　Odontogenic keratocyst
　Lateral periodontal cyst
　Gingival cyst
　Calcifying odontogenic cyst
Inflammatory
　Radicular cyst
　Residual cyst
　Paradental cyst
B. Nonodontogenic cysts (fissural cysts)
　Nasopalatine duct cyst
　Nasolabial cyst
　Globulomaxillary cyst
　Median cysts

ERUPTION CYSTS   This is a soft tissue analogue of the dentigerous cyst. It develops as a result of separation of dental follicle from the crown of an erupting tooth. Clinically it appears as a purplish swelling in the mucosa overlying an erupting tooth.

ODONTOGENIC KERATOCYST (PRIMORDIAL CYST)   The odontogenic keratocyst (OKC) is a distinctive form of odontogenic developmental cyst with a unique growth pattern, histopathologic features, and clinical behavior. It is believed to arise from the dental lamina. Unlike the dentigerous and radicular cysts, which enlarge as a result of osmotic pressure, the OKC grows by mural proliferation. Therefore marsupialization is not an effective treatment option.

These cysts usually occur in the second through fourth decades of life with a 2:1 male predominance. Seventy to 80% involve the mandible, particularly at the third molar region. Because of its unique growth pattern, the OKC—unlike other odontogenic cysts, which present with bony swelling—invades the bone and can reach a large size without causing bony expansion. Although the majority of OKCs present as solitary lesions, about 7% of the patients present with two or more cysts. Multiple OKCs are associated with the basal cell–nevus syndrome (Gorlin-Goltz syndrome), inherited as an autosomal-dominant trait with marked penetrance and variable expressivity. The stigmata of this syndrome are as follows:

1. Multiple OKCs
2. Multiple nevoid basal cell carcinomas, which can occur anywhere on the body
3. Skeletal deformities involving ribs and vertebrae
4. A typical facies with frontal bossing, hypertelorism, and mild mandibular prognathism
5. Calcification of the falx cerebri

Radiographically, OKCs appear as well-defined radiolucent areas that may be unilocular or multilocular. Resorption of adjacent roots is less common than with dentigerous cysts. OKCs contain thick, grayish, cheesy material with little free fluid. A preoperative diagnosis of OKC can be made with a high degree of accuracy from the cystic aspirate by identifying keratinizing squamous cells and soluble protein less than 4 g/dL. Although the presence of an OKC may be suspected on clinical or radiologic grounds, histopathologic confirmation is required for diagnosis. The cystic wall is thin and friable, consisting of five to ten cells; a thick, parakeratinizing stratified squamous epithelium; and a thin fibrous capsule. Small satellite cysts and epithelial residue are seen in the adjacent tissues.

Treatment consists of enucleation and aggressive curettage. Cryosurgical or chemical cauterization of the bony cavity following enucleation has been shown to decrease the incidence of recurrence. A 5 to 63% recurrence rate mandates follow-up for many years posttreatment.

LATERAL PERIODONTAL CYST   These rare cysts arise from rests of dental lamina. They often present as asymptomatic, well-circumscribed radiolucent areas located lateral to the roots of vital teeth. They occur in the premolar, canine region of the mandible. These cysts can be treated by conservative enucleation and preservation of the teeth.

GINGIVAL CYST   Gingival cysts are of little clinical significance. Gingival cysts of infants arise from remnants of dental lamina, which appear as small, multiple, whitish superficial cysts on the alveolar ridge. They spontaneously regress. Gingival cysts of adults present as painless bluish dome-like swellings, predominantly seen in the mandibular premolar region (60–75%). They are considered to be the soft tissue counterpart of the lateral periodontal cyst, arising from the dental lamina, and may erode cortical bone with saucerization. They usually occur in the mandibular cuspid, premolar region.

CALCIFYING ODONTOGENIC CYSTS   The calcifying epithelial odontogenic cyst is an uncommon lesion that shows diverse histopathologic features and clinical behavior. Despite the terminology, some authors group this under odontogenic tumors rather than cysts. Clinically, the lesion occurs over a wide range of age from infancy to old age, but it usually occurs in patients under 40 years of age. Even though it is predominantly an intraosseous lesion, about 20% appear as extraosseous lesions. The lesion shows equal predilection to the maxilla and mandible and is often seen anterior to the first molars. The lesion usually presents as a slowly enlarging but otherwise asymptomatic swelling. Extraosseous lesions may cause saucerization of cortical bone. Radiologically, the lesion appears as a well-defined unilocular or multilocular radiolucent region containing varying amounts of radiopaque areas. Histologically, the lesion is often cystic (90%), lined by epithelium containing the characteristic keratinized epithelial cells, which are usually referred to as "ghost" cells. Recurrence is rare following enucleation.

Inflammatory
RADICULAR CYSTS   This is the most common cystic lesion of the jaws (55 to 74%). Radicular cysts are always associated with nonvital teeth and arise from the cell rests of Malassez. Depending upon its relation to the root, such a cyst is described as either apical or lateral. The lesion often presents as a painless swelling in relation to a nonvital tooth. On imaging, it is round to ovoid and radiolucent, with well-defined sclerotic borders. Treatment consists of enucleation of the cyst and endodontic treatment of the offending tooth.

RESIDUAL CYST   The radicular cyst persists postextraction in 4 to 21% of cases as a well-defined radiolucent lesion in an edentulous area.

PARADENTAL CYST   This type of cyst arises alongside a partially erupted third molar tooth involved by pericoronitis. Radiologically, it appears as a well-defined radiolucency related to the neck of the tooth and the coronal third of the root. Treatment is by enucleation.

Nonodontogenic Cysts (Fissural Cysts)
NASOPALATINE DUCT (INCISIVE CANAL) CYST   This is the most common nonodontogenic cyst, occurring in about 1% of the population. The cyst is thought to arise from the remnants of the nasopalatine duct. It often presents in the fifth or sixth decade as a slowly enlarging swelling in the anterior region of the midline of the palate. Imaging shows the presence of a well-defined round, ovoid, or heart-shaped radiolucency, often with a sclerotic border. The cyst should be differentiated from the normal incisive fossa, which is generally accepted as a radiolucency not greater than 6 mm wide. The cyst is lined by either stratified squamous or pseudostratified ciliated columnar (respiratory) epithelium.

NASOLABIAL (NASOALVEOLAR, KLESTÄDT'S) CYST   This is a rare lesion, thought to arise according to the fissural hypothesis from epithelial inclusion during fusion of the globular, lateral nasal, and maxillary processes. Alternatively, it has been thought to arise from the remains of the lower part of the embryonic nasolacrimal duct. These cysts are usually lined by pseudostratified ciliated columnar (respiratory) epithelium. They are soft tissue cysts that occur on the floor of the vestibule, anterior to the inferior turbinate, presenting as slowly enlarging lesions that cause nasal obstruction, obliteration of the nasolabial fold, and elevation of the ala. Ten percent of patients have bilateral cysts.

GLOBULOMAXILLARY CYST   This is a rare cyst occurring between the roots of the maxillary lateral incisor and cuspid teeth. It was previously thought that the lesion arose from epithelium trapped during fusion of the globular process with the maxillary process. There is, however, little evidence to support this view, and the status of the cyst as a discrete entity is now questioned. It typically presents as an inverted pear-shaped radiolucency.

MEDIAN CYST   The median palatal cyst arises from epithelium trapped in the line of fusion of the palatal process. Midline mandibular cysts are called median mandibular cysts, thought to originate from epithelial inclusion between mandibular processes. Current concepts of embryogenesis, however, do not support a fissural origin, and this entity may well represent an odontogenic origin.

Malignant Change in Odontogenic Cysts

It is estimated that about 1 to 2% of all oral cavity carcinomas may originate from odontogenic cysts. Epithelial dysplasia, occasionally observed in odontogenic cysts, may be a precursor of carcinoma. The peak reported age is 60 years, with a 2 : 1 male predilection. Even though a ragged radiolucent lesion raises suspicion of a malignant process, diagnosis can be made only after histopathologic examination. About 25% of reported odontogenic carcinomas have arisen in dentigerous cysts.

Odontogenic Tumors

Odontogenic tumors comprise a complex group of lesions demonstrating varying inductive interactions between odontogenic epithelium and ectomesenchyme. They therefore exhibit diverse histopathologic features and clinical behavior. Some are true neoplasms, yet others are tumor-like malformations (hamartomas) or dysplastic lesions. Based on the principal tissue involved, odontogenic tumors can be classified into three groups: epithelial, ectomesenchymal, and mixed (Table 29-4).

Tumors of Odontogenic Epithelium without Odontogenic Ectomesenchyme

AMELOBLASTOMA   Ameloblastoma is the commonest odontogenic tumor, yet it accounts for only about 1% of all oral tumors. It is a benign but locally invasive neoplasm derived from odontogenic epithelium. It has three different clinicopathologic subtypes:

1. *Multicystic* ameloblastoma (86%)
2. *Unicystic* ameloblastoma (13%)
3. *Peripheral* (extraosseous) (1%)

Ameloblastomas usually occur in the fourth and fifth decades with equal gender predilection. About 80% of the tumors occur in the mandible, of which some 70% arise in the molar and ascending ramus regions, 20% in the premolar region, and 10% in the incisor region. The typical presentation is a gradually expanding, painless swelling. Radiographically, the lesion appears as a multilocular radiolucency with adjacent tooth roots showing varying degree of resorption. The unilocular lesion is often indistinguishable from an odontogenic cyst; how-

TABLE 29-4. CLASSIFICATION OF ODONTOGENIC TUMORS

Tumors of odontogenic epithelium without odontogenic ectomesenchyme
  Ameloblastoma
  Malignant ameloblastoma and ameloblastic carcinoma
  Calcifying epithelial odontogenic tumor
  Squamous odontogenic tumor
  Clear cell odontogenic tumor
  Primary intraosseous carcinoma
Tumors of odontogenic epithelium with odontogenic ectomesenchyme
  Ameloblastic fibroma and ameloblastic fibrosarcoma
  Ameloblastic fibro-odontoma
  Odontoameloblastoma
  Adenomatoid odontogenic tumor
  Complex odontoma
  Compound odontoma
Tumors of odontogenic ectomesenchyme
  Odontogenic fibroma
  Odontogenic myxoma
  Cementoma
Tumors of debatable origin
  Melanotic neuroectodermal tumor of infancy
  Congenital gingival granular cell tumor

ever, the extent of root resorption is an indication of a neoplastic process. Histopathologically, the neoplastic epithelial cells show two patterns of arrangement, plexiform and follicular, with no difference in clinical behavior. The tumor typically exhibits infiltrating islands of tumor in adjacent bone, with simple curettage resulting in a 50 to 90% incidence of recurrence. Surgical resection with a margin of normal bone is the treatment of choice. The unicystic variant, often seen in younger age groups, shows a lower incidence of recurrence; here, conservative enucleation is adequate. The rare extraosseous ameloblastoma is also less invasive, and local excision is the treatment of choice.

MALIGNANT AMELOBLASTOMA AND AMELOBLASTIC CARCINOMA   Less than 1% of ameloblastomas show malignant features with distant metastasis. The peak age is 30 years. The common sites of metastasis are lungs, cervical lymph nodes, and bone. This tumor has a poor prognosis.

SQUAMOUS ODONTOGENIC TUMOR   Squamous odontogenic tumor is a rare lesion presenting with local tenderness, tooth mobility, and a well-defined radiolucency; it is associated with the roots of the teeth. Treatment is local excision.

CALCIFYING EPITHELIAL ODONTOGENIC TUMOR   This is a benign but locally invasive, odontogenic epithelial neoplasm. The lesion is most commonly seen at the mandibular premolar and molar region. Imaging of the lesion shows an irregular radiolucent area with varying amount of radiopaque bodies. Histologically the tumor consists of sheets of polyhedral epithelial cells and a fibrous stroma. The presence of amyloid-like material, which may calcify, within the epithelial strands is a characteristic feature.

CLEAR CELL ODONTOGENIC TUMOR   This is a very rare intraosseous odontogenic tumor. The majority of reported cases occur in females over 50 years of age. Histologically, these lesions appear as poorly circumscribed tumors consisting of glycogen-rich sheets of cells. They are locally aggressive and have a high recurrence rate.

PRIMARY INTRAOSSEOUS CARCINOMA   This rare condition—unless related to a pre-existing cyst—is presumed to arise from odontogenic epithelium. Intraosseous tumors are unique to the jaws.

Tumors of Odontogenic Epithelium with Odontogenic Ectomesenchyme
In this group, both epithelial and mesenchymal components are neoplastic.

AMELOBLASTIC FIBROMA, AMELOBLASTIC FIBROSARCOMA, AMELOBLASTIC FIBRO-ODONTOMA, AND ODONTOAMELOBLASTOMA   In these tumors, unlike ameloblastoma, *both* epithelium and stroma are neoplastic. The ameloblastic fibroma consists of proliferating strands of odontogenic epithelium and cellular fibroblastic tissue. It is important to differentiate this lesion, as the lesions do not exhibit local invasion and have a low incidence of local recurrence. The exceedingly rare ameloblastic fibrosarcoma is a malignant counterpart of ameloblastic fibroma, in which the mesenchymal portion of the lesion shows features of malignancy. Those tumors in which dentin and enamel matrix are present are called ameloblastic fibro-odontomas. Most of these lesions occur in association with unerupted teeth in children younger than 10 years of age. Odontoameloblastomas are those tumors with ameloblastoma-like tissue combined with enamel and dentin as an ill-defined mass. This tumor behaves like an ameloblastoma.

ADENOMATOID ODONTOGENIC TUMOR   Adenomatoid odontogenic tumors are thought to represent a developmental anomaly (hamartoma) formed from an abortive attempt at enamel organ formation. It consists of strands and whorls of ameloblast-like epithelial masses with the central space containing eosinophilic material. These lesions usually present in patients less than 20 years of age and have a striking tendency to occur in the anterior maxilla.

COMPLEX/COMPOUND ODONTOMA   This is the most common odontogenic tumor. It is considered a hamartoma rather than a true neoplasm. The complex odontoma consists mainly of a mass of haphazardly arranged enamel, dentin, and cementum, whereas the compound odontoma consists of collections of numerous discrete, tooth-like structures with calcified structures in an orderly arrangement. Such odontomas often present in the first two decades of life as an incidental finding of an irregular, radiopaque mass. Treatment consists of local excision.

Tumors of Odontogenic Ectomesenchyme
ODONTOGENIC FIBROMA AND MYXOMA   Odontogenic fibroma is a well-demarcated and readily enucleated benign fibroblastic neoplasm comprising mature collagenous tissue containing varying amounts of apparently inactive odontogenic epithelium. There may be areas of cementum- and dentin-like structure within the tumor. Myxomatous lesions in the jaw are considered benign, whereas those arising in other parts of the body are considered malignant, thus giving rise to the idea that their origin may be different. Though benign, these tumors are locally invasive. Hence, wide local excision is essential. Radiographically, a unilocular or multilocular radiolucent lesion is seen.

CEMENTOMAS   These are a complex group of lesions containing cementum or cementum-like tissues. They include true neoplasms and dysplastic or reactive processes. The clinical, histopathologic, and radiographic features of cementomas of the jaws are identical to those of other bones. They may not, therefore, represent odontogenic tumors. This group consists of four different clinical subtypes.

1. *Benign cementoblastoma:* This is a true neoplasm, closely related to osteoblastoma of bone. It presents in young males as a slowly increasing radiopaque mass attached to the roots of mandibular premolar and molar teeth.

2. *Cemento-ossifying fibroma:* This lesion starts as a cellular fibroblastic lesion, which, radiologically, appears as a well-demarcated radiolucent area. As the lesion calcifies, cementum-like tissues are deposited. Radiologically, its appearance varies from a speckled to a radiopaque mass.

3. *Periapical cemental dysplasia:* This lesion resembles fibrous dysplasia of bone. It is most frequently seen in the mandibular incisor region in postmenopausal women. The lesion evolves from a cellular fibrous tissue at the apices of the teeth to a mature, cementum-like tissue. Involved teeth remain vital.

4. *Florid cemento-osseous dysplasia:* This is an extensive dysplastic lesion involving multiple teeth, commonly seen in middle-aged African-American women. It enlarges slowly and presents radiographically as a poorly defined radiopaque mass.

Tumors of Debatable Origin

MELANOTIC NEUROECTODERMAL TUMOR OF INFANCY   This is a rare tumor of infancy, occurring at less than 6 months of age in the anterior maxilla. Radiographically indistinct borders with alveolar destruction are seen. Local excision is often curative.

CONGENITAL GINGIVAL GRANULAR CELL TUMOR   This rare lesion is seen in newborn infants, predominantly female, at the anterior maxilla. It is probably more reactive than truly neoplastic.

Nonodontogenic Tumors and Tumor-like Lesions of the Jaw (Table 29-5)

Bone-Forming Tumors

OSTEOMA   Osteoma is a benign, slow-growing tumor consisting of well-differentiated mature bone. Multiple osteomas of the jaw are associated with Gardner's syndrome, consisting of epidermal sebaceous cysts, multiple cutaneous fibromas, polyposis coli (which may undergo malignant transformation (40%), and multiple impacted supernumerary teeth. This is a rare familial autosomal-dominant disorder.

OSTEOBLASTOMA   This is a rare benign tumor consisting of proliferating osteoblasts, multinucleated giant cells, and varying amounts of osteoid. It often presents as a dull, aching lesion of the jaw that, radiographically, appears as a well-circumscribed radiolucent or speckled area with peripheral sclerosis.

OSTEOSARCOMA   Osteosarcoma is the most common malignancy of bone but is rare in the jaws. It usually presents in the third decade, with a 2:1 male preponderance. Occasionally, the tumor can present in older patients when associated with Paget's disease or as a late sequel to radiotherapy. Clinically, the tumor appears as a rapidly growing bony swelling

TABLE 29-5. CLASSIFICATION OF NONODONTOGENIC TUMORS AND TUMOR-LIKE LESIONS OF THE JAWS

Bone-forming tumors
   Osteoma
   Osteoblastoma
   Osteosarcoma
Cartilage-forming tumors
   Chondroma
   Osteochondroma
   Chondrosarcoma
Tumors of fibrous connective tissue
   Fibrosarcoma
   Desmoplastic fibroma
Fibro-osseous and giant cell lesions of jaws
   Central giant cell granuloma
   Brown tumor
   Giant cell tumor
   Histiocytosis
   Fibrous dysplasia
   Cemento-osseous dysplasia
Other conditions
   Paget's disease
   Exostosis
   Cherubism
   Hemangiomas and vascular malformations
   Metastatic tumors
   Myeloma

with associated pain or numbness and mobile teeth. Variable radiographic appearance is observed, with lytic, poorly defined margins and radiopaque areas indicating neoplastic new bone formation. Differential diagnosis includes metastatic disease (prostate, lung). There is about a 13% incidence of metastasis, usually to the lungs. Treatment is ablative, with poorer prognosis in the jaws than in long bones due, in part, to a poorer response to adjuvant chemotherapy (20 to 35% 5-year survival).

Cartilage-Forming Tumors

CHONDROMA AND CHONDROSARCOMA   This is a rare head and neck malignancy. Anterior maxilla and posterior mandible (where there are cartilage remnants of the nasal capsule and Meckel's cartilage) are the common sites. Histologic differentiation of the two lesions is often difficult. An apparently benign tumor may pursue an aggressive clinical course. Therefore, wide surgical resection is advisable. Radiation-induced cases are reported.

OSTEOCHONDROMA   This is considered a developmental anomaly (hamartoma). Seen in young children, it consists of mature bone capped by hyaline cartilage, often found in relation to the coronoid process. Growth often stops with the cessation of skeletal growth.

Tumors of Fibrous Connective Tissue

DESMOPLASTIC FIBROMA   This is the osseous counterpart of the soft tissue desmoid tumor. The mandible is the fourth most commonly affected bone. The majority of these tumors are seen in patients less than 30 years old. Radiographically, a typical lesion is a unilocular radiolucency with resorption of associated tooth roots. Because of the locally aggressive nature of the tumor and soft tissue extension, recommended treatment is wide en bloc excision.

FIBROSARCOMA   This rare tumor can arise in either soft tissue or bone. The medullary lesion has a greater propensity for local recurrence and metastasis. The typical patient is over 40 years old, presenting with pain, pathologic fracture, and radiographic evidence of root resorption and a moth-eaten appearance. Treatment is wide local excision.

Fibro-osseous and Giant Cell Lesions of the Jaw

FIBROUS DYSPLASIA   This is a developmental tumor-like lesion involving a single bone (monostotic) or several bones (polyostotic). The former accounts for 80% of all cases. In about 3% of patients with *polyostotic* lesions, fibrous dysplasia is associated with the McCune-Albright syndrome, consisting of cutaneous pigmentation, autonomic hyperfunctioning endocrine glands, and precocious puberty. The lesion presents as a progressively enlarging, painless, bony swelling. The process typically becomes quiescent at puberty. Radiographic presentation varies from a radiolucent "ground glass" to a radiopaque appearance, depending on the lesions's stage of development. Conservative cosmetic recontouring is recommended. Sudden growth and pain may herald malignant transformation (less than 1%).

CENTRAL GIANT CELL GRANULOMA   This is a relatively common osseous lesion of the jaw. Of unknown etiology, it consists of large numbers of multinucleated osteoclast-like giant cells lying in a vascular stroma. It presents as a well-defined radiolucent lesion of the anterior part of the jaws in children and young adults. Its growth may be rapid. Curettage is curative.

BROWN TUMOR   This osteolytic lesion, composed of osteoclasts, is seen in primary hyperparathyroidism. Histologically, it is impossible to distinguish from central giant cell granuloma.

GIANT CELL TUMOR (OSTEOCLASTOMA)   In general, giant cell tumors of the jaws have a less aggressive clinical course than those of the long bones. Histologic differentiation of this rare tumor from the relatively common central giant cell granuloma is very difficult. The giant cell tumors usually present between 20 and 40 years of age, whereas the giant cell granuloma tends to occur in adolescents. Curettage is the treatment of choice.

HISTIOCYTOSIS   This is an idiopathic group of disorders in which there is infiltration of proliferating histiocytes (macrophages) admixed with eosinophils. These clinically present as three distinct groups:

1. Solitary eosinophilic granuloma; commonly seen in children and young adults
2. Multifocal eosinophilic granuloma (Hand-Schüller-Christian syndrome); commonly seen in children, which involves multiple bones and viscera.
3. Rapidly progressive disseminated histiocytosis (Letterer-Siwe disease): presents with fever, skin rash, hepatosplenomegaly, lymphadenopathy, pancytopenia, and diffuse osteolytic lesions; commonly occurs in infants and children. This is a fatal disorder.

Radiographically, the jaw lesions present as osteolytic areas with teeth appearing to "float in air." Treatment consists of curettage with sacrifice of adjacent teeth.

CHERUBISM   This rare autosomal-dominant disorder of the jaws is seen in young children. It manifests as a painless, bilateral expansion of the posterior mandible, resulting in the characteristic cherubic facies. It can also involve the maxilla. An association with Noonan syndrome has been reported. Radiographically, the lesion has typical multilocular, expansile radiolucencies. Histologically, it consists of giant cells within a fibrovascular stroma. The clinical progress is unpredictable. Some of the lesions regress spontaneously; however, others have a progressive course. Excellent results have been reported with early surgical curettage.

Other Related Lesions

PAGET'S DISEASE   This disorder is thought to be due to a slow virus infection. It is characterized by disorganized bone formation and resorption, resulting in deformation of the affected bone. The disease progresses from a predominantly osteolytic phase to an active stage of resorption and apposition and on to a sclerotic osteoblastic phase. It is predominantly seen in patients over 40 years of age, with high predilection in Anglo-Saxons. The jaw is involved in 10 to 15% of patients. There, it presents as a slowly enlarging bony mass causing facial deformity. Bone pain and sensory or motor deficit related to a pressure effect might be another presenting complaint. In addition to the pressure effect, extensive disease can cause high-output cardiac failure, and about 0.1 to 0.2% of patients may develop osteosarcoma. Autopsy series show a 3% incidence, suggesting that much of Paget's disease may be subclinical. Radiographic appearances vary with the stage of the disease. The typical lesion will have a cotton-wool appearance.

EXOSTOSES   These are nonneoplastic developmental bony outgrowths. Common sites are the palatal midline, called torus palatinus, and the mandibular lingual sulcus, called torus mandibularis. Other sites are the buccal sulcus of the maxilla and the region of the mandibular genial tubercle. Mandibular and maxillary tori are present in as many as 30% of the U.S. population. They appear after puberty and are left undisturbed unless they become symptomatic (mucosal ulceration, disturbed fit of denture prosthesis).

HEMANGIOMA   Although hemangiomas of bone are rare lesions, they are important to consider in the differential diagnosis of radiolucent lesions, as an unplanned operative intervention can cause considerable morbidity. Presenting symptoms include a slowly enlarging painless swelling, spontaneous gingival bleeding, tooth mobility, and dysesthesia. Radiographically, the hemangioma has a multilocular honeycomb appearance. Individualized treatment is based on angiographic findings.

EWING'S SARCOMA   Fewer than 1% of all Ewing's tumors are Ewing's sarcoma. Of these, 88% present from 6 to 20 years of age, typically with pain, swelling, fever, anemia, leukocytosis, and an elevated erythrocyte sedimentation rate. A variable radiographic appearance is seen. There is a rapid hematogenous spread, with 25% of tumors metastatic at diagnosis or treatment. A 75% 5-year survival rate with early adjuvant therapy (chemotherapy, radiotherapy) has been achieved consistently.

BURKITT'S LYMPHOMA   Maxillary involvement is most common in Burkitt's lymphoma, with rapid growth, distortion, and loosening of teeth. African and American forms are noted. An Epstein-Barr viral induction mechanism is proven. Cure or remission may be achieved in 90% of cases. The role of surgery is cytoreductive, to debulk massive lesions prior to definitive chemotherapy.

METASTATIC TUMORS   These account for about 1% of malignant tumors of the oral cavity, mandibular involvement being more common than maxillary. Even though most metastatic lesions are osteolytic, metastatic deposits from prostate and some breast carcinomas are *osteoblastic.* Common primary sites are breast, lungs, and kidney.

MYELOMA   Myeloma is a tumor of plasma cells. It presents either as multiple myeloma, involving many bones, or as a solitary lesion. The gnathic bones can be involved in either situation. Recognition of the monoclonal gammopathy often confirms the diagnosis. The classic radiographic appearance is the presence of multiple punched-out osteolytic lesions.

Bibliography

Carotid Body Tumors

Hodge KT, Byers RM, Peters LJ. Paragangliomas of the head and neck. *Arch Otolaryngol Head Neck Surg* 1988;114:872–877.

Leonetti JP, Donzelli JJ, Littooy FN, et al. Perioperative strategies in the management of carotid body tumors. *Otolaryngol Head Neck Surg* 1997; 117(1):111–115.

Ward PH, Liu C, Vinuela F, et al. Embolization: An adjunctive measure for removal of carotid body tumors. *Laryngoscope* 1988;98:1287–1291.

Vascular Anomalies

Edgerton MT. The treatment of hemangiomas: With special reference to the role of steroid therapy. *Ann Surg* 1976;183:517–530.

Jackson IT, Carreno R, Potparic Z, et al. Hemangiomas, vascular malformations, and lymphovenous malformations: Classification and methods of treatment. *Plast Reconstr Surg* 1993; 91:1216–1230.

Mulliken JB, Fishman SJ, Burrows PE. Vascular anomalies. *Curr Probl Surg* 2000;520–584.

Mulliken JB, Glowacki J. Classification of pediatric vascular lesions. *Plast Reconstr Surg* 1982;70: 120–121.

Zarem HA, Edgerton MT. Induced resolution of cavernous hemangiomas following prednisolone therapy. *Plast Reconstr Surg* 1967;39:76–83.

Melanoma and Pigmented Cutaneous Lesions

Anderson RG. Skin tumors: 11. Melanoma. *Selected Readings in Plastic Surgery,* 6th ed. Waco, TX: Baylor University Medical Center, November 1990, 1–24.

Balch CM. The revised melanoma staging system: Its use in the design and interpretation of melanoma clinical trials. *ASCO Proc* 2001;82–87.

Balch CM, Soong SJ, Bartolucci AA, et al. Efficacy of an elective regional lymph node dissection of 1 to 4 mm thick melanomas for patients 60 years of age and younger. *Ann Surg* 1996;224(3): 255–266.

Kaleya RN et al. Management of malignant melanoma—A symposium. *Contemp Surg* 1994;44: 241–254.

Kirkwood JM, Strawderman MH, Ernstoff MS, et al. Interferon alfa-2b adjuvant therapy of high-risk resected cutaneous melanoma: The Eastern Cooperative Oncology Group Trial EST 1684. *J Clin Oncol* 1996;14(1):7–17.

Manola J, Atkins M, Ibrahim J, Kirkwood J. Prognostic factors in metastatic melanoma: A Pooled Analysis of Eastern Cooperative Oncology Group Trials. *J Clin Oncol* 2000;18(22):3782–3793.

McMasters KM, Reintgen DS, Ross MI, et al. Sentinel lymph node biopsy for melanoma: Controversy despite widespread agreement. *J Clin Oncol* 2001;19 (11):2851–2855.

Myers JN. Value of neck dissection in the treatment of patients with intermediate thickness cutaneous melanoma of the head and neck. *Arch Otolaryngol Head Neck Surg* 1999;125:110–115.

O'Brien C, Uren RF, Thompson JF, et al. Prediction of potential metastatic sites in cutaneous head and neck melanoma using lymphoscintigraphy. *Am J Surg* 1995;170:461–466.

Rosenberg SA, et al. Treatment of 283 consecutive patients with metastatic melanoma or renal cell cancer using high-dose bolus interleukin-2. *JAMA* 1994;271:907–913.

Van de Vrie W, Eggermon AMM, Van Putten WLJ, et al. Therapeutic lymphadenectomy in melanomas of the head and neck. *Head Neck* 1993; 15:377–381.

Wells KE, et al. The use of lymphoscintigraphy in melanoma of the head and neck. *Plast Reconstr Surg* 1994;93:757–761.

Cysts and Tumors of the Jaws

Delgado R, et al. Osteosarcoma of the jaw. *Head Neck* 1994;16:246–252.

Ellis EE, Fonseca RJ. Management of odontogenic cysts and tumors. In: Thawley SE, Panje WR, eds. *Comprehensive Management of Head and Neck Tumors.* Philadelphia: Saunders, 1987, 1483–1509.

Greer RO, Rohrer MD, Young SK. Non-odontogenic tumors: Clinical evaluation and pathology. In: Thawley SE, Panje WR, eds. *Comprehensive Management of Head and Neck Tumors.* Philadelphia: Saunders, 1987, 1510–1559.

McDaniel RK: Odontogenic cysts and tumors: Clinical evaluation and pathology. In: Thawley SE, Panje WR, eds. *Comprehensive Management of Head and Neck Tumors.* Philadelphia: Saunders, 1987, 1446–1483.

Scott RF, Ellis EE. Surgical management of non-odontogenic tumors. In: Thawley SE, Panje WR, eds. *Comprehensive Management of Head and Neck Tumors.* Philadelphia: Saunders, 1987, 1559–1577.

The Nose and Paranasal Sinuses

30

I. SINONASAL EMBRYOLOGY

A. Nasal Embryology[1]

Olfactory placodes develop at about 3 weeks gestation, develop into nasal pits, and become cleft-like structures separated by a primitive septum at 5 weeks. The maxillary and ethmoid folds (later becoming turbinates) appear and the oronasal membrane opens at about 6 weeks. Palatal fusion separates the nasal cavity and stomodeum at about 3 months.

B. Paranasal Sinus Embryology[2–5]

1. Maxillary Sinuses

These grow laterally from a middle meatal infundibulum at about 3 months gestation and are about $7 \times 7 \times 4$ mm at birth. They are first visible on plain radiographs at about 5 to 6 months of age and undergo two periods of rapid growth (both coinciding with dental development) in the first 3 years of life and again at ages 7 to 12.

2. Ethmoid Sinuses

These appear as middle meatal outgrowths around the third to fourth months of gestation. Several are present at birth, but they are not visible on plain films until age 1 year. Near complete development occurs by age 12.

3. Frontal Sinuses

These develop from anterior ethmoid air cells and are usually not present at birth. Not visible on plain radiographs until after age 1 and development not complete until end of second decade of life.

4. Sphenoid Sinuses

Paired sphenoid sinuses develop separately at about 4 months gestation. They are of minimal size at birth, reach the sella turcica around age 7, and are fully grown at age 15.

II. PERTINENT SINONASAL ANATOMY[1,6–8]

A. Sinonasal Histology

1. Vestibule

Stratified squamous epithelium with sweat glands, sebaceous glands, vibrissae.

2. Internal Nasal/Sinus Mucosa

Pseudostratified, columnar, ciliated epithelium (respiratory epithelium).

3. Olfactory Epithelium

One square centimeter bilaterally on septal/lateral surface in uppermost nasal cavity. Include ciliated bipolar receptor cells, microvillar cells, supporting cells, basal cells. About 20 un-

682

myelinated fibers pass through cribriform plate foramina bilaterally to reach olfactory bulb, a 3- by 15-mm portion of rhinencephalon of brain.

B. Sinonasal Blood Supply[6,9–11]

1. External Nose

A. ARTERIAL SUPPLY

(1) Internal Carotid (Minor Contribution)   Via nasal branches of anterior ophthalmic and anterior ethmoidal arteries.

(2) External Carotid Artery via Facial Artery (Primary Supply)   Superior labial artery, lateral nasal artery, angular artery. Angular artery/vein are frequent sources of bleeding during external ethmoidectomy incision.

B. VENOUS DRAINAGE   Recall that the nose is in the "danger triangle area" of the face.

(1) Anterior Facial Vein   Drains through common facial vein to internal jugular; also communicates through infraorbital vein and pterygoid venous plexus to cavernous sinus.

(2) Angular Vein   Communicates via ophthalmic veins to cavernous sinus. Anterior facial vein.

C. LYMPHATICS   Follow anterior facial vein to submandibular nodes.

2. Nasal Cavity and Paranasal Sinuses

A. ARTERIAL SUPPLY

(1) Internal Carotid Artery System

(A) OPHTHALMIC ARTERY   Enters orbit to give off ethmoidal arteries, which traverse ethmoid sinuses near fovea ethmoidalis, enter anterior cranial fossa, then enter nose through cribriform plate.

(B) ANTERIOR AND POSTERIOR ETHMOIDAL ARTERIES   Supply, respectively, anterior/posterior regions of nasal cavity and sinuses.

(C) SUPRAORBITAL AND SUPRATROCHLEAR ARTERIES   To frontal sinuses.

(2) External Carotid Artery System

(A) SPHENOPALATINE ARTERY VIA SPHENOPALATINE FORAMEN   Major artery of nasal cavity/septum plus adjacent sinuses.

(B) DESCENDING PALATINE ARTERY   Posteroinferior nasal cavity.

(C) GREATER PALATINE ARTERY THROUGH INCISIVE FORAMEN FROM ORAL CAVITY.

(D) INFRAORBITAL, POSTEROSUPERIOR ALVEOLAR, ANTEROSUPERIOR ALVEOLARY. Supply maxillary sinuses.

(E) PHARYNGEAL ARTERY—POSTERIOR NASAL ROOF

(F) SUPERIOR LABIAL ARTERY OF FACIAL ARTERY   To Kiesselbach's plexus.

B. VENOUS DRAINAGE—LARGELY PARALLELS ARTERIES

(1) Supratrochlear, Supraorbital, Ethmoidal Veins   Drain via ophthalmic vein to cavernous sinus.

(2) Sphenoidal, Alveolar, and Palatine Veins   Drain via maxillary vein to posterior facial vein but communicate with cavernous sinus via pterygoid plexus.

C. LYMPHATIC DRAINAGE   Anterior third of nose drains to submandibular nodes. Posterior two-thirds of nose plus sinuses drain to retropharyngeal nodes (of Rouvière) and superior deep cervical nodes.

C. Innervation[6,9–11]

1. Sensory Innervation

A. EXTERNAL NOSE

(1) Ophthalmic Division (V_1) of Trigeminal Nerve

(A) INFRATROCHLEAR NERVE   Bony nasal dorsum.

(B) EXTERNAL NASAL NERVE   From anterior ethmoidal through superior nasal vault to caudal nose/tip.

B. MAXILLARY DIVISION (V_2) OF TRIGEMINAL NERVE—INFRAORBITAL NERVE

2. Nasal Cavity and Sinuses

A. OPHTHALMIC (V_1) DIVISIONS OF TRIGEMINAL NERVE

(1) Anterior Ethmoidal Nerve   Parallels anterior ethmoidal artery. Supplies anterosuperior nasal cavity/septum and ethmoid sinuses; terminates in external nasal nerve.

(2) Posterior Ethmoidal Nerve—Occasionally Present   Parallels posterior ethmoidal nerve to posterior nasal cavity and adjacent sinuses.

(3) Supraorbital and Supratrochlear Nerves   Frontal sinuses.

B. MAXILLARY (V_2) DIVISION OF TRIGEMINAL NERVE

(1) Sphenopalatine Nerve   Posterior and inferior portions of nasal cavity/septum plus ethmoid and sphenoid sinuses. Terminates at septum as nasopalatine nerve passing through incisive foramen to supply anterior hard palate.

(2) Anterior, Middle, Posterior Superior Alveolar Nerves   Maxillary sinuses.

B. Autonomic Innervation

1. Sympathetic Innervation

Spinal nerves T1 to T3, to superior cervical sympathetic ganglion, to deep petrosal nerve, joining greater superficial petrosal nerve in order to form vidian nerve canal. Distribute with branches of sphenopalatine nerve. Vasoconstrictive effect.

2. Parasympathetic Innervation

Superior salivatory nucleus, to nervus intermedius, to greater superficial petrosal nerve, to vidian nerve canal. Synapses at sphenopalatine ganglion (only parasympathetics synapse here) and distributes via branches of sphenopalatine nerve. Vasomotor stimulation.

III. SINONASAL PHYSIOLOGY[1,12–14]

A. Nasal Respiration

1. Four nasal sites produce 30 to 50% of nasal resistance:
   a. External nasal valve: ala, columella, nostril sill.
   b. Internal nasal valve: determined by angle between septal cartilage and upper lateral cartilages. Most significant in Caucasians.
   c. Inferior turbinates. Most significant in non-Caucasians.
   d. Septum—due to obstruction from deviation.
2. Some 70 to 80% of individuals demonstrate alternating respiration through the right and left nasal cavities due to cycles of inferior turbinate vasoconstriction/congestion lasting 30 minutes to 3 hours. Absent in those who have had laryngectomies.
3. Air inspired through the nose reaches body temperature and almost 100% humidification. The body reclaims about one-third of the heat and moisture on exhalation through the nose.
4. Nasal vibrissae capture larger inspired foreign particles, while smaller particulate matter adsorbs onto the mucous layer and is swallowed. Nasal mucus contains lysozyme and immunoglobulins, primarily IgA.
5. Debate exists regarding the presence of a nasopulmonary reflex that, theoretically, causes hypoventilation in response to nasal obstruction, and of a nasobronchial reflex in which nasal irritation causes bronchoconstriction.
6. Nasal obstruction aggravates snoring and obstructive sleep apnea.
7. Chronic nasal obstruction (ie, due to adenoid hypertrophy) may alter facial/dental development in children and produce a high arched palate, narrow dental arch, and crossbite.

IV. OLFACTION

See Sec. II.A.3, above.

V. PHONATION

Normal voice depends on the contribution of nasal resonance. *Rhinolalia aperta* is hypernasal speech. *Rhinolalia clauda* refers to hyponasal speech.

VI. SINONASAL EXAMINATION AND EVALUATION

A. Anterior Rhinoscopy

Examination should be performed before and after decongestion with attention to mucosal color, edema, nasal discharge, and effect of vasoconstriction. Allows viewing of septum and turbinates with limited visualization of posterior and superior nasal vault.

B. Nasal Endoscopy[15,16]

Nasal endoscopy supplements information gained by anterior rhinoscopy, particularly to examine the nose posterior to an obstruction. Either a flexible fiberoptic scope or a rigid Hopkins rod scope may be used. The flexible scope is more comfortable, particularly with fixed obstruction, while a rigid scope with a 30-degree lens may allow better examination of the middle meatus. Nasal endoscopy provides additional diagnostic information in 11 to 26% of cases, particularly in examining areas that are difficult to see. Included in the examination should be the inferior and middle meati, the nasopharynx with sphenoid ostia, and the roof of the nasal cavity.

C. Acoustic Rhinometry[17–19]

This technique uses a transducer and sound waves to generate a two-dimensional plot of the nasal cavity cross section relative to distance posteriorly into the nose. Its potential advantages include rapid acquisition of data, minimal invasiveness, independence from patient effort (eg, pediatric patients), and reproducibility of results. Unfortunately, this is presently more a tool for research, with limited usefulness in clinical practice. It offers less information than computed tomography (CT) scanning or nasal endoscopy. Subjects must avoid swallowing, moving, or breathing during data acquisition; serial measurements with data averaging are necessary. Accuracy of information declines in progressing from the anterior to the posterior nasal cavity. This technique requires further refinement before it will gain commonplace use in normal general otolaryngology practice.

D. Rhinomanometry[17,20,21]

This technique is perhaps better suited for research than for general clinical practice. It is often time-consuming, cumbersome, and subject to operator error. It may have up to 50% test-retest variability.

Unilateral nasal rhinomanometry correlates better with a subjective sensation of unilateral nasal airflow, while measurement of both nostrils simultaneously correlates poorly with the patient's sensation of obstruction.

1. Anterior Rhinomanometry

This technique is used most often. A face mask incorporates an airflow meter for the nostril being tested as well as an occluding pressure transducer for the other nostril, used to determine nasopharyngeal air pressure.

2. Posterior Rhinomanometry

The face mask measures unilateral or bilateral nasal airflow. Pharyngeal pressure is determined by a transducer held perorally and placed beneath the soft palate or passed along the nasal floor to the nasopharynx.

3. Active versus Passive Rhinomanometry

In *active rhinomanometry*, used most often, the patient breathes actively. *Passive rhinomanometry* involves air being blown through the nasal passages.

E. Sinonasal Imaging[22–24]

Plain radiographic views include the Caldwell (for frontal sinuses), Waters (maxillary sinuses) lateral, and submental vertex projections. These best demonstrate opacification or air-fluid levels in the large sinus but are less reliable for mucosal thickening. They offer little information on the osteomeatal complex and ethmoid sinuses. Limited/screening coronal sinus CT has replaced plain films in many places because it offers much more information while being of comparable cost.

Sinus CT has many imaging advantages, including good resolution of the osteomeatal complex and delineation of mucosal disease (particularly ethmoidal); it also provides a "road map" for surgery. The coronal view offers the most information, but some surgeons like to also obtain axial views to image the anterior/posterior walls of the frontal and sphenoid sinuses and *Onodi cells* of posterior ethmoids as well as to demonstrate anteroposterior dimensions. Adding axial views usually increases cost. Coronal films are obtained in a prone position with neck hyperextension. If patients cannot tolerate this, a supine "head-hanging" position may be used, but the views of the osteomeatal complex may be compromised by secretions in the now dependent maxillary infundibulum. Alternately, helical CT scanners may perform 2- to 3-mm volumetric data acquisition in the supine position and reconstruct fairly good coronal reformations. Three-millimeter slices are usually acquired for coronal views and 5-mm slices for axial views. Images are magnified 1.5 to 2 times.

1. Points of Interest on Sinus CT

A. NASAL CAVITY   Septal deviation, polyps/masses, concha bullosa (4 to 15% of population), paradoxic middle turbinates.

B. OSTEOMEATAL COMPLEX   Includes maxillary ostium/infundibulum, ethmoid infundibulum, frontoethmoidal recess, uncinate process, hiatus semilunaris, ethmoidal bulla, and middle meatus.

C. ETHMOID AIR CELLS

Haller cells—ethmoid cells extending along medial orbital floor (10% of patients).
Agger nasi cells—most anterior ethmoid cells, located anterior, lateral, and inferior to frontal recess. Represent pneumatized lacrimal bone.
Onodi cells—posterior/lateral ethmoid pneumatization around orbital apex, which places optic nerve at risk.

D. PREOPERATIVE CT EVALUATION   Surgeon and radiologist should review films with attention to features that increase operative risk:

Atelectatic uncinate—adherent to inferomedial orbit wall, placing lamina papyracea at surgical risk.
Dehiscent lamina papyracea—increases risk to orbital contents.
Fovea ethmoidalis, cribriform plate—if low-lying, asymmetric, or thin, increase risk to skull base.
Absence of middle turbinate—from prior surgery; increases risk to cribriform plate.
Onodi cells—pose surgical risk to orbital apex and optic nerves.
Sphenoid sinus—dehiscence of bony wall over optic nerves (10%) or carotid artery (22%). Manupulation of intrasphenoidal septum overlying carotid may breach bony covering over the artery.

Noncontrasted views are obtained for routine sinus studies. Contrast should be used and axial plus coronal views obtained when there is concern of neoplasm or infectious complications of sinusitis.

2. Comparison of Sinus CT and MRI

CT provides superior bony detail compared with magnetic resonance imaging (MRI) and, as it is often more readily available and cheaper, may be the initial study. MRI best shows intracranial complications, and MR venography can identify septic intracranial thrombosis. Sinus secretions and neoplasm often appear similar on CT but may often be differentiated on MRI. Sinus secretions and hypertrophic mucosa are hyperintense on T2 images, while tumors produce intermediate signals. Neither modality accurately separates benign and malignant processes, although secondary findings such as bony destruction and extension may be helpful with regard to this. Sinonasal polyposis (with or without fungal etiology) may also cause bony remodeling/erosion but often shows a heterogeneity of signal intensity on MRI, while tumors are more often homogeneous.

A-mode ultrasound has been used to a limited extent to demonstrate opacification of frontal and maxillary sinuses.

F. Nasal Cytology[25,26]

1. Specimen is best obtained by curetting the underside of the nonvasoconstricted inferior turbinate rather than nose-blowing into plastic wrap or from nasal lavage. Wright-Giemsa stain is used.
2. The presence of a large amount of eosinophils or basophils suggests allergic rhinitis or nonallergic rhinitis with eosinophilia (NARES). Neutrophils, bacteria, and fungal elements indicate infection.

VII. CONGENITAL DISORDERS

A. Choanal Atresia[27–29]

1. Believed to be due to persistence of bucconasal membrane beyond 6 weeks gestation.
2. Occurs in 1 per 7000 to 8000 births; two-thirds unilateral, one-third bilateral; right side more commonly involved; 90% bony/10% membranous only. Female predominance 2:1.
3. Bilateral atresia classically presents immediately at birth as cyclic apnea relieved by crying or mouth breathing. It is a life-threatening situation because infants are obligate nasal breathers for 2 to 6 weeks. Prompt recognition is essential. Initial treatment options include intubation, McGovern nipple (with a large opening for airflow), or an oropharyngeal airway. Orogastric feedings may be necessary.
4. Unilateral atresia presents later in infancy/childhood as chronic unilateral rhinorrhea, nasal obstruction, and/or anosmia.
5. Diagnosis at birth is suggested by inability to pass an 8 Fr catheter beyond 5–6 cm from nasal rim. Lack of fogging on a mirror placed at a nostril suggests airflow obstruction. CT scan has replaced contrasted plain lateral radiographs.
6. Some 20 to 50% of patients have associated congenital anomalies. Children should be evaluated for the CHARGE association [Coloboma, Heart anomaly, choanal Atresia, Retardation-development delay, Genital anomalies, Ear anomalies]. Some 10 to 15% of infants with Treacher-Collins syndrome have choanal atresia.
7. Bilateral atresia is treated shortly after birth while unilateral disease may be treated electively during childhood.
8. Surgical options include endoscopic repair, transpalatal approach, blind transnasal puncture, and drilling out with operating microscope. There is no standard treatment protocol.
9. Endoscopic repair with or without powered instrumentation offers good visualization and avoidance of the midpalatal suture. May be technically difficult due to small neonatal nasal cavity. Possibly associated with a higher recurrence rate than the transpalatal approach.
10. Transpalatal approach involves elevating hard palate mucosa and drilling away palatine bone anterior to greater palatine vessels, atresia plate, and portion of vomer. May be better for thicker plates, smaller neonates, and revision cases. One study reported 50% crossbite due to palatal narrowing as patients grew.
11. Stents are placed for 6 to 8 weeks with all techniques.

B. Midline Congenital Nasal Lesions

1. Common Features[30–35]

    a. Differential includes nasal encephalocele, glioma, and dermoid sinus cysts—all due to similar failure of embryologic separation of ectoderm and neuroectoderm.

    b. Occur in 1 per 40,000 to 1 per 20,000 births.

    c. Around gestation day 50 to 60, a dural diverticulum (+/− arachnoid or neural component) prolapses through the foramen cecum (anterior aspect of the anterior cranial fossa) and fonticulis frontalis (mesoderm separating frontal and nasal bones) to come into contact with skin. It runs between the more superficial nasal bone and underlying nasal cartilage capsule in the prenasal space.

    d. Incomplete regression of this diverticulum can leave neural or ectodermal tissue in the nasal root area. Intracranial connection may occur through a persistently patent foramen cecum.

    e. It is essential to rule out an intracranial connection preoperatively. CT and MRI both image the area well. CT may falsely suggest a central nervous system (CNS) connection; it is best to confirm this with MRI before performing craniotomy.

    f. Surgical approaches include vertical midline rhinotomy, lateral rhinotomy, transverse nasion incision, open rhinoplasty, and (for wide exposure) bicoronal flap. The reason for excision is avoidance of infection or nasal deformity/hypertelorism due to mass enlargement.

2. Nasal Dermoids[30–35]

    a. Account for 1 to 3% of all dermoids and 4 to 12% in the head and neck region.

    b. Classically seen as a midline cutaneous sinus with protruding hair and associated mass, but may be a dermal sinus or cyst and may have a fibrous cord with anterior CNS connection. Cord usually runs beneath nasal bones. Ostium reported in 40 to 80% and is usually on nasal dorsum but may be at nasal tip or columella. Often present after becoming infected.

    c. Occur mostly in children. Negative Furstenburg sign (no enlargement with crying, Valsalva maneuver, or jugular compression); noncompressible; do not transilluminate.

    d. Frequency of intracranial involvement debated, probably 20 to 40%.

    e. Histology: cyst lined with squamous epithelium containing keratinized debris and surrounded by mesodermal elements such as sebaceous glands, hair follicles, sweat glands.

3. Nasal Gliomas[30,33,36,37]

    a. Heterotopic glial tissue without patent intracranial connection.

    b. Firm, noncompressible masses that do not transilluminate and have a negative Furstenburg sign (do not enlarge with crying/Valsalva). Intranasal masses are reddish polypoid lesions. Overlying nasal skin may be discolored or telangiectatic. External gliomas arise at nasion area, intranasal gliomas arise from lateral nasal wall (unlike encephaloceles).

4. Encephaloceles[30,33]

    a. Similar to gliomas but have patent cerebrospinal fluid (CSF) connection to CNS. May be meningeal only (encephalocele), brain plus meninges (encephalomeningocele), or even with connection to ventricle (encephalomeningocystocele).

    b. Some 75 to 80% occur in posterior, occipital, or parietal regions, while the remainder are found around the nasal root or skull base.

    c.   Some 60% are extranasal, 30% intranasal, 10% combined; 15 to 20% have a fibrous connection to dura. Sincipital (nasal) encephaloceles are nasofrontal, nasoethmoidal, or nasoorbital and may be internal or external. Basal lesions are internal and are transethmoidal, sphenoethmoidal, transphenoidal, or sphenomaxillary.

    d.   These are soft, bluish, compressible masses that transilluminate. Positive Furstenburg sign. Classic history includes nasal mass, recurrent clear rhinorrhea, and recurrent meningitis.

    e.   Intranasal lesions arise medially in the nose, unlike gliomas.

C. Rathke's Pouch Cyst[38,39]

1. A portion of stomodeum ectoderm invaginates into adjacent mesoderm to form Rathke's pouch, which passes through the future site of the sphenoid bone during gestational week 3 or 4. This combines with the infundibular process of the neural tube and forms the anterior hypophysis. Rathke's pouch and the associated craniopharyngeal duct are normally obliterated by week 12 of gestation. Pituitary remnants occur in 12 to 33% of autopsies.

2. A nasopharyngeal remnant of Rathke's pouch is called a pharyngeal hypophysis and may result in a Rathke's pouch cyst located in the adenoid region. These cysts are typically asymptomatic but may become infected and require treatment by antibiotics or marsupialization.

D. Tornwaldt's Cyst[40]

1. Around gestation week 6, a transient communication may develop between notochord and pharynx. The pharyngeal bursa (distinct from Rathke's pouch) is a persistence of this attachment located above the superior pharyngeal constrictors around the level of Rosenmüller's fossa. It is caudad to Rathke's pouch. About 3% of adults have a persistent pharyngeal bursa.

2. A Tornwaldt's cyst is a midline or off-midline smooth, submucosal mass. If infected, it is treated with antibiotics and/or marsupialization.

E. Nasopalatine Duct Cyst[41,42]

1. Most common maxillary cyst of nonodontogenic origin; occurs in 1% of population.

2. Nasopalatine duct passes through incisive canal and facilitates olfaction by connecting the oral and nasal cavities in lower mammals. Located on nasal floor near septum approximately 2 cm posterior to columella. It may be associated with vomeronasal organ of humans.

3. Cyst appears most commonly in fourth through sixth decades of life, with palatal pain, swelling, and purulent discharge. Some 75% are less than 2 cm in diameter. Contains stratified squamous and/or respiratory epithelium.

4. Treatment is by excision, with recurrence reported in 0 to 11%.

F. Globulomaxillary Cyst[43]

1. Epithelial islands may become trapped in the area of fusion of the medial nasal, lateral nasal, and maxillary processes—the area between the lateral maxillary incisors and canines.

2. Typically an asymptomatic cyst is noted on routine radiographs; this appears as an inverted teardrop-shaped radiolucency between the maxillary canine and lateral incisors.

G. Nasolabial Cyst[44,45]

1. Rare cyst of nasal alar region. Origin debated but probably either from nasolacrimal duct system or from epithelium trapped between the fusing nasal and maxillary processes.
2. Smooth, mobile, soft tissue mass between pyriform aperture and upper lip. May protrude lip, elevate nasal ala, or erode bone. Most grow slowly but can become infected and drain into mouth or nose. Responds well to enucleation.

VIII. NASAL SKIN INFECTIONS

A. Cellulitis[46–49]

1. Infection of dermis and subcutaneous tissue with beta-hemolytic streptococci or *Staphylococcus aureus*. Streptococci may spread quickly through subcutaneous tissue due to production of hyaluronidase. *Haemophilus influenzae* may be seen in pediatric facial cellulitis.
2. May be associated with underlying sinusitis or dental infection.
3. Patients experience localized erythema, edema, warmth, and pain. Malaise, fever, and leukocytosis may be seen.
4. Cellulitis of the nasal and surrounding region is of concern because of the valveless venous communication between the facial vein, superior ophthalmic vein, pterygoid plexus, and cavernous sinus.
5. Erysipelas ("St. Anthony's fire") is a superficial skin infection with lymphatic involvement primarily due to group A beta-hemolytic streptococci, less often due to group G beta-hemolytic streptococci, and infrequently from *S. aureus* or other bacteria.
6. Treatment: topical mupirocin (Bactroban) is 90% effective for localized disease. Systemic beta-lactamase–stable antibiotics such as dicloxacillin or cephalosporins should be used for most cases. Pediatric facial cellulitis should also be treated with agents active against *H. influenzae*.

B. Impetigo[50–52]

1. Superficial skin infection caused by *S. aureus* or streptococci. More common in children.
2. Two forms: small vesicle with honey-colored crust (usually streptococcal) and bullous impetigo (usually staphylococcal). Bullae occur due to staphylococccal exotoxins. Contagion by topical bacterial transmission.
3. Topical mupirocin 90% effective in treating; alternatively use systemic beta-lactamase–resistant antibiotic.
4. Complications are rare. Post-streptococcal acute glomerulonephritis occurs 0.5 to 2% several weeks later. "Scalded skin syndrome" can occur in an extreme form of bullous impetigo and is found in patients under age 5.

C. Furunculosis[53]

1. Staphylococcal or streptococcal bacterial infection of skin in nasal vestibule, usually associated with injury due to manipulation.
2. Infection coalesces into abscess (furuncle), which may be incised and drained. Treatment includes topical mupirocin and/or a penicillinase-resistant antibiotic.

IX. RHINITIS

A. Viral Rhinitis[54]

1. Rhinovirus is responsible for about 50% of viral upper respiratory infection (URI), coronavirus causes 10 to 20%, and the remainder are due to influenza virus, adenovirus, and respiratory syncytial virus (RSV).
2. Children experience 6 to 10 colds per year, adults 2 to 3 per year.
3. Rhinovirus and coronavirus do not produce nasal epithelial damage, while influenza virus, adenovirus, and RSV produce cytopathic effects.
4. Symptoms of rhinorrhea, nasal obstruction, sneezing, pharyngitis, cough, and malaise last 5 to 10 days. Treatment is symptomatic.

B. Bacterial Rhinitis[55]

This uncommon entity may occur with or without a precursor of viral rhinitis. Symptoms include nasal obstruction, facial pain, crusting, and purulent drainage. *Streptococcus pneumoniae,* group A beta-hemolytic streptococci, and *H. influenzae* are the most common causative bacteria; anaerobes and fungi may be seen in chronic infections. Treatment includes a beta-lactamase–stable antibiotic, irrigation, decongestants, and analgesics.

C. Nasal Staphylococcal Carriage[56–58]

1. 10 to 30% of individuals are chronic nasal carriers in the anterior nares, with a higher number among health care workers. Some 30 to 70% are intermittent or occasional carriers.
2. Nasal carriage of *S. aureus* has been associated with surgical wound infection and access-site infection for patients undergoing hemodialysis and continuous ambulatory peritoneal dialysis. A correlation of about 40 to 60% between wound and nasal phage types of *S. aureus* has been shown.
3. Mupirocin nasal ointment used twice daily for 5 days has been shown to eradicate nasal colonization (both methicillin susceptible and resistant). Chronic use has demonstrated emergence of mupirocin resistance.
4. The indication for treatment of staphylococcal nasal carriage remains undefined but may include reservoir eradication in dialysis patients with infection as well as perioperative prophylaxis for major (eg, cardiothoracic) surgery and treatment of nasal carriage in health care workers.

D. Syphilis[59,60]

"He knows all of syphilis, knows all of medicine."—Sir William Osler.

1. *Treponema pallidum,* a spirochete bacterium, is demonstrated by dark-field microscopy. Laboratory studies include nonspecific serologic tests (RPR, VDRL), which may be false-negative in up to 30% of cases and may return to negative in tertiary syphilis. RPR or VDRL titers may be followed to monitor response to therapy. Specific treponemal tests (FTA-ABS, MHA-TP) remain positive for life, even after treatment. The primary painless chancre heals in 3 to 6 weeks and the variable skin manifestations of secondary syphilis appear 6 to 8 weeks later. Of untreated patients, one-third undergo remission, one-third remain in a latent stage, and one-third progress to tertiary syphilis.
2. *Congenital syphilis,* acquired via transplacental infection, may result in stillbirth or illness in the newborn, or illness in later childhood or adulthood. Mucocutaneous chancres occur due to exposure in an infected birth canal. Infants may have mucopurulent rhinitis

("snuffles") with upper lip excoriation. Other stigmata of congenital syphilis include frontal bossing, high arched palate, Hutchinson's triad (peg-shaped, notched incisors, interstitial keratitis, sensorineural hearing loss), mulberry molars, and "saber shin" tibial changes.

3. Primary nasal syphilis is rare but may present as an erosive or scabbed area at the muco-cutaneous junction of the nasal vestibule. There is often disproportionately prominent submandibular/preauricular lymphadenopathy.

4. Secondary nasal syphilis involves acute rhinitis with scant, thick discharge. Mucous erythema and scabbing, syphilitic pharyngitis, or nasal stenosis may be seen.

5. Tertiary syphilis is extremely uncommon and involves a nasal gumma (primarily on the septum) presenting as a smooth mass covered by an inflammatory mucosal reaction. Septal perforation, saddle-nose deformity, ulcerative destruction of the external nose, and even lateral nasal wall involvement may be seen. Other granulomatous processes of the nose must be excluded from the differential diagnosis.

E. Tuberculosis[61,62]

1. Uncommon entity caused by *Mycobacterium tuberculosis.* Primary nasal tuberculosis is uncommon and may occur from aerosol or digital inoculation; it is most often an extension of pulmonary TB.

2. Symptoms include unilateral/bilateral nasal obstruction, rhinorrhea, epistaxis, crusting, and malodorous discharge. There is a female predilection. Lesions may be ulcerative or granular and tend to be friable. The cartilaginous septum is the most common location (bony septum involvement is unusual), with nasal turbinates and nasal floor infection seen also.

3. Diagnosis is elusive, and other causes of granulomatous rhinitis should be considered. Biopsy specimens are often negative for acid-fast bacilli and caseating granulomas. Culture should be submitted as tissue specimen rather than swabs, and staining and culture done for fungus and *T. pallidum.* Diagnostic studies include FTA-ABS/MHA-TP, PPD, skin testing for suspected fungal agents, chest radiograph, and CT of sinuses. DNA probes and polymerase chain reaction (PCR) studies may be used in the future.

4. Treatment involves culture-directed multi-drug antituberculous therapy, as in pulmonary disease. Isolated nasal involvement is less contagious than pulmonary TB. Surgical excision is associated with at least a 50% recurrence.

F. Leprosy (Hansen's Disease)[63,64]

1. Caused by *Mycobacterium leprae.* Nasal symptoms occur in 97% of patients with lepromatous (generalized) leprosy, but a smaller percentage have localized disease. These include nasal obstruction, impaired smell, and a highly infectious discharge. The antero-inferior turbinates are classically involved, with subsequent involvement of nasal mucosa generally, the septum, and the paranasal sinuses. Deformity may occur due to destruction of the nasal bone/cartilage and nasal spine.

2. Special stains are used for biopsy specimens, and other causes of granulomatous rhinitis should be considered.

3. Dapsone is the therapeutic mainstay, with rifampin and clofazimine used also. Therapy is given for several years or life.

G. Rhinoscleroma[65–67]

1. This granulomatous bacterial infection is caused by *Klebsiella rhinoscleromatis.* Endemic in eastern Europe, north/central Africa, South America, Central America. Not highly contagious or hereditary but associated with poor hygiene, malnutrition, and crowded living conditions.

2. Slowly progressive, granulomatous process with a nasal predilection, but can involve upper and lower airway mucosa. Four stages: catarrhal (exudative), atrophic, granulomatous (proliferative), and fibrotic (cicatricial). Can cause significant midfacial destruction and is included in differential diagnosis of necrotizing midfacial lesions. Infected tissue almost always culture-positive.

3. Treatment is difficult, involving debridement and long-term antibiotics; therapy with topical (acriflavine, rifampin) and/or systemic antibiotics produces varying success and frequent relapse.

H. Rhinosporidiosis[65,68]

1. Fungal infection with *Rhinosporidium seeberi,* producing a chronic inflammatory disease. Transmission may be via contaminated water. It is mostly unilateral with a predilection for the nasal septum, floor, and inferior turbinates. Ocular disease is often present. The disease is endemic to south India and Sri Lanka.

2. Patients experience nasal obstruction, epistaxis, and serous rhinorrhea. Mucosa demonstrates a corrugated, strawberry-like appearance with or without polyposis. Other mucosal surfaces may also be involved. Light microscopy usually demonstrates the organism without special staining.

3. Treatment remains primarily surgical, with cauterization of the margins. Ketoconazole, clotrimazole, and dapsone have some reported efficacy.

I. Actinomycosis[69,70]

1. Granulomatous bacterial infection that may occur in any area of the head and neck, including the maxilla and sinuses, with a mean patient age in the 40s. Trauma (often dental) may have occurred. It usually presents as a perimandibular mass, often with a sinus tract. Sinonasal disease involves purulent nasal, sinus, or maxillary drainage.

2. Anaerobic or microaerophilic gram-positive bacillus. Diagnosis made by light microscopy of material from infection site with characteristic sulfur granules on Brown-Hopp or methenamine silver stain. Cultures are very slow-growing and should be specifically requested to include actinomyces.

3. Treatment involves surgical excision plus 2 to 3 weeks of IV penicillin G (tetracycline or erythromycin used for penicillin allergy).

J. Histoplasmosis[71,72]

1. Caused by *Histoplasma capsulatum,* this is the most common fungal infection in the United States. Endemic in Ohio/Mississippi River valleys and central states, where most people have had some subclinical infection. Head and neck manifestations occur primarily in patients with disseminated disease, and this may be the presenting site. Typical flat, nontender lesions that subsequently become ulcerated and painful may be confused with carcinoma or tuberculosis.

2. Diagnosis made by biopsy or culture. Wright-Giemsa/methenamine silver stain.

3. Acute pulmonary histoplasmosis usually requires no treatment. Disseminated disease is treated with amphotericin B followed by lifelong maintenance therapy of fluconazole or itraconazole.

K. Cryptococcosis[73]

1. Unusual infection caused by inhalation/ingestion of fungus *Cryptococcus neoformans.* Organism found in pigeon/bird feces.
2. Protean manifestations, usually with initial pulmonary infection and hematogenous dissemination, usually to brain and meninges. Otolaryngologic infection is unusual, and sinonasal involvement demonstrates a granulomatous mass.
3. Diagnosis is made by biopsy with stain for fungal organisms; and treatment is with amphotericin B.

L. Blastomycosis[72,74,75]

1. Uncommon fungal infection of *Blastomyces dermatitidis* from inhalation of spores in soil. Endemic in Ohio/Mississippi River valleys. Initial pulmonary infection with pneumonia-like presentation may lead to hematogenous spread to skin, bones, genitourinary system, and elsewhere. Highly variable presentation. Nasal lesions are often painless ulcerations that may be confused with carcinoma or other noncaseating granulomatous lesions.
2. Diagnosis made by histopathology of biopsies; success in culture is variable.
3. Amphotericin B used for severe disease, with subsequent ketoconazole and itraconazole. These azole agents are suitable alone for less severe infection.

M. Glanders[76]

1. Primarily an equine disease due to *Pseudomonas mallei,* with debated mode of inoculation—possibly inhalation, ingestion, or through broken skin or nasal mucosa.
2. Nasal infection results in ulcerating granulomatous lesions with mucopurulent discharge. Cervical adenopathy often seen. Systemic, septicemic infection may occur. Patients experience significant systemic symptoms. Diagnosis is by histology demonstrating gram-negative bacilli (usually scant), culture, and serology.
3. Treatment includes surgical drainage as needed, sulfadiazine, and/or pencillin.

X. SINUSITIS
A. Acute Bacterial Rhinosinusitis (ABRS)[77,78]

1. Approximately 20 million cases of ABRS annually in the United States. This diagnosis is the fifth most common reason for antibiotic prescription, accounting for 7 to 12% of antibiotic prescriptions. Annual health care costs for ABRS are over $3 billion. ABRS defined as up to 4 weeks in duration.
2. Viral rhinitis usually precedes ABRS, but other causative factors include allergy, trauma, and dental infection. Ostial impingement due to nasogastric tubes, septal deviation, enlarged/paradoxic middle turbinates, concha bullosa, nasal polyps, nasal neoplasm, or packing may predispose to sinusitis. Less frequent causes include impaired clearance due to ciliary dyskinesias (immotile cilia syndrome, Kartagener's syndrome) or abnormal mucus (cystic fibrosis). Impaired immune states such as HIV, diabetes, posttransplant immunosuppression, selective IgG subclass deficiency, and some connective tissue diseases may predispose to recurrent sinusitis.

3. Viral rhinitis and ABRS are differentiated on clinical grounds. ABRS is suggested with persistence beyond the typical 10-day duration of viral infection, worsening after 5 to 7 days, or if symptoms are more severe than expected from a virus. These include maxillofacial pain, dental pain, otalgia, increased malaise, and increased drainage. Change in drainage color is not a specific indicator of ABRS.

4. Causative organisms of ABRS includes *S. pneumoniae* (20–43%) *H. influenzae* (22–35%), *Moraxella catarrhalis* (2–10%), other streptococci (3–9%), anaerobes (0–9%), and *S. aureus* (0–8%).

5. Medical management (recommendations from the Sinus and Allergy Health Partnership).

    a. Penicillin resistance in *S. pneumoniae* increased to 28.6% in 1998, and occurs via a different mechanism than with beta-lactamase production. The latter occurs in about 40% for *H. influenzae* and 100% for *M. catarrhalis*.

    b. Mild disease without antibiotics in previous 6 weeks: amoxicillin 1.5 to 3.5 g/day, amoxicillin/clavulanate, cefpodoxime, or cefuroxime. Trimethoprim/sulfamethoxazole, doxycycline, azithromycin, clarithromycin, erythromycin, and cefprozil have up to a 25% failure rate.

    c. Moderate disease without preceding antibiotics or for patients with previous antibiotics in past 6 weeks: amoxicillin 3 to 3.5 g/day, amoxicillin/clavulanate, cefpodoxime, cefuroxime. Gatifloxacin, levofloxacin, and moxafloxacin are used for allergy or intolerance of the above medication.

    d. Moderate disease with recent antibiotic therapy: amoxicillin/clavulanate, gatifloxacin, levofloxacin, moxafloxacin, or combination therapy (amoxicillin or clindamycin plus cefpodoxime or cefixime).

    e. "Switch" therapy—may include amoxicillin/clavulante with an increased dosage of amoxicillin component to 3 to 3.5 g/day. However, this is not FDA-approved.

    f. Antibiotic therapy should be prescribed for 10 to 14 days.

    g. Adjunct therapy: nasal saline irrigation helps remove inspissated secretion and nasal obstruction. Hypertonic saline (1/2 tsp salt in 8 oz water) osmotically decreases mucosal congestion. Systemic decongestants improve nasal obstruction and decrease mucosal edema at sinus ostia. These should be used with caution in patients with hypertension, urinary retention, or coronary artery disease. Topical decongestant sprays are helpful in the same way but should not be used for more than 3 to 4 days. Antihistamines are helpful if an allergic component is present. Second-generation antihistamines have fewer anticholinergic effects and therefore are less likely to thicken mucus and impair drainage. Mucolytics (eg, guaifenesin) are helpful but should be used in full dose of 1200 mg bid.

    h. Antral puncture via canine fossa or inferior meatal route may be helpful for recalcitrant or particularly symptomatic maxillary sinusitis. Care is taken to remain posterior to the lacrimal duct opening with the intranasal approach. Frontal sinusitis may be followed *closely* on an outpatient basis but often requires hospitalization with intravenous antibiotics. For sinusitis treatment failure despite adequate antibiotic therapy, further diagnostic evaluation is necessary, including CT, sinus aspiration, and culture-directed therapy.

B. Pediatric Sinusitis[78-81]

1. Sinusitis is more difficult to differentiate from viral rhinitis and allergic rhinitis in children than in adults since children have more episodes of viral rhinitis and less specific

symptoms. Pediatric patients experience 6 to 10 URIs per year and 5 to 13% develop sinusitis. Symptoms of ABRS include nasal obstruction, rhinorrhea (clear or purulent), daytime cough, halitosis, headache, facial pain/swelling, or dental pain that persist beyond 10 days or are unusually severe. Physical examination is often unreliable in children age 10 or younger. The finding of middle meatal pus on endoscopy is helpful.

2. Recurrent ABRS ($\geq$ 4 per year) and chronic sinusitis are associated with allergy and asthma plus up to 14% immune deficiency.[80] In patients with recurrent sinusitis and bronchitis/pneumonia, consider IgG or IgA deficiency (total or subclass), immotile cilia syndrome, or cystic fibrosis. Other predisposing factors may include day care, cigarette smoke exposure, adenoid hypertrophy, and perhaps gastroesophageal reflux.

3. Causative organisms: *S. pneumoniae,* 35 to 42%; *H. influenzae,* 21 to 28%; *M. catarrhalis,* 21 to 28%; *Streptococcus pyogenes,* 3 to 7%; anaerobes, 3 to 7%.

4. Antibiotic therapy:
    a. Mild disease and no antibiotics in past 6 weeks: amoxicillin (45–90 mg/kg/day), amoxicillin/clavulanate, cefpodoxime, cefuroxime.
    b. Mild disease and recent antibiotic therapy: as above but amoxicillin 90 mg/kg/day.
    c. Mild disease with beta-lactam allergy: azithromycin, clarithromycin, erythromycin, trimethoprim/sulfamethoxazole. Up to 25% failure is reported with these.
    d. Moderately severe disease: amoxicillin/clavulanate; amoxicillin or clindamycin plus cefpodoxime or cefixime.
    e. "Switch" therapy for lack of improvement at 72 hours or high local incidence of resistant *S. pneumoniae:* amoxicillin/clavulanate with 80 to 90 mg/kg/day amoxicillin component may be considered.
    f. Topical decongestants, systemic decongestants, mucolytics, and saline irrigation are helpful.

5. Recurrent ABRS may be treated with episodic antibiotic therapy; chronic antibiotic prophylaxis has been suggested but is of concern due to the risk of resistance development. Also, similar chemoprophylaxis for recurrent otitis media has been abandoned. Children with chronic sinusitis are more likely to require functional endoscopic sinus surgery (FESS) for relief of disease.

C. Chronic Sinusitis[82–85]

1. Arbitrarily defined as greater than 12 weeks duration of symptoms.
2. Reports differ on microbiology of chronic sinusitis but also include coagulase negative staphylococci, anaerobes, and are often multibacterial.
3. Patients are treated with a beta-lactamase–resistant antibiotic for 4–6 weeks for maximal medical therapy prior to CT scanning.
4. CT scanning demonstrates anatomic variants predisposing osteomeatal compromise, extent of sinomucosal disease, and potential surgical hazards in order to provide a "road map" for the surgeon. The Task Force on Rhinosinusitis reviewed a number of radiographic staging systems for sinusitis and found the Lund-Mackay sinusitis scoring system to be the most consistent (Table 30-1).
5. Chronic sinusitis very frequently fails medical therapy. FESS is successful in many cases by promoting natural drainage and aeration of the sinuses. Previous external sinus surgery is felt to be less physiologic with regard to natural drainage. It is probably best reserved at present for failure of other surgical modalities (see Chapter 19).

TABLE 30-1. LUND-MACKAY SINUSITIS SCORING SYSTEM[85]

Sinus	Left	Right
Maxillary		
Anterior ethmoid		
Posterior ethmoid		
Sphenoid		
Frontal		
Osteomeatal complex	_____	_____
Total points for each side:		

Scoring (sinus): 0 = normal, 1 = partial opacification, 2 = total opacification; (osteomeatal complex): 1 = clear, 2 = occluded.

D. Fungal Sinusitis

1. Allergic Fungal Rhinosinusitis (AFRS)[86–89]

a. Hypersensitivity reaction to members of the family Dematiaciae: *Bipolaris spicifera* as well as *Drechslera, Alternaria, Curvularia, Exserohilium* spp., and others. Some 5 to 10% of sinus surgery patients have AFRS. It is more prevalent in warmer climates; 30 to 50% have asthma.

b. Disease is caused when atopic individuals inhale fungi that produce a noninvading infection. Gell and Coombs type I reactions (possibly type III also) produce mucosal edema, stasis of secretions, and ostial obstruction. Secondary bacterial infection may occur. Presentation is similar to that of ABRS. Patients often have nasal polyposis (almost 100%) and demonstrate dark, rubbery mucous secretions. Diagnostic criteria include type I hypersensitivity, polyps, CT scan findings, positive stain/culture, and allergic mucin with fungal elements.

c. Characteristic radiographic findings include proteinaceous allergic mucin-producing hyperattenuation on CT but MRI hypointensity on T1 and signal void on T2 images. Fungal disease is unilateral in about 50%. Bony erosion and remodeling may occur due to expansion of the fungal infection.

d. Allergic mucin contains eosinophils, Charcot-Leyden crystals, and possibly fungal hyphae. Laboratory evaluation may include total eosinophil count, IgE level, antigen-specific IgE, intraoperative stain and culture of mucin, and possibly fungal-specific IgG levels.

e. *Treatment:* Medical therapy has a limited role. Antifungals have a limited role, since this is an allergic rather than primarily infectious process. Effective immunotherapy is not presently available. Topical and systemic steroids are helpful, but therapy is primarily surgical. Goals of surgery include (1) complete removal of fungal elements and allergic mucin, (2) provision of permanent aeration and drainage of sinuses, and (3) ensuring postoperative access to affected sinuses. Systemic steroids are used perioperatively and afterward tapered. Topical steroids are continued to reduce recurrence.

2. Fungus Ball (Mycetoma)[87,90]

a. Noninvasive fungal infection with a mass of tangled hyphae usually involving one maxillary sinus or, less commonly, the sphenoid. Usually due to *Aspergillus fumigatus, Pseudallescheria boydii, Alternaria,* and some other species. *Mycetoma* is somewhat of a misnomer since it properly refers to an infection of the feet due to other fungi. Patients are usually immuno*competent,* without atopy.

  b. Symptoms are similar to those of ABRS, including nasal obstruction, discharge, and sometimes polyps. CT shows sinus opacification, bony sclerosis, and often central densities in the fungal ball due to calcification or protein.
  c. Treatment is surgical removal of the fungal ball to provide sinus ventilation. The fungal ball often has a clay-like or an onionskin consistency. Recurrence is not common.

3. Acute Invasive Fungal Sinusitis[87,91]
  a. Invasive fungal rhinosinusitis in immunocompromised host with prominent vascular invasion and duration less than 4 weeks. Prevalence increasing as more patients live with relative immunocompromise, as due to organ transplantation or HIV. Up to 70% of cases in patients with diabetic ketoacidosis (DKA). Caused by members of family Mucoraceae (hence name), with *Rhizopus oryzae* responsible for 90% of rhinocerebral mucormycosis.
  b. Diagnosis suggested by symptoms of rhinosinusitis, although their severity may be attenuated due to immunocompromise. The most common symptoms are fever (44%), nasal ulceration/necrosis (38%), periorbital facial swelling (34%), vision impairment (30%), and ophthalmoplegia (39%). Leukocytosis occurs as an early sign in less than 20%. Eighty percent of patients eventually develop a necrotic nasal or oral lesion. Infection usually begins on the inferior or middle turbinates. Tissue anesthesia may herald impending ischemic necrosis. Plain films are insensitive and may show only mucosal thickening. Radiographic evidence of bony destruction lags behind disease. Sinus aspirates and tissue biopsy should be evaluated immediately for the presence of fungal elements with hematoxylin/eosin or Gomori methenamine silver. Fungal cultures should not be used to determine the diagnosis of acute, fulminant disease because they take days to weeks to grow, may be positive in patients without invasive disease, and sometimes fail due to specimen mishandling. They should be obtained to guide antifungal selection.
  c. Treatment requires correction of the immunocompromise (if possible), radical surgical treatment, and systemic antifungal therapy. Multiple debridements may be required. Survival rates are 60 to 90% in diabetics (where the DKA can be controlled and immunocompromise corrected) but only 20 to 50% in leukemics.

4. Chronic Invasive Fungal Sinusitis[87,92]
  a. Rare fungal sinus infection defined as invasive disease of over 4 weeks duration that typically presents in immuno*competent* individuals. Due to *Aspergillus, Mucor, Alternaria, Curvularia, Bipolaris, Candida, Drechslera,* and other organisms. Symptoms may develop over months or years and present when the orbit or skull base is involved. Granulomatous and nongranulomatous forms have been described.
  b. Examination shows nasal congestion and polypoid mucosa. A soft tissue mass may be noted with either mucosal coverage or an ulcerated surface.
  c. CT scan shows typical fungal rhinosinusitis findings but also demonstrates invasion, often soft tissue infiltration around periantral fat pads. MRI is helpful for dural and intracranial involvement but cannot differentiate malignant disease.
  d. This condition must be differentiated from other chronic infections, granulomatous diseases, and neoplastic processes such as syphilis, TB, Wegener's granulomatosis, sarcoidosis, etc.
  e. No standardized treatment exists, but a prudent approach includes surgery to remove all disease, a 6-week course of amphotericin B, and possibly prolonged treatment with either amphotericin B or itraconazole.

E. Sinusitis and HIV[93,94]

1. Sinonasal disease is very common in HIV patients. Allergic rhinitis occurs twice as often as in non-HIV individuals because of excessive IgE due to immune dysregulation. Up to 68% of patients experience sinusitis. Nasal obstruction may be due to allergy, sinusitis, adenoid hypertrophy, or neoplasm. Kaposi's sarcoma or non-Hodgkins lymphoma present with nasal obstruction, rhinorrhea, or epistaxis. Allergic manifestations in HIV respond to nasal steroids and antihistamines. Adenoid hypertrophy in the adult raises the concern of HIV.

2. Acute sinusitis pathogens are similar in those in HIV-infected and normal patients. Chronic sinusitis in HIV involves *Staphylococcus, Pseudomonas,* anaerobes, and fungal organisms.

3. Therapy
   a. For CD4 counts >200/mm³: Amoxicillin/clavulanate, systemic decongestant, and guaifenesin 1200 mg bid for 3 weeks. Topical decongestant spray for 4 to 5 days.
   b. For CD4 counts <200/mm³ add coverage for *Staphylococcus, Pseudomonas,* and anaerobes (ciprofloxacin + clindamycin).
   c. Hospitalization, intravenous antibiotics, and possibly surgical drainage are required for severe infections.
   d. Middle meatal cultures should be used to direct therapy for treatment failure, which should be given for 4 to 6 weeks.
   e. Endoscopic sinus surgery is effective in appropriate HIV patients, though less so than in immunocompetent patients.

F. Sinusitis and Asthma[95–100]

1. The relationship between rhinosinusitis and asthma remains to be clearly defined, but 65 to 88% of asthmatic patients experience rhinitis. Twenty-five to 30% of asthma patients may develop nasal polyps, and vice versa.

2. Postulated causes include (a) aspiration of infected sinus secretions during sleep; (b) vagal stimulation from infected sinuses, causing bronchospasm; (c) infected sinus production of bacterial toxins, cytokines, and bronchoconstrictive mediators; and (d) lower airway drying resulting from mouth breathing due to nasal blockage.

3. Although further study is clearly warranted, subjective asthma improvement has been shown in 40 to 85% of patients undergoing endoscopic sinus surgery. Sinus disease (allergic or infectious) should be evaluated in patients with recalcitrant asthma. Aggressive medical management should be used first and endoscopic sinus surgery considered if this fails.

G. Complications of Sinonasal Disease[101–104]

1. Local Complications

a. *Primary mucocele* (mucus retention cyst): due to blockage of minor mucous gland, primarily in maxillary sinus. Usually asymptomatic unless obstructs maxillary infundibulum.

b. *Secondary mucocele:* due to blockage of sinus ostium. Occur primarily in the frontal sinus, with sphenoid and maxillary sinuses rarely involved. Patients experience a slow-growing expansile lesion with headache. Plain radiographs show sinus opacification and expansion as well as either bony erosion, sclerosis, or remodeling. CT defines anatomy relative to adjacent structures. MRI typically shows T2 enhancement of the mucocele fluid, helping to differentiate this from neoplasm. Mucoceles grow slowly and may displace or directly invade adjacent structures, such as the orbit and cranial cavity. Infection produces a mucopyocele and can also result in osteomyelitis. Frontal sinus mucoceles are treated with osteoplastic flap obliteration. Sphenoid, maxillary, and ethmoid mucoceles are amenable to endoscopic decompression and marsupialization.

c. *Osteomyelitis:* Thrombophlebotic spread via diploic veins or (less commonly) direct extension of sinusitis can result in marrow infection. Frontal bone osteomyelitis progressing to erosion of the anterior bony table and subperiosteal abscess has been called *Pott's puffy tumor.* Organisms usually are *S. aureus,* streptococci, and anaerobes. The infection is drained and intravenous antibiotic therapy instituted. Debridement of bone and frontal sinusectomy may be necessary. Gallium scanning may be used to follow disease resolution. CT scanning often lags 1 to 2 weeks behind disease progression. Maxillary osteomyelitis is unusual because of the lack of marrow space and the excellent local blood supply. Odontogenic origin is the most common cause of etiology here. Sphenoid osteitis is also rare but is dangerous, as it constitutes skull base infection. Intravenous antibiotics and surgical drainage are used.

2. Orbital Complications

Most common site of sinusitis extension due to close proximity to the ethmoid and other sinuses. The lamina papyracea is thin and often dehiscent. Valveless veins communicate between the nose, sinuses, pterygoid plexus, and orbits. More common in children than in adults. Contrasted axial and coronal sinus CT is required for evaluation. Orbital complications were classified by Chandler as follows:

a. *Inflammatory edema* (most common): Nontender eyelid edema with or without edema of orbital contents. No limitation in ocular movement or visual change. Thought to be due to impairment of venous outflow by inflammation due to sinusitis.

b. *Orbital cellulitis:* Diffuse orbital infection and inflammation without abscess formation. Findings include chemosis, impairment of extraocular movement, proptosis, and possibly visual impairment with disease progression. Antibiotic therapy usually produces rapid improvement.

c. *Subperiosteal abscess:* Collection of pus between medial periorbita and bone. Exophthalmos and chemosis are more pronounced than in stage 2. Extraocular movement is impaired, often with inferolateral displacement of the globe. Visual acuity decreases in later stages.

d. *Orbital abscess:* Discrete pus collection in orbital tissue. Exophthalmos/chemosis are more marked. Complete ophthalmoplegia is accompanied by severe visual impairment. Spontaneous drainage of pus through the lid may occur. Blindness may result.

e. *Cavernous sinus thrombosis:* Characterized by *bilateral* ocular symptoms and worsening of all other previously described findings. Edema of the mastoid emissary vein may be seen. Prostration, meningismus, and, often, frank meningitis occur.

Early, mild preseptal infection can be managed by *close follow-up* on an outpatient basis with a beta-lactamase–stable antibiotic. Topical/systemic decongestants, mucolytics, and nasal saline irrigation should be used. A low threshold is maintained for hospital admission. Ophthalmologic consultation is obtained in all but mild cases. Surgical exploration is advised for progression over 24 hours, failure of response to intravenous antibiotics in 48 to 72 hours, or for any patient with impaired visual acuity or frank orbital abscess. Subperiosteal abscess usually indicates the need for drainage. Pediatric patients appear to respond better to medical management than do adults. Endoscopic decompression is one option, although the significant mucosal edema and inflammation frequently require an external ethmoidectomy (Lynch) approach. Cavernous sinus thrombosis is treated with high-dose antibiotics and possibly drainage of sinusitis; use of heparin and steroids is debated. Mortality is 30%.

3. Intracranial Complications
Occur in up to 4% of patients who require hospitalization for sinusitis.

    a. *Meningitis:* Most common intracranial complication of sinusitis. Sphenoid/ethmoid sinuses are the usual origins. Contrasted CT should be performed to rule out a mass effect before lumbar puncture. Lumbar puncture is diagnostic for meningitis and Gram stain/culture should be obtained. Treat with high-dose antibiotics with known CSF penetration. Sinus surgery is indicated if meningitis cannot be controlled or sinusitis persists.

    b. *Epidural abscess:* Usually occurs due to frontal sinusitis because of the venous communication and loosely adherent dura. Often seen with frontal sinusitis. Symptoms are protean, often mild, and neurologic findings usually absent. Treatment involves antibiotics, drainage, and usually sinus obliteration.

    c. *Subdural abscess:* Unusual sinusitis complication due to thrombophlebitis. Frontal sinus edema, fever, meningeal signs are usually seen. High-dose antibiotics, sinus drainage, and neurosurgical consultation for drainage are required. Outcome often poor.

    d. *Brain abscess:* 15% are of sinugenic origin, usually through thrombophlebitis. Frontal abscesses are most common and present with headache and behavioral change. Antibiotics, sinus drainage, and neurosurgical consultation for drainage are required. Mortality is 20 to 30%.

XI. INFLAMMATORY CONDITIONS

A. Viral and Bacterial Rhinosinusitis
    See Sec. IX, above.

B. Allergic Rhinitis[105,106]
    1. Allergic rhinitis affects over 10% of Americans, with direct and indirect treatment costs in 1996 of over $5 billion. This includes both year round (perennial) allergy as well as seasonal allergic rhinitis ("hay fever"). Some 80% of patients will develop symptoms before age 20. History of parental allergy/atopy increases the risk for allergy. Classically there is an IgE-mediated Gel and Coombs–type I hypersensitivity reaction. Tree pollen predominates in spring, grasses in late spring/early summer, and weeds from late summer until early fall. Some molds are also seasonal and manifest in summer and fall. Perennial allergy occurs due to dust mites, cockroach allergens, perennial molds, and animal urine/saliva/dander. In the home, carpets, upholstery, drapes, and bedclothes are reservoirs for dander, dust mites, and cockroach allergens. Plants and soil are sources of fungus.

    2. Complaints include nasal obstruction, congestion, rhinorrhea/postnasal drip, nasal/ocular/palatal pruritus, anosmia, sneezing, sinus pain, and headache. Nasal mucosa often shows bluish discoloration and edema, although erythema may be seen. Clear, watery rhinorrhea is often seen. Turbinates are frequently edematous. Some patients manifest an

"allergic salute" by upward stroking of the nasal base, which can produce a transverse supratip crease. "Allergic shiners" probably arise because of venous stasis in the lower eyelid area due to nasal vascular congestion. A complete head and neck examination is performed to rule out other sources of nasal problems, such as polyps, adenoid hypertrophy, or neoplasia.

3. Diagnosis is usually based upon typical history and clinical findings without need for specific testing.
4. Allergy testing is performed for failure of medical therapy and for confusing cases.
    a. *Scratch testing:* Test antigen is placed on an area of skin scratched to remove keratinized layers. This lacks sensitivity and specificity and should not be used.
    b. *Skin-prick testing:* Antigen is placed upon skin and delivered by puncturing the skin with a lancet. This produces a relatively controlled dose of antigen. Although disagreement exists regarding its use versus intradermal testing, this remains a safe, fast, and reliable method.
    c. *Intradermal dilution testing:* Standard quantities of differing antigen dilutions are placed intradermally by injection. This allows identification of the correct starting dose but cannot predict the ultimate optimum therapeutic dose and is as good as or better than skin-prick testing. Disadvantages include increased time and personnel costs.
    d. *In vitro testing:* Serum is obtained for immunoassay testing of antigens specific for a geographic region. This is safe, effective, and independent of antihistamine/steroid use. It is less traumatic for young children, avoids the risk of anaphylaxis, can be used in patients with dermatographism, and may be used for testing severely allergic patients during a specific antigen's season.
    e. *Nasal cytology:* Increased eosinophils are seen with allergic rhinitis and nonallergic rhinitis with eosinophilia (NARES).
5. Treatment includes the following:
    a. *Environmental control:* Patients should reduce time outdoors during high pollen counts and minimize household pollen by closing windows and using air conditioning rather than window/attic fans. Outdoor molds grow on live and decaying vegetation and are increased during plowing, excavation, and harvesting. Household molds are found in basements, crawl spaces, humidifiers, cold outside walls, sinks, showers, and indoor plants. Fungicides such as Clorox and Lysol are helpful. Plastic vapor barriers help in crawl spaces. Carpeting, upholstery, stuffed toys, and bedding contain mold spores as well as dust mite feces and dander. Mites require ≥ 50% humidity. Living areas should be furnished without carpets or plants and with a minimum of upholstered furniture. Vacuuming and bed making should be avoided or at least done with an efficiently filtered vacuum and while wearing a face mask during these tasks and for 15 minutes afterward. Mattresses, box springs, and pillows should be covered with zippered vinyl casings. Cat dander is worse than dog dander, and pets should be excluded at least from the bedroom. Six months or more may be required for dander to clear. Patients are often resistant to this, however, and many would rather do without a spouse than a favorite family pet.
    b. *Pharmacologic therapy:* Antihistamines provide H_1-receptor blockage. First-generation antihistamines have significant sedating effects (that often improve after a week's medication) and can produce tachyphylaxis, which requires rotation among

different antihistamine groups. Second-generation antihistamines do not produce this problem. Aztemizole (Hismanal) and terfenadine (Seldane) were removed from the market due to QT prolongation producing torsades de pointes when taken with macrolide antibiotics and azole antifungals. Pseudoephedrine is effective for nasal obstruction; it is used alone or in combination with some fexofenadine (Allegra), cetirizine (Zyrtec), and loratadine (Claritin) preparations; it is the only systemic decongestant available since the withdrawal of phenylpropanolamine. Oral antileukotriene agents such as montelukast (Singulair) may be helpful but require further study. Topical steroid sprays are very effective for nasal allergy symptoms. Several new ophthalmic antihistamine and mast cell stabilizer drops are available. Azelastine (Astelin) is an intranasal antihistamine spray. Ipratropium (Atrovent) nasal spray is an anticholinergic agent useful for rhinorrhea. Cromolyn spray (Nasalcrom) is now available as an over-the-counter medication, but it is less effective than steroid and anticholinergic sprays.

c.   *Allergy immunotherapy (desensitization):* Indicated for individuals who fail environmental control and pharmacologic therapy, this may be combined with immunotherapy to enhance benefit. Therapy is based upon antigen sensitivity delineated by allergy testing, either on skin or in vitro. Disadvantages include the cost and inconvenience of treatment, which may require weekly injection for 2 to 5 years, plus risk of anaphylaxis. Possible contraindications include beta-blocker therapy, hypersensitivity to epinephrine, poorly controlled asthma, induction during pregnancy, and autoimmune disease. Long-term control of symptoms is 60%.

C. Vasomotor Rhinitis[106]

1. Inflammatory nasal condition unrelated to allergy, infection, or other etiology. Patients are sensitive to cold, dry air, perfumes, paint fumes, cigarette smoke, and other chemical irritants.
2. Patients may experience predominantly rhinorrhea or nasal obstruction.
3. Treatment options include nasal steroids, topical anticholinergics, decongestants, and perhaps antihistamines. Surgical treatments include turbinate reduction cautery; parasympathetic nerve section has been suggested by way of transnasal, transpalatal, or transantrial vidian neurectomy.

D. Nonallergic Rhinitis with Eosinophilia (NARES)[106,107]

1. Nasal disorder accounting for about 15% of rhinitis, associated eosinophil count >10% and negative allergy testing. Nasal smears show eosinophilia. Typically arises in third to fourth decade with a female predilection. Patients experience watery rhinorrhea +/− obstruction.
2. Topical steroids and ipratropium bromide sprays can be helpful, as may systemic decongestants. Turbinate cautery or cryotherapy are other options.

E. Nasal Polyposis[108–110]

1. Idiopathic perennial, reactive, inflammatory condition of mucous membranes of nose and paranasal sinuses. Most cases originate in the lateral aspect of the middle meatus. Polyp epithelium contains a large number of mast cells, eosinophils, and high histamine concentration. These are typically bilateral. Unilateral disease should prompt consideration of inverting papilloma or malignancy. One-third of aspirin-allergic patients have

nasal polyps. Samter's triad = nasal polyposis, aspirin sensitivity, and reactive airway disease.

2. Nasal polyposis causes symptoms of nasal obstruction, hyposmia/anosmia. Patients may have nonallergic rhinitis.

3. Topical corticosteroids are the drugs of choice, although the oral or intramuscular route may be necessary for initial treatment ("medical polypectomy"), with nasal steroid sprays used for maintenance. Oral steroids are often effective against anosmia, while topical steroids are not. Unfortunately, anosmia frequently recurs after cessation of oral steroids. Antibiotics plus systemic steroids should be used for polyposis associated with sinusitis.

4. Surgical options include polypectomy under local/topical anesthesia or general anesthesia as well as functional endoscopic sinus surgery (FESS). Topical steroid therapy is used for maintenance afterward. Recurrence is common, however.

F. Atrophic Rhinitis (Ozena)[111,112]

1. Idiopathic condition endemic in both tropical and temperate areas. Proposed etiologies include bacteria, nutritional deficiency, estrogen deficiency, excess sympathetic activity, chronic irritant exposure, and excessive nasal patency (developmental or iatrogenic). Predilection for females and for individuals of Asian, Hispanic, and African ethnicities. Often seen in females beginning at puberty and may worsen during menses. Associated with overresection of nasal turbinates.

2. Headache, nasal obstruction, epistaxis, anosmia, halitosis, malodorous crusting, and discharge.

3. Examination shows a widely patent nose with large, obstructing crusts. Crust removal leaves atrophied turbinates and bleeding, ulcerated mucosa. Diagnostic studies include nasal culture, sinus CT, syphilis serology, CBC, serum protein and iron levels.

4. Therapy is palliative. Regular nasal irrigation with saline or sodium bicarbonate solution helps. Application of oily lubricants such as menthol 2% in paraffin or glucose in glycerin may help. Systemic and local estrogen therapy has been recommended. Large doses of vitamin A have been prescribed. Surgical nasal blockage for 6 to 36 months demonstrates a good cure rate with high recurrence. Submucosal nasal implants to provide narrowing are frequently successful but often fail due to extrusion and absorption. The plethora of treatments attests to the paucity of definitively successful therapy.

G. Sarcoidosis[113,114]

1. Idiopathic granulomatous inflammatory condition; involves the head and neck in 10 to 15% of cases. Predilection for females and African Americans in the United States.

2. Initial manifestations mimic allergic rhinitis, with airway obstruction due to mucosal edema and inferior turbinate hypertrophy. Subsequently, crusting, submucosal granulomas, epistaxis, and pain develop. Later, ulceration, synechiae, cartilage destruction, nasal stenosis, and sinus involvement may occur. Nonhealing midfacial papular skin lesions often develop.

3. Diagnostic findings include hilar adenopathy on chest radiographs and elevated angiotensin converting enzyme (ACE) in 60 to 90%. The caseating granulomas frequently occur at nasal mucocutaneous junctions.

4. Depending on disease severity, intranasal steroid sprays, intralesional steroid injections, or systemic steroid therapy is required.

H. Lethal Midline Granuloma[115]

Confusing and obsolete terminology has included Wegener's granulomatosis, polymorphic reticulosis, idiopathic midline destructive disease, and non-Hodgkin's lymphoma. This is now consolidated as either Wegener's granulomatosis or angiocentric T-cell lymphoma.

I. Wegener's Granulomatosis (WG)[116–118]

1. Wegener's triad: necrotizing granulomas of upper/lower respiratory tract, vasculitis, and glomerulonephritis. "ELK" acronym to represent ENT, lung, and kidney.
2. Sinonasal complaints develop in 90% of patients and include nasal congestion, discharge, pain, and ulcerations as well as septal perforation, saddle-nose deformity, headache, and sinusitis. Other otolaryngologic manifestations are serous otitis, otalgia, hearing loss, oral ulcers, laryngeal ulcerations/lesions, and subglottic stenosis. Imaging studies usually demonstrate only soft tissue swelling.
3. Average age at initial presentation of this rare disease is 20 to 40 years, without sexual preference.
4. Biopsy classically includes necrosis, granulomas, and vasculitis. Unfortunately, biopsy specimens are often lacking all of these and are nonspecific. Pulmonary lesions are more likely to show "classic" findings. The erythrocyte sedimentation rate (ESR) is elevated. Coarsely staining antinuclear cytoplasmic antibody (c-ANCA) has over 90% specificity/sensitivity for generalized active disease—probably about 65% for active localized disease. Positive p-ANCA staining is not specific for WG. Serial ANCA testing is unhelpful in monitoring disease remission and recurrence.
5. Treatment includes corticosteroids and cyclophosphamide; it produces remissions in over 90% of patients and a 5-year survival over 75%. Methotrexate, cyclosporine, and trimethoprim-sulfamethoxazole may also have a role.

J. Angiocentric T-Cell Lymphoma

See Sec. XIII, below.

K. Lupus Erythematosus[119,120]

Multisystem inflammatory disease that involves skin, joints, nervous system, mucosa, and hematopoietic system. A characteristic "butterfly" malar rash may be seen with both discoid and systemic lupus. Lab findings include positive anti–double strand DNA antibody, anti-Sm antibodies (both ANA tests), positive lupus erythematosus (LE) cell preparation, and false-positive VDRL/RPR. Treatment involves steroids with or without azathioprine, cyclophosphamide, and methotrexate.

L. Scleroderma[121,122]

Idiopathic, multifactorial collagen vascular disease most significantly producing esophageal, joint, pulmonary, and renal pathology. Dysphagia and decreased mouth opening are the most common head and neck findings. Nasal involvement is rare and includes mucosal/skin telangiectasias and skin pigment irregularity and tightening. Treatment is nonspecific and symptom-directed.

M. Sjögren's Syndrome[123,124]

1. Idiopathic, autoimmune destruction of exocrine glands. Primary Sjögren's syndrome (sicca syndrome) is xerophthalmia and xerostomia; secondary Sjögren's syndrome includes these plus a connective tissue disorder, usually rheumatoid arthritis.

2. Nasal findings are uncommon but may include dryness, crusting, and decreased smell.

3. Diagnostic studies include salivary gland biopsy, antinuclear antibody, rheumatoid factor, and Sjögren's antibodies (SS-A, SS-B)

4. Symptomatic treatment. Sjögren's syndrome is associated with an increased incidence of non-Hodgkin's lymphoma.

N. Relapsing Polychondritis (RP)[125,126]

1. Condition of recurrent, often severe and acute inflammation of cartilaginous tissues. Auricular chondritis occurs in 90%, is often the presenting complaint, and is often misdiagnosed as infectious perichondritis. Sinonasal complaints include nasal pain, obstruction, epistaxis, crusting, and saddle-nose deformity. Other ENT symptoms include throat pain, hoarseness, and difficulty speaking. Diagnosis is made with three or more of the following features: bilateral auricular chondritis, nonerosive seronegative inflammatory arthritis, nasal chondritis, ocular inflammation, respiratory tract inflammation, and audiovestibular injury. Onset usually occurs at age 40 to 60 without sexual predilection. Vasculitides and other autoimmune phenomena may be associated with RP.

2. There are no pathognomonic histopathologic findings. Immune complex deposition at the fibrocartilaginous junction has been demonstrated. ESR and C-reactive protein are elevated.

3. Corticosteroids are the mainstain of therapy. Dapsone, cyclophosphamide, azathioprine, and methotrexate have also been used. Five-year survival is 75% and 10-year survival 55%, with pneumonia as the most common cause of death.

O. Churg-Strauss Syndrome[127,128]

1. Necrotizing vasculitis classically characterized by asthma and hypereosinophilia. Diagnostic criteria require four of the following: asthma, eosinophilia >10%, sinusitis, pulmonary infiltrate, histologically proven vasculitis, and mononeuritis multiplex.

2. ENT manifestations include initial sinusitis or history of sinusitis in 14 to 47%.

3. *Treatment:* Corticosteroids alone or with cyclophosphamide and/or plasma exchange. Good long-term prognosis.

P. Necrotizing Sialometaplasia[129,130]

Infarcted mucosal salivary gland producing deep, demarcated ulcer resembling squamous cell carcinoma. Classically noted on hard palate but occasionally presents in nose. Squamous metaplasia strongly resembles carcinoma. Heals spontaneously. Treatment is observation.

XII. BENIGN SINONASAL TUMORS

A. Nasal Polyposis

See Sec. XI, above.

B. Maxillary Mucous Retention Cysts[131,132]

1. Classically a rounded, dome-shaped radiopacity noted on the maxillary sinus floor on sinus radiographs and dental x-rays. Due to fluid collection in sinus mucous gland with blocked duct.

2. Rarely symptomatic unless they are obstructing the maxillary infundibulum, are filling and expanding the sinus, or are infected.

3. Specific treatment and workup usually not necessary unless symptomatic. MRI may help differentiate neoplasia. Treatment, if needed, by needle aspiration or endoscopic marsupialization/excision.

C. Sinonasal Papilloma[133,134]

1. Squamous Papilloma
a. Primarily seen in alar/nasal vestibular area.
b. Probable viral cause. Painless, friable warty growth arising on stratified squamous epithelium.

2. Schneiderian Papilloma
a. Arise from respiratory (schneiderian) epithelium and associated with human papillomaviruses 6 and 11. Malignant transformation in 10 to 15%.
b. Unilateral sinonasal mass/polyp producing nasal obstruction, epistaxis, rhinorrhea, sinusitis, facial pain, anosmia, anesthesia, and epiphora.
c. Three types:
Septal papilloma: 50% of schneiderian papilloma. Occur in exophytic, verrucoid, pedunculated, and sessile forms. Male predilection, with age 20 to 50 most common. Histology similar to squamous papilloma/verruca vulgaris.
Inverting papilloma: 47% of schneiderian papilloma. Bulky, red-gray polypoid mass that is usually found on lateral nasal wall. Ages 40 to 70. Epithelium invades surrounding stromal tissue, hence term *inverting.*
Cylindrical papilloma: 3% of cases. Red-brown papillary lesion of lateral nasal wall/sinuses. Histology similar to rhinosporidiosis. Male predilection, ages 40 to 70.
d. Treatment with surgical excision but significant recurrence rate. Traditional surgery involved open rhinotomy, medial maxillectomy, and maxillectomy, but trend now is toward endoscopic management.

C. Rhinophyma[135–137]

1. Slowly progressive nasal enlargement due to acne rosacea. Male predilection 3 : 1, with presentation usually after age 45. Previously associated with alcoholism, although there may be some association with spicy food, caffeine, and alcohol. Parasitic mite *Demodex folliculorum* may be etiology.
2. Histology shows sebaceous gland hypertrophy with ductal obstruction, fibrosis, and inflammation. Nodularity and telangiectasias seen. Association with basal cell carcinoma reported.
3. Primarily a cosmetic concern, although may produce nasal obstruction.
4. Medical treatment for rosacea may be used with early disease before establishment of fibrosis and scarring. Isotretinoin (Accutane) and oral/topical antibiotics may be used. Advanced cases require surgery with decortication, sculpting, and then allowing re-epithelialization. Cold scalpel, CO_2 laser, Shaw thermal scalpel, dermabrasion, and other modalities have been employed. Skin grafting may be used.

D. Juvenile Nasopharyngeal Angiofibroma[138–141]

1. Benign but locally aggressive vascular tumor of adolescent males; has been reported in females only very rarely. Accounts for 0.05% of head and neck tumors. Cause is unknown; may be hormonal.

2. Originates in posterolateral nasal wall near sphenopalatine foramen. Blood supply primarily from external carotid, although some feeding vessels from the internal carotid often exist. Tumor presents with nasal obstruction and recurrent epistaxis. Smooth, lobulated, red-gray mass in the posterolateral nasal cavity. Infiltrates nearby fissures and foramina in nasopharynx and skull base area. Diagnosis made by contrasted CT and MRI; MRI provides best delineation of tumor extent. Diagnostic angiography is not necessary but is performed with preoperative embolization. Several staging systems exist.

3. Treatment is primarily surgical, with 6 to 24% recurrence. Preoperative embolization 48 to 72 hours preoperatively reduces operative blood loss. Transpalatal, transmaxillary, sphenoethmoidal, and other skull base techniques may be used, depending on tumor size and location. Locally recurrent disease is amenable to revision surgery. Skull base involvement is frequently treated with radiation. Radiation is not used initially because of risk to structures such as the optic nerve, concern of malignant transformation during a patient's subsequent lifetime, and relative efficacy of surgery. If radiotherapy is necessary, gamma knife should be considered in order to spare adjacent structures.

E. Hemangioma[142–145]

1. Sinonasal hemangioma—uncommon tumor of sinonasal region. Bluish-red lesions may be up to 2 cm in size and cause nasal obstruction/epistaxis. Maxillary hemangiomas may also result in sinusitis and mass effect, dental symptoms, orbital symptoms. Contrasted CT shows inhomogenous enhancement and T2 MRI enhances brightly. Treatment is surgical excision with adequate mucosal and periochondrial/periosteal cuff to prevent recurrence.

2. Lobular capillary hemangioma (also known as pyogenic granuloma, pregnancy tumor, granuloma gravidarum). Unusual septal or turbinate lesion producing nasal obstruction, epistaxis, or a visible mass. Red-brown lesions, sessile or pedunculated, which are friable and often ulcerated. These generally resolve postpartum and may be observed, cauterized, or excised with local anesthesia.

F. Osteoma[146–149]

1. Uncommon benign bony tumor of sinuses. 0.4 to 3% found incidentally on sinus radiographs or CTs. Mostly in frontal sinus, often near duct. Most common in fifth to sixth decade of life. Symptoms include facial pain/headache, sequelae of frontal ostium obstruction, mass effect; usually asymptomatic and noted incidentally on radiographs.

2. Rate of growth is variable and may be up to 6 mm per year.

3. Surgical treatment required for symptomatic lesions and those causing obstructive or mass effect. Debate exists whether to remove small asymptomatic osteomas, which can probably be followed with serial radiographs. Small lesions may be removed by sinus trephination and endoscopic surgery, while larger osteomas require an open approach. Sinus ablation afterward is debated.

4. Osteomas in sinuses or anywhere else may be associated with *Gardner's syndrome*—an association of intestinal polyposis, soft tissue tumors, and osteomas. The polyps undergo malignant change in 40% of cases. The prevalence of Gardner's syndrome with isolated osteomas is unknown.

G. Fibrous Dysplasia[150–152]

1. Idiopathic, benign bony condition in which fibro-osseous tissue replaces the normal medullary bone. Three types: (a) *Monostotic form,* 70 to 80% of cases. Single bone

involved—usually rib, tibia, femur. (b) *Polyostotic form,* 20 to 25%. Two or more bones, usually ribs, pelvis, long bones of extremities. (c) *McCune-Albright syndrome*—polyostotic disease plus endocrine disorders and hyperpigmentation.

2. Onset in adolescents/young adults with female predilection in polyostotic disease. Monostotic form involves the craniofacial region on 25% and 40 to 60% in polyostotic disease. Patients experience painless expansile growth and bony deformity. It may involve the nose, sinuses, orbit, and internal auditory canal. Radiology is characteristic but biopsy may be necessary. Three radiologic forms: (a) pagetoid with "ground glass" appearance from both radiodense/radiolucent areas and usually involving calvaria, (b) sclerotic pattern usually found in maxilla, and (c) cystic form.

3. Surgery is indicated for expansile, disfiguring growth; involves recontouring. Radiation and chemotherapy are not used. Recurrence up to 25%.

H. Uncommon Sinonasal Tumors[153–157]

1. *Paraganglioma:* Neural crest cell origin. Rare appearance in nose arising from mucosa or from extension of nasopharyngeal tumor. Painless, red, pulsatile mass producing obstruction, epistaxis, or rhinorrhea. Excision is curative.

2. *Leiomyoma:* Although common in uterus, digestive system, and subcutaneous tissue, very rarely seen in nose. Symptoms are obstruction and epistaxis. Excision is curative.

3. *Schwannoma:* Also called neurinomas, neurilemmomas. Four percent of head and neck schwannomas present in sinonasal area, usually from nerve sheath of V_1 or V_2 divisions of trigeminal nerve. Patients experience obstruction, epistaxis, rhinorrhea, mass effect, and anosmia. Biopsy is avoided due to vascularity. Excision is curative.

XIII. MALIGNANT SINONASAL TUMORS

A. Carcinoma[158,159]

1. About 3% of head and neck tumors are sinonasal. Some 45 to 80% are squamous cell carcinomas; 4 to 15%, salivary carcinomas (adenoid cystic and adenocarcinomas); 4 to 6%, sarcomas; and the remainder other types. Maxillary sinus, 55 to 63%; nasal cavity, 27 to 35%; ethmoid sinus, 10%; and frontal/sphenoid, 1 to 2%. Unlike the case with other head and neck carcinomas, tobacco and alcohol are not risk factors. Hardwood dust is associated with ethmoid sinus adenocarcinoma; softwood dust and nickel exposure with squamous cell and anaplastic carcinoma of the nose and sinuses. Latent period, 18 to 36 years after exposure. Shoe industry, leather tanning, radium, and other chemical industry workers show an increased incidence of sinonasal malignancy. Patients tend to be male, aged 40 to 60.

2. Nasal obstruction, pain, epistaxis, nasal discharge, and cheek swelling are common presenting symptoms, and a 6- to 8-month delay to diagnosis is common. Cervical metastasis reported in 1 to 26% but probably about 10%.

3. En bloc resection by craniofacial approach is most desirable, but complete excision often limited by extent of spread and proximity of adjacent important structures. Radiation therapy is often used adjuvantly. Chemotherapy retains a role for palliation.

B. Angiocentric T-Cell Lymphoma[160–162]

1. Although uncommon in western populations, lymphomas may be the most common nonepithelial malignancy of the nose. Constitute 5.8 to 8% of extranodal head and neck

lymphomas. More common in Asia. Almost all associated with Epstein-Barr virus. Male predilection 2:1.

2. Maxillary antrum, nasal cavity, and ethmoid sinuses most often involved. Nasal discharge, obstruction, unilateral face/cheek/nasal swelling, headache, epistaxis, and occasionally diplopia. Midfacial destruction may be seen. Systemic symptoms of fever, chills, and weight loss less common.

3. Radiology demonstrates sinus opacification, bony erosion, and occasionally a defined mass.

4. Biopsy specimens should be sent *fresh* to allow flow cytometry and "touch prep" studies. Superficial biopsies are often falsely negative.

5. Radiotherapy alone provides local control but involves risk of distant recurrence. Combined radiation and chemotherapy are therefore preferred, with about a 50% 5-year survival.

C. Sinonasal Melanoma[163]

1. Represents 1% of melanoma overall and 7% of sinonasal malignancies. Present in patients age 60 and above without sexual predilection. No causative agent known; possibly associated with inhaled irritants.

2. Present with obstruction and epistaxis. May appear as a pink, benign-appearing polyp or a fungating dark neoplasm.

3. Treatment is surgical resection, as the role of radiation, chemotherapy, and immunotherapy is as yet undefined. Local and regional recurrence are also addressed with surgery. Five-year survival is about 30%.

D. Esthesioneuroblastoma[164–167]

1. Unusual neuroectodermal tumor arising from olfactory epithelium and comprising 3% of intracranial tumors. Arises high in the nasal vault and usually involves skull base by spreading through the cribriform plate.

2. Patients experience anosmia, nasal obstruction, epistaxis, pain, and mass effect. Some 8 to 10% have neck metastases.

3. Treatment is primarily surgical via craniofacial approach. Radiation is added for low-grade margins with close/positive margins, recurrent disease, and all high-grade lesions.

4. Most recurrences appear in 2 years but can be seen at 5 or 10 years. Survival is 74 to 78% at 5 years and 60 to 71% at 10 years.

E. Sinonasal Undifferentiated Carcinoma (SNUC)[168,169]

1. Rare sinonasal malignancy presenting with nasal obstruction, proptosis, epistaxis, rhinorrhea, and facial pain. Neurologic symptoms include cranial nerve palsies, headache, and impaired mentation. Onset of symptoms is usually rapid, but these are often less than would be expected based upon the usually considerable amount of disease. Local invasion of sinuses and cranial fossa is typical.

2. Treatment is usually multimodal but not standardized due to the rarity of SNUC. It is important to distinguish this from lymphoma, rhabdomyosarcoma, melanoma, and olfactory neuroblastoma. Prognosis is uniformly dismal due to the typical late presentation and aggressive nature of the tumor.

F. Chordoma[170,171]

1. Arise from primitive notochord remnant and comprise 1% of intracranial tumors; 35% sphenooccipital, 50% sacrococcygeal, 15% spinal column. Age prevalence 30–50 years.

2. Slow-growing, locally aggressive tumor. Head and neck complaints include headache, visual change, facial pain, hearing loss/tinnitis, and dizziness. Involve nasopharynx and adjacent areas; can invade skull base, brain stem, and neurovascular structures. Neck metastases occur sporadically and more often with recurrent disease.

3. Image with CT and MRI. Histology shows characteristic vacuolated *physaliferous cells* with a "soap bubble" appearance.

4. Surgical excision is treatment of choice, often using various skull base approaches. Complete removal usually not possible and postoperative radiotherapy is generally used. Five-year survival 62%.

G. Sarcoma[172]

1. Sarcomas comprise 1% of head and neck malignancies and 15% of paranasal sinus tumors. Prior radiation exposure is a risk factor. Often misdiagnosed initially as inflammatory conditions, with delayed diagnosis.

2. Worse prognosis than other head and neck sarcomas due to the proclivity for invasion of adjacent structures and the difficulty of obtaining adequate surgical margins in this area. Treatment is surgical, which may be used alone with low-grade lesions and clear tissue margins. High-grade lesions and positive margins are indications for radiotherapy. The usefulness of chemotherapy has not been shown. Treatment success is dependent on tumor grade and surgical margins. The N_0 neck does not require treatment.

3. *Rhabdomyosarcoma:* Considered separately, since the behavior is significantly different from other head and neck sarcomas. Comprises 75% of pediatric head and neck sarcomas. 70% of these are orbital. Although small lesions may be resected, radiotherapy usually used to avoid functional and cosmetic deformity. In localized disease, 80% cure, although some visual deficit common. Adjuvant chemotherapy always used.

H. Plasmacytoma[173]

1. Solitary plasmacytoma is a variant of multiple melanoma and normally appears in long bones. *Extramedullary* plasmacytoma occurs primarily in the head and neck and is usually in the submucosal lymphoid tissue in the nasopharynx or sinuses. Localized disease may be treated with excision or radiotherapy. Follow-up is essential to monitor for development of multiple myeloma.

XIV. MISCELLANEOUS CONDITIONS

A. Nasal Obstruction[14,20]

1. Causes of nasal obstruction
   a. *Mucosa and turbinates:* Allergy, rhinitis, and other inflammatory disease can cause inflammation and edema of the nasal mucosa and turbinates, particularly the inferior turbinate.
   b. *Septal deviation:* More common in Caucasians than in non-Caucasians. About 80% of Caucasians have some septal deviation. Septal perforation and crusting may produce obstruction.
   c. *Turbinate hypertrophy:* Primarily involves middle turbinate, but concha bullosa of middle turbinate may block airway. Hypertrophy may be due to soft tissue or bony component.
   d. *Narrow nasal vault:* External pyramid may be narrowed due to trauma, deviation, or reduction rhinoplasty. Patients occasionally have a narrow internal nasal cavity.

    e.   *Nasal soft tissue:* Narrowed or weak nasal valve may produce obstruction. Less commonly, there may be narrow nostrils or excess columellar width (due to splaying of feet of medial crura of lower lateral cartilages). Tip ptosis due to age may cause obstruction.

    f.   *Nasal masses:* Consider polyps, adenoid hypertrophy, intranasal tumors, and nasopharyngeal tumors.

    g.   *Functional:* Uncommonly, patients may experience subjective nasal restriction despite an adequate airway.

2. Assessment

    a.   Inquire about seasonal/perennial allergy, smoking, possible overuse of nasal decongestant spray.

    b.   Examine patient before/after nasal decongestant. Observe for inspiratory nasal valve collapse; distract nasal valve/cheek skin laterally (Cottle maneuver) to assess obstruction here. Nasal endoscopy allows evaluation for polyps, enlarged adenoid, masses, and posterior turbinate hypertrophy.

3. Treatment

    a.   *Medical management:* Decongestants, antihistamines, topical/submucosal intraturbinate steroids, topical anticholinergics, topical antihistamines, topical mast cell stabilizers, and allergy immunotherapy are options.

    b.   *Septoplasty:* Avoid submucosal resection (SMR) because of long-term risk of nasal collapse due to loss of support plus contractile forces where cartilage was removed. Also, SMR removes the firm septal surface, which may be necessary for nasal cycle. Current thought is for minimal cartilage/bone resection, with replacement of straightened cartilage if possible.

    c.   *Turbinate surgery:* Primarily involving inferior turbinate. Turbinate outfracture is rarely successful, since these structures usually resume original position. Soft tissue excess may be addressed by submucosal monopolar or bipolar cautery as well as cryosurgery and laser cautery. Surgical resection may involve submucosal turbinoplasty, simple resection of the inferior one-third to one-half of the turbinate, or resection with preservation of a medial mucosal flap to fold under the cut edge of turbinate bone. The anterior aspect of the turbinate near the pyriform aperture/nasal valve area is particularly important to address, although some patients have obstruction due to posterior "mulberry" turbinate hypertrophy. Complete resection is to be avoided due to concern over atrophic rhinitis.

    d.   *Rhinoplasty:* Functional rhinoplasty may address nasal deviation, valve collapse, and tip ptosis. Spreader graft and alar batten techniques may be used for valve collapse. Widened columellar base may be addressed with narrowing sutures. Reverse: "Weir" procedures can increase nostril width by lateral repositioning of ala.

B. Rhinitis Medicamentosa[55,174,175]

1. Two groups of topical vasoconstrictors. Sympathomimetic amines (phenylephrine, ephedrine, phenylpropanolamine) stimulate nasal mucosal vessel alpha receptors indirectly by stimulating the release of norepinephrine. Imidazole derivatives (oxy- and xylometazoline) directly stimulate alpha receptors and are more alpha-2 selective. Imidazole derivatives have been suggested to be less likely to cause addiction. Benzalkonium chloride (a preservative in topical decongestants) may produce nasal injury and edema with long-term use, further compounding the problem.

2. Pathophysiology of rhinitis medicamentosa is not known. Theories include increased parasympathetic tone, development of presynaptic negative feedback, exhaustion of vasopressor mechanism, and local tissue release of vasodilating chemical mediators.

3. Treatment involves discontinuation of the topical decongestant and use of hypertonic nasal saline plus nasal steroid sprays. Systemic decongestants and/or corticosteroids as well as submucosal turbinate injection with corticosteroids may also be considered.

4. Topical decongestant use should generally be limited to 3 to 5 days, although at least one study has suggested safety when used as a nighttime-only dose for up to 30 days.

C. Systemic and Endocrine-Related Nasal Problems

1. *Hypothyroidism*[106]: Nasal obstruction and or rhinorrhea have been associated with hypothyroidism, although the frequency and etiology remain undefined.

2. *Medications*[14,106]: See Table 30-2.

3. *Rhinitis of pregnancy*[14,106,176]

   a. Estrogen produced by pregnancy has a cholinergic effect (by inhibiting acetylcholinesterase), resulting in edema of the nasal mucosa and hypersecretion of mucus. Progesterone may cause vasodilation via relaxation of vascular smooth muscle. This may predispose to sinusitis. Up to 30% of pregnant women experience rhinitis. Typically begins around second month, persisting to term.

   b. Consider also allergic, nonallergic, and viral causes. Bacterial sinusitis may occur up to six times more frequently during pregnancy. These are all more common than rhinitis due to pregnancy.

   c. *Treatment:* Hypertonic saline nasal irrigation acts as an osmotic decongestant and is virtually without risk. Medications are best avoided during the first trimester. Intranasal cromolyn may be tried first, with nasal beclomethasone spray as a second choice if this is ineffective. Pseudoephedrine in the first trimester has been associated with gastroschisis, but it may be used afterward. Chlorpheniramine and tripelennamine are the preferred antihistamines. Penicillins and cephalosporins are the desired antibiotics.

D. Epistaxis[177–179]

1. Physiologic demands of nasal mucosa in warming, filtering, and humidifying air require a strong blood supply, with the attendant potential for hemorrhage.

2. Anything that injures or produces hyperemia in nasal mucosa predisposes to epistaxis. Epistaxis is common in winter months due to the drying effect of central heating and lowered humidity. Trauma, nose picking, and vigorous nose blowing can irritate mucosa. Sinusitis, upper respiratory infection, and allergy increase mucosal vascularity and fri-

TABLE 30-2. MEDICATIONS THAT PRODUCE RHINITIS

ACE inhibitors	NSAIDs
Reserpine	Oral contraceptives
Guanethidine	Alprazolam
Phentolamine	Hydralazine
Methyldopa	Thioridazine
Prazosin	Perphenazine
Chlorpromazine	Chordiazepoxide-amitriptyline (Limbitrol)
Beta blockers	

ACE, angiotensin converting enzyme; NSAID, nonsteroidal anti-inflammatory drug.

ability. Neoplasia may present with epistaxis. Septal deviation may disturb airflow and cause turbulence, thereby resulting in mucosal drying and epistaxis. Hypertension is a debated risk factor. Renal disease, hepatic failure, and heavy alcohol consumption predispose to nosebleeds.

3. Hemophilia, coagulopathies, and acquired thrombocytopenia (due to hematologic malignancy, chemotherapy, or HIV) increase epistaxis risk. Hereditary hemorrhagic telangiectasia (Osler-Weber-Rendu disease) is an autosomal-dominant disorder involving a defect in vessel walls. Patients characteristically have telangiectasias of the nasal septum, turbinates, lips, and tongue. Up to 33% will have pulmonary arteriovenous malformations, with up to 11% having them in the CNS. Warfarin, dipyridamole, nonsteroidal antiinflammatory drugs, and thioridazine are associated with nosebleeds. Medications with anticholinergic effects may cause mucosal drying and cracking. Nasal sprays such as decongestants and topical steroids can cause irritation and epistaxis. Cocaine has a similar effect.

4. Some 95% of nosebleeds occur in the anterior nasal cavity, and probably 90% are located at *Kiesselbach's plexus* in *Little's area*—a confluence of vessels at the anterior septum. In addition to often having prominent vessels, this area is most subject to drying, mechanical trauma, and exposure to irritants. Posterior epistaxis is often more severe and has a debated association with hypertension and atherosclerosis.

5. *Assessment:* Inquire whether bleeding was *initially* anterior or posterior, right or left. Although epistaxis is normally unifocal, patients will eventually note bleeding from the nostril and in the throat and often on both sides after bleeding for a while. Assess the duration and quantity of blood loss with regard to the possible need for fluid replacement. Address hypertension and potential for cardiac ischemia in patients with low hematocrit and coronary artery disease.

6. *Management*
   a. Protective eyewear, cover gown +/− mask for physician and assistant; cover patient's clothing with sheet or gown. Obtain desired equipment/supplies, including light and suction.
   b. Patient gently blows nose to expel clots; alternate suction and spraying of nose with decongestant/topical anesthetic. May be supplemented by nasal pledgets with decongestant/anesthetic. Local injection of lidocaine/epinephrine into mucosa may reduce bleeding. Greater palatine nerve block can provide posterior anesthesia and temporary hemostasis.
   c. Anterior rhinoscopy or endoscopy used to identify bleeding site. There is usually one epistaxis site; however, if a patient has had recent packing, *additional* bleeding may occur at excoriated mucosal areas, such as at septal spurs.
   d. Silver nitrate or suction electrocautery under direct vision or via endoscopic guidance. Cautery of opposing sides at the same area of septum may lead to septal perforation.
   e. Anterior packing is usually successful; failure more often indicates inadequate packing rather than posterior epistaxis. Traditional gauze with either petrolatum or antibiotic-impregnated ointment is probably the most secure form. Expandable nasal sponges such as Merocel or Rhino Rocket products are convenient and effective. These should be lubricated before insertion. Other helpful products for patients with coagulopathies include Gelfoam sponge, Surgicel gauze, or Avitene gauze applica-

tion. Patients should receive pain medication plus oral antibiotics with activity against *S. aureus* (because of toxic shock) and sinusitis pathogens.

    f.   A posterior pack is indicated for failure of an *appropriately placed* anterior pack or an obvious posterior bleed. Traditional posterior packs include use of gauze/wool tied to umbilical tape or a Foley catheter plus standard anterior packing. These have largely been supplanted by the more convenient double-lumen nasal catheter, similar to the Epistat device. Any of these *must* have padding at the nostril to avoid disastrous columellar or alar notching due to pressure necrosis.

    g.   Packs remain for 3 to 5 days to allow remucosalization and healing. Antibiotics and pain medication are provided. Sedation is used judiciously. Elderly, frail patients and those with posterior packing are typically hospitalized for pain control and to receive supplemental oxygen—also, and as clinically indicated, continuous pulse oximetry. The debated *nasopulmonary reflex* postulates respiratory depression due to posterior nasal packing.

  7. *Surgical management*

    a.   Endoscopy allows visualization and treatment (with suction cautery) of posterior bleeding. It allows avoidance of prolonged nasal packing and may reduce hospital stays and cost.

    b.   Traditional surgical management is usually used for failure of appropriately placed packing. Anterior and posterior ethmoidal artery ligation is indicated for anterior/superior epistaxis sites. Posterior and inferior sites are addressed by transantral (via Caldwell-Luc approach) ligation of branches of the internal maxillary artery. The surgical microscope is used, fat is dissected away from vessels behind the maxillary sinus, and surgical clips are applied to all visible vessels. Simple ligation of the external carotid artery usually fails due to the numerous distal anastomoses.

    c.   Selective embolization may be used when an interventional radiologist is available. It is extremely effective but does involve some low risk for emboli to the cerebral vasculature. It is difficult to perform after vessel ligation, since this occludes the access vessels necessary for embolization.

    d.   Septal dermoplasty and laser coagulation can be used for hereditary hemorrhagic telangiectasia, but this condition is notoriously prone to recurrence regardless of the treatment modality used.

E. Disorders of Smell[180–184]

  1. Over 2 million Americans experience disordered taste and smell.

  2. *Conductive anosmia* is due to impaired transport of airborne odorants to the olfactory cleft. *Neuronal anosmia* is due to impairment of olfactory epithelial function or disrupted neuronal pathways.

  3. *Anosmia:* Loss of sense of smell. *Dysosmia:* Impaired sense of smell. About 80% of individuals over age 60 have decreased smell. Seen also in patients with Alzheimer's disease and parkinsonism. *Parosmia:* Distorted sense of smell. *Phantosmia:* Smelling of nonexistent odors. Both parosmia and phantosmia are associated with post-URI olfactory loss, trauma, aging, temporal/uncal lobe lesions, temporal lobe epilepsy, and olfactory hallucinations of schizophrenia. *Hyperosmia:* Increased smell sensitivity, reported in Addison's disease or cystic fibrosis.

4. *Common chemical sense:* Cranial nerves V, IX, X able to sense noxious stimuli. Malingerers may pretend not to detect noxious stimuli, such as ammonia, in addition to normal odorants.

5. *Causes of olfactory dysfunction*
   a. *Obstructive nasal disease* (23%): Includes nasal polyposis, mucosal disease, tumors, and nasal deformity. Treatment is directed at improving obstruction to allow odorants to reach olfactory cleft. Anosmia associated with nasal polyps may persist even after appropriate surgery.
   b. *Postviral anosmia* (19%): Due to viral injury to olfactory epithelium and more common in those above age 40. Hyposmia more common than frank anosmia. About one-third recover some function over 3 to 6 months. No specific treatment.
   c. *Head trauma* (15%): Anosmia occurs in 0.5% of head trauma cases and is felt to be due to shearing force on olfactory filaments, olfactory bulb contusion, or frontal lobe injury. Onset usually immediate but may be delayed. No specific therapy. Recovery reported in 8 to 40%.
   d. *Toxins, drugs* (3%): Numerous chemical agents and drugs are reported to affect olfactory function (see references 183 and 184).
   e. *Miscellaneous* (21%): Aging, congenital, neoplastic, psychologic, and other cause.
   f. *Idiopathic* (21%)

6. *Evaluation:* History inquires about onset, duration, previous dysosmia, taste loss, episodic improvement, medication, infection, and chemical exposure. Complete head and neck examination to include nasal encoscopy. Quick, convenient smell testing may be done with vials containing water, ammonia, and fresh coffee. Taste assessment (for sweet, sour, salt, bitter) done with swish/spit with 1 M NaCl, 1 M sucrose, 1 M citric acid, and 0.001 M quinine. Neoplasm (if suspected) may be ruled out with contrasted coronal sinus CT. The University of Pennsylvania Smell Identification Test (UPSIT), Pocket Smell Test, and Brief Smell Identification Test are commercially available olfactory tests.

7. *Treatment:* Condition-specific treatment helpful for allergy, airway obstruction, or other identifiable problems. The efficacy of zinc is debated, but it is not harmful. Steroid sprays may help. Anosmic patients should be counseled on the need for smoke detectors, risk of natural gas/propane leakage, risk of food spoilage, and social concerns about body and household odors.

F. Nasal Fracture[185–187]

1. Prominent location makes nose the most commonly fractured facial bone. Depending on the mechanism of trauma, patients may have edema, deviation, ecchymosis, pain, nasal obstruction, crepitus, nasal mobility, and epistaxis. Remember to inquire regarding preexisting deformity.

2. Patients may be seen immediately (before edema develops) or in about 5 days, after swelling subsides. Open fracture or septal hematoma requires immediate treatment. Treatment becomes more difficult after 10 to 14 days in adults and 7 to 10 days in children, as the bones begin to set.

3. Radiographs are clinically unhelpful and serve only to provide medicolegal documentation of fracture.

4. Reduction is accomplished in the office with local/topical anesthetic; general anesthesia is required for children, uncooperative patients, or complicated injury. A protective dor-

sal splint is placed for about 7 days. Intranasal packing is used to prevent depression of unstable bone fragments. The patient is reassessed in 1 week, at which time the nasal bones usually remain sufficiently mobile for repeat reduction if shifting of bones occurred.

5. Rhinoplasty is indicated for fractures seen later than 2 to 3 weeks after injury or for persistent deformity.

6. Septal dislocation occurs in 0.6 to 1% of births and results in dislocation of the quadrilateral cartilage off the maxillary crest and vomer. Patients demonstrate tip deviation, leaning of the columella, and alar flattening. Treatment should be given within the first several days of life and involves use of an elevator to replace the septum into the maxillary crest.

G. Septal Hematoma[186,188]

1. Usually bilateral; both traumatic and iatrogenic causes.

2. Hematoma between cartilage and mucoperichondrium separates septum from its blood and may cause cartilaginous atrophy and necrosis. Blood provides excellent bacterial medium and result in septal abscess. Cartilage loss, thickening of septum, fibrosis, and saddle-nose deformity may ensue. Septal infection is of concern due to valveless venous communication with orbit and cavernous sinus.

3. Hematoma evacuation required—usually by incision and drainage. Bilateral incisions should be staggered to reduce risk of septal perforation. Reaccumulation is discouraged by nasal packing left for several days. The patient is given oral antibiotics effective against *S. aureus* (toxic shock syndrome) and sinusitis pathogens.

References

1. Geurkink N. Nasal anatomy, physiology, and function. *J Allergy Clin Immunol* 1983;72: 123.

2. Libersa C, Laude M, Libersa J. The pneumatization of the accessory sinuses of the nasal fossae during growth. *Anat Clin* 1981;2:265.

3. Maresh M. Paranasal sinuses from birth to late adolescence. *Am J Dis Child* 1989;60:55.

4. Hengerer A. Embryologic development of the sinuses. *Ear Nose Throat J* 1984;63:134.

5. Schaeffer J. The clinical anatomy and development of the paranasal sinuses. *Pennsylvania Med J* 1936;39:395.

6. Clemente C. *Gray's Anatomy,* 30th American ed. Philadelphia: Lea & Febiger, 1985.

7. Morrison E, Costanzo R. Morphology of the human olfactory epithelium. *J Comp Neurol* 1990;297:1.

8. Bailey B, Johnson J, Kohut R, et al. *Head & Neck Surgery—Otolaryngology*. Philadelphia: Lippincott, 1993.

9. Cummings C, Fredrickson J, Harker L, et al. *Otolaryngology—Head and Neck Surgery,* 2nd ed. St. Louis: Mosby, 1993.

10. Paff G. *Anatomy of the Head and Neck.* Philadelphia: Saunders, 1973.

11. Hollinshead W. *Anatomy for Surgeons.* Vol I. *The Head and Neck,* 2nd ed. New York: Harper & Row, 1968.

12. Courtiss E, Gargan T, Courtiss G. Nasal physiology. *Ann Plast Surg* 1984;13:214.

13. Shapiro P. Effects of nasal obstruction on facial development. *J Allergy Clin Immunol* 1988; 81:967.

14. King H, Mabry R. *A Practical Guide to the Management of Nasal and Sinus Disorders.* New York: Thieme, 1993.

15. Benninger M. Nasal endoscopy: Its role in office diagnosis. *Am J Rhinol* 1994;11:177.

16. Hughes R, Jones N. The role of nasal endoscopy in outpatient management. *Clin Otolaryngol* 1998;23:224.

17. Roithmann R, Cole P, Chapnik J, et al. Acoustic rhinometry, rhinomanometry, and the sensation of nasal patency: A correlative study. *J Otolaryngol* 1994;23:454.

18. Tomkinson A. Acoustic rhinometry; its place in rhinology. *Clin Otolaryngol* 1997;22:189.

19. Fisher E. Acoustic rhinometry. *Clin Otolaryngol* 1997;22:307.

20. Lund V. Objective assessment of nasal obstruction. *Otolaryngol Clin North Am* 1989;22:279.

21. Cole P. Rhinomanometry 1988: Practice and trends. *Laryngoscope* 1989;99:311.

22. Hudgins P. Sinonasal imaging. *Neuroimaging Clin North Am* 1996;6:319.

23. Zeifer B. Update on sinonasal imaging. *Neuroimaging Clin North Am* 1998;8:607.

24. Rao V, El-Noueam K. Sinonasal imaging. *Neuroimaging Clin North Am* 1998;8:921.

25. Meltzer E, Jalowayski A. Nasal cytology in clinical practice. *Am J Rhinol* 1988;2:47.

26. Piacentini G, Kaulbach H, Scott T, et al. Evaluation of nasal cytology: A comparison between methods. *Allergy* 1998;53:326.

27. Adam H. Choanal atresia. *Pediatr Rev* 1995; 16:475.

28. Park A, Brockenbrough J, Stankiewicz J. Endoscopic versus traditional approaches to choanal atresia. *Otolaryngol Clin North Am* 2000;33:77.

29. Friedman N, Mitchell R, Bailey C. Management and outcome of choanal atresia correction. *Int J Pediatr Otorhinolaryngol* 2000;52:45.

30. Harley E. Pediatric congenital nasal masses. *Ear Nose Throat J* 1991;70:28.

31. Sweet R. Lesions of the nasal radix in pediatric patients. *South Med J* 1992;85:164.

32. Cauchois R, Laccourreye O, Bremond D, et al. Nasal dermoid sinus cyst. *Ann Otol Rhinol Laryngol* 1994;103:615.

33. Fitzpatrick E, Miller R. Congenital midline nasal masses: Dermoids, gliomas, and encephaloceles. *J La State Med Soc* 1996;148:93.

34. Dennoyelle F, Ducroz V, Roger G, et al. Nasal dermoid sinus cysts in children. *Laryngoscope* 1997;107:795.

35. Rohrich R, Lowe J, Schwartz M. The role of open rhinoplasty in the management of nasal dermoid cysts. *Plast Reconstr Surg* 1999;104: 459.

36. Pensler J, Ivescu B, Ciletti S, et al. Craniofacial gliomas. *Plast Reconstr Surg* 1996;98:27.

37. Claros P, Bandos R, Claros A, et al. Nasal gliomas. Main features, management, and report of five cases. *Int J Pediatr Otorhinolaryngol* 1998;46:15.

38. Fuller G, Batsakis J. Pathology consultation. Pharyngeal hypophysis. *Ann Otol Rhinol Laryngol* 1996;105:671.

39. Brassier G, Morandi X, Tayiar E, et al. Rathke's cleft cysts: Surgical–MRI correlation in 16 symptomatic cases. *J Neuroradiol* 1999;26:162.

40. Weissman J. Tornwaldt's cysts. *Am J Otolaryngol* 1992;13:381.

41. Swanson K, Kaugars G, Gunsolley J. Nasopalatine duct cyst: An analysis of 334 cases. *J Oral Maxillofac Surg* 1991;49:268.

42. Jacob S, Zelano B, Gungor A, et al. Location and gross morphology of the nasopalatine duct in human adults. *Arch Otolaryngol Head Neck Surg* 2000;126:741.

43. D'Silva N, Anderson L. Globulomaxillary cyst revisited. *Oral Surg Oral Med Oral Pathol* 1993;76:182.

44. Wesley R, Scannell T, Nathan T. Nasolabial cyst: Presentation of a case with a review of the literature. *J Oral Maxillofac Surg* 1984:42:188.

45. Cure J, Osguthorpe J, Van Tassel P. MR of nasolabial cyst. *Am J Neuroradiol* 1996;17: 585.

46. Kimura C, Pien F. Head and neck cellulitis in hospitalized adults. *Am J Otolaryngol* 1993; 14:343.

47. Eriksson B, Jorup-Ronstrom C, Karkkonen K, et al. Erysipelas: Clinical and bacteriologic spectrum and serological aspects. *Clin Infect Dis* 1996;23:1091.

48. Chartier E, Grosshans E. Erysipelas: An update. *Int J Dermatol* 1996;35:779.

49. Veien N. The clinician's choice of antibiotics in the treatment of bacterial skin infection. *Br J Dermatol* 1998;139:30.

50. Malcolm B. Impetigo. *Practitioner.* 1998;242: 405.

51. Hogan P. Impetigo. *Aust Fam Physician* 1998;27:735.

52. O'Dell M. Skin and wound infections: An overview. *Am Fam Physician* 1998;57:2424.

53. Habif T. *Clinical Dermatology.* St Louis: Mosby, 1990.

54. Winther B, Gwaltney J, Mygind N, et al. Viral induced rhinitis. *Am J Rhinol* 1998;9:17.

55. Lucente F. Rhinitis and nasal obstruction. *Otolaryngol Clin North Am* 1989;22:307.

56. Wenzel R, Perl T. The significance of nasal carriage of *Staphylococcus aureus* and the incidence of postoperative wound infection. *J Hosp Infect* 1995;31:13.

57. Boyce J. Preventing staphylococcal infections by eradicating nasal carriage of *Staphylococ-*

cus aureus: Proceeding with caution. *Infect Control Hosp Epidemiol* 1996;17:775.

58. Casewell M. The nose: An underestimated source of *Staphylococcus aureus* causing wound infection. *J Hosp Infect* 1998;40:53.

59. McNulty J, Fassett R. Syphilis: An otolaryngologic perspective. *Laryngoscope* 1981;91:889.

60. Martinez S, Mouney D. Treponemal infections of the head and neck. *Otolaryngol Clin North Am* 1982;15:613.

61. Waldman S, Levine H, Sebek B, et al. Nasal tuberculosis: A forgotten entity. *Laryngoscope* 1981;91:11.

62. Goguen L, Karmody C. Nasal tuberculosis. *Otolaryngol Head Neck Surg* 1995;113:131.

63. Brazin S. Leprosy (Hansen's disease). *Otolaryngol Clin North Am* 1982;15:697.

64. Thami G, Baruah M, Sharmace S, et al. Nasal myiasis in leprosy leading to unusual tissue destruction. *J Dermatol* 1995;22:348.

65. Batsakis J, El-Naggar A. Rhinoscleroma and rhinosporidiosis. *Ann Otol Rhinol Laryngol* 1992;101:879.

66. Andraca R, Edson R, Kern E. Rhinoscleroma: A growing concern in the United States? Mayo Clinic experience. *Mayo Clin Proc* 1993;68: 1151.

67. Al-Serhani A, Al Qahtani A, Arafa M. Association of rhinoscleroma with rhinosporidiosis. *Rhinology* 1998;36:43.

68. Elgart M. Unusual subcutaneous infections. *Dermatol Clin North Am* 1996;14:105.

69. Richtsmeier W, Johns M. Actinomycosis of the head and neck. *Crit Rev Clin Lab Sci* 1979; 8:175.

70. Richtsmeier W, Johns M. Bacterial causes of granulomatous diseases. *Otolaryngol Clin North Am* 1982;15:473.

71. Gerber M, Rosdeutscher J, Seiden A, et al. Histoplasmosis: The otolaryngologist's perspective. *Laryngoscope* 1995;105:919.

72. Bradsher R. Histoplasmosis and blastomycosis. *Clin Infect Dis* 1996;22(suppl 2):S102.

73. Briggs D, Barney P, Bahu R. Nasal cryptococcosis. *Arch Otolaryngol* 1974;100:390.

74. Blitzer A, Lawson W. Fungal infections of the nose and paranasal sinuses: Part I. *Otolaryngol Clin North Am* 1993;26:1007.

75. Reder P, Neel H. Blastomycosis in otolaryngology: Review of a large series. *Laryngoscope* 1993;103:53.

76. Mandell G, Bennet J, Dolin R. *Principles and Practice of Infectious Diseases,* 4th ed. New York: Churchill Livingstone, 1995.

77. Osguthorpe J, Hadley J. Rhinosinusitis— current concepts in evaluation and management. *Med Clin North Am* 1999;83:27.

78. Sinus and Allergy Health Partnership. Antimicrobial treatment guidelines for acute bacterial rhinosinusitis. *Otolaryngol Head Neck Surg* 2000;123:S1.

79. Fireman P. Diagnosis of sinusitis in children: Emphasis on the history and physical examination. *J Allergy Clin Immunol* 1992;90:433.

80. Weinberg E, Brodsky L, Brody A, et al. Clinical classification as a guide to treatment of sinusitis in children. *Laryngoscope* 1997;107:241.

81. Hopp R, Cooperstock M. Medical management of sinusitis in pediatric patients. *Curr Probl Pediatr* 1997;27;178.

82. Lanza D, Kennedy D. Current concepts in the surgical management of chronic sinusitis and recurrent acute sinusitis. *J Allergy Clin Immunol* 1992;90:505.

83. Brook I. Microbiology and management of sinusitis. *J Otolaryngol* 1996;25:249.

84. Lund V, Kennedy D. Staging for rhinosinusitis. *Otolaryngol Head Neck Surg* 1997;117:S35.

85. Lund V, Mackay I. Staging in rhinosinusitis. *Rhinology* 1993;107:183.

86. Ponikau J, Sherris D, Kern E, et al. The diagnosis and incidence of allergic fungal sinusitis. *Mayo Clin Proc* 1999;74:877.

87. Ferguson B. Definitions of fungal rhinosinusitis. *Otolaryngol Clin North Am* 2000;33:227.

88. Houser S, Corey J. Allergic fungal rhinosinusitis: Pathophysiology, epidemiology, and diagnosis. *Otolaryngol Clin North Am* 2000;33:399.

89. Marple B. Allergic fungal rhinosinusitis: Surgical management. *Otolaryngol Clin North Am* 2000;33:409.

90. Ferguson B. Fungal balls of the paranasal sinuses. *Otolaryngol Clin North Am* 2000;33.

91. Ferguson B. Mucormycosis of the nose and paranasal sinuses. *Otolaryngol Clin North Am* 2000;33:389.

92. Stringer S, Ryan M. Chronic invasive fungal rhinosinusitis. *Otolaryngol Clin North Am* 2000; 33:375.

93. Tami T, Wawrose S. Diseases of the nose and paranasal sinuses in the human immunodefi-

ciency virus infected population. *Otolaryngol Clin North Am* 1992;25:1199.

94. Truitt T, Tami T. Otolaryngologic manifestations of human immunodeficiency virus infection. *Med Clin North Am* 1999;83:303.

95. Slavin R. Sinopulmonary relationships. *Am J Otolaryngol* 1994;15:18.

96. Park A, Lau J, Stankiewicz, et al. The role of functional endoscopic sinus surgery in asthmatic patients. *J Otolaryngol* 1998;27:275.

97. Senior B, Kennedy D, Tanabodee J, et al. Long term impact of functional endoscopic sinus surgery on asthma. *Otolaryngol Head Neck Surg* 1999;121:66.

98. Dunlop G, Scadding G, Lund V. The effect of endoscopic sinus surgery on asthma: Management of patients with chronic rhinosinusitis, nasal polyposis, and asthma. *Am J Rhinol* 1999; 13:261.

99. Peters E, Crater S, Phillips C, et al. Sinusitis and acute asthma in adults. *Int Arch Allergy Immunol* 1999;118:372.

100. Scadding G. The effect of medical treatment of sinusitis upon concomitant asthma. *Allergy* 1999;54(Suppl 57):136.

101. Chandler J, Langenbrunner D, Stevens E. The pathogenesis of orbital complications in acute sinusitis. *Laryngoscope* 1970;80:1414.

102. Clayman G, Adams G, Paugh D, et al. Intracranial complications of paranasal sinusitis: A combined institutional review. *Laryngoscope* 1991;101:234.

103. Wagenmann M, Naclerio R. Complications of sinusitis. *J Allergy Clin Immunol* 1992;90:552.

104. Stankiewicz J, Newell D, Parki A. Complications of inflammatory diseases of the sinuses. *Otolaryngol Clin North Am* 1993;26:639.

105. Fornadely J, Corey J, Osguthorpe J, et al. Allergic rhinitis: Clinical practice guideline. *Otolaryngol Head Neck Surg* 1996;115:115.

106. Dykewicz M, Fineman S, Skoner D, et al. Diagnosis and management of rhinitis: Complete guidelines of the joint task force on practice parameters in allergy, asthma, and immunology. *Ann Allergy, Asthma, Immunol* 1998;81:478.

107. Purello-D'Ambrosio F, Isola S, Ricciardi L, et al. A controlled study on the effeciveness on loratedine in combination with flunisolide in the treatment of nonallergic rhinitis with eosinophilia (NARES). *Clin Exp Allergy* 1999; 29:1143.

108. Holmberg K, Karlsson G. Nasal polyps: Medical or surgical management. *Clin Exp Allergy* 1996;26(Suppl 3):23.

109. Mygind N. Advances in the medical treatment of nasal polyps. *Allergy* 1999;54(Suppl):12.

110. Stammberger H. Surgical treatment of nasal polyps: Past and future. *Allergy* 1999;54 (Suppl):7.

111. Zohar Y, Talmi Y, Strauss M, et al. Ozena revisited. *J Otolaryngol* 1990;19:345.

112. Shehata M. Atrophic rhinitis. *Am J Otolaryngol* 1996;17:81.

113. Krespi Y, Kurliloff D, Aner M. Sarcoidosis of the sinosal tract: New staging system. *Otolaryngol Head Neck Surg* 1995;112:221.

114. Shah U, White W, Gooey J, et al. Otolaryngologic manifestations of sarcoidosis: Presentation and diagnosis. *Laryngoscope* 1997;107:67.

115. Hartig G, Montone K, Wasik M, et al. Nasal T-cell lymphoma and the lethal midline granuloma syndrome. *Otolaryngol Head Neck Surg* 1996;114:653.

116. Vartiainen E, Nuutinen J. Head and neck manifestations of Wegener's granulomatosis. *Ear Nose Throat* 1992;71:423.

117. Duna G, Galperin C, Hoffman G. Wegener's granulomatosis. *Rheum Dis Clin North Am* 1995;21:949.

118. O'Devaney K, Ferlito A, Huner B, et al. Wegener's granulomatosis of the head and neck. *Ann Otol Rhinol Laryngol* 1998;107:439.

119. Robson A, Burge S, Millard P. Nasal mucosal involvement in lupus erythematosus. *Clin Otolaryngol* 1992;17:341.

120. Pisetsky D, Gilkeson G, St. Clair E. Systemic lupus erythematosus. Diagnosis and treatment. *Med Clin North Am* 1997;81:113.

121. Weisman R, Calcaterra T. Head and neck manifestations of scleroderma. *Ann Otol* 1978; 87:332.

122. Tuffanelli D. Systemic scleroderma. *Med Clin North Am* 1989;73:1167.

123. Maran A. Sjogren's syndrome. *J Laryngol Otol* 1986;100:1299.

124. Rasmussen N, Brofeldt S, Manthorpe R. Smell and nasal finding in patients with primary Sjogren's syndrome. *Scand J Rheumatol* 1986; 61:142.

125. Rampelberg O, Gerard J, Namias B, et al. ENT manifestations of relapsing polychondritis. *Acta Otorhinolaryngol Belg.* 1997;51:73

126. Trentham D, Le C. Relapsing polychondritis. *Ann Intern Med* 1998;129:11.

127. Specks U, De Remee R. Granulomatous vasculitis, Wegener's granulomatosis, and Churg-Strauss syndrome. *Rheum Dis Clin North Am* 1990;16:377.

128. Guillevin L, Cohen P, Gayraud M, et al. Churg-Strauss syndrome: Clinical study and long-term follow-up of 96 patients. *Medicine* 1999;78:26.

129. Maisel R, Johnston W, Anderson H, et al. Necrotizing sialometaplasia involving the nasal cavity. *Laryngoscope* 1977;87:429.

130. Russell J, Friedmann I. View from beneath: Pathology in focus. Necrotizing sialometaplasia. *J Laryngol Otol* 1992;106:569.

131. Bohay R, Gordon S. The maxillary mucus retention cyst: A common incidental panoramic finding. *Oral Health* 1997;87:7.

132. Hadar T, Shvero J, Nageris B. Mucus retention cyst of the maxillary sinus: The endoscopic approach. *Br J Oral Maxillofac Surg* 2000;38:227.

133. Myers E, Fernau J, Johnson J, et al. Management of inverting papilloma. *Laryngoscope* 1990;100:481.

134. Pelausa E, Fortier M. Schneiderian papilloma of the nose and paranasal sinuses. The University of Ottawa experience. *J Otolaryngol* 1992;21:9.

135. Har-El G, Shapsha S, Bohigian K, et al. The treatment of rhinophyma. "Cold" vs laser techniques. *Arch Otolaryngol Head Neck Surg* 1993;119:628.

136. Hoasjoe D, Stucker F. Rhinophyma: Review of pathophysiology and treatment. *J Otolaryngol* 1995;24:51.

137. Nelson B, Fuciarelli K. Surgical management of rhinophyma. *Cutis* 1998;61:313.

138. Gullane P, Davidson J, O'Dwyer T, et al. Juvenile angiofibroma: A review of the literature and a case series report. *Laryngoscope* 1992;102:928.

139. Deschler D, Kaplan M, Boles R. Treatment of large juvenile nasopharyngeal angiofibroma. *Otolaryngol Head Neck Surg* 1992;106:278.

140. Ungkanont K, Byers R, Weber R, et al. Juvenile nasopharyngeal angiofibroma: An update of therapeutic management. *Head Neck* 1996; 18:60.

141. Tewfik T, Tan A, Al Noury K, et al. Juvenile nasopharyngeal angiofibroma. *J Otolaryngol* 1999;28:145.

142. McShane D, Walsh M. Nasal granuloma gravidarum. *J Laryngol Otol* 1988;102:828.

143. Sheppard L, Mickelson S. Hemangiomas of the nasal septum and paranasal sinuses. *Henry Ford Hosp Med J* 1990;38:25.

144. Lim A, Sing K, Prasad R, et al. "Pregnancy tumor" of the nasal septum. *Aust N Z J Obstet Gynaecol* 1994;34:109.

145. Miller F, D'Agostino, Schlack K. Lobular capillary hemangioma of the nasal cavity. *Otolaryngol Head Neck Surg* 1999;120:783.

146. Smith M, Calcaterra T. Frontal sinus osteoma. *Ann Otol Rhinol Laryngol* 1989;98:896.

147. Earwaker J. Paranasal sinus osteomas: A review of 46 cases. *Skeletal Radiol* 1993;22:417.

148. Hehar S, Jones N. Frontoethmoid osteoma: The place of surgery. *J Laryngol Otol* 1997; 111:372.

149. Koivunen P, Lopponen H, Fors P, et al. The growth rate of osteomas of the paranasal sinuses. *Clin Otolaryngol* 1997;22:111.

150. Beasley D, Lejeune F. Fibro-osseous lesions of the head and neck. *J La State Med Soc* 1996; 148:413.

151. Espinosa J, Elizalde A, Aquerreta J. Imaging case of the month—fibrous dysplasia of the maxilla. *Ann Otol Rhinol Laryngol* 1998;107:175.

152. Posnick J. Fibrous dysplasia of the craniomaxillofacial region: Current clinical perspectives. *Br J Oral Maxillofac Surg* 1998;36:264.

153. Tang S, Tse C. Leiomyoma of the nasal cavity. *J Laryngol Otol* 1988;102:831.

154. Watson D. Nasal paraganglioma. *J Laryngol Otol* 1988;102:526.

155. Kuhn J, Aronoff B. Nasal and nasopharyngeal paraganglioma. *J Surg Oncol* 1989;40:38.

156. Younis R, Gross C, Lazar R. Schwannomas of the paranasal sinuses. Case report and clinicopathologic analysis. *Arch Otolaryngol* 1991; 117:677.

157. Llorente J, Suarez C, Seco M, et al. Leiomyoma of the nasal septum: Report of a case and review of the literature. *J Laryngol Otol* 1996; 110:65.

158. Spiro J, Soo K, Spiro R. Squamous carcinoma of the nasal cavity and paranasal sinuses. *Am J Surg* 1989;158:328.

159. Carrau R, Myers E, Johnson J. Paranasal sinus carcinoma—diagnosis, treatment, and prognosis. *Oncology* 1992;6:43.

160. Davison S, Habermann T, Strickler J, et al. Nasal and nasopharyngeal angiocentric T-cell lymphomas. *Laryngoscope* 1996;106:139.

161. Fajardo-Dolci G, Magana R, Bautista E, et al. Sinonasal lymphoma. *Otolaryngol Head Neck Surg* 1999;121:323.

162. Vidal R, Devaney K, Ferlito A, et al. Sinonasal malignant lymphomas: A distinct clinicopathological category. *Ann Otol Rhinol Laryngol* 1999;108:411.

163. Brandwein M, Rothstein A, Lawson W, et al. Sinonasal melanoma. *Arch Otolaryngol Head Neck Surg* 1997;123:290.

164. Dulguerov P, Calcaterra T. Esthesioneuroblastoma—the UCLA experience, 1970–1990. *Laryngoscope* 1992;102:843.

165. Morita A, Ebersold M, Olsen K, et al. Esthesioneuroblastoma: Prognosis and management. *Neurosurgery* 1993;32:706.

166. Eden B, Debo R, Larner J, et al. Esthesioneuroblastoma long term outcomes and patterns of failure—the University of Virginia experience. *Cancer* 1994;73:2556.

167. Levine P, Gallagher R, Cantrell R. Esthesioneuroblastoma: Reflections of a 21 year experience. *Laryngoscope* 1999;109:1539.

168. Righi P, Francis F, Aron B, et al. Sinonasal undifferentiated carcinoma: A 10-year experience. *Am J Otolaryngol* 1996;17:167.

169. Houston G, Gillies E. Sinonasal undifferentiated carcinoma: A distinct clinicopathologic entity. *Adv Anat Pathol* 1999;6:317.

170. Weber A, Brown E, Hug E, et al. Cartilaginous tumors and chordomas of the cranial base. *Otolaryngol Clin North Am* 1995;28:453.

171. Al-Mefty O, Borba L. Skull base chordomas: A management challenge. *J Neurosurg* 1997; 86:182.

172. Sercarz J, Mark R, Tran L, et al. Sarcomas of the nasal cavity and paranasal sinuses. *Ann Otol Rhinol Laryngol* 1994;103:699.

173. Yacoub G, Dubaybo B. Plasmacytoma and upper airway obstruction. *Am J Otolaryngol* 1999;20:257.

174. Graf P. Rhinitis medicamentosa: Aspects of pathophysiology and treatment. *Allergy* 1997; 52(40 Suppl):28.

175. Yoo J, Seikaly H, Calhoun K. Extended use of topical nasal decongestants. *Laryngoscope* 1997;107:40.

176. Schatz M, Zeiger R. Diagnosis and management of rhinitis during pregnancy. *Allergy Proc* 1988;9:545.

177. Randall D, Freeman S. Management of anterior and posterior epistaxis. *Am Fam Physician* 1991;43:2007.

178. Haitjema T, Balder W, Disch F, et al. Epistaxis in hereditary haemorrhagic telangiectasia. *Rhinology* 1996;34:176.

179. Tan L, Calhoun K. Epistaxis. *Med Clin North Am* 1999;83:43.

180. Park R. Olfaction. *Otolaryngol Clin North Am* 1973;6:637.

181. Scott A. Clinical characteristics of taste and smell disorders. *Ear Nose Throat J* 1989;68: 297.

182. Deams D, Doty R, Settle R, et al. Smell and taste disorders: A study of 750 patients from the University of Pennsylvania Smell and Taste Center. *Arch Otolaryngol Head Neck Surg* 1991;117:519.

183. Cullen D, Leopold D. Disorders of smell and taste. *Med Clin North Am* 1999;83:57.

184. Bromley S. Smell and taste disorders: A primary care approach. *Am Fam Physician* 2000;61:427.

185. Renner R. Management of nasal fractures. *Otolaryngol Clin North Am* 1991;24:195.

186. Mathog R. *Atlas of Craniofacial Trauma.* Philadelphia: Saunders, 1992.

187. Hughes C, Harley E, Milmoe G, et al. Birth trauma in the head and neck. *Arch Otolaryngol Head Neck Surg* 1999;125:193.

188. Kryger H, Dommerby H. Haemotoma and abscess of the nasal spetum. *Clin Otolaryngol* 1987;12:125.

EMBRYOLOGY AND ANATOMY[1-5]

For embryologic explanations, see Chapter 10. The larynx consists of a framework of cartilages held in position by an intrinsic and an extrinsic musculature and lined by mucous membrane that is arranged in characteristic folds.[1-3]

The larynx is situated in front of the fourth to sixth cervical vertebrae. The upper portion of the larynx, which is continuous with the pharynx above, is almost triangular in shape; the lower portion, leading into the trachea, presents a circular appearance.

Laryngeal Cartilages

The laryngeal cartilages form the main framework of the larynx and consist of the following:

1. Thyroid cartilage (unpaired)
2. Cricoid cartilage (unpaired)
3. Epiglottis (unpaired)
4. Arytenoid cartilage (paired)
5. Corniculate cartilage (paired)
6. Cuneiform cartilage (paired)
7. Triticeous cartilage (not always present)

Thyroid Cartilage

The thyroid cartilage (hyaline cartilage) is the largest and encloses the larynx anteriorly and laterally, thus shielding it from all but the most forceful blows. This cartilage is composed of two alae, which meet anteriorly, dipping down from above to form the thyroid notch before meeting at the protuberance of the Adam's apple. Posteriorly, each wing has a superior cornu, extending upward about 2 cm, and a much shorter inferior cornu that articulates with the cricoid cartilage via the cricothyroid articulation. It is the only direct articulation of the thyroid cartilage, all other relations with contiguous structures being maintained by muscles or ligaments.

Cricoid Cartilage

The cricoid cartilage (hyaline cartilage) lies directly below the thyroid cartilage. It is the strongest of the laryngeal cartilages and is shaped like a signet ring. The flat portion of the ring, or lamina, is located posteriorly and extends upward to form the posterior border of the larynx. Because the cricoid cartilage forms the only complete annular support of the laryngeal skeleton, its preservation is essential for maintenance of the enclosed airways. In the adult, the cricoid cartilage is at the level of C6 to C7, and in the child it is at the level of C3 to C4.

Posterolaterally, the cricoid articulates with the inferior cornua of the thyroid cartilage, with which it shares true synovial joints. These joints permit a rocking action of the cricoid cartilage on the thyroid cartilage and a slight anteroposterior sliding motion. Also through synovial joints, the cricoid cartilage on its posterosuperior aspect supports the two arytenoid cartilages.

Epiglottis

The epiglottis (fibroelastic cartilage) is a leaf-shaped structure attached to the inside of the thyroid cartilage anteriorly and projecting superiorly and posteriorly above the laryngeal opening. The petiole is the small, narrow portion of the epiglottis that is attached to the internal aspect of the thyroid cartilage.

Arytenoid Cartilages

The arytenoid cartilages (mostly hyaline cartilages) are much smaller in size, yet they are primarily responsible for the opening and closing of the larynx. Roughly pyramidal in shape, they rest on the upper edge of the cricoid lamina at the posterior border of the larynx. The anterior projection of each arytenoid, or vocal process, receives the attachment of the posterior or membranous end of each vocal cord. The lateral prominence of each arytenoid cartilage is known as the muscular process because of the insertion of numerous intrinsic laryngeal muscles. The arytenoid cartilages articulate with the cricoid cartilage at the cricoarytenoid joint. Because the base of arytenoid cartilage has a concave configuration, the articulation of the arytenoid and cricoid cartilages permits a sliding or rocking movement of the arytenoid, not just rotation of the arytenoid. Rocking forward motion of the arytenoid cartilage is more important than rotation.

Corniculate Cartilages

The corniculate cartilages (fibroelastic cartilage), also called cartilages of Santorini, are small cartilages above the arytenoid and in the aryepiglottic folds. These cartilages provide rigidity to the aryepiglottic folds.

Cuneiform Cartilages

The cuneiform cartilages (fibroelastic cartilage), also called cartilages of Wrisberg, are elongated pieces of small yellow elastic cartilage in the aryepiglottic folds. These cartilages also provide rigidity to the aryepiglottic folds.

Triticeous Cartilage

The triticeous cartilage (cartilago triticea) is a small elastic cartilage in the lateral thyrohyoid ligament. When calcified, it could be mistaken for a foreign body on soft tissue x-ray films. It may be absent.

The Hyoid Bone

The hyoid bone is commonly described as part of the laryngeal framework, because it is an important point of attachment for the extrinsic muscles of the larynx. The hyoid bone has ligaments such as the stylohyoid and the thyrohyoid ligaments. These ligaments and the muscles of the pharynx help in maintaining the structural integrity of the pharynx and the vocal tract.

Ossification

1. Thyroid cartilage begins ossification at puberty and ossifies at 20 to 30 years of age. Ossification begins in the inferior margin and progresses cranially.
2. Cricoid cartilage ossifies after the thyroid cartilage. The first part to be calcified is the posterior superior portion and could be mistaken for a foreign body. Calcification progresses caudally.
3. Arytenoid cartilages calcify at the third decade.
4. The hyoid bone ossifies from six centers shortly after birth; ossification is complete by 2 years of age.

5.   Because hyaline cartilage may undergo calcification and even ossification changes with aging, significant portions of the larynx may undergo these processes. These areas must not be mistaken for intraluminal foreign bodies on soft tissue radiographs of the neck.[5]

Laryngeal Ligaments and Membrane

Extrinsic Ligaments

The extrinsic ligaments of the larynx bind the cartilages to the adjoining structures and to one another and round out the laryngeal framework.

1.   Thyrohyoid membrane and ligaments attach the thyroid cartilage to the hyoid bone. The thyrohyoid membrane is pierced on each side by superior laryngeal vessels and internal branch of superior laryngeal nerve. Median thyrohyoid ligament is the thickened median portion of the thyrohyoid membrane. Lateral thyrohyoid ligament forms the thickened posterior border of the thyrohyoid membrane on each side, and the cartilago triticea is often found in this ligament.
2.   Cricothyroid membrane and ligaments connect the thyroid and cricoid cartilages. This ligament may be pierced for emergency tracheotomy (cricothyrotomy) with little fear of bleeding. However, because of the proximity of the vocal cords, this space should not be used for prolonged tracheal intubation, as scar tissue may be produced, interfering with the mobility of the cords or producing subglottic stenosis.
3.   The cricotracheal ligament attaches the cricoid cartilage to the first tracheal ring.
4.   The thyroepiglottic ligament extends from the epiglottis anteriorly to its attachment on the thyroid cartilage just below the thyroid notch. The hyoepiglottic ligament connects the posterior surface of the hyoid bone and the lingual side of the epiglottis.

Intrinsic Ligaments

The intrinsic ligaments unite the cartilages of the larynx and perform an important role in the closure of this organ.

The elastic membrane is the fibrous framework of the larynx. It lies beneath the laryngeal mucosa and is divided into upper and lower parts by the ventricle of the larynx.

The quadrangular membrane is the upper part of the elastic membrane of the larynx, extending from the lateral margin of the epiglottis to the arytenoid and corniculate cartilages and inferiorly to the false cord. It forms part of the wall between the upper pyriform sinus and the laryngeal vestibule. The quadrangular membrane and the conus elasticus are separated by the ventricle of Morgagni.

Conus elasticus (cricovocal membrane) is the name given to the lower part of the elastic membrane of the larynx. It is composed mainly of yellow elastic tissue. It is attached to the superior border of the cricoid cartilage inferiorly, deep surface of angle of the thyroid cartilage superoanteriorly, and vocal process of the arytenoid cartilage superoposteriorly. It is also called the triangular membrane.

The median cricothyroid ligament is formed by the thickened anterior part of the conus elasticus.

The vocal ligament, which forms the framework of the vocal cord, is the free upper edge (the strongest part) of the conus elasticus. The anterior condensation of the vocal ligament inserts as the anterior macula flava at the anterior commissure as the Broyle's ligament. The posterior condensation of the vocal ligament thickens to attach on the vocal process of the arytenoid cartilage as the posterior macula flava. Differential thickness of the vocal ligament is an important consideration during phonomicrosurgery.

Cavity of the Larynx

The cavity of the larynx is divided into three parts—vestibule, ventricle, and subglottic space—by two folds of mucous membrane: (1) false cords and (2) true cords.

The vestibule lies between the inlet of the larynx and the edges of the false cords and is bordered as follows:

Anterior: Posterior surface of the epiglottis
Posterior: Interval between the arytenoid cartilages
Lateral: Inner surface of the aryepiglottic folds and upper surfaces of the false cord

The ventricle of the larynx (ventricle of Morgagni) is a deep, spindle-shaped recess between the false and true cords and is lined by a mucous membrane that is covered externally by the oblique, superior extension of the thyroarytenoid muscle.

The saccule is a conical pouch that ascends from the anterior part of the ventricle. It lies between the inner surface of the thyroid cartilage and the false cord. Numerous minor salivary glands open onto the surface of its lining mucosa for lubricating the vocal cords.

The glottis (rima glottidis) is the space between the free margin of the true vocal cords. This space is wide and triangular when the vocal cords are abducted (as during respiration) but assumes a slit-like appearance during adduction of the cords (during phonation). The length of the glottic chink in the adult is 18 to 19 mm. The total glottic chink in a newborn is 14 mm.

The false cords (false folds, ventricular bands) are the upper set of two horizontal folds on each side of the laryngeal cavity and extend from the angle of the thyroid cartilage anteriorly to the bodies of the arytenoid cartilages posteriorly. They have a primitive constricting function important during swallow and gestures involving forced glottal closure.

The true cords (true folds) are directly concerned with the production of voice and with protection of the lower respiratory passages. These folds stretch from the angle of the thyroid cartilage anteriorly to the vocal processes of the arytenoid cartilages posteriorly; the vocal folds include the epithelium, the specialized layered structure of the vocal fold mucosa called the vocal fold cover, the vocal ligament, and, a major portion of the vocalis muscle. The covering epithelium and transitional layers below are attached to the underlying vocal ligament, and the blood supply is poor—hence the pearly white appearance of the vocal cords in life.

Clinical Subdivisions

Clinically, the larynx is divided into three areas:

1. Supraglottis (from the tip of the epiglottis to the junction between respiratory and squamous epithelium on the floor of the ventricle). For practical reasons, the inferior boundary is commonly considered to be the junction between the lateral wall and the floor of the ventricle.
2. Glottis (surrounded by the anterior commissure, the true vocal cords, and the so-called posterior commissure). The anterior two-thirds of the vocal fold in adults is called the membranous vocal folds, as it is made of the vocal ligament, muscle, and the vocal cover. The posterior one-third of the glottis is called the cartilaginous larynx, as it is made of the arytenoid cartilages and the posterior interarytenoid soft tissue and interarytenoid muscle. The vocal folds do not meet posteriorly; consequently, the real posterior border is the arytenoid cartilages and the superior edge of the cricoid lamina.
3. Subglottis (from the junction of squamous and respiratory epithelium on the undersurface of the true vocal folds to the inferior edge of the cricoid cartilage). The superior

margin has been arbitrarily assigned to the point 5 mm below the free edge of the true vocal cords.

The epilarynx is that part of the epiglottis and aryepiglottic folds located above the hyoid bone. The vallecula (whose boundaries are the epiglottis posteriorly, the base of tongue anteriorly, and the glossoepiglottic folds laterally and medially), the pyriform sinus (pear-shaped recess between the thyroid cartilage laterally and the quadrangular membrane and arytenoid cartilage medially), and the posterior cricoid esophageal inlet regions are all parts of the hypopharynx, not the larynx proper.

Laryngeal Spaces

Compartments defined by laryngeal structures are as follows:

1. The paraglottic space (bounded by the thyroid cartilage lamina, conus elasticus, and quadrangular membrane)
2. The pre-epiglottis space (bounded by the vallecular mucosa, thyroid cartilage, thyro-hyoid membrane, and epiglottis)

Laryngeal Joints

Cricothyroid Joint

The cricothyroid joint is a synovial joint with a capsular ligament between the inferior cornu of the thyroid cartilage and the facet on the cricoid cartilage at the junction of the arch and the lamina. Two movements occur:

1. Rotation: through a transverse axis
2. Gliding: slightly

Cricoarytenoid Joint

The cricoarytenoid joint is a synovial joint with a capsular ligament between the base of the arytenoid cartilage and the facet on the upper border of the lamina of the cricoid cartilage. Because the arytenoid cartilage has a concave base, its articulation with the cricoid cartilage is a complex one that involves both a sliding and rocking movement of the arytenoid across the cricoid lamina, not just a rotation of the arytenoid cartilage around its vertical axis.

Laryngeal Muscles

The muscles of the larynx may be classified as follows:

1. Extrinsic (depressors and elevators of the larynx); these muscles arise from other sites and insert on the laryngeal skeleton.
2. Accessory (pharyngeal constrictors); these muscles arise from the pharynx and insert on the larynx.
3. Intrinsic (control the positions of the laryngeal cartilages with respect to one another); these muscles arise from within the larynx and insert on the larynx.

The extrinsic muscles of the larynx, concerned with the movement and fixation of the larynx as a whole, consist of elevator and depressor groups.[5–8]

The depressor group consists of the

1. Sternohyoid (C2, C3)
2. Thyrohyoid (C1)
3. Omohyoid (C2, C3)

The elevator group consists of the

1. Geniohyoid (C1)
2. Digastrics (anterior belly—cranial nerve V; posterior belly—nerve VII)
3. Mylohyoid (V)
4. Stylohyoid (VII)

The accessory muscles of the larynx are as follows:

1. *Middle pharyngeal constrictor.* This muscle encircles the hypopharynx and inserts upon the greater cornua of the hyoid bone. Contraction of this muscle pulls the larynx posteriorly and superiorly.
2. *Inferior constrictor.* This muscle has a similar arrangement and is attached to the oblique line of the thyroid cartilage. It also draws the larynx posteriorly and superiorly.
3. *Cricopharyngeus muscle.* This muscle surrounds the esophageal inlet and attaches to the cricoid cartilage. It functions as an upper esophageal sphincter, which releases its tonic state of contraction during swallow to allow bolus passage into the esophagus.

The intrinsic muscles of the larynx are as follows:

1. *Muscles of the quadrangular membrane* (the thyroarytenoid, thyroepiglottic, and aryepiglottic muscles). These form a sheet of striated muscle along the inner surface of the quadrangular membrane. The thyroarytenoid and thyroepiglottic muscles both originate from the posterior midline of the thyroid cartilage. The thyroarytenoid muscle extends nearly horizontally to the vocal process of the arytenoid cartilage. The lateral portion of the thyroarytenoid muscle is oblique. Its medial portion is nearly horizontal and forms the vocalis muscle. The thyroepiglottic muscle is oriented more vertically. The aryepiglottic muscle runs along the free edge of the aryepiglottic fold from the epiglottis to the arytenoid cartilage. The most posterior extensions of this muscle cross over the arytenoid cartilage as the oblique arytenoid muscle.
2. *Muscles of the arytenoid cartilage* (the interarytenoid, posterior cricoarytenoid, and lateral cricoarytenoid muscles). The interarytenoid muscle, also known as the arytenoid muscle, connects the two arytenoid cartilages. The posterior cricoarytenoid muscle originates from the posterior part of the cricoid lamina and inserts upon the posteromedial surface of the muscular process of the arytenoid cartilage. The lateral cricoarytenoid muscle originates from the lateral part of the cricoid arch and inserts upon the anterolateral surface of the muscular process of the arytenoid cartilage.
3. *The cricothyroid muscle.* This muscle arises from the arch of the cricoid cartilage anteriorly and inserts upon the inferior horn and body of the thyroid cartilage above.

Because of the complexity of the cricoarytenoid joint, it is incorrect to conceive of the actions of the intrinsic laryngeal muscles as simple abduction and adduction of the vocal folds.

1. Vocal cord abduction leads to lateral, superior, and posterior displacement of the vocal process of the arytenoid cartilage, while vocal cord adduction leads to medial, inferior, and anterior displacement of the vocal process of the arytenoid cartilage.
2. Each intrinsic laryngeal muscle acts in conjunction with the other intrinsic laryngeal muscles; vocal cord movement results from the net effect of the resultant diverse forces that act upon the arytenoid cartilages.

3. The intrinsic laryngeal muscles also help determine the vibratory characteristics (such as tension, mass per unit length, and cross-sectional contour) of the vocal folds.

With these caveats in mind, primary functions for the intrinsic laryngeal muscles nonetheless may be assigned.[9,10]

1. The posterior cricoarytenoid muscle primarily abducts the vocal cord. Contraction of this muscle pulls the muscular process of the arytenoid cartilage medially and thereby opens the glottis. In the process, the vocal cord is lengthened and its tension is increased.
2. The lateral cricoarytenoid and the thyroarytenoid muscles both adduct the vocal cord. The lateral cricoarytenoid muscle pulls the muscular process of the arytenoid cartilage laterally, narrowing the glottic opening. The length of the vocal cord is also increased by contraction of this muscle. The thyroarytenoid muscle also adducts and shortens the vocal cord. The interarytenoid muscle also theoretically contributes to vocal cord adduction; however, in vivo this muscle most likely contributes to the net position of the arytenoid cartilage, not true arytenoid movement. This muscle is important in approximating the vocal processes and closing of the cartilaginous glottis during phonation.
3. The cricothyroid muscle tenses and also lengthens the vocal cord. Cricothyroid contraction is coordinated with respiration to open the glottic opening so that effective airway resistance is minimized.
4. The vocalis portion of the thyroarytenoid muscle acts as a vocal cord tensor. This muscle also shortens the vocal cord and thickens its cross-sectional area. This muscle acts as an antagonist to the cricothyroid muscle during phonation by adjusting the length, tension, mass, and stiffness of the vocal folds.

Mucous Membrane

Stratified squamous epithelium is found over the vocal cords and the upper part of the vestibule of the larynx. Ciliated columnar epithelium lines the remainder of the cavity.

Mucous glands are found in:

1. False vocal folds, especially the surface facing the ventricles and the saccule
2. Posterior surface of epiglottis
3. Margins of aryepiglottic folds (none on the free edges of the vocal cords)
4. Infraglottic surface of the vocal fold

Vocal Fold Histology[7–14]

The true vocal fold alone participates in the vibratory movements of the larynx. This structure is limited to the membranous portion of the vocal folds and extends from the anterior commissure to the tip of the vocal process of the arytenoid cartilage. The vocal process of the arytenoid cartilage is not considered to be a part of the membranous vocal fold. The true vocal fold is a layered structure composed of the following:

1. Nonkeratinizing, stratified squamous epithelium
2. Superficial layer of the lamina propria (mostly amorphous material, corresponds to Reinke's space)
3. Intermediate layer of the lamina propria (mostly elastic fibers)
4. Deep layer of the lamina propria (mostly collagenous fibers)
5. Vocalis muscle

The intermediate and deep layers of the lamina propria form the vocal ligament, which is the superior free edge of the triangular membrane. The intermediate layer of the lamina propria is thickened anteriorly and posteriorly to form the anterior macula flava and the posterior macula flava, respectively.

Mechanically, the true vocal fold acts as three layers:

1. The cover (the squamous epithelium and superficial layer of the lamina propria)
2. The transitional zone (the intermediate and deep layers of the lamina propria)
3. The body (the vocalis muscle)

Nerve Supply

The larynx is supplied by two branches of the vagus nerve: the superior laryngeal and inferior (recurrent) laryngeal nerves. The superior laryngeal nerve (SLN) divides extralaryngeally into the internal branch (sensory) and the external branch (motor and sensory). Sensory innervation of the anterior subglottis by the external branch of the superior laryngeal nerve has been demonstrated only in the cat model. The larger internal branch supplies sensory innervation to those areas of the larynx above the glottis. This nerve has subdivisions that supply the epiglottis, arytenoid mucosa, and false vocal folds. The smaller external branch gives motor innervation to the cricothyroid muscle and sensory supply to the anterior infraglottic larynx at the level of the cricothyroid membrane. A recent study in dogs has shown that the external branch of the superior laryngeal nerve may provide some motor innervation to the thyroarytenoid muscle as well.[6]

The recurrent (inferior) laryngeal nerve (RLN) supplies motor innervation to all the intrinsic laryngeal muscles of the same side except for the cricothyroid. The anterior branch of the RLN innervates the lateral cricoarytenoid, thyroarytenoid, vocalis, and aryepiglottic muscles, while the posterior branch innervates the posterior cricoarytenoid and interarytenoid muscles. The interarytenoid muscle is the only intrinsic laryngeal muscle to receive bilateral innervation from the RLNs. Recent data suggest that the SLN may also contribute to interarytenoid muscle innervation.[4,5] The RLN also supplies sensory innervation to those portions of the larynx below the glottis. The cricothyroid muscle is innervated by the external branch of the ipsilateral superior laryngeal nerve. The proprioceptive information from the muscle spindles of all the intrinsic laryngeal muscles except the cricothyroid muscle is carried by the ipsilateral recurrent laryngeal nerve. The somatic motor nucleus for this nerve is the nucleus ambiguus, and its sensory component projects to the nucleus solitarius via the nodose ganglion.

Visceral motor input to the larynx is from the dorsal motor nucleus and is carried by the internal branch of the SLN and the RLN to the supraglottic mucosa and the infraglottic mucosa, respectively. The superior cervical ganglion gives rise to the sympathetic innervation.

The nerve of Galen (ramus communicans) connects the SLN and RLN. This nerve innervates the chemoreceptors and baroreceptors of the aortic arch and also gives visceral motor input to the tracheal mucosa, esophageal mucosa, and tracheal smooth muscle.[171]

The RLN has a much longer course on the left side than on the right. On the left side it turns around the arch of the aorta. On the right side it turns around the subclavian artery. In the neck it lies between the trachea and esophagus as it approaches the larynx. Its terminal part passes upward, under cover of the ala of the thyroid cartilage, immediately behind the inferior cricothyroid joint. Rarely, the right RLN does not loop around the right subclavian artery. In these cases, the nerve descends directly to the larynx, and a right retroesophageal subclavian artery, whose origin is distal to the ligamentum arteriosum, is always present.[13]

The nucleus ambiguus is the somatic motor nucleus of cranial nerves IX, X, and XI. The nucleus ambiguus is supplied by the posteroinferior cerebellar artery (branch of the vertebral) and the anteroinferior cerebellar artery (branch of the basilar).

Blood Supply

Upper Larynx

1. External carotid artery
2. Superior thyroid artery
3. Superior laryngeal artery

Lower Larynx

1. Subclavian artery
2. Thyrocervical artery
3. Inferior thyroid artery
4. Inferior laryngeal artery

Venous Drainage

Upper Larynx

1. Superior laryngeal vein
2. Superior thyroid vein
3. Internal jugular vein

Lower Larynx

1. Inferior laryngeal vein
2. Inferior thyroid vein
3. Innominate vein

Lymphatic Drainage

The lymphatics arising from the larynx drain mainly into the deep cervical group of lymph nodes. It is of great clinical importance that the vocal cords themselves contain scarcely any lymphatic channels. At the glottis, the lymphatics are sparse and drain anteriorly and posteriorly with little crossover to the contralateral neck. The lymphatic drainage of the supraglottic and subglottic area is more extensive and has bilateral drainage.

The lymphatic network of the supraglottic structures is extensive. The channels collect in a pedicle at the anterior end of the aryepiglottic fold, pass laterally, anterior to the anterior wall of the pyriform fossa, and leave the larynx with the neurovascular bundle through the thyrohyoid membrane. Almost all (98%) of the channels end in the upper deep cervical nodes between the digastric tendon and the omohyoid muscle. The remainder pass to the lower cervical chain or the spinal accessory chain.

The lymphatics of the infraglottic area have a more variable drainage pattern than those of the supraglottic network. These channels leave the area in three pedicles. The anterior pedicle passes through the cricothyroid membrane, and many vessels end in the prelaryngeal (Delphian) nodes in the region of the thyroid isthmus. Channels then leave these nodes with the remaining anterior channels to travel to the deep inferior cervical nodes. The two posterolateral pedicles leave the larynx through the cricotracheal membrane, with some channels going through the cricotracheal membrane to the paratracheal chain of nodes, whereas others pass to the inferior jugular chain.

Generally, lymphatic drainage from each half of the glottis is separate, and little crossover or mixing occurs. There is evidence that lymphatic channels do cross the midline in the supra- and infraglottic areas. Contralateral drainage is more likely to occur spontaneously from the infraglottic areas; thus lesions of this area may be associated with less consistent patterns of metastasis.

PHYSIOLOGY[7,8]

Basic Functions

Three basic functions of the larynx, in order of importance, are airway protection, respiration, and phonation.

1. Acting as a sphincter, the larynx prevents the entrance of anything but air into the lung.
   a. Closure of the laryngeal inlet
   b. Closure of the glottis
   c. Cessation of respiration
   d. Cough reflex, expulsion of secretions and foreign bodies
2. Respiration governed by active muscular dilation of the laryngeal aperture, assists in the regulation of gaseous exchange with the lung and in the maintenance of acid-base balance.
3. Phonation is voice produced by the vibration of the vocal cords, resulting in the sound source for voice production.
4. Other functions
   a. Fixation of the chest is also a function of the larynx.
   b. Closure of the glottis helps to increase intrathoracic and intra-abdominal pressure and aids in lifting, digging, defecation, vomiting, urination, or childbirth.
   c. The airway protective function of the adult human larynx is admittedly precarious by virtue of its low position in the neck.
      (1) The resting position of the human larynx has a variable position in the neck depending on age. In the newborn, the position of the larynx is high (C1–C2). In the adult, the position of the larynx migrates to C5–C6. During senescence, the larynx may further descend to T1–T2. This puts the larynx at greater risk for aspiration in the elderly.
      (2) The human newborn exhibits a nasolaryngeal connection by approximation of the epiglottis with the posterior surface of the palate, thereby ensuring against aspiration by forming a continuous upper and lower airway. Obligate nasal breathing during the newborn period (1 through 6 months) is related to this anatomic configuration.
      (3) The epiglottis in the adult serves as a laryngeal shield to direct swallowed food laterally into the pyriform fossae and away from the midline laryngeal aperture. This protective function is enhanced by elevation of the larynx toward the nasal cavity during the height of deglutition. The corniculate and cuneiform cartilages are contained in the aryepiglottic folds to provide stiffness and support to these structures.
      (4) Because of their structural configuration, the false cords prevent egress of air from the lungs (providing an expectorative function), whereas the true cords

with their upturned margins are capable of impeding its ingress (protective function).

Neuromuscular Physiology

Afferent System

The density of sensory innervation is greatest in the laryngeal inlet and especially the mucosal surfaces overlying the arytenoid and corniculate cartilages, an observation consistent with its protective function of the distal respiratory tract. Afferent impulses are delivered through the ganglion nodosum to the brain stem tractus solitarius.

Efferent System

Motor distribution to the intrinsic laryngeal musculature originates in the medulla in the nucleus ambiguus. The interarytenoid muscles receive bilateral motor innervation from both RLNs.

The sole abductor is the posterior cricoarytenoid, which is a muscle extending from the posterior aspect of the cricoid plate to the muscular process of the arytenoid. The major laryngeal adductors are the thyroarytenoid and lateral cricoarytenoid muscles. The cricothyroid muscle adducts and tenses the vocal cord, passively lengthening it by 30%. The interarytenoid muscles close the posterior gap in the glottis.

Paralysis of the SLN leads to denervation of the ipsilateral cricothyroid muscle, resulting in rotation of the posterior commissure toward the inactive side from unopposed contraction of the contralateral cricothyroid muscle. Injury to the RLN results in a paramedian vocal cord position because of the adductor action of the intact SLN contracting the ipsilateral cricothyroid muscle.

Position of the Vocal Folds

The position of the vocal folds may be described as being in various positions. These are:

1. Abducted position 30 to 45 degrees from the midline. This is the position of maximal abduction during inspiration.
2. Cadaveric position, or intermediate, 15 to 20 degrees from the midline. This is the position of immediate total denervation of both the SLN and RLN nerves, as in high vagal paralysis.
3. Paramedian position. Just off midline. The resting position of vocal folds after long-term RLN injury.
4. Median position. The position of SLN paralysis and normal larynx during phonation.

Neurophysiology of Protective Function

Humans do not possess a crossed adductor reflex; that is, stimulation of one SLN does not produce simultaneous activation of the contralateral adductor musculature. Therefore, unilateral SLN paralysis may lead to aspiration (failure of ipsilateral cord closure) despite the integrity of both RLNs.

There are three sphincteric tiers of airway protection:

1. Contraction of the superior division of the thyroarytenoid muscles contained in the aryepiglottic folds.
2. Contraction of middle thyroarytenoid fibers in the false cords.
3. Contraction of inferior division of the thyroarytenoid at the level of the true cord. This barrier to aspiration is the most significant one owing to the upturned border of the cord margin.

Stimulation of the SLN—as well as all major cranial afferent, special sensory, and spinal somatic sensory nerves—produces strong laryngeal adductor responses, emphasizing the primitive role of respiratory protection from a wide variety of potentially noxious stimuli. Laryngeal spasm is mediated solely by the SLN. Superior laryngeal nerve stimulation also produces inhibition of laryngeal abductor activity, resulting in various degrees of reflex apnea.

Respiratory Function

Widening of the glottis occurs with rhythmic bursts of activity in the RLN. The glottis opens a fraction of a second before air is drawn in by the descent of the diaphragm. Electromyelographic (EMG) studies show that phasic inspiratory abduction, via muscular contraction of the posterior cricoarytenoids, is synchronous with respiration. The degree of abductor activity varies directly with the degree of ventilatory resistance (eg, decreases with tracheotomy). Phasic inspiratory contraction of the cricothyroid muscle (vocal cord adductor and isotonic tensor) increases the anteroposterior diameter of the glottic chink. Therefore, both the posterior cricoarytenoid and cricothyroid muscles are driven by the medullary respiratory center.

Phonation

Speech results from the production of a fundamental tone at the level of the true vocal folds of the larynx. This initial speech signal is then modified by the resonating chambers of the upper aerodigestive tract.

Two theories have been produced to explain human speech production:

1. The myoelastic-aerodynamic theory
2. The neuromuscular theory (also known as the neurochronaxic theory)

Myoelastic-Aerodynamic Theory

During expiration, the air current flowing through the glottis is unidirectional and the vocal cords vibrate, cutting off the airflow and then permitting airflow. This results in the vocal folds serving to direct airflow to an alternating airflow modulator. The sequence of events is as follows. The laryngeal muscles first position the vocal cords (various degrees of adduction) and place them under the appropriate longitudinal tension. Next, muscular and passive forces of exhalation cause the subglottic air pressure to increase. Subglottic air pressure reaches a point where it exceeds muscular opposition, and the glottic chink is forced open. When the vocal cords start opening from complete closure, they open in an inferior to superior direction. After the release of the puff of air, there is a reduction of subglottic pressure, and the vocal cords approximate each other again. The myoelastic forces are the deformed vocal folds' natural tendency to resume their natural configuration. (The myoelastic forces of the vocal cords exceed the aerodynamic forces.) The myoelastic forces are enhanced because air current flowing through a narrow channel exerts a negative pressure on the channel walls (Bernouilli effect). This effect is combined with the myoelastic forces of the vocal folds to close the vocal folds. The vocal cords are thus sucked back together in an approximated state until the subglottic air pressure can overcome the myoelastic forces of the reapproximated cords, and the cycle is thereby repeated.

The resulting waveform of the vocal cords is not sinusoidal but sawtooth in type and can be classified as a relaxation oscillator. The oscillation frequency is quasi-periodic and accounts for the ability to produce a clear tone with sound production. An unvoiced output (glottis opened) has no such oscillatory properties and is essentially a noise.

Neuromuscular or Neurochronaxic Theory

This theory, now disproved, suggested that each new vibratory cycle is initiated by central neuronal impulses via the vagus nerve to the appropriate laryngeal muscles. According to this theory, the rate of impulses delivered to the larynx determines the frequency of vocal cord vibration. Physiologic and audiometric analyses have led us to believe that this theory is untrue (eg, voice is still produced in a patient with bilateral vocal cord paralysis).

Vocal Tract Components

The human vocal tract may be divided into multiple components[14]:

1. *Activator.* The pulmonary system, including the lungs and the muscles of respiration, produce the airflow that powers the true vocal fold vibrations.
2. *Sound source generator.* The true vocal folds act as vibrators.
3. *Resonator.* The cavities of the supraglottis, hypopharynx, oropharynx, and nasopharynx modulate the sound signal by acting as resonance chambers whose fundamental resonant frequency may be finely adjusted by altering the three-dimensional configuration of these spaces.
4. *Articulators.* The palate, tongue, teeth, and lips are used to further modulate the sound signal.

Glottic Closure Reflex: Control Mechanisms

Reflex laryngeal closure is produced by rapid contraction of the thyroarytenoid muscle in response to SLN stimulation. Exaggerated reflex glottic closure leads to laryngospasm, which is maintained well beyond the cessation of mucosal irritation. Obstructive apnea secondary to prolonged laryngospasm may produce death by acute hypoxia and hypercapnia. The body's fail-safe mechanism in dealing with this phenomenon is that laryngospasm is inhibited by (1) increased arterial carbon dioxide pressure (Pco_2), (2) decreased arterial oxygen pressure (Po_2), (3) positive intrathoracic pressure, and (4) inspiratory phase of respiration. The most common causes of laryngospasm are inhaled irritants, gastric acid refluxed into the larynx, manipulation of the upper aerodigestive tract (eg, extubation), foreign bodies, and mucus or blood in the glottic chink.

Arrhythmia, bradycardia, and occasionally cardiac arrest may result from stimulating the larynx.[7,15] The mechanism appears to be related to stimulation of nerve fibers that arise in aortic baroreceptors and, in some individuals, travel to the central nervous system (CNS) by way of the RLN, ramus communicans, and SLN. They can result from light anesthesia, prolonged laryngoscopy, repeated attempts at intubation, respiratory obstruction, and tracheal irritation. The reflex cardiac effects can be controlled by atropine and are enhanced by morphine.

SELECTED DISORDERS

Inflammatory Diseases

Acute Epiglottitis

Acute epiglottitis[16–23] is a special form of rapidly progressive acute laryngitis in which the inflammatory changes primarily involve the epiglottis. It occurs mainly in children aged 2 to 7 years, although infants, older children, and even adults may be affected.[23,24]

Etiology is *Haemophilus influenzae* type B. Symptoms include the following:

1. Rapidly progressive dyspnea, especially in children, may be fatal within a few hours of onset unless immediately diagnosed and treated. This is a medical emergency.
2. Dysphagia starts with sore throat, difficulty in swallowing, then refusal of oral feedings.
3. Dehydration, fever, tachycardia, restlessness, and exhaustion with respiratory and circulatory collapse may be present.
4. The voice usually is not hoarse but may present as a "hot potato voice."
5. Patient prefers the upright position and leaning slightly forward. Do not place the patient in a recumbent position.
6. The most important clinical feature is the swollen, bright red epiglottis obstructing the pharynx at the base of the tongue.
7. A patient who is already in extreme respiratory distress may develop total airway obstruction when an attempt is made to visualize the epiglottis. A quick look at the epiglottis in the emergency room with a tongue blade is to be condemned. In the adult patient, transnasal fiberoptic laryngoscopy may be performed to safely visualize the supraglottic larynx. In cases of acute epiglottitis, a grossly swollen and erythematous ("cherry red") epiglottis will be seen. Soft tissue radiographs of the neck will be diagnostic in children and adults. Typical findings include "thumbprinting" of the epiglottis and effacement of the valleculae.
8. Blood culture may show *H. influenzae* type B.

Changes have occurred in the management of acute epiglottitis. Data suggest that orotracheal intubation is the preferred method of treatment for acute epiglottitis. The following steps of management are recommended:

1. The patient suspected of acute epiglottitis is evaluated in the emergency room by a team consisting of a pediatrician, anesthesiologist, and otolaryngologist.
2. A lateral extended neck x-ray film is obtained with a physician in attendance. Oral examination with a tongue depressor is not advised.
3. The patient is immediately taken to the operating room if the x-ray film is diagnostic or progressive epiglottitis is suspected.
4. Orotracheal intubation is performed with an anesthesiologist and an otolaryngologist present, and the patient is prepared for immediate bronchoscopy and/or tracheotomy.
5. The otolaryngologist examines the epiglottis by direct laryngoscopy, and the epiglottis and blood are cultured. The endotracheal tube is replaced by a nasotracheal tube, which is firmly secured by tape and a string around the neck.
6. The patient is transferred to the intensive care unit (ICU) for close observation. Restraints to prevent accidental self-extubation may be necessary.
7. Antibiotic therapy with adequate coverage for beta-lactamase–producing *H. influenzae* must be instituted. (In certain regions of the United States, some 20% or more of *H. influenzae* isolates produce beta-lactamase.) Antibiotics of choice include ampicillin/sulbactam, cefuroxime, and ceftriaxone. Aztreonam and chloramphenicol may be used in patients with penicillin or cephalosporin allergies.
8. Steroids may be of value in limiting the progression of inflammation and edema.
9. Extubation is done 24 to 48 hours after intubation if direct laryngoscopy at bedside shows a decrease in the supraglottic edema.

10. The patient is observed for an additional 24 to 48 hours and discharged with appropriate antibiotic therapy for a total of 10 days.

11. It is important to emphasize that skilled nursing staff familiar with the management of acute cardiorespiratory problems is necessary following nasotracheal intubation, and that the anesthesiologist and otolaryngologist should always be available in the event of self-extubation. In an institution where the special 24-hour pediatric ICU is not available or for those responsible for the occasional case, it is safer to rely on the time-tested tracheotomy.

12. Because complete obstruction can occur with alarming suddenness, nasotracheal intubation or tracheotomy should be performed as soon as the diagnosis of acute epiglottitis is made. When possible, this should be done after secured orotracheal intubation is done.

13. In regard to acute epiglottitis in the adult, a study has shown that patients who present within 8 hours from the onset of symptoms usually require airway intervention[23,24] in the form of orotracheal intubation or tracheotomy. Most patients who present more than 8 hours after the onset of symptoms do not develop acute respiratory obstruction and are treated medically. An artificial airway is indicated in all patients who have significant drooling. Studies have shown a significant decrease in the incidence of epiglottitis in children with the widespread use of *H. influenzae* B vaccine. However, the relative incidence of acute epiglottitis in adults appears to be increasing.[18–20,22]

Adult Supraglottitis[21,23]

Adult supraglottitis differs from the pediatric form of the disease in that it is caused by different infectious organisms. Multiple sites in the larynx and oropharynx are inflamed, but the epiglottis may not be the most involved area. Acute supraglottitis is a potentially fatal process, and early in the course, a rapidly developing severe sore throat may be the most reliable indicator of an impending airway obstruction.[21] In the study by Shapiro and associates, *H. influenzae* was not found in any patient, nor did any patient experience respiratory compromise. Epiglottitis is apparently an erroneous term for this disorder. The non–*H. influenzae* adult type of supraglottitis appears to follow a less pernicious course than classic epiglottitis. While supraglottitis in adults is sometimes associated with *H. influenzae,* many other bacterial agents have been implicated. Despite the variety of etiologic organisms, antibiotic therapy that covers *H. influenzae* is recommended. Broad-spectrum antibiotics that cover *H. influenzae* include ampicillin/sulbactam, cefuroxime, ceftriaxone, aztreonam, and chloramphenicol.

Acute Laryngotracheobronchitis ("Croup")

Laryngotracheobronchitis is an acute infection of the lower respiratory passages, extending from the larynx into the smaller subdivisions of the bronchial tree. It is endemic throughout the year but may react in epidemic proportions in any locality during the winter season.

Etiology is probably a virus. Parainfluenza types 1 to 4 have been isolated frequently. *H. influenzae,* streptococci, staphylococci, and pneumococci are commonly cultured. The disease occurs in children, especially between the ages of 1 and 3 years.

Pathology is descending inflammation of the mucous membrane lining the lower respiratory tract, followed by congestion, edema, and exudation of a thick, tenacious secretion. Anatomically, the conus elasticus is the most involved site.

Symptoms are as follows:

1. At the onset, the disease is like an ordinary cold except for the early presence of a croupy cough.

2. Hoarseness is noted shortly thereafter.
3. As the swelling increases, inspiratory stridor develops.
4. Retractions then occur.
5. Circumoral pallor and cyanosis usually precede a decrease in breath sounds, which, in turn, is an indication that death may be imminent. Immediate establishment of an airway is mandatory.
6. In addition to these symptoms of respiratory embarrassment, anorexia and fever are common in the early stages, and restlessness, dehydration, and exhaustion may be noted later.
7. Agitation and an increased pulse (to 140) and respiration rate (to 80) are signs of increasing levels of CO_2.
8. An anteroposterior soft tissue radiograph of the neck will reveal the "steeple" sign (subglottic narrowing due to edema).

Treatment regimen is as follows:

1. Hospitalization and close observation.
2. Ultrasonic humidification (an important treatment).
3. Antibiotic coverage is similar to that for acute epiglottitis. Ampicillin/sulbactam, cefuroxime, or ceftriaxone may be used. Aztreonam or chloramphenicol is indicated in patients with histories of penicillin or cephalosporin allergies. Lastly, the combination of cefazolin and sulfonamide, or the combination of nafcillin and sulfonamide, are possible alternatives.
4. Racemic epinephrine via intermittent positive-pressure breathing (IPPB).
5. Corticosteroids (100 mg hydrocortisone IM on admission) may be helpful.
6. Sedation is contraindicated, as it may compromise the airway.
7. Parenteral fluids.
8. Oxygen.
9. Timely endotracheal intubation or tracheotomy. When in doubt, do it. Progressive retraction associated with agitation, cyanosis, lethargy, and an increased pulse (to 140), respiration rate (to 80), and CO_2 level is an indication for immediate nasotracheal intubation or tracheotomy.

Aspecific Membranous Laryngitis
1. Rare but serious complication of viral infections.
2. Mucopus and sloughed epithelium from a pseudomembrane in the supraglottis, which may cause obstruction.
3. Differential diagnosis includes diphtheria, epiglottitis, viral or bacterial croup, and laryngotracheal bronchitis.
4. Treatment is endoscopy and antibiotics.

Bacterial Tracheitis
1. Rare but serious complication of viral and laryngotracheal bronchitis.
2. Offending organisms are staphylococcus, streptococcus, and *Streptococcus pneumoniae*.
3. Presents with high fever, stridor, and symptoms of upper airway obstruction.
4. Tracheal cast of sloughed debris may cause obstruction.
5. There is a high incidence of progression to pneumonia.
6. Treatment is by bronchoscopy, lavage, and intubation.

Tuberculous Laryngitis[25,26]

Tuberculous laryngitis is almost always secondary to active pulmonary tuberculosis.
Pathology is as follows:

1. Cellular infiltration.
2. Tuberculous granuloma in the subepithelial tissue. The avascular tubercle consists of an area of central caseation surrounded by epithelial cells and a peripheral zone of mononuclear cells. The individual nodules coalesce into larger lesions.
3. The tubercles are surrounded by fibrous tissue (capsule).
4. Perichondritis and cartilage necrosis.
5. Granulation tissue or multiple small superficial ulcers in the interarytenoid space, false and true cords, and the epiglottis.

Symptoms include the following:

1. Hoarseness.
2. Cough (late) with production of blood-streaked sputum.
3. Pain and referred earache are fairly common.
4. In advanced cases, dyspnea from edema of the larynx and scar contraction or destruction of underlying cartilages.
5. Direct laryngoscopy and biopsy are essential in order to establish the diagnosis. Of note, both tuberculous granuloma and the pemphigoid lesion share many histopathologic features; however, tuberculous granuloma is subepithelial, while the pemphigus lesion is intraepithelial.
6. The most common site of tuberculosis of the larynx is the posterior larynx (interarytenoid fold). The next most common site is the laryngeal surface of the epiglottis.

Some studies, however, show no predisposition for posterior laryngeal involvement. In a study of 15 patients with laryngeal tuberculosis by Thaller and associates,[26] involvement of true vocal cord was noted in 10 patients, epiglottic lesions in 4 patients, and arytenoid and interarytenoid areas in only 2 patients.
Treatment is as follows:

1. Isoniazid and rifampin. The emergence of mycobacteria with multiple drug resistances requires at least consideration of the inclusion of additional antibiotics in the treatment regimen. Possibilities include ethambutol and pyrazinamide. More aggressive antibiotic treatment is also required for all patients infected with HIV.
2. Treatment of pulmonary lesion.
3. Voice rest.
4. Narcotics for pain.
5. Injection of the superior laryngeal nerve with procaine (Novocaine) or alcohol for relief of pain.
6. Tracheotomy for obstruction.
7. Surgery for secondary stenosis if indicated.

If diagnosed and treated early, prognosis is good. If the local manifestations include cartilaginous involvement, the prognosis is more serious, as irreparable harm may have been inflicted on the framework or soft tissues of the larynx.

Syphilitic Laryngitis

Etiology of syphilitic laryngitis is *Treponema pallidum.* The disorder is extremely rare in the congenital form and now rare also in the acquired form.

The larynx is never affected in the primary stage of the disease. During the secondary stage, infection and mild edema of the larynx are common and mucous patches may be observed; these lesions are temporary and disappear with the resolution of this phase. The gummas are characteristic of laryngeal involvement in the tertiary stage. Ultimate breakdown of these lesions results in the development of ulcerations, perichondritis, and fibrosis.

Symptoms include the following:

1. Mild hoarseness is often the only symptom. Gummas and ulcerations may lead to varying degrees of hoarseness.
2. There is no pain.
3. As the swelling increases or fibrosis develops, symptoms of respiratory embarrassment may occur.

The diagnosis is confirmed by serologic tests (RPR, VDRL, and FTA-ABS) and biopsy. Treatment is as follows:

1. Penicillin or tetracycline. (Prolonged antibiotic treatment may be required in patients infected with HIV.)
2. Supportive measures.
3. Tracheotomy for respiratory obstruction.
4. Reconstructive operation for severe laryngeal stenosis.

With early lesions, the prognosis is quite favorable, but destruction of cartilage causes permanent changes.

Scleroma of the Larynx[27]

Klebsiella rhinoscleromatis (von Frisch bacillus) causes scleroma of the larynx, which is rare in the United States.

Symptoms are as follows:

1. Hoarseness, cough, and increasing dyspnea.
2. The most common site of sclerosis of the larynx is the subglottic region.
3. Many present with subglottic and/or glottic stenosis or granulomas.[27]
4. Pale pinkish swelling may be seen below the vocal cords.

Treatment is as follows:

1. Oral tetracycline.
2. Steroids.
3. May require endoscopy, dilation, or laser excision.
4. Tracheotomy may be needed.

Perichondritis of the Larynx

There are several causes of perichondritis of the larynx.

1. Infection (eg, tuberculosis, syphilis, septic laryngitis)
2. Trauma
3. High tracheotomy

4. Radiotherapy
5. Neoplasm with secondary infection

Perichondritis leads to subperichondrial abscess, necrosis of cartilage, and later stenosis. Perichondritis of the thyroid cartilage is more common than perichondritis of the epiglottis because the epiglottis is fibroelastic cartilage, whereas the perichondrium adheres to the cartilage.

Symptoms are as follows:

1. Insidious or of sudden onset
2. Fever and malaise (acute form)
3. Local pain and tenderness
4. Enlargement of laryngeal framework, swelling of the neck
5. Abscess and fistula
6. Hoarseness, cough, dysphagia, dyspnea

Diagnosis requires that syphilis, malignant disease, or an unsuspected foreign body be ruled out.

Treatment is as follows:

1. Hospitalization.
2. Systemic antibiotics and steroids.
3. Tracheotomy.
4. Incision and drainage of intralaryngeal fluid collection.
5. Dilation for stenosis.
6. Laryngofissure for debridement.
7. Laryngectomy for extensive necrosis of a cartilage.
8. Some patients with perichondritis after radiation therapy benefit with use of hyperbaric oxygen therapy.

Glanders
Glanders is a serious infectious disease marked by the occurrence of multiple granulomatous abscesses throughout the body caused by *Pseudomonas (Actinobacillus) mallei.* Perichondritis and cartilage destruction may complicate the laryngeal disease.

Leprosy
Leprosy of the larynx is rare. The disease affects the larynx in 10% of the cases and is caused by *Mycobacterium leprae,* or Hansen's bacillus. It is treated as follows:

1. DDS (diaminophenylsulfone; dapsone) for 1 to 4 years
2. Corticosteroids
3. Tracheotomy

Diphtheritic Laryngitis
Diphtheritic laryngitis is rare. It is caused by *Corynebacterium diphtheriae.*
Its symptoms are as follows:

1. Onset is insidious.
2. Hoarse, croupy cough is the first symptom.
3. Grayish-white membrane appears on the larynx. Its removal is followed by bleeding.

Treatment is as follows:

1. Antitoxin
2. Penicillin
3. Tracheotomy

Mycotic Infection of the Larynx

Fungal infections of the larynx are rare. Blastomycosis, histoplasmosis, and candidiasis are the most commonly encountered.

BLASTOMYCOSIS[28]   Blastomycosis is seen in endemic proportions in North America (southwestern United States) and is mainly a disease of the skin and lungs. However, primary involvement of the larynx does occur. It is caused by *Blastomyces dermatitidis* and is characterized by diffuse nodular infiltration of the larynx, vocal cord fixation, ulcer, and stenosis.

The epithelium undergoes marked hyperplasia of the pseudoepithelial type and may be mistaken for carcinoma. Microabscesses containing the organisms, giant cells, and mononuclear cells occur in the epidermis and dermis and are characteristic of this disease. Definitive diagnosis is made by isolating the yeast forms on culture.

Symptoms include the following:

1. Hoarseness and cough occur early.
2. Dyspnea and dysphagia are late symptoms.
3. In the early stage, the laryngeal mucosa is diffusely inflamed and granular.
4. Tiny miliary nodules may be seen on the vocal cords.
5. In the advanced stage, mucosal ulceration is covered with foul-smelling, greenish exudate, under which is a bright red granular bed.
6. Later, fibrosis, fixation of arytenoids, or stenosis develops.

Treatment is intravenous amphotericin B. Less severe infection may be treated with ketoconazole or itraconazole.

HISTOPLASMOSIS   Histoplasmosis is caused by *Histoplasma capsulatum* and is usually associated with pulmonary histoplasmosis. Treatment is with amphotericin B. *H. capsulatum* has a worldwide distribution and is endemic to the Ohio, Mississippi, and Missouri River valleys in the United States. Acute pulmonary histoplasmosis may not require antifungal therapy. When symptoms are severe, treatment may include amphotericin B, ketoconazole, fluconazole, or itraconazole. With disseminated histoplasmosis, immune compromise is often present. Treatment in these cases should be with amphotericin B. The "azole" antifungals may be less effective in these cases.

CANDIDIASIS (MONILIASIS)   The etiologic organism is *Candida albicans.* This disease is characterized by white patches on a bright red mucosa. Patients with candidiasis are commonly immunocompromised (infected with HIV or receiving chemotherapy). Immunocompetent individuals who are receiving broad-spectrum antibiotics also may develop candidiasis. Another etiology contributing to development of laryngeal candidiasis is the use of inhaled corticosteroids. Treatment is with topical nystatin, clotrimazole, or miconazole. Withholding of the offending steroid spray is effective. Oral antifungal agents, such as fluconazole or ketoconazole, may be required. Rarely, intravenous amphotericin B may be necessary.

ACTINOMYCOSIS   Actinomycosis, caused by *Actinomyces bovis,* is characterized by a yellowish, granulomatous infiltration that suppurates. It involves the neck and perilaryngeal structures. Treatment is with penicillin or tetracycline.

COCCIDIOIDOMYCOSIS   Caused by *Coccidioides immitis,* coccidioidomycosis is endemic in the southwestern United States. It is more often seen in nonwhite races. The lesion consists of nodular masses of granulomatous tissue.

Benign Tumors of the Larynx

Benign tumors of the larynx[1-4] are relatively uncommon. They occur in the following order of frequency: papilloma, chondroma, neurofibroma, leiomyoma, angiofibroma, myoma, hemangioma, and chemodectoma.

Papilloma

Papilloma[30-39] is the most common benign tumor of the larynx and occurs in patients of all ages. The causative agent is thought to be human papillomavirus. It seems to be related to hormonal changes. Papillomas usually regress during puberty.

The pathology is as follows:

1. Papillary epithelial tumor usually involving the true cords but may affect supraglottic and subglottic regions.
2. May also involve the trachea and bronchus.
3. Papilloma in juveniles is more often multiple and recurs more frequently than in adults.
4. Papillomas in adults are usually single but may undergo malignant change. This may be seen with specific subtypes, ie, HPV 16.
5. Malignant transformation is more common with papilloma subtypes 6 and 11.
6. In an analog study of 113 patients with laryngeal papillomatosis by Quiney and coworkers,[33] 26 patients had juvenile-onset disease and 87 acquired the disease as adults. About half of the patients with juvenile-onset disease were women; most patients with adult-onset disease were men. Seventy-three percent of single lesions were on the true vocal cord and more than 50% of lesions that spread to more than one site involved the vocal cord. Multiple discrete lesions were more likely to appear on both vocal cords. The true vocal cord predominated as the initial site in men; distribution was more random in women. In juvenile-onset disease the initial sites were much more random and more likely to involve both vocal cords, the anterior commissure, and supraglottis from the onset. Multiple and confluent lesions were more common in women with juvenile-onset disease than in men. Single-site lesions in adults had the best prognosis, and multiple confluent lesions in girls had the worst prognosis.

Symptoms are as follows:

1. Aphonia or weak cry is usually the first sign in infants.
2. Dyspnea and stridor are seen.
3. Hoarseness is the most common symptom in adults.

Treatment includes the following:

1. Suspension microlaryngoscopy with CO_2 laser excision is the most commonly employed treatment modality. Multiple excisions are usually required. The laser is favored because

of its hemostatic properties, and its precision allows for vaporization of the lesion without harming the underlying vocal fold.[172]

2. Tracheotomy is occasionally necessary but should be avoided due to concern about subglottic spread. If a tracheotomy is necessary, early decannulation after debridement is recommended.

3. Cryosurgery.[33]

4. Photodynamic therapy.

5. Autogenous vaccine.

6. Avidano and Singleton[37] have shown that significant benefit is seen using adjuvant therapy with systemic interferon, and methotrexate for recalcitrant cases. In their study, juvenile-onset disease had a slightly higher response to interferon than adult-onset disease. Studies evaluating the benefits of intralesional alpha-interferon are also in progress.

7. In view of a high incidence of recurrence, thyrotomy and pharyngotomy are not recommended.

8. Cidofovir, a new antiviral agent approved for ocular cytomegalovirus (CMV) infections, has shown promise as a local injection in adjuvant therapy.

9. Irradiation is contraindicated because of its carcinogenic effects.

Chondroma

Chondroma[1–4,40–42] is a slow-growing lesion composed mainly of hyaline cartilage. It affects men more often than women.

The most frequent site of origin is the internal aspect of the posterior plate of the cricoid cartilage, followed by the thyroid, arytenoid, and epiglottis.

Symptoms include the following:

1. Hoarseness, dyspnea, and dysphagia (in that order) are the presenting symptoms.

2. A full sensation within the throat may be present.

3. The symptoms are insidious.

4. Dyspnea and hoarseness are prominent with a subglottic mass arising from the internal aspect of the cricoid.

5. The dysphagia is more common in lesions arising from the posterior aspect of the cricoid.

6. Hoarseness is due to restriction of cord mobility by the mass.

7. Laryngoscopic examination shows a smooth, firm, round, or nodular, fixed tumor covered by normal mucosa. Currently the imaging modality of choice is computed tomography (CT).

8. Chondroma of the thyroid, cricoid, or tracheal cartilage may be present as a hard neck mass.

9. A soft tissue film, laminogram, and laryngogram delineate the extent and site of the lesion.

10. Calcification is commonly seen on x-ray film.

Treatment is as follows:

1. Surgical excision: the site of origin determines the approach.

2. Thyrotomy for tumors of the anterior aspect of the cricoid.

3. A lateral external approach, with or without pharyngotomy, for chondromas of the thyroid, posterior aspect of the cricoid, or the arytenoid cartilages.

4. Recurrence is common if the tumor is not removed completely. Peroral removal is not advised.
5. Total laryngectomy may be necessary for treatment of recurrences.
6. Reconstruction of cricoid cartilage defect by suturing the inferior cornu of the thyroid cartilage to the first tracheal ring obviates the need for total laryngectomy in selected cases.[42]

Neurofibroma
Neurofibroma is a rare tumor arising from Schwann cells. The tumor most commonly arises from the aryepiglottic fold. The incidence favors women 2 to 1.

Granular Cell Myoblastoma
Granular cell myoblastomas are thought to be of neurogenic origin. They occur in any age group and preponderantly affect men. The lesion usually occurs at the posterior aspect of the true cords or arytenoids. The lesion is small, sessile, and gray. Hoarseness is often the only symptom. The mucosa may show pseudoepitheliomatous hyperplasia. Treatment is excision by direct laryngoscopy.

Adenoma
Adenomas are rare. They arise from the mucous glands. The most common site is the false cord or ventricle. Treatment is excision perorally or by thyrotomy.

Chemodectoma
Chemodectomas arise from paraganglion tissue. They usually are seen in the false cord and aryepiglottic fold, and are smooth, cystic, and red. Biopsy may be associated with bleeding. Treatment is surgical excision via lateral pharyngotomy.

Lipoma
Lipoma is a rare, pedunculated or submucosal tumor that usually arises from the aryepiglottic fold, epiglottis, true cord, and pharyngeal wall. Treatment is (1) excision via laryngoscope for a pedunculated lesion or (2) lateral pharyngotomy for a submucous tumor.

Hemangioma[43–48]
Hemangiomas are more common in children than in adults. They occur on vocal cords, subglottic regions, and the pyriform sinus. Subglottic hemangioma is the most common neoplasm of the infant airway. Treatment is excision, which is best handled by suspension microlaryngoscopy with CO_2 or Nd:YAG laser (for a small angioma) or lateral pharyngotomy (for a large angioma). Intralesional or systemic steroids are a useful adjuvant to laser therapy. With massive or life-threatening hemangiomas, daily subcutaneous alpha-interferon has been shown to hasten their involution.[43–48]

Pseudoepithelial Hyperplasia
Pseudoepithelial hyperplasia is a benign epithelial change that may resemble carcinoma. It can be caused by the following:

1. Tuberculosis
2. Syphilis
3. Granular cell myoblastoma
4. Blastomycosis
5. Pachyderma laryngis

6. Radiation
7. Papillary keratosis (premalignant)

When a diagnosis of pseudoepithelial hyperplasia is made, further biopsy or studies may be necessary to rule out blastomycosis, granular cell myoblastoma, and so forth.

Cysts and Tumor-like Lesions of the Larynx

Retention Cyst

Retention cysts occur most often where mucous glands are abundant. The false cord, ventricle, epiglottis, and aryepiglottic fold are potential sites. Treatment is (1) laryngoscopic removal or (2) marsupialization.

Prolapse of the Ventricle

Ventricular prolapse is protrusion of ventricular mucosa between the true and false cords. It is frequently associated with chronic bronchitis, and the presenting symptom is hoarseness. A sessile pink mass arising between the false and true cords is seen. Treatment is laryngoscopic removal with a forceps.

Laryngocele

Laryngocele is an air-filled dilation of the appendix of the ventricle. There are three types:

1. External laryngocele. In the more common form, the sac protrudes above the thyroid cartilage and the thyrohyoid membrane and presents as a mass in the neck.
2. Internal laryngocele. Less common, in which the sac remains within the thyroid cartilage.
3. A combined type may also be present.

The etiology is unknown. Symptoms may include the following:

1. External laryngocele presents as a swelling in the neck which increases in size with increased intralaryngeal pressure.
2. Internal laryngocele presents with hoarseness and dyspnea.
3. Laryngoscopy may show a smooth dilation at the false cord level involving the false cord and aryepiglottic fold.

Diagnosis is as follows:

1. Characteristic clinical history (as outlined above).
2. Typical appearance of a bulging laryngeal mass, visualized during indirect laryngoscopy, fiberoptic laryngoscopy, or direct laryngoscopy.
3. CT or magnetic resonance imaging (MRI). Because these imaging modalities provide excellent anatomic detail, they help distinguish among the three subtypes of laryngocele and guide surgical therapy.

Treatment is (1) laryngoscopic decompression for small lesions, (2) lateral external approach for larger lesions, or (3) laser endoscopy.[49,50]

Miscellaneous Benign Lesions

Contact Ulcer of the Larynx

Contact ulcers and granulomas[51] appear to be caused by vocal abuse or nonlinguistic laryngeal trauma, such as repeated harsh coughing or persistent throat clearing. Allergic rhinosinusitis causing postnasal drip may also be a factor. Many patients have a hiatal hernia or extraesophageal reflux disease, predisposing to reflux of gastric contents and acid into the pharynx, with resulting coughing, laryngospasm, and harsh throat clearing. Contact ulcers and granulomas heal when the hiatal hernia, gastric reflux, and peptic esophagitis are treated adequately.[51]

The most common site of the lesion is the vocal process of the arytenoid. Symptoms include the following:

1. Hoarseness
2. Pain on phonation
3. Typical ulceration

Treatment consists of the following:

1. Absolute voice rest.
2. Vocal re-education.
3. Eradication of chronic sinusitis and gastroesophageal reflux.
4. Antibiotics/decongestants/nasal steroids and antireflux therapy.
5. If conservative methods fail, endoscopic removal may be needed.

Vocal Nodules (Singer's Nodules)

Vocal nodules may be considered localized traumatic laryngitis. They are caused by the following:

1. Vocal overuse: Screaming (children), harsh talking (adults), and faulty techniques in singers.
2. Predisposing factors: Ectomorphic and athletic body type, vociferous and aggressive personalities.
3. Precipitating factors: Allergy, thyroid and emotional imbalance, upper respiratory infection, sinusitis.
4. Aggravating factors: Cigarette smoking and alcohol.

Pathologically there are two types.

1. Acute or fresh type (soft, reddish, vascular, edematous).
2. Chronic or mature type (hard, white, thickened, fibrosed).

The site of vocal injury is the epithelium and the basement membrane of the vocal fold.

Clinical features include the following:

1. Found more often in women, children (more often in boys), professional singers, lecturers.
2. Hoarseness.
3. The most common site is at the junction of the anterior and middle thirds, usually bilateral (Table 31-1). (The middle part of the membranous vocal cord has the greatest amplitude of vibration and hence is most likely to develop singer's nodule.)

Treatment for children includes the following:

1. Parent counseling
2. Psychotherapeutic rehabilitation using behavioral modification
3. Vocal reeducation
4. Microlaryngoscopic excision in rare cases unresponsive to voice therapy

TABLE 31-1. THE MOST COMMON SITES OF BENIGN LARYNGEAL LESIONS

Lesion	Most Common Site	Side
Contact ulcer	Vocal process of arytenoid	Unilateral or bilateral
Laryngeal polyp	Junction of anterior and middle third	Usually unilateral
Vocal cord nodule	Junction of anterior and middle third	Bilateral
Intubation granuloma	Vocal process of the arytenoid	About 50% bilateral

Treatment for adults includes the following:

1. Voice rest.
2. Voice therapy.
3. Microlaryngoscopic excision or laser vaporization followed by voice therapy. Voice surgery must be done with attention to avoid the consequences of scar.[173]

Intubation Granuloma

The cause of intubation granuloma is endotracheal incubation. It appears only in adults. The incidence is higher in women, 4 to 1. Because of the relatively smaller size of the female larynx, the tube falls more to the posterior commissure. It is invariably seen on the vocal process of the arytenoid.

Treatment includes the following:

1. Excision when pedunculated.
2. Medical treatment with antibiotics, antacids, and steroids may be effective in reducing the intubation granuloma.
3. Attempts to remove during the sessile stage are avoided, as recurrence is likely.
4. Microlaryngoscopic laser excision appears to be more effective than surgical excision. Intubation granuloma may make extubation of the patient with prolonged intubation very difficult. In cases where extubation failure is attributed to intubation granuloma, empiric therapy with a 3- to 5-day course of a first-generation cephalosporin antibiotic and corticosteroids may be instituted prior to a second extubation attempt.

Sarcoidosis

Sarcoidosis[1-4,52-54] is a systemic granulomatous disease of unknown etiology. It affects primarily the lung and mediastinal nodes, but laryngeal involvement may occur in 1 to 5% of all patients with sarcoidosis.

A diagnosis of sarcoidosis is established by biopsy evidence of noncaseating granulomas and exclusion of fungal infections and other granulomatous diseases. Serum levels of angiotensin-1 converting enzyme and gallium scanning have been shown to be of value in the diagnosis and follow-up of patients with sarcoidosis. The Kveim skin test, although rarely used today, supports the diagnosis when positive.

The lesion is characterized by a noncaseating granuloma. The lack of caseation distinguishes sarcoidosis from tuberculosis pathologically. Because the disease occurs submucosally, ulcerations are rare.

Symptoms include the following:

1. Hoarseness is the prominent feature.
2. Pain usually is not present.

3. If the lesion is large, dyspnea may be present.
4. The epiglottis is most often involved, typically with small nodules at the free margin that can become a confluent, indurated swelling. Other areas commonly affected are the aryepiglottic folds, arytenoids, false cords, and subglottic areas. The true vocal cords are rarely involved.
5. Diffuse edema and exophytic masses may cause airway obstruction.
6. A characteristic "honking" voice with pink, edematous turban-like enlargement of the supraglottic structures is pathognomonic for laryngeal sarcoid.

Treatment is as follows:

1. Systemic and/or local injection of steroids may relieve airway obstruction by decreasing edema.
2. External radiation therapy has proved to be ineffective and is not recommended.
3. Tracheotomy, with surgical removal of bulky obstructing lesions, is a safe, conservative approach.

Overall prognosis probably is determined by the pattern of systemic and pulmonary involvement of the sarcoidosis.

Chronic Nonspecific Diseases

Gastroesophageal Reflux Laryngitis[1,4,55]

Almost two-thirds of otolaryngology patients with laryngeal and ??MS 974 voi?? disorders have gastroesophageal reflux as the primary cause or as a significant cofactor.[55] Gastroesophageal reflux laryngitis (GERL) or laryngopharyngeal reflux (LPR), also called acid laryngitis, is the most common manifestation of GERD in the upper airway. The signs and symptoms of reflux laryngitis are quite different from those of gastroenterology patients.[174] Patients with classic GERD characteristically have heartburn. Patients with LPR present with a variety of symptoms that include hoarseness, chronic throat clearing, excessive phlegm, globus pharyngeus, and throat discomfort. In a large series of ear, nose, and throat patients with LPR, Koufman found that dysphonia (not heartburn) was the most common symptom (92%), and 10% had granuloma of the vocal process.[55]

Conditions in which gastroesophageal reflux is the cause or a causative cofactor include reflux laryngitis (GERL), subglottic stenosis, carcinoma of the larynx, endotracheal injury, contact ulcer and granuloma, posterior glottic stenosis, arytenoid fixation, laryngospasm, globus pharyngeus, nodules, polypoid degeneration, laryngomalacia, pachyderma laryngis, and leukoplakia. The highest association (92%) is with subglottic stenosis in children and adults.[55]

Symptoms of GERL

1. Dysphonia (hoarseness) (most common)
2. Dysphagia
3. Chronic throat clearing and cough
4. Excessive throat mucus
5. Vocal fatigue
6. Heartburn

DIAGNOSTIC TESTS

1. Complete ear, nose, and throat examination
2. Fiberoptic laryngoscopy with photographic documentation
3. Ambulatory 24-hour double-probe pH monitoring
4. Barium esophagography

CLINICAL MANIFESTATION OF LPR

1. Posterior laryngitis with "characteristic" red arytenoids and piled-up interarytenoid mucosa. According to Koufman, however, edema and not erythema is the most common finding.[55]
2. Diffuse edema/Reinke's edema.
3. Diffuse erythema with granular mucosa.
4. Mucosal swelling without erythema.
5. Granuloma of vocal process of the arytenoid, unilateral or bilateral.

TREATMENT FOR LARYNGOPHARYNGEAL GERD[175]

Level I
1. Dietary modification (avoid fatty foods, chocolate, cigarettes, coffee)
2. Lifestyle modification (elevation of head of the bed)
3. Use of liquid antacid

Level II Antireflux medication
1. H_2 blockers (decrease acid secretion)
   Ranitidine (Zantac)
   Cimetidine (Tagamet)
   Famotidine (Pepcid)
2. Prokinetic drugs (increase lower esophageal sphincter tone and promote gastric emptying)
   Bethanecol (Urecholine)
   Metoclopramide (Reglan)
3. Cytoprotective agents (form protective coating)
   Sucralfate (Carafate)
4. Hydrogen pump blocker used as single- or double-dose regimen.
   Omeprazole (Prilosec, more effective than H_2 blockers)
   Lanzoprazole (Prevacid)

Level III
1. Antireflux surgery laparoscopic Nissen fundoplication.
2. Nissen fundoplication

The results of empiric treatment and pH probe result-directed therapy in the larynx are based on symptom resolution and endoscopic documentation of resolution of laryngeal and pharyngeal inflammation. The symptoms of LPR often improve well before the finding of tissue response to medical therapy.[176]

Pachyderma Laryngis

Pachyderma laryngis is a specific entity in which the posterior commissure and the posterior third of the true cords are the site of a localized hyperplastic and keratinizing process. Histologically, acanthosis, parakeratosis, keratosis, and hyperkeratotic papilloma are noticed.

There is no dyskeratosis, and it is not a premalignant condition. Diagnosis is made by biopsy. The contributing etiology includes smoking, LPR, and chronic throat clearing due to postnasal drip. The symptoms are hoarseness and chronic throat clearing. Treatment is by removal or reversal of the suspected irritant.

Keratosis of the Larynx

Keratosis of the larynx is a term used to denote a group of premalignant epithelial lesions in which an abnormality of growth and/or maturation has occurred. The exact cause is unknown, but smoking, vocal abuse, chronic laryngitis, GERD, and vitamin deficiencies contribute.

Hoarseness is the only symptom. A raised reddish area of mucosal irregularity overlying a portion of one or both cords with chronic inflammation may be seen during examination.

Treatment is as follows:

1. Cessation of use of tobacco and other causative agents
2. Antireflux therapy with H_2 blockers or H^+ proton pump inhibitors
3. Direct laryngoscopy with excision
4. Periodic examination

Leukoplakia of the Larynx

Laryngeal leukoplakia is a pathologic premalignant process characterized by a thick whitish layer of hyperkeratotic epithelial cells. It is caused by vocal abuse, excessive smoking and intake of alcohol, and an irritative environment. The differential diagnosis is between a benign condition such as benign keratosis to mild, moderate, or severe dysplasia to carcinoma in situ and invasive squamous cell carcinoma. It is not possible to differentiate between these entities except with histologic examination and biopsy. The major symptom is hoarseness. White patches may be seen on the vocal cords. Treatment is as follows:

1. Laryngoscopic examination and excision. Endoscopic diagnosis with contact endoscopy has been reported by Andrea as helpful in the diagnosis.[177] Intravital staining using DNA stains such as toluidine blue has been used to stain dysplastic areas and facilitate complete removal.
2. Removal of causative factors.
3. Periodic examination.

Some patients will have repeated recurrence of the white to red lesions of the larynx, which may result in need for repeated excisions. The risk of malignant degeneration is low but real: 10 to 25%.[178] Repeated vocal fold stripping by complete excision or partial excision for diagnosis have been used to manage recurrences. Repeated vocal fold stripping may result in long-term voice deterioration.

ARTHRITIS OF THE CRICOARYTENOID JOINT. The etiology of cricoarytenoid joint arthritis is as follows. Rheumatoid arthritis is by far the most common cause (about 25% of cases are due to rheumatoid arthritis). Other causes include gout, collagen disease (lupus erythematosus), Crohn's disease, and ankylosing spondylitis. Gonorrhea, tuberculosis, and syphilis are rare causes. Trauma may also be a factor.

Symptoms are as follows:

1. Sensation of lump in throat
2. Throat pain aggravated by swallowing or speaking

3. Referred otalgia
4. Hoarseness, stridor, and dyspnea
5. Striking, bright red swelling over the arytenoid
6. Palpation of the arytenoid produces severe pain

Physical examination (including laryngoscopy) reveals the following:

1. Striking bright red swelling over the arytenoid.
2. Palpation of the arytenoid produces severe pain.
3. Arytenoid fixation and glottic narrowing (chronic cases).
4. Vocal cord may be fixed in the paramedian or intermediate position.
5. Direct laryngoscopy and palpation of the arytenoids or laryngeal electromyography is necessary to differentiate fixation from paralysis.

Diagnosis is established as follows:

1. Typical laryngoscopic examination—ie, erythematous, swollen arytenoids, normal or slightly edematous vocal cords, variable vocal cord mobility, with immobility of arytenoid cartilage on palpation[4]
2. Serology (elevated erythrocyte sedimentation rate, rheumatoid factor, decreased complement levels, abnormal lupus panel)
3. High-resolution CT scan (erosion and subluxation of the cricoarytenoid joint with soft tissue swelling)[56,57]
4. Laryngeal electromyography showing normal innervation and recruitment

Treatment includes the following measures:

1. Medical control of systemic rheumatoid arthritis or related conditions.
2. Salicylates.
3. Corticosteroids.
4. Tracheotomy.
5. Arytenoidectomy or arytenoidopexy for midline fixation of both vocal cords; unilateral fixation rarely requires therapy.

Acquired Stenosis of the Larynx

Injury to the larynx leading to acquired stenosis[58,59] can involve the supraglottis, glottis, subglottis, or any combination of these structures. GERD is also a major cause of laryngeal stenosis, including subglottic and posterior stenosis. Clinical features and evaluation include the following:

1. Careful history taking.
2. Thorough physical examination of head and neck, with special attention to the neck, larynx, and pharynx.
3. Radiologic examination includes x-ray films of the chest and lateral neck. CT scan has been found to be of great value in the evaluation of laryngeal trauma.
4. Endoscopy.[60]
   a. Fiberoptic flexible nasopharyngolaryngoscope (Machida or Olympus) is a useful atraumatic diagnostic tool for evaluation of laryngeal trauma. It also can be used to evaluate the subglottic region via the tracheotomy stoma and eliminates the need for direct laryngoscopy in some cases.

    b.   Rigid telescope with right-angle lens (excellent tool for photographic documentation).[61]

    c.   Direct laryngoscopy.

    d.   Esophagoscopy.

    e.   Tracheoscopy.

    f.   Bronchoscopy.

Supraglottic Stenosis

Supraglottic stenosis may be caused by external crushing trauma (in the region of the hyoid bone, inflicted during an automobile accident or by a penetrating wound), caustic ingestion, or severe infection.

With supraglottic injuries, the blow often leads to fractures of the thyroid ala transversely with detachment of the epiglottis and false cords. The most common injury seen is rupture of the thyroepiglottic ligament with superior retraction of the epiglottis and herniation of the soft tissues of the pre-epiglottic space into the laryngeal lumen. There is often an associated tear in the posterior pharyngeal wall,[59] and the arytenoid cartilages may be dislocated. The epiglottis is easily seen on tongue depression in these cases (a useful clinical sign).

Direct laryngoscopy reveals that the false cords are splayed apart, and necrotic granulation tissue is present between the true and false cords.

Tracheotomy may be a lifesaving measure. Intubation prior to tracheotomy should be avoided.

The transhyoid or thyrotomy approach is used for repair of lacerations and for replacing various structures to their normal positions. Epiglottidectomy and arytenoidectomy may be necessary. These procedures may also be performed endoscopically using a laser.

Glottic Stenosis

Glottic stenosis may be classified into three varieties[58]:

1.   Anterior stenosis (web)

    a.   With laryngeal function

    b.   With bilateral paralysis

2.   Posterior stenosis

3.   Complete stenosis

    a.   With laryngeal function

    b.   With bilateral laryngeal paralysis

Anterior Glottic Stenosis

There are two types of anterior glottic stenosis: (1) anterior web results from traumatic endoscopy, lye burns, infections, or foreign body and (2) more extensive (thick) stenosis usually results from external trauma. Symptoms from anterior webs may be minimal. Hoarseness and varying degrees of respiratory distress may be present.

Treatment for thin webs is endoscopic section followed by dilations. For thick stenosis, treatment is as follows:

1.   Vocal cords are not paralyzed.

    a.   Endoscopic section with insertion of a keel without thyrotomy, as described by Dedo and Sooy.[62]

    b.   External thyrotomy approach with insertion of a keel (McNaught).

2. Bilateral paralysis complicates the glottic stenosis.
   a. External thyrotomy approach with arytenoidectomy, lateralization of the vocal cord, and insertion of a conforming silicone stent (instead of a keel).

Posterior Glottic Stenosis

Posterior glottic stenosis may be caused by external trauma or intubation or by infection (tuberculosis, diphtheria).

Diagnosis is made by indirect, fiberoptic, or direct laryngoscopy. Dyspnea may be seen on exertion, and hoarseness may be present.

Treatment is resection of the posterior web via the thyrotomy approach. Montgomery[58] recommends use of a superiorly based mucous membrane flap from the interarytenoid space. Cartilage grafting and stenting combined with arytenoidectomy may be used in combination in treatment of a thick posterior glottic web.

Complete Glottic Stenosis

External laryngeal trauma may cause complete glottic stenosis. Treatment includes the following measures:

1. Anterior midline vertical thyrotomy approach with incision of the stenotic area in the midline.
2. Use of local mucosal flap, buccal or nasal septal mucosal grafts, or split-thickness skin grafts.
3. Insertion of a conforming intralaryngeal stent.
4. The stent is left in position for 4 to 8 weeks.
5. When bilateral vocal cord paralysis accompanies complete glottic stenosis, arytenoidectomy is necessary.
6. Multistaged laryngeal reconstruction using cervical skin, cartilage graft, and flaps has been reported by Conley.[69a]
7. Laryngeal transplantation has been performed in one patient.

Subglottic Stenosis[1–4,62–69]

Etiology

1. Long-tern endotracheal intubation (most frequent cause). The incidence reported by several authors varies between 0.9 and 3.0%. This problem occurs most frequently in children because the subglottis is the narrowest part of the child's upper airway. Consequently, pressure from an endotracheal tube inflicts the most damage to this area.
2. External trauma (penetrating wound).
3. Internal trauma (high tracheotomy, traumatic endoscopy, foreign body, burns).
4. Neoplasm (chondroma, fibroma, and carcinoma are most common).
5. Irradiation.
6. Severe infection (laryngotracheal bronchitis with pneumonia).
7. Congenital stenosis and tracheomalacia.

Clinical Features

1. Dyspnea on exertion—presenting symptom.
2. Wheezing is common and is often misinterpreted as asthma or a chronic tracheobronchial infection.
3. Nonproductive cough and voice change.

4. Children may present with respiratory distress syndrome: tachypnea, increased ventilatory effort, expiratory grunting, and cyanosis.

5. Other symptoms include stridor, with or without cyanosis, and an inability to be extubated or decannulated.

6. The diagnosis can be made by laryngoscopy. However, it is difficult to determine the exact level of the stenosis with the laryngeal mirror examination. A lateral neck x-ray film resolves this problem by indicating more exactly the size of the lesion. The lesion is even more accurately outlined in a CT scan. The inferior extent may be evaluated by a flexible fiberoptic endoscope passed retrogradedly via a tracheotomy stoma.

Prevention

Use of an appropriate (in size and shape) endotracheal tube, proper humidification, control of infection, as well as length and repetition of intubation are significant factors in the prevention of acquired subglottic stenosis.

Treatment

1. Dilation may be helpful but may also be harmful, as it may denude the mucosa, thereby worsening stenosis.

2. Local steroid injection is of benefit in some cases.

3. A low tracheotomy may be used. It should be considered when an effective laryngeal airway cannot be maintained after attempts at endoscopic removal, dilations, or other surgery (eg, cricoid split).

4. Some subglottic granulomas, webs, and adhesions can be removed by endolaryngeal laser microsurgery. Stenosis of less than 1 cm is amenable to laser surgery, while thickness greater than 1 cm will need open laryngotracheoplasty.

5. In Rethi's procedure,[63] the anterior and posterior rings of the cricoid are split in a sagittal plane. This maneuver enlarges the diameter of the subglottic lumen without disturbing the esophageal mucosa. A Montgomery's stent is inserted with or without a mucosal graft to ensure maintenance of anterior and posterior diastasis of the cartilage fragments. Although Rethi did not originally describe keel insertion to prevent anterior commissure webbing, this approach is currently considered preferable. The keel is inserted at the time the internal stent is removed through a laryngofissure. The keel is then removed 2 weeks later.

6. Hyoid arch transposition has been described by Druck and associates[64] as a method of treatment for subglottic stenosis in which the anterior arch of the cricoid is removed and an autogenous bone graft from the midportion of the hyoid is interposed between the cut edges of the cricoid, thereby externally widening the subglottic diameter.

7. Cricoid excision with thyrotracheal anastomosis, described by Conley[69a] in 1953, introduced the concept of segmental resection of the stenotic subglottis with end-to-end anastomosis; and it has subsequently[65,66] been reported by several authors.

8. Laryngotracheoplasty, as reported by Evans and Todd,[67] introduces the use of a surgical approach for relief of subglottic stenosis in children. In this procedure the laryngofissure is modified in a "stepped-off" fashion, producing cartilaginous interdigitations of the cricoid and upper tracheal rings on each side. These interdigitations are distracted, and the open position is maintained by suturing the cartilage externally and stenting internally with rolled silicone elastomer sheeting. The internal stent is then removed after

6 weeks by the endoscopic approach. Good results have been reported with use of this method.

9. Anterior cartilage splitting with or without autogenous cartilage grafts using either costal cartilage or auricular cartilage may be performed. This may be coupled with a posterior cartilage split.[70–77]

10. Endoscopic treatment by radial incision and dilation (Shapshay and coworkers[69]).

Congenital Anomalies

Congenital Web

A congenital web develops as a band that extends over part (web) or all (atresia) of the glottis; the anterior two-thirds of the glottis is the most susceptible site. The symptoms are as follows:

1. Depend on degree of glottic closure.
2. Atresia present as severe dyspnea at birth. Death may follow if not promptly recognized and treated.
3. Small web may be asymptomatic.
4. Mainly weak or hoarse cry and cough.

Treatment includes the following measures:

1. Immediate insertion of a bronchoscope or a tracheotomy tube for atresia
2. Thyrotomy and insertion of a McNaught's tantalum plate between the vocal cords

Congenital Laryngeal Cyst

The congenital laryngeal cyst occurs most commonly in the supraglottic area (lateral wall of the supraglottis or on the epiglottis) or in association with a laryngocele, producing inspiratory stridor and weak cry. Diagnosis is made by direct laryngoscopy. Treatment is (1) emergency treatment by aspiration and (2) endoscopic excision later.

Congenital Subglottic Stenosis

The subglottic region 2 to 3 mm below the true cord is the site of predilection for congenital subglottic stenosis.[73] Subglottic stenosis is considered to be congenital when there is no other obvious cause—ie, endotracheal incubation. This is usually due to a cartilaginous stenosis, which may be from a trapped first tracheal ring, elliptical cricoid cartilage, or an abnormally small cricoid cartilage.[79] Symptoms are (1) severe barking stridor and (2) expiratory stridor if subglottic. Some 40 to 50% of patients need tracheotomy, although dilation is sufficient in some.

VOCAL CORD PARALYSIS   Etiology of vocal cord paralysis is as follows:
1. Trauma at birth (unilateral).
2. Platybasia (bilateral).
3. Arnold-Chiari syndrome (bilateral).
4. Left vocal cord paralysis may result from stretching of the left recurrent nerve due to a congenital cardiovascular lesion.

The symptoms are as follows:

1. Unilateral: weak cry.
2. Bilateral: crowing inspiration, severe stridor, but often with a normal voice or cry.

Treatment includes the following:

1. Unilateral: no treatment.
2. Bilateral: (1) tracheotomy; (2) arytenoidectomy or arytenoidopexy (best delayed until age 5 or 6).

Subglottic Hemangioma

Subglottic hemangioma[1-4,43-48] is a rare anomaly of early infancy that may be associated with a skin hemangioma (50% of cases). The anterior subglottic area is the most susceptible site.
Symptoms are as follows:

1. Inspiratory stridor is noted at birth or soon thereafter.
2. There may be a history of repeated episodes of croup.
3. Hoarseness is not a common symptom.
4. Direct laryngoscopy reveals a pink to blue, easily compressible subglottic tumor.
5. A biopsy is never done, as the ensuing hemorrhage may be fatal.
6. The tumor can be seen on a lateral neck x-ray film.

Treatment includes the following:

1. Tracheotomy for respiratory obstruction.
2. Systemic administration of steroids: A course of prednisone (20 mg) daily for 1 month, repeated one or two times as indicated. It may be the least hazardous therapy.
3. Intralesional injection of steroid.
4. Use of CO_2 laser excision appears to be a safe, effective treatment for subglottic capillary hemangiomas and is recommended by Healy and colleagues.[43] It is not used for cavernous-type lesions. Intense humidification is necessary during the immediate postoperative period to prevent crust formation.
5. Daily subcutaneous injections of alpha$_{2a}$-interferon have been shown to be effective in hastening the involution of symptomatic or life-threatening hemangiomas that have not responded to other treatment modalities.[44-46,48]
6. Because of the possibility of injury to developing laryngeal cartilage and the risk of thyroid carcinoma, radiation therapy is not recommended.
7. Surgical excision via a midline tracheal incision and an intraluminal stent.

Subglottic Cysts

1. May be acquired in newborns after long-term intubation.
2. Usually in the posterior subglottic larynx.
3. May present with stridor.
4. Cysts may be submucosal within a soft tissue subglottic stenosis.
5. Diagnosis usually made with endoscopy.
6. Treatment with endoscopic excision, cupped forceps, or laser.
7. If associated with a subglottic stenosis, may require an anterior cricoid split or tracheostomy.[80-82]

Laryngomalacia

Laryngomalacia[78,83-85] is the most common laryngeal abnormality of the newborn and is due to unusual flaccidity of the laryngeal tissues, especially the epiglottis. Symptoms are as follows:

1. Inspiratory stridor and noisy respiration noted soon after birth, usually worse when the infants are on their backs than when on their stomachs.

2. Diagnosis requires flexible or direct laryngoscopy, which reveals a flaccid, curled epiglottis that is drawn over the glottis on inspiration. Airway fluoroscopy demonstrates the flaccidity of the laryngeal and tracheal cartilages.
3. The vocal cords are normal in appearance and mobility.
4. Rule out lower respiratory tract anomalies by bronchoscopy.

Treatment is generally observation (stridor usually disappears by 12 to 16 months of age). Tracheotomy is performed in rare cases. Aryepiglotticoplasty or laser laryngoplasty may also be required in children with failure to thrive due to poor oral intake or poor airway.

Cri-du-Chat Syndrome
A nasologic entity called the cri-du-chat syndrome has been described[86] in which the larynx has the same appearance as that seen in laryngeal chondromalacia. The cri-du-chat syndrome is caused by partial deletion of a no. 5, group B chromosome and is characterized by a weak, wailing cry, like that of a kitten. Other accompanying features of the syndrome include severe mental retardation, rounded facies, a beak-like profile, microcephaly, hypotonia, hypertelorism, antimongoloid palpebral fissures, epicanthal folds, strabismus, and a variety of visceral abnormalities.

Laryngeal Clefts[87]
Laryngeal clefts are rare. Irregular and incomplete fusion of the laryngotracheal septum results in a tracheoesophageal fistula or cleft of the larynx. These anomalies manifest soon after birth. Symptoms include the following:

1. Cyanosis with feeding
2. Stridor
3. Abnormal cry
4. Pneumonia

The disorder is usually fatal unless diagnosed and corrected early. Diagnosis is made by direct laryngoscopy.

Laryngeal Atresia
Laryngeal atresia results from failure of the developing larynx to recanalize after the normal epithelial fusion that takes place toward the end of the third month of gestation. Atresia may be at the supraglottic, glottic, or subglottic levels, either separately or combined. Clinical features include aphonia if atresia is complete or a hoarse, stridorous voice if atresia is incomplete.
Treatment is as follows:

1. Immediate tracheotomy.
2. When the laryngeal skeleton is preserved: Partial resection of the atretic portion in the transverse plane with reanastomosis of the distal portion of the laryngotracheal tube to the proximal part.
3. When the entire laryngeal lumen is filled with scar: A hollowed groove for the future respiratory tube is created, lined with a free skin graft, and later implanted with cartilage.

Congenital Supraglottic Webs
If they are relatively thin and membranous, supraglottic webs may be treated by direct incision of the web through the laryngoscope. Thicker webs may require subsequent dilation to maintain an adequate lumen.

Congenital Glottic Stenosis (Webs)

Glottic stenosis occurs in three forms: (1) a thin, transparent, membranous sheet covering the superior aspect of the true vocal cords and the anterior part of the intervening glottis; (2) a web of variable thickness lying between portions of the membranous cords; and (3) fusion of the anterior half of the true vocal cords.[88]

Treatment for a thin web is endoscopic section followed by dilations. For a thick web, it involves endoscopic section with insertion of a tantalum or silicone keel; tracheotomy is required. The external thyrotomy approach may be tried with insertion of a silicone keel; the keel is left in for 2 weeks.

Acute Laryngeal Trauma

Blunt trauma to the neck is being seen with increasing frequency. Severe laryngeal injury[89-91] may occur without open neck injuries. The patient with undiagnosed laryngeal trauma may succumb early from laryngeal obstruction or develop late laryngeal stenosis that requires permanent wearing of a tracheotomy tube.

Three poor prognostic features in acute blunt laryngeal injuries include (1) early airway obstruction requiring tracheotomy, (2) the presence of bare cartilage in the laryngeal lumen, and (3) fracture and collapse of the cricoid.

In any patient who has sustained a possible laryngeal injury, the following symptoms are indicative of some derangement of laryngeal structure:

1. Increasing airway obstruction with dyspnea and stridor
2. Dysphonia or aphonia
3. Cough
4. Hemoptysis
5. Neck pain
6. Dysphagia and odynophagia

Distinctive clinical signs indicative of laryngeal injuries are the following:

1. Deformities of the neck, including alteration in contour and swelling
2. Subcutaneous emphysema
3. Laryngeal tenderness
4. Crepitus over the laryngeal framework

Diagnosis is based on the following:

1. Indirect and direct laryngoscopy. Direct laryngoscopy may precipitate airway obstruction in a patient with an acute laryngeal injury. In cases not requiring tracheotomy, indirect mirror laryngoscopy or flexible fiberoptic laryngoscopy gives a comprehensive and undisturbed view of the larynx.
2. Roentgenograms of the neck and chest must be taken to detect laryngeal fractures, tracheal injuries, and pneumothorax.
3. The CT scan is an excellent method of diagnosing hyoid fractures, fracture dislocation of thyroid and cricoid cartilages, and distortion of laryngeal structures.

Treatment

1. Conservative management is recommended when blunt trauma has resulted in soft tissue injuries (eg, small lacerations, ecchymoses, or submucosal hematomas) without

evidence of laryngeal fracture or a compromised airway. Conservative management includes voice rest, humidification, bed rest, and systemic steroids.

2. Indications for exploration include displaced laryngeal fracture, open injury with exposed cartilage, and fracture associated with upper airway obstruction.

3. Studies indicate improved functional outcome in patients who can be repaired immediately. If the larynx cannot be immediately repaired for any reason, it may be helpful to administer steroids and antibiotics (such as first-generation cephalosporin or clindamycin), so that granulation tissue and collagen deposition are reduced, thereby facilitating an anatomic repair.

4. For establishment of an airway, tracheotomy is the preferred means of management in these patients (avoid high tracheotomy). Premature intubation can obscure important diagnostic considerations as well as precipitate life-threatening airway obstruction.

5. Cricothyrotomy may be indicated in a dire emergency. In such cases, remove the tracheotomy as soon as possible and convert it to a standard tracheotomy.

6. Many of these patients have multiple injuries; yet suspicion and recognition of the acute laryngeal injury is imperative.

7. Surgical exploration is indicated for any neck injury with symptoms of stridor, voice change, cartilage disruption, and cervical emphysema.

8. Exploration of laryngeal structure is best performed through a horizontal incision to minimize scarring of the anterior neck.

9. Tears of the pyriform sinuses, hypopharynx, posterior larynx, and thyroarytenoid ligament and muscle are repaired.

10. When repairing laryngeal injuries, all mucosa must be sutured carefully. Local flaps or free mucosal grafts taken from the epiglottis or buccal mucosa should be used to close defects. All cartilaginous and submucosal tissues must be covered with epithelium.

11. If an arytenoid cartilage is completely avulsed and displaced, it is better to remove it than attempt to reposition it. Partial arytenoid disruption can be treated with repositioning and mucosal repair.

12. Laryngeal cartilage fractures, like any other fracture, must be reduced and immobilized. Repair should be done within 7 to 10 days of the time of injury.

13. Splint a laryngeal fracture by means of a mold or stent in the laryngeal lumen. A rubber finger cot filled with sponge may be used. Preformed Silastic stents that conform to the larynx are helpful to establish a preformed airway during initial healing.

14. The stent is usually inserted through a thyrotomy or infrahyoid laryngotomy and fixed above and below by stainless steel sutures passed through the skin.

15. The stent is fixed in such a position that the upper end is at the level of the aryepiglottic folds and the lower end just above the tracheotomy site. It is left for 4 to 8 weeks. Duration of stenting varies from 2 weeks to longer. Prolonged laryngeal stenting is appropriate for severely injured laryngeal skeleton but is hampered by more granulation tissue.

Foreign Bodies in the Larynx and Tracheobronchial Tree

1. Choking on food causes 2500 to 3000 deaths per year in the United States. It is the sixth most common cause of accidental death. Fifty-five percent of aspirated foreign bodies involve the respiratory tract in children 6 months to 4 years of age. The accident is neither observed nor suspected in more than one-third of these cases.

2. All techniques used for aiding the obstructed patient in an emergency, such as pounding on the back, Heimlich maneuver, and finger probing of the throat, are dangerous and are discouraged unless the airway obstruction is unrelieved by the patient's own reflexes. These techniques may result in further impaction and the possibility of a total obstruction that was not present before these attempts.

3. In the series of Cohen and associates,[91a] nuts were the most common type of foreign body aspirated (55%), followed by food particles (20%) and metallic objects (16.7%). Forty-three percent were found in the left bronchial tree (contrary to the common belief based on anatomic details), 38% in the right bronchial tree, and 4% in the larynx.

4. General anesthesia is recommended. Oxygen standby without any anesthesia may have to be used in cases where the airway obstruction is severe and the airway cannot be adequately controlled. Jet ventilation may be required.

5. The most common postoperative problem is subglottic laryngeal edema, treated with humidification and systemic steroids. Bronchitis, pneumonia (impaction with long-standing foreign bodies), and laryngotracheobronchitis may be seen. Complications of foreign bodies include bronchial suppuration, bronchial ulceration, granulation tissue, bronchial stenosis, peribronchial and peritracheal lymphadenopathy with compression of bronchi, pneumonitis, atelectasis, obstructive emphysema, pneumomediastinum, and pneumothorax.

6. Encapsulated dry vegetable substances can swell in the presence of moisture and may have to be broken into smaller pieces to avoid total obstruction of the trachea during removal.

7. A serious intraoperative complication can result from the removal of a large obstructive foreign body from the bronchus and having it get stuck at the level of the larynx. Attempts should be made to remove it from the glottis; if this is not possible, the foreign object is pushed back down into one of the bronchi so that ventilation can proceed with the unobstructed lung.

8. Preanesthesia medications (narcotics and sedatives) are contraindicated because they may depress respirations. The apneic relaxant technique allows sufficient time for atraumatic manipulation of the bronchoscope. It consists of a light plane of anesthesia accompanied by a muscle relaxant.

9. Intravenous dexamethasone phosphate (4–8 mg) is given before endoscopy to minimize subglottic edema.

10. Foreign body removal is facilitated by the use of the ventilating rigid bronchoscope and optical forceps, which may be used in conjunction with rigid fiberoptic telescopes.[92]

Paralysis of the Larynx

1. The larynx is supplied by two branches of vagus nerve: the SLN and RLN. The SLN divides extralaryngeally into (a) the internal branch, which supplies sensory innervation to the laryngeal cavity above the glottis, and (b) the external branch (motor), which supplies the cricothyroid muscle. A recent study in dogs has shown that the external branch of the superior laryngeal nerve may provide some innervation to the thyroarytenoid muscle as well.[6] The RLN supplies motor innervation to all the intrinsic laryngeal muscles of the same side except for the cricothyroid and to the interarytenoid muscle of both bodies. It also supplies sensory innervation to those portions of the larynx below the glottis.

2. Paralysis of the laryngeal muscles[1–4,93,94] originates in one of two areas: the CNS or the peripheral motor nerves. In most cases (90%), laryngeal paralysis is the result of peripheral nerve involvement. The anterior branch of the RLN innervates the cricoarytenoid, thyroarytenoid, vocalis, and aryepiglottic muscles while the posterior branch innervates the posterior cricoarytenoid and interarytenoid muscles. The interarytenoid muscle is the only intrinsic laryngeal muscle to receive bilateral innervation from the RLNs. Recent data suggest that the SLN may also contribute to interarytenoid muscle innervation.[57] Arising from the nucleus ambiguus in the midbrain, motor impulses to the intrinsic laryngeal muscles travel via the vagus nerve into the chest, where they enter the RLN. On its passage back to the larynx the right RLN crosses the right subclavian artery, and the left RLN winds around the arch of the aorta in close relation to the heart. The ascent of the RLN occurs in a groove between the trachea and the esophagus in close relation to the mediastinal lymph nodes, thyroid gland, and esophagus; thus the swelling of any of these structures may cause pressure on one of the RLNs and disrupt neural signals to the involved side. Depending on the nerve fibers involved and the muscles they supply, many types of paralysis may occur.

3. Paralyzed vocal cords are best described by their position: median, paramedian, intermediate or cadaveric, extreme abduction (lateral). In the median position, the paralyzed cord remains in the midline. This position of a paralyzed vocal cord is a frequent one, as the abductor muscles are weaker and more vulnerable than the adductor fibers. The intermediate position, often called cadaveric, is midway between the midline and a position of complete abduction. The paramedian position is between the median and intermediate positions.

4. Regardless of the type of paralysis, it is difficult to predict the permanent position of the vocal cord because of the following:
    a. Continued function of remaining muscles
    b. Partial reinnervation of the paralyzed muscles
    c. Muscle fibrosis
    d. Tone of the autonomic system
    e. Cricoarytenoid joint fibrosis
    f. Tension of the conus elasticus

5. Unilateral midline paralysis is the most frequent, the left more than the right. The paralyzed vocal cord usually lies lower than the normal cord.

6. Diagnostic evaluation
    a. Careful history and physical examination.
    b. Inspection. Indirect mirror examination of the larynx is the time-honored standard for evaluating the larynx. A flexible fiberscope passed through the nose and nasopharynx or a rigid telescope introduced through the oral cavity provides a better view of laryngeal movement and allows prolonged study of the larynx during phonation. These laryngoscopes are adaptable to the television camera, giving permanent records of the patient's laryngeal function.
    c. Laryngostroboscopy complements the endoscopic examination of the larynx.[9,95–100] Stroboscopic laryngeal examination was first performed by Oertel in 1878. By using a rotating disk spinning in synchrony with the patient's phonatory frequency, the laryngeal image viewed by indirect laryngoscopy could be "frozen." With further advances in electronic stroboscopy, the diagnostic value of the stroboscope

has been greatly improved. To perform stroboscopy, the nasal and intraoral mucosa are topically anesthetized. A contact microphone is placed on the patient's neck to determine the fundamental vocal frequency. The fundamental frequency is transmitted electronically to a xenon lamp, which flashes an intermittent beam of light at the same frequency. The strobe light gives the laryngologist the optical illusion that the vocal folds are moving slowly or not at all, which permits thorough study of the vocal folds throughout their vibratory cycle. Examination may be performed using indirect, fiberscopic, and telescopic methods. Videotape recording should always be done for documentation and later playback analysis. The laryngeal images are studied from the videotape recording, with observations made of shape, movement, vibratory pattern, and timing relationships between opening and closing. Videostroboscopic rating forms are very useful for analyzing the stroboscopic findings and include parameters such as symmetry, periodicity, glottic closure, amplitude of vibration, mucosal wave, and stiffness.[95] The diagnostic areas where stroboscopic examination is especially useful are in (1) early diagnosis of small lesions of the vocal fold, (2) analysis of phonatory vibratory patterns that result in poor glottal efficiency, (3) evaluation on the depth of early glottic cancer invasion, (4) evidence of early reinnervation after vocal cord paralysis, and (5) analysis of dysphonia of uncertain origin. Both flexible fiberscopic and rigid telescopic examinations provide excellent visualization of stroboscopic images. The advantages of the flexible fiberscope are that (1) normal speech can be documented, (2) the subglottic region can be examined if the patient is well anesthetized, and (3) it is better tolerated and can be performed even in hypersensitive adults and uncooperative children. The disadvantages of the fiberscope are that (1) the image is dark and of limited resolution; and (2) image distortion may occur because the fiberscope is introduced laterally through the nostril, particularly in a patient with deviated nasal septum. The Olympus ENF-L fiberscope, which has a larger (4.4-mm) diameter, provides better illumination and larger image.[101] Advantages of the rigid telescope are that (1) the images are consistently of better quality than those of the fiberscope, with excellent color and resolution, and (2) minimal image distortion occurs because the telescope is introduced in a midline position. Disadvantages of the rigid telescope are (1) more difficult examination in patients with hypersensitive gag reflex and (2) normal speech impossible with tongue held by examiner. Videostrobolaryngoscopy has been increasingly used by otolaryngologists interested in structural and functional disorders of the larynx, and its use in laryngeal evaluation is becoming more widespread. Videostrobolaryngoscopy is of great value for precise evaluation of the paralyzed cord(s) and may help to predict the prognosis of laryngeal paralysis. It is also helpful in diagnosis of very small laryngeal cancer, scarred vocal folds, laryngeal cysts vs. polyps, and sulcus vocalis.

d. Electromyography (EMG). With the patient awake under topical anesthesia, EMG can be done with monopolar or concentric bipolar needle electrodes through an external approach. This technique gives a precise indication of the function of the intrinsic muscles of the larynx but requires experience and special skill in placement of these electrodes. Hirano and Ohala[102] claimed that it can be done without affecting normal speech and articulation and that muscle activity can be recorded during normal speech. Although it has a great deal to offer in exactly delineating the extent of laryngeal nerve paralysis, it is still a research tool in most institutions. Laryngeal electromyography is useful in (1) differentiating ankylosis from paralysis in patients with unilateral vocal fold immobility, (2) distinguishing subtle vocal fold paresis from vocal fold paralysis, and (3) predicting return of vocal function to determine timing and type of surgical rehabilitation.

    e.   Laboratory studies to be considered are the following:

        (1) Chest x-ray films.

        (2) An MRI or CT scan of the chest and neck to rule out mass lesions invading or compressing the RLN. CT scan may also be needed to rule out erosion of jugular foramen.

        (3) CF3C, urinalysis.

        (4) Barium swallow.

        (5) Thyroid scan.

        (6) VDRL, FFA.

        (7) Glucose tolerance test.

        (8) Lumbar puncture (LP).

        (9) Lyme titer.

      (10) Erythrocyte sedimentation rate (ESR), complement level (to rule out collagen vascular disease).

      (11) Angiotension converting enzyme (ACE) level (elevated in 50–80% of patients with sarcoidosis).

      (12) Mono spot (Epstein-Barr virus infections).

      (13) Arsenic, lead, mercury levels.

    f.   Endoscopy. Endoscopy should be done as the last step in evaluating vocal cord paralysis. It should include nasopharyngeal examination to rule out neoplasm and direct laryngoscopy to palpate the arytenoid to differentiate vocal cord paralysis from fixation of the cricoarytenoid joint. Bronchoscopy and esophagoscopy may help to rule out a mass lesion or occult neoplasm.

    g.   Radiologic evaluation can be of value in the detection and evaluation of vocal cord paralysis. With RLN paralysis, four distinctive x-ray findings have been reported: (1) the vocal cord takes a triangular shape, (2) the laryngeal ventricle is dilated, (3) the cross-sectional area of the vocal cord is diminished, and (4) the normal subglottic shoulder is replaced by a straight line. In addition, a loss of abduction can be seen on inspiration. A CT scan of the larynx is also of help in the evaluation of laryngeal paralysis.

Unilateral Paralysis

    Unilateral paralysis of the vagus or RLNs can be the result of one of the following:

1. Tumor in the thyroid gland, mediastinum, esophagus, or larynx
2. Surgical trauma (most commonly by thyroidectomy)
3. Mediastinal compression (cardiac hypertrophy, aortic aneurysm, mediastinal and lung masses)
4. Toxic neuritis following influenza, alcohol, lead or arsenic poisoning
5. Collagen vascular diseases
6. Sarcoidosis (diagnosed by ACE level)

7. Lyme disease (diagnosed by Lyme titer)
8. Syphilis (FTA-ABS, VDRL)
9. Infectious mononucleosis
10. Diabetic neuropathy
11. Central lesion (rare)
12. Unknown (about 20%)

With modern diagnostic techniques such as LEMG and the increasing use of interventional surgery, there has been a shift in the demographics of etiology of vocal fold paralysis. Whereas the idiopathic type of vocal fold paralysis was a large percentage in previous reported series, reports of vocal fold paralysis secondary to iatrogenic injuries have increased.[179]

Symptoms

Hoarseness is usually the only symptom of unilateral laryngeal paralysis. Initially, some patients have aspiration of liquids during swallow, and this symptom improves with time. Vocal complaints include breathy dysphonia, vocal fatigue, and dyspnea with speaking. Even this symptom often gradually disappears as the healthy vocal fold increases its excursion beyond the median line. The feebleness of the cough mechanism parallels the degree of hoarseness. Severe glottal incompetence in the postoperative patient may result in poor pulmonary toilet, which prolongs patient morbidity.

Treatment

Treatment may be nonsurgical (ie, voice therapy) or surgical. Surgical therapy includes the following:

1. *Vocal fold injection.*[103,104] Intracordal injection of the vocal cord was first performed by Brunings in 1911.[91] He used paraffin for injection, but because it resulted in paraffin granulomas, the technique has been discontinued. Arnold,[105] using Teflon mixed with glycerin, revived injection of the vocal cord for treatment of paralysis. Largely through his work and that of Lewy,[106] Teflon injection became a mainstay of treatment for hoarseness associated with unilateral laryngeal paralysis, but granuloma formation has been a problematic complication. Long-term inflammatory response to Teflon injection may result in progressive voice loss. Gelfoam, cross-linked bovine collagen, and autogenous fat are other materials used for vocal fold augmentation.[107] More recently, the use of autologous collagen has been described, with results comparable to those from injectable bovine collagen but without the risk of a hypersensitivity reaction.[104] Gelfoam paste may be injected initially to judge whether vocal augmentation will be effective. This technique is usually performed under local anesthesia. Gelfoam paste also has been used as a temporary material for injection laryngoplasty. Using a Brunings syringe, Teflon is injected posterior and lateral to the paralyzed vocal fold, along the lateral aspect of the thyroarytenoid muscle. Collagen must be injected in a more superficial plane, ideally into the deep lamina propria. Deeper injections into muscle lead to rapid resorption. Teflon injection may be complicated by Teflon granuloma of the vocal fold.

2. *Medialization thyroplasty.*[108–113] Isshiki popularized thyroplasty as a means to medialize the paralyzed vocal fold without disrupting the mucosal surface of the vocal fold. Under local anesthesia, a thyroid cartilage window is removed from the lower half of the thyroid ala (at the level of the vocal fold) and a Silastic implant is inserted, thereby

medializing the paralyzed vocal fold. Simultaneous observation of the larynx with a fiberscope permits precise visualization of the extent of medialization. There are many modifications of the Isshiki procedure. Cummings has recently advocated the use of preformed. Hydroxylapatite implants of various sizes for medialization. These are currently under investigation. Montgomery has a prefabricated implant that comes in various sizes.[180] Advantages of medialization thyroplasty include (a) precise positioning of vocal fold; (b) vocal fold structure remains undisturbed; (c) potentially reversible; and (d) local anesthesia, with short surgical time. Disadvantages include (a) open approach; (b) perioperative edema or bleeding may compromise airway; and (c) implant may extrude.

3. *Arytenoid adduction.*[114–115] Isshiki proposed arytenoid adduction under local anesthesia as a means of reducing large posterior glottic gaps, especially when the vocal folds lie at different levels.[181] The muscular process of the arytenoid cartilage is identified, sometimes necessitating removal of the inferior cornu and posterior border of the thyroid cartilage. Sutures are placed through the muscular process and passed through the anterior thyroid ala. Traction on these sutures results in simulation of the adductor vectors of the lateral cricoarytenoid and the thyroarytenoid muscles. The result is medial rotation of the arytenoid and vocal fold adduction. Once the desired tension and placement are obtained, the sutures are tied to each other. The main disadvantage of this procedure is that it is technically difficult to perform. In patients with a large posterior gap and where the vocal folds are in a different plane, the use of arytenoid adduction suture along with a medialization laryngoplasty is essential to correct the open posterior biomechanical unit.[182]

4. *Laryngeal reinnervation.* Reinnervation techniques aid in improving the resting tone and mass of the phonatory muscles. Few studies have documented functional voluntary movement in the denervated and reinnervated muscle. Neuromuscular pedicle, popularized by Tucker, is indicated in patients with unilateral paralysis with involvement of superior and recurrent laryngeal nerves, posterior glottic defects less than 3 to 4 mm, and a bowed vocal fold.[116] The ansa hypoglossi is traced to the omohyoid muscle, where a 1-cm block of muscle is harvested. In unilateral paralysis, a thyroid cartilage window is removed, with suture placement of the neuromuscular pedicle into the thyroarytenoid muscle. An alternative technique is the ansa cervicalis–recurrent laryngeal nerve anastomosis popularized by Crumley.[117] The ansa cervicalis is identified medial to the sternocleidomastoid muscle, and a tension-free end-to-end anastomosis is then performed with 10-0 nylon sutures to the previously RLN. Unlike injection or thyroplasty, where immediate results are seen, these techniques involve a period of at least several months before final results are obtained. To allow for more specific reinnervation without the problem of synkinesis, some surgeons combine a RLN reinnervation with selected denervation of the adductor or abductor branches. In patients with bilateral vocal fold paralysis, reinnervation is done in conjunction with cutting of the RLN branch to the adductor muscles. This prevents aberrant reinnervation.[183]

Bilateral Abductor Paralysis

Bilateral abductor paralysis is the most common form of bilateral motor paralysis and is of great clinical importance. In almost all instances it is caused by extensive thyroid surgery, with injury to both RLNs. Bilateral abductor paralysis of the vocal cords is manifest by a paralysis of both vocal cords near the median line.

Patients who do not have an iatrogenic cause of bilateral vocal fold paralysis from thyroid surgery should be worked up for

1. Neuromotor weakness (myasthenia gravis), muscular dystrophy, multiple sclerosis, syringobulbia, Arnold-Chiari malformation, hydrocephalus
2. Vocal fold fixation due to intubation resulting in pseudoparalysis
3. Arytenoid ankylosis from inflammatory arthritis such as rheumatoid arthritis

Symptoms
1. Destruction of or injury to both RLNs is usually followed by transient hoarseness.
2. Weakness of voice is usually prolonged.
3. Cough mechanism is less forceful.[4] As the vocal cords approach the median line, respiratory embarrassment may become increasingly severe; progressive dyspnea with exertion may result in upper airway obstruction requiring immediate establishment of an adequate airway.

Treatment
A tracheotomy is performed for immediate respiratory difficulty. The long-term management of this condition requires lateralization of one of the paralyzed vocal cords to an appropriate position so that the airway is adequate for removal of the tracheotomy and the voice is not weakened excessively. A 5-mm glottic chink provides an adequate airway but may result in a weak voice. Four millimeters seems to be ideal if the treated paralyzed cord is at a lower level than the nonlateralized cord. There are three major techniques:

1. Endolaryngeal arytenoidectomy.[118,119] In 1948, Thornell[118] first described the oral approach to arytenoidectomy for lateralization of one or both vocal cords. A contraindication to this procedure is severe cardiopulmonary disease, where adequate respiratory function requires a normal glottic airway of a tracheotomy tube. This procedure has been regarded as technically difficult; use of the surgical microscope and CO_2 laser has made it easier. Ossoff and colleagues[119] established endoscopic laser arytenoidectomy for the treatment of bilateral vocal cord paralysis.
2. Extralaryngeal arytenoidectomy
   a. Posterior approach. King[120] first described an extralaryngeal approach to improve respiratory obstruction and to maintain the voice. Today this procedure or a modification thereof is an effective surgical approach for the treatment of respiratory obstruction due to bilateral vocal cord paralysis. The arytenoid is exposed through the external approach. The body of the arytenoid is cut from the vocal process and removed. The suture is placed through the vocal process and then tied around the inferior cornu of the thyroid cartilage, while the surgeon, using a laryngoscope, directs the securing of the structure to allow lateralization of the vocal cord 4 to 5 mm and a downward positioning of 1 to 2 mm below the opposite cord level. A 5-mm chink can be reduced to 4 mm by placing one vocal cord lower than the other. The success rate of decannulation is 75 to 95%.
   b. Thyrotomy approach. This is the procedure of choice of many laryngologists for bilateral abductor vocal cord paralysis. It offers direct surgical visualization and exact placement of the vocal cord. The disadvantages of a thyrotomy lie in the need for tracheotomy and the risk of laryngeal stenosis and web using a thyrotomy approach.

3. Transverse cordotomy using the CO_2 laser as described by Kashima is a safe and effective means of enlarging the posterior glottic aperture to restore the airway and preserve close approximation of the anterior cords for phonation.[121]

4. Nerve-muscle transposition
   a. The technique of nerve–muscle pedicle transposition was described by Tucker.[110] The advantages stated by Tucker are as follows:
      (1) It restores an adequate airway without further loss of voice.
      (2) There is a return of function within 6 to 12 weeks.
      (3) There is selective reinnervation of abductor muscles only that avoids crossed or inappropriate return of function.
      (4) This procedure does not interfere with potential spontaneous reinnervation.
      (5) It is technically less difficult than nerve anastomosis. The procedure is based on the assumption that the strap muscles are accessory muscles of respiration and contract during deep inspiration.
   b. By transposing a nerve-muscle pedicle into the posterior cricoarytenoid muscle, one would expect contraction of this muscle and resultant abduction of the vocal cords during deep inspiration.
   c. The indication for this operation is bilateral vocal cord paralysis with airway obstruction. Contraindications are as follows: (1) Preexisting traumatic or neurologic loss of the branch of the ansa hypoglossi to the anterior belly of the omohyoid muscles and (2) fixation of the cricoarytenoid joints.
   d. The controversies over the nerve-muscle transposition are as follows:
      (1) It is technically difficult to achieve vocal fold mobility.
      (2) A prolonged period of time is necessary for reinnervation.
      (3) There may be failure to achieve an airway adequate to allow for decannulation after the above.

5. Some authors have tried implantable pacemakers in the management of bilateral vocal fold paralysis, but this should be considered still an experimental procedure.

6. In patients who are dependent on an excellent voice, the choice between excellent airway versus voice may need to be addressed. With static methods, there are no surgical procedures that can result in both. In these patients, a trial of a tracheotomy button with a Passy Muir valve is an alternative.

Superior Laryngeal Nerve Paralysis

Superior laryngeal nerve paralysis is usually secondary to thyroidectomy or supraglottic laryngectomy. Its symptoms include the following:

1. Lowered voice.
2. Posterior commissure deviating to the paralyzed side.
3. Paralyzed side has a vocal cord that is bowed, flabby, and lower. Guttman's test: frontal pressure on the thyroid cartilage in the normal subject lowers the voice while lateral pressure raises the voice. With paralysis of the cricothyroid muscle, the opposite is true.

As a rule, no therapy is necessary, although vocal therapy may be helpful. A surgical procedure to narrow the cricothyroid space may be of benefit if symptoms are severe. Arnold[105] described suturing the thyroid to the cricoid cartilage to elevate the cartilage during phonation.

Dysphonia[3]

Dysplastic Dysphonia

Dysplastic dysphonia refers to chronic hoarseness due to structural malformation of the larynx (asymmetry of larynx, congenital webbing, vocal cord sulcus).

Habitual Dysphonia

1. Vocal nodules and polyps: Unilateral polyps cause different vibratory patterns of the two vocal cords, leading to diplophonia. Polypoid degeneration of the entire cord is known as Reinke's edema. Speech therapy and surgical ablation (CO_2 laser is especially useful here) are the modalities of treatment.

2. Chronic hypertrophic laryngitis is the end result of chronic laryngeal irritation secondary to vocal abuse, smoking, excessive alcohol use, allergies, or nasal obstruction.

3. Dysphonia plicae ventricularis or ventricular dysphonia[122] is faulty participation of the false cords in phonation. There are two types. The primary type is a functional voice disorder can be the end stage of chronic hyperkinetic dysphasia from continuous vocal abuse. The other type is a compensatory type and is seen in response of the larynx to use supraglottic structures as a secondary oscillatory source. This can be seen in some cases of laryngeal paralysis, after hemilaryngectomy, after vocal fold scarring, and due to CNS disorders.

Treatment of ventricular dysphonia is dependent on the etiology. The functional type of ventricular dysphonia is best treated by speech therapy, whereas the compensatory type is best addressed by surgery to improve glottic insufficiency.

Functional, Psychogenic Dysphonia of Emotional Origin

Some voice disorders are characterized by hoarse voice with a lack of physical etiology. This is called functional dysphonia. Functional dysphonia may be classified as follows:

1. Hyperfunctional or hypofunctional voice disorder. The patient habitually produces too much voice volume and uses too much effort—or the opposite. This is usually treated by speech therapy.

2. Psychogenic dysphonia. Voice may be lost as part of a conversion disorder. *Hysterical aphonia* is a term sometimes used to describe this. It is treated by psychological evaluation and speech therapy.

3. Puberphonia describes the failure of change of voice in the male with puberty. This can occur despite a good development in laryngeal structures. It is treated by speech therapy.

4. Dysphonia for secondary gain. Some patients develop dysphonia for secondary gain as part of an occupational voice loss or trauma. This requires a multidisciplinary evaluation using forensic medicine, speech therapy, and otolaryngology.

Endocrine Dysphonia

1. Gonadic disorders: eunuchoid voice, laryngopathia gravidarum

2. Thyroid and parathyroid disorders: cretinism, myxedema, hyperthyroidism, calcium imbalances affecting speech musculature

3. Adrenal disorders: Addison's disease leads to progressive aphonia secondary to muscular weakness; adrenocortical hyperfunction leads to vocal virilization, particularly in women.

4. Pituitary disorders: acromegaly leads to vocal virilization; pituitary hypogenitalism results in the eunuchoid voice of dwarfism.

Paralytic Dysphonia
See "Paralysis of the Larynx," above.

Dysarthric Dysphonia of Central Origin
Dysarthric dysphonia may result from cerebral palsy, stroke, parkinsonism, chorea, multiple sclerosis, cerebellar disease, or bulbar paralysis.

Myopathic Dysphonia from Muscular Disease
Sternothyroid muscle paralysis secondary to injury of the ansa hypoglossi and myasthenia gravis pseudoparalytica can result in myopathic dysphonia.

Traumatic Dysphonia after Laryngeal Injury
Hematomas, joint articulation injuries, and lesions of the extrinsic laryngeal muscles are the cause of traumatic dysphonia.

Spasmodic Dysphonia

Spasmodic dysphonia is a discrete vocal disorder characterized by strained, choked vocal attacks (laryngeal stuttering) and associated with increased tension of the entire phonatory system. The voice characteristics of spasmodic dysphasia include glottic stammering, hoarseness, monopitched voice, and reduced volume. The secondary characteristics associated with this disorder include facial and neck grimacing, fatigue of chest musculature, tic-like contractions of the upper torso and face, and facial flushing. The onset usually follows some stressful period in middle life, and there is no gender predominance. The etiology is unknown. It is classified as a focal dystonia or movement disorder involving the subcortical structures of the basal ganglia and the subcortical regulatory circuits. Spasmodic dysphonia is not a vocal expression of psychoneurotic behavior. Other authors have thought it to be secondary to a CNS or proprioceptive disorder of the larynx.

Laryngeal findings are those of hyperadduction of the vocal cords with the patient attempting to phonate against a closed glottis.

Treatment modalities are as follows:

1. Psychotherapy and speech therapy are reported to have uniformly poor results after long periods of intervention.
2. Surgical therapy, first proposed by Dedo,[24] was to deliberately section the RLN to prevent hyperadduction of the vocal cords. It was done after temporary paralysis with lidocaine (Xylocaine) produced significant improvement in voice quality. Sectioning of the RLN in spasmodic dysphonia patients has resulted in greater ease and improved quality of phonation, with reduction or elimination of facial and neck grimaces in most patients. Other authors suggest selective sectioning of the adductor branch of the RLN.[124]
3. One study[125] showed a high rate of recurrence of spasmodic dysphonia symptoms (39%) 1.5 years after RLN sectioning. This problem can be treated in some cases by deliberate paralysis of the ipsilateral superior laryngeal nerve.
4. Blitzer and coworkers[126] reported the successful use of botulinum toxin (Botox) for the treatment of spasmodic dysphonia. They treated more than 100 patients with dystonia, including 5 with laryngeal dystonia. All of the patients' laryngeal dystonia improved dramatically after 48 to 72 hours; the benefit lasted 3 to 9 months for each injection period. Botox injection can be performed on awake, ambulatory patients. Bilateral treatment and titration of dose can achieve the desired degree of weakness. Miller,[127] Lud-

low,[128] and their associates also reported favorable results using Botox to treat spasmodic dysphonia. Techniques of Botox injection have included translaryngeal injections using needle EMG, indirect injection using a curved needle, and fiberscope-guided translaryngeal and endoscopic needle injections. Some controversy continues as to whether unilateral versus bilateral injection techniques result in better voice.

5. Isshiki and then Tucker have reported success in the management of adductor spasmodic dysphonia with a laryngoplasty approach. Lateralization laryngoplasty (thyroplasty type II) creates a bowed and less competent glottal aperture, resulting in a less pressed phonation.[184]

Intractable Aspiration

Intractable aspiration resulting from loss of protective laryngeal function is seen with severe deficits in the brain stem or cranial nerves IX, X, and XII. Aspiration pneumonia can be a devastating and fatal complication of an otherwise debilitating but nonfatal illness, often a neurologic disorder. Numerous nonsurgical and surgical techniques have been proposed to prevent this intractable life-threatening condition.

1. Nonsurgical techniques
    a. Nasogastric tube supplemented by IV feeding provides a temporary solution for obtaining nutrition. Long-term use of the tube may result in rhinosinusitis, postcricoid ulceration, and chondritis of the larynx.
2. Surgical techniques
    a. Cuffed tracheotomy tube for temporary relief from aspiration. Long-term use of cuffed tubes may result in stomal infection, tracheal stenosis, esophageal erosion, and innominate artery fistulization. Tracheotomy may predispose to aspiration as follows:
        (1) Tracheotomy interferes with anterior displacement and elevation of the larynx during swallowing.
        (2) The tracheotomy tube is a foreign body that promotes crust formation and the pooling of secretions.
        (3) Tracheotomy compromises the normal cough mechanism.
        (4) Tracheotomy disrupts normal laryngeal reflexes, such as vocal fold adduction during swallowing.
        (5) The tracheotomy tube cuff may compress the esophagus, hindering bolus transport. On the other hand, tracheotomy facilitates pulmonary toilet and nursing care in these patients.[129]
    b. Vocal cord augmentation with injection laryngoplasty or medialization laryngoplasty with or without arytenoid adduction (in cases of unilateral vocal cord paralysis).
    c. Cricopharyngeal myotomy to facilitate passage of food and minimize pooling of secretions (in cases of cricopharyngeal spasm, which may be documented by a modified barium swallow).
    d. Bilateral chorda tympani and tympanic nerve sections to reduce saliva production.
    e. Percutaneous endoscopic gastrostomy (better tolerated than nasogastric tubes on a long-term basis).
    f. Separation of the larynx and trachea by creation of a tracheostoma and closure of the larynx at the level of the first tracheal ring.[126]
    g. Use of epiglottic flap to arytenoids.[130]

h. Linderman's diversion procedure with tracheoesophageal anastomosis and creation of a tracheotome[127,128]; with this technique, aspirated saliva and food are diverted into the esophagus. This procedure may be reversible.

i. Montgomery's glottic closure procedure.[131] The vocal cords are sutured together via a laryngofissure, a theoretically reversible procedure. Sasaki and coworkers described a modified method of laryngeal closure.[132]

j. Total laryngectomy.

VOICE RESTORATION AFTER LARYNGECTOMY

See references 133 to 135 for further discussion.

Esophageal speech and artificial electrolarynx are two nonsurgical alternatives after total laryngectomy for speech restoration. The esophageal speech requires an intensive course of treatments with a speech pathologist and success rates vary depending on the motivation of the patient and the skill and experience of the therapist. Electrolarynx has been used as a method of communication, but its role in human communications is limited due to the mechanical nature of the sound, limited by a set fundamental frequency and poor simulation of the resonance structure of the vocal tract.

In 1931, Guttman described a technique that restored voice in several patients. He created a fistula between the trachea and the pharynx using an electrocautery needle. Since then numerous methods of surgical restoration of voice after laryngectomy have been described, including Asai's laryngoplasty,[136] air bypass voice prosthesis, and the pseudoglottis procedure.[137,138]

In 1980, Singer and Blom[134] described a technique of voice restoration that created a fistula between the top of the tracheal stoma and the tube. A soft silicone elastomer device was inserted in the fistula to maintain its patency and allow shunting of air from the trachea into the hypopharynx without aspiration. In 1981, they described 129 patients, 88% of whom had achieved fluent voices.[135] They noted that the esophageal voice is profoundly affected by the residual function of the pharyngeal constrictor musculature. Selective division of these muscles enhances voice acquisition in most cases of failed esophageal speakers. Candidates for Singer and Blom's tracheoesophageal puncture include any motivated patient who, after total laryngectomy, fails to achieve fluent esophageal speech. An adequate-sized tracheostoma as well as a patent pharyngoesophageal lumen are important considerations in the preoperative assessment of these patients. Prior radiation therapy or partial or total pharyngectomy is not a contraindication. Postoperative complications include bleeding and crusting around the fistula site, leakage of saliva (especially in previously irradiated patients), pain secondary to improper fitting of a prosthesis, and failed tracheoesophageal speech, usually secondary to poor volume or lack of fluency.

Second-generation tracheoesophageal prostheses have improved the success rate of this procedure. They have obviated the need for daily changing of the prosthesis as well as offering less resistance to airflow. In addition to the Blom-Singer prostheses, currently available are the Panje button, the Henley-Cohn prosthesis, and the Blaise-Rapheal voice prosthesis developed by K. J. Lee. External valves are now being developed that preclude the need to cover the stoma with the thumb or finger during speech production. Despite some minor postoperative problems, it appears that at the present time this type of surgery is the procedure of choice for vocal rehabilitation of the total laryngectomy patient.

TRACHEOTOMY

Tracheotomy is done to form a temporary opening in the trachea. Tracheostomy, in which the trachea is brought to the skin and sewn in place, provides a permanent opening.

Tracheotomy is indicated for three groups of patients:

1. Those who have an obstruction at or above the level of the larynx (mechanical obstruction)
2. Those who have no actual obstruction to the airway but cannot raise secretions (secretional obstruction)
3. Those who have need for prolonged mechanical ventilation

Tracheotomy in the second and third group is becoming increasingly common.

Elective tracheotomy may be necessary when respiratory problems are anticipated during the postoperative period in patients being subjected to major head and neck or thoracic operations or in those with chronic pulmonary insufficiency. Therapeutic tracheotomy is indicated in any case of respiratory insufficiency due to alveolar hypoventilation in order to bypass an obstruction, remove secretions, or provide for the use of mechanical artificial respiration.

Clinical signs of upper airway obstruction include the following:

1. Retraction (suprasternal, supraclavicular, intercostal)
2. Inspiratory stridor
3. Restlessness, apprehension, disorientation leading to coma
4. Rising pulse and respiratory rates
5. Pallor (earlier sign) and cyanosis (late danger sign)
6. Fatigue and exhaustion due to excessive efforts to breathe through an obstructed airway

The patient's exhaustion must not be regarded as a sign of improvement but rather as a danger sign. It is a mistake to wait for late clinical signs of obstruction to appear before performing a tracheotomy. The time to proceed with the operation is whenever the need is first considered. Surgical manipulation in hypoxemic patients is often associated with cardiac arrest.

Function of a Tracheotomy

In addition to bypassing an upper airway obstruction, tracheotomy has several other physiologic functions:

1. Decreasing the amount of dead space in the tracheobronchial tree, usually by 70 to 100 mL. The decrease in dead space may vary from 10 to 50%, depending on the individual's physiologic dead space.
2. Reduction of resistance to airflow, which in turn reduces the force required to move air. It results in increased total compliance and more effective alveolar ventilation provided that the tracheotomy opening is large enough.
3. Protection against aspiration.
4. Enables swallowing without reflex apnea, which is important in respiratory patients.
5. Access to the trachea for cleaning.
6. Pathway to deliver medication and humidification to the tracheobronchial tree, with or without intermittent positive-pressure breathing.

7. Decreasing the power of the cough, thereby preventing peripheral displacement of secretions by the high negative intrathoracic pressure associated with the inspiratory phase of normal cough.

Tracheotomy in Infants and Children

Tracheotomy in infants and children[139-141] should always be done after a bronchoscope, endotracheal tube, or catheter has been inserted to provide an airway and some rigidity to the trachea. It converts an emergency tracheotomy to an orderly one. It is easy in these small patients to carry dissection too deeply and laterally to the trachea, with resulting damage to the recurrent laryngeal nerve, common carotid artery, apex of the pleura, or cervical esophagus. Caution must be used when incising the tracheal wall not to insert the tube too deeply and lacerate the posterior wall. When the child's head is turned or keeps moving, the trachea may be entered laterally. A bronchoscope or endotracheal tube in the trachea helps eliminate these complications.[140] A needle cricothyroidotomy may be performed initially in order to establish an emergency airway in the pediatric patient.

Tracheotomy Indications

1. Mechanical obstruction
   a. Obstructive tumors involving the larynx, pharynx, upper trachea and esophagus, and the thyroid gland
      (1) When in advanced stage
      (2) Edema from radiotherapy
      (3) As adjunct to surgery
   b. Inflammation of larynx, trachea, tongue, and pharynx
      (1) Acute epiglottitis
      (2) Viral croup
      (3) Ludwig's angina
   c. Congenital anomalies obstructing larynx or trachea
      (1) Laryngeal web or atresia
      (2) Tracheoesophageal anomalies
   d. Trauma to larynx and trachea
      (1) Cartilaginous framework and soft tissue
      (2) Inhalation of steam or fumes (burn)
   e. Maxillofacial trauma with extensive bone and soft tissue damage
      (1) LeFort II and III, multiple fractures of mandible and maxilla
      (2) Hemorrhage
      (3) As adjunct to surgery
   f. Bilateral vocal cord paralysis
   g. Foreign bodies
   h. Sleep apnea syndrome
2. Secretional obstruction
   a. Retained secretions and inadequate cough
      (1) Thoracic and abdominal surgery
      (2) Bronchopneumonia
      (3) Burns about face, neck, and respiratory tree
      (4) Conditions producing coma (eg, diabetes mellitus, uremia, septicemia, and liver failure)

    b.   Alveolar hypoventilation
- (1) Drug intoxication and poisoning
- (2) Flail chest, fractured ribs, surgical emphysema
- (3) Paralysis of chest wall
- (4) Chronic obstructive pulmonary disease (emphysema, chronic bronchitis, atelectasis, bronchiectasis, and asthma)

    c.   Retained secretions and alveolar hypoventilation
- (1) CNS disease (eg, stroke, encephalitis, Guillain-Barré syndrome, poliomyelitis, and tetanus).
- (2) Eclampsia.
- (3) Massive head and chest injuries.
- (4) Neurosurgical postoperative coma.
- (5) Air and fat embolism.
- (6) Several of the conditions noted in a and b, above, may include both alveolar hypoventilation and retained secretions.

Postoperative Considerations

1. Immediate postoperative chest x-ray films (anteroposterior and lateral) are important to ascertain the length and position of the tracheotomy tube and to rule out complications such as pneumomediastinum or pneumothorax.
2. The inner cannula of the tracheotomy tube is removed and cleaned every 1 to 2 hours for the first 2 to 3 days to prevent obstruction by dried mucus. It is especially important in infants.
3. A tracheotomy tube in a fresh tracheotomy is left in place 2 to 5 days before it is changed. By this time a permanent tract exists and there is little danger of being unable to reinsert the tube. Changing a tube before this time may result in loss of the tracheal opening into the neck wound, with possible fatality.
4. A string around the neck should never be loosened "for comfort." The tube may slip out of the fresh tracheotomy wound.
5. Suctioning must be done often, especially during the first few days after tracheotomy, because of the increase in tracheobronchial secretions secondary to tracheal irritation.
6. A tracheotomy is left in place no longer than necessary, especially in children. Removal as soon as safely possible helps reduce the incidence of tracheobronchitis, tracheal ulceration, tracheal stenosis, tracheomalacia, and persistent tracheocutaneous fistula.

Complications

Complications of tracheotomy[140,142–149] may be summarized as follows:

1. Immediate complications
   - a. Apnea
   - b. Hemorrhage
   - c. Pneumothorax and pneumomediastinum
   - d. Subcutaneous emphysema
   - e. Malpositioned tube
   - f. Tracheoesophageal fistula
   - g. Recurrent laryngeal nerve paralysis
   - h. High tracheotomy (injury to the cricoid cartilage)

      i.   Aerophagia
      j.   Aspiration of gastric contents
2. Delayed complications
    a.   Delayed hemorrhage (innominate artery erosion)
    b.   Tracheoesophageal fistula (following decannulation)
    c.   Tracheocutaneous fistula
    d.   Displacement or obstruction of a tube and cuff
    e.   Atelectasis and pulmonary infection
    f.   Tracheomalacia
    g.   Dysphagia
    h.   Difficult decannulation
    i.   Problems with neck scar
    j.   Tracheal stenosis

Apnea

When tracheotomy is performed on a patient with a history of chronic hypoxia, the patient may take one or two breaths right after the procedure and then suddenly become apneic. This phenomenon is due to physiologic denervation of the peripheral chemoreceptors by the sudden increase of Po_2; moreover, because hypoxia may be largely responsible for the respiratory drive in these patients, apnea results. Some form of respiratory assistance is necessary until enough Co_2 is removed to allow a return of sensitivity of central chemoreceptors. The patient should never be left unattended after an emergency tracheotomy.

Tracheoesophageal Fistula

Inadvertent perforation of the trachea during surgery may occur when the tracheostomy is placed through the tracheal wall instead of following the tracheal lumen. Another mechanism of injury may occur during surgery if the surgeon incises too deep into the trachea, causing a tracheal incision of the posterior tracheal wall into the esophagus or approaching the trachea from the side. Recurrent laryngeal nerve injury rarely occurs. These complications can be avoided by dissecting the midline of the neck and inserting a rigid endotracheal airway.

Aerophagia

Aerophagia[148] is seen most often in infants and young children and should be recognized as a cause of persistent dyspnea. It is treated with nasogastric tube decompression of the swallowed air. Death of an infant secondary to aerophagia with respiratory compromise has been reported.

Delayed Hemorrhage

Delayed hemorrhage[142,149,150] is most often due to erosion of a major vessel by pressure necrosis from the cuff or occasionally the tip of the tracheotomy tube. Any bleeding that occurs 4 to 5 days postoperatively should be given careful and immediate attention because of the threat that it may represent erosion into a major vessel. The innominate artery is the vessel most commonly involved,[141] but the common carotid, inferior and superior thyroid arteries, aortic arch, or occasionally the innominate vein may also be involved.

Hemorrhage

Hemorrhage may occur if hemostasis is not secured at operation.

Pneumothorax

Pneumothorax may be caused by injury to the copula of the pleura, which rises into the neck in infants and young children and is subject to injury during the operative procedure. It usually occurs when tracheotomy is done without prior establishment of an airway by a bronchoscope or an endotracheal tube.

Pneumomediastinum

Pneumomediastinum may result from air being sucked through the wound in a severely obstructed child having violent respiratory movements, or it may result from excessive coughing, which forces air into the deep tissue planes of the neck and then dissects into the mediastinum. Should the parietal pleura rupture, pneumothorax results. Pneumomediastinum may require no surgical therapy, but pneumothorax often requires placement of chest tubes with an underwater seal.

Malpositioned Tube

Malpositioned tubes are a frequent complication. Careful preoperative selection of a tube followed by postoperative roentgenographic evaluation prevents this complication. Tubes of excessive length may impinge on the anterior wall of the trachea or the carina, producing partial tracheal obstruction as well as ulceration and possible rupture of the innominate artery. The tube may extend down one bronchus, with resultant atelectasis of the opposite lung. A tube that is too short may predispose to displacement of the tube out of the trachea, especially when the neck is flexed in obese individuals or small children. Patients who are obese or have distorted anatomy are more at risk. The use of customized tracheostomy tubes may be necessary. The use of a vertical incision in the neck will allow the tube's position to be directed by the proper placement in the trachea and not by the skin incision.

Prevention of Complications

Mathog and coworkers[146] proposed possible preventive measures, including the following: (1) adequate skin incision to allow visualization or palpation of abnormal vessels; (2) avoidance of a "low" tracheotomy (ie, minimal extension of the head, gentle traction with a tracheal hook, and the stoma placed in the second and third tracheal rings); (3) elimination of metal tubes, with the use of plastic or silicone rubber tubes without a cuff and roentgenographic guidance to be certain the position and length of tubes are appropriate; and (4) high humidity and aseptic care of the tracheotomy.

Delayed Complications

Tracheoesophageal Fistula

A delayed tracheoesophageal fistula is usually fatal and results from severe pressure necrosis from an overinflated cuff or from the tip of a malpositioned tube, the erosion occurring through the posterior tracheal wall and the anterior wall of the esophagus. Typically, aspiration through the fistula results in severe pneumonitis.

Difficult Decannulation

Difficult decannulation is a frequent complication in children. A tracheotomy tube is decannulated within 8 to 10 days (or sooner) whenever possible. If not, decannulation becomes difficult because (1) the child becomes accustomed to less resistance and less effort (tracheotomy decreases the dead space), (2) the child forgets the apneic reflex during deglutition, and (3) tracheal collapse develops.

Neck Scar

The use of a vertical skin incision is the most frequent cause of unsightly scar formation. The duration of tracheotomy is also important to scarring, which is lessened by early removal of the tube. Vertical contracture and widening scar requires a Z-plasty for repair.

Tracheal Stenosis

Stenosis of the larynx follows injury and perichondritis of the cricoid cartilage, which is the only circular tracheal support. Tracheal stenosis is most common in children and is thought to result from excision of cartilage from the anterior tracheal wall. Exuberant granulations may develop on the anterior tracheal wall owing to delayed epithelialization when there is a large defect in the anterior tracheal wall, and they may cause obstruction and bleeding.

Subglottic Stenosis

Tracheotomy-related subglottic stenosis may be related to bacteriologic pathogenesis via tracheostomal contamination. Therefore, the ability to control stomal contamination with topical and/or systemic antibiotics may play a role in the prevention of a wound infection leading to cicatricial scar and stricture.[151]

Endotracheal Intubation

Nasotracheal intubation has been recommended for treating acute epiglottitis. A smooth polyvinyl chloride tube of somewhat smaller caliber than that corresponding to the patient's age is used. After intubation, children are placed in a cool mist/oxygen tent. The tube is tolerated well. Duration of intubation is usually 24 to 48 hours. Because most children with acute epiglottitis must be intubated to be tracheotomized and because the critical period for airway obstruction is at most 48 hours, nasotracheal intubation may be preferable to acute tracheotomy in a severely ill child.[16] However, for those who are responsible for the occasional case, and where nursing care in a pediatric ICU is not available, it is safer to rely on the time-tested tracheotomy. Endotracheal intubation should be done only by an experienced anesthesiologist or otolaryngologist.

There has been renewed interest in prolonged endotracheal intubation. Autopsy studies have shown the following:

1. Total damage and laryngeal ulceration in the intubated larynx and trachea were statistically related to duration of intubation but not to age or sex of the patient.
2. Significant ulcerations were confined to the posterior half of the larynx and the anterior and lateral aspects of the trachea between the third and tenth rings.
3. Intubation beyond 48 hours was associated with significant laryngeal ulceration, increasingly severe vocal process perichondritis, and frequent infection by microorganisms.
4. Intubation beyond 96 hours was associated with severe damage to the vocal processes and the subglottis as well as a high incidence of inferior vocal fold ulceration.
5. Tracheal damage in patients with multiple intubations or extubation before death was similar to that in continuously intubated patients, but inflammation was more widespread and deeper.
6. Orotracheal intubation of adults for more than 96 hours may cause permanent damage.

Causes of inadequate ventilation with intubation include the following:

1. Mucus or clot obstruction
2. Herniation of the cuff down over the end of the tube

3. Collapse of the beveled end of the tube so as to block the lumen
4. Lodging of the open portion of the beveled tube against the tracheal wall so as to occlude its lumen
5. Kinking of the proximal unarmored end of the tube at its attachment to the adaptor
6. Collapse of the endotracheal tube lumen by the inflated cuff[153]

Tracheotomy and Laryngeal Function

Prolonged tracheotomy may result in aspiration owing to a weakened, ill-coordinated adductor reflex response resulting from behavioral alterations of medullary adductor motor neurons. Experimental evidence has shown that phasic abductor activity in the posterior cricoarytenoid muscles diminishes as ventilatory resistance decreases. When airflow is shunted through a tracheotomy, abductor activity not only gradually diminishes but completely disappears. The longer the duration of decreased ventilatory resistance, the more difficult it is to re-establish the abductor function once it is lost. This fact helps to explain the difficulty encountered in tracheotomy decannulation when laryngeal abductor activity is lost, resulting in the absence of phasic inspiratory abduction.

Neurologically Intact Larynx before Tracheotomy

Vocal cords abduct and elongate on inspiration secondary to activation of the posterior cricoarytenoid (PCA) muscle (producing abduction) and cricothyroid muscle (producing elongation). During expiration, the cords close to the median position (cricothyroid muscle adduction).

Neurologically Intact Larynx after Tracheotomy

Vocal cords remain in the intermediate position in both phases of the respiratory cycle. Decreased airway resistance produced by tracheotomy abolishes the physiologic activity of both the PCA and cricothyroid muscles. Therefore, tracheotomy can and does cause lateralization of a paralyzed cord (in acute low vagal or RLN paralysis), which should be considered when determining the neuroanatomic site of injury.

LASERS IN LARYNGEAL SURGERY

Four types of lasers have been used in laser surgery of the larynx: (1) the CO_2 laser, (2) the argon laser, (3) the Nd:YAG laser, and (4) the potassium titanyl phosphate laser (KTP-532). The CO_2 laser has been the most frequently used wavelength in the larynx, while the KTP-532 laser is the most recent addition to laryngeal laser surgery.[42,97,155–163]

Laser and Tissue Interaction

Lasers produce coherent light energy that is in phase, has a discrete wavelength, and interacts with tissue in specific ways by its wavelength. When it hits the tissue, laser light may be transmitted, absorbed, or reflected. When the laser energy is absorbed, the concentration of laser energy that is absorbed determines the laser–tissue interaction. In all soft and hard tissues, thermal, optical, physical, and chemical changes may occur. For application of lasers in otolaryngology, thermal effect has been the most often applied. Thermal effects on tissue depend largely on the amount of laser energy applied over time. The amount of laser energy is expressed as W/cm^2 and is called power density. The amount of energy applied over time is expressed as the number of joules. At power density of $1000 \ W/cm^2$, the thermal effect is coagulation; at $10,000 \ W/cm^2$, the thermal effect on soft tissue is vaporization.

With a power density of 100,000 W/cm^2, the laser effect is cutting. Because the laser energy is focused to a very small spot size, the spot size plays an important role in the understanding of laser energy delivery.

Carbon Dioxide Laser

The CO_2 laser, which emits an invisible beam of light of 10.6 μm, is absorbed by glass and water and reflected by mirrors or metallic substances. Because the CO_2 laser beam is invisible, the surgeon uses an aiming beam (a red or green dot) to direct the laser. It is imperative to make sure that this aiming beam is aligned with the real laser beam before use. It is also important that protective glasses be worn by the surgeon at all times when using the CO_2 laser, so that a misdirected ray from the laser will be absorbed by the glass and not injure the eye. Contact lenses or acrylic lenses are not sufficiently protective.[51,156,159]

Due to its specific wavelength and beam coherence capability, the CO_2 laser vaporizes tissues precisely with minimal surrounding thermal damage and is therefore frequently used for microlaryngeal surgery. A major disadvantage of the CO_2 laser is that fiberoptic transmission is not possible. A relative disadvantage is that most delivery systems are capable of a 7000-μm minimum spot size at the 400-mm focal length usually employed during laser microlaryngoscopy. The Ultraspot micromanipulator delivery system, however, allows a spot size of 200 μm at a 400-mm focal distance.[156]

The radiant waves from the CO_2 laser at 10.6 μm are ideal for surgical removal of tissue for four reasons:

1. They are strongly absorbed by all solids (except metals and certain metallic compounds) and by liquids, notably water, which is the major constituent of most living cells. In water, nearly all the radiant energy is absorbed within a depth of 100 μm from the irradiated surface.
2. They are not significantly scattered laterally from the target point.
3. Their absorption is not dependent on the color of the tissue.
4. When deliberately defocused, they can be used to coagulate blood and seal small vessels in vascular tissue without vaporizing the cells.

Argon Laser

The argon laser, unlike the CO_2 laser, is a visible beam of light of 0.5-μm wavelength in the blue-green spectrum. It is absorbed only by the color red and is transmitted through water, glass, and those tissues that are not red. For this reason, simple glasses are not adequate protection when using the argon laser; a stray argon laser beam would simply pass through regular glasses to the eyes, most likely damaging the retina. It is for this reason that the argon laser is used to treat retinal hemorrhages; the argon laser passes safely through the clear cornea and is absorbed only by the red pigment in the retina. Therefore, amber glasses must be worn at all times during this procedure, because a stray laser ray would be absorbed by the amber-colored glass and, being unable to pass through, would not damage the eyes.[159]

Unlike the CO_2 laser, the argon laser is not absorbed by glass and hence can be transmitted through fiberoptic cables. This is a distinct advantage to the surgeon because it eliminates the cumbersome articulated arm used with the CO_2 laser. The disadvantage is that the argon laser operates on a 220-V energizer and an open cooling system, requiring both a voltage adapter and an exterior plumbing and cooling system.

Like the CO_2 laser, the argon laser is precise; it causes minimum penetration, minimum edema, and minimum scarring.

The argon laser is capable of delivery via a fiberoptic system with beam sizes as small as 0.15 mm, and it has been utilized for selected laryngeal pathology, including hemorrhagic nodules, polyps, and vascular granulomas.[156]

YAG Laser

The Nd:YAG laser emits an invisible beam of light of 1.06 μm. As with the argon laser, the beam is transmitted through nonred tissues and glass. However, it is absorbed by water and dark pigments; thus, green glasses are worn for protection. Like the argon laser, the Nd:YAG laser utilizes a 220-V energizer and needs an exterior cooling device.

The Nd:YAG laser is an excellent photocoagulator, even better than the argon laser. It can be transmitted through fiberoptic cables. However, unlike both the CO_2 and argon lasers, it is not precise, having a 20 to 40% scatter, and it penetrates deeply. The Nd:YAG laser also causes more edema and scarring than the other two lasers. Because of its excellent ability to evaporate and coagulate, it is used for vascular tumors and tumors of the tracheobronchial area, to control gastrointestinal bleeding, and to destroy gastric tumors.

With the advent of sapphire tips that are available in different sizes and shapes, the scatter and poor predictability of depth penetration have been minimized. The frosted tips are for coagulation while the clear tips are for cutting. The sapphire tips have also made the Nd:YAG laser a fine dissecting tool with good hemostasis.[156,159]

Because most tissues have a low coefficient absorption of Nd:YAG laser energy (with the exception of hemoglobin and other dark pigments), most tissues produce a high degree of scattering, which results in low precision in terms of cutting and vaporization. For this reason, the Nd:YAG laser has not been used frequently in the larynx and has been reserved for obstructive malignant lesions of the tracheobronchial tree.[156]

KTP-532 Laser

The potassium titanyl phosphate (KTP-532) laser has been applied to laryngeal lesions. This laser system produces visible light with a wavelength of 532 μm. The KTP-532 laser does not vaporize as precisely as the CO_2 laser; however, it has the advantage of combining a very small spot size (200 μm) with delivery through a fiberoptic system. Another advantage of this system is the sharp edge of the aim beam, which is an attenuated version of the surgical beam. The KTP-532 laser has been useful for such lesions as papillomas and carcinomas and for phonosurgical procedures. The surgical results have been reported to be superior to or comparable to those of the CO_2 laser.

Clinical Applications

The laser has been used in a variety of benign and malignant lesions affecting the larynx. The precision afforded by a nontouch technique has been the main advantage of the use of lasers. Unintended lateral thermal effects may cause scarring and stiffness in the vocal folds. In recent papers, there is controversy as to the role of the CO_2 laser in the management of certain benign mucosal lesions such as vocal fold nodules and vocal fold cysts.

1. Excision of benign lesions
    a. Polyps
    b. Cysts
    c. Granulomas
    d. Recurrent papillomas
    e. Subglottic hemangioma

      f.   Laryngoceles

      g.   Contact ulcers

      h.   Lymphagiomas

2. Excision and palliation of malignant lesions

      a.   Early cancer (T_1 lesions, carcinoma in situ) can be cured by laser excision.[160,162,163]

      b.   Use of laser for malignant lesions is for diagnosis (biopsy), debulking, improved airway, and cure.

      c.   Recent studies reported in the literature have demonstrated that when T_1 glottic carcinomas were treated with CO_2 laser excisional biopsy, cure rates (80–90%) matched those produced either by conservation laryngeal surgery or radiotherapy.[156,157,161,164] Blakeslee and coworkers[155] established rigid criteria that must be met before CO_2 laser excisional biopsy can be considered a "cure" (no further therapy needed).

          (1)   The lesion must be completely visualized at the time of laser microlaryngoscopy.

          (2)   The lesion must not extend to involve the anterior commissure or vocal process.

          (3)   The lesion must involve the mucous membrane only.

          (4)   Further tumor is not visible at $\times25$ magnification.

          (5)   Frozen-section biopsy of the wound edges must show them to be free of disease.

          (6)   The final permanent section should show freedom of disease at the margin. It is important to note that incomplete laser excisional biopsy does not preclude further treatment (conservation surgery or radiotherapy) if these criteria are not met. CO_2 laser excisional biopsy can also be considered a diagnostic procedure for evaluation of the degree of invasive tumor.

      d.   Kaufman[157] reported that 16 patients with anterior commissure extension who underwent laser excisional biopsy were tumor-free 38 to 66 months postoperatively. Wetmore and associates[164] noted 2 recurrences in 8 patients (total series of 21 patients) originally diagnosed with anterior commissure involvement.

      e.   Krespi and Meltzer[158] concluded that anterior commissure carcinomas are not completely excised via the CO_2 laser due to the following:

          (1)   The mechanical constraints of the laser when operating in the three-dimensional anatomy of the anterior commissure

          (2)   The possible and unrecognized presence of tumor invasion into the anterior commissure ligament

      They believe that laser excisional biopsy for attempted cure is contraindicated for tumors that involve or approach the anterior commissure.

      f.   Laser excisional biopsy, when properly done, has several advantages.

          (1)   The procedure establishes the diagnosis and can be curative for small lesions removed with clear margins.

          (2)   Laser excisional biopsy with positive margin establishes the need for further treatment (conservation surgery or radiotherapy).

          (3)   Complete excisional biopsy is accomplished in the outpatient setting.

          (4)   Operative morbidity is equal to that of laryngoscopy and biopsy.

      g.   Hirano and colleagues[88] compared vocal function in patients who had undergone laser excisional biopsy with or without radiotherapy with that of patients subjected to radiotherapy only. The phonatory function tests included psychoacoustic evaluation of hoarseness, videolaryngostroboscopy, measurement of maximum phonation time, measurement of mean airflow rate during phonation, measurement of physiologic fundamental frequency range of phonation, measurement of intensity range of phonation, and measurement of the intensity–flow ratio. Evaluation of hoarseness revealed that laser surgery results in a hoarse voice more frequently than does radiotherapy. Videostroboscopic analysis showed incomplete glottal closure and decreased vocal fold vibration following laser excisional biopsy. The remainder of the parameters showed no appreciable difference between patients subjected to laser excisional biopsy and radiotherapy. Overall, the authors concluded that vocal function following laser excisional biopsy is nearly comparable to that after radiotherapy in terms of conversational voice.[156,165]

   h.   Davis and associates[165] used the CO_2 laser in 20 highly selected patients to perform transoral epiglottic resection or partial supraglottic resection of tumor. The procedures were performed for the following:

      (1)   Laser excisional biopsy on limited epiglottic cancers, especially tumors involving the suprahyoid epiglottis.

      (2)   Removal of benign epiglottic lesions obstructing the airway.

      (3)   Laser resection of the epiglottis for adequate visualization of the true vocal folds on previously treated cancer patients via indirect mirror examination.

   i.   Steiner has treated a large series of glottic, supraglottic, and hypopharyngeal squamous carcinoma using the laser as a primary modality of treatment by endoscopic excision. The surgery is not limited to T_1 or early T_2 glottic cancers but may be extended to selected T_3 carcinomas. Specialty instruments designed for tissue retraction and laryngeal distention help to alleviate the problems reported by prior authors. The treatment consists of oncologic excision with margin control. The long-term cure rate has been reported to be comparable to that of radiation with total laryngectomy and other open surgical approaches.[185]

3.   Treatment of airway obstruction

   a.   Vocal fold paralysis; endoscopic laser arytenoidectomy

   b.   Bilateral vocal fold motion impairment with airway obstruction; endoscopic laser transverse cordotomy[2]

   c.   Anterior and posterior glottic web

   d.   Subglottic stenosis

   e.   Obstructing malignant neoplasms

   f.   Laryngomalacia (excision of obstructive supraglottic tissue including aryepiglottic folds and cuneiform cartilages)

4.   Phonosurgical applications

   a.   Reinke's edema (polypoid corditis)

   b.   Dysphonia plica ventricularis

   c.   Vocal fold nodules (laser excision of nodules is controversial)

Advantages, Disadvantages, and Complications of Laser Surgery

Advantages

1.   Precise excision
2.   Rapid tissue destruction
3.   Reach inaccessible sites
4.   Excellent hemostasis

5. Minimal postoperative edema, pain, and scarring
6. Avoid tracheotomy
7. Minimize hospitalization

Disadvantages
1. Costly.
2. Time-consuming.
3. May be harmful to patients and operating room personnel if proper precautions are not taken.

Precautions
1. Protect eyes.
2. Protect adjacent tissues.
3. Avoid flammable anesthetics.
4. Protect endotracheal tubes.
5. Keep protective gauze wet.

Anesthetic Management of Endolaryngeal CO_2 Laser Surgery
1. A properly protected red rubber endotracheal tube or flexible metal endotracheal tube is used.
2. Venturi technique. A smaller catheter is placed in the laryngoscope above the level of the vocal cords. The high-pressure passage of oxygen out of the needle causes room air to flow down the laryngoscope. The pressure produced inflates the lungs. This type of anesthetic management is contraindicated in the obese patient and the patient with severe restrictive pulmonary disease.
3. Jet insufflation anesthesia. This is similar to the Venturi technique. In this case, a small catheter is placed at the level of the vocal cords or beneath it. An intermittent burst of high-pressure oxygen is jet-insufflated through the catheter to ventilate the patient.

Complications
1. Complications of CO_2 laser microlaryngoscopy are generally associated with striking unprotected material in the airway and unprotected tissues of the patient or operating room personnel. To reduce the risk of ocular damage, the patient's eyes are covered by moistened eye pads, and all operating room personnel wear plastic protective glasses. The radiation emitted by the CO_2 laser is predominantly absorbed in the cornea, not the retina, and gross corneal opacification can result from thermal denaturation and coagulation of proteins.
2. Precautions are taken to avoid endotracheal tube ignition during CO_2 laser surgery. These measures involve the use of specialized laser-retardant endotracheal tubes, wrapping the tube with reflective aluminum tape (it is advisable to test the tape before use), and placing moist neurologic cottonoids over the entire balloon. Oxygen concentration used during the anesthesia should be monitored. The use of oxygen levels of greater than 50% is contraindicated during laser surgery. Because nitrous oxide also supports combustion, the use of nitrous oxide should also be limited to total concentrations of O_2 and NO_2 of less than 50%.
3. Results of irradiating polyvinyl chloride and red rubber tubes indicate that red rubber is less flammable and therefore safer to use in conjunction with the CO_2 laser. Management of endotracheal tube ignition involves the following:

a. Remove the damaged tube while the patient is paralyzed to facilitate reintubation without laryngospasm.

b. Intravenous steroids and antibiotics are given as if treating a tracheal or pulmonary burn.

c. Intraoperative bronchoscopy is performed to remove any charred debris and assess the extent of the damage.

d. Delayed extubation with reexamination of the subglottis and trachea may be needed to assess the extent of further airway compromise.

Photodynamic Therapy[156,166–170]

Photodynamic therapy involves the systemic administration of a photosensitizing agent to living tissues. The photosensitizing agent is then activated by a specific laser wavelength, which causes destruction of target tissue. Hematoporphyrin derivative is concentrated preferentially in tumor cells and is activated by the argon laser.[156,167] Kelley and colleagues[169] utilized photodynamic therapy to treat 32 head and neck (3 of them laryngeal cancers) and pulmonary carcinomas in 30 patients. Tumor response was variable, with superficial tumors showing a more consistent response than deep infiltrating tumors. Another promising chemosensitizing agent for the argon laser appears to be rhodamine 123.[166,167] A specific advantage of rhodamine 123 versus hematoporphyrin derivative is the absence of generalized photosensitivity. Further investigations are needed to define the role of photodynamic therapy in the treatment of laryngeal disease.

References

1. Bailey BJ, Johnson JT, Kohut RI, et al. *Head and Neck Surgery—Otolaryngology.* Philadelphia: Lippincott, 1993.

2. Cummings CW, Fredrickson JM, Harker LA, et al, eds. *Otolaryngology—Head and Neck Surgery,* 2nd ed. Vol III. St. Louis: Mosby, 1993.

3. Fried MP. *The Larynx—A Multidisciplinary Approach,* 2nd ed. St. Louis: Mosby, 1996.

4. Rubin JS, Sataloff RT, Korovin GS, Gould WJ. *Diagnosis and Treatment of Voice Disorders.* New York: Igaku Shoin, 1995.

5. Holingshead WH. *Anatomy for Surgeons.* Vol I. *The Head and Neck,* 2nd ed. New York: Harper & Row, 1968.

6. Nasri S, Beizai P, Ye M, et al. Cross-innervation of the thyroarytenoid muscle by a branch from the external division of the superior laryngeal nerve. *Ann Otol Rhinol Laryngol* 1997;106:594–598.

7. Kirchner JA. Physiology of the larynx. In: Paparella MM, Shumrick DA, eds. *Otolaryngology.* Philadelphia: Saunders, 1980.

8. Sasaki CT. Physiology of the larynx. In: English GM, ed. *Otolaryngology.* Vol III. New York: Harper & Row, 1977.

9. Hirano M. *Clinical Examination of Voice.* New York: Springer-Verlag, 1981.

10. Hirano M. Phonosurgical anatomy of the larynx. In: Ford CN, Bless DM, eds. *Phonosurgery: Assessment and Surgical Management of Voice Disorders.* New York: Raven, 1991, 25–41.

11. Hirano M, Kurita S, Kiyokawa K, Sato K. Posterior glottis: Morphological study in excised human larynges. *Ann Otol Rhinol Laryngol* 1986;95:576–581.

12. Suzuki M, Kirchner JA. Afferent nerve fibers in the external branch of the superior laryngeal nerve in cat. *Ann Otol Rhinol Laryngol* 1968; 77:1059–1070.

13. Work WP. Unusual position of the right recurrent laryngeal nerve. *Ann Otol Rhinol Laryngol* 1941;50:769–775.

14. Baer T, Gore JC, Gracco LC, et al. Analysis of vocal tract shape and dimensions using magnetic resonance imaging: Vowels. *J Acoust Soc Am* 1991;90:799–828.

15. Strong MS et al. Cardiac complications of microsurgery of the larynx: Etiology, incidence and prevention. *Laryngoscope* 1974;84:908.

16. Tos M. Nasotracheal intubation in acute epiglottitis. *Arch Otolaryngol* 1973;97:373.

17. Bottenfield GW et al. Diagnosis and management of acute epiglottitis—Report of 90 consecutive cases. *Laryngoscope* 1980;90:822.

18. Berg S, Trollfors B, Nylen O, et al. Incidence, aetiology, and prognosis of acute epiglottitis in children and adults in Sweden. *Scand J Infect Dis* 1996;28:261–264.

19. Hickerson SL, Kirby RS, Wheeler JG, Schutze GE. Epiglottitis: A 9-year review. *South Med J* 1996;89:487–490.

20. Madore DV. Impact of immunization on *Haemophilus influenzae* type B disease. *Infect Agents Dis* 1996;5:8–20.

21. Deeb ZE. Acute supraglottitis in adults—Early indicators of airway obstruction. *Am J Otolaryngol* 1997;18:112–115.

22. Senior BA, Radkowski D, MacArthur C, et al. Changing patterns in pediatric supraglottitis: A multi-institutional review, 1980–1992. *Otolaryngol Head Neck Surg* 1994;110:203–210.

23. Shapiro J, Eavey RD, Baker AS. Adult supraglottitis: A prospective analysis. *JAMA* 1988;259:563–567.

24. Dedo HH. Recurrent laryngeal nerve section for spastic dysphonia. *Ann Otol Rhinol Laryngol* 1976;85:451.

25. Levenson MJ et al. Laryngeal tuberculosis: Review of twenty cases. *Laryngoscope* 1984;94:1094.

26. Thaller SR, Gross JR, Pilch BZ, Goodman ML. Laryngeal tuberculosis as manifested in the decades 1963–1983. *Laryngoscope* 1987;97:848–850.

27. Amoils CP, Shindo ML. Laryngotracheal manifestations of rhinoscleroma. *Ann Otol Rhinol Laryngol* 1996;105:336–340.

28. Reder PA, Neel HB. Blastomycosis in otolaryngology—Review of a large series. *Laryngoscope* 1993;103:53–58.

29. Gerber ME, Rosdeutscher JD, Seiden AM, Tami TA. Histoplasmosis: The otolaryngologist's perspective. *Laryngoscope* 1995;105:919–923.

30. Gissman L, Diehl V. Schultz-Coulton HJ, et al. Molecular cloning and characterization of human papilloma virus DNA derived from a laryngeal papilloma. *J Virol* 1982;44:393–400.

31. Leventhal B, Kashima H, Levine A. Treatment of recurrent laryngeal papillomatosis with an artificial interferon inducer (poly ICLC). *J Pediatr* 1981;99:14.

32. Lusk RP, McCabe BF, Mixon JH. Three-year experience of treating recurrent respiratory papilloma with interferon. *Ann Otol Rhinol Laryngol* 1987;96:158–162.

33. Quiney RE, Hall D, Croft CB. Laryngeal papillomatosis: Analysis of 113 patients. *Clin Otolaryngol* 1989;14:217–225.

34. Quiney RE, Wells M, Lewis FA, et al. Laryngeal papillomatosis: Correlation between severity of disease and presence of HPV 6 and 11 detected by in situ DNA hybridization. *J Clin Pathol* 1989;42:694–698.

35. Singleton GT, Adkins WY. Cryosurgical treatment of juvenile laryngeal papillomatosis: Eight-year experience. *Ann Otol Rhinol Laryngol* 1972;81:784.

36. Strong MS et al. Recurrent respiratory papillomatosis: Management with the CO_2 laser. *Ann Otol Rhinol Laryngol* 1976;85:508.

37. Avidano MA, Singleton GT. Adjuvant drug strategies in the treatment of recurrent respiratory papillomatosis. *Otolaryngol Head Neck Surg* 1995;112:197–202.

38. Bujia J, Feyh J, Kastenbauer E. Photodynamic therapy with derivatives from hematoporphyrines for recurrent laryngeal papillomatosis of the children—Early results. *Ann Otorrinolaryngol Ibero Am* 1993;20:251–259.

39. Lie ES, Karlsen F, Holm R. Presence of human papillomavirus in squamous cell laryngeal carcinomas—A study of thirty nine cases using polymerase chain reaction and in situ hybridization. *Acta Otolaryngol (Stockh)* 1996;116:900–905.

40. Hyams VJ, Habuzzi DD. Cartilaginous tumors of the larynx. *Laryngoscope* 1970;80:755.

41. Swerdlow RS et al. Cartilaginous tumors of the larynx. *Arch Otolaryngol* 1974;100:269.

42. Daminani KK, Tucker HM. Chondroma of the larynx. *Arch Otolaryngol* 1981;107:399.

43. Healy G et al. Treatment of subglottic hemangioma with the carbon dioxide laser. *Laryngoscope* 1980;90:809.

44. Bauman NM, Burke DK, Smith RJ. Treatment of massive or life-threatening hemangiomas with recombinant alpha(2a)-interferon. *Otolaryngol Head Neck Surg* 1997;117:99–110.

45. MacArthur CJ, Senders CW, Katz J. The use of interferon alpha-2a for life-threatening heman-

giomas. *Arch Otolaryngol Head Neck Surg* 1995;121:690–693.

46. Olms LA, Jones DT, McGill TJ, Healy GB. Interferon alpha-2a therapy for airway hemangiomas. *Ann Otol Rhinol Laryngol* 1994; 103:1–8.

47. Sie KC, Mcgill T, Healy GB. Subglottic hemangioma—Ten years' experience with the carbon dioxide laser. *Ann Otol Rhinol Laryngol* 1994;103:167–172.

48. Soumekh B, Adams GL, Shapiro RS. Treatment of head and neck hemangiomas with recombinant interferon alpha-2b. *Ann Otol Rhinol Laryngol* 1996;105:201–206.

49. Komisar A. Laser laryngoscopic management of internal laryngocele. *Laryngoscope* 1987; 97:368–369.

50. Myssiorek D, Persky M. Laser endoscopic treatment of laryngoceles and laryngeal cysts. *Otolaryngol Head Neck Surg* 1989;100:538–541.

51. Ward PH et al. Contact ulcers and granulomas of the larynx: New insights into their etiology as a basis for more rational treatment. *Otolaryngol Head Neck Surg* 1980;88:262.

52. Weisman R et al. Laryngeal sarcoidosis with airway obstruction. *Ann Otol Rhinol Laryngol* 1980;89:58.

53. Benjamin B, Dalton C, Croxson G. Laryngoscopic diagnosis of laryngeal sarcoid. *Ann Otol Rhinol Laryngol* 1995;104:529–531.

54. Gallivan GJ, Landis JN. Sarcoidosis of the larynx—Preserving and restoring airway and professional voice. *J Voice* 1993;7:81–94.

55. Koufman JA. Gastroesophageal reflux and voice disorders. In: Rubin JS, et al, eds. *Diagnosis and Treatment of Voice Disorders.* New York: Igaku Shoin, 1995, chap 11.

56. Brazeau-Lamontagne L, Charlin B, Levesque RY, et al. Cricoarytenoiditis: CT assessment in rheumatoid arthritis. *Radiology* 1986;158: 463–466.

57. Futran ND, Sherris D, Norante JD. Cricoarytenoid arthritis in children. *Otolaryngol Head Neck Surg* 1991;104:366–370.

58. Montgomery WW. *Surgery of the Upper Respiratory System.* Vol II. Philadelphia: Lea & Febiger, 1973.

59. Ogura J. Management of traumatic injuries of the larynx and trachea including stenosis. *J Laryngol Otol* 1971;85:1250.

60. Benjamin B. Endoscopy in congenital tracheal anomalies. *J Pediatr Surg* 1980;15:164.

61. Yanagisawa E, Casuccio JR, Suzuki M. Videolaryngoscopy using a rigid telescope and home video system color camera: A useful office procedure. *Ann Otol Rhinol Laryngol* 1981; 90:346–350.

62. Dedo HH, Sooy CD. Endoscopic (laser) repair of posterior glottic, subglottic and tracheal stenosis by division or micro-trapdoor flap. *Laryngoscope* 1984;94:445–450.

63. Rethi A. An operation for cicatricial stenosis of larynx. *J Laryngol Otol* 1956;70:283.

64. Druck NS, Alonso WA, Ogura JH. Hyoid arch transportation. *Trans Am Acad Ophthalmol Otolaryngol* 1976;82:175–187.

65. Gerwat J, Bryce DP. The management of subglottic laryngeal stenosis by resection and direct anastomosis. *Laryngoscope* 1974;84:940.

66. Pearson FG et al. Primary tracheal anastomosis after resection of the cricoid cartilage with preservation of recurrent laryngeal nerves. *J Thorac Cardiovasc Surg* 1975;70:806.

67. Evans JNG, Todd GB. Laryngotracheoplasty. *J Laryngol Otol* 1974;88:589.

68. Fearon B, Cotton R. Subglottic stenosis in infants and children: The clinical problem and experimental surgical correction. *Can J Otolaryngol* 1972;1:281.

69. Shapshay SM, Beamis JF, Hybels RL, Bohigian RK. Endoscopic treatment of subglottic and tracheal stenosis by radical laser incision and dilatation. *Ann Otol Rhinol Laryngol* 1987; 96:661–664.

69a. Conley JJ. Reconstruction of the subglottic air passage. *Ann Otol Rhinol Laryngol* 1953;62: 477.

70. Cotton RT, Gray SD, Miller RP. Update of the Cincinnati experience in pediatric laryngotracheal reconstruction. *Laryngoscope* 1985;99: 1111–1115.

71. Cotton R, Myer CM, Bratcher GO, Fitton CM. Anterior cricoid split, 1977–1987. *Arch Otolaryngol Head Neck Surg* 1988;114:1300–1302.

72. Grundfast KM, Camilon FS, Barber CS, et al. Prospective study of subglottic stenosis in intubated neonates. *Ann Otol Rhinol Laryngol* 1990;99:390–395.

73. Healy GB. Subglottic stenosis. *Otolaryngol Clin North Am* 1989;22:599–606.

74. Holinger LD. Subglottic stenosis. *Curr Ther Otolaryngol Head Neck Surg* 1990;369–373.

75. Holinger LD, Stankiewicz JA, Livingston GL. Anterior cricoid split—The Chicago experience with an alternative to tracheotomy. *Laryngoscope* 1987;97:19–24.

76. Lusk R, Kang D, Muntz H. Auricular cartilage grafts in laryngotracheal reconstruction. *Ann Otol Rhinol Laryngol* 1993;102:247–254.

77. Seid AB, Pransky SM, Kearns DB. One-stage laryngotracheoplasty. *Arch Otolaryngol Head Neck Surg* 1991;117:408–410.

78. Holinger LD, Konior RJ. Surgical management of severe laryngomalacia. *Laryngoscope* 1989;99:136–142.

79. Holinger LD, Oppenheimer RW. Congenital subglottic stenosis—The elliptical cricoid cartilage. *Ann Otol Rhinol Laryngol* 1989;98:702–706.

80. Smith JD, Cotton R, Meyer CM. Subglottic cysts in the premature infant. *Arch Otolaryngol Head Neck Surg* 1990;116:479–482.

81. Smith SP, Berkowitz RG, Phelan PD. Acquired subglottic cysts in infancy. *Arch Otolaryngol Head Neck Surg* 1994;120:921–924.

82. Toriumi DM, Miller DR, Holinger LD. Acquired subglottic cysts in premature infants. *Int J Pediatr Otorhinolaryngol* 1987;14:151–160.

83. McClurg FLD, Evans DA. Laser laryngoplasty for laryngomalacia. *Laryngoscope* 1994;104:247–252.

84. Polonovski JM, Contencin P, Viala P, et al. Aryepiglottic fold excision for the treatment of severe laryngomalacia. *Ann Otol Rhinol Laryngol* 1990;99:625–627.

85. Zalzal GH, Anon JB, Cotton RT. Epiglottoplasty for the treatment of laryngomalacia. *Ann Otol Rhinol Laryngol* 1987;96:72–76.

86. Ward PH, Engel E, Nance WE. The larynx in cri du chat (cat cry) syndrome. *Laryngoscope* 1968;78:1716.

87. Myer CM, Holmes DK, Cotton RT, Jackson RK. Laryngeal and laryngotracheoesophageal clefts—Role of early surgical repair. *Ann Otol Rhinol Laryngol* 1990;99:98–104.

88. Holinger PH, Brown WT. Congenital webs, cysts, laryngoceles, and other anomalies of the larynx. *Ann Otol Rhinol Laryngol* 1967;76:744.

89. Brandenburg J. Management of acute blunt laryngeal injuries. *Otolaryngol Clin North Am* 1979;12:741.

90. Olson N. Surgical treatment of acute blunt laryngeal injuries. *Ann Otol Rhinol Laryngol* 1978;87:716.

91. Sofferman R. Management of laryngotracheal trauma. *Am J Surg* 1981;141:412.

91a. Cohen S et al. Foreign bodies in the airway: Five-year retrospective study with special reference to management. *Ann Otol Rhinol Laryngol* 1980;89:437.

92. Holinger LD. Diagnostic endoscopy of the pediatric airway. *Laryngoscope* 1989;99:346–348.

93. Schechter GL, Kostianovsky M. Vocal cord paralysis in diabetes mellitus. *Trans Am Acad Ophthalmol Otolaryngol* 1972;76:729–740.

94. Sessions DG et al. Surgical management of bilateral vocal cord paralysis. *Laryngoscope* 1976;86:559.

95. Bless DM, Hirano M, Feder RJ. Videostroboscopic evaluation of the larynx. *Ear Nose Throat J* 1987;66:289–296.

96. Kitzing P. Stroboscopy—A pertinent laryngological examination. *J Otolaryngol* 1985;14:151–157.

97. Hirano M, Hirade Y, Kawasaki H. Vocal function following carbon dioxide laser surgery for glottic carcinoma. *Ann Otol Rhinol Laryngol* 1985;94:232–235.

98. Wendler J. Stroboscopy. *J Voice* 1992;6:149–154.

99. Yanagisawa E, Yanagisawa R. Laryngeal photography. *Otolaryngol Clin North Am* 1991;24:999–1022.

100. Yanagisawa E, Yanagisawa K. Stroboscopic videolaryngoscopy: A comparison of fiberscopic and telescopic documentation. *Ann Otol Rhinol Laryngol* 1993;102:255–265.

101. Yanagisawa E, Owens TW, Strothers G, Honda K. Videolaryngoscopy: A comparison of fiberscopic and telescopic documentation. *Ann Otol Rhinol Laryngol* 1983;92:430–436.

102. Hirano M, Ohala J. Use of hooked-wire electrodes for electromyelography of the intrinsic laryngeal muscles. *J Speech Hear Res* 1969;12:362.

103. Varvares MA, Montgomery WW, Hillman RE. Teflon granulomas of the larynx—Etiology, pathophysiology and management. *Ann Otol Rhinol Laryngol* 1995;104:511–515.

104. Ford CN, Staskowski PA, Bless DM. Autologous collagen vocal fold injection—A preliminary study. *Laryngoscope* 1995;105:944–948.

105. Arnold GE. Vocal rehabilitation of paralytic dysphonia IX. Technique of intratracheal injection. *Arch Otolaryngol* 1962;76:358.

106. Lewy RB. Experience with vocal cord injection. *Ann Otol Rhinol Laryngol* 1976;85:440.

107. Meurmann Y. Operative mediofixation of the vocal cord in complete unilateral paralysis. *Arch Otolaryngol* 1952;55:554.

108. Benninger MS, Crumley RL, Ford CN, et al. Evaluation and treatment of the unilateral paralyzed vocal cord. *Otolaryngol Head Neck Surg* 1994;111:497–508.

109. Isshiki N, Morita H, Okamura H, et al. Thyroplasty as a new phonosurgical technique. *Acta Otolaryngol (Stockh)* 1974;78:451–457.

110. Isshiki N, Taira T, Kojima H, et al. Recent modifications in thyroplasty type I. *Ann Otol Rhinol Laryngol* 1989;98:777–779.

111. Montgomery WW. Cricoarytenoid arthrodesis. *Ann Otol Rhinol Laryngol* 1966;75:380.

112. Montgomery WW, Blaugrund SM, Varvares MA. Thyroplasty: A new approach. *Ann Otol Rhinol Laryngol* 1993;102:571–579.

113. Cummings CW, Purcell LL, Flint PW. Hydroxylapatite laryngeal implants for medialization: Preliminary report. *Ann Otol Rhinol Laryngol* 1993;102:843–851.

114. Isshiki N, Tanabe M, Sawada M. Arytenoid adduction for unilateral vocal cord paralysis. *Arch Otolaryngol* 1978;104:555–558.

115. Netterville JL, Stone RE, Civantos FJ, et al. Silastic medialization and arytenoid adduction—The Vanderbilt experience. *Ann Otol Rhinol Laryngol* 1993;102:413–424.

116. Tucker HM. Human laryngeal reinnervation: Long-term experience with the nerve-muscle pedicle technique. *Laryngoscope* 1978;88:598.

117. Crumley R, Izdebski K. Voice quality following laryngeal reinnervation by ansa hypoglossi transfer. *Laryngoscope* 1986;96:611–616.

118. Thornell WC. Intralaryngeal approach for arytenoidectomy in bilateral abductor vocal cord paralysis. *Arch Otolaryngol* 1948;47:505.

119. Ossoff RH, Duncavage JA, Shapshay SM, et al. Endoscopic laser arytenoidectomy revisited. *Ann Otol Rhinol Laryngol* 1990;99:764–771.

120. King BT. New and function-restoring operation for bilateral abductor cord paralysis. *JAMA* 1939;112:814.

121. Kashima HL. Bilateral vocal fold motion impairment—Pathophysiology and management by traverse cordotomy. *Ann Otol Rhinol Laryngol* 1991;100:717–721.

122. Von Doersten PG, Krzysztof I, Ross JC, et al. Ventricular dysphonia—A profile of 40 cases. *Laryngoscope* 1992;102:1296–1301.

123. Biller H, Som M, Lawson W. Laryngeal nerve crush for spastic dysphonia. *Ann Otol Rhinol Laryngol* 1979;88:531.

124. Carpenter RJ II, Snyder GG II, Henley-Cohn JL. Selective section of the recurrent laryngeal nerve for the treatment of spastic dysphonia: An experimental study and preliminary clinical report. *Otolaryngol Head Neck Surg* 1981; 89:986.

125. Aronson AE, DeSanto LW. Abductor spastic dysphonia: 1-1/2 years after recurrent laryngeal nerve resection. *Ann Otol Rhinol Laryngol* 1981;90:2.

126. Blitzer AB, Brin MF, Fahn S, Lovelace RE. Localized injections of botulinum toxin for the treatment of focal laryngeal dystonia (spastic dysphonia). *Laryngoscope* 1988;98:193–197.

127. Miller RH, Woodson GE, Jankovic J. Botulinum toxin injection of the vocal fold for spasmodic dysphonia: A preliminary report. *Arch Otolaryngol Head Neck Surg* 1987;113: 603–605.

128. Ludlow CL, Naunton RF, Sedory SE, et al. Effects of botulinum toxin injections on speech in abductor spasmodic dysphonia. *Neurology* 1988;38:1220–1225.

129. Eibling DE, Johnson JJ, Bacon GW. *Understanding and Treating Aspiration.* Alexandria, VA: American Academy of Otolaryngology—Head and Neck Surgery Foundation, 1993, 31–33.

130. Lindeman RC. Diverting the paralyzed larynx: A reversible procedure for intractable aspiration. *Laryngoscope* 1975;85:157.

131. Montgomery WW. Surgery to prevent aspiration. *Arch Otolaryngol* 1975;101:679.

132. Sasaki CT et al. Surgical closure of the larynx for intractable aspiration. *Arch Otolaryngol* 1980;106:422.

133. Johns ME, Cantrell RW. Voice restoration of the total laryngectomy patient: The Singer-Blom technique. *Otolaryngol Head Neck Surg* 1981;89:82.

134. Singer MI, Blom ED. An endoscopic technique for restoration of voice after total laryngectomy. *Ann Otol Rhinol Laryngol* 1980;89:529.

135. Singer MI, Blom ED, Hamaker RC. Further experience with voice restoration after total laryngectomy. *Ann Otol Rhinol Laryngol* 1981; 90:498.

136. Asai R. Laryngoplasty after total laryngectomy. *Arch Otolaryngol* 1972;95:114.

137. Sisson GA, Goldman ME. Pseudoglottis procedure: Update and secondary reconstruction techniques. *Laryngoscope* 1980;90:1120.

138. Staffieri M, Serafini I. La riabilitazione chirurgica della voce e della respirazione dopo laryngectomia totale. *29th National Congress of the Associazione Otologi Ospedalieri Italiana.* Bologna: Associazione Otologi Ospedalieri Italiana, 1956, 57–111.

139. Gaudet PT et al. Pediatric tracheostomy and associated complications. *Laryngoscope* 1978; 88:1633.

140. Hawkins DB, Williams EH. Tracheotomy in infants and young children. *Laryngoscope* 1976;86:331–340.

141. Tucker JA, Silberman HD. Tracheotomy in pediatrics. *Ann Otol Rhinol Laryngol* 1972; 81:818.

142. Biller HF, Ebert PA. Innominate artery hemorrhage complicating tracheotomy. *Ann Otol Rhinol Laryngol* 1970;79:301.

143. Chew JY, Cantrell RW. Tracheotomy: Complications and their management. *Arch Otolaryngol* 1972;96:538.

144. Glas WW et al. Complications of tracheotomy. *Arch Surg* 1962;85:56.

145. Grillo HC. Tracheal reconstruction: Indications and techniques. *Arch Otolaryngol* 1972;96: 31–39.

146. Mathog RH et al. Delayed massive hemorrhage following tracheostomy. *Laryngoscope* 1971;81:107.

147. Rabuzzi DD, Reed GF. Intrathoracic complications following tracheotomy in children. *Laryngoscope* 1971;81:939.

148. Rosnagle RS, Yanagisawa E. Aerophagia: Unrecognized complications of tracheotomy. *Arch Otolaryngol* 1969;89:537.

149. Utley JR et al. Definitive management of innominate artery hemorrhage complicating tracheostomy. *JAMA* 1972;220:577.

150. Margolis CZ et al. Routine tracheotomy for *Haemophilus influenzae* type B epiglottis. *J Pediatr* 1971;81:1150.

151. Sasaki CT et al. Tracheostomy-related subglottic stenosis: Bacteriologic pathogenesis. *Laryngoscope* 1979;89:857.

152. Hilding AC. Laryngotracheal damage during intratracheal anesthesia: Demonstration by staining unfixed specimen with methylene blue. *Ann Otol Rhinol Laryngol* 1971;80:565.

153. Pearson KD. Defective endotracheal tube demonstrated on chest roentgenogram: A case report. *Radiology* 1970;95:304.

154. Sasaki CT et al. The effect of tracheostomy on the laryngeal closure reflex. *Laryngoscope* 1977;87:1428.

155. Blakeslee D, Vaughn CW, Shapshay SM, et al. Excisional biopsy in the selective management of T_1 glottic cancer—A three-year follow-up study. *Laryngoscope* 1984;94:488–494.

156. Crockett DM, Reynolds BN. Laryngeal laser surgery. *Otolaryngol Clin North Am* 1990; 23:49–66.

157. Kaufman JA. The endoscopic management of early squamous carcinoma of the vocal cord with the carbon dioxide laser: Clinical experience and a proposed subclassification. *Otolaryngol Head Neck Surg* 1986;95:531–537.

158. Krespi Y, Meltzer CJ. Laser surgery for vocal cord carcinoma involving the anterior commissure. *Ann Otol Rhinol Laryngol* 1989;98: 105–109.

159. Lee KJ, Lee KE. The laser in otolaryngology—Head and neck surgery. In Lee KJ, ed. *Textbook of Otolaryngology and Head and Neck Surgery.* New York: Elsevier, 1989.

160. McGuirt WF, Koufman JA. Endoscopic laser surgery: An alternative in laryngeal cancer treatment. *Arch Otolaryngol Head Neck Surg* 1987;113:501–505.

161. Ossoff RH, Sisson GA, Shapshay SM. Endoscopic management of selected early vocal cord carcinomas. *Ann Otol Rhinol Laryngol* 1985;94:560–564.

162. Shapshay SM, Hybels RL, Bohigian RK. Laser excision of early vocal cord carcinoma: Indications, limitations, and precautions. *Ann Otol Rhinol Laryngol* 1990;99:46–50.

163. Wolfensberger M, Dort JC. Endoscopic laser surgery for (early glottic) carcinoma: A clini-

cal and experimental study. *Laryngoscope* 1990;100:1100–1105.

164. Wetmore SJ, Key JM, Suen JY. Laser therapy for T_1 glottic carcinoma of the larynx. *Arch Otolaryngol Head Neck Surg* 1986;112:853–855.

165. Davis RK, Shapshay SM, Strong MS, Hyams VJ. Transoral partial supraglottic resection using the CO_2 laser. *Laryngoscope* 1983;93:429–432.

166. Brodsky L, Yoshpe N, Ruben RJ. Clinical-pathological correlates of congenital subglottic hemangiomas. *Ann Otol Rhinol Laryngol* 1983;92(suppl 105):4–18.

167. Castro DJ, Saxton RE, Markley J, et al. Argon laser phototherapy of human malignancies using rhodamine-123 as a new laser dye: The intracellular role of oxygen. *Laryngoscope* 1990;100:884–891.

168. Gluckman JL. Hematoporphyrin photo-dynamic therapy: Is there truly a future in head and neck oncology? Reflections on a 5-year experience. *Laryngoscope* 1991;101:36–42.

169. Keller GS, Doiron DR, Fisher GU. Photo-dynamic therapy in otolaryngology—Head and neck surgery. *Arch Otolaryngol* 1985;111:758–761.

170. Biel MA. Photodynamic therapy and the treatment of neoplastic diseases of the larynx *Laryngoscope* 1994;104:399–403.

171. Nasri S et al. Cross-innervation of the thyro-arytenoid muscle by a branch from the external division of the superior laryngeal nerve. *Ann Otol Rhinol Laryngol* 1997;106(7 Pt 1):594–598.

172. Ossoff RH, Duncavage JA, Dere H. Microsub-glottoscopy: An expansion of operative micro-laryngoscopy. *Otolaryngol Head Neck Surg* 1991;104(6):842–848.

173. Benninger MS et al. Vocal fold scarring: Current concepts and management. *Otolaryngol Head Neck Surg* 1996;115(5):474–482.

174. Bobin S, Attal P. Laryngotracheal manifestations of gastroesophageal reflux in children. *Pediatr Pulmonol Suppl* 1999;5:1873–1875.

175. Beck IT et al. The second Canadian consensus conference on the management of patients with gastroesophageal reflux disease. *Can J Gastroenterol* 1997, B7b–B20b.

176. Belafsky PC, Postma GN, Koufman JA. Laryngopharyngeal reflux symptoms improve before changes in physical findings. *Laryngoscope* 2001;111(6):979–981.

177. Andrea M, Dias O, Santos A. Contact endoscopy of the vocal cord: Normal and pathological patterns. *Acta Otolaryngol* 1995; 115(2):314–316.

178. Fiorella R, Di Nicola V, Resta L. Epidemiological and clinical relief on hyperplastic lesions of the larynx. *Acta Otolaryngol Suppl* 1997;52777–52781.

179. Benninger MS, Gillen JB, Altman JS. Changing etiology of vocal fold immobility. *Laryngoscope* 1998;108(9):1346–1350.

180. Montgomery WW, Montgomery SK. Montgomery thyroplasty implant system. *Ann Otol Rhinol Laryngol Suppl* 1997;16:1701–1716.

181. Woodson GE et al. Arytenoid adduction: Controlling vertical position. *Ann Otol Rhinol Laryngol* 2000;109(4):360–364.

182. Woo P. Arytenoid adduction and medialization laryngoplasty. *Otolaryngol Clin North Am* 2000;33(4):817–840.

183. Zheng H et al. Update: Laryngeal reinnervation for unilateral vocal cord paralysis with the ansa cervicalis. *Laryngoscope* 1996;106(12 Pt 1):1522–1527.

184. Tucker HM. Laryngeal framework surgery in the management of spasmodic dysphonia. Preliminary report. *Ann Otol Rhinol Laryngol* 1989;98(1 Pt 1):52–54.

185. Steiner W. Results of curative laser micro-surgery of laryngeal carcinomas. *Am J Otolaryngol* 1993;14(2):116–121.

Obstructive Sleep Apnea   32

Obstructive sleep apnea is a common but not new disorder. Health care providers are becoming increasingly aware of this entity and its health impact. Dickens,[1] in his *Posthumous Papers of the Pickwick Club* (1837), described the obese and somnolent Joe, who "goes on errands fast asleep and snores as he waits on the table." Besides the classic "Pickwickian syndrome," obstructive sleep apnea may afflict both obese and nonobese individuals. Up to 24% of males and 9% of females meet the polysomnographic criteria to diagnose the condition. When the polysomnographic data are combined with symptoms of sleep apnea (obstructive sleep apnea syndrome, or OSAS), the prevalence rate is around 4 and 2% in males and females, respectively.[2] Obstructive sleep apnea is dangerous for the patient and others. It is easily recognizable and is treatable.

DEFINITIONS

Sleep-disordered breathing refers to a group of disorders caused by abnormal breathing patterns that disrupt sleep. It includes habitual snoring, upper airway resistance syndrome, and obstructive sleep apnea. The hallmark symptom of sleep-disordered breathing is snoring.

Apnea (from the Greek *ápnoia,* meaning "want of breath") is defined as the cessation of airflow for 10 or more seconds.[3,4] Controversy exists about the definition of hypopnea. The most widely used definition, however, is a more than 50% drop in airflow for 10 or more seconds, which results in either arousal from sleep or a greater than 4% drop in oxyhemoglobin saturation.[5] The apnea index (AI) is the number of apneas per hour of sleep, while the hypopnea index is the number of hypopneas per hour of sleep. Since hypopnea has similar clinical effects to apnea, a more commonly used index is the apnea/hypopnea index (AHI) or the respiratory disturbance index (RDI), which refers to the total number of apneas and hypopneas per hour of sleep. An RDI (or AHI) ≥5 respiratory events per hour of sleep indicates sleep apnea. An RDI of <5 events per hour of sleep is considered normal.

There are three characteristic patterns of apnea. Central apnea is the absence of airflow due to the lack of ventilatory effort. Obstructive sleep apnea (OSA) is defined by the absence of airflow despite persistent ventilatory effort, demonstrated by contraction of the respiratory muscles, such as the diaphragm. Obstructive sleep apnea syndrome (OSAS) refers to findings of OSA in combination with symptoms related to sleep deprivation or cardiopulmonary dysfunction. A mixed apnea includes both central and obstructive components, usually with an initial central component followed by the obstructive component.

Upper airway resistance syndrome (UARS) refers to increased ventilatory effort due to upper airway narrowing, leading to sleep fragmentation, arousals, and daytime somnolence but without apnea, hypopnea, or oxyhemoglobin desaturation.[6] The clinical significance and criteria essential for the diagnosis of UARS are controversial.

Subjects with habitual snoring seek medical care for loud snoring that disrupts the sleep of the bed partner. However, they do not meet the criteria for UARS or OSA.

PATHOPHYSIOLOGY OF OBSTRUCTIVE SLEEP APNEA

The portion of the airway in the regions of the oropharynx and hypopharynx in humans has little or no bony or rigid support and is dependent on the function of the pharyngeal dilator muscles to maintain its patency. The most prominent of these muscles are the genioglossus (GG) and tensor palatini (TP).

Patients with OSAS have anatomic narrowing of the upper airway. Inspiring through a narrow passageway leads to acceleration of airflow (Venturi effect). Negative pressure is generated at the edges of this current of flowing air. The faster the airflow, the greater the partial vacuum or negative pressure (Bernoulli principle). This negative pressure is countered during wakefulness by the increased activity of GG and TP muscles in patients with OSAS, as demonstrated by electromyographic (EMG) studies, which keeps the airway patent. During sleep, this neuromuscular compensation is lost and the muscle activity returns to the same level as seen in individuals without OSAS.[7,8] The loss of muscle tone is most pronounced during the rapid-eye-movement (REM) phase of sleep. The combination of anatomic narrowing and loss of neuromuscular control leads to airway collapse and cessation of airflow.

Nasal obstruction has been implicated in the pathogenesis of sleep-disordered breathing, including OSAS.[9–11] The switch to the oral route for breathing changes the dynamics of the upper airway, predisposing to its collapse. The stimulating effect of nasal airflow on breathing is lost. In addition, nasal blockage increases the negative inspiratory pressure, thus augmenting the collapse of an anatomically compromised airway.

Snoring is generated by vibrations of the pharyngeal soft tissues created by the resistance met by a fast-moving column of air. The force of air being drawn in and the resistance met determine the loudness of snoring, while the pitch is determined by the thickness and consistency of the tissues that are vibrating.[12,13] The posterior edge of the soft palate, the uvula, and the tonsillar pillars are the most common locations where the snoring sound is generated.

Hypoxia and hypercapnia result from the cessation or reduction of airflow during apneic or hypopneic events. Increased inspiratory effort is needed to overcome the airway resistance during these respiratory events. The combination of hypoxia, hypercapnia, and increased ventilatory effort causes sleep fragmentation and arousals. Once the patient arouses, the pharyngeal muscle activity is restored, and the airway opens. The patient then hyperventilates to correct the blood gas derangements, returns to sleep, and the cycle begins again (Figure 32-1).

CLINICAL CONSEQUENCES OF SLEEP APNEA

Sleep can be severely disrupted by the repetitive arousals needed to end the apneas and hypopneas and the episodes of cyclic hypoxia and hypercapnia. These events lead to the observed clinical consequences (Table 32-1).

Daytime Somnolence

Sleep-disordered breathing causes multiple awakenings each night. The involved subjects are usually not aware of these events, because they are brief. However, they lead to disruption of the restorative effect of sleep. As a result, patients complain of excessive daytime somnolence and fatigue despite what should be adequate (and sometimes excessive) amounts of time in bed. This daytime somnolence can have significant consequences. Patients with OSAS have an increased incidence of motor vehicle accidents,[14] work-related injuries, poor job performance, depression, family discord, and overall decreased quality of life.[15]

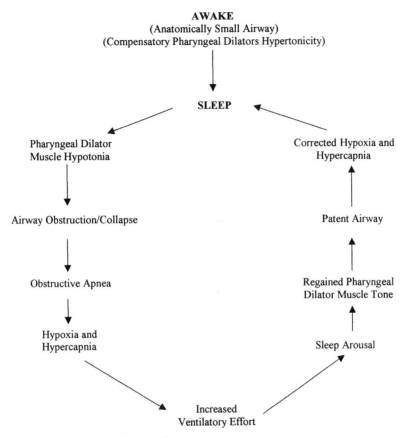

Figure 32-1. Pathophysiology of obstructive sleep apnea.

TABLE 32-1. CLINICAL CONSEQUENCES OF OBSTRUCTIVE SLEEP APNEA

Sleep fragmentation
  Daytime somnolence
  Daytime fatigue
  Morning headache
  Motor vehicle accidents
  Job-related injuries and poor job performance
  Depression
  Family discord
Cardiovascular consequences
  Systemic hypertension
  Coronary artery disease
  Cardiac arrhythmia
  Cerebrovascular accidents
  Pulmonary hypertension and cor pulmonale
  Polycythemia
Shorter life expectancy/increased mortality

Symptoms of excessive daytime somnolence can be objectively measured by multiple sleep latency testing (MSLT). MSLT is typically performed after an all-night polysomnogram. A four- or five-nap opportunity is given in a quiet darkened room. Sleep latency is defined as the elapsed time from lights out to the beginning of sleep in any state.[16] The mean sleep latency in normal persons is between 10 and 15 minutes for the four- to five-nap opportunity. Patients with sleep apnea or narcolepsy exhibit a sleep-onset latency average of 5 minutes or less. The stages of sleep during these naps help to differentiate the various sleep disorders that may cause daytime somnolence.

Cardiovascular Consequences

The second major category of morbidity from sleep apnea is cardiovascular dysfunction.

Systemic hypertension has been reported in up to 50% of patients with OSAS.[17] Mean morning blood pressure has been shown to increase almost linearly with increased apneic activity in both obese and nonobese patients.[18] Hypertension was recently associated with all forms of sleep-disordered breathing, including habitual snoring.[19]

Cardiac arrhythmia has also been associated with OSAS.[20] Bradycardic arrhythmia is more common, but tachyarrhythmia may be noted with severe hypoxemia. Hypoxemia, arrhythmia, and the rise in systemic blood pressure may induce myocardial ischemia and possibly myocardial infarction.[21]

Pulmonary hypertension, polycythemia, and cor pulmonale can be precipitated by both hypercapnia and hypoxemia in cases of severe OSAS.[22] In addition, patients with sleep-disordered breathing are at increased risk for stroke even in the absence of OSAS.[23]

The end result is increased mortality and shorter life expectancy of patients with OSAS, especially those with RDI > 20 events per hour of sleep.[24]

RISK FACTORS FOR OBSTRUCTIVE SLEEP APNEA

Obesity is the most common risk factor linked to OSAS. This mainly relates to upper body fat distribution, which is reflected in the neck circumference. A neck circumference of >17 inches in males and 16 inches in females is associated with the development of OSAS.[25] A measure of obesity is the body-mass index (BMI), which is calculated by dividing the weight in kilograms by the square of the height in meters.

Males are more at risk for developing OSAS, with a male-to-female ratio ranging between 2:1 and 10:1.[26] On the other hand, OSAS is more prevalent in both sexes with increasing age, especially those older than 65 years.[27]

Anatomic abnormalities that narrow the upper airway predispose to OSA. Examples of such abnormalities are nasal obstruction, adenotonsillar hypertrophy, macroglossia, micrognathia, and retrognathia.

A family history of sleep apnea increases an individual's risk of developing it. The risk increases with the number of affected family members and is fourfold greater if three relatives are affected.[28]

Sedatives have been shown to induce or worsen sleep apnea. They reduce the muscle tone of pharyngeal dilators. In addition, they prolong the apneas by elevating the arousal threshold.[29] Similar effects are reported with alcohol consumption.[30] Cigarette smoking is also a risk factor for the development of sleep apnea, with current smokers being at a greater risk than former smokers, while both are at greater risk than individuals who never smoked.[31]

Endocrine abnormalities such as hypothyroidism[32] and acromegaly[33] predispose to the development of OSA. Thyroid hormone replacement therapy can reduce the degree of apnea independent of weight change. Other conditions that increase the risk for OSA include amy-loidosis (mainly through macroglossia),[34] Marfan syndrome,[35] Down syndrome,[36] and neuromuscular disorders such as post-polio syndrome, muscular dystrophy, and kyphosco-liosis[37] (Table 32-2).

CLINICAL EVALUATION
History

The first step in evaluating individuals suspected of having sleep apnea is a detailed med-ical history. Patients are asked about their sleep habits, daytime somnolence, and fatigue. It is important to differentiate between sleepiness and fatigue or tiredness, which can be due to other medical problems such as depression, anemia, or heart failure. Loud, long-lasting snoring, especially when associated with nocturnal arousal and choking or gasping episodes, suggests sleep apnea.[38] Information concerning risk factors such as weight gain, alcohol con-sumption, smoking, intake of sedative or sleeping medications, predisposing medical con-ditions, and family history should be obtained as well. History of multiple automobile- or job-related accidents is relevant and should be elicited. The Epworth Sleepiness Scale, in which subjects are asked about the likelihood of falling asleep in eight situations, is a use-ful adjunct in quantifying daytime somnolence.

Patients tend to minimize their symptoms and are often unaware of what happens dur-ing sleep. A bed partner's description of witnessed apneas and the quality of the patient's sleep (including loudness of snoring) is highly suggestive of the presence of sleep apnea. Moreover, family members can provide valuable information about daytime sleepiness.

Physical Examination

The physical examination may be divided into a general examination and another specific to the upper airway. The general examination aims at detecting findings that predispose to

TABLE 32-2.   RISK FACTORS FOR OBSTRUCTIVE SLEEP APNEA

Obesity
Male gender
Age
Anatomic facial abnormalities
   Nasal obstruction
   Adenotonsillar hypertrophy
   Macroglossia
   Micrognathia
   Retrognathia
Family history of sleep apnea
Sedatives and alcohol
Smoking
Endocrine abnormalities
   Hypothyroidism
   Acromegaly
Systemic disorders/chromosomal syndromes
   Down's syndrome
   Marfan's syndrome
   Neuromuscular disorders (such as postpolio syndrome)
   Muscular dystrophy
   Kyphoscoliosis
   Amyloidosis

OSAS or are associated with it, such as obesity, hypertension, and features of endocrine abnormalities or systemic disorders. Obesity, especially upper body fat, is associated with the presence and severity of sleep apnea.[39] Weight, height, and neck circumference are recorded and BMI is calculated.

The upper airway examination aims at determining the cause and site of airway narrowing and detecting anatomic abnormalities that are amenable to surgical correction. Retro- and micrognathia places the tongue in a more posterior position that narrows the pharyngeal airway. Similarly, other craniofacial anomalies predispose to sleep apnea. Since airway obstruction during apnea commonly occurs at multiple levels, a detailed examination of the nasal passages, pharynx, and larynx is needed. The nasal passages are assessed by anterior rhinoscopy and fiberoptic endoscopy to rule out obstruction caused by septal deviation, turbinate hypertrophy, polyps or masses, intranasal synechiae, or nasal valve collapse. The nasopharynx is examined for adenoid hypertrophy or masses.

The retropalatal region is a common site for airway collapse. This may be precipitated by tonsillar hypertrophy, a long and thick uvula, excessive pharyngeal mucosal folds (including webbing of the posterior tonsillar pillar), and a long, low-lying soft palate. Poor visualization of the uvula or posterior edge of the soft palate, even with downward displacement of the tongue with a tongue depressor, suggests an oropharyngeal/retropalatal site of airway obstruction. The relative size and position of the tongue are evaluated. Lingual tonsillar hypertrophy and macroglossia (such as caused by amyloidosis) can narrow the airway.

The hypopharynx and larynx are examined for pathologies that can compromise the airway. Fiberoptic transnasal endosocopy provides valuable information and is an essential component of the physical examination.

A particularly helpful dynamic assessment of the airway involves Müller's maneuver. A flexible fiberoptic laryngoscope is passed through the nostril and positioned directly above the segment to be evaluated. The patient is then asked to inhale forcefully at end-expiration against occluded oral and nasal passages. The site and degree of airway collapse is determined. This is performed with the patient in both the sitting and supine positions. The main disadvantages of the test are its subjectivity and dependence on patient cooperation. The Müller maneuver is more useful in predicting failures of palatopharyngeal surgery than surgical success. A greater than 40% narrowing of the airway at the level of tongue base/hypopharynx suggests poor outcome with uvulopalatopharyngoplasty.[40,41]

A minority of patients with significant OSAS are thin, have no apparent anatomic abnormalities on physical examination, and have an oropharyngeal inlet that appears widely patent.

Imaging

The role of imaging in the workup of patients suspected of having sleep apnea is controversial. Imaging studies are not routinely obtained because of their cost and the fact that they frequently do not add to the airway assessment provided by the physical examination.

Cephalometry is the most commonly obtained imaging study for this purpose. It offers both bone and soft tissue measurements and is used for surgical planning and predicting outcome. Its main drawback is lack of normative data, especially for soft tissue measurements. Findings that correlate with the diagnosis of sleep apnea are low hyoid bone position, long and thick soft palate, diminished size of the posterior airway space, increased distance from the tip of tongue to the base of vallecula, and facial skeletal abnormalities (such as micrognathia).[42,43]

Computed tomography (CT) provides excellent resolution for soft tissue, airway, and bone. It offers an accurate determination of upper airway cross-sectional area and volume and is helpful in evaluating the efficacy of dental appliances and maxillomandibular advancement in patients with sleep apnea. Spiral CT provides direct three-dimensional volumetric reconstruction of the images.[44]

Magnetic resonance imaging (MRI) offers superior soft tissue resolution, multiplane imaging, three-dimensional reconstruction, ultrafast imaging techniques, and lack of radiation exposure. MRI is useful in evaluating the efficacy of soft tissue surgery but not in predicting surgical outcome in sleep apnea patients.[45]

However, both MRI and CT are not routinely used in the clinical evaluation of patients with sleep apnea because of cost, supine imaging, poor prediction of surgical outcome, and the additional risk of radiation exposure with CT.

Polysomnography

Polysomnography (sleep study) is essential for the diagnosis of sleep apnea. It serves to confirm the presence of sleep apnea and exclude other causes of excessive daytime somnolence, such as narcolepsy, insufficient amount of sleep, and periodic limb movement disorder. Moreover, polysomnography determines the severity of the sleep apnea, since the information obtained from the medical history and physical examination in any particular patient is a poor indicator of disease severity.[46]

Polysomnography may be obtained in the laboratory or at home. Home studies, in general, collect data pertaining to oxyhemoglobin saturation, nasal and oral airflow, heart rate, and loudness of snoring. More convenient and less expensive, they test the patient in a more natural environment than studies performed in the laboratory. Laboratory polysomnography is more comprehensive and is considered the "gold standard" for the diagnosis of OSA and determination of its severity. In addition, it allows for continuous positive airway pressure (CPAP) titration and initiation of therapy. A sleep technician observes the individual being tested during sleep to correct problems with recording, guaranteeing that quality signals are obtained throughout the study. The technician may also detect the presence of other sleep disorders.

A standard in-the-laboratory polysomnogram consists of an electroencephalographic tracing (EEG) that determines stage of sleep, an electro-oculogram (EOG) that differentiates REM and non-REM phases of sleep, an electrocardiogram (ECG) to monitor cardiac arrhythmia, and measurement of arterial oxygen saturation, nasal-oral airflow, chest and abdominal wall motion, and leg movements.[47]

In-the-laboratory polysomnograms may be all-night or split-night studies. A full-night study allows for a more complete evaluation of the sleep disorder. In a split-night study, the first half of the study is diagnostic, while the second half is devoted to CPAP titration and initiation of therapy. Even though the diagnostic time is limited in a split-night study, patients are tested only once and the cost is reduced.

Particularly useful data to be gathered from polysomnography includes RDI, lowest oxyhemoglobin saturation and the duration of the desaturation events, associated cardiac arrhythmia, and associated arousal (sleep fragmentation as determined by EEG). Respiratory events are more common during REM sleep. The average of both REM and non-REM RDI—ie, total sleep—is calculated. The diagnosis of OSA can be made if the RDI is greater than 5 events per hour of sleep. However, the health impact of OSA with an RDI between 5 and 20 is controversial. Most agree that an RDI > 20 and oxyhemoglobin desaturation lower than 86% are associated with increased mortality and morbidity and therefore need to be treated.[17,20–22,24] Further useful information is the presence of positional component to the sleep-disordered breathing.

TREATMENT OF OBSTRUCTIVE SLEEP APNEA

Once the diagnosis is confirmed by polysomnography, treatment is initiated without delay, especially if the RDI is >20 events per hour of sleep and lowest oxyhemoglobin saturation is less than 86%. The nature and aggressiveness of the treatment are guided by the signs and symptoms of the patient, in particular daytime somnolence and signs of cardiovascular dysfunction, and the results of the polysomnogram, including RDI, extent of arterial oxygen desaturation, sleep disruptions, and arrhythmia.

The goals of the treatment are the reduction of morbidity and mortality and improvement of the quality of life. Patients should be counseled regarding their increased risk of motor vehicle accidents, on-the-job injuries, and impaired judgment. The treatment may include behavioral, medical, and surgical interventions.

Behavioral Interventions

Weight loss should be encouraged in all obese patients. Weight loss can be very effective and, in some cases, even curative.[48] Unfortunately, weight loss is difficult to achieve and maintain. Therefore, other forms of treatment should not be withheld until weight loss is achieved.

Alcohol and sedatives should be avoided. In addition, smoking cessation is to be encouraged. Since sleep deprivation may by itself worsen both snoring and apnea,[49] patients are advised to obtain regular and adequate hours of sleep.

In many instances, sleep apnea is worse in the supine position, and avoidance of that position may reduce the severity of apnea. Patients may benefit from sleep-position training, which is designed to prevent sleeping in the supine position.[50] One method for achieving this is sewing a tennis ball into the back of the patient's pajama top or nightshirt. However, the presence of a position-dependent breathing disturbance should be demonstrated during polysomnography before this form of treatment is initiated.

Medical Intervention

Pharmacologic Treatment

Pharmacologic treatment has a limited role in the treatment of OSAS. Nasal decongestants, intranasal steroids, and antihistamines are helpful in relieving nasal symptoms, including blockage, particularly when related to the use of positive pressure devices.

Protriptyline or fluoxetine may reduce the number of apneas in some patients. Treatment with those agents is limited by a high rate of side effects.[51]

Supplemental Oxygen

Supplemental oxygen is beneficial in patients with severe oxyhemoglobin desaturation, especially those with arrhythmia, and those who will not accept more definitive treatment. It may reduce the frequency of apnea-related cardiac arrhythmia.[52] Oxygen therapy, however, does not prevent nocturnal respiratory events and the resultant sleep fragmentation. In addition, supplemental oxygen therapy may prolong the apneas by abolishing the ventilatory stimulus of hypoxia; it should be used with caution in patients with chronic obstructive pulmonary disease.

Oral/Dental Appliance

Oral appliances may be effective in the treatment of patients with habitual snoring or mild OSAS. The most common appliance is the mandibular repositioning device, which causes the mandible to move forward and the bite to open slightly. This enlarges the airway and decreases airway resistance.[53] The use of an oral appliance may lead to some side effects, such as temporomandibular joint discomfort, increased salivation, and dental misalignment.

Positive Airway Pressure

Continuous positive airway pressure (CPAP) is the mainstay of therapy for OSAS because it is effective in the majority of patients. CPAP serves as pneumatic stent for the upper airway, preventing its collapse. The pressure requirement is determined during polysomnography, when the pressure is titrated until the majority of the respiratory events are abolished. CPAP is applied via devices that are portable, fit on a nightstand, and can be easily transported outside of the home.

When properly applied, CPAP reduces the mortality and morbidity associated with OSAS, including excessive daytime somnolence.[54,55]

Several side effects are associated with CPAP use. They include discomfort with the mask, air leaks, nasal skin breakdown, nasal congestion, rhinorrhea, dry nose and throat, and claustrophobia. Many patients find CPAP inconvenient and noisy. This leads to a low compliance rate for its long-term use. Only half the patients are regular CPAP users, defined by the use of their CPAP for 4 hours or more at least five nights a week, while only 20% use it all night.[56,57] The most consistent factor associated with improved compliance is patient and family recognition of improvement in the sensations of sleepiness and alertness.[58]

Compliance with CPAP can be improved by addressing the underlying cause for its discontinuation. Nasal congestion may respond to decongestants, topical corticosteroids, or nasal airway surgery. Adding a humidifier can alleviate airway dryness. The type of mask may be changed to improve patient comfort and decrease air leak. Mouth air leak is addressed by applying a chin strap. Nasal pillows may be helpful for people who find the mask too uncomfortable or who complain of claustrophobia. A bilevel pressure device (Bi-PAP) improves the acceptance of airway pressure therapy for those who complain of difficulty exhaling against a high expiratory pressure.[59] Bi-PAP devices allow the application of different pressure levels during inspiration and expiration. The airway is less likely to collapse during expiration, which reduces the level of needed positive pressure. By adjusting the pressure, the patient can exhale against a lower positive pressure. On the other hand, patients who have problems falling asleep due to the high pressure benefit from the use of the ramp feature, which gradually increases the CPAP pressure to the treatment pressure over a defined period of time, allowing the patient to fall asleep before maximal pressure is achieved.[60]

Surgical Intervention

Many surgical procedures are available for the treatment of patients with OSAS. The operations are designed either to bypass the obstructive area or to prevent collapse of the soft tissues at the obstructive site. The kind and extent of surgery are tailored to the severity of sleep apnea, the findings on physical examination, and, in some instances, imaging studies. Airway closure during sleep commonly occurs at multiple levels, which limits the effectiveness of site-specific surgery.

Nasal Surgery

Nasal obstruction may cause or worsen sleep-disordered breathing, including obstructive sleep apnea. Accordingly, nasal surgery is often necessary to treat patients with OSAS. In addition, some patients require nasal surgery to improve comfort and compliance with CPAP use. The nature of the operation is determined by the physical examination (anterior rhinoscopy and nasal endoscopy). Depending on the etiology of the obstruction, the surgery may involve septoplasty, inferior turbinate volume reduction, and polypectomy, alone or in combination.

Palatopharyngeal Surgery

The retropalatal region is the most common site for airway collapse in patients with OSAS. Furthermore, vibrations of the mucosal folds at the posterior edge of the soft palate, uvula, or tonsillar pillars generate the snoring sound. Palatopharyngeal surgery is indicated when the clinical evaluation points to the retropalatal region as the primary site of airway obstruction. This is commonly based on the physical examination, including flexible fiberoptic endoscopy (Müller maneuver). The presence of a >30 to 40% narrowing in the hypopharynx/tongue base region on the Müller maneuver predicts a poor outcome with palatopharyngeal surgery. However, a narrowing of <30% in that region does not guarantee surgical success.[40,41] There are a variety of operations designed to treat the airway at this level.

LASER-ASSISTED UVULOPALATOPLASTY (LAUP).   LAUP was introduced in 1993 to treat snoring and OSAS.[61] The procedure is performed in the office under local anesthesia. It involves amputating the uvula and making two lateral incisions in the soft palate, which induce retraction of the soft palate and stiffening of the soft tissues. The current indications for this procedure are habitual snoring or mild OSAS, defined as RDI <15 events per hour of sleep and lowest arterial oxygen saturation >86%.[62] Therefore, a polysomnographic study is recommended prior to the procedure. LAUP cures or improves snoring in approximately 80% of such patients.[63] The main disadvantages of the procedure are the frequent need for multiple treatments, cost, and postoperative pain requiring narcotics. Potential complications include infection, laser burns, and velopharyngeal insufficiency (VPI). The risk of VPI may be reduced with conservative tissue resection and palatal incisions during each treatment, even though this leads to an increase in the number of treatments.

RADIOFREQUENCY VOLUME REDUCTION OF SOFT PALATE (SOMNOPLASTY).   Somnoplasty uses low-temperature energy to produce submucosal coagulation necrosis and later scar formation, which results in volume contraction and soft tissue stiffening. The soft tissue effect is gradual over the course of approximately 12 weeks. Somnoplasty was introduced in 1998 for the treatment of sleep-disordered breathing.[64] This is an office procedure performed under local anesthesia. Typically, three "lesions" are created in the soft palate during each treatment: one in the midline and one on each side. Most patients require more than one treatment.[64] Somnoplasty has the same indications as LAUP, with similar surgical success. Its main advantage, however, is the minimal postoperative pain, rarely requiring analgesics.

Potential complications include palatal fistula, uvular edema, and local infection. The risk of palatal fistula and ulcerations may be reduced by infiltrating the "lesion" site with an adequate amount of ionic solution (local anesthetic and saline), which acts as a heat sink while improving the therapeutic efficacy of radiofrequency ablation, and by delivering less energy per lesion. The main drawbacks are cost and the need for multiple treatments.

TONSILLECTOMY.   Adenotonsillar hypertrophy is a common cause of OSAS in the pediatric population, and tonsillectomy with adenoidectomy is effective for its cure. In adults with OSAS, however, tonsillar hypertrophy is rarely the main cause of airway obstruction. Tonsillectomy in adults is typically performed in conjunction with uvulopalatopharyngoplasty. The surgical technique and potential complications for tonsillectomy are discussed in other chapters in this textbook and are not reviewed here.

UVULOPALATOPHARYNGOPLASTY (UPPP).   UPPP is designed to treat OSAS by preventing oropharyngeal obstruction through the excision of excessive soft tissue at the free margin of the soft palate (sparing the underlying muscle) and posterior lateral pharyngeal wall and uvulectomy. It was first described by Ikematsu in 1964[65] and popularized by Fujita et al. in 1981.[66] When present, the tonsils are excised, excessive tissues along the posterior tonsillar pillar are removed, and the anterior and posterior pillars are sutured together (Figure 32-2). Patients generally require narcotics for pain control in the immediate postoperative period.

The surgery is particularly effective when the site of airway obstruction is only or mainly at the retropalatal region. The major dilemma is the inability to determine which patients will benefit from the surgery. Various criteria have been used to predict surgical outcome, including preoperative weight, objective evidence of anatomic obstruction on physical examination, and site of airway collapse as judged by the Müller maneuver. Cephalometry has also been utilized to aid in this determination. Both cephalometry and the Müller maneuver are more helpful in predicting which patients fail UPPP than in predicting surgical success. Evidence of airway obstruction at the hypopharynx/tongue base region (such as >30 to 40% narrowing with the Müller maneuver) indicates poor outcome with UPPP, while the lack of obstruction in that area (<30% narrowing on Müller maneuver) does not guarantee good prognosis.

UPPP eliminates snoring in approximately 90% of patients. However, its surgical success for curing sleep apnea, defined as >50% reduction of apnea index and drop of RDI to below 20 events per hour of sleep, is on the order of 40 to 50%. A meta-analysis by Sher et al. demonstrated that there was only a 41% response rate, defined as a reduction in the RDI to less than 20 events per hour of sleep following surgery. The more severe the apnea, the lower the likelihood of achieving a surgical cure utilizing this procedure.[67] Accordingly, a follow-up sleep study should be performed following UPPP to ensure that OSAS has been adequately treated.

Potential complications of the operation include bleeding, velopharyngeal insufficiency (VPI), nasopharyngeal-palatal stenosis, mild dryness in the throat, a sensation of persistent mucus in the throat, and dysphagia.

VPI may occur initially for a few weeks in the immediate postoperative period, but permanent significant palatal incompetence is unusual unless an excessive resection is performed. Accordingly, conservative soft tissue resection is recommended, especially along the middle third of the posterior edge of the soft palate. Persistent symptomatic VPI can be treated with speech therapy, palatal prosthesis, or palatopharyngeal flap.

Nasopharyngeal-palatal stenosis is rare but should be avoided at all costs because it is difficult to repair. This is more likely to occur with excessive resection of the posterior tonsillar pillars, excessive use of cautery (especially in the adenoid bed by performing a concomitant adenoidectomy), undermining the mucosa of posterior pharyngeal wall, wound dehiscence, infection, and necrosis.[68] Initial treatment of symptomatic nasopharyngeal-palatal stenosis includes dilatation with stenting. Resection of the scar tissue and resurfacing of the stenotic

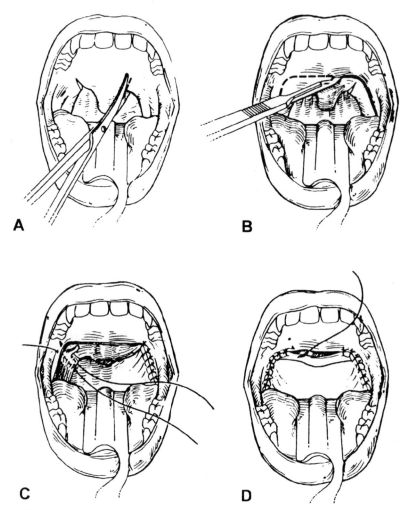

Figure 32-2.   Uvulopalatopharyngoplasty. **A.** Incision is made on the soft palate and extended along the base of the uvula. **B.** The incision is extended to the anterior tonsillar pillars. **C.** The posterior tonsillar pillar as a flap is rotated anteriorly and sutured to the anterior pillar. **D.** The dorsal soft palate mucosa is advanced and sutured to the ventral mucosa, closing the soft palate incision. [*Reproduced with permission from Fujita S. Pharyngeal surgery for obstructive sleep apnea and snoring. In: Fairbanks DNF et al, eds.* Snoring and Obstructive Sleep Apnea. *New York: Raven, 1987, 162–165.*]

area is needed for those who fail conservative treatment. Resurfacing (epithelialization) may be achieved with local rotational flaps. Free tissue transfer, such as a radial forearm free flap, is occasionally necessary.

Hypopharyngeal/Tongue Base Surgery
Widening a narrow airway at the level of the hypopharynx and tongue base and preventing its collapse during sleep is frustrating despite the multitude of procedures described for that

purpose. Operations on this part of the airway have a low overall long-term success rate for curing OSAS. Such operations may be performed alone or in conjunction with palatopharyngeal or nasal surgery.

This surgery is indicated for patients with significant OSAS and airway collapse in the hypopharynx/tongue base region as determined by physical examination (including the Müller maneuver) supplemented with imaging studies (commonly cephalometry).

LINGUAL TONSILLECTOMY.   Lingual tonsillectomy is indicated for patients with lingual tonsil hypertrophy that contributes to airway narrowing as judged by the physical examination. This surgery is associated with a high level of morbidity and technically cumbersome. Patients require narcotics for an extended period. Bleeding is a common complication. The risk of bleeding can be reduced by limiting the resection to the middle part of the tongue, staying more than 1 cm away from the lateral tongue margin so as to avoid the neurovascular bundle.

MIDLINE GLOSSECTOMY.   Midline glossectomy involves the resection of the midline of the base of tongue to reduce tongue volume and hence prevent its posterior displacement during sleep. It may be considered for patients who have failed UPPP and are noted to have significant hypopharyngeal collapse on physical examination, including flexible fiberoptic endoscopy. In a series of 12 patients reported by Fujita et al., the apnea index improved in 42%.[66] Potential complications are bleeding as well as speech and swallowing problems.

HYOID MYOTOMY AND SUSPENSION WITH GENOID TUBERCLE ADVANCEMENT.   This surgery aims at anterior displacement of the tongue to prevent airway collapse in the hypopharynx. The infrahyoid muscles are transected, allowing the hyoid bone to be advanced anteriorly. The hyoid bone is anchored in its new position by suturing it to the mandible or thyroid cartilage. Concomitantly, the genoid tubercle, where the genioglossus muscle inserts, is advanced to pull this muscle and hence the tongue base forward (Figure 32-3). The continuity of the mandible and dental occlusion are maintained, obviating the need for intermaxillary fixation.[69] Preserving an adequate bony rim inferior to the osteotomy can reduce the risk of mandibular fracture.

MANDIBULAR ADVANCEMENT.   Retrognathia and micrognathia are not uncommon in patients with OSAS. This places the tongue in a more posterior position, compromising the airway. Several surgical procedures have been described and reported to address this issue. Total mandibular advancement is an alternative to genoid tubercle advancement and hyoid myotomy and suspension as a primary treatment or for UPPP failures in patients with demonstrated retrognathia. This is performed through bilateral mandibular osteotomies posterior to the last molar. The mandible is then advanced anteriorly and held in position with intermaxillary fixation.

For such surgery to be beneficial, patients must have documented retrognathia. Since retrognathia might not be obvious on physical examination, cephalometric studies should be obtained to document the presence of retrognathia and narrowing of the hypopharyngeal airway prior to recommending the surgery.[70,71]

The main disadvantages of the surgery are the need for intermaxillary fixation, the resultant change in occlusion, and the lack of large enough experience with it to demonstrate its effectiveness.

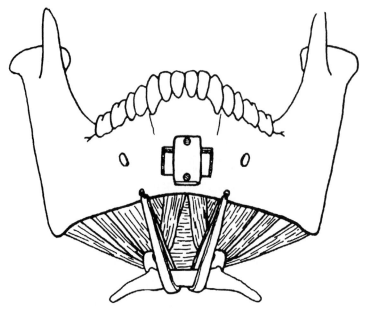

Figure 32-3.   Inferior sagittal osteotomy of the mandible, with hyoid myotomy and suspension. (*Reproduced with permission from Riley RW, Powell NB, Guilleminault C. Maxillofacial surgery and obstructive sleep apnea: a review of 80 patients. Otolaryngol Head Neck Surg 1989;101:354.*)

Maxillomandibular Advancement (MMA)

MMA is designed to address narrowing in the entire upper airway (retropalatal region and hypopharynx). A Le Forte I maxillary osteotomy is performed in conjunction with bilateral mandibular osteotomies (Figure 32-4). The maxilla and mandible are then advanced anteriorly and fixed in a position that maximally increases the size of the airway while maintaining function and esthetics.[72]

This procedure requires substantial commitment from the patient. The postoperative cosmetic change should also be considered. MMA is indicated for patients with OSAS who have failed nasal surgery, UPPP, and genoid tubercle advancement with hyoid myotomy and suspension and those who refuse CPAP or tracheotomy.

The results of MMA are comparable to those of optimal CPAP treatment as measured by RDI, lowest oxyhemoglobin desaturation, and the number of desaturations to below 90%.[73]

Tracheotomy

Tracheotomy as a surgical treatment for OSAS is designed to bypass the entire upper airway. It is indicated for patients with severe OSAS, especially when it is associated with significant oxyhemoglobin desaturation, life-threatening cardiac arrhythmia, or marked cardiopulmonary dysfunction. It may be utilized as a permanent treatment or as a temporary stabilizing measure until a cure is achieved by other upper airway surgery, such as those described earlier in this chapter.

Tracheotomy is highly successful for treating OSAS. However, few patients accept it due to the associated morbidity and the need for long-term care.

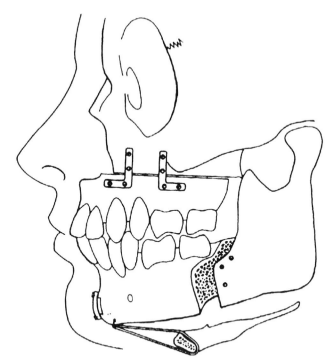

Figure 32-4.   Maxillary mandibular and hyoid advancement. (*Reproduced with permission from Riley RW, Powell NB, Guilleminault C. Maxillofacial surgery and obstructive sleep apnea: a review of 80 patients.* Otolaryngol Head Neck Surg *1989;101:354.*)

CONCLUSION

In conclusion, obstructive sleep apnea is a common disorder with a significant health and socioeconomic impact on the affected individuals and their family members. Fortunately, it is easily recognizable. The diagnosis is based on the medical history, physical examination, and polysomnography. The morbidity of obstructive sleep apnea can be reduced or averted by appropriate treatment. The therapy is multidisciplinary and involves behavioral, medical, and surgical interventions.

References

1. Dickens C. *Posthumous Papers of the Pickwick Club.* London: Chapman & Hall, 1837.
2. Young T, Palta M, Dempsey J, et al. The occurrence of sleep-disordered breathing among middle-aged adults. *N Engl J Med* 328:1230, 1993.
3. Sleep Disorders Classification Committee. Diagnostic classifications of sleep and arousal disorders. *Sleep* 2:1, 1979.
4. American Thoracic Society. Indications and standards for the use of nasal continuous posi-

tive airway pressure (CPAP) in sleep apnea syndrome. *Am J Respir Med* 150:1738, 1994.
5. Moser NJ, Phillips BA, Berry DTR, Harbison L. What is hypopnea anyway? *Chest* 105:426, 1994.
6. Guilleminault C, Stoohs R, Clerk A, et al. A cause of excessive daytime sleepiness. The upper airway resistance syndrome. *Chest* 104(3):781, 1993.
7. Mezzanote WS, Tangel DJ, White DP. Waking genioglossal electromyogram in sleep apnea patients versus normal controls (a neuromuscular

compensatory mechanism). *J Clin Invest* 89(5): 1571, 1992.

8. Remmers JE, de Groot WJ, Sauterland EK, Anch AM. Pathogenesis of upper airway obstruction during sleep. *J Appl Physiol* 44:931, 1978.

9. Busaba NY. The nose in snoring and obstructive sleep apnea. *Curr Opin Otolaryngol Head Neck Surg* 7:11, 1999.

10. Levine P, Rubin AE. Effects of nasal occlusion on respiration in sleep: evidence of inheritability of sleep apnea process. *Acta Otolaryngol (Stockh)* 97:127, 1984.

11. Gleeson K, Zwillich CW, Bendrick TW, White DP. Effect of inspiratory nasal loading on pharyngeal resistance. *J Appl Physiol* 60:1882, 1986.

12. Sullivan CE, Issa FG. Pathophysiological mechanisms in obstructive sleep apnea. *Sleep* 3:235, 1980.

13. Lugaresi E, Cirignotta F, Coccagna G, Baruzzi A. Snoring and the obstructive sleep apnea syndrome. *Electromyogr Clin Neurophysiol (Suppl)* 35:421, 1982.

14. Findley LU, Unverzagt ME, Suratt PM. Automobile accidents involving patients with obstructive sleep apnea. *Am Rev Respir Dis* 138:337, 1988.

15. Roth T, Roehrs TA, Conway WA. Behavioral morbidity of apnea. *Semin Respir Med* 9:554, 1988.

16. Carskadon MA, Dement WC, Mitler MM, et al. Guidelines for the multiple sleep latency test (MSLT): a standard measure of sleepiness. *Sleep* 9:519, 1986.

17. Fletcher EC. The relationship between systemic hypertension and obstructive sleep apnea: facts and theory. *Am J Med* 98(2):118, 1995.

18. Strohl KP, Novak RD, Singer W, et al. Insulin levels, blood pressure and sleep apnea. *Sleep* 17(7):614, 1994.

19. Nieto FJ, Young TB, Lind BK, et al. Association of sleep-disordered breathing, sleep apnea, and hypertension in a large community-based study. *JAMA* 283:1829, 2000.

20. Guilleminault C, Connolly SJ, Winkle RA. Cardiac arrhythmia and conduction disturbances during sleep in 400 patients with sleep apnea syndrome. *Am J Cardiol* 52:490, 1983.

21. Hung J, Whitford EG, Parsons RW, Hillman DR. Association of sleep apnoea with myocardial infarction in men. *Lancet* 336(8710):261, 1990.

22. Rapoport DM, Garay SM, Epstein H, Goldring RM. Hypercapnia in the obstructive sleep apnea syndrome. A reevaluation of the "Pickwickian syndrome." *Chest* 89(5):627, 1986.

23. Palomaki H. Snoring and the risk of ischemic brain infarction. *Stroke* 22:1021, 1991.

24. He J, Kryger MH, Zorick FJ, et al. Mortality and apnea index in obstructive sleep apnea. *Chest* 94:9, 1988.

25. Davies RJ, Stradling JR. The relationship between neck circumference, radiographic pharyngeal anatomy, and the obstructive sleep apnoea syndrome. *Eur Respir J* 3(5):509, 1990.

26. Strohl KP, Redline S. Recognition of obstructive sleep apnea: *Am J Resp Crit Care Med* 154:279, 1996.

27. Ancoli-Israel S, Klauber MR, Kripke DF, et al. Sleep apnea in female patients in a nursing home. Increased risk for mortality. *Chest* 96(5):1054, 1989.

28. Redline S, Tishler PV, Tosteson TD, et al. The familial aggregation of obstructive sleep apnea. *Am J Resp Crit Care Med* 151:682, 1995.

29. Dolly FR, Block AJ. Effect of flurazepam on sleep-disordered breathing and nocturnal oxygen desaturation in asymptomatic subjects. *Am J Med* 73(2):239, 1982.

30. Bonora M, Shields GI, Knuth SL, et al. Selective depression by ethanol of upper airway respiratory motor activity in cats. *Am Rev Respir Dis* 130(2):156, 1984.

31. Wetter DW, Young TB, Bidwell TR, et al. Smoking as a risk factor for sleep-disordered breathing. *Arch Intern Med* 154(19):2219, 1994.

32. Rajogopal KR, Abbrecht P, Derderian SS, et al. Obstructive sleep apnea in hypothyroidism. *Ann Intern Med* 101:491, 1984.

33. Paritnen M, Telakivi T. Epidemiology of obstructive sleep apnea syndrome. *Sleep* 15:S1, 1992.

34. Kales A, Bela-bueno A, Kales JD. Sleep disorders: sleep apnea and narcolepsy. *Ann Intern Med* 106:434, 1987.

35. Cistulli P, Sullivan CE. Sleep apnea in Marfan's syndrome. *Am Rev Respir Dis* 147:645, 1993.

36. Redline S, Tishler PV. Familial influences on sleep apnea. In: Lenfant C, Saunders N, eds. *Lung Biology in Health and Disease: Sleep Related Breathing Disorder.* New York. Marcel Decker 1994, 363.

37. Guilleminault C. Clinical features and evaluation of obstructive sleep apnea. In: Kryger MH, Roth T, Dement WC, eds. *Principles and Practice of Sleep Medicine,* 2nd ed. Philadelphia: Saunders, 1994, 667.

38. Stradling JR, Crosby JH. Predictors and prevalence of obstructive sleep apnoea and snoring in 1001 middle aged men. *Thorax* 46:85, 1991.

39. Millman RP, Carlisle CC, McGarvey ST, et al. Body fat distribution and sleep apnea severity in women. *Chest* 107:362, 1995.

40. Sher AE, Thorpy MJ, Shprintzen RJ, et al. Predictive value of Muller maneuver in selection of patients for uvulopalatopharyngoplasty. *Laryngoscope* 95:1483, 1985.

41. Katsantonis GP, Maas CS, Walsh JK. The predictive efficacy of the Muller maneuver in uvulopalatopharyngoplasty. *Laryngoscope* 99:677, 1989.

42. Petri N, Suadicani P, Wildschiodtz G, Bjorn-Jorgensen J. Predictive value of Muller maneuver, cephalometry, and clinical features for the outcome of uvulopalatopharyngoplasty: evaluation of predictive factors using discriminant analysis in 30 sleep apnea patients. *Acta Otolaryngol (Stockh)* 114:565, 1994.

43. Woodson BT, Conley SF. Prediction of uvulopalatopharyngoplasty response using cephalometric radiographs. *Am J Otolaryngol* 18:179, 1997.

44. Ryan CF, Lowe AA, Li D, Fleetham JA. Three-dimensional upper airway computed tomography in obstructive sleep apnea. *Am Rev Respir Dis* 144:428, 1991.

45. Sudo Y, Matsuda E, Noue Y, et al. Sleep apnea syndrome: comparison of MR imaging of the oropharynx with physiologic indices. *Radiology* 201:393, 1996.

46. Viner S, Szalai JP, Hoffstein V. Are history and physical examination a good screening test for sleep apnea? *Ann Intern Med* 115:356, 1991.

47. American Thoracic Society. Indications and standards for cardiopulmonary sleep studies. *Am Rev Respir Dis* 139:559, 1989.

48. Smith PL, Gold AR, Meyers DA, et al. Weight loss in mildly to moderately obese patients with obstructive sleep apnea. *Ann Intern Med* 103:850, 1985.

49. Neilly JB, Kribbs NB, Maislin G, Pack AI. Effects of selective sleep deprivation on ventilation during recovery sleep in normal humans. *J Appl Physiol* 72(1):100, 1992.

50. Cartwright R, Ristanovic R, Diaz F, et al. A comparative study of treatments for positional sleep apnea. *Sleep* 14(16):546, 1991.

51. Hanzel DA, Proia NG, Hudgel DW. Response of obstructive sleep apnea to fluoxetine and protriptyline. *Chest* 101:416, 1991.

52. Fletcher EC, Munafo DA. Role of nocturnal oxygen therapy in obstructive sleep apneas. When should it be used? *Chest* 98(6):1497, 1990.

53. Schmidt-Nowara W, Lowe A, Wiegand L, et al. Oral appliances for the treatment of snoring and obstructive sleep apnea: a review. *Sleep* 18(6):501, 1995.

54. He J, Kryger MH, Zorick FJ, et al. Mortality and apnea index in obstructive sleep apnea. *Chest* 94:9, 1988.

55. Findley L, Levinson MR, Bonnie RJ. Driving performance and automobile accidents in patients with sleep apnea. *Clin Chest Med* 13(3):427, 1992.

56. Nino-Murcia G, McCann CC, Bliwise DL, et al. Compliance and side effects in sleep apnea patients treated with nasal continuous positive airway pressure. *West J Med* 150(2):165, 1989.

57. Kribbs NB, Pack AI, Kline LR, et al. Objective measurement of patterns of nasal CPAP use by patients with obstructive sleep apnea. *Am Rev Respir Dis* 147:887, 1993.

58. American Thoracic Society. Indications and standards for the use of nasal continuous positive airway pressure (CPAP) in sleep apnea syndromes. *Am J Respir Crit Care Med* 150:1738, 1994.

59. Strollo PJ Jr, Sanders MH, Stiller RA. Continuous and bi-level positive airway pressure therapy in sleep disordered breathing. *Oral Maxillofac Surg Clin North Am* 7:221, 1995.

60. Pressman MR, Peterson DD, Meyer TJ, et al. Ramp abuse, a novel form of patient noncompliance to administration of nasal continuous positive airway pressure for treatment of obstructive sleep apnea. *Am J Respir Crit Care Med* 151(5):1632, 1995.

61. Kamami YV. Outpatient treatment of sleep apnea syndrome with CO_2 laser: laser assisted UPPP. *J Otolaryngol* 23:395, 1994.

62. American Sleep Disorders Association. Practice parameters for the use of laser-assisted uvulopalatoplasty. *Sleep* 17:744, 1994.

63. Walker RP, Grigg-Damberger MM, Gopalsami C, Totten MC. Laser-assisted uvulopalatoplasty for snoring and obstructive sleep apnea: results in 170 patients. *Laryngoscope* 105:938, 1995.

64. Powell NB, Riley RW, Troell RJ, et al. Radio-frequency volumetric tissue reduction of the palate in patients with sleep-disordered breathing. *Chest* 113:1163, 1998.

65. Ikematsu T. Study of snoring—fourth report: therapy. *J Jpn Otorhinolaryngol* 64:434, 1964.

66. Fujita S, Conway W, Zorick F. Surgical correction of anatomic abnormalities in obstructive sleep apnea syndrome. Uvulopalatopharyngoplasty. *Otolaryngol Head Neck Surg* 89:923, 1981.

67. Sher AE, Schechtman KB, Piccirillo JF. The efficacy of surgical modifications of the upper airway in adults with obstructive sleep apnea syndrome. *Sleep* 19(2):156, 1996.

68. Katsantonis GP et al. Nasopharyngeal complications following uvulopalatoplasty. *Laryngoscope* 97:309, 1987.

69. Riley RW, Powell NB, Guilleminault C. Inferior sagittal osteotomy of the mandible with hyoid myotomy suspension: a new procedure for obstructive sleep apnea. *Otolaryngol Head Neck Surg* 94:589, 1986.

70. Riley RW et al. Cephalometric analyses and flow-volume loops in obstructive sleep apnea patients. *Sleep* 6:303, 1983.

71. Burstone CJ et al. Cephalometrics for orthognathic surgery. *J Oral Surg* 36:269, 1978.

72. Riley RW, Powell NB, Guilleminault C, Nino-Murcia G. Maxillary-mandibular and hyoid advancement: an alternative to tracheostomy in obstructive sleep apnea. *Otolaryngol Head Neck Surg* 94:584–588, 1986.

73. Riley RW, Powell C, Guilleminault C. Obstructive sleep apnea syndrome: a review of 306 consecutively treated surgical patients. *Otolaryngol Head Neck Surg* 108:117–125, 1993.

Pediatric Otolaryngology 33

This chapter focuses on otolaryngologic issues unique to or characteristic of the pediatric population. It is not an exhaustive compendium of pediatric otolaryngology. Topics covered in other chapters are referenced. The chapter is divided into five sections: (1) "Airway/Upper Aerodigestive Tract," (2) "Ears and Hearing," (3) "Head and Neck," (4) "Syndromes of the Head and Neck," and (5) "Other/Miscellaneous."

AIRWAY/UPPER AERODIGESTIVE TRACT

The airway and upper digestive tract share a common space and therefore are closely related. This relationship is particularly important in infants and children.

Symptoms of airway compromise in infants and children:

Noisy breathing
Abnormal cry
Cough
Color change
Increased work of breathing
Feeding difficulties
Mental status changes

Signs of airway compromise:

Stridor or stertor
Hoarseness/voice change
Cyanosis
Retraction of neck and/or chest with inspiration
Tachypnea
O_2 desaturation
CO_2 retention
Failure to thrive
Right heart failure

Assessment of a child with airway compromise should include systematic consideration of the entire upper aerodigestive tract. The upper aerodigestive tract is divided into its anatomic components in this section. The pertinent developmental anatomy, signs and symptoms, common diagnoses, and treatments specific to the anatomic sites are discussed.

Nose/Nasopharynx

I. Developmental anatomy

Development of the nose is closely related to craniofacial development.

    A. Prenatal development of the nasal cavities[1]

        1. Nasal placodes become the nasal pits at about 30 days gestation.

        2. Each nasal pit is surrounded by the medial and lateral nasal prominences.

        3. Nasal septum forms from the fused nasofrontal process and medial nasal prominences.

        4. Turbinates form as swellings of the lateral nasal wall, starting at about 38 days.

        5. Maxillary prominences grow toward the nasal pits, ultimately fusing to form the intermaxillary segment (about 48 days gestation).

        6. Intermaxillary segment is the precursor of the philtrum, premaxilla, and primary palate.

        7. Nasal pits deepen to become the nasal sacs and ultimately the nasal cavities.

        8. Primitive choana is posterior to the primary palate and is patent at about 7 weeks.

        9. With development of the secondary palate, the choana is located at the junction of the nasal cavity and the pharynx.

        10. Nasolacrimal groove separates the lateral nasal prominence from the maxillary prominence (at about 10 weeks gestation).

        11. The floor of the nasolacrimal groove thickens to form the nasolacrimal duct.

    B. Postnatal development[2]

        1. The vomer and perforated portions of the cribriform ossify by 3 years of age.

        2. Adenoids peak in size between 3 and 5 years of age and start to regress by 8 years of age.

        3. Nasal cavity grows rapidly in the first 6 years of life.

        4. External nasal dimensions are generally mature by 13 years of age in females and 15 years of age in males.

        5. Normal nasal flora includes *Staphylococcus, Haemophilus influenzae, Moraxella catarrhalis, Streptococcus pneumoniae.*

II. Signs and symptoms

    A. Clinical manifestations of pathology are usually related to nasal airway obstruction or epistaxis.

    B. Infants are obligate nose breathers for several weeks postnatally.

    C. After infants are able to breathe through their mouths, the clinical signs and symptoms of nasal pathology may be limited to sleep (obstructive sleep symptoms) and feeding.

III. Clinical assessment

    A. Complete head and neck examination is important.

    B. Dysmorphic features should be noted.

    C. Anterior rhinoscopy, often performed with an otoscope, is helpful in assessing the vestibule and anterior nasal cavity.

    D. Flexible fiberoptic nasendoscopy is required to assess the entire nasal passage and nasopharynx.

    E. Radiographic imaging studies may be helpful in further delineating the pathology. Specific imaging studies are discussed as appropriate.

IV. Pathology/treatment/complications
    A. Congenital
        1. Choanal atresia/stenosis[3]
            a. Clinical features:
                (1) 1 per 5000 live births.
                (2) $F:M = 2:1$.
                (3) Unilateral : bilateral = $2:1$.
                (4) About 50% of patients have other congenital anomalies.
                (5) Atresia may be bony, bony-membranous, or membranous (most are bony-membranous).[4]
                (6) Failure of resorption of the nasobuccal membrane.
                (7) Associated with "CHARGE" association:

                    C: Coloboma of retina
                    H: Heart defects
                    A: Atresia choanae
                    R: Retardation of growth and development and CNS anomalies
                    G: Genitourinary anomalies
                    E: Ear abnormalities, including hearing loss

                (8) Can be seen in Treacher Collins syndrome (mandibulofacial dysostosis).
                (9) "Cyclical cyanosis," with airway obstruction and cyanosis at rest and resolution with crying and agitation (when the child is in the open-mouth position), is typical of infants with bilateral choanal atresia.
              (10) Unilateral atresia associated with unilateral purulent rhinorrhea and obstruction.
              (11) Infants who do not respond appropriately to airway management should be suspected of having other airway lesions.
            b. Diagnosis
                (1) Classic clinical finding of inability to pass 8 French catheters from nose into oropharynx.
                (2) Fiberoptic examination of the nasal passages allows direct visualization of the choanae.
                (3) Computed tomography (CT) scan of the choanae confirms the diagnosis and characterizes the nature of the atresia.
                (4) CT scan should be performed using a bone algorithm with the gantry of the scanner tilted at 30 degrees cephalad from the plane of the nasal floor in a modified axial plane.[5]
            c. Management
                (1) Oral airway may be helpful in maintaining a patent airway while the infant is an obligate nose breather.
                (2) Early surgical repair for bilateral choanal atresia is advocated.
                (3) Unilateral atresia can be repaired later in childhood, usually prior to starting to school.

       (4)   Surgical approaches include endoscopic, transpalatal, transnasal, and transseptal. Stents are generally placed intraoperatively.

       (5)   Infants with syndromic choanal atresia may have poor outcome after repair of choanal atresia, and may require tracheotomy for definitive airway management.[6,7]

2. Congenital pyriform aperture stenosis (or nasal obstruction without choanal atresia)

   a. Clinical features

       (1)   Presentation similar to choanal atresia.

       (2)   Related to overgrowth of nasal process of the maxilla causing obstruction of the pyriform apertures.[8]

       (3)   Associated with single central incisor, holoprosencephaly, and pituitary abnormalities (hypodevelopment and dysfunction).[9]

   b. Diagnosis

       (1)   Based upon physical examination and confirmed on CT scan.

       (2)   CT as described for choanal atresia is helpful in delineating anatomy of the maxilla.

       (3)   Magnetic resonance imaging (MRI) of the head may be helpful in infants with pituitary dysfunction.

   c. Management

       (1)   Most patients do not require any intervention.

       (2)   Patients with significant airway compromise may require surgical management.

       (3)   Surgery involves sublabial incision and opening of the pyriform apertures.

3. Nasolacrimal duct obstruction/cysts

   a. Clinical features

       (1)   Results from failure of the caudal nasolacrimal duct to canalize.

       (2)   90% are unilateral.

       (3) $F:M = 1:1$.

       (4)   Usually associated with epiphora, medial canthal discharge, and noninjected conjunctiva.

       (5)   Partial nasal obstruction in the neonate.

       (6)   Symptoms generally present at 1 to 3 weeks of age.[10]

       (7)   Persistent distal lacrimal valve (valve of Hasner).[10]

   b. Diagnosis: Appearance of a cystic lesion in the inferior meatus[10]

   c. Management

       (1)   Many cases resolve spontaneously with rupture of the cyst into the nasal passage.

       (2)   Marsupialization of the cyst can be performed in the clinic setting.[11]

       (3)   Associated nasolacrimal duct (NLD) stenosis may require dilatation.

4. Nasal encephalocele/glioma/dermoid

   a. Clinical features

       (1)   Encephaloceles and gliomas arise from failure of closure of the foramen caecum at about the third week of gestation. The skin of the forehead and nasal dorsum is intact with these lesions.

        (2)   Encephalocele; includes dura, organized neural elements, and communication with the subarachnoid space.
            (a) $1:35{,}000$ live births.
            (b)   30 to 40% have other abnormalities.[12]
            (c)   Sincipital encephaloceles present as a mass at the nasal dorsum (nasoethmoid), orbits (naso-orbital), or glabella (nasofrontal).
            (d)   Basal encephaloceles usually present as intranasal masses.
        (3)   Gliomas
            (a)   Intranasal or extranasal, based upon the relationship with the nasal skeleton.
            (b)   Approximately 15% of gliomas have a fibrous stalk continuous with the dura.
        (4)   Nasal dermoids
            (a)   Often associated with a pit in the midine nasal dorsum.
            (b)   Composed of ectodermal elements.
            (c)   May have communication with floor of anterior cranial fossa through the foramen caecum.
    b.   Diagnosis
        (1)   Physical signs which are helpful in distinguishing one from another include location, change with respiration, transillumination.
        (2)   Radiographic imaging is important to assess possible communication with intracranial space.
    c.   Management
        (1)   Infection should be treated with antibiotics.
        (2)   Elective surgical excision is required for definitive management.
        (3)   Neurosurgical consultation may be required for those lesions with an intracranial extent.
5.   Nasal deformity associated with cleft lip. See Chapter 11.
6.   Tornwaldt's disease[13]
    a.   Clinical features
        (1)   Persistence of pharyngeal bursa.
        (2)   May present as chronic crusting in the midline of the nasopharynx or as a cystic lesion in the same area.
    b.   Diagnosis: communication with the underlying cervical vertebrae can be demonstrated with CT or MRI.
    c.   Management: lesions should be removed or marsupialized through a transpalatal approach.
7.   Immotile cilia syndrome (primary ciliary dyskinesia)
    a.   Clinical features
        (1)   The functional abnormality results from defective dynein arms.
        (2)   May be familial.
        (3)   Kartagener's syndrome
            (a)   Sinusitis.
            (b)   Situs inversus.
            (c)   Bronchiectasis.
            (d)   May be associated with infertility.

        b.   Diagnosis requires ciliary biopsy to examine ciliary motility and ultra-structure.

        c.   Management is symptomatic.

B.   Trauma

   1.   Septal deviation

        a.   Neonatal septal deviation is relatively common.[14]

           (1)   Most cases of neonatal septal deviation will improve spontaneously.

           (2)   Severe deviations associated with airway compromise should be corrected early.[15]

        b.   Acquired septal deviation is related to nasal trauma.

           (1)   Impact of early surgical management of nasoseptal deformities on facial growth is controversial.[16,17]

           (2)   Conservative therapy, with minimal removal of cartilage, has been advocated.[18]

        c.   Septal hematoma may result from nasal trauma. Commonly presents with nasal obstruction and rhinorrhea after nasal trauma.

           (1)   Symptoms of septal hematoma with fever and nasal pain are suggestive of septal abscess.[19]

           (2)   Septal abscess is commonly associated with cartilage loss and nasal deformity.

           (3)   Requires drainage and antibiotic management.

           (4)   Usual organisms are *S. pneumoniae* and group A beta-hemolytic streptococci.

           (5)   Septal hematoma or abscess in children under 2 years of age is suggestive of nonaccidental trauma (child abuse).

   2.   Nasal fractures

        a.   Clinical features

           (1)   Most common facial fracture in childhood.

           (2)   May occur after relatively minor nasal trauma.

           (3)   Greenstick fractures may occur.

        b.   Diagnosis—radiographs may not be helpful in the pediatric population.

        c.   Treatment—closed reduction is preferred for fractures associated with deformity of the nasal dorsum.

   3.   Nasoethmoid fractures[20]

        a.   Relatively uncommon in children.

        b.   Must rule out intracranial and cervical spine injuries.

        c.   May require major reconstructive surgery.

   4.   Nasal foreign body

        a.   Associated with malodorous rhinorrhea; often unilateral.

        b.   Intranasal buttons or disc batteries are associated with liquefaction necrosis of the nasal mucosa and resultant septal perforation.[21,22] These must be removed emergently.

C.   Infectious/inflammatory

   1.   Allergic rhinitis (see Chapter 12)

        a.   Very common in childhood.

      b. Positive family history of atopy in 50 to 75% of pediatric patients with environmental allergies.

      c. Associated with "allergic shiners" and transverse crease in midnasal dorsum.

      d. IgE-mediated allergic response (type I).

      e. Should be managed medically (nasal sprays, antihistamines, immunotherapy).

  2. Viral rhinitis—very common in childhood

Common viral pathogens include rhinovirus, coronavirus, adenovirus, and respiratory syncytial virus.

  3. Bacterial rhinitis

      a. Diphtheria—pseudomembrane formation on the nasal septum.

      b. Pertussis—associated with prolonged cough.

      c. *Chlamydia*—fiery red nasal mucosa in neonate with rhinorrhea; vertica transmission.

      d. Syphilis—congenital infection.

          (1) First stage—presents in first 3 months of life with watery rhinorrhea that progresses to mucopurulent drainage.

          (2) Second stage—presents later in childhood with "snuffles" and gumma formation in the nasal cavity.

  4. Rhinitis of infancy[23]

      a. May cause significant airway obstruction and associated feeding difficulties in infants.

      b. Onset of symptoms at birth or within the first month of life.

      c. Seasonal variation, more common in the fall and winter.

      d. Management: bulb suction, Neo-Synephrine for 3 days, and nasal saline drops. If no improvement in 5 days, steroid drops should be added.

          (1) CT scan reserved for patients who do not respond to medical management.

          (2) Culture may be helpful.

  5. Adenoid hypertrophy

      a. Associated with nasal obstruction, hyponasal speech, rhinorrhea, and eustachian tube dysfunction.

      b. May contribute to chronic rhinosinusitis in young children.

D. Neoplasm—most nasal tumors in children are benign.

  1. Nasopharyngeal teratomas: usually present at birth

      a. May be associated with nasal obstruction and cleft palate.

      b. Composed of tissue from all three germ layers.

      c. Require surgical excision.

      d. Benign, with low malignant potential.

  2. Juvenile nasopharyngeal angiofibroma (JNA)

      a. Clinical features

          (1) Most common benign nasopharyngeal tumor.

          (2) Incidence between 1 per 5000 and 1 per 60,000.

          (3) Most commonly affects prepubescent males, with peak incidence at 14 to 18 years.

      (4) Early signs include nasal obstruction and epistaxis.

      (5) May progress to cause facial deformity and proptosis.

      (6) Vascular mass may be visible in nasal cavity and nasopharynx.

   b. Diagnosis is clinical; biopsy is usually not required.

      (1) Tumor originates in the sphenopalatine recess; it may extend laterally to the pterygomaxillary space and superiorly to the cavernous sinus and middle cranial fossa.

      (2) CT, MRI, and magnetic resonance angiography (MRA) are helpful in defining extent of the lesion.

      (3) Angiography is diagnostic.

   c. Treatment

      (1) Surgical excision is mainstay of therapy.

      (2) Preoperative embolization is helpful in minimizing intraoperative blood loss.

      (3) Surgical approach depends upon extent of lesion. Approaches include

         (a) Endoscopic

         (b) Le Fort I osteotomy and midface degloving

         (c) Lateral rhinotomy

         (d) Transpalatal

         (e) Lateral infratemporal fossa

      (4) Tumors with significant intracranial extension require neurosurgical consultation and may ultimately be more appropriately managed with radiation therapy.

      (5) Role of hormonal therapy (estrogens or testosterone blockers) remains unclear.

      (6) Spontaneous regression has been reported but is uncommon.

   d. Close follow-up is required for patients with

      (1) Large tumors

      (2) Incomplete resection

      (3) Intracranial disease

      (4) Radiation treatment

   e. Malignant transformation has been reported and may be more common in patients treated with radiation therapy.

  3. Rhabdomyosarcoma (see "Head and Neck," below)

  4. Lymphoma (see "Head and Neck," below)

E. Idiopathic

  1. Wegener's granulomatosis—triad of acute necrotizing granulomas of upper respiratory mucosa, vasculitis of small to medium vessels, and glomerulonephritis.

   a. DX: Elevated c-ANCA

   b. TX: Immunosuppressive therapy

  2. Systemic lupus erythematosus—autoimmune vasculitis—may be associated with an extrinsic trigger.

  3. Sarcoid—characterized by noncaseating granulomas. Can involve any organ system.

  4. Pemphigus—characterized by intraepidermal blisters, positive Nikolsky sign; treated medically.

Paranasal Sinuses

I. Developmental anatomy[1]
   A. Prenatal development
      1. Maxillary sinuses form as furrows in the lateral nasal wall at 65 to 70 days.
      2. Ethmoid sinuses begin to form in the second trimester. The basal lamella of the middle turbinate separates the anterior and posterior ethmoid cells.
   B. Postnatal development
      1. The floor of the maxillary sinus is superior to the floor of the nose at birth, at about the same level as the nasal floor by 8 to 9 years, and 4 to 5 mm below the floor by adulthood.
      2. Anterior and posterior ethmoid air cells grow postnatally.
      3. Sphenoid sinuses start to pneumatize at about 2 years of age. They continue to grow postnatally.
      4. Frontal sinuses are generally evident by 7 years of age.
II. Signs and symptoms
   A. Infection, purulent rhinorrhea
   B. Obstruction
   C. Mass effect
III. Clinical assessment
   A. Physical examination findings may be fairly limited.
   B. Radiographic imaging helpful in assessing sinuses.
IV. Pathology/treatment/complications
   A. Congenital—asymmetric aeration of the sinuses is relatively common.
   B. Neoplastic
      1. Fibrous dysplasia
         a. Clinical features
            (1) Commonly involves maxilla and mandible.
            (2) Histologically benign.
            (3) Most commonly monostotic.
            (4) Polyostotic lesions may be associated with McCune-Albright syndrome.
               (a) Multiple café au lait spots
               (b) Precocious puberty
               (c) Involvement of lower extremities
      2. Diagnosis—typical "ground glass" appearance of bony lesion on CT scan. Often an incidental finding. Histology confirms diagnosis.
      3. Management—monostotic lesions will tend to slow in progression during puberty. Lesions that are symptomatic should be excised if possible. High recurrence rate when treated with curettage.
   C. Infectious/inflammatory
      1. Acute rhinosinusitis[24]
         a. Clinical features
            (1) Defined as purulent rhinorrhea lasting more than 10 days, associated with fever.
         b. Most common pathogens:
            (1) *S. pneumoniae* (20–30%)

        (2) *M. catarrhalis* (15–20%)

        (3) *H. influenzae* (15–20%)

        (4) *Streptococcus pyogenes* (5%)

  c. Diagnosis

        (1) Based upon clinical symptoms, as radiographic sinus opacification is nonspecific in young children.

        (2) Nasal cultures do not correlate with sinus cultures.

        (3) Plain radiographs of the sinuses may be helpful in management of maxillary sinusitis in children.

  d. Treatment

        (1) Empiric management with oral antibiotics for 10 to 14 days.

        (2) Oral amoxicillin remains the first choice.

        (3) Symptoms should improve within 72 hours of starting antibiotic therapy.

        (4) If no improvement occurs, antibiotics should be changed to include a beta-lactamase–stable agent.

            (a) A beta-lactamase–stable agent should be used as a first agent if the child has severe symptoms.

2. Recurrent acute rhinosinusitis

  a. Clinical features—symptoms clear completely for at least 2 weeks between infections.

  b. Diagnosis

        (1) Consideration should be given to contributing factors, such as immunodeficiency, cystic fibrosis, immotile cilia syndrome, and gastroesophageal reflux disease (GERD).

        (2) Adenoid size can be assessed based upon flexible fiberoptic nasopharyngoscopy, lateral neck x-ray, or sinus CT scan.

  c. Treatment—each acute episode may be treated with oral antibiotics. Adenoidectomy may be helpful in management of rhinosinusitis in children with an obstructive adenoid pad.

3. Chronic rhinosinusitis

  a. Clinical features

        (1) Symptoms include nasal congestion, rhinorrhea, headache, irritability, cough, postnasal drip, and halitosis.

        (2) Low-grade symptoms lasting more than 12 weeks.

        (3) Most common pathogens:

            (a) *S. aureus*

            (b) Alpha-hemolytic *Streptococcus*

            (c) *M. catarrhalis*

  b. Diagnosis

        (1) Cultures taken from the middle meatus/ethmoid bulla may be helpful.

        (2) Cultures are necessary in the following situations:

            (a) Child is systemically ill.

            (b) Progression of symptoms despite appropriate therapy.

        (c)   Immunocompromised host.

        (d)   Suppurative complications.

   c.   Treatment should include beta-lactamase–stable antibiotic for 4 to 6 weeks.

4.   Treatment of uncomplicated rhinosinusitis

   a.   Antibiotic therapy (oral or IV, as appropriate)

   b.   Adenoidectomy may be helpful in younger children.

   c.   Nasoantral windows have been largely supplanted by endoscopic sinus surgery. They may still play a role in managing patients with ciliary dysfunction and/or cystic fibrosis.

   d.   Endoscopic sinus surgery

       (1)   Usually limited to the involved sinuses, most commonly anterior ethmoids and maxillary sinuses.

       (2)   More likely to be required in children with immune deficiency, ciliary dysmotility, allergy, asthma, cystic fibrosis.

       (3)   Absolute indications

           (a)   Intracranial complications

           (b)   Cavernous sinus thrombosis

           (c)   Mucopyocele

           (d)   Subperiosteal or orbital abscess

           (e)   Allergic or invasive fungal sinusitis

           (f)   Antrochoanal polyp

           (g)   Complete nasal obstruction

           (h)   Tumors of the nasal cavities or sinuses

           (i)   Cerebrospinal fluid (CSF) leaks

       (4)   Relative indications

           (a)   Subacute or chronic rhinosinusitis after failure of aggressive medical management.

           (b)   Recurrent acute rhinosinusitis for which the child requires frequent courses of oral antibiotics.

5.   Complications of sinusitis

   a.   Extracranial

       (1)   Periorbital cellulitis

       (2)   Subperiosteal abscess

       (3)   Orbital cellulitis—associated with chemosis

       (4)   Orbital abscess

       (5)   Pott's puffy tumor

   b.   Intracranial

       (1)   Meningitis

       (2)   Cavernous sinus thrombosis

       (3)   Abscess (subdural, epidural, or brain)

6.   Treatment of complicated rhinosinusitis

   a.   Intravenous antibiotics with excellent soft tissue and CNS penetration.

   b.   Consultation of ophthalmology and/or neurosurgery

   c.   Drainage of abscesses with culture

   d.   Decompression of involved sinuses with culture

7. Nasal polyps
   a. Cystic fibrosis (CF)
      (1) Clinical presentation
         (a) Children under 10 years old with nasal polyps should be suspected of having CF.
         (b) Associated with chronic sinusitis.
         (c) Children with significant GI symptoms are generally diagnosed early.
      (2) Pathophysiology/diagnosis
         (a) Defect in cell membrane chloride transport associated with genetic mutation at deltaF508 (CFTR). Role of genetic testing is evolving.
         (b) Affects the respiratory and GI epithelium and exocrine function.
         (c) Immunoreactive trypsinogen levels used as screening test for CF.
         (d) Elevated sweat chloride level has long been the "gold standard" for diagnosis.
         (e) Fat malabsorption may result in coagulopathy (vitamin K deficiency).
         (f) Classic radiographic findings of medialized medial wall of the maxillary sinus and bilateral pansinusitis.
      (3) Treatment
         (a) Medical management
            i. Nasal steroid sprays
            ii. Oral antibiotics for acute exacerbations
            iii. Role of topical antibiotics evolving
         (b) Surgical management
            i. Indicated for patients who fail medical management and those who seem to have exacerbation of pulmonary disease related to rhinosinusitis.
            ii. Check coagulation studies preoperatively.
            iii. Can expect improvement in symptoms for 2 to 3 years.
         (c) Endoscopic sinus surgery and/or nasoantral windows may be recommended prior to lung transplant.
   b. Antrochoanal polyps
      (1) Clinical features
         (a) Originate in the antrum of the maxillary sinus and frequently extend into the middle meatus through the maxillary ostium.
         (b) Most commonly unilateral.
         (c) More common in children.
      (2) Treatment
         (a) Require surgical removal.
         (b) Endoscopic removal and Caldwell-Luc approaches have been described.
         (c) Propensity for recurrence.

D. Traumatic
   1. Orbital floor fracture
      a. History of antecedent trauma.
      b. Complications of injury.
         (1) Hypesthesia of infraorbital nerve
         (2) Entrapment of inferior rectus muscle
         (3) Associated injuries to the globe
         (4) Enophthalmos
      c. Diagnosis confirmed on CT scan of sinuses.
      d. May require surgical repair.

Oral Cavity/Oropharynx

I. Developmental anatomy
  A. Prenatal development[1]
    1. Development of the oral cavity is defined by the development of the palate (see Chapter 11), the tongue, and the mandible.
    2. Median tongue bud (tuberculum impar) arises in the pharynx, rostral to the foramen caecum (about end of the fourth week).
    3. Two distal tongue buds (lateral lingual swellings) are derived from the first branchial arches and arise on either side of the median bud.
    4. The lateral tongue buds fuse in the midline to form the anterior two-thirds of the tongue.
    5. The posterior third of the tongue is comprised of the copula (from the second branchial arch) and the hypobranchial eminence (from the third and fourth arches).
    6. The mandible forms from the first branchial arch between the fifth and eighth weeks.
  B. Postnatal development: All structures of the oral cavity grow postnatally. Tonsils are generally small at birth, usually peak in size by 5 to 8 years of age.
II. Signs and symptoms
  A. Mass lesion
  B. Airway obstruction
  C. Feeding difficulties
  D. Sialorrhea
  E. Altered speech
  F. Bleeding
III. Clinical assessment: Careful intraoral examination can generally be performed on children of any age.
IV. Pathology/treatment/complications
  A. Congenital
    1. Ankyloglossia—may interfere with feeding or speech
      a. Release of ankyloglossia is usually performed for feeding or speech issues.
      b. Specific indications for release of frenulum are not well established.
    2. Cleft lip/palate—(see Chapter 11)

3. Ranula
    a. Clinical features
        (1) Obstruction of the sublingual gland.
        (2) May present at any age.
        (3) Usually seen as unilateral cystic lesion in the floor of mouth.
        (4) May pierce the mylohyoid and extend into the submandibular triangle, ie, "plunging ranula."
    b. Diagnosis
        (1) Clinical appearance is usually diagnostic.
        (2) Main distinction is with lymphatic malformation. Lymphatic malformations tend to be multicystic, while ranulas are usually composed of a single cyst.
        (3) Distinction is made on pathology.
    c. Treatment
        (1) Marsupialization
            (a) Avoids extensive dissection of floor of mouth.
            (b) High incidence of recurrence.
        (2) Surgical excision
            (a) Requires removal of sublingual gland.
            (b) Lower incidence of recurrence.
4. Lingual thyroid
    a. Clinical features
        (1) Results from abnormal descent of the thyroglossal tract into the neck.
        (2) Increases in size with age.
        (3) Symptoms related to mass effect at base of tongue.
        (4) May include all of the patient's functioning thyroid tissue.
    b. Evaluation should include radionuclide thyroid scan to determine whether there is any other functioning thyroid tissue lower in the neck.
    c. Treatment dictated by symptoms.
        (1) Observation for asymptomatic or minimally symptomatic patients.
        (2) Thyroid suppression.
        (3) Surgical therapy may be indicated for failure of medical management or suspicion of malignancy.
5. Midline rhomboid glossitis
    a. Presents as soft tissue mass in the posterior midline of the tongue, in the region of the embryonic tuberculum impar.
    b. Defect in posterior lingual development.
6. Branchial cleft anomalies (see Chapter 11)
7. Glossoptosis—often seen with micrognathia.
    a. Clinical syndromes
        (1) Pierre-Robin sequence
            (a) Micrognathia
            (b) U-shaped cleft of the secondary palate
            (c) Associated with significant mandibular growth in the first 4 to 6 months of life (with subsequent improvement of upper airway patency)

        (2)   Stickler syndrome
            (a)   Autosomal dominant
            (b)   Myopia before 10 years of age; retinal detachments
            (c)   Micrognathia/glossoptosis
            (d)   Midfacial hypoplasia
            (e)   Hearing loss, mixed
        (3)   Nager's syndrome—acrofacial dysostosis
            (a)   Auricular anomalies, including aural atresia
            (b)   Micrognathia/glossoptosis
            (c)   Hypoplasia of thumb
        (4)   Treacher Collins syndrome—mandibulofacial dysostosis
            (a)   Malar hypoplasia with deficient zygomatic arches
            (b)   Lid colobomas
            (c)   Severe mandibular deficiency
            (d)   Bilateral microtia and atresia
            (e)   Choanal atresia
    b.   Management
        (1)   Dependent on degree of airway obstruction
        (2)   Range of interventions
            (a)   Prone positioning
            (b)   Nasopharyngeal airway
            (c)   Tongue lip adhesion
            (d)   Distraction osteogenesis of the mandible
            (e)   Tracheotomy
        (3)   Monitoring of nutritional status and weight gain
  8.   Macroglossia
    a.   May be associated with:
        (1)   Beckwith-Wiedemann syndrome
            (a)   Macrosomia (birthweight over 10 pounds)
            (b)   Neonatal hypoglycemia
            (c)   Macroglossia—usually does not cause significant airway obstruction
            (d)   Omphalocele
            (e)   Hepatosplenomegaly
            (f)   Auricular pits
        (2)   Trisomy 21 (Down's syndrome)
        (3)   Congenital hypothyroidism
            (a)   Part of neonatal screening.
            (b)   Early detection and adequate thyroid replacement will allow the patient to have normal growth and development.
            (c)   Macroglossia caused by myxedema of the tongue.
        (4)   Mucopolysaccharidoses
    b.   Main indication for tongue reduction surgery is airway obstruction. Effect of tongue reduction on speech is difficult to assess.
B. Neoplastic
  1.   Rhabdomyosarcoma—(see "Head and Neck," below)

2. Lymphoma—(see "Head and Neck," below)
3. Squamous cell carcinoma
    a. Rare in children.
    b. Lesions tend to grow rapidly.
    c. Regional metastases occur early.
    d. Most commonly involves the tongue.
    e. Lip, palate, and gingiva may be involved.
    f. Treatment similar to that recommended for adults.
4. Epulis—heterogenous group of benign lesions involving the gingiva.
    a. May be fibrous, vascular, or granular in histologic appearance.
    b. Congenital epulis:
        (1) More commonly involves maxilla.
        (2) F:M = 4:1
    c. Treated with surgical excision.
5. Epignathus: congenital lesion of the maxilla or mandible. Includes hamartomas, choristomas, teratomas. Surgical excision indicated.

C. Infectious/inflammatory
1. Tonsillitis
    a. Most commonly viral in nature.
    b. Group A beta-hemolytic *Streptococcus* is most common bacterial pathogen.
        (1) May be associated with rheumatic fever or acute poststreptococcal glomerulonephritis.
        (2) Diagnosis requires culture.
        (3) Should be treated with antibiotics to avoid complications.
2. Peritonsillar abscess—usually forms at the superior pole of the tonsil.
    a. Clinical presentation
        (1) History
            (a) Antecedent pharyngitis
            (b) May have been partially treated with oral antibiotics
            (c) Odynophagia
        (2) Physical findings
            (a) Fever
            (b) Unilateral palatal edema and fullness
            (c) Asymmetric tonsils
            (d) Deviation of the uvula to the contralateral side
            (e) Trismus
    b. Diagnosis
        (1) Clinical examination may be diagnostic.
        (2) Distinction between peritonsillar cellulitis and abscess may be challenging, especially in younger children.
        (3) Response to intravenous antibiotic therapy may be helpful in making the distinction between cellulitis and abscess.
        (4) CT scan with contrast may provide further information.

      c.   Treatment
- (1) Abscess formation generally requires drainage by needle aspiration, incision and drainage, or tonsillectomy.
- (2) Intravenous antibiotics.

3.   Tonsillar hypertrophy

      a.   Clinical features
- (1) Associated with airway and feeding difficulties.
- (2) Airway difficulties most commonly manifest as obstructed sleep.
- (3) Often associated with adenoid hypertrophy.
- (4) Associated symptoms include
  - (a) Excessive daytime somnolence
  - (b) Short nap latency
  - (c) Enuresis
  - (d) Failure to thrive
- (5) Behavioral disturbance and poor school performance have also been attributed to chronic sleep deprivation.

      b.   Diagnosis of obstructed sleep
- (1) Based upon history (snoring and gasping while asleep) provided by the child's caregiver.
- (2) Sleep study may be helpful in quantitating degree of obstruction and ruling out central apnea.

      c.   Treatment
- (1) Indications for tonsillectomy
  - (a) More than six episodes of tonsillitis in one year.
  - (b) More than five episodes per year for 2 years.
  - (c) Recurrent peritonsillar abscess.
  - (d) Acute management of peritonsillar abscess.
  - (e) Asymmetric tonsils.
  - (f) Tonsillar hypertrophy or asymmetry in immunosuppressed children to rule out lymphoproliferative disorder.
  - (g) Obstructive adenotonsillar hypertrophy—consideration should be given to adenoidectomy when indications are primarily for obstruction.
- (2) Complications of adenotonsillectomy
  - (a) Bleeding: 0.1 to 3 per 100
  - (b) Aspiration pneumonia
  - (c) Velopharyngeal insufficiency
  - (d) Nasopharyngeal stenosis
  - (e) Torticollis
  - (f) Injury of the carotid artery
  - (g) Death
  - (h) Airway obstruction—more common in children under 3 years of age with significant obstruction and history of pulmonary compromise

4. Retropharyngeal abscess
   a. Suppurative infection of lymph nodes between the posterior pharyngeal wall and prevertebral fascia (present in younger children).
   b. Infection may extend inferiorly to the mediastinum.
   c. History of antecedent upper respiratory infection (URI) is common.
   d. Clinical presentation may be associated with
      (1) High fever
      (2) Progressive sialorrhea
      (3) Torticollis
      (4) Anorexia/dysphagia
      (5) Airway obstruction
      (6) Edema or mass of the posterior pharyngeal wall
   e. Most common organisms
      (1) Beta-hemolytic streptococci
      (2) Anaerobic streptococci
      (3) *S. aureus*
   f. Diagnosis
      (1) Lateral neck film shows thickening of the prevertebral soft tissue. Air-fluid level is diagnostic of abscess. Artifact may be related to crying patient or rotation.
      (2) CT scan of the neck with contrast may be helpful in distinguishing cellulitis from abscess.
   g. Treatment should include
      (1) Surgical drainage
      (2) Intravenous antibiotics and fluids
5. Parapharyngeal abscess
   a. Similar to retropharyngeal abscess.
   b. Patients tend to be older than those presenting with retropharyngeal abscess.
   c. These patients are more likely to have trismus because of involvement of the pterygoid musculature.
   d. Treatment involves surgical drainage.
D. Traumatic
1. Penetrating trauma of the oral cavity[25,26]
   a. Clinical features
      (1) Impalement of the oropharynx and palate are relatively common accidental injuries in the pediatric population.
      (2) Proximity to the carotid sheath and possible injury cause great consternation. Injuries lateral to the anterior tonsillar pillar may have higher likelihood of injury to the carotid sheath.
   b. Management
      (1) Children with this history should be carefully observed, either as outpatients or in the hospital setting.
      (2) Intraoral trauma in infants who are not yet walking should alert the clinician to the possibility of nonaccidental trauma.
      (3) Most injuries do not require repair.

Larynx/Subglottis

I. Developmental anatomy
   A. Prenatal development[1]
      1. The larynx and tracheobronchial tree are derived from the primitive foregut starting at about 25 days gestation.
      2. The larynx, trachea, and esophagus are formed by the eighth week of gestation.
      3. Epiglottis is derived from the hypobranchial eminence, related to the third and fourth branchial arches.
      4. The laryngeal musculature derives from the fourth and sixth arches.
      5. Laryngeal movement can be detected by the third month of gestation.
   B. Postnatal development[27]
      1. The neonatal glottis measures approximately 7 mm in the anteroposterior and 4 mm in the lateral dimensions.
      2. Subglottis is the narrowest part of the neonatal airway, measuring about 4 to 5 mm in diameter.
      3. The larynx continues to descend in the neck, with the inferior aspect of the cricoid cartilage positioned at
         a. C4 at birth
         b. C5 at 2 years of age
         c. C6 at 5 years of age
         d. C6-7 at 15 years of age
II. Signs and symptoms
   A. Laryngeal pathology is generally characterized by
      1. Inspiratory (supraglottic) or biphasic (glottic) stridor
      2. Change in voice
      3. Feeding difficulties, including aspiration
      4. Tachypnea
      5. Tachycardia
      6. Use of accessory muscle of respiration
   B. Subglottic pathology is generally associated with
      1. Biphasic stridor
      2. Croupy cough
      3. Feeding difficulties
III. Clinical assessment
   A. Auscultation over the large airway may help to detect and characterize the stridor.
   B. Careful inspection of the neck and chest during respiration is important.
   C. Flexible fiberoptic laryngoscopy in the awake child is generally the most effective way to assess laryngeal function.
   D. Direct laryngoscopy may be required to delineate laryngeal pathology.
   E. Visualization of the subglottis requires laryngoscopy and bronchoscopy under general anesthesia.
   F. O_2 (oxygen) saturation and serum electrolytes.
IV. Pathology/treatment/complications
   A. Laryngomalacia
      1. Clinical features
         a. Most common cause of stridor in infants.
         b. Usually presents as inspiratory stridor within the first 6 weeks of life.

    c.   Stridor may be variable and usually resolves when the infant is crying.

    d.   90% of patients will have spontaneous resolution of symptoms, usually by 12 months of age.

    e.   Children with neurologic impairment may have progressive laryngomalacia.

    f.   Severe laryngomalacia may be associated with more severe airway compromise (ie, stridor, retractions, and desaturation), feeding difficulties, and failure to thrive.

2.   Diagnosis: confirmed upon flexible fiberoptic laryngoscopy with findings of prolapse of supraglottic tissue into the laryngeal inlet on inspiration.

3.   Management

    a.   Most patients do not require any intervention because of high rate of spontaneous improvement.

    b.   There is 10 to 20% incidence of synchronous airway lesions and therefore patients with more severe or atypical symptoms should undergo direct laryngoscopy and bronchoscopy to assess the entire tracheobronchial tree.

    c.   Infants with severe laryngomalacia (ie, significant airway obstruction with/without failure to thrive) may benefit from supraglottoplasty.

    d.   Patients with other medical conditions in addition to laryngomalacia may not respond to supraglottoplasty.

    e.   Gastroesophageal reflux may exacerbate laryngomalacia and should be treated medically.

B.   Vocal cord dysfunction[28,29]

1.   Clinical features

    a.   Second most common laryngeal anomaly of infancy.

    b.   Most commonly idiopathic in infants.

    c.   Most commonly iatrogenic in older children.

    d.   Left vocal cord more commonly affected.

2.   Etiology

    a.   Congenital

        (1)   Complex congenital heart disease

        (2)   CNS anomalies

            (a)   Hydrocephalus

            (b)   Spinal cord anomalies

            (c)   Nucleus ambiguus dysgenesis (usually familial and bilateral)

            (d)   Kernicterus

        (3)   Other associations

            (a)   Möbius' syndrome—associated with bilateral facial nerve palsy

            (b)   Trisomy 21 (Down's syndrome)

            (c)   Mediastinal anomalies

            (d)   Trauma—usually improves in 4 to 6 months

            (e)   Diaphragmatic hernia

            (f)   Erb's palsy

    b.   Acquired

        (1)   Arnold-Chiari malformation[30]

            (a)   May be associated with uni- or bilateral paresis.

            (b)   May also include central sleep apnea.

            (c)   Role of posterior fossa decompression is unclear.

       (2)   Infectious

            (a)   Poliomyelitis

            (b)   Guillain-Barré

            (c)   Botulism

            (d)   Diphtheria

            (e)   Syphilis

       (3)   Iatrogenic

            (a)   Cardiac surgery

            (b)   Thyroidectomy

            (c)   Intubation injury

   3.   Management

      a.   Dependent upon degree of airway compromise.

      b.   Spontaneous recovery may occur up to several years later.

      c.   May require tracheotomy; bilateral paresis more likely to require tracheotomy than unilateral paresis.

C.   Subglottic stenosis (SGS)

   1.   Congenital

      a.   May be membranous (fibrous thickening in the subglottis) or cartilaginous (abnormal cricoid cartilage).

      b.   May present with stridor at birth; less severe cases present with recurrent croup.

      c.   Patients who are intubated may present with failure to extubate.

      d.   Management depends upon severity of symptoms.

   2.   Acquired

      a.   May be exacerbated by GERD.

      b.   Associated with prolonged intubation.

      c.   Infants often require tracheotomy because of underlying bronchopulmonary dysplasia (which necessitated the prolonged ventilatory support).

      d.   Patients with congenital subglottic stenosis (SGS) may be at greater risk for acquired SGS.

      e.   Definitive management often requires airway reconstruction.

   3.   Treatment options

      a.   Endoscopic management (dilatation, laser treatment)

      b.   Anterior cricoid split

      c.   Laryngotracheal reconstruction

      d.   Cricotracheal resection

   4.   Timing of airway reconstruction is controversial; surgery should be undertaken when the pulmonary function is adequate.

D.   Laryngeal clefts[31]

   1.   Clinical features

      (a)   Incomplete separation of the foregut extending cephalad to include the interarytenoid space.

      (b)   Classification system based upon inferior extent of the cleft.

         (1)   Type 1—interarytenoid musculature

         (2)   Type 2—into cricoid

         (3)   Type 3—through entire posterior cricoid

         (4)   Type 4—extending through membranous trachea

   2.   Diagnosis—laryngoscopy and bronchoscopy

   3.   Treatment

      a.   Milder clefts may be amenable to endoscopic repair.

      b.   Deeper clefts generally require open surgical repair.

E. Vallecular cyst

   1.   Presents with dysphonia, dysphagia, and airway obstruction.

   2.   Diagnosis is made upon visualizing a cystic lesion in the vallecula.

   3.   Endoscopic marsupialization is usually therapeutic.

F. Subglottic hemangioma (SGH)—most common neoplasm of the pediatric airway

   1.   Clinical features

      a.   Onset of croup-like symptoms at 4 to 8 weeks of age; 85% present by 6 months of age.

      b.   F:M = 2:1.

      c.   Diagnosis is frequently delayed.

      d.   Associated with biphasic stridor.

      e.   Airway symptoms associated with progressive enlargement of the lesion through the proliferative phase of the hemangioma.

      f.   50% have a cutaneous hemangioma of the head and neck.

      g.   Expect spontaneous involution of the lesion by 2 years of age.

   2.   Diagnosis

      a.   Soft tissue radiographs of the neck demonstrate subglottic fullness.

      b.   Diagnosis made upon characteristic appearance of vascular lesion in the subglottis. Biopsy not required but may be helpful.

      c.   CT and MRI scans may be helpful in assessing patients with hemangiomas involving the neck and airway.

   3.   Management options

      a.   Tracheotomy

      b.   Intubation

      c.   Steroid injection

      d. CO_2 laser—mainstay of therapy

      e.   Open surgical excision

      f.   Systemic alpha interferon

G. Granular cell tumor—may be similar in appearance to SGH; requires excision.

H. Neurofibroma—benign tumor of Schwann cell origin with low malignant potential.

   1.   May be associated with neurofibromatosis.

   2.   Usually involves arytenoids or aryepiglottic folds.

   3.   Requires surgical management.

   4.   Complete excision may be difficult; repeated local excision may be required.

I. Malignant laryngeal tumors

   1.   Rare lesions; require total laryngectomy.

   2.   Adjuvant therapy depends upon tumor type.

J. Infectious/inflammatory

   1.   Laryngotracheobronchitis or croup

      a.   Clinical features

        (1)   Usually starts as viral infection, most commonly parainfluenza.

        (2)   Bacterial superinfection (*H. influenzae* or *S. aureus*) may occur.

        (3)   Usually affects children under 2 years of age.

        (4)   Children present with barky cough and biphasic stridor.

        (5)   Degree of airway compromise is variable.

    b.   Diagnosis—Plain soft tissue neck films [anteroposterior (AP) projection] show "steeple sign" of the subglottis.

    c.   Treatment is supportive and includes humidification, hydration, supplemental oxygen, and racemic epinephrine. Steroids may be helpful as well. Intubation should be avoided if at all possible.

  2.   Epiglottitis

    a.   Clinical features

        (1)   Usually caused by *H. influenzae* type B

        (2)   Incidence has fallen dramatically since introduction of HiB vaccine.

        (3)   Associated with rapid onset of symptoms, including sore throat, fever, inspiratory stridor, airway distress, and drooling.

        (4)   Patients typically position themselves in the "sniffing" position to optimize their airway.

        (5)   Once the diagnosis is considered, measures should be taken to avoid irritating the child (ie, intraoral examination, starting an IV, etc.).

    b.   Diagnosis

        (1)   Lateral plain film of the neck may show a widened epiglottis. (The child should be accompanied to the radiology suite by someone who can manage an airway emergency.)

    c.   Definitive diagnosis and management should be performed in the operating room.

        (1)   An inhalation anesthetic should be administered.

        (2)   Induction of anesthesia will be prolonged because of the airway obstruction.

        (3)   Visualization of an edematous and erythematous epiglottis is diagnostic.

        (4)   Intubation is critical.

        (5)   After the airway has been secured, cultures of the epiglottis and blood can be taken.

  3.   Recurrent respiratory papillomatosis[32]

    a.   Clinical features

        (1)   Most common benign neoplasm of the pediatric larynx.

        (2)   Second most common cause of hoarseness in childhood.

        (3)   Most commonly involves larynx.

        (4)   May involve any part of the aerodigestive tract.

        (5)   Most commonly diagnosed between 2 and 4 years of age.

        (6)   1500 to 2500 new cases diagnosed in the United States each year.

        (7)   Estimated incidence of 4.3 per 100,000.

    b.   Classification

        (1)   Juvenile (less than 12 years of age)

      (a)   Tends to be more aggressive.

      (b)   Vertical transmission.

      (c)   Human papillomaviruses (HPV) 6 and 11 most common (same subtypes cause genital condylomata).

      (d)   Extralaryngeal involvement in 30% of patients. Sites involved (decreasing frequency):

         i.   Oral cavity

         ii.   Trachea

         iii.   Bronchi

      (e)   May be manifestation of sexual abuse when symptoms present in children older than 7 years of age.

    (2)   Adult

      (a)   Tends to be less aggressive.

      (b)   Peak incidence 20 to 40 years of age.

      (c)   Extralaryngeal involvement in 16%.

  c. Diagnosis

    (1)   Children with hoarseness and any sign of airway obstruction require visualization of the larynx.

    (2)   Characteristic appearance of papillomatous lesions.

    (3)   Biopsy will confirm diagnosis.

    (4)   Polymerase chain reaction may be used to identify specific viral subtypes.

  d. Management

    (1)   Tracheotomy thought to be associated with extralaryngeal spread. Avoid tracheotomy if possible or decannulate as soon as possible.

    (2)   Goals of treatment are to

      (a)   Ensure airway patency

      (b)   Avoid long-term injury to airway

    (3)   Treatment generally requires multiple procedures to debulk the mass lesion. Multiple modalities have been used. CO_2 laser is most commonly used.

    (4)   Potassium titanium phosphate (KTP) laser may be useful for tracheo-bronchial lesions.

    (5)   Adjuvant therapy may be indicated for patients requiring more than four surgical procedures per year, for distal spread, and for rapid recurrence.

      (a)   Alpha-interferon

      (b)   Photodynamic therapy using m-tetrahydroxyphenyl chloride (Foscan) currently being studied.

      (c)   Other medications with uncertain benefit:

         i.   Indole-3-carbinol

         ii.   Ribavirin

         iii.   Acyclovir

         iv.   Intralesional cidofovir

         v.   Antireflux medications

    K. Iatrogenic
        1. Intubation injury[33]
            a. Acute
                (1) Edema
                (2) Granulation tissue
                (3) Ulceration
            b. Chronic
                (1) Tongues of granulation tissue
                (2) Ulcerated troughs
                (3) Healed furrows
                (4) Healed fibrous nodules
    L. Idiopathic
        1. Paroxysmal vocal fold dysfunction
            a. More common in girls with significant social stressors.
            b. Frequently misdiagnosed as asthma.
            c. Diagnosis made upon flexible laryngoscopy with adduction of vocal fold on inspiration.
            d. Associated with GER.
            e. Management may include biofeedback, management of GER, botulinum toxin injections.

Tracheobronchial Tree

  I. Developmental anatomy
    A. Prenatal development[1]
        1. Derives from the distal laryngotracheal tube.
        2. The lung bud grows at the distal end of the laryngotracheal tube.
        3. The lung bud divides into two bronchial buds, which form the primitive primary bronchi.
        4. Bronchial buds continue to divide to form the branching airway and associated lung parenchyma.
        5. Surfactant is secreted at 23 to 24 weeks and is sufficient in quantity to prevent lung collapse at 28 to 32 weeks.
    B. Postnatal development
        1. Normal ratio of tracheal cartilage to membranous wall is approximately $4:1$.
        2. The trachea continues to grow in length and descends deeper into the mediastinum.
        3. The trachea is approximately 4 cm at birth and grows to 12 cm in the adult.
        4. The neonatal trachea is more compliant than the adult trachea and is therefore more likely to collapse.
        5. Postnatal growth of the lungs, with further division of the bronchioles and alveoli, continues for at least 8 years after birth.
 II. Signs and symptoms
    A. Dyspnea
    B. Cough, grunting
    C. Failure to thrive
    D. Aspiration

III. Clinical assessment
   A. Auscultation.
   B. Chest x-ray (PA and lateral).
   C. Fluoroscopy.
   D. CT and MRI scanning.
   E. Laryngoscopy and bronchoscopy—bronchoscopy requires general anesthesia in infants and children.
   F. Oxygen saturation and serum electrolytes
IV. Pathology/treatment/complications
   A. Congenital
     1. Tracheomalacia
       a. Clinical features
         (1) Presents with grunting, expiratory stridor
         (2) May include recurrent pneumonia
         (3) Classification
           (a) Intrinsic—ratio of cartilage to membrane about 2 : 1
           (b) Extrinsic—normal ratio with extrinsic compression
             i. Vascular anomalies (aberrant subclavian, innominate artery compression, etc.)
             ii. Mediastinal masses
       b. Diagnosis
         (1) Airway fluoroscopy may be helpful.
         (2) Definitive diagnosis is made upon inspection of the trachea while the patient is spontaneously ventilating.
       c. Management—dependent upon degree of airway obstruction. May include
         (1) Observation
         (2) Continuous positive airway pressure
         (3) Tracheotomy
         (4) Aortopexy
         (5) Repair of vascular anomalies
     2. Tracheoesophageal fistula
       a. Clinical features
         (1) 1 per 2500 live births
         (2) More common in males
         (3) Incomplete separation of the foregut at 4 to 5 weeks gestation
         (4) May be associated with polyhydramnios
         (5) Associated with VACTERL syndrome, which includes

           V: Vertebral/vascular
           A: Anorectal
           C: Cardiac
           T: Tracheo-
           E: Esophageal
           R: Radial/renal
           L: Limb deformities

       b. Diagnosis—based upon contrast studies of the GI tract. Four main types:
         (1) Proximal esophageal atresia with distal tracheoesophageal fistula near bifurcation (approximately 90% of cases).

        (2) H-type fistula—may be very difficult to diagnose.

        (3) Proximal tracheoesophageal fistula with distal esophageal atresia.

        (4) Proximal esophageal atresia with tracheoesophageal fistula and distal esophageal atresia with second tracheoesophageal fistula.

    c. Management requires surgical repair.

  3. Tracheal stenosis

    a. Clinical features

        (1) Result of unequal partitioning of the foregut into the trachea and esophagus.

        (2) May be associated with tracheoesophageal fistula or complex congenital heart disease.

    b. Diagnosis based upon bronchoscopy. Location, degree, and extent of stenosis should be assessed. Radiographic imaging studies (CT or MRI) may be helpful.

    c. Management—dependent upon degree of airway compromise and characteristic of stenosis. Options include:

        (1) Dilatation

        (2) Sleeve resection and reanastomosis

        (3) Slide tracheoplasty

B. Infectious/inflammatory

  1. Allergic bronchopulmonary aspergillosis[34]

    a. History of reactive airway disease or cystic fibrosis is common; presents with wheezing, mucus production, pulmonary infiltrates, and elevated serum IgE.

    b. May cause unilateral symptoms and therefore be difficult to distinguish from foreign-body aspiration.

    c. Diagnosis is made upon retrieval of a cast of the bronchial tree.

    d. Treatment includes removal of plugs and systemic treatment of the atopic disease.

  2. Tuberculosis

    a. Granulomas may be seen in the tracheobronchial tree.

    b. Diagnosis based upon biopsy of the lesion.

    c. Treatment is based upon pharmacologic management of tuberculosis (TB).

C. Foreign-body (FB) aspiration

  1. Clinical features

    a. Accounts for over 1000 deaths per year in the United States.

    b. Most common cause of accidental death in children less than 1 year of age.

    c. 25% of airway foreign bodies have been present for over 2 weeks. These are more likely to be associated with chronic lung infection and bronchiectasis.

    d. Frequently associated with an episode of cough, gagging, or sputtering.

    e. Symptoms related to level and degree of obstruction.

    f. Sites of airway FB in decreasing order:

        (1) Right mainstem (60%)

        (2) Left mainstem (30%)

        (3) Hypopharynx (2–5%)

          (4)   Trachea (3–12%)

          (5)   Larynx (1–7%)

   2.   Diagnosis

      a.   History

      b.   Physical findings

          (1)   Laryngeal—change in voice, cough, and odynophagia. May be associated with complete airway obstruction.

          (2)   Tracheal—an audible slap; palpable thud and expiratory wheeze.

          (3)   Bronchial—cough, unilateral wheeze.

      c.   Radiographic changes

          (1)   Laryngeal—soft tissue neck films may demonstrate an FB.

          (2)   Bronchial FB—inspiratory and forced expiratory chest x-ray

              (a)   Hyperinflation ipsilateral to FB (seen in approximately 50% of patients with bronchial FB).

              (b)   Mediastinal shift away from FB.

              (c)   Postobstructive collapse if FB has been present for some time.

              (d)   Elevation of hemidiaphragm on contralateral side.

              (e)   Radiopaque lesion may be seen (less than 25%).

          (3)   Other concerning findings

              (a)   Pneumomediastinum

              (b)   Pneumothorax

           (4)   Videofluoroscopy may be helpful.

      d.   Definitive diagnosis made upon bronchoscopy.

   3.   Management

      a.   Bronchoscopic removal of FB under direct visualization

      b.   Sequential endoscopy may be required for retained foreign bodies or associated inflammatory response.

      c.   Requires close communication with anesthesia team.

      d.   FB may become dislodged from the optical forceps upon removal. This most commonly occurs as the FB is being delivered through the glottis. The FB should be pushed back into the bronchus from which it came, and repeat attempt should be made for removal.

      e.   FB may be removed in piecemeal fashion.

      f.   Occasionally tracheotomy is required for removal of large foreign bodies.

Esophagus

   I.   Developmental anatomy

      A.   Prenatal development

         1.   Derived from the foregut when the tracheoesophageal septum separates the trachea from the esophagus, as described in tracheal development.

         2.   The esophagus elongates until the seventh week of gestation.

      B.   Postnatal development—the esophagus elongates to a length of 18 to 20 cm at maturity.

   II.   Signs and symptoms

      A.   Esophageal obstruction usually manifests as feeding difficulties.

      B.   May be associated with airway obstruction.

III. Clinical assessment
   A. Passage of a naso- or orogastric tube can demonstrate the patency of the upper aerodigestive tract.
   B. Barium swallow may be helpful in defining esophageal anomalies.
IV. Pathology/treatment/complications
   A. Congenital
      1. Tracheoesophageal fistula (see "Tracheobronchial Tree")
      2. Esophageal stenosis can occur anywhere along the length of the esophagus but is most commonly found in the distal third.
      3. Achalasia—rare in children
         a. Clinical features
            (1) Children present with failure to thrive and chronic pulmonary disease related to chronic aspiration.
            (2) Characterized by decreased ganglion cells in the enteric nervous system within the smooth muscle of the esophagus.
         b. Diagnosis
            (1) X-ray—Mediastinum may be widened on plain film, and barium swallow demonstrates "bird-beak" deformity with dilated proximal esophagus and tapering of the distal esophagus.
            (2) Manometry shows increased tone in the lower esophageal sphincter (LES), failure of the LES to relax on swallow, and absence of peristalsis in the esophagus.
         c. Treatment
            (1) Medical management to improve peristalsis and decrease LES tone.
            (2) Dilatation or esophageal myotomy may be indicated for patients who do not respond to medical management.
   B. Neoplastic lesions of the esophagus are rare in children.
   C. Infectious/inflammatory
      1. Stevens-Johnson syndrome may involve the GI mucosa.
      2. Dermatomyositis.
   D. Traumatic
      1. Foreign-body ingestion
         a. Clinical features
            (1) Present with dysphagia, increased drooling, history of choking episode.
            (2) May cause compression of the membranous trachea and airway obstruction.
            (3) Diagnosis may be delayed.
         b. Diagnosis
            (1) Neck and chest radiographs (AP and lateral views) are useful to identify radiopaque objects.
            (2) Contrast esophagogram may be necessary to rule out radiolucent foreign-body ingestion.
         c. Treatment
            (1) Removal of esophageal foreign bodies is most safely done endoscopically with the assistance of optical forceps.

        (2)   Esophagoscopy is usually performed under general anesthesia in young children.

        (3)   Esophageal disc batteries should be removed emergently. These batteries contain sodium or potassium hydroxide solutions that rapidly cause liquefaction necrosis in the moist environment of the esophagus.

        (4)   Batteries that have passed into the stomach can generally be followed radiographically until they pass spontaneously.

        (5)   Coins most commonly lodge at the thoracic inlet.

2. Caustic ingestion

   a.   Clinical features

        (1)   Accidental ingestion is more common during childhood and is most common in the first 3 years of life. (Adults tend to ingest caustic substances during suicide attempts and therefore tend to have more severe injuries.)

        (2)   Types of corrosives

            (a)   Alkali (most commonly $NaOH$, KOH, NH_4OH) commonly used in drain cleaners and disc batteries; cause liquefaction necrosis; tend to diffuse into deep tissue layers.

            (b)   Acids (most commonly HCL, H_2SO_4, HNO_3) cause coagulation necrosis; degree of injury tends to be more superficial.

            (c)   Phenol (Lysol)

            (d)   Hypochlorous acid ($HClO$) is the active ingredient in bleach. It forms hydrochloric acid when the oxygen is released.

        (3)   Degree of injury related to:

            (a)   Type of corrosive

            (b)   Concentration of corrosive

            (c)   Amount of corrosive

            (d)   Duration of mucosal contact

   b.   Assessment

        (1)   It is important to identify the substance that was ingested.

        (2)   Intraoral involvement does not correlate with esophageal exposure. Absence of intraoral lesions does not preclude the presence of significant esophageal injury.

        (3)   The entire patient must be assessed to rule out airway involvement and perforated viscus.

   c.   Management

        (1)   Dependent upon the degree of exposure suspected.

        (2)   Patients with few symptoms and benign physical examination may be observed without any intervention.

        (3)   Clear liquid diet during observation, with intravenous hydration if necessary.

        (4)   Steroids may be helpful in minimizing injury if administered in the first 8 hours. If severe esophageal injury is noted at endoscopy, the steroids should be discontinued to minimize the risk of esophageal perforation.

(5) Esophagoscopy, if indicated, should be done 24 to 72 hours after the incident in order to delineate the areas of injury. Earlier endoscopy may underestimate the degree of injury. The scope should not be advanced beyond an area of significant injury in order to minimize the chance of esophageal rupture.

(6) Nasogastric tube should be passed under direct vision if severe esophageal injury is noted at endoscopy.

(7) Feeding gastrostomy may be required.

(8) Antibiotics may hasten re-epithelialization.

(9) Esophageal stricture may develop and require management with dilatation, bypass procedures, or reconstruction.

E. Idiopathic

   1. Gastroesophageal reflux—regurgitation of stomach contents into esophagus.

      a. Very common in infants

      b. May cause apnea, laryngospasm, cough, bronchospasm, hoarseness

      c. Diagnostic tests include:

         (1) Barium swallow

         (2) PH probe

         (3) Radionuclide study

         (4) Esophagogastroduodenoscopy

         (5) Esophageal biopsy

      d. Treatment

         (1) Physical measures

            (a) Elevate head of bed

            (b) Thicken feeds

            (c) Small, frequent feeds

         (2) Pharmacologic measures

            (a) Acid suppression

               i. Antacids

               ii. Ranitidine

               iii. Famotidine

               iv. Omeprazole

            (b) Prokinetic agents

               i. Metoclopramide

               ii. Cisapride

         (3) Surgery

            (a) Fundoplication

            (b) Feeding gastrojejunostomy

EARS AND HEARING

Ear/Outer (Pinna, External Auditory Canal, and Tympanic Membrane)

  I. Developmental anatomy

    A. Prenatal development[1]

      1. Auricle develops from the six hillocks of His, derived from the first and second branchial arches, starting at about 6 weeks gestation.

2. The lobule is the last part of the auricle to form.
3. The concha cavum, derived from the first branchial groove, invaginates at about 8 weeks gestation to form the lateral cartilaginous external auditory canal (EAC).
4. The EAC starts as the external acoustic meatus, which invaginates as a solid epithelial core, the meatal plug. At about 6 months gestation, the epithelial cells of the plug degenerate, causing canalization of the medial bony EAC.
5. The tympanic membrane (TM) is derived from the membrane between the first branchial groove and the first pharyngeal pouch. Ultimately the TM is composed of ectoderm from the meatal plug, endoderm of the tubotympanic recess, and mesenchyme from the first and second branchial arches.

B. Postnatal development
1. The medial EAC ossifies within the first 2 years of life.
2. The EAC reaches adult size by about 9 years of age.
3. TM is almost adult size by birth, but it is almost horizontal in orientation. As the EAC grows, the TM assumes a more vertical position.
4. The cartilaginous pinna continues to grow for 10 to 12 years, achieving approximately 80% of adult height by 8 years of age. Thereafter the lobule may continue to grow.

II. Signs and symptoms—visible lesion or abnormality of the pinna, EAC, TM
III. Clinical assessment—careful inspection of the pinna, otoscopic examination, and otomicroscopy
IV. Pathology/treatment/complications

A. Congenital
1. Preauricular pit
   a. Probably related to failure of fusion of the first and second hillocks.
   b. Pits below the tragus generally represent remnants of the first branchial cleft.
   c. Not considered a risk factor for hearing loss.
   d. Acutely infected lesions should be managed with antibiotics; abscesses require drainage.
   e. Excision is recommended for lesions that have been infected. Ideally the procedure is performed after the acute inflammation has resolved.
2. Preauricular tag
   a. Remnant of one of the hillocks.
   b. Probably not a risk factor for hearing loss.
   c. Associated with multiple craniofacial syndromes.
   d. May be removed electively.
   e. Facial tags may be associated with the facial nerve.
3. Microtia
   a. Clinical features
      (1) Approximately 1 per 7000
      (2) Unilateral : bilateral = 3 : 1
      (3) Males more commonly affected.
      (4) Right ear more commonly affected.
      (5) Classification schemes based upon degree of abnormality.

        (6)   Associations
- (a) Frequently associated with hemifacial microsomia
- (b) Aural atresia and maximal conductive hearing loss (see below)
- (c) Bilateral microtia suggestive of craniofacial syndrome (Treacher Collins, Nager's syndromes)
- (d) Facial nerve palsy

        (7)   Absence of lobule is unusual and is associated with retinoic embryopathy.

b. Assessment
- (1) Clinical examination to rule out syndromic diagnosis
- (2) See below (atresia)

c. Management
- (1) Reconstruction is generally initiated when the child is at least 5 to 6 years of age.
- (2) Reconstructive surgery should be performed prior to any attempt at atresia repair.
- (3) Surgical reconstruction
  - (a) Autogenous rib graft
    - i. Stage 1: harvest rib graft and place framework at microtic site.
    - ii. Stage 2: lobule transposition.
    - iii. Stage 3: skin graft to create postauricular sulcus.
  - (b) Advantages
    - i. Requires no special care once the reconstruction has been completed.
  - (c) Risks and disadvantages
    - i. Bleeding
    - ii. Infection
    - iii. Loss of skin
    - iv. Loss of the cartilage
    - v. Pneumothorax (if autogenous rib used)
    - vi. Unsatisfactory cosmetic result
  - (d) Other implant materials
    - i. Medpore
    - ii. Irradiated rib
- (4) Prosthetic management
  - (a) Osseointegrated implant
    - i. Requires removal of the vestigial pinna and placement of skin graft to create immobile recipient bed.
    - ii. Prosthetic ear is created and anchored upon the implants.
  - (b) Tissue adhesives—a prosthetic ear is placed over the remnant.
  - (c) Advantages
    - i. Prosthetic ear may be more normal in configuration.
    - ii. Does not require extensive surgery.
  - (d) Risks/disadvantages
    - i. Infection at the osseointegration sites.

          ii.   Potential for the ear to become dislodged.

          iii. The ear must be removed at night and reapplied in the morning.

4. Aural atresia

    a.   Clinical spectrum

       (1) Stenosis—high risk of canal cholesteatoma[35]

       (2) Medial atresia

       (3) EAC atresia

    b.   Assessment

       (1) Ear-specific audiologic assessment is critical at the earliest possible time.

       (2) Audiologic monitoring.

       (3) Monitor speech and language development.

       (4) High-resolution CT scan of the temporal bones to assess status of middle and inner ear.

    c.   Management[36,37]

       (1) Treat occult ear infections.

       (2) Carefully monitor patent ear.

       (3) Amplification and early intervention if appropriate.

       (4) Patients with bilateral microtia should be fitted with bone-conduction hearing aid as soon as possible (as long as there is normal cochlear reserve).

       (5) Atresia repair

          (a) Likelihood of achieving significant improvement in hearing can be assessed by careful evaluation of the CT scan using Jahrsdorfer's criteria[38]:

             i.   Stapes (2 points)

             ii.   Patent oval window (1)

             iii. Patent round window (1)

             iv. Aerated middle ear space (1)

             v.   Position of facial nerve (1)

             vi. Lateral ossicular complex (1)

             vii. Incudostapedial connection (1)

            viii. Mastoid pneumatization (1)

             ix. Appearance of external ear (1)

          (b) Atresia repair should be done only after reconstruction of the microtia.

          (c) Role of surgery in patients with normal hearing in the contralateral ear is somewhat controversial.

          (d) Main risks of surgery include facial nerve palsy, hearing loss, and canal stenosis.

5. Prominent ear deformity

    a.   Usually associated with absence of the superior crus of the triangular fossa or the antihelix.

    b.   Otoplasty is generally very successful at creating normal appearance of the ear.

　　　　B.　Traumatic
　　　　　　1.　Auricular hematoma
　　　　　　　　a.　Often associated with wrestling.
　　　　　　　　b.　Requires incision and drainage to minimize risk of auricular deformity.
　　　　　　　　c.　Occurrence in nonambulatory infant should raise the possibility of non-accidental trauma (child abuse).

Ear/Middle

　　I.　Developmental anatomy
　　　　A.　Prenatal development[1,39]
　　　　　　1.　The distal aspect of the tubotympanic recess of the first pharyngeal pouch becomes the tympanic cavity.
　　　　　　2.　The proximal portion of the tubotympanic recess becomes the auditory tube, and later the eustachian tube.
　　　　　　3.　Mastoid air cells form as a result of expansion of the tympanic cavity in late fetal development.
　　　　　　4.　Stapes footplate and annular ligament arise from the otic capsule.
　　　　　　5.　Ossicles start to develop in the first 4 to 6 weeks of gestation.
　　　　　　6.　Ossicles are derived from
　　　　　　　　a.　Head of malleus, short process and body of incus from the cartilage of the first arch (mandibular).
　　　　　　　　b.　Manubrium of malleus, long process of incus, stapes suprastructure from the cartilage of the second arch (hyoid).
　　　　　　7.　Ossicles are of adult size and shape by 6 months gestation.
　　　　B.　Postnatal development
　　　　　　1.　The eustachian tube doubles in length between birth and adulthood.
　　　　　　2.　Mastoid tip is poorly developed at birth.
　　　　　　3.　The mastoid air cells grow significantly in the first 2 to 3 years of life.
　　　　　　4.　Stylomastoid foramen assumes a more medial position with development of the mastoid tip.
　　II.　Signs and symptoms
　　　　A.　Conductive hearing loss
　　　　B.　Middle ear dysfunction
　　　　C.　Otorrhea
　　　　D.　Otalgia
　　　　E.　Dysequilibrium
　　　　F.　Systemic symptoms common in young children
　III.　Clinical assessment
　　　　A.　Otoscopic examination, including pneumatic otoscopy
　　　　B.　Audiological tests, including tympanometry
　　　　C.　CT scan
　IV.　Pathology/treatment/complications
　　　　A.　Congenital
　　　　　　1.　Congenital cholesteatoma[40]
　　　　　　　　a.　Clinical features
　　　　　　　　　　(1)　Result of persistent epithelial rests in the middle ear space.

          (2)   Most commonly presents as "closed" keratotic cyst medial to the anterior superior tympanic membrane.

          (3)   Less commonly presents as an "open" infiltrative lesion which is more extensive.

          (4)   Diagnosis may be obscured by history of eustachian tube dysfunction.

          (5)   Average age of diagnosis between 2.5 and 5 years of age.

          (6)   Bilateral in 3% of patients with congenital cholesteatoma.

          (7)   F:M = 1:3.

    b.   Diagnosis

          (1)   Characteristic appearance of lesion with intact TM.

          (2)   Absence of significant middle ear disease.

          (3)   CT scan of temporal bones may be helpful in large or atypical lesions.

    c.   Management

          (1)   Surgical removal is mainstay of therapy.

          (2)   Small anterior lesions can usually be removed through a modified tympanomeatal flap.

          (3)   Larger lesions may require tympanomastoidectomy.

          (4)   Recurrence is higher for the infiltrative type.

  2.   Vascular anomalies of the petrous apex

    a.   High jugular bulb—may be visible through the TM.

    b.   Aberrant carotid artery—may be associated with pulsatile tinnitus.

  3.   Ossicular anomalies

    a.   Congenital footplate fixation—stable hearing loss present at birth. Bilateral in 75%.

          (1)   Syndromic—associated with craniofacial anomalies, osteogenesis imperfecta, X-linked progressive mixed hearing loss with perilymphatic gusher, branchiotorenal syndrome.

          (2)   Nonsyndromic

    b.   Juvenile otosclerosis—up to 15% of patients with otosclerosis have onset of symptoms before 20 years of age.

          (1)   Progressive hearing loss starting at about 10 years of age.

          (2)   90% are bilateral.

          (3)   Family history in half of patients.

B. Neoplastic lesions of the temporal bone

  1.   Benign

    a.   Glomus tumors—extremely rare in children; may be confused with eustachian tube dysfunction

    b.   Histiocytosis (see "Head and Neck," below)

    c.   Dermoid

    d.   Adenomatous tumor—originate from middle ear mucosa

  2.   Malignant

    a.   Rhabdomyosarcoma

    b.   Adenocarcinoma

    c.   Leukemia

    d.   Ewing's sarcoma

     e.   Chondrosarcoma

     f.   Fibrosarcoma

     g.   Endodermal sinus

C. Infectious (see Chapter 23)

  1. Acute otitis media (AOM)

     a.   AOM is the most common bacterial infection of childhood.

     b.   About 60% of children will have one ear infection by 1 year of age; 80% have had AOM by 3 years of age.

     c.   Most common organisms

       (1) *S. pneumoniae*

       (2) *H. influenzae*

       (3) *M. catarrhalis*

     d.   Incidence of beta-lactamase–producing organisms is about 20 to 30%.

     e.   Neonates are more likely to have gram-negative organisms causing AOM.

     f.   Risk factors for recurrent AOM

       (1) Smokers in the home

       (2) Day care with more than 6 children

       (3) Sibling with history of recurrent AOM

       (4) Onset of infection less than 6 months

       (5) Male gender

       (6) Not breast-fed

     g.   Indications for tympanocentesis

       (1) Febrile neonate with middle ear effusion.

       (2) Inadequate response to empiric antibiotic coverage.

       (3) Complications of otitis media; may also benefit from placement of tympanostomy tube for drainage of middle ear space.

       (4) Toxic child with AOM.

  2. Complications of otitis media

     a.   Intracranial

       (1) Meningitis—children with recurrent associated with AOM should be evaluated for possible cochlear malformation.

       (2) Sigmoid sinus thrombosis

       (3) Otitic hydrocephalus

       (4) Epidural abscess

       (5) Subdural abscess

       (6) Intracranial abscess

     b.   Extracranial

       (1) TM perforation

       (2) Cholesteatoma

       (3) Facial nerve palsy

       (4) Labryinthine fistula

       (5) Bezold's abscess

       (6) Zygomatic root abscess

  3. Treatment of otitis media

     a.   Immunizations

           (1)   While HiB vaccine has dramatically affected incidence of HiB meningitis, it has not affected incidence of AOM because the *H. influenzae* causing AOM is usually nontypable.

           (2)   Effect of streptococcal vaccine on AOM is not yet clear. Currently a heptavalent conjugate vaccine is recommended and seems to have a positive effect on incidence of AOM.[41]

    b.   Antibiotic therapy

    c.   Tympanostomy tube placement

    d.   Adenoidectomy

    e.   Tympanomastoidectomy

    f.   Tympanoplasty

    g.   Management of complications

D. Traumatic

  1.   Temporal bone fractures less common in children; fractures more likely to be oblique; less likely to be associated with facial palsy or sensorineural hearing loss.

  2.   Impalement of middle ear

    a.   Most traumatic perforations of the TM will heal spontaneously.

    b.   May be associated with perilymphatic fistula.

    c.   Children with vertigo or sensorineural hearing loss should have audiologic assessment; consideration should be given to middle ear exploration.

Ear/Inner

I. Developmental anatomy

  A. Prenatal development

    1.   Otic placode appears at about 4 weeks gestation.

    2.   Otic placode forms the otic pit, which forms the otic vesicle.

    3.   The otic vesicle is the precursor of the membranous labyrinth.

    4.   The endolymphatic duct and sac emanate from the otic vesicle.

    5.   The otic vesicle has two parts:

      (a)   Dorsal (utricular)—utricle, semicircular and endolymphatic ducts

      (b)   Ventral (saccular)—saccule and cochlear duct

    6.   Organ of Corti forms in the wall of the cochlear duct.

    7.   Otic capsule is formed from mesenchyme around the otic vesicle.

    8.   The perilymphatic space forms around the cochlear duct, contributing to the scala tympani and vestibuli.

    9.   Inner ear is mature in size and function at birth.

  B. Postnatal development—the endolymphatic sac and duct grow after birth.

II. Signs and symptoms

  A. Speech delay

  B. Behavioral problems

  C. Dysequilibrium

III. Clinical assessment

  A. History

    1.   Risk factors for congenital hearing loss

      a.   Birth weight under 1.5 kg

      b.   Family history of childhood hearing loss

      c.   In utero infection (cytomegalovirus, rubella, syphilis, herpes, *Toxoplasma*)

        d.   Craniofacial anomalies
        e.   Hyperbilirubinemia requiring exchange transfusion
        f.   Ototoxic exposures
        g.   Bacterial meningitis
        h.   Apgar scores 0 to 4 at 1 minute and 0 to 6 at 5 minutes
        i.   Mechanical ventilation for 5 days or more
        j.   Stigmata or other findings associated with a syndrome known to include hearing loss

B. Auditory function tests (see Chapter 2)
    1. Physiologic tests
        a.   Evoked otoacoustic emissions
        b.   Auditory brain stem responses
        c.   Tympanometry—tests middle ear status. Not useful in infants because of compliance of the external auditory canal.
    2. Behavioral tests
        a.   Visual reinforcement of audiometry responses in the sound field; used for children 6 to 24 months of age.
        b.   Conditioned play audiometry—ear-specific responses; used for children 24 to 48 months of age.
        c.   Conventional audiometry—ear-specific air- and bone-conduction thresholds.

C. Vestibular testing (see Chapter 4)
D. Radiographic imaging of temporal bones
    1. High-resolution CT scan remains the standard to define cochlear morphology
    2. MRI scan may be helpful in delineating status of the contents of the IAC, the endolymphatic sac, and the patency of the cochlear duct (ie, the soft tissue/fluid compartments of the temporal bone).

IV. Pathology/treatment/complications
  A. Congenital hearing loss (see Chapter 5)
    1. Genetic—several hundred genes have been associated with hearing loss.
        a.   Autosomal recessive
           (1) Connexin mutations GJB2—most common single cause of genetic nonsyndromic sensorineural hearing loss. 35delG accounts for approximately 80% of connexin mutations.
          (2) Usher's syndrome—most common autosomally inherited cause of syndromic deafness.
              (a) Type I—congenital bilateral profound hearing loss, absent vestibular function, retinitis pigmentosa with progressive visual loss. MYO7A.
              (b) Type 2—mild to severe congenital, bilateral hearing loss; may have progression of hearing loss; vestibular impairment variable; progressive visual impairment. USH2A.
          (3) Pendred's—PDS; second most common cause of autosomally inherited syndromic deafness.
              (a) Associated with euthyroid goiter.
              (b) Diagnostic test is perchlorate uptake test.

          (c)   Defect in iodine organification.

          (d)   Associated with enlarged vestibular aqueduct syndrome.

     (4)   Jervell and Lange-Nielsen—third most common type of autosomally inherited syndromic deafness.

          (a)   Prolonged QT interval. Associated with recurrent syncope or early death.

     (5)   Refsum's hearing loss and retinitis pigmentosa—defect in phytanic acid metabolism; diagnosed by measuring serum phytanic acid levels.

  b.   Autosomal dominant

     (1)   Branchiootorenal—EYA1

     (2)   Stickler—COL2A1, COL11A1, COL11A2

     (3)   Waardenburg's

          (a)   Type 1—lateral displacement of medial canthi (dystopia canthorum); pigmentary changes in hair, skin, and irides. PAX 3.

          (b)   Type 2—absence of dystopia canthorum. Sensorineural hearing loss and heterochromia irides are most common features.

     (4)   Neurofibromatosis II (NF2)

          (a)   Bilateral vestibular schwannomas

          (b)   Onset of hearing loss usually in the third decade

     (5)   Autosomal-dominant nonsyndromic hearing loss; multiple genes identified; may be progressive.

  c.   X-linked recessive

     (1)   Alport's—progressive sensorineural hearing loss, progressive glomerulonephritis, and variable ophthalmologic findings

     (2)   DFN1—nonsyndromic, progressive, postlingual hearing loss

  d.   Mitochondrial disorders—may predispose to susceptibility to ototoxicity

2. Infectious

  a.   Congenital—TORCH [toxoplasmosis, other (congenital syphilis and viruses), rubella, cytomegalovirus, herpes]

     (1)   Toxoplasmosis

     (2)   Other—syphilis—potentially treatable cause of SNHL

     (3)   Rubella

          (a)   Eye (cataracts, retinopathy, glaucoma)

          (b)   Cardiovascular (patent ductus arteriosus, pulmonary artery stenosis)

          (c)   Neurologic (developmental delay, meningoencephalitis)

          (d)   Sensorineural hearing loss

     (4)   Cytomegalovirus—most common infection causing congenital hearing loss. Congenital syndrome varies widely, with most infants asymptomatic. Infants with severe congenital infection (5%) may have

          (a)   Intrauterine growth retardation (IUGR)

          (b)   Jaundice

          (c)   Thrombocytopenia (purpura)

          (d)   Hepatosplenomegaly

           (e)   Microcephaly

           (f)   Intracerebral calcification

           (g)   Retinitis

           (h)   Hearing loss—varies in degree and may be progressive

        (5)   Herpes

  B. Acquired

      1. Ototoxic

          a.   Cisplatin

          b.   Carboplatin

          c.   Furosemide

          d.   Aminoglycoside

          e.   Noise

      2. Postnatal

          a.   Meningitis—any organism can cause hearing loss.

          b.   Mumps.

          c.   Traumatic—temporal bone fracture.

      3. Diagnosis (see Chapter 2)

      4. Management

          a.   Early identification is critical.

          b.   Universal newborn hearing screening programs are being implemented across the country.

          c.   Identification and enrollment in early intervention programs by 6 months of age associated with more favorable language and cognitive outcomes.

          d.   Amplification.

          e.   Family chooses language/communication system.

             (1)   American Sign Language

             (2)   Signed Exact English

             (3)   Auditory Verbal

             (4)   Cued Speech

             (5)   Pidgin Signed English

          f.   Cochlear implant (see Chapter 6).

HEAD AND NECK

Developmental Anatomy (See Chapter 10)

Signs and Symptoms

    I.   Signs and symptoms generally associated with mass effect.

   II.   Airway and feeding may be compromised.

Clinical Assessment

    I.   Complete head and neck examination, including cranial nerve examination.

   II.   Radiographic imaging studies are often helpful in defining extent of mass lesions.

Pathology/Treatment/Complications

    I.   Congenital

      A. Hemangioma

1. Clinical features
   a. Most common neoplasm of childhood.
   b. Mesodermal rests of vasoproliferative tissue.
   c. May occur anywhere on the body; head and neck is most common site of involvement.
   d. Occurs in 10 to 12% of Caucasians.
   e. More common in preterm infants.
   f. $F:M = 3:1$.
   g. Usually not familial.
   h. Lesion is generally small at birth, with proliferative phase starting several weeks after birth and continuing for about 1 year.
   i. Spontaneous involution usually starts at 6 to 9 months of age and takes several months, depending upon the size of the lesion.
   j. Deeper lesions may not be associated with any cutaneous changes.
2. Diagnosis
   a. History and physical examination should be adequate for diagnosis. Sequential examination is often helpful.
   b. Biopsy may be indicated in atypical lesions.
   c. Imaging studies may be necessary for deep lesions.
3. Treatment
   a. Most lesions may be followed clinically because of the high rate of spontaneous involution.
   b. Therapeutic intervention should be considered when there is airway compromise, interference with visual axis, resectable cosmetically deforming lesion, compromise of cartilage, systemic disease.
   c. Therapeutic modalities include
      (1) Systemic steroid therapy
      (2) Intralesional steroid therapy
      (3) Alpha-interferon therapy
      (4) Laser therapy—pulsed dye laser (CO_2 laser for airway lesions)
      (5) Surgical excision
   d. May require reconstructive surgery to address residual cutaneous changes.
B. Vascular malformations and tumors
   1. Clinical features
      a. Classification
         (1) Venous
         (2) Lymphatic
         (3) Lymphaticovenous malformation
         (4) Arteriovenous malformations—usually associated with palpable thrill, bruit, hypertrichosis, hyperthermia, hyperhidrosis
         (5) Kasabach-Merritt phenomenon—hemangioendothelioma and thrombocytopenic coagulopathy
      b. Lymphatic and venous lesions are typically present at birth and grow in proportion to the child. Fluctuation in size may be related to infection or hemorrhage.

       c.   Arterial lesions may present later in life; onset may be related to hormonal changes.

  2. Diagnosis

       a.   CT scan with contrast, MRI scan with contrast, and MRA may be helpful in making the distinction between the different malformations.

  3. Treatment

       a.   Venous and lymphatic malformations should generally be resected with care to preserve normal structures.

       b.   Arteriovenous malformation should be treated definitively with pre-operative embolization and surgery. Sequential embolization will not be effective in managing the lesion.

       c.   Recurrence and complications are generally associated with the location of the lesion.

       d.   Sclerosing agents and laser therapy may be used as adjuvant therapy.

C. Branchial remnants (see Chapter 10)

  1. Branchial cleft cyst—most common cystic lesion of the anterior triangle of the neck in children.

  2. Branchial cleft fistulas or sinus tracts—external pit may be located at any point along the anterior border of the sternocleidomastoid (SCM); internal communication defined by embryologic origin.

  3. First branchial cleft remnants:

       a.   Type 1—ectodermal origin; duplication of membranous EAC.

       b.   Type 2—contains ecto- and mesoderm; may consist of fistula from the EAC to the upper neck.

  4. Pharyngeal pouch remnants.

  5. Branchial arch remnants—cartilaginous rests along the length of the SCM.

D. Thyroglossal duct cyst

  1. Clinical features

       a.   Midline lesion anywhere between foramen caecum and thyroid gland.

       b.   Moves with protrusion of tongue.

       c.   May contain ectopic thyroid tissue.

       d.   May contain all of the functioning thyroid.

       e.   Superior aspect often has projections into base of tongue musculature.

       f.   Malignant changes rare but reported.

  2. Diagnosis

       a.   Should be distinguished from dermoid if possible.

       b.   Ultrasound of thyroid gland can confirm presence of thyroid gland in normal position in the neck.

       c.   Thyroid scans may also be used.

  3. Treatment

       a.   Surgical excision should include resection of midportion of hyoid (Sistrunk procedure) to minimize chance of recurrence.

E. Dermoid

  1. Clinical features

       a.   Presents as asymptomatic lesion in the midline of the neck.

       b.   Usually attached to the skin.

2. Diagnosis—gross appearance of the lesion is characteristic.
3. Treatment—simple surgical excision.

II. Neoplastic

  A. Rhabdomyosarcoma

    1. Clinical features

      a. Most common soft tissue malignancy of childhood.

      b. Arises from mesenchymal tissue.

      c. 40% present by 5 years of age.

      d. 70% present by 12 years of age.

      e. Most common sites of origin, in decreasing frequency:

        (1) Orbital—best prognosis, presents with rapid onset of proptosis in child less than 10 years of age.

        (2) Nasopharyngeal—presents with unilateral eustachian tube dysfunction, nasal obstruction, and rhinorrhea. Associated with late diagnosis.

        (3) Middle ear/mastoid—unilateral otorrhea with aural polyp.

        (4) Sinonasal—symptoms of sinonasal obstruction. Associated with late diagnosis.

    2. Diagnosis

      a. Diagnosis requires biopsy.

      b. Staging requires

        (1) Skeletal survey

        (2) Radionuclide bone scan

        (3) Bone marrow biopsy or aspirate

      c. Pathologic types:

        (1) Embryonal (including botyroid)—more common in young children.

        (2) Pleomorphic—usually seen in adults.

        (3) Alveolar and undifferentiated—poor prognosis.

        (4) Metastases occur through hematogenous and lymphatic routes.

    3. Treatment

      a. Determined by clinical stage of disease.

      b. Most patients benefit from adjuvant chemotherapy.

      c. Radiation therapy is appropriate for orbital and incompletely resected tumors.

      d. Resectable lesions should be excised to avoid long-term sequelae of craniofacial radiation.

      e. Parameningeal lesions more likely to have meningeal involvement and less likely to be amenable to complete resection.

    4. Outcome

      a. Dependent on site of lesion, clinical stage, and pathology.

      b. Two-year survival rates range from 85 to 40%.

  B. Lymphoma

    1. Hodgkin's lymphoma

      a. Clinical features

        (1) Malignancy of lymphoreticular system affecting adolescents and young adults.

        (2) Rarely occurs in children less than 5 years of age.

         (3)   F:M = 1:2.
         (4)   Arises in lymph nodes in 90% of cases.
         (5)   Extranodal involvement usually associated with progression of disease; spleen is most common extranodal site.
         (6)   Cervical and supraclavicular nodes are most common.
         (7)   Waldeyer's ring is rarely involved.

   b.   Diagnosis
         (1)   Lymph node biopsy; specimen should be sent fresh.
         (2)   Pathologic diagnosis based upon presence of Reed-Sternberg cells (multinucleated giant cells).
         (3)   Four subtypes:
             (a)   Lymphocyte-predominant
             (b)   Nodular sclerosis—most common type
             (c)   Mixed cellularity
             (d)   Lymphocyte-depleted—rarely seen in children
         (4)   Staging
             (a)   Chest x-ray or chest CT
             (b)   Abdominal CT scan; possibly staging laparotomy
             (c)   Skeletal survey or bone scan
             (d)   Bone marrow aspirate and biopsy
             (e)   Lumbar puncture

   c.   Treatment
         (1)   Dependent upon stage of disease at presentation.
         (2)   Role of surgery is in diagnosis and staging.
         (3)   Radiation therapy is used for early stages of disease.
         (4)   Radiation and chemotherapy are used for more advanced stages.

   d.   Outcome
         (1)   90% of patients have good initial response to therapy regardless of stage.
         (2)   Long-term survival ranges from 90% for early stages to 35% with advanced stages of disease.
         (3)   Significant risk for second malignancies.

 2.   Non-Hodgkin's lymphoma
   a.   Clinical features
         (1)   Occurs most commonly in 2- to 12-year-old range in the pediatric population.
         (2)   Males more commonly affected.
         (3)   Increased incidence in immunosuppressed children.
         (4)   Cervical and supraclavicular nodes are most common presenting site.
         (5)   Usually presents as asymptomatic adenopathy.
         (6)   May involve Waldeyer's ring.
         (7)   Children more commonly present with advanced disease.

   b.   Diagnosis
         (1)   Pathologic diagnosis required.
         (2)   Heterogenous pathologic appearance.
         (3)   Staging same as for Hodgkin's.

    c.   Treatment
      (1) Radiation alone for early disease.
      (2) Radiation and chemotherapy for advanced disease.
    d.   Outcome
      (1) Prognosis associated with stage at presentation.
      (2) Patients with CNS involvement do worse.

3.   Burkitt's lymphoma
    a.   Clinical features
      (1) A type of non-Hodgkin's lymphoma
      (2) Associated with Epstein-Barr virus (EBV) infection
      (3) Almost exclusively seen in children
      (4) Males more commonly affected
      (5) Potential for rapid proliferation
      (6) African disease:
        (a) Commonly affects maxilla; may affect mandible.
        (b) Usually present with loose dentition, facial distortion, proptosis, and trismus.
      (7) North American disease:
        (a) Present with abdominal mass.
        (b) Some 25% have involvement of the head and neck; asymptomatic adenopathy is most common presenting feature; nasopharyngeal and tonsillar involvement has been reported.
    b.   Diagnosis
      (1) Pathologic appearance—diffuse proliferation of uniform, undifferentiated cells with small nuclei. Classically described as a "starry sky pattern" because of interspersed large macrophages.
      (2) Staging—similar to non-Hodgkin's lymphoma.
    c.   Treatment
      (1) Chemotherapy.
      (2) Surgical debulking indicated for bowel obstruction.
    d.   Outcome
      (1) About 90% have complete response to therapy initially.
      (2) Overall 2-year survival about 50%.
      (3) Children presenting at less than 12 years of age have a more favorable prognosis.
      (4) North American patients with high anti-EBV antigen titers also have a more favorable prognosis.

C. Histiocytosis
  1. Clinical features
    a.   Consists of Langerhans' cells.
    b.   Clinical subtypes
      (1) Eosinophilic granuloma—monostotic lesion, most commonly involving the calvarium; 50% diagnosed by age 5 years; excellent prognosis.
      (2) Hand-Christian-Schüller disease—multifocal lesions presenting in early childhood; may have extraskeletal disease; commonly takes a more chronic course with resultant morbidity.

          (3) Letterer-Siwe disease—disseminated histiocytosis with multiple organ involvement; usually presents by 3 years of age; often has a rapidly progressive course.

     c. Some 20% present with otologic involvement.

     d. Males more commonly affected.

  2. Diagnosis

     a. Pathologic diagnosis—nonneoplastic proliferation of Langerhans' cells; Birbeck granules (organelles within the nuclear cytoplasm) define Langerhans' cells.

     b. Clinical workup should include complete physical examination, skeletal survey or bone scan, serum electrolytes, and urine specific gravity.

  3. Treatment

     a. Surgical debridement and curettage may adequately treat focal lesions.

     b. Adjuvant therapy may be required for systemic involvement.

     c. Radiation therapy may be useful for lesions that are not surgically accessible.

     d. Monitor urine specific gravity to rule out diabetes insipidus.

III. Infectious/inflammatory

  A. Cervical lymphadenitis—very common in childhood; most commonly reactive lymphadenopathy that does not require intervention. May represent other disease entities, such as:

    1. Cat scratch

     a. History of exposure to cats, usually kittens.

     b. Usually asymptomatic; may have systemic involvement.

     c. *Bartonella henselae* (gram-negative bacillus) is causative agent.

     d. Responsive to clarithromycin and azithromycin.

     e. Suppurative infection may require drainage.

    2. Atypical mycobacteria

     a. Associated with erythema of overlying skin.

     b. May suppurate and drain spontaneously.

     c. Most commonly caused by *Mycobacterium avium intracellulare* or *Mycobacterium scrofulaceum.*

     d. Identification can be made with polymerase chain reaction techniques.

     e. Diagnosis supported by identification of caseating granulomas. Confirmation requires identification of the organism.

     f. Curettage may be therapeutic.

    3. Kawasaki disease—mucocutaneous lymph node syndrome

     a. Clinical features

        (1) Multisystem vasculitis of unknown etiology.

        (2) Usually seen in children less than 5 years of age.

        (3) Most common cause of acquired heart disease in children.

        (4) Associated with coronary artery aneurysm.

     b. Diagnosis

        (1) Fever lasting at least 5 days and four or more of the following clinical features:

        (2) Nonexudative conjunctivitis

        (3) Fissured lips or strawberry tongue

        (4)   Polymorphous exanthem

        (5)   Palmar erythema, nonpitting edema of extremities, periungual desquamation

        (6)   Nonsuppurative cervical adenopathy of greater than 1.5 cm

    c. Treatment—to prevent coronary complications

        (1)   Aspirin

        (2)   Intravenous immunoglobulin therapy

IV. Traumatic

    A. Congenital torticollis/fibromatosis colli

      1. Clinical features

        a. Associated with breech position in utero.

        b. Associated with congenital hip dysplasia.

        c. Presents as asymptomatic neck mass within the first 6 weeks of life.

        d. Neck mass is located within the body of the SCM.

        e. May be associated with torticollis.

      2. Diagnosis—based upon clinical history and physical findings

      3. Treatment

        a. Physical therapy may be indicated for infants with torticollis.

        b. Observation is adequate in most cases, as spontaneous resolution is expected.

        c. More severe cases may require release.

    B. Arteriovenous fistulas

      1. Associated with trauma (as opposed to congenital arteriovenous malformation).

      2. May be treated angiographically if there is a single site of communication between the arterial and venous system.

      3. May require surgery.

SYNDROMES OF THE HEAD AND NECK

See Chapter 9.

OTHER/MISCELLANEOUS

Facial Nerve Palsy

I. Congenital

    A. Traumatic[42]

      1. Risk factors

        a. Primiparous mother

        b. High birth weight

        c. Prolonged labor

        d. Assisted (forceps or vacuum) vaginal delivery

        e. Signs of trauma, ecchymosis, fractures, laceration

      2. Diagnosis based upon history and physical examination. Sequential facial nerve conduction studies starting in the first 3 days of life may be helpful in distinguishing traumatic from developmental congenital facial palsy.

      3. About 90% recover spontaneously.

    B. Syndromic
        1. Congenital lower lip palsy[43]
            a. May be familial
            b. May be associated with congenital heart disease
            c. Unclear whether pathology is related to nerve palsy or absence of the muscle (depressor anguli oris).
        2. Möbius syndrome
            a. Bilateral multiple cranial nerve palsies
            b. Most commonly involves cranial nerves VI and VII
        3. Other syndromes with facial nerve palsy
            a. "CHARGE"
            b. Myotonic dystrophy
  II. Acquired
    A. Infectious
        1. Otomastoiditis
        2. Herpes zoster oticus
        3. Bell's palsy
            a. Prognosis in children is better than for adults.
            b. Treatment with steroids is controversial because of the excellent prognosis.
    B. Temporal bone pathology
  III. Management (see Chapter 8)

Salivary Gland Disease

  I. Salivary gland tumors in childhood
    A. Most common tumors of the parotid in children are hemangiomas.
    B. Solid tumors of the salivary glands are unusual.
        1. Pleomorphic adenoma is the most common.
        2. Mucoepidermoid and acinar cell carcinoma may present in childhood.
        3. High-grade malignancies have been reported; usually associated with nerve palsies and fixation to surrounding tissue.
  II. Lymphadenitis is a common cause of parotid mass.
  III. Sarcoid is a common cause of bilateral parotid enlargement in young black patients; Heerfordt disease is uveoparotid fever associated with sarcoid.
  IV. Submandibular glands commonly enlarged in patients with cystic fibrosis.
  V. Recurrent parotitis of childhood
        1. Related to sialectasia.
        2. Clinical course unpredictable.
        3. Often progresses to involve both sides.
        4. Treatment includes supportive care and antibiotics; avoid surgery.

Velopharyngeal Insufficiency (VPI)

  I. Clinical features
    A. Nasal air escape on consonant sounds.
    B. Hypernasality on vowel sounds.
    C. Associated with compensatory misarticulations.
    D. Sounds that do not require velopharyngeal closure: m, n, ng, w, r, l, h.
    E. 25 to 40% of patients with cleft palate will have VPI after closure of the cleft.

   II. Diagnosis
      A. Perceptual speech evaluation
      B. Nasendoscopy
      C. Multiplanar videofluoroscopic speech study
   III. Management
      A. Dental appliance
         1. Palatal lift
         2. Obturator
      B. Surgery
         1. Furlow palatoplasty
         2. Sphincter pharyngoplasty
         3. Posterior pharyngeal flap
      C. Speech therapy—indicated to treat sound-specific VPI and compensatory misarticulations associated with VPI.

References

1. Moore K. *The Developing Human: Clinically Oriented Embryology.* Philadelphia: Saunders, 1982, 479.
2. Beck JC, Sie KC. The growth and development of the nasal airway. *Facial Plast Surg* 1999; 7:257–262.
3. Hengerer AS, Strome M. Choanal atresia: a new embryologic theory and its influence on surgical management. *Laryngoscope* 1982; 92:913–921.
4. Brown OE, Pownell P, Manning SC. Choanal atresia: a new anatomic classification and clinical management applications. *Laryngoscope* 1996; 106:97–101.
5. Chinwuba C, Wallman J, Strand R. Nasal airway obstruction: CT assessment. *Radiology* 1986; 159:503–506.
6. Asher BF, McGill TJ, Kaplan L, et al. Airway complications in CHARGE association. *Arch Otolaryngol Head Neck Surg* 1990; 116:594–595.
7. Roger G, Morisseau-Durand MP, Van Den Abbeele T, et al. The CHARGE association: the role of tracheotomy. *Arch Otolaryngol Head Neck Surg* 1999; 125:33–38.
8. Brown OE, Myer CM III, Manning SC. Congenital nasal pyriform aperture stenosis. *Laryngoscope* 1989; 99:86–91.
9. Van Den Abbeele T, Triglia JM, Francois M, Narcy P. Congenital nasal pyriform aperture stenosis: diagnosis and management of 20 cases. *Ann Otol Rhinol Laryngol* 2001; 110:70–75.
10. Mazzara CA, Respler DS, Jahn AF. Neonatal respiratory distress: sequela of bilateral nasolacrimal duct obstruction. *Int J Pediatr Otorhinolaryngol* 1993; 25:209–216.
11. Lusk RP, Muntz HM. Nasal obstruction in the neonate secondary to nasolacrimal duct cysts. *Int J Pediatr Otorhinolaryngol* 1987; 13:315–322.
12. Hengerer AS, Yanofsky S. Congenital malformations of the nose and paranasal sinuses. In: Bluestone CD, Stool SE, Kenna MA, eds. *Pediatric Otolaryngology.* Vol 1. Philadelphia: Saunders, 1996, 831–842.
13. Miyahara H, Matsunaga T. Tornwaldt's disease. *Acta Otolaryngol Suppl* 1994; 517:36–39.
14. Kent SE, Reid AP, Nairn ER, Brain DJ. Neonatal septal deviations. *J R Soc Med* 1988; 81:132–135.
15. Emami AJ, Brodsky L, Pizzuto M. Neonatal septoplasty: case report and review of the literature. *Int J Pediatr Otorhinolaryngol* 1996; 35:271–275.
16. Healy GB. An approach to the nasal septum in children. *Laryngoscope* 1986; 96:1239–1242.
17. Bejar I, Farkas LG, Messner AH, Crysdale WS. Nasal growth after external septoplasty in children. *Arch Otolaryngol Head Neck Surg* 1996; 122:816–821.
18. Healy GB, McGill T, Strong MS. Surgical advances in the treatment of lesions of the pediatric airway: the role of the carbon dioxide laser. *Pediatrics* 1978; 61:380–383.
19. Canty PA, Berkowitz RG. Hematoma and abscess of the nasal septum in children. *Arch Otolaryngol Head Neck Surg* 1996; 122:1373–1376.

20. Alcaraz N, Lawson W. Trauma of the nose and nasoethmoid complex in children and adolescents. *Facial Plast Surg* 1999; 7:175–183, viii.

21. McRae D, Premachandra DJ, Gatland DJ. Button batteries in the ear, nose and cervical esophagus: a destructive foreign body. *J Otolaryngol* 1989; 18:317–319.

22. Gomes CC, Sakano E, Lucchezi MC, Porto PR. Button battery as a foreign body in the nasal cavities. Special aspects. *Rhinology* 1994; 32: 98–100.

23. Nathan CA, Seid AB. Neonatal rhinitis. *Int J Pediatr Otorhinolaryngol* 1997; 39:59–65.

24. Lusk RP, Stankiewicz JA. Pediatric rhinosinusitis. *Otolaryngol Head Neck Surg* 1997; 117:S53–S57.

25. Radkowski D, McGill TJ, Healy GB, Jones DT. Penetrating trauma of the oropharynx in children. *Laryngoscope* 1993; 103:991–994.

26. Hellmann JR, Shott SR, Gootee MJ. Impalement injuries of the palate in children: review of 131 cases. *Int J Pediatr Otorhinolaryngol* 1993; 26:157–163.

27. Isaacson G. The larynx, trachea, bronchi, lungs, and esophagus. In: Bluestone CD, Stool S, Kenna M, eds. *Pediatric Otolaryngology*. Vol 2. Philadelphia: Saunders, 1996, 1202–1211.

28. Daya H, Hosni A, Bejar-Solar I, et al. Pediatric vocal fold paralysis: a long-term retrospective study. *Arch Otolaryngol Head Neck Surg* 2000; 126:21–25.

29. de Jong AL, Kuppersmith RB, Sulek M, Friedman EM. Vocal cord paralysis in infants and children. *Otolaryngol Clin North Am* 2000; 33:131–149.

30. Choi SS, Tran LP, Zalzal GH. Airway abnormalities in patients with Arnold-Chiari malformation. *Otolaryngol Head Neck Surg* 1999; 121:720–724.

31. Benjamin B, Inglis A. Minor congenital laryngeal clefts: diagnosis and classification. *Ann Otol Rhinol Laryngol* 1989; 98:417–420.

32. Derkay CS. Recurrent respiratory papillomatosis. *Laryngoscope* 2001; 111:57–69.

33. Benjamin B. Prolonged intubation injuries of the larynx: endoscopic diagnosis, classification, and treatment. *Ann Otol Rhinol Laryngol Suppl* 1993; 160:1–15.

34. Cockrill BA, Hales CA. Allergic bronchopulmonary aspergillosis. *Annu Rev Med* 1999; 50:303–316.

35. Cole RR, Jahrsdoerfer RA. The risk of cholesteatoma in congenital aural stenosis. *Laryngoscope* 1990; 100:576–578.

36. Declau F, Cremers C, Van de Heyning P. Diagnosis and management strategies in congenital atresia of the external auditory canal. Study Group on Otological Malformations and Hearing Impairment. *Br J Audiol* 1999; 33: 313–327.

37. Chandrasekhar SS, De la Cruz A, Garrido E. Surgery of congenital aural atresia. *Am J Otol* 1995; 16:713–717.

38. Jahrsdoerfer RA, Yeakley JW, Aguilar EA, et al. Grading system for the selection of patients with congenital aural atresia. *Am J Otol* 1992; 13:6–12.

39. Kenna MA. The ear and related structures. In: Bluestone CD, Stool SE, Kenna MA, eds. *Pediatric Otolaryngology*. Vol 1. Philadelphia: Saunders, 1996, 113–126.

40. McGill TJ, Merchant S, Healy GB, Friedman EM. Congenital cholesteatoma of the middle ear in children: a clinical and histopathological report. *Laryngoscope* 1991; 101:606–613.

41. Eskola J, Kilpi T, Palmu A, et al. Efficacy of a pneumococcal conjugate vaccine against acute otitis media. *N Engl J Med* 2001; 344: 403–409.

42. Hughes CA, Harley EH, Milmoe G, et al. Birth trauma in the head and neck. *Arch Otolaryngol Head Neck Surg* 1999; 125:193–199.

43. Kobayashi T. Congenital unilateral lower lip palsy. *Acta Otolaryngol* 1979; 88:303–309.

Facial Plastic Surgery 34

Facial plastic surgery encompasses both cosmetic and reconstructive procedures in the head and neck; it overlaps significantly with the specialties of plastic surgery, head and neck reconstructive surgery, and dermatology. The clinical problems encountered in this subspecialty revolve around two broad themes: modification of the facial changes associated with aging and the resculpturing of undesirable facial features, either congenital or acquired.

FACIAL ANALYSIS

In order to communicate effectively about facial features, it is critical to have a fundamental understanding of normal and aesthetic facial proportions, and the terms used to define them. This guides discussions among surgeons in communicating techniques and facilitates communication with patients regarding contemplated interventions.

Facial width: Five equal parts, each the width of one eye. Nasal base width should equal intercanthal distance.

Facial length: Three equal parts. Hairline to glabella represents the *upper third*. Glabella to nasal tip represents the *middle third*. Nasal tip to menton represents the *lower third*.

Frankfort horizontal line: An imaginary line drawn from the upper aspect of the cartilaginous external auditory canal (roughly the top of the tragus) through the infraorbital rim. In performing facial photography, it is important to establish this line in the mind's eye when the lateral photographs are being taken and to position the patient's head so that this line runs parallel to the floor. This assures standardization of facial position.

Facial Landmarks (Figure 34-1)

Trichion: Hairline in the midsagittal plane

Glabella: Most prominent portion of forehead in the midsagittal plane

Nasion: Deepest point in the nasofrontal angle and the beginning of the nasal dorsum

Radix: Root, or "origin," of the nose. Uppermost segment of the nasal pyramid

Rhinion: Junction of the bony and cartilaginous nasal dorsum, where skin is thinnest

Nasal tip: Anterior most point of the nose

Nasal base: Area of nose defined by lateral crura of the lower lateral cartilages and their conjoined medial crura, forming the columella

Pogonion: Anterior most point on chin

Menton: Inferior most point of chin

Facial Angles

Nasofacial angle   Angle between the plane of the face and the nasal dorsum; normally 36 degrees

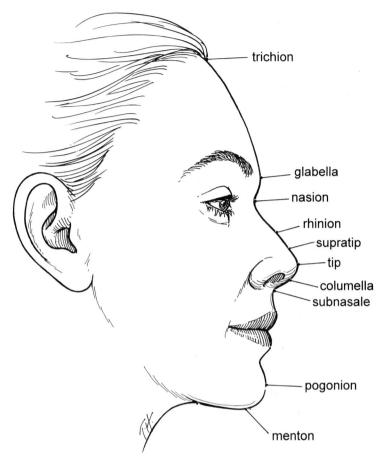

Figure 34-1. Facial anatomic landmarks. *(From Cheney ML, ed.* Facial Surgery, Plastic and Reconstructive. *Baltimore: Williams & Wilkins, 1997, with permission.)*

Nasolabial angle	Angle between upper lip and nasal tip; normal range is 90 to 95 degrees in men and 95 to 105 degrees in women

Other Terms and Relationships

Nasal projection	The degree to which the nasal tip extends from the plane of the face.
Nasal rotation	The plane of the nostril openings with respect to the plane of the face; underrotation implies a drooping tip, whereas overrotation gives a snout nose appearance.
Ears	A 2:1 length-to-width ratio, 20 degree projection from the mastoid.
Pogonion projection	Normally extends to a vertical line dropped from the nasion through the lower lip.

While variations in normal facial anatomy exist, these definitions facilitate identification of facial disproportions and potential modifications that patients may desire.

THE AGING FACE

With aging, predictable skin changes occur that result in skin laxity and variable degrees of wrinkling (rhytids). Collagen synthesis by fibrocytes in the dermis declines 3% per year in adult life, resulting in a thinning of the papillary dermis. There is also a reduction in elastic fibers in aging skin. The cumulative effects of sun exposure, referred to as *photoaging,* include dermal atrophy, a decrease in subdermal fat, loss of elastic fibers, and a homogenization of collagen fibers.

Precise examination of each zone of the face will assist in identifying individual problem areas, so that therapy can be tailored appropriately.

Issues in the upper third:

1. The sagging brow line, horizontal forehead rhytids
2. Prominent glabellar wrinkling, furrowing
3. "Crow's feet"; rhytids lateral to the eyes
4. Upper eyelid fat accumulation, laxity
5. Lower lid fat accumulation, laxity

Inspection of the upper third of the face during rest and with facial expression will identify which of these conditions exist and to what degree. The brow area, historically overlooked, is now recognized as critical to the final facial rejuvenation result.

Brow Lifting

Brow-lifting techniques can address the ptotic brow, the horizontal forehead rhytids, and to a limited degree the crow's feet lateral to the lateral canthi. Correct brow position lies at the supraorbital rim in males and just above the rim in females. The highest point of the brow should be vertically up from the lateral limbus and should be more prominent in females than in males. The medial and lateral aspects of the brows should sit at the same horizontal height. There are currently five commonly employed surgical techniques for correction of the sagging brow.

1. Coronal Forehead Lift

The coronal forehead lift is a common approach that offers excellent exposure and predictable results. It requires a coronal incision 4 to 6 cm behind the anterior hairline, parallel to it, through the galea. The incision is beveled to parallel the hair shafts so as to minimize hair loss. The anterior tissues are dissected in a subgaleal, supraperiosteal plane to the level of the supraorbital rims, with care not to damage the neurovascular bundles that emanate there. Laterally, the plane of dissection is immediately on the deep temporalis fascia, to protect the frontal branch of the facial nerve, which courses in the temporoparietal fascia. The frontalis, corrugator, and procerus musculature can be scored or partially excised to address glabellar rhytids and forehead rhytids as appropriate. The skin is then draped superoposteriorly, a 2- to 4-cm ribbon of skin and soft tissue is excised along the entire length of the incision, and the incision is closed.

Advantages: No visible scar (do not use in the alopecic male)
Unparalleled exposure
Ability to precisely address different muscle groups

Disadvantages: Most extensive procedure (highest average blood loss)
Elevates the hairline
Results in scalp hypesthesia

2. High Forehead Lift

The high forehead lift is performed similarly to the coronal forehead lift, but the incision is placed either just inferior to the hairline (pretrichial lift) in a forehead crease or 2 mm posterior to the hairline (trichophytic lift), tapering into the hairline laterally. The elevation plane is subgaleal, and any problematic musculature is addressed in the same way as in the coronal lift. The wound must be meticulously closed, since it has the potential to be visible at the hairline.

Advantages: Excellent exposure
Will not alter the height of the hairline, so a good choice for individuals with a high hairline, in whom increasing the vertical height of the forehead would not be appropriate
Disadvantages: Potentially visible scar
Scalp hypesthesia

3. Midforehead Lift

A midforehead lift is performed through an incision made along existing horizontal rhytids in the midforehead. The incision can course in one rhytid, or a Z-plasty into an adjacent rhytid at both lateral aspects can be employed for further camouflage and to prevent wound depression. The flap is elevated above the galea, then dropped into the subgaleal plane as the supraorbital rim is approached. This preserves sensation to the area while allowing access to the musculature for scoring and excision. It is appropriate in males with prominent forehead wrinkles, a receding hairline, or very thin hair.

Advantages: Less extensive procedure
Does not alter hairline, or may lower it if desired
Allows precise brow elevation
Disadvantages: Visible scar
Difficult to achieve excellent lateral elevation

4. Direct Brow Lift

The procedure of direct brow lifting is now infrequently employed. It involves the excision of two separate wedges of skin and subcutaneous tissue, one above each eyebrow, with the inferior aspect of the incision running along the superior edge of the eyebrow. It does allow correction of severely asymmetric brows and has application in the very elderly, where the risk of more extensive procedures is not warranted. It is also appropriate in the patient with functional brow ptosis (restriction of the visual field) in whom cosmesis is not important.

Advantages: Short, simple procedure with minimal blood loss
Able to tightly control brow position and shape
Disadvantages: Visible scar
Unable to address lateral rhytids
Unable to manipulate underlying musculature

5. Endoscopic Brow Lifting

The most recent approach to brow lifting is through a minimally invasive approach which requires small scalp incisions and endoscopic guidance. The procedure is performed by placing four to six 1-cm incisions several centimeters behind the anterior hairline, oriented perpendicular to the hairline. Periosteal elevators are inserted through these incisions to perform dissection anteriorly to the supraorbital rims and laterally on the temporalis fascia. An endoscope is introduced through an adjacent incision to allow visualization and avoidance of the neurovascular bundles. Long, curved grasping instruments can be inserted, advanced to the glabellar region, and utilized to resect procerus and corrugator musculature. Four- or 6-mm screws are placed into the cranium at the incision sites and permanent sutures affixed from the screws to the anterior flap, from subdermis through periosteum, to suspend the brow in its new position. This procedure involves significantly less blood loss, given the absence of long scalp incisions.

Advantages: Least invasive, minimal blood loss
Able to address brow and muscle issues
Disadvantages: Occasional problem with permanent screws (infection, or persistently palpable)
May be unable to achieve same degree of pull as coronal lift

Complications of Brow Lifting
Hematoma
Infection
Asymmetry
Nerve injury (frontal branch of cranial nerve VII, supraorbital and supratrochlear nerves)
Alopecia
Recurrent brow ptosis

Upper Lid Blepharoplasty
Excess upper eyelid skin laxity (dermatochalasis) is a common consequence of aging and, in severe cases, can lead to visual field impairment. Variable degrees of fat protrusion in the central and medial fat compartments can also contribute to upper lid fullness. *Blepharochalasis* refers to a specific, uncommon condition involving recurrent episodes of marked eyelid edema, ultimately resulting in atrophic, thinned eyelid skin.

It is important not to overlook the contribution of brow ptosis versus upper lid laxity to the overall appearance of aging eyes. Often patients will not recognize the duality of the problem and will request a procedure that will not fully address their complaint.

Surgical Approach
The procedure begins with precise skin markings; the lower marking is made at the superior border of the tarsal plate, in the naturally formed skin crease. This should fall 7 to 10 mm from the lash line. At the midpupillary line, a caliper is used to mark a point 8 to 10 mm superior to this marked line and at the lateral canthus 5 mm superior to the line. An elliptoid marking is then completed to encompass these points, with care never to extend medially onto nasal skin, since this will result in hooding. Laterally, the marks can be gently curved upward, into the sulcus between the orbital rim and the eyelid. In men, the incision stops at the lateral canthus, since these patients do not employ postoperative cosmetics to camouflage the visible scar. The skin ellipse is excised, revealing the orbicularis oculi muscle. A strip of muscle is removed, and a strip of the underlying orbital septum is excised. Gentle pressure on the eye allows prolapse of the excess fat, which is sharply removed following bipolar cautery. The medial fat compartment must not be overlooked. With the patient in

the supine position, it is easy to underrecognize the presence of excess fat in this location and thus to underresect it.

Complications of Blepharoplasty

Orbital hematoma	Rare but potentially catastrophic. Key is prompt recognition, immediate decompression by opening the incision, evacuating clot, cantholysis if necessary, and ophthalmologic consultation. Hematoma causing optic nerve compression may result in permanent vision loss.
Poor scarring	Erythema, milial deposits. Milia may be uncapped or treated with needle-tip cautery.
Ptosis	Existing preoperative unilateral ptosis may be unmasked by the correction of upper lid laxity. Minimal ptosis (<2 mm) can be treated with transconjunctival resection of Müller's muscle. Larger degrees of ptosis are addressed best with levator resection or levator aponeurosis dehiscence repair.
Lagophthalmos	Usually resolves with time, but if persistent, requires full-thickness skin grafting for correction. This is the result of overzealous skin excision.

Lower Lid Blepharoplasty

Preoperative evaluation is critical when contemplating lower lid surgery. The lid distraction test should allow less than 10 mm of play in the lower lid tissues. Lower lid weakness must be identified to avoid postoperative ectropion. Fat herniation occurs above the infraorbital rim, whereas fluid retention occurs along and beneath it and would not be corrected by blepharoplasty.

There are several commonly employed approaches to lower lid blepharoplasty, each appropriate for specific clinical scenarios.

Skin–Muscle Flap

Indicated for fat pseudoherniation; this is the most common approach.

Performed through a subciliary incision 2 to 3 mm below lash line
Extends from 1 mm lateral to inferior punctum to 8 to 10 mm lateral to lateral canthus
Retention suture placed for retraction, skin-muscle flap raised to level of orbital rim
Fat removed
Skin–muscle flap redraped superotemporally, redundancy excised, with blade beveled caudally to excise 1 to 2 mm more muscle than skin to avoid bulging ridge of muscle at incision line
Single-layer closure

Skin Flap

Indicated in patients with excess skin laxity only.

Subciliary incision through skin only
Skin flap raised to level just below infraorbital rim
Flap redraped, excess skin trimmed, leaving 1 mm of redundancy to avoid postoperative ectropion
Single-layer closure

Transconjunctival Approach

Indicated when excess fat is the dominant issue, not skin excess.

> Retraction with Demarres retractor and a shoehorn lid plate with gentle pressure on the globe
> Transverse incision through the conjunctiva and lower lid retractors
> Fat compartments unroofed and debulked following cautery
> Closure with 6-0 fast-absorbing gut (optional)

The significant advantages of the transconjunctival approach are that there is no risk of postoperative ectropion, since the healing forces are pulling in a favorable direction, and that there is no postoperative facial scar.

Complications of Lower Lid Blepharoplasty

> Eyelid malposition
> Hematoma
> Epiphora
> Milia/inclusion cysts
> Extraocular muscle palsy

The Middle and Lower Face

Analysis of the aging face by zones allows for proper management of each segment. The lower two-thirds of the face is host to a series of age-related abnormalities, which can be categorized and addressed as needed.

Issues in the lower two-thirds:

1. Generalized skin laxity, rhytids
2. Prominent nasolabial creases
3. Jowling (fullness along mandible)
4. Submental sagging, fat accumulation

The middle and lower face can be rated according to the degree of severity of these issues. *Class I* patients have minimal laxity and are not good surgical candidates. *Class II* involves skin laxity alone, where *class III* implies a degree of submental jowling and excess fat. *Class IV* patients have anterior platysmal banding, and *class V* patients have either congenital or acquired micrognathia, which might benefit from adjunctive chin augmentation. The *class VI* patient has a low-lying hyoid bone. This is important to identify and point out in preoperative counseling, as rhytidectomy procedures will not correct the cervicomental contour in this group.

The aging middle and lower face is addressed through various facelifting techniques (also termed rhytidectomy, rhytidoplasty). Each has advantages and disadvantages, the highlights of which are outlined below.

1. Superficial Musculoaponeurotic System (SMAS) Plication Techniques

The most common approach to rhytidectomy involves plication of the SMAS layer. The standard procedure involves elevation of anterior (temporal and preauricular) and posterior (postauricular and cervical) skin flaps. The incision is marked from the temporal region into a preauricular crease, around the lobule, and onto the postauricular surface of the auricle. It is extended into the posterior hairline and turned upward at its most posterior aspect to avoid the appearance of a dog-ear upon redraping. The skin is elevated just deep to the hair follicles in the hair-bearing portions of the flap and more superficially just deep to the subdermal plexus in the remaining portions. The skin is elevated a distance of 2.5 to 6 cm and, in the neck, can be elevated near or to the midline. The SMAS is then plicated with permanent sutures to provide appropriate deep suspension, and the skin flaps are redraped and trimmed for the closure. Suction drainage is commonly employed.

2. Deep-Plane Facelift Techniques

Over the past 10 to 15 years, more aggressive facelifting techniques have been described to achieve repositioning of both facial skin and several key underlying structures. The concept that prominent nasolabial folds result from inferior displacement of the cheek fat pad and that malar bags represent ptotic orbicularis oculi musculature leads to the desire to reposition these structures for proper facial recontouring.

SMAS dissection techniques begin in the same way as the superficial facelift procedure, described above. Once the SMAS is exposed on its superficial surface, the SMAS itself is elevated fully off the parotidomasseteric fascia. A segment is then excised and redraped with tension, followed by skin redraping and closure. This allows more thorough platysmal repositioning when necessary.

Deep-plane rhytidectomy follows a similar course, but the deep plane lies directly on the anterior surface of the zygomaticus major and minor muscles. Because these muscles are innervated from their deep surfaces, the risk of facial nerve injury is minimized. This deeper plane allows thorough repositioning of the cheek fat pad and thus has a more dramatic effect on the nasolabial region.

Composite rhytidectomy, the most aggressive of the described techniques, is an extension of the deep-plane technique, where the plane is dropped deep to the orbicularis oculi muscle, so that the muscle itself is contained in the elevated flap, much like the platysma inferiorly. The flap is elevated in the subperiosteal plane, and the orbicularis oculi is thus suspended in a higher position, eliminating malar bagging.

Revision Rhytidectomy

Secondary facelifting is occasionally desired years after an initial procedure, when laxity reappears. The flap elevation is generally easier than in primary rhytidectomy, and flap survival is excellent even with tension, as it is, in fact, a delayed flap from the initial procedure. In order to reposition the skin appropriately, the flaps are rotated superiorly rather than pulled laterally, as in primary procedures.

Complications of Rhytidectomy

1. *Hematoma.* Occurs in 3 to 15% of cases, manifests with unilateral severe pain. If untreated, necrosis of overlying skin flaps and interstitial blood may cause permanent scarring or nodularity. Prompt evacuation is required.

2. *Skin necrosis.* Occurs when tension on skin flaps is excessive. Postauricular area is most common site. Skin slough manifests with dark eschar at wound edges. Most often, complete healing occurs with satisfactory result. Occasional poor scarring can be revised at later date. Reassurance is critical.

3. *Hair loss.* Alopecia may occur in the hair-bearing regions if the dissection jeopardizes the hair follicles in the subdermal plane. Loss of hair at the incision lines can be avoided by appropriate beveling of the incisions parallel to the shafts of the hairs, so that minimal loss of follicles occurs.

4. *Nerve injury.* The great auricular nerve and the branches of the facial nerve are both at risk. It is more common to injure the great auricular nerve, but much more serious to damage the facial nerve. The frontal, buccal, and mandibular branches of the facial nerve have each been cited as the most commonly injured branch in different sources, so the branch with the highest injury rate likely varies with individual technique.

5. *Other complications.* Infection, prolonged edema, hypertrophic scarring, and ear lobe deformities have also been described, though their incidence is low. These are treated with antibiotic therapy, facial massage, steroid injections, and minor revision procedures, respectively, as necessary.

Facial Skin Rejuvenation/Resurfacing

For skin texture problems, superficial lesions, and generalized shallow and medium-depth facial rhytids, nonsurgical resurfacing procedures are employed. They can also be used as adjunctive procedures when rhytidectomy is planned, though the timing must be such that multiple simultaneous insults to the dermis do not occur. There are both mechanical (dermabrasion) and chemical (chemexfoliation) approaches to injuring the epidermis and superficial (papillary) dermis, so that regenerative restructuring of this layer will yield tighter, younger-looking skin.

Skin Layers

Epidermis	Contains keratinocytes, melanocytes, Langerhans' cells, Merkel cells
Dermis	*Papillary dermis*—thin, loose collagen surrounding adnexal structures, abundant elastic fibers.
	Reticular dermis—thick, compact collagen. Damage to this layer results in permanent scar.
Superficial fascia	

Classification of Skin Types (Fitzpatrick Scale)

Class I:	very white +/− freckles, always burns
Class II:	white, usually burns
Class III:	white to olive, sometimes burns
Class IV:	brown, rarely burns
Class V:	dark brown, very rarely burns
Class VI:	black, never burns

Dermabrasion

Dermabrasion is a technique in which the epidermis is removed, the papillary dermis entered, and the reticular dermis left undamaged. The procedure is accomplished using either wire brushes, diamond fraises, or most recently the CO_2 laser. Facial tissues are ideal for resurfacing this way, since they are rich in sebaceous glands, which are the primordial follicles for the re-epithelialization process.

Patients with a history of herpes simplex virus (HSV) are treated with preoperative antiviral agents. All patients receive 0.5% tretinoin to accelerate healing. The classic procedure is performed by pretreatment of a patch of skin with a refrigerant spray, followed by dermabrasion with a hand-held device. Adjacent areas are treated until all desired areas have been addressed. Occlusive dressings or biosynthetic dressings that promote rapid re-epithelialization are then placed.

Laser dermabrasion for facial resurfacing has become increasingly popular. The method is simple, the depth consistency predictable, and good results can be achieved without extensive experience. The drawback is equipment expense and maintenance.

Indications:

Surgical scars
Acne scarring
Tattoo removal
Telangiectasias
Melasma
Wrinkles
Milia

Pigmentation changes can result from dermabrasion. Hyperpigmentation is treated with topical hydroquinone, though preoperative tretinoin usually prevents this complication.

Chemexfoliation (Chemical Peeling)

Chemical peeling involves the application of a caustic agent to the facial skin for a variable period, followed by removal. Depending upon the substance used and the length of application, different depths of skin removal are possible. Depth of peel is classified as superficial, medium, or deep, and each has a slightly different clinical application. Ideal candidates for chemical peels are fair-skinned Caucasian patients with Fitzpatrick type I to III nonoily skin.

Superficial Peels

Penetration level	Papillary dermis, partial epidermolysis
Effects	Rejuvenates skin, addresses very fine rhytids, treats pigment changes, actinic damage
Solutions	Glycolic acid
	Tretinoin
	Trichloroacetic acid (TCA) 10 to 25%
	Jessner's solution: 14 g resorcinol, 14 g salicylic acid, 14 mL lactic acid in 100 mL ethanol (breaks intracellular bridges between keratinocytes, allows other agents to penetrate more deeply)

These can be used with all Fitzpatrick skin types and may be performed serially, every 1 to 2 weeks, until the desired effect is achieved. Heals in 3 to 5 days.

Medium-Depth Peels

Penetration level	Superficial reticular dermis
Effects	Removes actinic keratoses, pigmentary changes, flattens depressed scars
Solutions	TCA 35 to 50%
	Full-strength unoccluded phenol (88%)

The depth of exfoliation can be controlled by the concentration of TCA; peel can be repeated every 6 to 12 months as needed. TCA is not systemically toxic and can be used in patients with medical problems. It has no significant bleaching effect so may be used in darker-skinned patients. Heals in 7 to 10 days.

Deep Peels

Penetration level	Mid-reticular dermis
Effects	Corrects most severe actinic damage, rhytids, acne scarring, pre-malignant skin lesions
Solutions	Baker's phenol (phenol USP 88%, 2 mL tap water, 3 drops croton oil, 8 drops soap solution)

With these peels, it is important to avoid the neck skin, as it lacks adnexal structures to promote re-epithelialization. Systemic toxicity is a risk (cardiac and renal). Not for use in Fitzpatrick IV to VI skin. Concentration of phenol is inversely proportional to depth of peel, because higher concentrations yield more protein coagulation (frosting), inhibiting further penetration of the agent.

Complications of Chemical Peeling

Pigmentary changes
Scarring
Infection
Prolonged erythema
Milia
Cardiac arrhythmias (phenol)

ESTHETIC NASAL SURGERY

Alteration of nasal appearance is a very well developed field. Critical to the outcome is a solid understanding of nasal anatomy and function, precise nasal analysis with respect to esthetic proportions, and patient preferences.

Additional anatomic terms and relationships (also see earlier discussion and Figure 34-1):

Supratip	Below rhinion, just cephalic to tip
Lobule	On basal view, triangular area anterior to nostrils, with apex at nasal tip
Columella	Soft tissue and medial crura separating nostrils
Alae	Lateral walls of the nostrils
Subnasale	Point of junction of columella with upper lip
Nasofrontal angle	Between nasal dorsum and forehead—ideally 120 degrees.
Nasal height	Should represent 47% of the height of the face from menton to radix.
On lateral view	Distance from vermilion border to subnasale should equal distance from subnasale to tip.
	Distance from alar crease to midpoint of nares should equal the distance from midpoint of nares to tip.
Skin of the nose	Most critical factor for final result. Thin skin is best; thick, sebaceous skin may yield poor result even when underlying structures are appropriately contoured.

Based on these terms and relationships and review of photographs and/or digital morphing programs with the patient, an operative plan is developed. There are both closed and open surgical approaches, dictated by planned intervention, surgeon preference, and clinical setting.

Closed Approach

Intercartilaginous incisions are made between upper and lower lateral cartilages, and the skin and soft tissue overlying the nasal dorsum are elevated. An Aufrecht retractor exposes the bony and cartilaginous dorsum for alterations. The nasal tip structures can also be modified in limited fashion. Increased exposure is provided, if necessary, by delivering the lower lateral cartilages through additional marginal incisions at their caudal borders.

Advantages:

Minimizes tip edema
No external incision
Short operative time

Disadvantages:

Limited tip modification possible.
Distortion of normal anatomy can lead to surgical error.

Open Approach

Open rhinoplasty techniques involve a transcolumellar incision, which allows complete exposure of the nasal tip structures as well as the cartilaginous and bony dorsum. The incision is usually shaped like a "gull wing," or an inverted V. The skin is elevated off the medial crura and connected to marginal incisions along the lateral crura. The entire tip and supratip skin–soft tissue envelope (SSTE) is elevated along with that of the nasal dorsum. This approach provides unparalleled exposure for both diagnostic and therapeutic purposes and is strongly advocated as the best teaching approach.

Advantages:

Excellent exposure
Ability to make precisely controlled surgical manipulations

Disadvantages:

Visible scar (rarely a patient complaint)
Prolonged tip edema
Longer operative time

Regardless of surgical approach, maneuvers to alter specific features of the nose are similar. Usually, when the closed approach is employed, the tip work is performed first and the dorsal work is performed to match it, whereas in the open approach, the nasal dorsum is contoured first, followed by the tip work.

Nasal Dorsal Hump

The cartilaginous dorsum is brought down to the appropriate height with a #15 blade. This entails removal of a segment of the septal cartilage, with or without a strip of the medial portion of the upper lateral cartilages. The bony dorsum is likewise reduced, using the Rubin osteotome and/or nasal rasps. Rasps with smaller teeth are serially used to create a smooth surface. The thickness of the overlying skin varies, being thickest at the nasofrontal angle and thinnest at the rhinion, so it is desirable to leave a subtle hump in the area of the rhinion to achieve a straight profile with the overlying soft tissue.

Tip Modifications

The key to modifying the nasal tip is to achieve the appropriate nasal tip shape and position without losing significant tip support. Major sources of tip support include the medial and lateral crura of the lower lateral cartilages, the medial crural attachments to the septal cartilage, and the attachment of the upper to the lower lateral cartilages. Minor contributions to tip support are offered by the ligament spanning the domes of the lower lateral cartilages, the cartilaginous septal dorsum, the sesamoid complex, the attachments of the alar cartilages to the overlying skin, and the nasal spine.

1. ALAR CARTILAGE SHAPING   The reduction of tip bulbosity is accomplished by excising a portion of the lateral crura of the lower lateral cartilages along their cephalic margins. The amount of cartilage removed depends upon the degree of desired tip width reduction. In some cases a complete strip of the lateral crus is removed to achieve the desired reduction. The reduced crura can then be approximated to one another in the midline to render more support and more refined tip definition.

2. TIP PROJECTION   Strategies to enhance tip projection include transdomal suturing, lateral crural steal, cartilage tip grafts (either infratip lobule or domal onlay), and the placement of a columellar strut. For the latter two maneuvers, septal cartilage is the most popular grafting material. Shield tip grafts are sculpted into the shape of a shield and secured to the medial crura using 6-0 clear nylon, so that the top of the graft creates new, projected tip definition. A columellar strut can be placed by first creating a pocket between the medial crura. A cartilaginous strut is fashioned, inserted into the pocket, and secured with chromic suture. The strut is trimmed to an appropriate length in order to provide adequate midline tip support and projection.

3. TIP ROTATION   The nasal tip can be thought of as a tripod, with the medial crura of the lower lateral cartilages constituting one limb and each lateral crus constituting the other two limbs. Tip rotation can be accomplished by lengthening or shortening whichever of these limbs will yield the desired rotation. For example, upward rotation of the nose can be accomplished by shortening the lateral crura and holding the length of the medial crura constant. The nose can be deprojected by shortening all three limbs equally, yielding no overall change in tip rotation.

4. COLUMELLAR SHOW   To decrease the amount of columellar show, the caudal border of the septum and/or the medial crura can be trimmed by several millimeters. In severe cases, a segment of the membranous septum may also be removed to decrease columellar show.

5. NARROWING AND STRAIGHTENING THE BONY PYRAMID   Osteotomies are utilized to narrow or straighten the bony pyramid. These are often required after removal of a dorsal hump leaves an open roof deformity. In the absence of an open roof, medial osteotomies are required in addition to lateral osteotomies. Medial osteotomies are initiated between the upper lateral cartilages and the nasal septum and continue through the nasal bones, curving slightly laterally. Lateral osteotomies are performed through intranasal incisions at the anterior attachments of the inferior turbinates. A soft tissue pocket is first created over the ascending process of the maxilla, followed by osteotomies using a Park osteotome. The bony segments are then medialized to the appropriate position, either with the osteotome or manually.

Special Problems in Nasal Reconstruction

The Saddle-Nose Deformity

Augmentation of the nasal dorsum is a difficult undertaking. Many augmentation materials have been utilized in this location, with variable success. The current "gold standard" is autologous bone or cartilage, with common donor sites including the outer table calvarium, iliac crest, rib, and conchal cartilage. The advantage of bone grafts over other materials is that direct bone-to-bone contact promotes fixation of the graft, resulting in an immobile graft and minimal resorption. Silicone implants and more recently Gore-tex implants have been utilized for the correction of saddle nose deformity, with good success in some hands.

The Extremely Large Nose

The extremely large nose can be a challenge to alter without causing nasofacial mismatch. The dorsum and tip can be reduced as described above, and the base can be narrowed through Weir excisions of the lateral nostrils. Care must be taken not to overresect, since external nasal valve collapse may result. It is most important, in this group, to be certain the patient has realistic expectations about what is surgically possible.

Revision Rhinoplasty

The previously operated nose presents unique challenges. Poor cosmetic results, resulting from over- or underresection or healing complications, must be corrected. Frequently, the poor rhinoplasty result is accompanied by functional problems, such as internal or external nasal valve collapse. The goal of revision surgery is to restore or provide adequate function and address the cosmetic problem simultaneously.

Internal nasal valve collapse is addressed by the placement of spreader grafts between the upper lateral cartilages and the cartilaginous septum. External valve collapse, usually caused by weakened or overresected lower lateral cartilages, is corrected by batten grafting to stiffen the lateral crura or by excising the concave segments, turning them 180 degrees and resecuring them in place, thus creating convexity that serves to open the external valve.

SURGERY FOR ALOPECIA

The surgical correction of male-pattern baldness has become more sophisticated over the past several decades. Two approaches to the problem include hair transplantation and the rotation of hair-bearing flaps into the areas of alopecia. Baldness can be classified according to several scales, the most popular of which is the Norwood classification scheme (Table 34-1). The specific areas to be addressed are outlined, and the operative plan is developed accordingly.

TABLE 34-1. NORWOOD CLASSIFICATION OF MALE-PATTERN BALDNESS

Classification	Description
Type I	Minimal or no recession of the hairline.
Type II	Areas of recession at the frontotemporal hairline.
Type III	Deep symmetrical recession at the temples, which are bare or only sparsely covered.
Type IV	Hair loss is primarily from the vertex; limited recession of the frontotemporal hairline.
Type V	Vertex hair loss region is separated from the frontotemporal region but is less distinct; the band of hair across the crown is narrow.
Type VI	Frontotemporal and vertex regions are joined together.
Type VII	Most severe form. A narrow band of hair remains, in a horseshoe shape.

Hair Transplantation

The technique of hair transplantation has undergone marked refinement in the last two decades. Traditional techniques involved harvesting 4- to 5-mm punches of occipital scalp skin and transferring them into the anterior alopecic areas. This resulted in a "corn row" appearance of the new hairline. This has been replaced with minigrafting, micrografting, and follicular unit grafting, in which harvested grafts are divided into half grafts; quarters (minigrafts), each containing 3 to 8 hairs; sixteenths (micrografts), each containing 1 to 3 hairs; or follicular units, each containing 1 to 3 hairs. A series of minigrafts and micrografts are placed in random fashion along the anterior hairline to create a natural, unoperated appearance. This technique, termed *feathering,* yields a far more natural appearance than older techniques. Mini- and micrografts are currently inserted through simple stab incisions rather than removing a circular core of recipient bed skin. This method, termed *incisional slit grafting,* enhances vascularity, thereby improving graft survival.

The actual technique involves three sessions; in the first, 40 to 70 micrografts are placed, along with 50 to 70 half grafts, leaving 2-mm tissue bridges in between. In the anterior region, micrografts are commonly implanted, whereas posteriorly, larger grafts are preferred. Four weeks later, a similar number of grafts are placed to increase hair density. The final session is executed 4 months later, when the grafts are fully established. Roughly the same number of grafts are used, depending upon graft yield from the first two sessions.

After grafting, the hair follicles uniformly lose their shafts. The follicles, if viable, begin to redevelop hair shafts after several weeks.

Scalp Reduction, Juri Flaps, Scalp Lifting

The treatment of choice in crown balding is scalp-reduction surgery, where the alopecic area is excised and closed with local flaps. Flap design follows one of four patterns; the midline sagittal ellipse, the Y pattern, the paramedian pattern, and the circumferential pattern. Closure is accomplished by extensive undermining. These techniques frequently require serial excisions to achieve the final result. Tissue expansion can be used to decrease the number of procedures required.

The Juri flap is a pedicled temporoparietal-occipital transposition flap based upon the superficial temporal vessels. It can be used bilaterally to cover frontal baldness, and modifications involving delaying the flap have resulted in covering large frontal areas of balding.

Scalp lifting is a newer technique, where extensive skin elevation below the nuchal line results in the ability to excise a large area of bald skin. Surgical refinements have decreased the complication rates of skin necrosis, making it another viable option.

OTOPLASTY

The correction of prominent ears is ordinarily performed prior to school age (4–6 years old). The specific deformity must be identified: generalized auricular prominence, lack of an antihelical fold, prominent lobule, or other abnormality, so that surgical therapy can be individualized.

Two basic corrective techniques exist. The *Mustardé technique* involves decreasing auricular prominence by creating an antihelical fold. This is done by excising an ellipse of skin in the region of the postauricular crease, elevating the skin off the back of the auricular cartilage, and passing several permanent sutures through the cartilage and anterior perichondrium, so that tying them creates a gentle buckling of the cartilage, mimicking an antihelix. The second method, termed *cartilage sculpting,* involves elevating the anterior skin off the region of the proposed antihelix and scoring, excising, or otherwise weakening the cartilage until it conforms to an appropriate geometry. It is then secured with stitches and the skin ellipse closed. With either method, care must be taken to preserve at least 15 mm of skin from the helical rim to the outer rim of the ellipse to avoid secondary distortion. The final auriculomastoid angle should be at least 30 degrees.

Complications
Infection

Hematoma

Suture extrusion

Postoperative asymmetry, poor cosmetic result

Infection and hematoma must be aggressively treated to avoid perichondritis or chondritis, which can lead to cauliflower ear deformity.

SURGERY TO ALTER THE BONY FACIAL SKELETON

Alteration of the bony facial skeleton to achieve a more esthetic facial contour is performed either by altering the existing bony structure or by changing the contour with the addition of autologous, allogeneic, or synthetic implants.

Properties of the ideal synthetic implant include the ability to withstand mechanical forces while maintaining shape, low tissue reactivity, nonallergenicity and noncarcinogenicity, resistance to breakdown, and the ability to be customized at the time of surgery. Useful autologous materials include dermis, fat, cartilage, and bone. Membranous (ie, calvarium) bone grafts revascularize twice as rapidly as endochondral (ie, iliac) bone grafts and thus maintain much higher viability rates.

Recently, allogeneic bone stock, cartilage, and dermis have become popular.

GENIOPLASTY

Chin augmentation can be performed alone or in conjunction with rhinoplasty. Inadequate chin projection is due either to microgenia (diminished chin eminence) or retrognathia, where the entire mandible is posteriorly displaced, resulting in poor occlusal relationships.

Augmentation Genioplasty

Implant materials for the chin include silicone, polyamide, and polyethylene materials, among others. They can be inserted via an intraoral or a submental approach. A pocket closely matched to the implant size is created either subperiosteally or supraperiosteally, and the implant is inserted. Some studies show more underlying bony resorption with subperiosteal implantation. Complications include implant malposition, displacement, infection, and bony resorption, even to the point of tooth root interference.

Sliding Genioplasty

Sliding genioplasty requires a horizontal osteotomy of the mandibular symphysis, advancement of the mobilized segment, and rigid lag-screw fixation in the new position. This technique can also be employed to set back an overly prominent chin. Narrowing of the segment to reduce a wide chin is also possible. The technique requires precise rigid fixation and is usually performed under general anesthesia. Complications include mental nerve injury, bleeding, malposition of the symphysis, poor bony union, and damage to tooth roots during osteotomy.

MALAR AUGMENTATION

Malar augmentation to provide stronger cheekbone appearance can be performed through an intraoral or subciliary approach. For the intraoral approach, a canine fossa incision is used and a precise pocket created. The implant is inserted subperiosteally and held by the confines of the pocket rather than with sutures. Care is taken to avoid the infraorbital nerve. In the subciliary approach, an incision is made 2 to 3 mm below the lash line and a skin flap elevated. When the infraorbital rim is reached, the plane is dropped subperiosteally and the pocket is created. The implant is inserted, and a tarsal stitch to the periosteum is placed to avoid ectropion. Complications include initial malalignment, movement of the implant, hematoma, nerve injury, and infection. Infection mandates removal and antibiotic therapy.

ORTHOGNATHIC SURGERY

Cephalometric analysis can assist in identifying inappropriate maxillomandibular relationships, and techniques exist for repositioning of either of these structures for the improvement of facial appearance and dental occlusion.

Mandibular Prognathism

Two available techniques for setback of the protruded mandible are the vertical-subcondylar osteotomy (either intraoral or external) and the sagittal split osteotomy. The vertical subcondylar osteotomy involves bilateral oblique osteotomies from the sigmoid notch to the angle of the mandible, posterior to the inferior alveolar nerve bundles. The proximal segments are reflected laterally, allowing the anterior mandible to slide posteriorly. The sagittal split approach involves a horizontal osteotomy through the medial cortex in the subcondylar region and a vertical osteotomy in the lateral cortex at the second molar. The osteotomies are connected along an oblique line, and a vertical segment of bone is then removed from the proximal bony segment to achieve the desired position of the anterior segment. This approach carries a higher risk to the inferior alveolar nerve bundle. With either approach, intermaxillary fixation (IMF) is necessary for 6 to 8 weeks.

Mandibular Retrognathism

Retrognathism can be addressed using sliding genioplasty or implant techniques described above. But if the occlusal relationship is poor, mandating significant mandibular dental advancement, a sagittal split osteotomy technique is employed, similar to that described for mandibular setback. However, the anterior segment is moved anteriorly into an appropriate position, and IMF or rigid fixation is used to secure the anterior segment in its new position.

Maxillary Retrusion, Dysplasia, and Transverse Deficiency

Inappropriate maxillary position or dimension is usually addressed by a Lefort I osteotomy. A gingivobuccal sulcus incision from one second molar to the other is performed, and the mucoperiosteum is elevated to the pyriform apertures. The osteotomy is performed and the maxilla downfractured for complete mobilization. The maxilla can then be moved to its appropriate position, placed into proper occlusion with the mandible, and fixed via IMF and/or miniplates. If vertical mandibular height is required, bone grafts can be inserted into the osteotomy site. If there is maxillary hypoplasia with transverse deficiency, this can be addressed by an additional midline osteotomy of the mobilized maxillary segment, with the insertion of a spreading bone graft.

Distraction osteogenesis, where external fixators are placed onto the bone segments following osteotomy and serially repositioned to promote new bone formation at the osteotomy sites, is another evolving option for orthognathic procedures. Devices that allow movement in two planes are under development to make this a more attractive option.

FACIAL SCAR REVISION

Scar revision aims to camouflage or improve the appearance of an existing scar. Knowledge of the relaxed skin tension lines (RSTLs) is critical in planning management of an unsightly scar. These lines generally fall perpendicular to the underlying facial musculature and parallel to facial rhytids (Figure 34-2). Scars that are not aligned along the RSTLs may require irregularization with techniques that change the orientation of the scar (ie, Z-plasty).

Wound healing proceeds with an inflammatory phase (5–7 days); followed by a proliferative phase (6 weeks), during which collagen formation occurs and wound strength becomes maximal; and finally a maturation phase (12–24 months), during which type III collagen is replaced by type I collagen and the scar ordinarily becomes softer, paler, and smaller. Therefore, scar revision is delayed until the maturation phase is well under way or complete (6–12 months).

Approaches to Scar Revision
Excision
This involves excision of the scar along RSTLs, normal facial creases, and the junctions between distinct facial esthetic units, with meticulous everted closure. Serial excision of larger scars may be performed in stages according to these principles.

Irregularization
The term *Z-plasty* refers to the elongation of a scar by the addition of two limbs, one at either end of the existing scar, similar to the length of the scar and at 60-degree angles to it. The skin flaps are then undermined, elevated, and transposed to change the scar's orientation. Using 30-degree angles will elongate the scar by 25%, 45-degree angles by 50%, and 60-degree angles by 75%. Angles less than 30 degrees may result in flap tip necrosis. Multiple Z-plasties can be employed along a single long scar, to break up the line.

W-plasty, also termed *zig-zag plasty,* refers to the technique of scar excision with a series of interdigitating triangles on either side of the scar. A running W-plasty can be used to treat a single elongated scar. It does not add significant additional length to the scar but does not favorably alter scar orientation.

Geometric broken-line closure (GBLC) involves outlining one side of the scar to be excised with an irregular composite of rectangular, triangular, and semicircular shapes and creating a complementary template for interdigitation on the other side. The scar is excised according to this complex pattern, and the new scar carries an irregularly irregular pattern that is less eye-catching.

Abrasion Techniques
Scalpel abrasion refers to superficial cross-hatching of the epidermal layer of a scar. The creation of these micro Z-plasties prevents some degree of wound contracture.

Mechanical or laser dermabrasion, described previously, creates controlled injury to the papillary dermis and allows re-epithelialization from adnexal structures in the reticular dermis. This can serve as a primary scar treatment modality or as a planned adjunct to scar

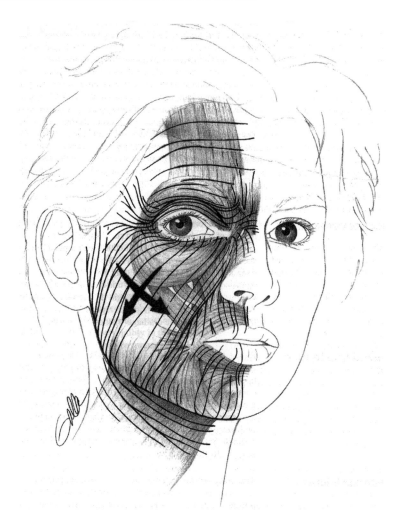

Figure 34-2.   Patterns of relaxed skin tension lines, perpendicular to facial musculature. *(From Cheney ML, ed.* Facial Surgery, Plastic and Reconstructive. *Baltimore: Williams & Wilkins, 1997, with permission.)*

revision. Crater-type wounds respond nicely, as the sharp borders can be beveled by dermabrasion, so that shadowing is less obvious and the lesion less conspicuous.

Following any scar revision, immobilization of the wound, protection from sun exposure, and massage to promote soft collagen formation all promote optimal final results.

ADJUNCTIVE AND MINOR THERAPIES

Collagen Injection

The injection of bovine collagen into facial tissues for the correction of facial skin depressions, prominent rhytids, and enhancement of the vermilion border has become increasingly popular. Preparations of 35 or 65 mg/mL are available for injection into the dermis. A test injection is mandatory, since 3% of the population develop an allergic reaction to the preparation. The treatment must be repeated on an ongoing basis, since the material is resorbed over a 6- to 12-month period.

Botulinum Toxin

Botulinum toxin has also become an extremely popular injection therapy for facial rhytids. The toxin acts to block the release of acetylcholine from the presynaptic membrane of nerve endings, resulting in temporary paralysis of affected muscle fibers. The effect lasts 3 to 9 months, so reinjection is required for the desired effect. Paralysis of glabellar musculature and other muscles of the forehead using botulinum can cause the disappearance of overlying rhytids. It is an extremely useful adjunct in the management of synkinesis and facial muscle imbalance following facial paralysis (see Chapter 8).

Bibliography

Cheney ML, ed. *Facial Surgery, Plastic and Reconstructive.* Baltimore, Williams & Wilkins, 1997.

Hamra S. *Composite Rhytidectomy.* St Louis: Quality Medical Publishing, 1993.

Johnson C, Toriumi D, eds. *Open Structure Rhinoplasty.* Philadelphia: Saunders, 1990.

Papel ID, Nachlas NE, eds. *Facial Plastic and Reconstructive Surgery.* St Louis: Mosby–Year Book, 1992.

Sheen JH, Sheen AP. *Aesthetic Rhinoplasty.* St. Louis: Mosby–Year Book, 1987.

Reconstructive Head and Neck Surgery

35

INTRODUCTION AND HISTORICAL PERSPECTIVE

Reconstructive surgery of the head and neck patient has experienced tremendous advancement over the last three decades, fueled largely by the increased application of microneurovascular free tissue transfer techniques to ablative and traumatic acquired and congenital defects. This era has been preceded by the fundamental contributions of many surgeons from the fields of plastic and reconstructive surgery, otolaryngology—head and neck surgery, neurosurgery, oral and maxillofacial surgery, and general surgery. The concepts of immediate reconstruction[1] and the contribution of the deltopectoral fasciocutaneous flap[2] were followed by the application of the newly defined myocutaneous flaps of the mid-1970s—in particular, the pectoralis major myocutaneous flap.[3]

Despite the report of the successful microvascular transfer of a jejunal interposition flap in 1959,[4] the modern era of clinical reconstructive microsurgery began in the early 1970s with increased refinement in instrumentation and technique, the description of new transfers, and the search for new applications of previously described flaps. This characterized the next decade with the reports of large series of the free jejunum interposition,[5] the radial forearm fasciocutaneous flap for oral reconstruction,[6] and, in particular, the fibula free flap for oro-mandibular reconstruction.[7] The recognition of the superiority of these techniques and the development of multidisciplinary teams and simultaneous interdependent operative procedures have resulted in aesthetic and functional restoration of the head and neck patient to a heretofore unprecedented level.

The availability of an increased armamentarium of reliable reconstructive options has given the head and neck surgeon increased confidence in the application of radical ablative or intensive therapeutic approaches to advanced and recurrent disease. It has also given surgeons increased responsibility in anticipating and planning the reconstructive requirements for a particular procedure and for choosing appropriate support teams to achieve the highest possible level of form and function in returning the patient toward his or her premorbid existence. General principles of defect analysis and of flap design, anatomy, and physiology apply across all techniques and must be emphasized.

The traditional concept of the *reconstructive ladder* begins defect analysis with a hierarchical approach to the suitability of techniques to a particular defect, emphasizing simplicity, ascending from simple to complex. It begins at the bottom rung with primary closure reconstruction, ascending from skin grafting to local flaps, through regional flaps, distant flaps, and on to the microneurovascular free tissue transfer of composite blocks of tissue at the top of the ladder. Surgeons must realize, however, that they are not obligated to push their patients though all or most of these steps and that many times the concept of the reconstructive *elevator*, advancing directly to microsurgical technique from the initial preoperative planning phase,

882

is most appropriate (eg, anterior oromandibular reconstruction after composite resection). Conversely, the surgeon must not be extravagant in the application of advanced technique and must always have multiple contingency plans in place in the event of flap failure or recurrence of disease. Defect considerations include volume, composition (soft tissue, bone), location (proximity to vital structures, need for external/internal surfaces), and general status (ie, previously operated, irradiated, infected, need for oronasocranial or oropharyngocervical separation, and the like). Functional considerations include the provision of sensibility, bone stock for skeletal framework and osseointegration, secretory mucosal surface, pliability, and so forth. Flap donor sites have been largely well defined and chosen for acceptability of residual functional or aesthetic deficit.

SKIN GRAFTS

Skin grafts have primary application in small defects of the oral cavity and ear, maxillectomy cheek flap, temporalis fascia flap, coverage of muscle or omental free flaps in scalp reconstruction, and coverage of the radial forearm and fibula free-flap donor sites. They allow the surgeon to overcome tethering and restriction of mobility, which can result from primary closure and critically affect orolingual function. Skin grafts generally heal well over fat, muscle, perichondrium, and fascia. They will heal over meninges or periosteum but afford neither adequate protection nor stable coverage in these contexts. Inasmuch as such grafts are completely dependent upon the recipient bed for survival via neovascularization, they are unsatisfactory for many previously operated, irradiated, or frankly infected sites, which are variably characterized by ischemic scar tissue, relative soft tissue hypovascularization, and inflammatory response. Such grafts are harvested with a dermatome in split-thickness (split-thickness skin graft, or STSG) fashion, usually from the lateral thigh or buttock. Thickness should vary according to need, from about 12 to 15/0.001 inch; thinner grafts exhibit easier take but also more contracture than thicker grafts. Meshing allows expansion of a sheet graft to larger dimensions and is generally restricted to scalp resurfacing contexts in the head and neck region.

Donor sites in smaller harvests are best managed with an occlusive semipermeable dressing left in place for about a week and larger donor sites covered by xeroform gauze until separation. Vacuum-assisted closure (VAC) devices have also been used. Topical anesthetic creams (EMLA) may ease donor site discomfort, which may well overshadow the larger cephalic procedure! Successful graft take is characterized by effective immobilization (to allow vascular ingrowth) utilizing a nonadherent antibiotic-impregnated bolster, intraoral prosthodontic device, and/or quilting sutures or staples. Additional requirements for success include meticulous hemostasis (avoidance of hematoma) and infection control (enzymatic dissolution), which includes timely removal of bolsters prior to significant bacterial colonization.

Full-thickness skin grafts (FTSGs) are appropriate to many small, externally visible facial defects. They are characterized by generally superior color match, contour, and texture; less contracture (secondary) potential; and poorer take than STSGs. Common donor sites include postauricular and upper eyelid (thin) and preauricular, nasolabial, and supraclavicular skin for thicker grafts. Templates should be slightly oversized due to primary contracture when FTSGs are harvested. Such grafts are usually taken with scalpel and subsequently thinned of subcutaneous fat (parasitic to new dermal blood supply) with scissors. Composite grafts of acellular dermal allograft plus the patient's STSG offers yet another approach to soft tissue resurfacing.

Local Skin Flaps

Local skin flaps are primarily applied in the reconstruction of external facial defects and are characterized by superior color match (in comparison to grafts), contour, texture, and ease of application/availability. Commonly used designs include advancement, rotation, bilobe, island transposition, and rhomboid transposition (Figure 35-1). In situ tubing of such flaps can be useful in recreating specialized structures (helical rim, alar rim, columella).

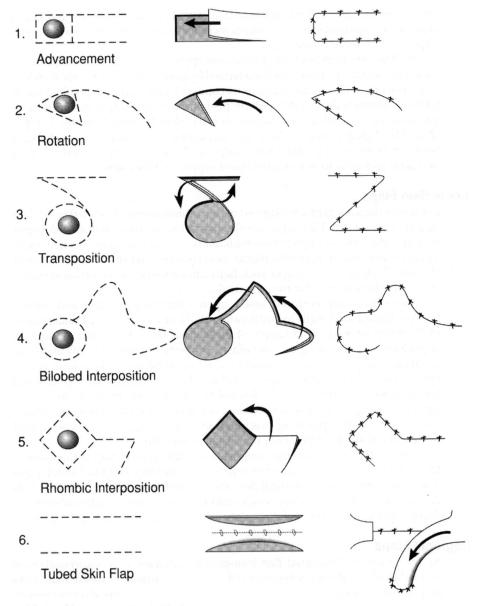

1. Advancement

2. Rotation

3. Transposition

4. Bilobed Interposition

5. Rhombic Interposition

6. Tubed Skin Flap

Figure 35-1. Six common local skin flaps.

These flaps are perfused based upon subdermal plexuses and generally observe traditional length-to-width ratios of 3:1 or less. Improved understanding of the microvascular blood supply of the face has refined our understanding and application of these designs.[8] Viscoelastic properties of skin and soft tissues such as creep, stretch, and stress relaxation are important concepts in local skin flap applications and will often require a balanced contribution from flap, donor site, and recipient site to achieve the desired result. Tension, infection, and cigarette smoking all impact upon wound healing in this type of flap and mandate attention to detail in operative planning, execution, and counseling. The reader is referred to two excellent atlases in planning the design of such flaps.[9,10]

One of the most common applications of this type of flap is the nasolabial flap.[11] Rhomboid flap designs can transfer hair-bearing scalp to frontotemporal defects and are also good general designs, inasmuch as six different rhomboid flap designs can be devised for any single defect. The Mustardé rotation-advancement flap for cheek and lower eyelid reconstruction also relies on these principles.

Regional Flaps

As the distance of required flap transposition increases, the incorporation of a defined axial blood supply becomes critical. This is further discussed in the section on myocutaneous flaps later in this chapter yet becomes a critical consideration in the paramedian forehead (supratrochlear), Abbé, Abbé-Estlander (superior labial), and facial artery myomucosal (FAMM) flaps.[12] The paramedian forehead flap remains a fundamental tool for major nasal reconstruction as refined by Burget and Menick[13] as well as for medial cheek reconstruction. Abbé designs transfer not only skin but also labial mucosa to compensate for soft tissue deficiency in lip reconstruction. The Washio postauricular flap and Mutter or epaulet flap are of historical interest and have largely been supplanted by free tissue transfer techniques.

The temporal fasciae (superficial or temporoparietal and deep) may be transferred as a bilobate flap pedicled on the superficial temporal system and may be thought of as a transferable bed for STSG placement in auricular reconstruction in both posttraumatic and complex congenital microtia reconstructions. The layers are highly vascular and pliable. This flap also has potential intraoral application (cheek, palate) independently and as part of temporalis muscle transfers and may be transposed either pre- or retrozygomatically. Accurate knowledge of facial nerve anatomy and of the nuances of the anatomy of this region is critical to confident surgery without complication. This anatomy has been described in detail by Stuzin.[14–15] The deltopectoral and forehead flaps are of historical importance.[16]

The recognition of defined territories of overlying skin, perfused by perpendicularly oriented myocutaneous perforating vessels, fueled many of the advancements in head and neck reconstructive work through the 1970s. This vascular orientation allowed circumferential suture around skin islands to be transferred with such flaps without compromising viability. Although the pectoralis major myocutaneous flap, described in 1978, was the most significant of this genre of flaps, the latissimus dorsi and trapezius flaps have also been explored in various head and neck applications. Myocutaneous flaps allowed the transfer of significant volumes of soft tissue (skin island, subcutaneous fat, and muscle) into major ablative head and neck defects. Such flaps demonstrated reliability and consequent versatility of application far in excess of their regional cutaneous and fasciocutaneous counterparts and allowed extension of the scope of ablative surgery and of functional reconstruction of the era. Sinocranial, orocervical, and pharyngocutaneous separation could now be reliably achieved.

Single-stage major reconstructions became the norm. Primary closure reduced donor site morbidity significantly, in contrast to previous fasciocutaneous designs. The application of these flaps as vehicles for the transfer of vascularized segments of bone (trapezius-scapular, pectoralis-rib, latissimus-rib, sternocleidomastoid-clavicle) was an important historical step toward the microvascular transfer of bone.

The concept of angiosomes[17] has challenged and extended the dogma that such flaps could reliably transfer only skin directly overlying the muscle component of a myocutaneous flap. The angiosome is a volume of tissue supplied by a single source artery and vein. Adjacent angiosomes are connected by a system of "choke" arteries (oscillating). Adjacent angiosomes may be captured in tissue transfer after interruption of the adjacent source artery through the reversal of physiologic blood flow. Once harvested tissue is extended *beyond* adjacent angiosomes (once removed), the incidence of necrosis is significantly increased.

Pectoralis Major

The pectoralis major myocutaneous flap remains the major myocutaneous–pedicled tissue transfer in head and neck reconstruction and continues to be a workhorse in selected applications. Its ease of development and application remains a fundamental part of the armamentarium of the contemporary head and neck surgeon. The flap is based upon the pectoral branch of the thoracoacromial artery off the second portion of the axillary artery. The architecture of the axial supply follows that generally observed throughout the body, namely that the axial pedicle enters the muscle from its undersurface, running in a fat plane up to its intramuscular course. While traditional incisional designs have avoided crossing the horizontally disposed deltopectoral flap and required flap dissection beneath a bridge of uninterrupted skin, the increased difficulty of flap dissection is obviated by a continuous serpiginous incision (burning an historical bridge) joining the vertical limb of a neck dissection incision. (It is highly unlikely that a deltopectoral fasciocutaneous flap would be called upon anymore to salvage a failed pectoralis major flap, thus invalidating this carryover of dogma from the early and unproven days of the pectoralis flap.) The contribution of the lateral thoracic artery to this flap is insignificant in the final analysis of most transfers.

Refinements in technique include developing the entire flap as an island design, allowing the transposition of a minimal amount of tissue over the clavicle and thus reducing external deformity. Section of the pectoral nerve branches to the muscle will ensure that the pedicle is not compressed against it when rotated into a defect and also that the flap muscle component will atrophy and contour to external defects more acceptably.

Transfer of the flap through the neck most easily follows radical lymphadenectomy procedures where the sternocleidomastoid muscle is sacrificed, the transposed pectoralis muscle affording reliable coverage to exposed critical neurovascular structures. The arc of rotation of the flap allows it to reliably reach the levels of the hard palate and superior helix. The flap may be applied to defects of nearly any configuration in structures inferior to these levels. Simultaneous harvest without patient repositioning is a significant advantage. The flap may be tubed upon itself to form an interposition conduit for pharyngoesophageal reconstruction in salvage situations.

A medially based generic curvilinear lunar skin paddle design facilitates primary closure of the donor site and minimizes the transfer of breast parenchyma and deformity in female patients. Preoperative marking should include the horizontal level of the contralateral nipple so as to minimize vertical deformity upon closure. Flap dissection is based upon the direct visualization of the pedicle, which is directed inferolaterally.

Disadvantages include the potential transfer of hair-bearing skin into the oral cavity and the sheer bulkiness of this flap. This will sometimes mandate the transfer of the flap as a muscle-only design, which can be used for the coverage of external defects in combination with other techniques and then skin grafted. Transposition of the flap, as with all pedicled designs, is limited by the arc of rotation of the flap pedicle over the clavicle. Such inferiorly pedicled flaps all exhibit an often relentless tendency toward dehiscence and/or fistulization the more superior the insetting requirement. In addition to the geometric contribution to this phenomenon, it is the fact that the most distal aspect of the skin paddle (and most poorly perfused and vulnerable) is necessarily inset into the superiormost and often most critical coverage requirement areas. Partial flap loss, dehiscence, stricture (through the requirement for secondary wound healing and ischemic scar contracture), fistulization, and the like are not uncommon phenomena despite the significant possibilities of myocutaneous flaps.

Latissimus Dorsi

This muscle is based upon the thoracodorsal pedicle from the versatile subscapular system of flaps. It is a broad, thin muscle that can be transposed into the head and neck region either subcutaneously or via a transaxillary approach.[18] Although its range of application as a pedicled flap and transferred soft tissue volume are similar to the pectoralis, decubitus positioning, decreased reliability, and a high incidence of donor site morbidity make this a tertiary choice to the pectoralis and free tissue transfer techniques.

The latissimus dorsi flap is a first-line choice, however, as a muscle flap for the reconstruction of massive scalp defects. As a free tissue transfer, it is characterized by a huge available surface area, thin, pliable consistency, a long, large caliber, and an anatomically consistent vascular pedicle, allowing ease of anastomosis in the neck. A meshed STSG completes the reconstruction.

Trapezius

Both vertically and transversely oriented skin paddle designs may be taken with this flap, which is based upon the occipital and descending cervical branches of the external carotid and transverse cervical vessels, respectively.[19] Applications of this flap and its variations were explored throughout the 1970s and 1980s. Although these were capable of reaching the midline neck, posteriorly situated defects were best suited to reconstruction with this method. Elegant anatomic studies have accurately documented variations in the vascular anatomy of these vessels.[20] Previous neck dissection status is an important consideration, inasmuch as the exact status of the transverse cervical vessels is often unmentioned in the operative notes of previously treated patients. Significant disadvantages are those of the pedicled latissimus transfer above, in addition to the occasional requirement for donor site skin grafting, making this flap a tertiary option.

Other Flaps

Myocutaneous flaps based on the platysma and sternocleidomastoid muscles have been described but offer little advantage in contemporary reconstruction. A more common potential application is that of the sternocleidomastoid muscle as a superiorly pedicled muscle flap to bolster oral and laryngopharyngeal suture lines. Rotation is limited by the spinal accessory nerve's entry into the anterior border of the muscle. In the context of staging supraomohyoid neck dissection or modified radical techniques, this is particularly facilitated. High-stage neck disease as well as extracapsular extension of metastatic disease would be contraindications to this application.

Similarly, the levator scapulae and posterior scalene muscles may be detached from their insertions as superiorly based muscle flaps for similar applications. Bipedicled and inferiorly unipedicled strap muscle flaps (eg, omohyoid) survive via microvascular supply transmitted through their origins and insertions and from neovascularization by surrounding tissues more centrally. These muscles are occasionally useful for reconstruction of partial laryngeal defects after conservation and extended conservation procedures.

FREE MICRONEUROVASCULAR TISSUE TRANSFER

Clinical microsurgery has provided the single most important contribution to reconstruction of the head and neck patient in the last two decades, restoring patients to a heretofore unprecedented degree of form and function. It is now possible to replace resected or missing tissues with nearly identical tissue types (eg, mucosa, bone, sensate skin, composites), volumes, and character. Many of the most significant drawbacks inherent to pedicled myocutaneous transfers can be more than adequately addressed through the thoughtful selection of microsurgical techniques.

The "free flap" is a composite block of tissue (fascia, muscle, fat, bone, skin, visceral conduit) perfused by a defined anatomic vascular pedicle and its subsequent myocutaneous or fasciocutaneous perforating vessels. It is geometrically "free" of limitations imposed by the requirements of an attached pedicle. In another sense, such transfers are "free" of limitations imposed by restricted tissue types that could be reasonably transferred to the head and neck region via available locoregional pedicles. Properly executed flap design and development will usually produce a reconstruction with a vascularity that is superior to its historical counterparts or alternatives. This, in addition to the advantages above, has decreased the incidence of dehiscence, fistulization, partial flap loss, stricture, and the like. Microsurgery has allowed ablative surgeons to extend their resective techniques in more radical directions in both curative- and palliative-intent procedures through providing unprecedented reliability and versatility of design. Despite numerous papers on multiple simultaneous free-flap reconstructions, such microsurgical tours de force rarely offer significant advantage over a well-planned single-flap design due to a very real increase in risk and morbidity.

The discipline of reconstructive microsurgery demands a degree of discipline and experience as well as applied technical expertise mandating significant additional training and commitment. It is the responsibility of the head and neck surgeon to foster the development of the simultaneous two-team approach.

As important as the actual microsurgical anastomosis is the preoperative planning, flap selection, flap development, and perioperative care of the microsurgical patient. Characteristics of the ideal donor site include

- Long, large-caliber, anatomically consistent vascular pedicle
- Minimal donor site morbidity—functional, aesthetic
- Simultaneous two-team approach
- Where applicable:
  Provision for functional motor capability
  Sensibility
  Secretory mucosa
  Bone stock capable of accepting osseointegrated implants

Patient Selection

The most significant application of microsurgical technique to reconstructive head and neck surgery is in post–tumor ablation. In general, most patients who are candidates for curative-intent resective procedures that will produce defects that would benefit from free-flap reconstruction are candidates for this technique. Numerous publications have documented the safety and efficacy of such procedures in the elderly. The general principle of "keep it simple" must prevail, however, over the desire to reconstruct a posterolateral composite mandible defect with a fibula in a edentulous septuagenarian diabetic with severe coronary artery disease, just for the sake of re-establishing bony continuity. Prohibitive or prognostic comorbid factors must be respected and considered in the planning phase. Age, chronic obstructive pulmonary disease (COPD), hypertensive vasculopathy and arteriosclerotic vascular disease, malnutrition, alcoholism, and active smoking all undoubtedly contribute to a potentially compromised outcome regardless of technique and are common denominators in the patient population with head and neck cancer. None of these factors, however, are absolutely prohibitive to the application of these techniques. Similarly, many of these entities will have systemic impact and donor site considerations in terms of donor vessels and wound healing, particularly the fibula donor site of the lower extremity.

Microsurgical techniques are also safe in the pediatric population but demand a very high level of expertise and capability. Applications to posttraumatic injuries are perhaps more straightforward and tend to occur in patients in their 20s and 30s who are otherwise healthy. Middle-aged patients present a similar physical health profile: postsuicide attempt mandibular and midface defects as well as unusual malignant ablative challenges are characteristic of this age group.

Previous treatment history is of critical importance in preoperative planning, with particular reference to recipient vessels. This is amplified if the patient has been treated "elsewhere," given the ambient lack of detail pertinent to microsurgical issues present in most operative notes. Vein grafts are usually avoidable through careful planning with regard to flap choice and contingency planning in such cases. Irradiation affects not only the microcirculation but also major vessels in terms of accelerating atherosclerotic degeneration, intimal and media thickening, and endothelial friability and dehiscence. Attention to technical detail is of the utmost importance in such cases, which provide a significant challenge to even the most experienced team. Previous surgery—either independent of radiation history or in addition to it—adds an additional degree of difficulty in terms of recipient vessel dissection, quality, and choice.

Points of Technique

Many aspects of resective surgery should be modified when a microsurgical transfer is anticipated. Routine sacrifice of the external jugular vein destroys a potential recipient vein or vein graft conduit and can usually be thoughtfully avoided. Major arterial and venous vessels that are to be transected should be handled with the utmost technical care and sacrificed somewhat away from their takeoff to allow a satisfactory stump for end-to-end anastomosis. This includes the internal jugular vein stump in radical dissections, where end-to-side techniques can be applied to a stump of satisfactory length in creating a functional end-to-end flow configuration.

Flap ischemia times are generally to be minimized but are rarely defining issues in flap survival. Most times are under 1 hour with the exception of osseous transfers, which require osteosynthesis in setting of skeletal components prior to revascularization. Enteric (jejunum), muscle, and osteocyte components of flaps are most sensitive to ischemia. Complete dissection of the flap in situ and microscopic positioning and recipient vessel preparation *prior* to pedicle transection maximize success and minimize overall ischemic time. Flap cooling with iced saline throughout the ischemic period significantly reduces the tissues' metabolic demand and extends available time (warm vs. cold ischemia time) prior to the onset of critical and irreversible changes.

Complications

In the most expert of hands, flap failure should occur in about 5% of cases or fewer, including the most complex of reconstructions. Free-flap loss is usually but not always an all-or-none phenomenon. Most failures will occur within the first 72 hours of revascularization. The majority of anastomotic failures should be successfully salvaged through timely recognition and revision.[21] A myriad of philosophies of perioperative management and monitoring techniques exist, but this is largely an individual, idiosyncratic, and theoretical art. It may be that specialized instrumentation for free-flap monitoring serves to improve survival only through increasing the vigilance of the nursing staff caring for the patient rather than because of some intrinsic superiority to clinical observation alone.[22]

Vessel wall dissection, disruption, and suture puncture result in endothelial discontinuity and exposure of thrombogenic subendothelial collagen. Platelet aggregation is enhanced through the production of the prostaglandin thromboxane-A_2 by activated platelets. Acute thrombosis is largely based upon this physiologic phenomenon, in addition to unfavorable mechanical factors (endothelial flaps, valves, adventitial inclusion, leaks, pleating, size mismatch, etc.) that may be present. This forms the basis for postoperative aspirin administration and for acute infusions of low-molecular-weight dextran-40 after revascularization. Bolus doses of 1000 to 3000 units of heparin are typically given just before pedicle transection and again just before flap reperfusion. Systemic heparinization does not occur and is not continued. Minidose heparin infusions are sometimes continued in cases requiring vein grafts or in revision cases. Restoration of endothelial continuity occurs over the ensuing 2 weeks.

Maintenance of perfusion through normal blood pressures is ensured by euvolemic status and by not attempting to overly modulate blood pressure in hypertensive patients. Similarly, the maintenance of normothermia will minimize peripheral vasoconstriction and sympathetic outflow, which are generally deleterious to microvascular blood flow. Attention to detail in flap design and insetting (pedicle geometry, tension, kinking) should minimize the need for special head positioning. Reverse Trendelenburg to about 15 to 30 degrees is preferred and relatively favorable with regard to general edema, intracranial pressure, and venous outflow; it is relatively unfavorable with regard to arterial inflow, cerebrospinal fluid (CSF) leak, and maintenance of slight neck extension.

The irreversible failure of reperfusion through a microvascular anastomosis is termed the "no-reflow phenomenon" and has as its basis ischemia and endothelial cell swelling, luminal occlusion, and the release of toxic free radicals with ongoing distal soft tissue damage and necrosis.

Subsequent sections will address commonly used flap transfers and issues of selection and design.

Radial Forearm Flap

This flap is a fasciocutaneous design with sensate capabilities based upon the *radial* vessels. It was one of the first flaps commonly applied to head and neck reconstruction (intraoral) and represents one of the most common transfers in contemporary reconstruction. Fasciocutaneous vessels are transmitted to the skin paddle via the lateral intermuscular (brachioradialis–flexor carpi radialis) septum. The flap may incorporate a monocortical segment of the radius bone (up to 10 cm) by including a cuff of flexor pollicis longus muscle. Sensate capabilities are provided by the *lateral and medial antebrachial cutaneous nerves.* The phenomenon of "sensory upgrading" has been observed in sensate reconstruction of the oral cavity, where the transferred forearm flap, anastomosed to the recipient lingual nerve, demonstrates greater fidelity in two-point discriminatory capability *after* transfer into the mouth than when *in situ* in the forearm *prior to* transfer.[23] This is believed to be due to a greater cortical representation devoted to orolingual structures subserved by the lingual nerve.

In addition to the capabilities above, the flap's most intrinsic advantage is its thin, pliable soft tissue component, which has made it outstanding for intraoral reconstruction. This has facilitated tongue mobility in particular and allowed reconstitution of contours, sulci, vestibules, and the like with relative ease. Inclusion of the palmaris longus tendon with the flap offers some theoretical advantage in suspending the flap laterally in palatal and total lower lip reconstruction.[24] The flap is also well suited to pharyngeal, laryngeal, and esophageal defects as a patched or tubed flap and to complex external defects such as cheek, forehead, and nose. Drawbacks to this flap center around its distal and outwardly obvious donor-site deformity, with mandatory skin grafting in most applications. In long-term follow-up, the impact is greatly diminished and well accepted by most. The bone stock provided by this transfer is usually inadequate and far inferior to alternatives where osseointegrated implantation is anticipated for oromandibular rehabilitation.[25] The combination of reconstruction plate plus fasciocutaneous flap, while apparently an attractive alternative to composite bone containing free flaps, is usually an inferior choice in anterior reconstruction. In application, it is often neither time- nor resource-conserving.

Lateral Arm Flap

This flap is a fasciocutaneous design with sensate capabilities based on the posterior branches of the *radial collateral* vessels. Fasciocutaneous perforators are transferred to the overlying skin through the lateral intermuscular (brachialis, brachioradialis-triceps) septum. It may incorporate the *posterior cutaneous nerve of the arm* for sensate capability and/or the *posterior cutaneous nerve of the forearm* for vascularized interpositional grafting. Transfer of a portion of the humerus and fascia-only designs have been described. The skin and subcutaneous tissues of this region of the arm are somewhat thicker and less pliable than their forearm counterparts. Pedicle caliber is similar to that of the radial forearm vessels. Flap geometry involving pedicle entry in the midportion of the cutaneous paddle complicates application to certain defects. Flap pedicle dissection is more difficult, and it is of shorter length than that of the radial forearm flap. This flap has advantages in that the donor site may be closed primarily with a single linear scar positioned in a location easily camouflaged by clothing, including short sleeves. This may be more appropriate to female and younger patients. In the male patient, this area of the arm may bear less hair than the forearm, making this flap a better choice for intraoral reconstructions in such patients.

Latissimus Dorsi

The latissimus dorsi is most commonly transferred as a muscle-only flap for the reconstruction of massive scalp defects. It is skin grafted with a meshed STSG for final resurfacing. The flap is based upon the *thoracodorsal* pedicle, which is part of the subscapular system of flaps.

The branch to the serratus anterior may be sacrificed, producing a very long pedicle of large caliber and facilitating anastomosis in the neck. The muscle is broad and thin, facilitating insetting over the calvarial contour. This flap does offer sensate capability, although motor reconstruction has been described. A lateral decubitus harvesting requirement usually mandates intraoperative position change and is a relative disadvantage.

Rectus Abdominis

This flap is based upon the deep inferior epigastric vascular pedicle and is generally transferred as a myocutaneous flap or as a muscle-only flap. It does not support sensate needs and is usually not applied as a functional motor reconstruction. The flap may be designed in a multitude of orientations but is usually oriented vertically or horizontally (TRAM, for transverse rectus abdominis muscle). This transfer has found particular application in the reconstruction of skull base defects, where the muscle component may be used to reliably seal off the subarachnoid space and the overlying soft tissue to pad and resurface massive scalp and forehead soft tissue and skeletal defects. The flap is capable of supporting a large volume of overlying soft tissue and finds additional application in massive combined head and neck defects.

Simultaneous flap harvest and resection are conducted with ease. Unilateral transfers may result in measurable abdominal wall weakness, which is well compensated by retained obliques, contralateral rectus, and muscle-sparing harvest techniques. This weakness is not noticed in the vast majority of individuals. Herniation potential should be minimal with attention to detail in closure and with muscle-sparing harvest.

Fibula

This transfer has revolutionized functional and aesthetic oromandibular reconstruction and rehabilitation since its application to the mandible. Subsequent refinements in technique have extended its application and usefulness. The flap is based upon the *peroneal* vessels of the tibial-peroneal trunk and the cutaneous component is perfused primarily by septocutaneous vessels transmitted via the posterior crural septum. Skin and muscle (flexor hallucis longus) may be reliably transferred with the bone and may be critical components in intraoral and external resurfacing (skin) and in submandibular contouring (flexor). These soft tissue components may be differentially inset, adding flexibility in the application of this flap.

The osseous component may be used to reconstruct the entire mandible. Its dimensions are aesthetically ideal for mandibular reconstruction and functionally ideal for osseointegrated implant placement. Simultaneous and independent maxillary reconstruction has also been accomplished with this flap.[26] More recent refinements of this transfer have included the *lateral sural cutaneous nerve,* adding sensate capability to the skin paddle.

Disadvantages of this flap are occasional difficulties in soft tissue wound healing, characteristic of the lower extremity, and the potential involvement of pedicle vessels with atherosclerotic vascular disease. Studies of postoperative function have demonstrated no significant long-term donor site morbidity and only short-term ankle stiffness.[27] An STSG is occasionally required to resurface the donor site in larger reconstructions.

The potential for osseointegrated implantation of dental prostheses represents a significant technical advancement over tissue-borne prosthodontics with the direct transfer of masticatory force to the underlying bone. It is important to realize, however, that this is an expensive and multistaged series of procedures, out of reach financially for most head and neck patients. In most series, fewer than one-quarter of patients complete this rehabilitative sequence.

Iliac Crest

This flap is based upon the *deep circumflex iliac system* (DCIA) and is capable of transferring large amounts of soft tissue and bone into massive defects. The composite flap may include skin, subcutaneous tissue, iliac crest, and the internal oblique muscle. Disadvantages have centered around the sheer volume of tissue and potential donor site morbidity. The capability of differential insetting of flap components is an attractive feature of this transfer.[28] Except for the most demanding situations, this flap has been relegated to a secondary role behind the fibula flap for most oromandibular defects. Simultaneous flap harvest and resection are conducted with ease. This flap does not support motored or sensate reconstructions.

Jejunum

Interposition reconstruction of segmental pharyngoesophageal or high cervical esophageal defects is well suited to this flap, which is based upon the accompanying *mesenteric* arcade vessels. The transverse cervical vessels are particularly good for recipient anastomosis if preserved in neck dissection procedures. A "sentinel loop" may be developed and brought out through the neck incision for monitoring of this otherwise buried flap.[29] The attractiveness of transferring a secretory mucosal surface to the oral and pharyngeal axis is real, particularly in the context of radiation. In such instances, the flap may be divided along its antimesenteric border and inset as a patch graft.

Potential disadvantages are those of laparotomy and enteric anastomosis. Endoscopic flap harvest may minimize donor site morbidity. A feeding jejunostomy is required. An advantage of this flap over the gastric transposition is the ability to superiorly inset the flap to *any* level defect, whereas the transposed, pedicled stomach often has difficulty reaching above the tongue base.[30,31] The superior vascularity of the transferred jejunum may reflect a lower dehiscence and fistulization rate than the relatively distal and ischemic stomach at this level of insetting. The jejunal transfer is limited by the level at which it is easy and safe to perform anastomosis to the remaining esophagus (thoracic inlet) without the need for thoracotomy and/or additional risk of intrathoracic anastomotic leak or fistula (inferior level *not* an issue for gastric transposition). Additional disadvantages include two circumferential enteric anastomoses in the neck (stomach—one anastomosis only), the propensity to anastomotic stricture requiring dilation therapy, and the lack of total esophagectomy recognizing the increased risk profile for synchronous and metachronous carcinomas, submucosal direct extension, and skip metastasis from more inferiorly positioned primaries. The mesenteric vessels must be respected for their friability and tendency toward rosetting and intimal separation.

MICROSURGICAL RECONSTRUCTION OF FACIAL PARALYSIS

Long-standing cases of facial paralysis are characterized by end-organ (mimetic musculature) atrophy and fibrosis. Similar loss of function follows radical ablative cases, in which these muscles of facial expression are resected. Dynamic rehabilitation of such patients may be achieved through free tissue transfer techniques, centering on the reconstruction of lower-third movements, more specifically smile. The sequence begins with the identification of contralateral buccal branches of the facial nerve and cross-face nerve grafting utilizing a reversed sural nerve graft. After clinical evidence of the arrival of fibers to the affected side (about 1 year), the microsurgical transfer of gracilis *(medial femoral circumflex—obturator),* serratus *(subscapular—long thoracic),* or pectoralis minor *(subclavian branches)* muscle may be performed with microvascular and microneural anastomosis. Muscle insetting is from zygoma to commissure, emphasizing smile reconstruction. Advantages of this dynamic functional reconstruction include volitional and symmetric emotive firing of the reconstructed hemiface. Disadvantages include the requirement for multistaged procedures and additional procedures for periocular and upper facial rehabilitation.

THE FUTURE

Prefabrication through tissue engineering promises to extend our current spectrum of flaps with the potential to customize flap tissue types and composition and is a logical outgrowth of microsurgical technique. Similarly, the potential for organ transplantation has been realized, with laboratory and clinical investigation in progress.

RECONSTRUCTION OF THE SCALP

The specialized hair-bearing tissues of the scalp are generally unyielding and require careful planning in reconstruction of midsized defects. Small defects may be closed with a variety of local rotation-advancement flap designs incorporating galeotomy and skin-grafted donor site defects that are small and easily camouflaged by neighboring hair. Large defects are similarly straightforward, with avulsion requiring microsurgical reattachment with a near mandatory vein graft requirement. Failure will produce a wig-dependent patient. Microsurgical technique has also aided this area of reconstruction in cases of scalp loss or ablation through skin-grafted latissimus dorsi transfer to reliably cover exposed calvarium with durable, easily contoured soft tissue. Midsized defects may be handled by skin grafting pericranium and later tissue expansion of adjacent scalp, with its attendant morbidity in terms of cranial deformity and discomfort while under expansion. The Orticochea three- and four-flap designs are of great use in these defects and have been applied to defects as large as 20 cm².

Aesthetic reconstruction of the frontal hairline is optimally performed with microsurgical transfer of a contralateral superficial temporal vessel–based Juri flap, providing a normodirectional hairstream.

ALLOPLASTIC IMPLANTATION AND THE MODULATION OF WOUND HEALING

The science of alloplastic implantology continues to evolve, and its application to aesthetic surgery should be sought in separate texts. Major reconstruction of the head and neck involves primarily implant systems for osteosynthesis and reconstruction of bony discontinuity as well as biomaterials aimed at decreasing donor-site morbidity (eg, bone extenders such as hydroxyapatite cement; soft tissue replacement and regeneration, acellular dermal allograft). Titanium is the basic rigid internal fixation material and is eminently biocompatible as a permanent implant. Absolute attention to detail in the proper application of these systems is essential and must resist an oft prevalent "hardware store mentality."[32] Autogenous bone grafts remain the material of choice for craniomaxillofacial reconstruction, and in these cases calvarial bone, rigidly fixated to adjacent skeletal components, has essentially replaced rib and iliac crest. A clear understanding of issues surrounding the surgery and healing of bone is essential to success.[33] Continuity defects of the mandible spanning 4 to 6 cm in relatively favorable recipient beds (eg, nonunion, comminution) may be grafted with tricortical grafts from the iliac crest. Longer defects or hostile recipient beds mandate revascularized free tissue transfer techniques if they are to be predictably reconstructed.

References

1. Edgerton MT. Replacement of lining to oral cavity following surgery. *Cancer.* 1951;4:110.

2. Bakamjian VY. Total reconstruction of pharynx with medially based deltopectoral skin flap. *NY State J Med.* 1968;1:2771.

3. Ariyan S. The pectoralis major myocutaneous flap. A versatile flap for reconstruction in the head and neck. *Plast Reconstr Surg.* 1979; 63:73.

4. Seidenberg B, Rosznak SS, Hurwittes, et al. Immediate reconstruction of the cervical esophagus by a revascularized isolated jejunal segment. *Ann Surg.* 1959;149:162.

5. Coleman JJ, Searles JM, Hester TR, et al. Ten years experience with free jejunal autograft. *Am J Surg.* 1987;154:394–398.

6. Soutar DS, McGregor IA. The radial forearm flap in intraoral reconstruction: The experience of 60 consecutive cases. *Plast Reconstr Surg.* 1986;78:1.

7. Hidalgo D. Fibula free flap: A new method of mandible reconstruction. *Plast Reconstr Surg.* 1989;84:71.

8. Whetzel TP. Arterial anatomy of the face: An analysis of vascular territories and perforating cutaneous vessels. *Plast Reconstr Surg.* 1992; 89:591–603.

9. Baker SR, Swanson NA. *Local Flaps in Facial Reconstruction.* St Louis: Mosby, 1995.

10. Jackson LT. *Local Flaps in Head and Neck Reconstruction.* St Louis: Mosby, 1985.

11. Shumrick KA. The anatomic basis for the design of forehead flaps in nasal reconstruction. *Arch Otolaryngol Head Neck Surg.* 1992;118:373–379.

12. Pribaz J. A new intraoral flap: Facial artery musculomucosal (FAMM) flap. *Plast Reconstr Surg.* 1992;90:421–429.

13. Burget GC, Menick FJ. *Aesthetic Reconstruction of the Nose.* St Louis: Mosby, 1994.

14. Stuzin JM. The anatomy and clinical applications of the buccal fat pad. *Plast Reconstr Surg.* 1990;85(1):29–37.

15. Stuzin JM. Anatomy of the frontal branch of the facial nerve: The significance of the temporal fat pad. *Plast Reconstr Surg.* 1989;83(2): 265–271.

16. Schuller DE, Mountain RE. Head and neck reconstructive surgery. In Lee KJ, ed. *Essential Otolaryngology,* 6th ed. Norwalk, CT: Appleton & Lange, 1995, 941–967.

17. Taylor G, Palmer J. The vascular territories (angiosomes) of the body: Experimental study and clinical applications. *Br J Plast Surg.* 1987; 40:113.

18. Sabatier RE, Bakamjian VY. Transaxillary latissimus dorsi flap reconstruction in head and neck cancer. *Am Surg.* 1985;50:427–434.

19. Urken ML, Naidu R, Lawson W, et al. The lower trapezius island musculocutaneous flap revisited. Report of 45 cases and a unifying concept of the vascular anatomy. *Arch Otolaryngol Head Neck Surg.* 1991;117:502.

20. Netterville JL, Wood D. The lower trapezius flap: Vascular anatomy and surgical technique. *Arch Otolaryngol Head Neck Surg.* 1991;117:73.

21. Hidalgo DA, Jones CS. The role of emergent exploration in free-tissue transfer: A review of 150 consecutive cases. *Plast Reconstr Surg.* 1990;86(3):492–498.

22. Jones NF. Discussion of monitoring of free flaps with surface-temperature recordings: Is it reliable? *Plast Reconstr Surg.* 1992;89(3):500–502.

23. Boyd B, Mulholland S, Gullane P, et al. Reinnervated lateral antebrachial cutaneous neurosome flaps in oral reconstruction: Are we making sense? *Plast Reconstr Surg.* 1994;93(7):1350–1362.

24. Sadove R, Luce E, McGrath P. Reconstruction of the lower lip and chin with the composite radial forearm-palmaris longus free flap. *Plast Reconstr Surg.* 1991;88:209.

25. Frodel JL, Funk GF, Capper DW, et al. Osseointegrated implants: A comparative study of bone thickness in four vascularized bone flaps. *Plast Reconstr Surg.* 1993;92(3):449–458.

26. Sadove R, Powell L. Simultaneous maxillary and mandibular reconstruction with one free osteocutaneous flap. *Plast Reconstr Surg.* 1993;92:141.

27. Anthony JP, Rawnsley JD, Benhaim P, et al. Donor leg morbidity and function after fibula free flap mandible reconstruction. *Plast Reconstr Surg.* 1995;96(1):146–152.

28. Urken ML, Vickery C, Weinberg H, et al. The internal oblique-iliac crest osseomyocutaneous free flap in oromandibular reconstruction: Report of 20 cases. *Arch Otolaryngol Head Neck Surg.* 1989;115:339.

29. Bradford CR, Esclamado RM, Caroll WR. Monitoring of revascularized jejunal auto-grafts. *Arch Otolaryngol Head Neck Surg.* 1992;18: 1042–1044.

30. Spiro RH. Gastric transposition for head and neck cancer: A critical update. *Am J Surg.* 1991; 162:348–352.

31. Inoue Y. A retrospective study of 66 esophageal reconstructions using microvascular anastomoses: Problems and our methods for atypical cases. *Plast Reconstr Surg.* 1994;94(2): 277–284.

32. DeLacure MD, Friedman CD. Metal plate and screw technology. *Otolaryngol Clin North Am.* 1994;27:983–1000.

33. DeLacure MD. The physiology of bone healing and bone grafts. *Otolaryngol Clin North Am.* 1994;27:859–874.

Anesthesia for Head and Neck Surgery 36

LOCAL ANESTHESIA

Local anesthesia is the blockade of sensation in a circumscribed area. Local anesthetic drugs have the common ability to block conduction of nerve impulses at the level of the axonal membrane when applied in sufficient concentration at a proposed site. All of the clinically useful agents belong to either the aminoester or aminoamide groups.[1] In addition, they have the following properties:

1. The nerve blockade is reversible.
2. There is a predictable time of onset and duration of blockade of the nerve fiber.
3. No local tissue irritation occurs when the drug is applied.
4. The drug is permeable and able to diffuse into tissue to attain its desired site of action.
5. The therapeutic index is high (ie, the ratio of therapeutic index to toxic effects is large), allowing for a greater margin of safety.
6. The drug is water soluble and clinically stable.

Mechanism of Action

Local anesthetics interfere with the functioning of the sodium channels, thereby decreasing the sodium current.[2–4] When a critical number of channels are blocked, propagation of a nerve impulse (action potential) is prevented, as in the refractory period following depolarization.

Chemistry

Local anesthetics consist of three parts: tertiary amine, intermediate bond, and an aromatic group. The intermediate bond can be of either of two types: ester (R-COO-R) or amide (R-NHCO-R); local anesthetics are therefore classified as aminoesters or aminoamides.[5]

In general there are three basic properties that will influence their activity[6]:

1. *Lipid solubility.* This will affect the potency and duration of effect.
2. *Degree of ionization.* According to the Henderson–Hasselbach equation, the local hydrogen ion concentration will determine where chemical equilibrium lies. The greater the pKa, the smaller the proportion of nonionized form at any pH. The ester pKa values are higher than the amide, accounting for their poor penetrance. The nonionized form is essential for passage through the lipoprotein diffusion barrier to the site of action. Therefore, decreasing the ionization by alkalinization will increase the initial concentration gradient of diffusible drug, thereby increasing the drug transfer across the membrane. Thus, the decreased pH found in infected tissues causes less nonionized drug to be present (or more ionized drug), and therefore a lesser concentration of drug at the site of action, resulting in a poor or nonexistent block.
3. *Protein binding.* A higher degree is seen with the longer-acting local anesthetics.

Uptake, Metabolism, and Excretion

Most local anesthetic agents diffuse away from the site of action in the mucous membranes and subcutaneous tissues and are rapidly absorbed into the bloodstream. Factors that affect this process are the physicochemical and vasoactive properties of the agent. The site of injection, dosage, presence of additives such as vasoconstrictors in the injected solution, factors related to the nerve block, and pathophysiologic features of the patient all enter into this equation.[7] Certain sites of particular interest to the otolaryngologist (eg, laryngeal and tracheal mucous membranes) are associated with such a rapid uptake of local anesthetics that the blood levels approach those achieved with an intravenous injection.

Amide local anesthetics are metabolized by the liver in a complex series of steps beginning with N-dealkylation. Ester drugs are hydrolyzed by cholinesterases in the liver and plasma. Both degradation processes depend on enzymes synthesized in the liver; therefore, both processes are compromised in a patient with parenchymal liver disease. Many of the end products of catabolism of both esters and amides are excreted to a large extent by the kidneys. Of note is that these by-products may retain some activity of the parent compound and may, therefore, contribute to toxicity.

Toxicity

Local Toxicity

Local toxicity is a reaction of tissue at the site of injection. It includes reactions of the skin and mesenchymal tissues (cellulitis, ulceration, abscess formation, and tissue slough) as well as lesions of the peripheral nerves (neuropathy). The most common causes of local tissue reactions include the following:

1. Faulty technique—contamination of the local anesthetic agents and traumatic administration.
2. Reactions from the local anesthetic agent itself.
3. Reactions from the preservatives added to the local anesthetic (methylparaben or metabisulfite).[8–10]
4. Reaction to the vasoconstrictor agents (epinephrine).

Systemic Toxicity

Systemic toxicity includes reactions that occur because of absorption of a given drug into the general circulation (Table 36-1). Reactions may be due to an excessively high blood level of local anesthetic, high blood levels of epinephrine added to the local anesthetic solution, allergy, or miscellaneous causes.

A toxic blood level can be achieved by rapid absorption, excessive dose, and/or inadequate metabolism and redistribution. Most often a toxic reaction is the result of administration of an excessive dose or inadvertent intravascular injection, as opposed to a true allergy.[10–13]

TABLE 36-1.   RATE OF TOPICAL ABSORPTION IN DECREASING ORDER

Tracheobronchial tree
Nose
Pharynx
Larynx
Esophagus

Significant symptoms of local anesthetic–induced toxicity are predominantly confined to the central nervous and cardiovascular systems (Tables 36-2 and 36-3). The CNS responses to local anesthetic toxicity begin with an excitatory phase, followed by depression. The extent of these symptoms is concentration-dependent.[14,15] Clinically, patients appear agitated, with feelings of lightheadedness or dizziness and disorientation, and confused and rambling speech. Shivering and twitching of the muscles of the face and distal extremities may progress to tonic-clonic seizures[16] and eventual coma, indicating the phase of CNS depression. This can then lead to respiratory depression and respiratory arrest.

Local anesthetics exert direct dose-related depressive effects on the cardiovascular system. Both myocardial contractility and peripheral vascular tone are diminished by increasing levels of local anesthetic agents. As local anesthetic potency increases, so does the ability to cause myocardial depression,[17] although this may not be the case for bupivacaine and etidocaine, which appear to be relatively more cardiotoxic.[18]

An important relationship exists for local anesthetics, the CC/CNS ratio. This is the ratio between the dosage necessary to cause cardiovascular collapse and that which causes central nervous system toxicity (eg, convulsions). The lower this ratio, the less time and dosage required to pass from initial CNS symptoms to irreversible cardiovascular collapse. For example, bupivacaine has a significantly lower CC/CNS ratio than lidocaine.[19]

As with most iatrogenic complications, the most effective treatment of local anesthetic toxicity is avoidance. This requires care in the choice of agent and its administration. For all but the most minor of procedures, an intravenous cannula should be secured prior to beginning, because this may become more difficult once attention must be turned to the management of toxic manifestations. Resuscitative equipment must be immediately available and fully functional, and skilled personnel must be present to assist.

When preliminary signs of toxicity appear, the ABC's of resuscitation are begun: Airway, Breathing, Circulation. These steps may range from placing supplemental oxygen on the patient and feeling for a pulse to intubation, mechanical ventilation, and pressor therapy.[20] Initial symptoms of excitement can be treated with benzodiazepines such as diazepam (Valium) or midazolam (Versed) or barbiturates, always remembering that they too can exacerbate respiratory depression. Should seizures ensue, symptomatic therapy should continue with the above-mentioned drugs and an adequate airway and ventilation must be assured.

Epinephrine is often added to local anesthetic mixtures to increase the duration of the nerve block, decrease systemic absorption of the local anesthetic, and decrease operative blood loss. In commercially prepared solutions of local anesthetics, epinephrine is usually

TABLE 36-2. LOCAL ANESTHETIC TOXIC SYMPTOMS

Central nervous system: *Excitation*
   Cerebral cortex → excitement, disorientation, rambling speech → seizures
   Brain stem → tachycardia, hypertension, vomiting, sweating
Central nervous system: *Depression*
   Cerebral cortex → coma
   Brain stem → bradycardia, hypotension, apnea
Cardiovascular system: *Depression*
   Bradycardia
   Hypotension
   Shock
Cardiorespiratory arrest
Death

TABLE 36-3. PREVENTION AND TREATMENT OF LOCAL ANESTHETIC TOXICITY

1. Prophylaxis
    a. Avoid overdose
    b. Diazepam (Valium) premedication
2. Maintain verbal contact with patient throughout surgery; must be alert to early signs and symptoms of excitation.
3. Have an IV in place before administration of local anesthetics.
4. When toxic symptoms appear, stop surgery, give oxygen.
5. Maintain airway and ventilation.
6. Avoid giving further depressants if possible. However, IV diazepam or pentothal may be required to terminate seizure.
7. Apply fluid or pressor resuscitation as required.

found in a 1 : 100,000 (1 mg/100 mL) or 1 : 200,000 (1 mg/200 mL) concentration. Epineph-rine toxicity can produce restlessness, nervousness, a sense of impending doom, headache, palpitations, respiratory distress, hypertension, and tachycardia. These symptoms may progress to ventricular irritability and seizures. Treatment of epinephrine toxicity is as out-lined above for local anesthetic toxicity. In addition, alpha- or beta-adrenergic blocking drugs (such as propranolol, labetalol, or esmolol) may be helpful.

True allergic reactions to local anesthetics are an infrequent occurrence (< 1% of adverse reactions)[11] and most commonly are attributed to the methylparaben or metabisulfite preser-vative found in the multidose or epinephrine-containing vials.[9] True allergy to local anes-thetics is observed most frequently among ester derivatives; it is extremely rare among the amide local anesthetics.[21] Allergic reactions may run the gamut from an innocuous rash to ana-phylactic shock. Strategies for treatment of allergic reactions to local anesthetic agents are the same as for any allergic reaction.

Choosing the anesthetic technique for a patient with a history of local anesthetic allergy is a not-infrequent clinical problem. A careful history with documentation, if possible, should help sort out those with toxic reactions from those with true allergy. If allergy is suspected, provocative intradermal testing has been advocated by some authorities.[10] However, others have pointed out the general unreliability of these results.[22] Alternatively, some authors sug-gest using the opposite class of local anesthetic from that suspected—for example, amide if ester was previously used (without preservative)—as a relatively safe approach. Dyclonine (piperidinopropriophenone), which is neither an ester nor an amide, may be safely tried in those extremely rare cases where allergy to both classes of drugs is suspected. If doubt still exists, one must consider alternative techniques, such as general anesthesia.

Miscellaneous reactions include those adverse reactions not specific to the local anes-thetic itself. These include neuromuscular blocking and ganglionic blocking properties and anticholinergic activity. However, they do not appear to be of clinical significance during routine use. A unique adverse reaction occurs with the local anesthetic prilocaine. When used in excess of approximately 600 mg in an adult, a significant fraction of the patient's hemoglobin is reduced to the methemoglobin state.[23] Methemoglobin has a diminished abil-ity to transport oxygen to the peripheral tissues. (*Note:* A pulse oximeter cannot measure methemoglobin. If significant quantities of methemoglobin are present, the oxygen satura-tion will read 85% regardless of what the actual saturation is, and therefore may be grossly in error and unreliable.) The treatment of methemoglobinemia is slow intravenous admin-istration of a 1% methylene blue solution to a total dose of 1 to 2 mg/kg. (*Note:* Methylene blue will also cause an error in the pulse oximeter reading.)[24]

Local Anesthetic Agents

Table 36-4 gives an overview of local anesthetic agents.

Aminoester Agents

COCAINE. Cocaine was the earliest recognized local anesthetic and is the only agent that occurs naturally.[25] It is an ester of benzoic acid present in the leaves of *Erythroxylon coca,* a tree growing in the Andes mountains. It was introduced into clinical practice for topical anesthesia by Sigmund Freud and Karl Koller in 1884, and for nerve trunk blockade by William Halsted in 1885.

Cocaine is unique among local anesthetic agents in its ability to block the re-uptake of norepinephrine and dobutamine at adrenergic nerve endings. It is this excess accumulation of neurotransmitter that accounts for cocaine's side effects of vasoconstriction, tachycardia, hypertension, mydriasis, cortical stimulation, addiction, and sensitization of the myocardium to catecholamines. Other drugs that interfere with catecholamine catabolism (eg, monoamine oxidase inhibitors) may interact with cocaine and cause a hypertensive crisis. Also, because cocaine is detoxified by plasma and liver cholinesterases, there may be an increased risk of toxic effects in patients with cholinesterase deficiency.

Cocaine is an extremely potent topical anesthetic agent but one with a low therapeutic ratio and very addictive potential. Despite these drawbacks, it is a valuable clinical tool. The maximum recommended dose is 2 to 3 mg/kg. The usual concentration is a 4% solution. Onset of action is relatively slow, and duration of action is 30 to 60 minutes. It is decomposed by autoclaving.

TABLE 36-4. CONCENTRATION AND MAXIMUM SAFE DOSES OF LOCAL ANESTHETICS

Anesthetic	Topical		Infiltration	
	Concentration	Maximum Dose	Concentration	Maximum Dose
Esters				
Cocaine	4–10%[a]	3 mg/kg	. . . Not used . . .	
Procaine (Novocain)	. . . Not effective . . .		1–2%	14 mg/kg in adults 5 mg/kg in children
Tetracaine (Pontocaine)	0.5–2%	1 mg/kg	0.10–0.25%	1–1.5 mg/kg
Chloroprocaine (Nesacaine)	. . . Not effective . . .		2%	14 mg/kg
Benzocaine (Americaine)	20%	200 mg	. . . Not used . . .	
Amides				
Lidocaine (Xylocaine)	2–4%	3 mg/kg	1–2%	3 mg/kg (without epinephrine) 7 mg/kg (with epinephrine)
Mepivacaine (Carbocaine)	. . . Not effective . . .		1–2%	7 mg/kg
Prilocaine (Citanest)	. . . Not effective . . .		1–2%	7 mg/kg
Bupivacaine (Marcaine)	. . . Not effective . . .		0.25–0.75%	3 mg/kg
Ropivacaine (Naropin)	. . . Not effective . . .		0.2–1%	1–3 mg/kg (250 mg)
Etidocaine (Duranest)	. . . Not used . . .		0.25%	4 mg/kg (300 mg)
Dibucaine (Nupercaine)	1.0%	50 mg	. . . Not used . . .	
Piperidine				
Dyclonine (Dyclone)	0.5%	4 mg/kg	. . . Not used . . .	
Epinephrine[b]	1 : 1000–1 : 100,000	1 mg	1 : 1000–1 : 100,000	1 mg

[a] 10% solution = 100 mg/mL; 1% solution = 10 mg/mL.

[b] With halothane anesthesia, 10 mL of 1 : 100,000 (0.1 mg) can be used over a 10-minute period or 30 mL over 1 hour (0.3 mg).

PROCAINE HYDROCHLORIDE (NOVOCAIN).   Procaine was first synthesized in 1905 by Einhorn as a result of a concerted effort to discover a safe substitute for cocaine. Procaine is a relatively weak ester-type local anesthetic agent with no surface activity (ineffective when applied topically). When used for infiltration, it is associated with a rapid onset (2–5 minutes) and a brief duration of action (30–90 minutes). It has relatively low toxicity, and the maximum recommended dose is 1000 mg. Procaine is rapidly hydrolyzed by plasma cholinesterase, and therefore may prolong the effect of succinylcholine (Anectine), which is also catabolized by cholinesterase. Its most common uses are a 2% solution for infiltration and differential nerve blocks.

CHLOROPROCAINE (NESACAINE).   Chloroprocaine is a halogenated derivative of procaine and has similar pharmacologic properties. It is hydrolyzed more rapidly than procaine and has relatively low potency, contributing to its low systemic toxicity. It is not useful for topical anesthesia. Chloroprocaine can be used for infiltration and peripheral nerve blockade, usually in a 2% concentration. However, duration of blockade is limited to 30 to 60 minutes. The maximum recommended dose is 800 mg with a non-epinephrine-containing solution, to 1000 mg with an epinephrine-containing solution.

TETRACAINE (PONTOCAINE).   Tetracaine is a potent ester local anesthetic possessing a potency and toxicity approximately 10 times that of procaine. Tetracaine is an excellent topical anesthetic and can be applied topically in a concentration of 1 to 2%. It is commonly used for anesthesia of the endotracheal surface via aerosol. It has a rather delayed onset (6–12 minutes) and prolonged duration of action (90–120 minutes). The maximum recommended single dose is 20 mg. Therefore, only 1 mL of a 2% solution (which contains 20 mg/mL) should be used for topical anesthesia of the upper respiratory tract because of its rapid uptake from this area.

BENZOCAINE (AMERICAINE).   Benzocaine is an ester of para-amino benzoic acid and structurally similar to procaine. However, its very low water solubility and relatively high oil solubility make it excellent for suspension in ointments and oily solutions for topical administration on raw or ulcerated surfaces. Its uptake in this situation is extremely slow, and risk of toxicity is minimal. It is available commercially as a 20% solution. Onset is slow, and duration of action is 30 to 60 minutes. The maximum recommended single dose is 200 mg.

Hurricaine is a solution containing 20% benzocaine in a flavored, water-soluble polyethylene glycol base. Its advantages are that it provides excellent topical anesthesia to all accessible mucous membranes, has a rapid onset and short duration of action, and tastes good.

Aminoamide Agents

LIDOCAINE (XYLOCAINE).   Lidocaine was the first aminoamide local anesthetic useful in clinical practice.[26] It has excellent penetrating powers and is effective by all routes of administration, providing a rapid onset and a moderate duration of action (1–3 hours when used for regional anesthesia) as well as effective topical anesthesia. The action may be prolonged by the addition of epinephrine in various concentrations. For infiltration or peripheral nerve block, 0.5 to 2% solutions are used. A 4% solution is used for topical anesthesia of the oropharynx and tracheobronchial tree. Transtracheal anesthesia of the trachea is performed by injecting 4 mL of a 4% lidocaine solution through the cricothyroid membrane after aspiration of air from a 20 gauge catheter. The maximum recommended doses are 5 mg/kg (without epinephrine) and 7 mg/kg (with epinephrine). Lidocaine (1.5 mg/kg) can be given intravenously during the induction of anesthesia to blunt the response to tracheal intubation. It acts by interrupting the vagal afferent pathway and thereby also helps to prevent bronchospasm.

The enhanced ability of lidocaine to suppress automaticity in ectopic myocardial foci has encouraged its use in the acute management of ventricular arrhythmias. A dose of 1 to 1.5 mg/kg intravenous bolus is used.

Anestacon is 2% lidocaine hydrochloride in a viscous solution for topical anesthesia.

MEPIVACAINE (CARBOCAINE).   Mepivacaine is an amide with properties similar to those of lidocaine: a relatively rapid onset of anesthesia, moderate duration of action, and dense blockade. It is effective for infiltration and peripheral nerve blockade; however, it is less effective than lidocaine for topical anesthesia. Mepivacaine produces somewhat less vasodilation than lidocaine, and therefore tends to have a slightly longer duration of action when both agents are used without epinephrine. A special 3% mepivacaine solution is available for dental anesthesia.

PRILOCAINE (CITANEST).   Prilocaine has a similar anesthetic profile to lidocaine but is more rapidly metabolized. It has a rapid onset, moderate duration of action, and profound depth of anesthesia. It also produces less vasodilation, making it useful without epinephrine. A particularly undesirable side effect of prilocaine is methemoglobinemia when a dose of approximately 600 mg is used.

The only current preparation available is EMLA cream, a mixture of lidocaine 2.5% and prilocaine 2.5% in an emulsion.[27] It has been shown to be effective in lessening the pain associated with venipuncture and catheter placement, and has been successfully employed in the harvesting of split-thickness skin grafts.[28,29] Satisfactory anesthesia is achieved by placing the cream under an occlusive dressing at least 1 hour prior to the procedure. Maximum anesthesia is attained at 2 to 3 hours, and duration persists 1 to 2 hours after removal.

BUPIVACAINE (MARCAINE, SENSORCAINE).   Bupivacaine, another aminoamide, combines several desirable properties: moderate onset, long duration of action, and separation of motor and sensory blockade. It can be used for infiltration, peripheral nerve blockade, and spinal and epidural anesthesia. Concentrations range from 0.125 to 0.75%. The duration of action averages from 3 to 10 hours depending on the type of block (the longest being brachial plexus blockade, which can last as long as 10–12 hours).

Bupivacaine is tightly bound to tissue and plasma protein, and does not produce high blood levels when appropriately administered. However, severe CNS and cardiovascular signs (intractable seizures and cardiovascular collapse) ensue if toxicity develops. As mentioned above, bupivacaine has a low CC/CNS ratio. The maximum recommended dose is 2 to 3 mg/kg.

ROPIVACAINE (NAROPIN).   This is the newest amide local anesthetic. It is chemically similar to bupivacaine but exists as a single isomer instead of a racemic mixture. Its pharmacologic profile is also similar to bupivacaine with regard to sensory blockade, but it exhibits a lesser motor blockade at equivalent concentrations. Ropivacaine is supplied in 0.2 to 1.0% solutions and can be administered to produce epidural anesthesia, major nerve blocks, or field blocks.

Duration can be from 2 to 8 hours. Preliminary reports show it to be less cardiotoxic at lower doses, although these benefits are lost at higher concentrations. Dosage is 1 to 3 mg/kg (*Note:* As with all local anesthetics, administration should be incremental with attention paid to possible symptoms of toxicity.) Further clinical use will determine what role ropivacaine will play.

ETIDOCAINE (DURANEST).   Etidocaine is an amide that is chemically similar to lidocaine. It shares the long duration of action of bupivacaine but differs in that the onset of action of etidocaine is more rapid. It also induces both a sensory and intense motor blockade, contrary to the differential blockade of bupivacaine. The usual concentrations for infiltration and peripheral nerve blockade are 0.5 and 1%. Its clinical profile includes a rapid onset and prolonged duration of action (from 2–12 hours). Maximum recommended dose is 300 mg (without epinephrine) to 400 mg (with epinephrine).

DIBUCAINE (NUPERCAINE).   Dibucaine is a potent aminoamide used mainly for spinal anesthesia outside the United States.[30] It has been used for both topical and infiltration, but has fallen out of common use because of a reported high incidence of local toxicity.

The dibucaine number is a determination of the percentage of inhibition of plasma cholinesterase (pseudocholinesterase) by dibucaine. Normal plasma cholinesterase is inhibited in vitro by dibucaine and will have a dibucaine number between 70 and 85. Heterozygotes have dibucaine numbers from 30 to 65, and those who are homozygote for the atypical enzyme are between 16 and 25. Therefore, those individuals with plasma cholinesterase deficiency (low dibucaine number) will have a prolonged response to any drugs requiring it for their metabolism (eg, succinylcholine).

MISCELLANEOUS AGENTS.   Cetacaine is a topical anesthetic agent designed to anesthetize accessible mucous membranes. It contains benzocaine, butyl aminobenzoate, and tetracaine hydrochloride. Cetacaine produces rapid anesthesia in 30 seconds. Maximum recommended dose is approximately 400 mg. (*Note*: A 1-second spray of cetacaine delivers 200 mg of anesthetic. Therefore, a duration of spray in excess of 2 seconds is contraindicated.)

Dyclonine (Dyclone) is 4'-butoxy-3-piperindinopropiophonone. Because it is neither an ester nor an amide, it may be used if allergy to both these classes has been documented. It has a rapid onset (2–10 minutes) and brief duration of action (30 minutes). It is used in a 0.5% topical solution. The recommended maximum adult dose is 300 mg. Dyclonine is highly irritating to tissues when injected, and is therefore used topically almost exclusively.

PREMEDICATION

The anesthetic begins at the time of the preoperative interview. A majority of patients have some degree of apprehension concerning an upcoming surgical procedure, and more often than not, the "anesthesia" figures prominently in this anxiety. It is therefore crucial that the anesthesiologist devote the necessary time (if the situation allows) to explain the sequence of events comprising the anesthetic, and to thoroughly answer any questions that patients or their family may have. It is important to gain the trust and confidence of patients within this short meeting, and at the same time reassure them of your competence and ability to see them through this trying time.

One central aspect is the unwillingness of patients to relinquish "control" of the situation. It is here where, in addition to adequate psychologic preparation, pharmacologic adjuncts may be of benefit. No "ideal" premedicant regimen exists. The various combinations depend many times on the experience of the anesthesiologist (Table 36-5). However, there are certain goals in mind when any premedication is ordered. These include anxiolysis, amnesia, antiemesis, sedation with or without analgesia, decreasing airway secretions, and decreasing gastric volume and acidity. Because the premedication is a prelude to the main anesthetic, it should be chosen with the same thoughts and concerns as was the anesthetic technique and individualized to each unique situation. One of the authors (KJ Lee) uses Seconal 100 mg p.o. 2 hours preoperatively, followed by morphine 8 to 10 mg IM and diazepam 8 to 10 mg IM on call to the operating room. However, in these days of ever-decreasing length of stay, much ear, nose, and throat surgery occurs on an outpatient basis (ie, admission and discharge on the same day). Most people are admitted within the hour prior to surgery and discharged after 2 hours of recovery following a general anesthetic—sooner if monitored anesthesia care was used. We must, therefore, employ medication which has a rapid onset and allows the patient to recover in a sufficiently fast manner following the procedure so that discharge can be accomplished in a timely fashion.

The following is an attempt to briefly outline the more commonly used classes of premedicant drugs.

Sedative Hypnotics/Tranquilizers

Benzodiazepines

These drugs have enjoyed widespread popularity because of their ability to reliably provide amnesia, reduce anxiety, and increase the seizure threshold without undue respiratory or

TABLE 36-5. COMMON PREOPERATIVE MEDICATIONS

Drug	Dosage
Tranquilizers	
Diazepam	5–10 mg p.o.
Midazolam	0.5–1.0 mg/kg IM
Lorazepam	2–4 mg p.o.
Hydroxyzine	25–100 mg p.o.
Droperidol	2.5–5.0 mg IM
Barbiturates	
Pentobarbital	50–100 mg p.o. or IM
Secobarbital	50–100 mg p.o. or IM
Narcotics	
Morphine	2–10 mg IM (0.1–0.2 mg/kg)
Meperidine	25–100 mg IM
Fentanyl	0.025–0.100 mg IM
Anticholinergics	
Atropine	0.2–0.5 mg IM
Scopolamine	0.2–0.4 mg IM
Glycopyrrolate	0.2–0.4 mg IM
Antacids	
Cimetidine	400 mg p.o./300 mg IM or IV
Ranitidine	150 mg p.o./50 mg IV
Famotidine	40 mg p.o./20 mg IV
Nizatidine	150 mg p.o.
Sodium citrate	15–30 mL p.o.
Gastrokinetics	
Metoclopramide	10 mg p.o./IM/IV

cardiovascular depression.[31] Protection against seizures may be of benefit when local anesthetics are employed.

The three most commonly used benzodiazepines are diazepam (Valium), midazolam (Versed), and lorazepam (Ativan). Midazolam has several advantages: It is water soluble, which reduces the pain of both intramuscular and intravenous injection associated with diazepam; it is approximately twice as potent as diazepam, with a more rapid peak onset (30–60 minutes) and an elimination half-time of 1 to 4 hours. It is therefore well suited to shorter procedures where extubation is anticipated or for sedation during local anesthesia (0.5–1 mg/kg IM or titration of 1–2 mg IV). The specific benzodiazepine antagonist is flumazenil (Romazicon), which is supplied in solutions containing 0.1 mg/mL (100 μg/mL). The recommended dose is 200 μg IV over 15 seconds, which can be repeated every 60 seconds for four doses (1 mg total). No more than 3 mg over 1 hour is advised.[32]

Barbiturates

The barbiturates have been safely used for many years to provide preoperative sedation and can be administered both orally and parenterally. However, when pain is present, patients may become disoriented without being sedated. Also, barbiturates are contraindicated in certain types of porphyria. The commonly used barbiturates are secobarbital (Seconal) and pentobarbital (Nembutal). Secobarbital is usually administered orally in doses of 50 to 200 mg (adult), with onset in 60 to 90 minutes and a duration of 4 or more hours. Pentobarbital can be administered both orally or intramuscularly in doses of 50 to 200 mg. It is important to note that both drugs are relatively long acting, and therefore may be less suitable for shorter procedures.

Butyrophenones

Droperidol (Inapsine) can be administered in doses of 2.5 to 7.5 mg to produce what is seemingly a sedated patient. However, the patient may in fact be agitated but unable to express it. While this is not the ultimate goal of droperidol administration, it does allow certain procedures (eg, awake fiberoptic intubation) to be accomplished with a reduced risk of oversedation and subsequent airway compromise. It is also very useful as an antiemetic in small doses (up to 2.5 mg IV). Another preparation, Innovar (fentanyl citrate/droperidol), is available as a premedicant or for sedation (neuroleptanalgesia). One milliliter of Innovar contains (in a 1:50 ratio) the equivalent of 50 μg of fentanyl and 2.5 mg of droperidol. Note that droperidol may cause extrapyramidal effects (because it is a dopamine antagonist) and that it also has alpha-blocking properties.

Haloperidol (Haldol) is a long-acting antipsychotic medication that may be useful as a premedicant if a patient has been maintained on it chronically. However, its routine use is not recommended.

Chloral Hydrate

Chloral hydrate produces both amnesia and anxiolysis and has been used extensively in the pediatric and geriatric age groups. Doses range from 20 to 40 mg/kg p.o. every 8 hours in children, to 500 to 1000 mg p.o. in adults. Recently, though, the benzodiazepines have supplanted much of chloral hydrate's role.

Antihistamines

Hydroxyzine (Vistaril, Atarax) is an antihistamine and antiemetic and is mainly used to potentiate the effects of opioids. The dose is 25 to 100 mg p.o. or IM.

Diphenydramine (Benadryl), another antihistamine, has sedative and anticholinergic as well as antiemetic properties. The usual dose is 25 to 50 mg p.o., IM, or IV. Because it blocks histamine release, it can be used in conjunction with steroids and H_2-blockers as prophylaxis for potential allergic reactions.

Phenothiazines

The phenothiazines are useful preoperative medications, with excellent sedative, antiemetic, and anticholinergic properties. They can be given orally as well as parenterally for preoperative medication. Commonly used premedicants in this group include promethazine (Phenergan) 25 to 50 mg, chlorpromazine (Thorazine), perphenazine (Trilafon), and prochlorperazine (Compazine) 5 to 10 mg.

Opioids

The opioid narcotics, especially morphine and meperidine (Demerol), are the most frequently used intramuscular premedications of this class. They are specifically designed to relieve pain, and therefore theoretically should not be used if no pain exists. In point of fact, however, they can be employed as adjuncts to other classes of premedications (eg, the benzodiazepines) to produce a calm, relaxed state. The opioids also provide for relative cardiovascular stability. One must keep in mind, though, that side effects of these drugs include CNS and respiratory depression and also nausea and vomiting. The elderly may be more sensitive to their effects, and caution should be used in this group of patients. Morphine should not be used in patients with asthma because of its ability to cause release of histamine with concomitant increase in central vagal tone and the possibility of bronchospasm. The usual dose of morphine is 0.1 to 0.15 mg/kg IM and meperidine 0.5 to 1 mg/kg IM.

Fentanyl (Sublimaze), sufentanil (Sufenta), and alfentanil (Alfenta), the synthetic opioids, can be given as premedications, although in general they are given intravenously in small amounts at the induction of general anesthesia or titrated to effect for conscious sedation or postoperative pain relief. Sufentanil is 5 to 10 times more potent than fentanyl, and alfentanil is one-quarter as potent as fentanyl (but 30 to 50 times more potent than morphine). This also provides a relative comparison of doses. For example, grossly, morphine 1 mg is equivalent to fentanyl 50 μg, sufentanil 5 to 10 μg, or alfentanil 200 μg.

A new ultra-short-acting selective micro-opioid receptor agonist, remifentanil (Ultiva), has recently been released. It is about 15- to 30-fold more potent than alfentanil in humans,[33] with similar pharmacologic effects. Remifentanil is rapidly hydrolyzed by nonspecific plasma and tissue esterases, making onset rapid and recovery brief after cessation of administration with no cumulative effects. Because of these characteristics, remifentanil appears to be easily titratable to achieve a desired level of anesthesia. However, this rapid return to consciousness is accompanied by a lack of postoperative analgesia; thus consideration must be given to other means if significant postoperative pain is anticipated. Similarly, it exhibits side effects common to other micro-opioid agents, but these are also attenuated in duration.[34]

Dosage should be calculated on ideal body weight, since both clearance and distribution correlate best with lean body mass[35] and appear not to be affected by impaired renal clearance or hepatic function.[36] A final concentration of remifentanil (*Note:* it must be reconstituted before use) should be 25 to 250 μg/mL after reconstitution depending upon age, type of anesthesia (ie, general vs. conscious sedation), and technique (ie, bolus vs. continuous infusion). As with all opioids, administration should be by trained personnel able to treat the potential adverse effects such as respiratory depression and hypotension.

Remifentanil offers some new approaches because of its unique properties and may be useful in such areas as neurosurgery, outpatient surgery, and painful procedures or in the emergency room and intensive care units where a rapid return to consciousness is desirable.

Combined agonist/antagonist drugs also exist, such as pentazocine, butorphanol, and nalbuphine. They do, however, exhibit a ceiling effect with regard to analgesia, and therefore may be less useful. The specific opioid antagonist is naloxone (Narcan). It is provided in ampules of 0.4 mg/mL (400 μg/mL) but, unless an emergency situation exists, can be titrated in doses of 20- to 40-μg increments to achieve the desired level of sedation. Naloxone has been associated with flash pulmonary edema when administered rapidly, usually in larger doses.

Belladonna Derivatives

Atropine sulfate 0.4 to 0.8 mg IM or IV, scopolamine 0.2 to 0.4 mg IM, or glycopyrrolate 0.2 to 0.4 mg are the most commonly employed belladonna derivatives. Used for their antimuscarinic properties, glycopyrrolate and scopolamine are potent antisialagogues. Atropine and scopolamine, because of their tertiary amine structure, penetrate the blood–brain barrier and act centrally to produce either sedation or excitation. Atropine is the most potent vagolytic of the three and will, therefore, produce the greatest increase in heart rate.

Histamine-2 Receptor Antagonists

Cimetidine (Tagamet) 400 mg p.o. or 300 mg IM or IV, ranitidine (Zantac) 150 mg p.o. or 50 mg IV, famotidine (Pepcid) 40 mg p.o. or 20 mg IV, and nizatidine (Axid) 150 mg p.o. are frequently administered as part of the premedicant regimen. They are used to raise the pH of secreted gastric acid above the critical level of 2.5, thereby reducing the pulmonary sequelae should aspiration occur. Note that they will have no effect on gastric acid that has already been secreted.

Gastrokinetics

Metoclopramide (Reglan) 10 mg p.o., IM, or IV, is a dopamine antagonist that may be administered to hasten gastric emptying and increase gastroesophageal sphincter tone.

Nonparticulate Antacids

Sodium citrate (Bicitra) 15 to 30 mL just prior to induction of anesthesia will be effective in raising the pH of gastric contents already present in the stomach. This, combined with H_2 blockers and metoclopramide, may help reduce the risk of aspiration in susceptible individuals.

INTRAVENOUS SEDATION

Intravenous (IV) or "conscious sedation," as coined by Bennett, has become a popular adjunct to local anesthesia.[37] As discussed above with premedication, the specific goals of IV sedation must be kept clearly in mind when selecting a technique. Sedation cannot substitute for an adequate local anesthetic block. However, the bounds of these procedures are ever expanding as newer, shorter-acting drugs are introduced. Conscious sedation should produce a patient who is calm and relaxed, can respond appropriately (not necessarily verbally) to simple commands (eg, "take a deep breath"), and is able to maintain protective airway reflexes.[38]

The anesthesiologist monitors the level of consciousness by frequent verbal contact as well as objective signs provided by ECG, end-tidal CO_2 monitoring, and pulse oximetry used to measure oxygen saturation (pulse oximetry has now become a standard of care). The technique selected will depend on several factors, such as type and length of the procedure, location of the surgery, the influences of coexisting patient disease, and the specific wishes of the surgeon. Obviously, patient safety must supercede all other concerns.

Those medications discussed earlier as premedications can all be used for conscious sedation. Usually, combinations of the various drugs, such as benzodiazepines and opioids, can be titrated to the desired effect. Other drugs that can be used include propofol (Diprivan), sodium thiopental (Pentothal), ketamine, and etomidate (Amidate). All of these are IV agents for the induction of anesthesia. However, when used in small, incremental amounts, they can produce degrees of conscious sedation. Of these agents, propofol, the newest drug, has probably had the greatest impact on expanding these possibilities.

Propofol is an IV sedative hypnotic agent that rapidly produces hypnosis, usually within about 40 seconds. It is also associated with several important side effects: arterial hypotension (about 20–30% decrease), apnea, airway obstruction, and oxygen desaturation. Propofol has been associated with local pain on injection, which can be decreased by prior injection of 1 mL of 1.0% lidocaine.

When a bolus technique is used, plasma propofol levels rapidly decline following injection secondary to accelerated metabolic clearance and rapid redistribution into tissues. Because of this rapid decrease, accumulation after repeated doses or continuous infusion is minimal. Boluses of propofol 10 to 20 mg (10 mg/mL) or a continuous infusion of 25 to 75 μg/kg per minute (1.5 mg/kg per hour) can be used once an adequate level of sedation has been established. As always, this dose should be carefully titrated to the desired effect. It should also be noted that there is a lesser incidence of nausea and vomiting with propofol.

BLOCK TECHNIQUES

With virtually all blocks, eliciting an appropriate paresthesia before injection of the agent helps assure success.

Laryngoscopy, Tracheoscopy

The larynx and trachea receive their sensory nerve supply from the superior and inferior laryngeal nerves, which are branches of the vagus nerve.

Anesthesia may be provided to the larynx by the topical application of local anesthesia (using a laryngeal syringe) to the mucous membrane of the pyriform fossa (deep into which runs the superior laryngeal nerve) and to the laryngeal surface of the epiglottis and the vocal folds (Figure 36-1). Local anesthesia of the larynx and trachea also may be accomplished by the percutaneous infiltration of local anesthetic solution around the superior laryngeal nerve and the transtracheal application of local anesthetic to the tracheal mucosa. For percutaneous infiltration, the superior laryngeal nerve is located as it pierces the thyrohyoid membrane (Figure 36-2). The transtracheal application of local anesthesia requires insertion of a 25 gauge needle through the cricothyroid membrane in the midline (Figure 36-3).

Reduction of Dislocated Temporomandibular Joint

In the common presentation of temporomandibular dislocation, the condyle rests on the anterior slope of the articular eminence (Figure 36-4). There is intense pain and severe spasm of

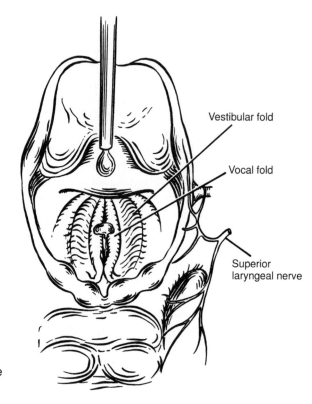

Figure 36-1. Topical anesthesia to the larynx.

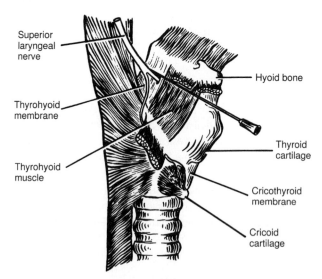

Figure 36-2. (1) Palpate the greater cornu of the hyoid bone. (2) Insert a 25 gauge needle approximately 1 cm caudal to this landmark. (3) The needle is inserted to a depth of approximately 1 cm until the firm consistency of the thyrohyoid membrane is identified. (4) Inject 3 mL of local anesthetic solution.

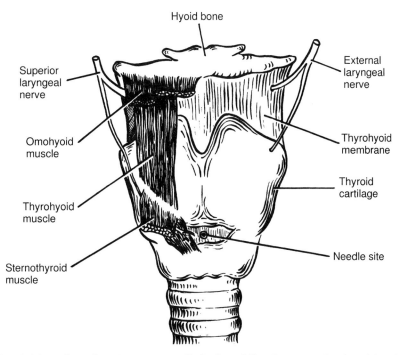

Figure 36-3.   (1) Introduce the 25 gauge needle in the midline between the thyroid and cricoid cartilages. (2) Puncture the cricothyroid membrane. It is readily felt as a "pop." Free aspiration of air with the attached syringe verifies the intratracheal position of the needle tip. (3) Instill 4 mL of local anesthetic solution. In addition to anesthesia of the larynx and trachea (steps 1 and 2), the topical application of local anesthesia to the oropharynx is required for adequate visualization for laryngoscopy and tracheoscopy.

the surrounding mandibular musculature. Reduction of this dislocation may frequently be accomplished by unilateral intracapsular injection of local anesthesia.

Reduction and Fixation of Mandibular Fracture

Complete anesthesia for reduction and fixation of a mandibular fracture requires adequate anesthesia of the maxillary and mandibular branches of the trigeminal nerve and superficial branches of the cervical plexus (Figure 36-5).

The mandibular branch of the trigeminal nerve is readily anesthetized near its exit from the skull through the foramen ovale (Figure 36-6). Anesthesia of the maxillary division of the trigeminal nerve may be accomplished in the pterygopalatine fossa near the foramen rotundum, where the nerve exits from the skull (Figure 36-7). The most frequent complication of mandibular and maxillary nerve block is hemorrhage into the cheek, which usually is managed conservatively. Subarachnoid injections and facial nerve blocks are two other rarely reported complications.

The superficial branches of the cervical plexus are easily blocked as they emerge along the posterior margin of the sternocleidomastoid muscle; infiltration is accomplished along the posterior margin of this muscle using 10 to 15 mL of anesthetic solution.

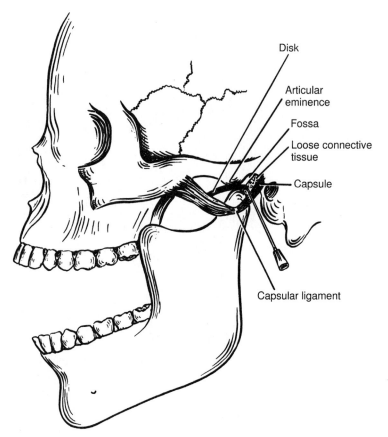

Figure 36-4.   (1) With the head of the condyloid process locked anteriorly, the depression of the glenoid fossa is easily palpated. (2) The needle is inserted into the depression of the glenoid fossa and directed anteriorly toward the head of the condyloid process. (3) When the condyloid process is contracted, the needle is slightly withdrawn. (4) Instill 2 mL of local anesthetic solution into the capsule.

Otology

The sensory innervation of the external ear is illustrated in Figure 36-8. The middle ear receives its sensory innervation through the tympanic plexus (cranial nerves V_3, IX, and X).

- V_3 Auriculotemporal nerve
- IX Jacobson's nerve
- X Auricular nerve

Myringotomy

For myringotomy, inject the cartilaginous and bony junction of the external auditory canal. Instead of introducing local anesthetic through the classic 12, 3, 6, and 9 o'clock infiltration, infiltrate at 12, 2, 4, 6, 8, and 10 o'clock. After the first injection, the subsequent injection sites are already anesthetized before the needle prick. For myringotomy alone it is not nec-

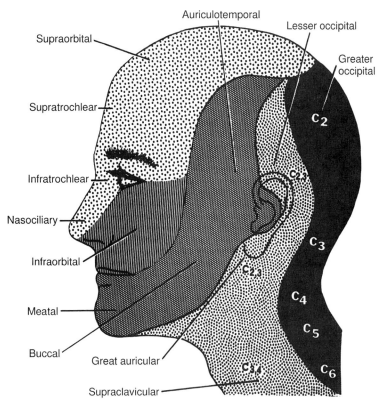

Figure 36-5.   Cutaneous innervation of the head and neck.

essary to infiltrate the skin of the bony canal wall and no local anesthetic agent should infiltrate into the middle ear cavity. (See "Complications" below.)

Stapedectomy

In addition to the technique described for myringotomy, with stapedectomy it is necessary to infiltrate the tympanomeatal flap. This technique ensures adequate anesthesia while providing vasoconstriction (1% lidocaine with epinephrine 1 : 100,000) for hemostasis.

Complications

Two transient complications have been reported from local anesthetic infiltration for stapedectomy. These result from diffusion of the local anesthetic from the tympanomeatal flap to the middle ear cavity.

1. Temporary facial nerve paralysis results from the local anesthetic coming into contact with the dehiscent facial nerve. Patience and reassurance for a few hours resolve the problem.
2. Violent vertigo with nystagmus (similar to Ménière's attack) can occur 45 minutes after infiltration. Provided no damage has been done to the vestibular labyrinth, this problem is secondary to the effect of lidocaine on the membranous labyrinth through the oval or round windows.

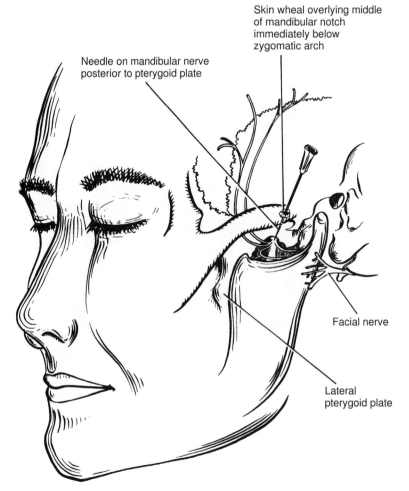

Skin wheal overlying middle
of mandibular notch
immediately below
zygomatic arch

Needle on mandibular nerve
posterior to pterygoid plate

Facial nerve

Lateral
pterygoid plate

Figure 36-6.   (1) A skin wheal is raised at the midpoint between the condyle and coronoid process of the mandible and just below the zygoma. (2) An 8-cm needle is introduced perpendicular to the skin until contact with the pterygoid plate occurs, usually at a depth of 4 cm. (3) The needle is withdrawn and then reinserted slightly posterior to a depth of approximately 6 cm. (4) When paresthesia in the mandibular division is elicited, the needle is fixed, and approximately 5 mL of anesthetic solution is administered.

These complications are particularly distressing if they occur after an office myringotomy. Therefore, we recommend that there be no infiltration of local anesthetic into the skin of the bony canal wall. Local anesthetic applied at the junction of the bony and cartilaginous canal is adequate and does not risk migrating into the middle ear cavity.

Tympanoplasty and Mastoidectomy (Canalplasty, Meatoplasty)

Tympanoplasty and mastoidectomy are usually performed under general anesthesia, although they may be done under local anesthesia. In addition to the stapedectomy infiltration,

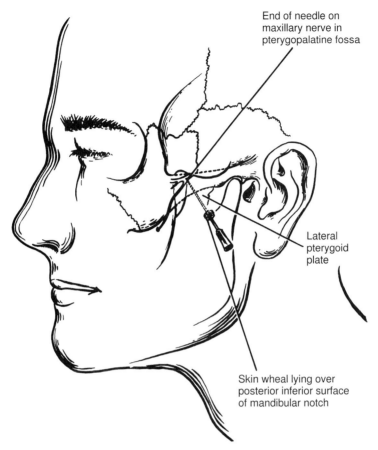

End of needle on
maxillary nerve in
pterygopalatine fossa

Lateral
pterygoid
plate

Skin wheal lying over
posterior inferior surface
of mandibular notch

Figure 36-7.   (1) A skin wheal is raised just over the posterior inferior surface of the mandibular
notch. (2) An 8-cm needle is inserted transversely and slightly anterior to a depth
of 4 to 5 cm, where it comes into contact with the lateral pterygoid plate. (3) The needle is withdrawn slightly and directed in a more anterosuperior direction to pass anterior to the pterygoid plate into the pterygopalatine fossa. (4) The needle is advanced
another 0.5 to 1.5 cm until paresthesia is elicited. A total of 5 to 10 mL
of local anesthetic solution is deposited.

postauricular and conchal infiltration are necessary (Figure 36-8) for sensory innervation.
The skin of the anterior canal wall needs to be anesthetized if surgery is to include that
anatomic site.

Nasal Surgery
Nasal Polypectomy
Cocaine pledgets along the mucosal surfaces, as well as those in contact with the sphenopalatine ganglion, supply adequate anesthesia for polypectomy. Occasionally it is necessary to
supplement this anesthesia with infiltration, as for rhinoplasty.

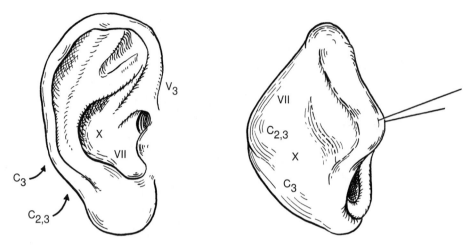

Figure 36-8.   Sensory innervation of the external ear.

Septoplasty and Rhinoplasty

The sensory innervation of the septum and external nose is illustrated in Figures 36-9 to 36-13 and in Tables 36-6 to 36-8. In addition to local infiltration, as shown in Figure 36-13, cocaine pledgets along the mucosal surfaces and sphenopalatine ganglion are used for septoplasty and rhinoplasty. For the best hemostasis and anesthesia result, it is wise to wait at least 20 minutes before performing the surgery.

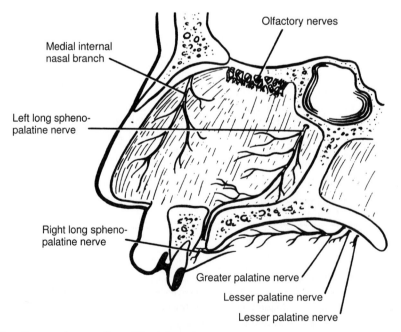

Figure 36-9.   Sensory innervation of the internal nose.

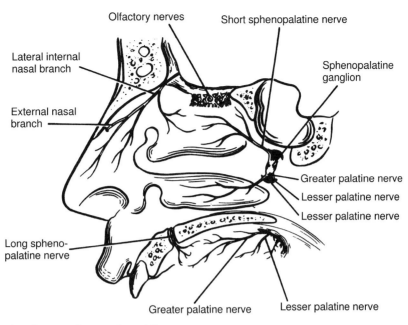

Figure 36-10. Sensory innervation of the nose.

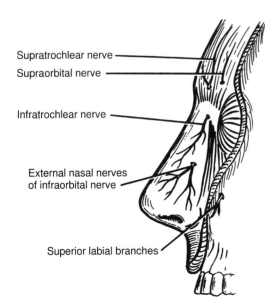

Figure 36-11. Sensory innervation of the nose.

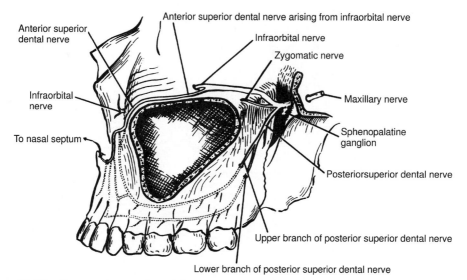

Figure 36-12. Sensory innervation of the nose.

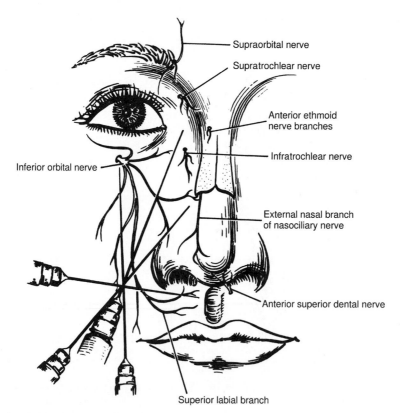

Figure 36-13. Infiltration for rhinoplasty.

TABLE 36-6. NASAL SENSORY INNERVATION

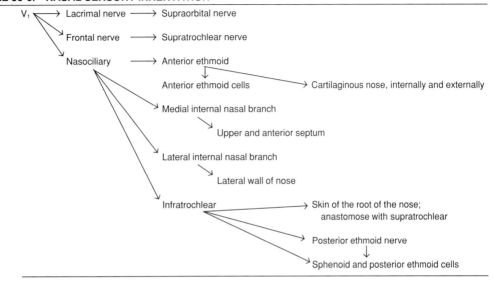

TABLE 36-7. NASAL SENSORY INNERVATION

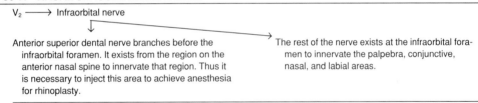

$V_2 \longrightarrow$ Infraorbital nerve

Anterior superior dental nerve branches before the
infraorbital foramen. It exists from the region on the
anterior nasal spine to innervate that region. Thus it
is necessary to inject this area to achieve anesthesia
for rhinoplasty.

The rest of the nerve exists at the infraorbital foramen to innervate the palpebra, conjunctive,
nasal, and labial areas.

TABLE 36-8. NASAL SENSORY INNERVATION

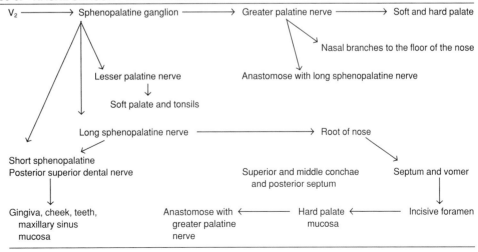

Sinus Surgery

Caldwell–Luc Operation

To achieve good anesthesia for sinus surgery, one needs to block the infraorbital nerve, the sphenopalatine ganglion, and the posterior superior dental nerve. The posterior superior dental nerve exists from the maxillary nerve adjacent to the sphenopalatine ganglion. To block the sphenopalatine ganglion and posterior superior dental nerve, introduce local anesthesia through the greater palatine foramen via a curved needle.

Further topical anesthesia is with cocaine pledgets applied intranasally against the sphenopalatine ganglion. Local infiltration of the mucosa in the canine fossa supplies the hemostasis needed over the line of incision.

Ethmoid Sinuses

The sensory innervation of the ethmoid sinuses is intertwined with that of the nose and septum. In addition, they are innervated by the anterior ethmoid nerve (branch of the nasociliary, V_1) and the posterior ethmoid nerve (branch of the infratrochlear, VI).

Sphenoid Sinuses

The sensory innervation of the sphenoid sinuses is from the pharyngeal branch of the maxillary nerve as well as the posterior ethmoid nerve.

GENERAL ANESTHESIA

General anesthesia is the ability to render a reversible state of unconsciousness, analgesia, muscle relaxation, and depression of reflexes. There is both an art and a science involved in this achievement. Although the exact mechanism of action of general anesthesia is not known, several theories have been advanced to explain this state. In general, it is thought that anesthetics act by reversibly inhibiting neurosynaptic function of various regions or components of the cell membrane, either through action on membrane proteins or lipids, or through modulation of the inhibitory neurotransmitter gamma-amino butyric acid (GABA). Because these compounds are involved in a number of multisynaptic pathways, they have repercussions far beyond their local sites of action. By altering sympathetic tone, these agents affect almost all organ systems, especially the cardiovascular system.

General Anesthetic Agents

Inhalation Agents

The inhalation anesthetics are those volatile agents that are administered by way of the lungs. They are administered by mask or through an endotracheal tube, attain a certain concentration in the alveoli, diffuse across the alveolar–capillary membrane, and are transported by the blood to their sites of action in the CNS. Many factors affect the uptake and distribution of the volatile agents, including agent concentration, minute ventilation, diffusion capacity across the alveolar membrane, blood–gas partition coefficient (solubility), cardiac output, alveolar–arterial gradient, and the blood–brain partition coefficient.

The potency of the inhalation anesthetics is usually described in terms of minimal alveolar concentration (MAC; Table 36-9). This is defined as the concentration of anesthetic at one atmosphere that will prevent movement in response to a surgical stimulus (surgical incision) in 50% of individuals. This allows for a somewhat quantitative assessment of the amount of anesthetic delivered. It should be noted that MAC is additive; for example, if one-half MAC of two agents is delivered simultaneously, this is equivalent to one MAC of a single agent. It

TABLE 36-9. INHALATION ANESTHETIC AGENTS

Agent	Minimal Alveolar Concentration (MAC) (%)
Halothane	0.77
Enflurane	1.7
Isoflurane	1.15
Sevoflurane	2
Desflurane	6
Nitrous oxide	104

is this concept that allows for a "balanced anesthetic technique," meaning that lesser amounts of several anesthetic agents (eg, a potent inhalation agent and a narcotic) can be combined to provide adequate anesthesia with reduced side effects from large doses of only one agent.

The inhalation agents in common use today are isoflurane (Forane), enflurane (Ethrane), halothane (Fluothane), desflurane (Suprane), and sevoflurane (Ultane). These are examples of halogenated hydrocarbons, with desflurane, isoflurane, and sevoflurane being ethers and halothane an alkane (which predisposes it to causing arrhythmias).

Desflurane and sevoflurane, although only of recent introduction, have made great inroads into the older entrenched volatile anesthetics, with sevoflurane all but replacing halothane for the induction of children in many practices. Because of the lack of pungency, lower solubility, lower MAC-awake (the concentration permitting voluntary response to command in 50% of patients), and less arrhythmogenic potential, it is easy to see why sevoflurane has gained so quickly in popularity.[41] It can also be administered using a standard vaporizer. A potential drawback to sevoflurane use in longer procedures is the biodegradation to a toxic substance, compound A, which can cause renal damage. To minimize this possibility, one should limit its use to short- to moderate-length procedures and use adequate fresh gas flows (> 2 L/min).

Desflurane, a very insoluble agent requiring a heated vaporizer because of its partial pressure, has also made great strides since its introduction. It tends to have a more pungent odor and, therefore, is less amenable to an inhalation induction than sevoflurane, but recovery from desflurane is more rapid. It produces similar hemodynamic effects to sevoflurane with relative heart rate and blood pressure stability.

Isoflurane is probably the most widely used inhalation anesthetic for adults, although the newer agents may change this in the future. It is more soluble than desflurane and, therefore, will not exit as quickly, producing a somewhat longer time (approximately three times longer) to MAC-awake.

Halothane is probably the most commonly used anesthetic worldwide but was used almost exclusively, until recently, in children in the United States. Because of a rare entity, halothane hepatitis, halothane has all but disappeared from use in adults in the United States. Halothane hepatitis is thought to have a certain genetic predisposition, which causes an allergic-type hepatocellular destruction.

Nitrous oxide (NO_2) is among the oldest inhalation agents in use today and remains a valuable part of our repertoire. It is mainly used as an adjunct to general anesthesia because, in contrast to the potent volatile agents, it is considered a weaker agent. This is because its MAC exceeds 100% (104), and therefore, one MAC of NO_2 cannot be delivered, except in a hyperbaric chamber. It is usually employed in a concentration of 50 to 70% in oxygen. Because of the relative insolubility of desflurane, NO_2 need not be used with this agent.

Intravenous Anesthetics

Many of the intravenous agents have already been discussed above. The agents that are specifically designed for the induction of anesthesia include thiopental (Pentothal), propofol (Diprivan), etomidate (Amidate), methohexital (Brevitol), and ketamine. Each of these drugs has advantages and disadvantages in its clinical profile, so that no one drug can be considered the "ideal" agent in all circumstances.

Thiopental is an ultra-short-acting thiobarbiturate that has enjoyed widespread and time-tested usage. It is associated with cardiac and respiratory depression and may accumulate after repeated doses, which may prolong wake-up. The usual induction dose is 3 to 5 mg/kg IV.

Propofol, the newest of these agents, has rapidly become a useful choice for induction. It is quickly eliminated with minimal accumulation after repeated doses, which allows for a more rapid return to consciousness. Propofol has also been associated with a lesser incidence of nausea and vomiting. These are particularly advantageous during outpatient surgery. The dose for induction ranges from 1.5 to 2.5 mg/kg IV. However, all of these agents, except etomidate and ketamine, will cause myocardial depression, which must be taken into consideration.

Ketamine, a phencyclidine derivative, induces a peculiar state, called dissociative anesthesia, in which patients are unresponsive to noxious stimuli but may appear to be awake, with eyes open and spontaneous movement. Pharyngeal and laryngeal reflexes also remain intact until very deep levels of anesthesia are attained. Of significance, ketamine is associated with dysphoric reactions, and therefore is not usually a drug of first choice in an otherwise healthy patient.

Muscle Relaxants

Neuromuscular blocking drugs are capable of interrupting nerve impulse conduction at the neuromuscular junction. This allows for muscle relaxation, which is used to facilitate intubation of the trachea and to provide for optimum surgical working conditions. They can be classified as either depolarizing muscle relaxants, of which succinylcholine is the only clinically available example, or nondepolarizing muscle relaxants, which include D-tubocurarine, pancuronium (Pavulon), metocurine (Metubine), vecuronium (Norcuron), atracurium (Tracrium), mivacurium (Mivacron), doxacurium (Nuromax), pipecuronium (Arduan), rocuronium (Zemuron), and cisatracurium (Nimbex). The nondepolarizing agents can be further subdivided into short-, intermediate-, and long-acting drugs (Table 36-10).

TABLE 36-10.   MUSCLE RELAXANTS

Depolarizing
Succinylcholine
Nondepolarizing
Short-acting
Mivacurium
Intermediate-acting
Atracurium
Vecuronium
Rocuronium
Cisatracurium
Long-acting
D-tubocurarine
Doxicurium
Metocurine
Pancuronium
Pipecuronium

Succinylcholine is the standard by which all other muscle relaxants are measured in regard to the rapidity of achieving adequate intubating conditions (45–60 seconds). Attempts at developing new nondepolarizing drugs with this rapid an onset and without a prolonged duration have yet to be successful. However, research in this domain continues. Rocuronium (Zemuron) is a new, nondepolarizing muscle relaxant which has been recently introduced. It is an intermediate-acting agent similar to vecuronium, but with a shorter onset of action. In a dose of 0.6 to 1 mg/kg, intubation can be achieved in approximately 60 to 90 seconds. Therefore, this nondepolarizer may be appropriate in situations where a rapid-sequence induction is necessary but where succinylcholine may be contraindicated.

Monitoring of neuromuscular blockade is accomplished by a supramaximal electric stimulation delivered to a muscle via a neuromuscular stimulator. Decreased twitch height (depolarizing relaxants) or fade (nondepolarizing relaxants) to either train-of-four (four 2-Hz impulses in 2 seconds) or tetanus (50–100 Hz for 5 seconds) is proportional to the percentage of neuromuscular blockade. In this way, with at least one twitch of a train-of-four present, reversal of the blockade can be reliably achieved. Reversal is accomplished with either edrophonium (Tensilon) 1 mg/kg, neostigmine (Prostigmin) 40 to 75 µg/kg, or pyridostigmine (Mestinon, Regonol) 0.2 mg/kg. These acetylcholinesterase inhibitors cause accumulation of acetylcholine at the neuromuscular junction, thereby facilitating impulse transmission and reversal of the blockade. Of importance, anticholinergic drugs (atropine or glycopyrrolate) must accompany administration of the reversal agents to avoid the undesirable muscarinic effects (only the nicotinic, cholinergic effects are necessary).

Postoperative Pain Management

During recent years there have been significant developments in the realm of postoperative analgesia. Patient-controlled analgesia (PCA) has become a well-established method of delivering traditional pain medications (usually morphine or meperidine) to postoperative surgical patients. It is generally well accepted by patients because it provides them with some degree of control over their situation. It is also readily adaptable to all age groups from pediatric to geriatric.

Other analgesics—such as dezocine (Dalgan), a mixed agonist/antagonist, and ketorolac (Toradol), a potent, nonsteroidal anti-inflammatory drug that can be administered either p.o. or IM—have become useful adjuncts to control postoperative pain. In addition, the nerve blocks used for surgical procedures may provide relief in the immediate postoperative period.

Complications

This discussion of complications of general anesthesia is confined to those that are of relevance to otolaryngologists. However, one should not lose sight of the fact that anesthesia affects all organ systems, which may be a source of potential complications.

Aspiration pneumonitis (Mendelson syndrome) may occur during general anesthesia, either during intubation of the trachea or on extubation. Gastric contents of > 25 mL with a pH < 25 are associated with a high risk of aspiration syndrome, although there are no published data to support this.[39] Of particular concern is that aspiration can also occur with a properly positioned, cuffed endotracheal tube and may be as high as 5%. Foreign matter (blood, secretions, or gastric contents) which is permitted to accumulate may gain access to the respiratory tree when the protective airway reflexes are obtunded. Close attention to airway management in those individuals at risk is of great importance in preventing this most serious complication.

Many of the inhalation anesthetics (most notably halothane) are associated with sensitization of the myocardium to catecholamines.[40] In the presence of excess endogenous or exogenous catecholamines, patients may develop cardiac arrhythmias (ventricular ectopy or fibrillation). It is therefore recommended that the dose of epinephrine administered not exceed 10 mL of a 1 : 100,000 solution (ie, 100 μg) in any 10-minute period when these anesthetics are in use.

Malignant hyperthermia (MH) is a rare (incidence of 1 : 10,000 to 1 : 50,000 anesthetics), potentially lethal entity that was first formally reported in 1960. It is triggered by the potent inhalation agents and succinylcholine and is associated with a genetic predisposition. Once triggered, MH causes a massive increase in intracellular calcium and uncoupling of metabolic pathways, resulting in an extreme elevation of temperature, increase in CO_2 production, metabolic acidosis, cardiac arrhythmias, and, if untreated, eventual cardiovascular collapse.[42] The specific treatment is dantrolene, which blocks intracellular calcium release. If a patient has a known history of MH or MH susceptibility—associated with masseter muscle rigidity (MMR), positive family history, or concurrent muscular dystrophy—a "nontriggering technique" or conduction anesthetic should be used.

Nitrous oxide–induced elevation of middle ear pressure may be seen. Because of its increased solubility relative to nitrogen (34 times more soluble), the use of nitrous oxide may cause a significant expansion of the closed middle ear space and potential disruption of a tympanic graft. This distention is readily reversible if the nitrous oxide is discontinued and 100% oxygen is administered.[43]

Hepatotoxicity is a potential problem with virtually all anesthetic techniques, because they all decrease hepatic blood flow to some degree. A preexisting subclinical hepatitis may be aggravated by exposure to anesthetic agents and mistakenly attributed to these drugs.

With the advent of electrocautery and lasers in surgery, the potential for airway fires has increased.[44] The oxygen-enriched and/or nitrous oxide–enriched atmosphere created in the oropharynx will readily support combustion of flammable materials such as an endotracheal tube. For this reason several precautions must be undertaken to ensure patient and personnel safety. It is important to realize that there are different types of lasers that produce varying degrees of energy.[45] This energy will determine how much time is necessary to ignite an object, which also depends on the material of which it is made. First, the lowest possible concentration of oxygen should be used (21–40% FiO_2) that will maintain adequate oxygen saturation. Next, the placement of an endotracheal tube constructed of materials with a high ignition point, or a tube wrapped with reflective material to reduce the amount of energy absorbed, is advantageous. Placement in the area surrounding the surgical field of saline-soaked pads will also help dissipate excess heat energy as well as any misdirected laser bursts. Limiting the bursts to a short duration and filling the endotracheal tube cuff with methylene-blue-colored saline will help to reduce the risk of an airway fire.[46] Should an airway fire become a reality, it is recommended that the endotracheal tube be immediately removed, any additional burning material extinguished and removed from the airway, and the patient reintubated. A protocol should be devised and readily available to deal with such emergencies.[47]

CONCLUSION

Anesthesia for head and neck surgery may provide some of the most challenging and stressful moments in the operating room. Although many of the procedures may be considered "minor" because they do not involve the major organs or cavities of the body, the access required and manipulation of the airway constantly test the limits of an anesthesiologist's ability to foresee and prevent potentially serious complications. It is, therefore, of supreme importance that the anesthesiologist and otolaryngologist work in tandem to ensure a successful outcome.

References

1. Strichartz GR, Covino BG. Local anesthetics. In Miller RD, ed. *Anesthesia*, 3rd ed. New York: Churchill Livingstone, 1990, 437.

2. Ritchie JM. Mechanism of action of local anesthetic agents and biotoxins. *Br J Anaesth.* 1975; 47:191.

3. Taylor RE. Effect of procaine on electrical properties of squid axon membrane. *Am J Physiol.* 1959;196:1071.

4. Hille B. The common mode of action of three agents that decrease the transient change in sodium permeability in nerves. *Nature.* 1966; 210:1220.

5. Strichartz GR, Covino BG. Local anesthetics. In Miller RD, ed. *Anesthesia,* 3rd ed. New York: Churchill Livingstone, 1990, 438.

6. Strichartz GR, Covino BG. Local anesthetics. In Miller RD, ed. *Anesthesia,* 3rd ed. New York: Churchill Livingstone, 1990, 438–440.

7. Stoelting RK. Local anesthetics. In *Pharmacology and Physiology in Anesthesia Pratice,* 2nd ed. Philadelphia: Lippincott, 1992, 150.

8. Aldrete AJ, Johnson DA. Allergy to local anesthetics. *JAMA.* 1969;207:356.

9. Nagel JE, Fuscaldo JT, Fireman P. Paraben allergy. *JAMA.* 1977;237:1594.

10. Aldrete JA, Johnson DA. Evaluation of intracutaneous testing for investigation of allergy to local anesthetic agents. *Anesth Analg.* 1970;49:173.

11. Adriani J. Reactions to local anesthetics. *JAMA.* 1966;196:119.

12. Brown DJ, Beamish D, Wildsmith JAW. Allergic reaction to an amide local anesthetic. *Br J Anaesth.* 1981;53:435.

13. Incaudo G, Schatz M, Patterson R, et al. Administration of local anesthetics to patients with a history of prior adverse reaction. *J Allerg Clin Immunol.* 1978;61:339.

14. Liu PL, Feldmen HS, Giasi R, et al. Comparative CNS toxicity of lidocaine, etidocaine, bupivacaine and tetracaine in awake dogs following rapid IV administration. *Anesth Analg.* 1983; 62:375.

15. Wagman IH, deJong RH, Prince DA. Effects of lidocaine on the central nervous system. *Anesthesiology.* 1967;28:155.

16. deJong RH, Robles R, Corbin RW. Central actions of lidocaine-synaptic transmission. *Anesthesiology.* 1969;30:19.

17. Block A, Covino BG: Effect of local agents on cardiac conduction and contractility. *Reg Anaesth.* 1981;6:55.

18. deJong RH, Ronfeld RA, DeRosa R. Cardiovascular effects of convulsant and supraconvulsant doses of amide local anesthetics. *Anesth Analg.* 1982;61:3.

19. Morishima HO, Pederson H, Finster M, et al. Bupivacaine toxicity in pregnant and nonpregnant ewes. *Anesthesiology.* 1985;63:134.

20. Moore S, Bridenbaugh LD. Oxygen: The antidote for systemic toxic reactions from local anesthetic drugs. *JAMA.* 1960;174:842.

21. Strichartz GR, Covino BJ. Local anesthetics. In Miller RD, ed. *Anesthesia*, 3rd ed. New York: Churchill Livingstone, 1990, 465.

22. Fisher MMcD. Intradermal testing in the diagnosis of acute anaphylaxis during anesthesia—Results of five years experience. *Anesth Intensive Care.* 1979;7:58.

23. Climie CR, McLean S, Starmer GA, et al. Methaemoglobinemia in mother and foetus following continuous epidural analgesia with prilocaine. *Br J Anaesth.* 1967;39:155.

24. Lund PC, Cwik PC. Propitocaine (Citanest) and methemoglobinemia. *Anesthesiology.* 1965;26: 569.

25. Bull CS. The hydrochlorate of cocaine as a local anaesthetic in ophthalmic surgery. *N Y Med J.* 1884;40:609.

26. Covino BG. Clinical pharmacology of local anesthetic agents. In Cousins MJ, Bridenbaugh PO, eds. *Neural Blockade in Clinical Anesthesia and Management of Pain*, 2nd ed. Philadelphia: Lippincott, 1988, 137.

27. Evers H, VonDardel O, Juhlin L. Dermal effects of compositions based on the eutectic mixture of

lignocaine and prilocaine (EMLA). *Br J Anaesth.* 1985;57:997.

28. Hallen B, Uppfeldt A. Does lidocaine-prilocaine cream permit pain-free insertion of IV catheters in children? *Anesthesiology.* 1982;57:340.

29. Ohlsen L, Englesson S, Evers H. An anaesthetic lidocaine/prilocaine cream (EMLA) for epicutaneous application tested for split skin grafts. *Scand J Plast Reconstr Surg.* 1985;19:201.

30. Covino BG. Clinical pharmacology of local anesthetic agents. In Cousins MJ, Bridenbaugh PO, eds. *Neural Blockade in Clinical Anesthesia and Management of Pain*, 2nd ed. Philadelphia: Lippincott, 1992, 139.

31. Moyers JR. Preoperative medication. In Barash PG, Cullen BF, Stoelting RK, eds., *Clinical Anesthesia*, 2nd ed. Philadelphia: Lippincott, 1992.

32. Kantor GSA. Flumazenil: A review for clinicians. *Am J Anesth.* 1997;26:2.

33. Glass PSA, Hardman D, Kamiyama Y, et al. Preliminary pharmacology and pharmacodynamics of an ultra-short opioid: Remifentanil (GI87084B). *Anesth Analg.* 1993; 77:1031–1040.

34. Egan TD. The clinical pharmacology of the new fentanyl congeners. IARS 1997 Review Course Lectures.

35. Egan TD, Gupta SK, Sperry RJ, et al. The pharmacokinetics of remifentanil in obese versus lean elective surgery patients. *Anesth Analg.* 1996; 82:S100.

36. Egan TD: Remifentanil pharmacokinetics and pharmacodynamics: A preliminary proposal. *Clin Pharmacokinet.* 1995;29: 80–94.

37. Bennett CR. *Conscious Sedation in Dental Practice,* 2nd ed. St. Louis: CV Mosby, 1978, 12.

38. Wetchler BV. Outpatient anesthesia. In Barash PG, Cullen BF, Stoelting RK, eds. *Clinical Anesthesia*. Philadelphia: Lippincott, 1989, 1347–1348.

39. Gibbs CP, Modell JH. Management of aspiration pneumonitis. In Miller RD, ed. *Anesthesia*, 3rd ed. New York: Churchill Livingstone, 1990, 1297.

40. Moore M, Weiskopf RB, Eger EI II. Arrhythmogenic doses of epinephrine are similar during desflurane or isoflurane anesthesia in humans. *Anesthesiology.* 1993;79:943–947.

41. Eger EI II. New inhaled anesthetics: Sevoflurane and desflurane. IARS 1997 Review Course Lectures, p 39.

42. Denborough MA. The pathopharmacology of malignant hyperpyrexia. *Pharmacol Ther.* 1980; 9:357.

43. Casey WF, Drake-Lee AB. Nitrous oxide and middle ear pressure. *Anesthesia.* 1982;37:896.

44. Bailey MK, Bromley HR, Allison JG, et al. Electrocautery-induced airway fire during tracheostomy. *Anesth Analg.* 1990;71:702.

45. Cork RC. Anesthesia for otolaryngologic surgery involving use of a laser. In Brown BR, ed. *Anesthesia and ENT Surgery—Contempory Anesthesia Practice*. Philadelphia: FA Davis Co., 1987.

46. Fried M. A survey of the complication of laser microlaryngoscopy. *Arch Otolaryngol.* 1984; 110:31.

47. Fein A, Leff A, Hopewell PC. Pathophysiology and management of the complications resulting from fire and the inhaled products of combustion. *Crit Care Med.* 1980;8:94.

Head and 37
Neck Radiology

Radiographic examination of the head and neck region will be divided into two categories:

1. Conventional radiography
2. Cross-sectional anatomy and imaging, which will include both computed tomography (CT) and magnetic resonance imaging (MRI)

CONVENTIONAL RADIOGRAPHY

The radiographic views to delineate the skull anatomy are described in other chapters. Table 37-1 summarizes the best view to visualize the skull base foramina and describes the content of the foramina.

Transorbital View

The transorbital view (Figure 37-1) is obtained with the patient's occiput to the film to magnify the orbit. The chin is slightly flexed until the orbitomeatal line is perpendicular to the film.[2,3]

In this view the petrous pyramid, especially the internal auditory canal, is clearly visualized through the radiolucency of the orbit. It also shows the cochlea, vestibule, and semicircular canals[7,8] (Figure 37-2).

Towne's View

Towne's view (Figure 37-3) is the anteroposterior projection with a 30° tilt (from "above and in front"). This view allows comparison of both petrous pyramids and mastoids on the same film. The petrous apex, internal auditory canals, arcuate eminence, mastoid, antrum, and mastoid process can be clearly identified. This view is useful for evaluation of apical petrositis, acoustic neuroma, and cerebellopontine angle tumor (Figure 37-4).[3,5,7,8]

Waters' View (Occipitomental, "Chin-Nose" Position)

This posteroanterior occipitomental projection is taken with the patient's head tilted upward so that the nose and chin are against the film surface (Figure 37-5). The petrous portion of the temporal bone is projected below the level of the maxillary sinus.[3]

The maxillary sinuses are best shown in this view, followed by the frontal sinuses. The ethmoid sinuses are not well shown. A good view of the sphenoid sinus and its septum is obtained through the open mouth (Figure 37-6).

This view also shows such maxillofacial structures as nasal bones, frontal process of the maxilla, zygomatic arch, and the mandible (especially the coronoid process).

Other structures to be recognized include the oblique orbital line, the rim and floor of the orbit, superior orbital fissure (cranial nerves III, IV, V_1, VI; ophthalmic vein), foramen

TABLE 37-1. FORAMINA IN BASE OF SKULL

Foramina	Contents	Best View
Anterior Cranial Fossa		
Foramen cecum	Emissary vein from nose to superior sagittal sinus	—
Anterior ethmoidal foramen	1. Anterior ethmoid vessels	Lateral
	2. Nasociliary nerve	
Foramina in cribriform plate	Olfactory nerves	—
Posterior ethmoidal foramen	Posterior ethmoidal vessels and nerves	Lateral
Middle Cranial Fossa		
Superior orbital fissure	1. Ophthalmic vein	1. Caldwell's
	2. Orbital branch of middle meningeal artery	2. Waters'
	3. Oculomotor nerve (III)	
	4. Trochlear nerve (IV)	
	5. Ophthalmic division of trigeminal nerve (V)	
	6. Abducens nerve (VI)	
	7. Recurrent branch of lacrimal artery	
Optic foramen	1. Optic nerve	Oblique orbital
	2. Ophthalmic artery	(Rhese)
Foramen rotundum	Maxillary division of trigeminal nerve (V)	1. Caldwell's
		2. Waters'
Foramen ovale	Mandibular division of trigeminal nerve (V)	1. Base
	Acessory meningeal artery	2. Waters'
Foramen lacerum (carotid canal)	1. Internal carotid artery	
	2. Sympathetic carotid plexus	
	3. Superficial petrosal nerve	Base
	4. Vidian nerve	
	5. Meningeal branch of ascending pharyngeal artery	
Foramen spinosum	1. Middle meningeal artery	Base
	2. Recurrent branch of mandibular nerve	
Posterior Cranial Fossa		
Internal auditory canal	1. Facial nerve (VII)	1. Transorbital
	2. Auditory nerve (VIII)	2. Towne's
	3. Internal auditory vessels	3. Base
Jugular foramen	1. Internal jugular vein	
	2. Inferior petrosal sinus	
	3. Meningeal branch from occipital and ascending pharyngeal arteries	1. Base
		2. Towne's
	4. Glossopharyngeal nerve (IX)	
	5. Vagus nerve (X)	
	6. Spinal accessory nerve (XI)	
Stylomastoid foramen	1. Facial nerve (VII)	Base
	2. Stylomastoid artery	
Hypoglossal canal	1. Hypoglossal nerve (XII)	Towne's
	2. Meningeal branch of ascending pharyngeal artery	
	3. Emissary vein from transverse sinus	
Foramen magnum	1. Medulla oblongata and spinal cord	
	2. Spinal accessory nerve	1. Base
	3. Vertebral arteries	2. Towne's
	4. Anterior and posterior spinal arteries	
	5. Membrana tectoria	
	6. Apical alignment	

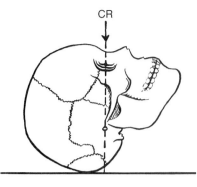

Figure 37-1. Position of the skull for temporal bone x-ray films: Transorbital view.

rotundum (V_2 maxillary nerve), foramen ovale (V_3 mandibular nerve), zygomaticofacial foramen, infraorbital foramen, nasal ala, and upper lip.

Lateral View

In this view (Figure 37-7) the sphenoid sinuses are shown to best advantage, followed by the frontal, ethmoidal, and maxillary sinuses, in that order (Figure 37-8).

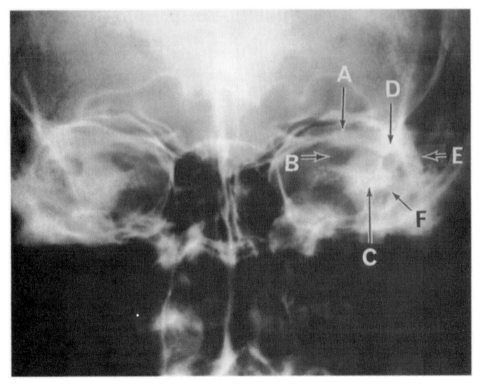

Figure 37-2. Transorbital view. (A, petrous pyramid; B, internal auditory canal; C, cochlea; D, vestibule; E, horizontal semicircular canal; F, promontory.)

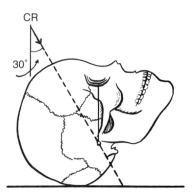

Figure 37-3. Position of the skull for temporal bone x-ray films: Towne's view.

The view also shows such maxillofacial structures as nasal bones, frontal sinus walls, the zygomatic process of the maxilla, the posterior wall of the maxillary sinus, the pterygoid plates, and the mandible. Other structures to be recognized in this view include anterior walls of the middle cranial fossa, roof of the sphenoid sinus, cribriform plate, inferior turbinate, coronoid process of the mandible, zygomatic recess, pterygomaxillary fissure, caroticoclinoid foramen, carotid sulcus, and soft tissues (tonsils, adenoids, earlobe, soft palate, and base of the tongue).[9–11]

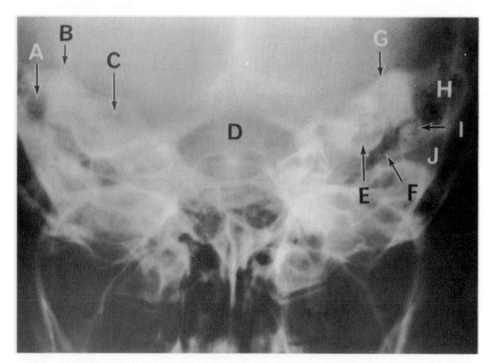

Figure 37-4. Towne's view. (A, antrum; B, arcuate eminence; C, internal auditory canal; D, foramen magnum; E, cochlea; F, tympanic cavity; G, superior semicircular canal; H, mastoid cells; I, ossicular mass; J, external auditory canal.)

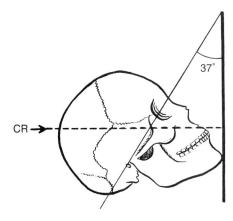

Figure 37-5.   Position of the skull for sinus x-ray films: Waters' view.

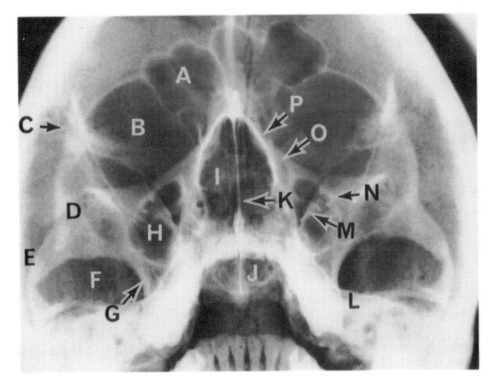

Figure 37-6.   Waters' view. (A, frontal sinus; B, orbit; C, zygomaticofrontal suture; D, zygoma; E, zygomatic arch; F, infratemporal fossa; G, maxilla; H, maxillary sinus; I, nasal cavity; J, sphenoid sinus; K, septum; L, petrous ridge; M, superior orbital fissure; N, infraorbital foramen; O, frontal process of maxilla; P, nasal bone.)

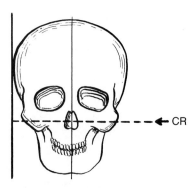

Figure 37-7. Position of the skull for sinus x-ray films: Lateral view.

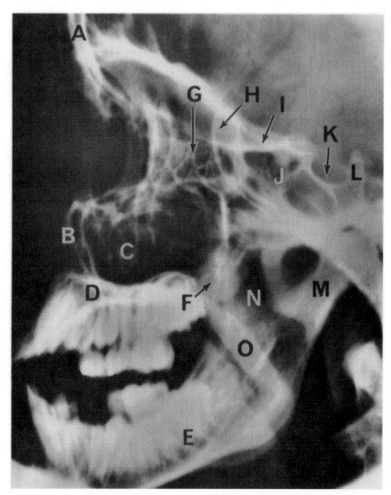

Figure 37-8. Lateral view. (A, frontal bone; B, anterior wall of maxillary sinus; C, maxillary sinus; D, alveolar process of maxilla; E, mandible; F, posterior end of inferior turbinate; G, ethmoid sinuses; H, anterior wall of middle cranial fossa; I, roof of sphenoid sinus; J, sphenoid sinus; K, sella turcica; L, posterior clinoid process; M, condyle of mandible; N, nasopharynx; O, soft palate.)

Submentovertical View (Basal or Base View)

This view (Figure 37-9) is obtained by passing x-rays at right angles through the base of the skull with the orbitomeatal line perpendicular to the central ray. In this view the sphenoid sinuses are shown best, followed by the posterior ethmoidal, maxillary, and frontal sinuses, in that order (Figure 37-10).[3]

The view shows such maxillofacial structures as the zygomatic arch, body of the zygoma, and mandible (especially the condyle).

Other structures to be recognized include pneumatization of the pterygoid process and the greater wing of the sphenoid; the lateral three lines, which include (1) the orbital line (a straight line formed by the lateral wall of the orbit), (2) the antral line (an S-shaped line formed by the lateral wall of the antrum), and (3) the middle cranial fossa line (a C-shaped curve with concavity backward formed by the anterior wall of the middle cranial fossa); the pterygoid plate and pterygoalar bar; nasal cavity; lacrimal canal; incisive foramen; greater and lesser palatine foramina; inferior orbital fissure; choana; foramen ovale (V_3 mandibular nerve); foramen spinosum (middle meningeal artery); foramen lacerum; carotid canals; eustachian tube; internal and external auditory canals and jugular foramen; and soft tissues (nasal turbinates, adenoids, uvula, lateral wall of the nasopharynx, and membranous external auditory canal).[7–9,12–15]

Caldwell View ("Forehead-Nose" Position)

The Caldwell view (Figure 37-11) is obtained by positioning the nose and forehead against the cassette with the external auditory meatus and outer canthus of the eye forming a line perpendicular to the cassette. The x-ray tube is tilted caudally 15 to 20°.[3]

In this view the frontal sinuses are best shown. The ethmoidal sinuses, particularly the orbital margin (lamina papyracea), are also well shown. The main cavity and lateral extensions of the sphenoid sinuses are recognizable. The posteromedial and inferolateral portions of the maxillary sinuses are usually visible (Figure 37-12).

The view shows such maxillofacial structures as the orbital margins, zygoma, zygomaticofrontal suture, maxilla, and mandible.

Other structures to be recognized include the nasal cavity and its contents, floor and rim of the orbit, infraorbital canal, superior orbital fissure, supraorbital foramen, Hyrtl's foramen (opthalmomeningeal vein), lambdoidal suture, foramen rotundum (always inferolateral to the lowermost portion of the superior orbital fissure), and soft tissues (palpebral fissures and "ponytail" hairstyle).[10,11]

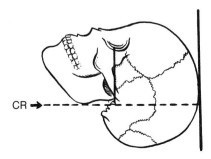

CR ➤

Figure 37-9. Position of the skull for sinus x-ray films. Submentovertical view.

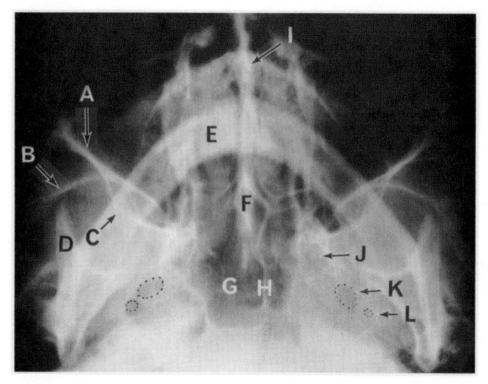

Figure 37-10. Submentovertical view. (A, lateral wall of orbit; B, anterior wall of middle cranial fossa; C, posterolateral wall of antrum; D, coronoid process of mandible; E, body of mandible; F, vomer; G, sphenoid sinus; H, intraseptum of sphenoid sinus; I, nasal septum; J, pneumatized pterygoid process; K, foramen ovale; L, foramen spinosum.)

Larynx and Neck

Radiographic examination of the larynx consists of anteroposterior (AP) and lateral views.[1,4,8]

Anteroposterior View

The AP view is of limited value for evaluation of the larynx itself because of the superimposition of the cervical spine. However, masses of the neck lateral to the larynx and distortion

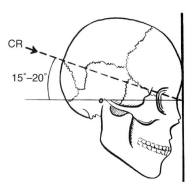

Figure 37-11. Position of the skull for sinus x-ray films. Caldwell's view.

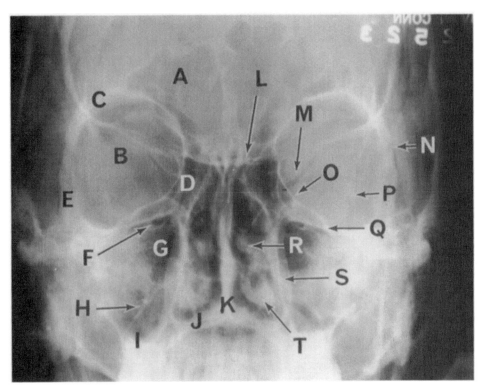

Figure 37-12. Caldwell's view. (A, frontal sinus; B, orbit; C, superior orbital margin; D, ethmoid sinus; E, frontal process of zygoma; F, foramen rotundum; G, pneumatized pterygoid process; H, lateral pterygoid plate; I, floor of maxillary sinus; J, floor of nasal sinus; K, nasal septum; L, limbus sphenoidalis; M, superior orbital fissure; N, frontozygomatic suture; O, lamina papyracea; P, oblique orbital line; Q, floor of orbit; R, middle turbinate; S, lateral wall of nasal cavity; T, inferior turbinate.)

and/or displacement of the upper airway are shown. Narrowing of the subglottic airway is visible.

Lateral View

The lateral view is of greater value and shows the outline of the base of the tongue and epiglottis, the vallecula, hyoid, aryepiglottic folds and arytenoids, ventricles, thyroid and cricoid cartilages, subglottic space, and prevertebral soft tissues (Figure 37-13). This view is useful for evaluation of tumors and fractures of the larynx; a foreign body in the larynx, hypopharynx, or upper esophagus; detection of calcification of normal and abnormal tissues; and evaluation of acute inflammatory conditions such as acute epiglottitis and retropharyngeal abscess. It also is useful for pre- and postoperative evaluation of a thyrotomy and tracheotomy. The accuracy of the stent or mold placement for a fractured larynx is also determined in this view.

Differential diagnosis of a foreign body in the larynx, hypopharynx, and upper esophagus includes:

1. Sialolith
2. Tracheal rings

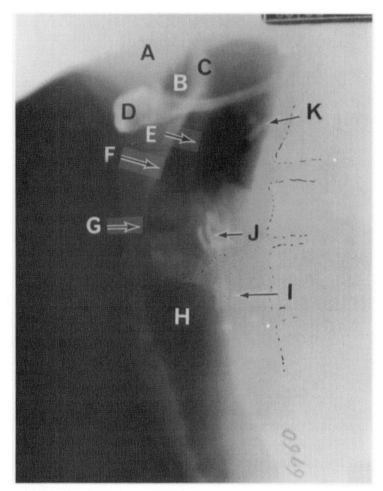

Figure 37-13.   Lateral view of the larynx. (A, base of tongue; B, vallecula; C, tip of epiglottis; D, hyoid bone; E, aryepiglottic fold; F, laryngeal surface of epiglottis; G, ventricle; H, trachea; I, inferior cornu of thyroid cartilage; J, calcified arytenoid cartilages; K, cartilago triticea.

3. Osteophytes of the cervical spine
4. Calcareous streaks in scar tissues
5. Ossification centers of the hyoid bone
6. Calcified cervical nodes
7. Residual dye from arteriography
8. Calcification in the laryngeal cartilages
9. Accessory ossification centers in the cervical spine
10. Calcified stylohyoid ligaments
11. Sesamoid laryngeal cartilages
12. Calcification in the vessels of the neck

Facial Bone Injuries

For the evaluation of the nasal bones, the right and left lateral, superoinferior axial occlusal, and Waters' views are usually taken. Lateral views reveal depression or elevation of nasal bone fragments, whereas superoinferior axial views show medial or lateral displacements of nasal fractures. The Waters' view also shows fracture and displacement of each nasal bone and the frontal process of the maxilla.[16]

A facial bone series should include, in addition to the four standard sinus projections, an underexposed submentovertical view of the zygomatic arches and the exaggerated Waters' view to demonstrate fracture of the infraorbital rim and fracture dislocation of the zygoma and zygomatic arch.[1,6,8,16–18]

CROSS-SECTIONAL ANATOMY

Computed tomography and MRI have revolutionized head and neck imaging. Their cross-sectional display of anatomy added new dimensions in the diagnostic workup. Knowledge of the anatomic spaces and their appearance in cross section is of paramount importance in the differential approach and understanding of head and neck disease. It is convenient to subdivide the neck into a suprahyoid and infrahyoid neck.

Suprahyoid Neck

Mucosal Space of the Nasopharynx

The nasopharynx stretches from the skull base to the hard and soft palate and is anteriorly bordered by the nasal choanae and posteriorly by the first two cervical vertebrae.[19] The mucosal space contains the mucosa (squamous and columnar epithelium), minor salivary glands, lymphoid tissue of the adenoids within the pharyngobasilar fascia, superior and middle constrictor muscles, levator veli palatini, torus tubarius, and fossa of Rosenmüller. The pharyngobasilar fascia serves as attachment of the constrictor muscles and therefore forms the outer border of the nasopharynx. The torus tubarius contains the orifice of the eustachian tube and therefore connects the nasopharynx with the middle ear (Table 37-2).

Parapharyngeal Space

The parapharyngeal space is a fat space located lateral to the mucosal space, medial to the masticator and parotid space, and anterior to the carotid space. Its inferior extent reaches to the submandibular gland and its upper extent to the base of the skull. The parapharyngeal space primarily contains fat. The third division of the trigeminal nerve enters the parapharyngeal space superiorly. The internal maxillary artery and parapharyngeal veins are the major vascular components in the parapharyngeal space. Salivary gland remnants occur in the parapharyngeal space. The parapharyngeal space serves as a major indicator for the origin of masses. Lesions arising within the parapharyngeal space widen the space, whereas adjacent lesions compress it.[1,20] Parotid lesions would compress the parapharyngeal space from the lateral aspect; lesions in the nasopharyngeal mucosal space from the medial aspect. Masticator space lesions impinge on the parapharyngeal space anteriorly; carotid space lesions posteriorly (Table 37-2; Figure 37-14).

Masticator Space

The masticator space is anterior and lateral to the parapharyngeal space. It extends from the insertion of the temporalis muscle (temporal fossa) at the calvarium to the mandible.

TABLE 37-2. ANATOMIC SPACE, ANATOMIC CONTENTS, AND PATHOLOGY OF THE SUPRAHYOID NECK

Anatomic Space and Contents	Pathology/Significance
Mucosal Space Nasopharynx	
Superior and middle constrictor muscle	Barrier to spread of tumor
Pharyngobasilar fascia	
Sinus Morgagni	Levator veli palatini and eustachian tube enter into nasopharynx; weak spot for spread of tumor
	Benign:
Tornwaldt cyst	Midline cyst
Adenoids	Hypertrophy infancy and adolescence, AIDS
Encephalocele	Dysraphism
Minor salivary gland	Ranula, benign mixed tumor
	Malignant:
Mucosa, minor salivary glands, torus tubarius	Squamous carcinoma (90%), adenoid cystic carcinoma (10%)
Lymphoid tissue	Non-Hodgkin's lymphoma
Torus tubarius	Obstruction by nasopharyngeal carcinoma leading to middle ear effusion and mastoiditis
Parapharyngeal Space	
	Benign
Salivary gland remnant, fat	Pleomorphic adenoma, lipoma
	Malignant
	Mucoepidermoid carcinoma, adenoid cystic carcinoma, direct spread of tumor into adjacent spaces
Trigeminal nerve (3rd portion)	Neurinoma, schwannoma
Atypical branchial cleft	Cyst, infected branchial cleft cyst
Maxillary artery, ascending pharyngeal artery	Traumatic aneurysm
Masticator Space	
	Congenital
	Hemangioma, lymphangioma
	Benign
	Leiomyoma
	Malignant
	Non-Hodgkin's lymphoma, invasion of squamous cell carcinoma from oral cavity retromolar trigone, anterior tonsillar pillar
Medial and lateral pterygoid muscle	Rhabdomyosarcoma
Masseter muscle, temporalis muscle	
Trigeminal nerve (3rd portion)	Neurinoma, schwannoma, malignant schwannoma
	Infection
Mandible	Odontogenic infection spreading throughout masticator space, subtemporal abscess
	Malignant
	Chondrosarcoma, osteosarcoma, squamous cell carcinoma from oropharynx (retromolar trigone)
Oral Cavity and Related Spaces:	**Congenital**
Sublingual Space	Hemangioma, lymphangioma, cystic hygroma, epidermoid, dermoid, lingual thyroid
	Infectious
Sublingual gland, deep submandibular gland	Ludwig's angina, ranula, abscess
	Benign
	Benign mixed tumor
	Malignant
	Mucoepidermoid carcinoma, adenoid cystic carcinoma
Submandibular gland	Stone with resulting sialadenitis or abscess
Hypoglossal muscle of tongue	**Benign**
	Pseudotumor secondary to twelfth nerve palsy
	Malignant
	Squamous cell carcinoma
Neurovascular pedicle tongue	Important route of spread of tumor

TABLE 37-2. *Continued*

Anatomic Space and Contents	Pathology/Significance
Submandibular Space	**Congenital**
	Second branchial cleft cyst, suprahyoid thyroglossal duct cyst
Submandibular gland superior portion	**Benign**
	Pleomorphic adenoma, ranula, epidermoid, dermoid, lipoma
	Malignant
	Adenoid cystic carcinoma, mucoepidermoid carcinoma, adenocarcinoma, squamous cell carcinoma
Submandibular nodes	Drainage oral cavity, submandibular gland, lymphoma
Hypoglossal nerve inferior loop	Neurinoma, schwannoma
Oropharynx	**Malignant**
Tongue base/vallecula	Squamous cell carcinoma
Palatine tonsils, lingual tonsils	**Infectious**
	Tonsillitis, tonsillar abscess
	Malignant
Retromolar trigone	Squamous cell carcinoma, lymphoma
Parotid Space	**Congenital**
	Branchial cleft cyst type I
Facial nerve	Neuroma, schwannoma, neurogenic spread of tumor
Retromandibular vein, external carotid artery	Marker for deep and superficial lobe of parotid
Parotid gland	**Inflammatory**
	Sjögren's syndrome, abscess, sarcoid
	Benign
	Pleomorphic adenoma, Warthin's tumor
	Malignant
	Mucoepidermoid tumor, adenoid cystic carcinoma, acinic cell carcinoma, adenocarcinoma, carcinoma ex pleomorphic adenoma, malignant mixed tumor, squamous cell carcinoma, lymphoepithelial cysts (AIDS)
Carotid Space	
Internal carotid	Aneurysm, dissection, glomus tumor
Internal jugular vein	Jugular vein thrombosis
Cranial nerves IX to XI	Neurinoma, schwannoma, paraganglioma
Sympathetic plexus	Paraganglioma
Lymph nodes (deep cervical chain)	Reactive and metastatic, non-Hodgkin's lymphoma
Retropharyngeal Space	
Fat	Retropharyngeal abscess
Medial retropharyngeal nodes	Enlargement most commonly seen in neonates and young children
Lateral retropharyngeal nodes	Drainage for nasopharynx, posterior oropharynx, paranasal sinuses, middle ear, postpalate and nasal cavity
Prevertebral Space	
Anterior prevertebral space proper	Space of spread for prevertebral abscesses
Pre- and paravertebral muscles, scalene muscles	
Vertebral artery and vein	Aneurysm, AV fistula
Brachial plexus, phrenic nerve	Neurinoma, schwannoma

Adapted from Hudgins PA. The nasopharynx and related spaces. *ASHNR 26th Annual Conference and Postgraduate Course.* Vancouver: ASHNR, 1993, 73–80.

It contains the mandible and masticator muscles (masseter, temporalis, medial and lateral pterygoid muscles). The masticator space contains the third portion of cranial nerve V, which enters the space via the foramen ovale, connecting the masticator space to the cavernous sinus. The inferior alveolar nerve is a branch of the third portion of the trigeminal nerve. It is in close proximity to the alveolar artery and vein (Table 37-2; Figures 37-14 and 37-15).

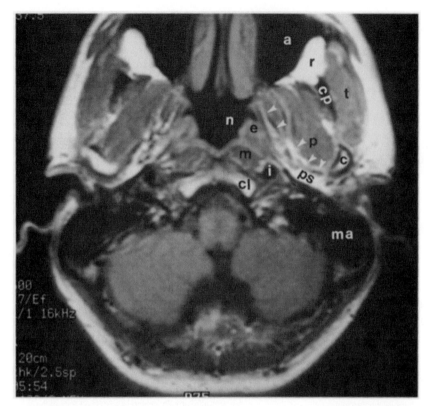

Figure 37-14. Normal nasopharyngeal space, masseteric space, and sinuses. Axial T_1W MRI. Arrowheads indicate nasopharyngeal space, (cl, clivus; m, longus colli muscle; e, torus tubarius; n, nasopharynx; ps, nasopharyngeal space; p, medial pterygoid muscle; c, mandibular condyle; t, temporalis muscle; r, retromaxillary fat space; a, antrum; ma, mastoids; i, internal carotid; cp, coronary process of mandible.)

Carotid Space

The carotid space is medial to the deep lobe of the parotid and posterior to the parapharyngeal space. It extends from the skull base at the carotid foramen and jugular foramen to the aortic arch. It contains the internal carotid artery, jugular vein, and cranial nerves IX to XII at the level of the nasopharynx. The vagus nerve continues in the carotid space to the aortic arch. The sympathetic plexus and the deep cervical lymph nodes are part of the carotid space (see Table 37-2).

Retropharyngeal Space

The retropharyngeal space is a potential midline space formed by the middle and deep layers of the deep cervical fascia. It is anterior to the prevertebral space, posterior to the nasopharyngeal mucosal space, and medial to the carotid space. It extends from the base of the skull at the clivus to the T4 vertebral body. The retropharyngeal space has only a few contents, as it is primarily a potential space. It therefore contains only fat and, above the hyoid bone, the medial and lateral retropharyngeal nodes (see Table 37-2).

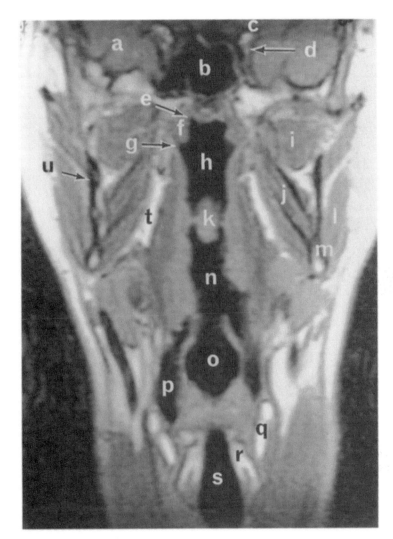

Figure 37-15.   Coronal MR image of the neck to demonstrate normal anatomy of the pharynx; larynx, and related structures. (a, temporal lobe; b, sphenoid sinus; c, lesser wings of
sphenoid; d, cavernous sinus; e, fossa of Rosenmüller; f, torus tubarius;
g, eustachian tube orifice; h, nasopharynx; i, lateral pterygoid muscle; j, medial pterygoid muscle with fascial planes; k, uvula; i, masseter; m, mandible; n, oropharynx;
o, supraglottis; p, pyriform sinus; q, thyroid cartilage; r, cricoid cartilage; s, subglottis;
t, parapharyngeal space; u, pterygomandibular space.)

Prevertebral Space

The prevertebral space extends from the skull base at the clivus to about the vertebral body.
It lies behind the retropharyngeal space, posteromedial to the carotid space, and medial to
the posterior cervical space. It contains the vertebral artery and vein, and the prevertebral,
paraspinal, and scalene muscles. It also contains the vertebral bodies with the brachial

plexus and phrenic nerve along the anterior scalene muscle and the sympathetic trunk anterior to the prevertebral muscles. Between the retropharyngeal space and prevertebral space is another potential space known as the *danger space.* It is formed by two leaves of the deep layer of the deep cervical fascia. It cannot be visualized by imaging methods, but reaches deeper into the mediastinum than the retropharyngeal space (see Table 37-2; Figure 37-16).

Sublingual and Submandibular Space

The sublingual space is located superomedial to the mylohyoid muscle in the oral cavity lateral to the geniohyoid and genioglossus complex. It contains the anterior hyoglossus muscle, lingual nerve, and lingual artery and vein, forming the neurovascular pedicle to the tongue, deep portion of the submandibular gland, and submandibular gland duct (Wharton's duct) as well as the sublingual glands and ducts. Posteriorly the sublingual space is in open connection to the submandibular space around the free edge of the mylohyoid muscle.

The submandibular space is located inferolaterally to the mylohyoid muscle and superior to the hyoid bone. It contains the anterior belly of the digastric muscle, superficial portion of the submandibular gland, submandibular lymph nodes, facial vein and artery, and inferior loop of the hypoglossal nerve. Superiorly the submandibular space borders the inferior nasoparapharyngeal space (see Table 37-2; Figure 37-15).

Parotid Space

The parotid space is lateral to the parapharyngeal space and behind the masticator space and mandible. It is lateral to the carotid space and contains the parotid gland, retromandibular vein, and external carotid artery (see Table 37-2).

Oropharynx

The oropharynx includes the tongue base, tonsillar fossa and tonsillar pillars, soft palate, and a portion of the posterior pharyngeal wall between the pharyngoepiglottic folds and the nasopharynx (Table 37-2; Figure 37-16).

Infrahyoid Neck

The infrahyoid neck is traditionally divided into triangles. The major division is the anterior and posterior triangle separated by the sternocleidomastoid muscle. Suprahyoid and infrahyoid compartments are differentiated.

The posterior belly of the digastric muscle superiorly, the sternocleidomastoid muscle anteriorly, and the omohyoid muscle medially and inferiorly form the carotid triangle.

Medial to the sternocleidomastoid muscle and omohyoid muscle is the muscular triangle.

The infrahyoid posterior triangle is subdivided into an occipital triangle formed by the sternocleidomastoid muscle anteriorly, omohyoid muscle inferiorly, and trapezius muscle posteriorly.

Inferior to the occipital triangle is the subclavian triangle, formed by the sternocleidomastoid muscle medially, omohyoid muscle superiorly, and clavicle inferiorly.

These traditional triangles are not well suited for cross-sectional imaging, and therefore a space-oriented approach is preferred. The superficial cervical fascia completely surrounds the neck containing the cutaneous structures and platysma. There are three layers of the deep cervical fascia cleaving the infrahyoid neck.[21,22]

- *Superficial (investing) layer:* Encloses the sternocleidomastoid, trapezius, and inferior omohyoid muscles, surrounding them by a fascial sling. It also contributes to the carotid sheath.

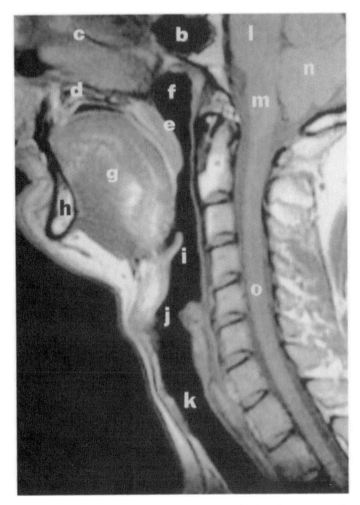

Figure 37-16.   Sagittal MR image of the pharynx, larynx, and related structures. (b, sphenoid sinus; c, turbinates, middle and inferior; d, hard palate; e, soft palate; f, nasopharynx; g, tongue; h, mandible; i, epiglottis; j, larynx; k, trachea; l, pons; m, medulla; n, cerebellum (vermis); o, spinal cord.)

- *Middle (visceral) layer:* The fascia envelopes the anterior infrahyoid strap muscles, and encircles the thyroid and parathyroid glands, larynx, trachea, esophagus, recurrent laryngeal nerves, and paraesophageal nodes.
- *Deep (prevertebral) layer:* The fascia encircles the prevertebral and paravertebral musculature, phrenic nerve, cervical plexus, vertebrae, and vertebral arteries and veins.[21,22]

Superficial Space

The superficial space lies between the superficial cervical fascia and the superficial layer of the deep cervical fascia. It extends from the skull base, mastoids, and mandible to the mediastinum. It contains the platysma, sternocleidomastoid muscle, trapezius, and inferior belly of the omohyoid muscles. Lymph nodes and the external jugular vein are in this space.

Visceral Space

The visceral space is formed by the middle layer of the deep cervical fascia. The space contains the thyroid and parathyroid glands, larynx, pharynx, trachea, esophagus, recurrent laryngeal nerves, juxtavisceral lymph node chain, and infrahyoid strap muscles.

Posterior Cervical Space

The posterior cervical space is not a fascially defined space. It is bordered anteriorly by the carotid space and medially by the deep layer of the deep cervical fascia enveloping the paravertebral and scalene muscles. Posterolaterally the space is bordered by the superficial layer of the deep cervical fascia enveloping the sternocleidomastoid muscle. The space extends from the skull base to the clavicle. It contains fat, the spinal accessory lymph node chain, spinal accessory nerve, preaxillary brachial plexus, and dorsal scapular nerves and arteries.

Anterior Cervical Space

The anterior cervical space also has complex fascial boundaries. Anteromedially the anterior cervical space is bordered by the middle layer of the deep cervical fascia; laterally the border is formed by the superficial layer of the deep cervical fascia; and posteriorly by the carotid space. It extends from the hyoid bone to the clavicle.

Infrahyoid Carotid, Retropharyngeal, and Prevertebral Spaces

These spaces traverse the supra- and infrahyoid neck and were described in the "Suprahyoid Neck" section earlier in the chapter.

LYMPH NODES

The numerous head and neck lymph nodes were according to the classic nomenclature related to regions. They were divided into ten groups by the French anatomist Rouvière: occipital, mastoid, parotid, facial, submandibular, submental, sublingual, retropharyngeal, anterior cervical, and lateral cervical nodes.[23]

The anterior cervical nodes are divided into superficial and deep nodes. The superficial nodes are anterior to the strap muscles. The deep division is comprised of the juxtavisceral nodes anterior to the larynx, thyroid gland, and trachea.

The lateral cervical group serves as common drainage to all regional nodes. They are divided in superficial and deep divisions. The superficial nodes follow the external jugular vein. The deep nodes are subdivided into three categories: *spinal accessory nodes (posterior triangle), internal jugular (deep cervical nodes)*, and *transverse cervical chains (supraclavicular nodes)*.

The spinal accessory chain drains the occipital and mastoid nodes as well as the lateral neck and shoulder.

The internal jugular chain follows the internal jugular vein anteriorly. At the point where the jugular vein is crossed by the posterior belly of the digastric muscle there is a single node larger than the surrounding nodes. It is called the jugulodigastric node. The submandibular nodes, palatine tonsil, and lateral oropharyngeal wall drain into these nodes. A similar larger node is present at the junction of the omohyoid muscle and the jugular vein. This node is called the jugulo-omohyoid node, which receives drainage from the tongue. It should be noted that internal jugular nodes are usually anterior to the jugular vein superior to the crossing of the omohyoid muscle. Inferior to the omohyoid muscle, the internal jugular nodes may be located anterior, medial, or posterior to the jugular vein.

The transverse cervical chain follows the course of the great cervical vessels in the lower neck. These nodes receive the drainage from the anterior cervical chains, internal jugular chain, and spinal accessory chain and also receive drainage from the arms and upper thorax.

In general, normal nodes in the neck should not exceed 1 cm in size, except for the jugulodigastric node, which can measure up to 1.5 cm normally.

A new, simplified classification of abnormal lymph nodes is related to the level of the nodes rather than the anatomic group of nodes (Table 37-3).

CROSS-SECTIONAL IMAGING

Computed Tomography

Over the years CT scanners have markedly improved, with increased detector sensitivity resulting in better soft tissue contrast resolution. The speed of image acquisition can be as fast as 0.5 second per slice, and the slice thickness can be as little as 0.5 mm. Recent developments allow continuous acquisition of data using spiral rather than axial slice-by-slice scanning. This permits high-speed examinations over a wide area of coverage.[24,25] If the patient can cooperate, direct coronal and sagittal imaging can be performed.[26] Otherwise electronic reconstruction techniques allow a multiplanar display of anatomy acquired with axial slices only. Three-dimensional surface reconstruction of bone or soft tissue is possible from axial slices.

Magnetic Resonance Imaging

Magnetic resonance imaging, or nuclear magnetic resonance (NMR), is a noninvasive, non-x-ray imaging technique with no known biologic hazards. Like CT, it is a cross-sectional technique; however, it offers a superior soft tissue contrast unmatched by other imaging techniques. Therefore, it is particularly suited for otolaryngological imaging.

TABLE 37-3. LYMPH NODE CLASSIFICATION

Anatomic Area	Level	Drainage
Submandibular, submental nodes	Level 1	Oral cavity, submandibular gland
Internal jugular chain nodes: skull base to carotid bifurcation, or suprahyoid internal jugular chain	Level 2	Nasopharynx, oropharynx, parotid, supraglottic larynx
Internal jugular chain nodes from carotid bifurcation to intersection of the omohyoid muscle or infrahyoid internal jugular chain nodes above cricoid cartilage	Level 3	Oropharynx, hypopharynx, supraglottic larynx
Infraomohyoid portion of the internal jugular chain nodes or infracricoid internal jugular chain nodes	Level 4	Subglottic larynx, hypopharynx, esophagus, thyroid
Posterior triangle lymph nodes	Level 5	Nasopharynx, oropharynx
Parathyroid nodes	Level 6	Thyroid, larynx
Tracheoesophageal groove nodes, superior mediastinal nodes	Level 7	Thyroid, larynx, lung

Adapted from Holiday RA. Neck nodes and masses. *ASHNR 26th Annual Conference and Postgraduate Course.* Vancouver: ASHNR, 1993, 87–97.

Magnetic resonance imaging can be performed in multiple planes without the need to move the patient or to rely on computer-reformatted images with their assorted lower spatial resolutions.

Certain nuclei, when placed into a strong magnetic field, absorb and subsequently release energy at specific radio frequencies if they are stimulated with radio frequency (RF) electromagnetic energy.[27] Detection and spatial encoding of the released energy then allow reconstruction of an image. Almost all MRI in humans has been based on proton imaging, because hydrogen ions are present in high concentration in all parts of the body.

Contrast in MRI imaging is a composite of several factors, including proton concentration, proton relaxation times (the period for a stimulated nucleus to resume its base energy state), and also flow. The two kinds of relaxation are T_1 and T_2. T_1 relaxation measures the time it takes a proton which is deflected away from the main magnetic field lines to go back to its original longitudinal alignment. The T_1 time (longitudinal or spin lattice relaxation) is dependent on the physical state of the proton-bearing material. The T_2 relaxation measures the time it takes for protons deflected into a plane transverse to the magnetic field lines to lose their coherence. Over the time period T_2 the protons lose their coherence in the transverse plane. As each proton precesses like a spinning top in the transverse plane, loss of coherence means that the protons have a slightly different precession frequency and therefore get out of phase, resulting in signal loss. The T_2 signal decay is referred to as transverse or spin-spin relaxation. It is dependent on the interaction between the spins and also on field inhomogeneity.

Every tissue in the body can be characterized by its T_1 and T_2 values. These can be altered by a disease process. There is, however, a wide overlap of T_1 and T_2 times in different diseases, so that there is no one characteristic T_1 or T_2 time for a particular disease or tissue. As the signal is, however, dependent on at least four factors—proton concentration, T_1 time, T_2 time, and flow—MRI is superior in soft tissue contrast to x-rays including CT, as contrast in x-rays is based solely on the different attenuation of x-rays by the different tissues.

Basic Considerations

General Advantages

One of the major advantages of MRI in head and neck imaging is its superior display of soft tissue detail in any plane: coronal, axial, or sagittal without moving the patient (Table 37-4). The soft tissue contrast is superior to CT. Magnetic resonance imaging also displays the vascular anatomy without the help of intravenous contrast; however, it is inferior to CT in its evaluation of bony structures.

TABLE 37-4. GENERAL ADVANTAGES AND DISADVANTAGES OF MRI

Advantages	Disadvantages
1. Better soft tissue contrast than CT	1. Prolonged data collection times
2. Multiplanar capability (axial, coronal, sagittal)	2. Higher sensitivity to patient motion
3. Clear delineation of arteries and veins as well as major cranial nerves	3. Scanning not possible in patients with a history of pacemakers, certain implants, or metallic foreign bodies
4. Less invasive than CT, although paramagnetic contrast may be necessary	4. Inferior display of bone detail
5. Absence of ionizing radiation	5. Claustrophobia may prohibit examination
6. Absence of beam-hardening artifacts from dental implants	6. Higher equipment cost, hence higher examination cost

Contrast Behavior

One should be familiar with the signal intensity produced by different anatomic structures and the relation of that signal to various pulse sequences used.

It is important to recognize what type of contrast a particular pulse sequence is highlighting. One can differentiate between T_1-weighted (T_1W), proton density–weighted (PDW), T_2-weighted (T_2W), and flow-enhanced contrast. Which contrast is highlighted depends on physical parameters during the acquisition. The main parameters are the pulse repetition time (TR) and the echo time (TE), which determine the weighting of the contrast. The most common technique applied is the spin-echo technique, and the discussion is mainly limited to this rather standard technique (Table 37-5).

Short of analyzing the physical parameters, one can determine the type of contrast by analyzing the signal of water. Water is low signal (dark) on T_1W images, intermediate signal on PDW images, and high signal (bright) on T_2W images (Table 37-6).

Fat is generally high signal on T_1W images and low signal on T_2W spin-echo images. The type of pulse sequence used may, however, affect the signal on T_2W images. When fast spin-echo techniques are used, fat is relatively high signal on T_2 due to J-coupling effects.

Signal characteristics vary depending on the water and fat content. However, in MRI these characteristics are especially dependent on the interaction of water and fat with the molecular environment (Table 37-7).[28] Free water acts as it was described; however, if water is bound, the T_1 and T_2 relaxation are markedly affected and as a result, the signal changes. Protein will shorten the T_1 time and increase the signal of water it is dissolved in.[29] Paramagnetic substances will have a similar but more pronounced effect on the signal. The molecular structure has a marked effect on the signal characteristics. Myelin, for instance, contains a large amount of fatty molecules; however, fat molecules are structured in a membranous fashion so that molecular motion is affected. Myelin, therefore, gives much less signal on T_1W images than does body fat. The amount of structuring is very important for the signal.[30] Cells with a low nucleocytoplasmatic ratio in general have a higher signal than cells with a high nucleocytoplasmatic ratio. Therefore, primitive tumors, which generally have a high nucleocytoplasmatic ratio, have a relatively low signal on T_2, whereas other tumors mostly have a high signal on T_2W images. The signal is also related to the amount of protein synthesis. Intracellular water is affected significantly by bonding to cellular macromolecules, shortening T_1 and T_2. (Shortening of T_1 results in an increased signal, shortening of T_2 in a decreased signal.) Cellular tissues therefore have a shorter T_1 and T_2 relaxation time than tissues primarily composed of extracellular water. Collagen-rich tissues (ligaments, tendons, fibrocartilage, or fibrosis) have relatively low signal on T_1- and T_2-weighted images, primarily due to a short T_2 as a result of anisotropic motion of the adsorbed water molecules relative to the magnetic field. The signal of tendinous structures also depends on the orientation of the tendon to the magnetic field.[31]

TABLE 37-5. PHYSICAL PARAMETERS IN SPIN-ECHO IMAGING

Contrast	Pulse Repetition Time (TR)	Echo Time (TE)
T_1 (T_1 weighting or T_1W)	Short; <600 msec	Short; <20 msec
Proton density (PDW) or spin density	Long; >2000 msec	Short; <20 msec
T_2 (T_2 weighting or T_2W)	Long; >2000 msec	Long; >80 msec

TABLE 37-6. MRI SIGNAL OF WATER AND FAT IN VARIOUS PULSE SEQUENCES

Pulse Sequences	Water	Fat
T_1W	Low signal (dark)	High signal (bright)
Proton density (PDW)	Intermediate signal (gray)	Intermediate to high signal (gray to white)
T_2W	High signal (bright)	Low signal (dark)[a]

[a]On fast spin-echo imaging the fat remains bright due to J-coupling effects.

Blood has markedly different signal characteristics depending on the age of the blood clot and its biochemical composition. As blood is changing from oxyhemoglobin (Oxy-Hb) to deoxyhemoglobin (Deoxy-Hb) and subsequently to methemoglobin (Met-Hb), a marked change in signal behavior is noted. The signal will also depend on the integrity of the blood cells. Methemoglobin has a markedly different signal depending on whether a blood clot has lysed or not (Table 37-8).[32,33]

Another factor affecting the signal in MRI imaging is motion. If blood flows fast enough, it appears as a signal void in spin-echo imaging. There are, however, flow-sensitive techniques that will show blood flowing into an imaging volume or section as high signal. This is primarily achieved by a time of flight and a phase-contrast technique.[34-36] Flow can also be quantified.[37-39] Both time of flight and phase contrast techniques can be used to reconstruct an angiographic image of rather high detail. For these MRI angiograms no contrast is necessary. Jugular venous flow and carotid flow can be imaged.

Air-containing structures are always black and without signal, as there are no water protons. Cortical bone is similar in its behavior, as there are fewer water protons and as they are too tightly bound to give off any signal. Though the T_1 time is within the imaging range, the T_2 decay is too fast to obtain any significant signal. However, it is possible to see the bone marrow signal. On T_1W imaging, fatty bone marrow is very bright, whereas hematopoietic bone marrow is intermediate in its signal (Table 37-9).

Noncalcified hyaline cartilage in the larynx has a high to intermediate signal and resembles fat on T_1. Calcified laryngeal cartilage, however, has low signal on T_1- and T_2-weighted images. Marrow within the cricoid is seen as increased signal with T_1W. With aging there is

TABLE 37-7. MRI SIGNAL CHARACTERISTICS FOR VARIOUS TISSUES (SPIN-ECHO IMAGING)

	T_1W			T_2W		
	Low	*Intermediate*	*High*	*Low*	*Intermediate*	*High*
Air	X			X		
Fast flow	X			X		
Cortical bone	X			X		
Calcified cartilage	X			X		
Ligaments/fascia	X			X		
Inner ear fluid	X					X
Cerebrospinal fluid	X					X
Nasopharyngeal mucosa		X				X
Fat			X		X	
Lymphoid tissue		X			X	
Cranial nerves		X			X	
Muscles		X		X		
Salivary gland		X			X	
Thyroid gland		X			X	

TABLE 37-8. MRI SIGNAL OF BLOOD CLOTS

Type of Blood Clot	Hemoglobin	Cell Integrity	T_1W	T_2W
Acute bleed (1–3 days)	Deoxy Hb	Intact	Intermediate signal	Low signal
Subacute bleed (3–10 days)	MetHb	Intact	High signal	Low signal
Chronic bleed (>10 days)	MetHb	Lysed	High signal	High signal
Hemosiderin	Hemosiderin		Low to intermediate signal	Low signal

increasing calcification of the laryngeal bones, decreasing overall signal. The signal of laryngeal skeleton is therefore highly variable, depending especially on the amount of calcification, which is age-dependent.[40]

The signal overall is rather variable due to the complex factors affecting the signal behavior. Muscle tissue in general is intermediate in signal intensity on T_1- and T_2-weighted images. Lymphoid tissue is slightly higher in signal intensity on T_1- and T_2-weighted images than muscle.

Magnetic resonance imaging has benefited markedly from the introduction of paramagnetic contrast materials, mainly based on gadolinium, which is a paramagnetic agent. It is very safe and has a very low allergy rate. The paramagnetic contrast has similar distribution characteristics to the iodine-based radiographic contrast. Lesions in the brain enhance when there is a breakdown of the blood-brain barrier.[41] The enhancement is based on shortening of the T_1 relaxation times, which results in a high signal if a lesion accumulates gadolinium.

Safety

Magnetic resonance imaging has the great advantage of not using ionizing radiation. There are no known biologic hazards. It is, however, potentially harmful in patients with a pacemaker, cochlear implants, certain other implants, neurostimulators, metal injury (especially of the eye), and certain aneurysm clips used in brain surgery. Careful screening, therefore, should be conducted by both the referring physician and the radiologist performing the MRI. A complete listing of magnet compatibility of different devices is given by Shellock and associates.[42]

There has been a reluctance to use MRI for patients who have had a stapedectomy. According to the study of Applebaum and Valvassori,[43] however, there is no apparent danger of certain commonly employed stapes prostheses to become displaced when subject to MRI, with the exception of the McGee stapedectomy piston prosthesis manufactured during mid-1987.[42]

Clinical Application

Sinuses

Computed tomography added a new dimension to sinus imaging by very accurate delineation of the highly variable sinus anatomy. Its primary use is in the workup of chronic or recurrent sinusitis. It accurately delineates the presence and extent of the inflammatory dis-

TABLE 37-9. MRI SIGNAL OF BONE MARROW

Bone Marrow Type	T_1W	T_2W
Fatty bone marrow	High signal	Low signal[a]
Hematopoietic	Intermediate signal	Intermediate to high signal

[a]On fast spin-echo imaging the fat remains bright due to J-coupling effects.

ease. It depicts possible underlying anatomic abnormalities, which potentially interfere with the nasal or osteomeatal air passages. The examination is done in the axial and coronal plane. Pneumatized normal anatomic structures often obstruct the osteomeatal passage due to their air expansion. The most common variants of pneumatization include concha bullosa (36%), representing a pneumatized turbinate; Haller cells (10%), representing extension of ethmoid air cells along the orbital floor lateral to the uncinate process; prominent ethmoid bulla (8%); and uncinate bulla (0.4%). Other anatomic variants readily depicted by CT include nasal septal deformity (21%), uncinate process deviation (3%), and paradoxical middle turbinate (15%) (Figure 37-17).[44–47]

Computed tomography outlines the full extent of the disease very accurately and therefore should be the first cross-sectional imaging study. In tumor cases it demonstrates bone destruction and in that respect is superior to MRI. Chronic inflammation will result in bony thickening of the sinus wall, more readily appreciated on CT than on MRI. Disadvantages of sinus CT, especially when done without contrast, are that it is difficult to differentiate retention of fluid or inflammatory change from tumor. As tumors in the sinuses lead to obstruction of the ostium, the tumor extent may be overestimated due to the retained fluid.

Magnetic resonance imaging is a very accurate way of differentiating retained fluid from tumor (Figure 37-18). As about 95% of the sinus tumors have an intermediate to low signal on T_2W images, the tumor contrasts very well to the retained fluid and inflammatory mucosa,

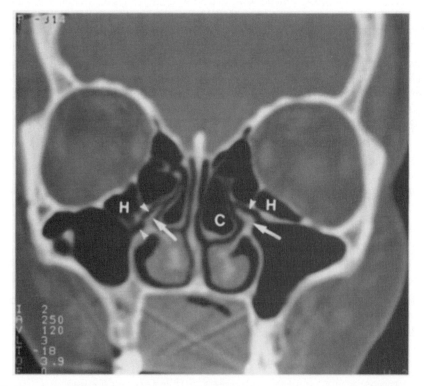

Figure 37-17.   Coronal CT scan of sinuses with Haller cells and concha bullosa. (H, Haller cell; C, concha bullosa; arrowhead, infundibulum; arrow, uncinate process.)

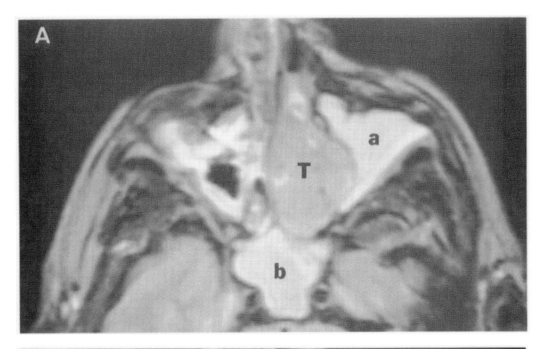

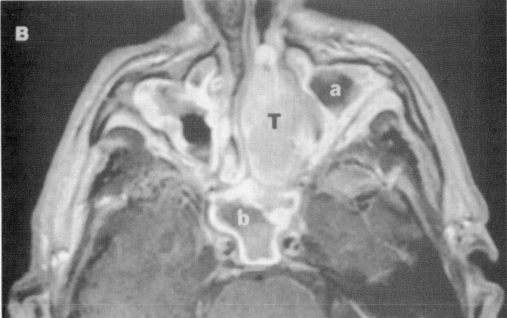

Figure 37-18.   Poorly differentiated squamous cell carcinoma of the nasal cavity. **A.** Axial T$_2$-weighted image showing clear separation of the tumor from the retained fluid in the maxillary and sphenoid sinuses (a and b). **B.** Axial T$_2$-weighted image showing enhancement of the tumor, separating it from the obstructed maxillary and sphenoid sinuses. (T, tumor; a, maxillary sinus; b, sphenoid sinus.)

which generally are high in signal on T_2W images. The relatively low signal on T_2 results from the fact that squamous carcinomas independent of their differentiation are highly cellular lesions with little interstitial fluid and vascularity. Squamous cell carcinomas represent about 80% of all sinus tumors. The other rare tumors, such as lymphomas, esthesioneuroblastomas, sarcomas, and fibrous histiocytomas, have a high nucleocytoplasmatic ratio, are very cellular, and therefore show relatively low signal on T_2W images. Ten percent of the tumors are of minor salivary gland origin. Half of these have large stromal components containing seromucinous secretions, resulting in a high signal on T_2W imaging, obscuring the borders to surrounding inflammatory mucosa or retained fluid. Intravenous gadolinium may help to delineate the adenoid cystic tumor from retained fluid. In summary, MRI is the modality of choice for tumor mapping.[48–53]

Although MRI shows inflammatory disease very well, one has to be aware of potential pitfalls. Entrapped secretions in mucoceles or obstructed sinuses usually have low-to-high T_1W signal intensity and high-to-low T_2W signal intensity. The signal is dependent on the protein content and viscosity of the lesion. Protein will shorten T_1 and T_2 time, therefore increasing signal on T_1W images and decreasing signal on T_2W images. The T_1 effect is more pronounced with lower concentrations of protein. With higher concentrations of protein, the T_2 shortening predominates, resulting in signal loss on T_2W and eventually also T_1W images. Very thick inspissated mucus simulates on MRI an air-filled sinus. It is for this reason primarily that MRI is not recommended as primary examination in inflammatory sinus disease. In CT, chronic secretions will be readily visible, have slightly higher attenuation than fluid, and therefore be slightly hyperintense. There usually is a hypodense seam along the bony wall representing markedly thickened mucosa. The appearance of thick secretions can be identical to mycetomas and fungal disease on CT as well as MRI imaging (Table 37-10; Figure 37-19).[54–56]

Given the excellent resolution and thin slices on CT as well as the exquisite bone detail, CT is the standard for imaging of facial trauma. Fractures are easily demonstrated. Three-dimensional display technology is increasingly becoming available, facilitating preoperative planning.[57]

In cases of cerebrospinal fluid (CSF) rhinorrhea, a CT cisternogram is the procedure of choice. Radiographic contrast is injected intrathecally in a Trendelenburg position and CT slices are obtained in axial, coronal, or side-dependent positions. Extravasation of contrast can be identified by the high attenuation of radiographic contrasts in the sinus air cells. Not only does CT cisternography establish the diagnosis of a CSF leak but it also helps to precisely localize the leak for surgical intervention. The underlying reasons for CSF leaks, such as fractures, congenital pits, arachnoid diverticula, and empty sella, are easily recognized (Figure 37-20).[58]

Magnetic resonance imaging without contrast using high-resolution heavily T_2W techniques with submillimeter resolution in all imaging planes plays an increasing role in the

TABLE 37-10. SIGNAL OF NASAL SECRETIONS

Type of Mucous Secretion	T_1W	T_2W
Low protein and viscosity	Low signal	High signal
Intermediate protein and viscosity	High signal	High signal
High protein and viscosity	High signal	Low signal
Very high protein, inspissated mucus	Low signal	Low signal

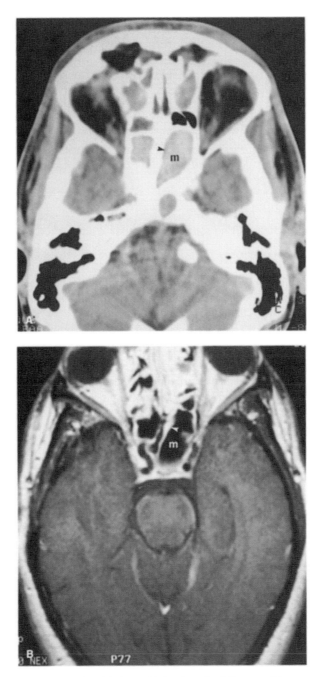

Figure 37-19. Sphenoid mucocele with fungal infection. **A**. CT scan without contrast showing obstructed sphenoid sinuses filled with proteinaceous high-attenuation secretions. (m, mucocele; arrowhead, thickened lucent mucosa.) **B**. MRI scan with T₁ weighting and gadolinium. (m, obstructed sphenoid sinus with low signal secondary to inspissated secretions simulating an air-filled sinus; arrowhead, enhancement of thickened mucosa with gadolinium.)

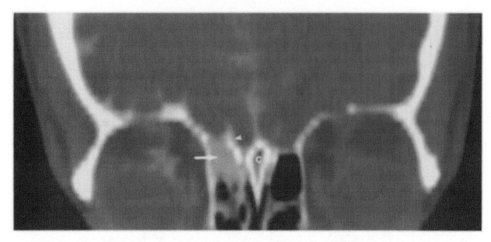

Figure 37-20. Ethmoid dehiscence with arachnoid herniating into an anterior ethmoid air cell resulting in CSF rhinorrhea. Secondary coronal reconstruction from axial CT slices. (Arrow, arachnoid diverticulum herniating into anterior ethmoid diverticulum filled with intrathecal contrast; arrowhead, cribriform plate elevated by arachnoid diverticulum; C, crista galli.)

work-up of CSF leaks. Cerebrospinal fluid "streets" connecting subarachnoid space to sinus cavities in areas of bony dehiscence can be visualized, especially when there is opacification of the sinuses, which makes the separating bone visible as thin dark line.[59]

Petrous Bone

Examination of the temporal bone has been revolutionized by CT and MRI. Conventional tomography has been largely abandoned. Computed tomography offers very high-resolution images with a slice thickness of about 1 mm. This allows good visualization of the bony anatomy, ossicular anatomy, and inner ear anatomy.[60] Congenital abnormalities such as an aberrant internal carotid artery in the middle ear or a jugular dehiscence can be appreciated by CT alone. Soft tissue abnormalities in the middle ear, mastoid air cells, and antrum are clearly seen by CT in relation to the middle and inner ear structures. Bony erosions by soft tissue masses are well delineated. There is very good contrast present on CT between bone, soft tissue, and air. On MRI, soft tissue disease is very well appreciated; however, there is no contrast between cortical bone and air, as both will have no signal. Bone is only appreciated if it contains marrow. Therefore, MRI is inferior to CT for evaluation of the middle ear. However, due to its high soft tissue contrast, it is the ideal method for evaluation of the inner ear. It is almost impossible in CT to demonstrate an intracanalicular small tumor, such as a small acoustic neurinoma (Figure 37-21). In order to obtain high resolution in the temporal bone, reconstruction algorithms have to be used, which degrade contrast resolution markedly. Therefore, enhancement with iodinated intravenous contrast may not be visible or may be confused with bone, as both bone and enhancement show as an area of high attenuation. Another disadvantage of CT in the posterior fossa is beam hardening artifacts, and as a result soft tissue detail and contrast can be negatively affected. Therefore, in the evaluation of the inner ear internal auditory canal, or cerebellopontine angle, MRI is the preferred method (Figure 37-22).[61–64]

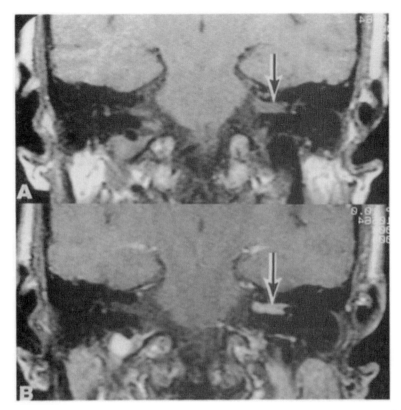

Figure 37-21.   Coronal MR scans of the temporal bone demonstrating a left intracanalicular acoustic neuroma. A. T_1-weighted image without gadolinium showing acoustic neuroma noted in the left internal auditory canal (*arrow*). B. T_1-weighted image of the same patient with gadolinium showing a brightened acoustic neuroma (*arrow*).

With MRI it is possible to demonstrate small neurinomas of only a few millimeters in size within the canal or even cochlear schwannomas. It is therefore the method of choice for the evaluation of sensorineural hearing loss. As there is a marked contrast of an enhancing structure against the background of air and bone, MRI has the capability of showing contrast enhancement in facial nerve neuritis (Bell's palsy)[65] and also labyrinthitis in the inflamed portion of the cochlear and vestibular nerve and labyrinth.[66] Facial nerve neurinomas (Figure 37-23) can be distinguished by their mass-like appearance, whereas inflammatory conditions only slightly distort the anatomy by edema.[67–70]

As the resolution of MRI is already in the submillimeter range, especially when using phase array coils, the anatomy of the inner ear is shown in high detail on T_2W images.[71] The fluid signal of the membranous inner ear and internal auditory canal gives a high signal on T_2W images, whereas the facial nerve in its intrapetrous portion gives an intermediate signal. Within the internal auditory canal one can differentiate the superior and inferior division of the vestibular nerve as well as the facial and cochlear nerve using sagittal imaging through the canal.[72] Congenital malformations can be diagnosed equally well with CT and MRI. The

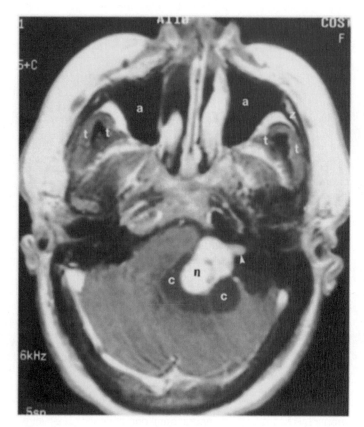

Figure 37-22.   Large partially cystic acoustic neurinoma in CP angle. Gadolinium-enhanced T_1W
MRI. (n, solid portion of acoustic neurinoma; c, cystic portion of acoustic neurinoma;
arrowhead, solid tumor within internal auditory canal; a, antrum; t, temporalis muscle;
z, zygomatic arch.)

Mondini malformation, as the most common congenital abnormality, is characterized most
commonly by a wide vestibular aqueduct, plumb deformed vestibule, and semicircular canals
or cochlear deformities (Figure 37-24)[73–76] The normal loops of the anterior-inferior cerebellar artery within the canal can be seen with high-resolution MRI.

For the workup of acute otomastoiditis and its complications, MRI is well suited, especially when evaluating for associated parameningeal abscesses, jugular vein thrombosis,
meningitis, and brain abscesses. For the evaluation of jugular vein patency, MR angiography is indicated and easy to perform. This allows differentiation of jugular vein compression by epidural empyemas along the jugular sinus vs. thrombosis. Petrous apicitis and its
effect on the nervous structures in the cavernous sinus can be shown with MRI, and less well
with CT. The strength of MRI is therefore in the evaluation of the structures surrounding
the temporal bone.

In the evaluation of chronic otomastoiditis CT is the prime modality used. Erosions of the
ossicular chain can occur in chronic otitis media with or without a cholesteatoma; however,
erosions are far more common with a cholesteatoma. Ossicular destruction is the most fre-

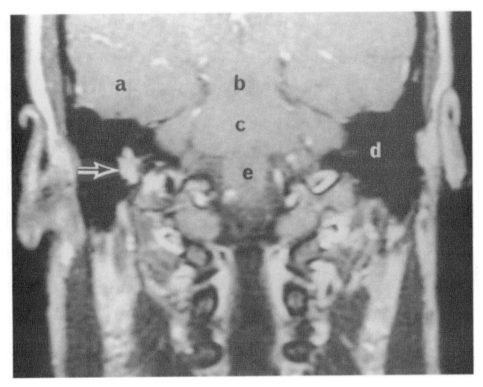

Figure 37-23.   Coronal T_1-weighted MR image with gadolinium showing right facial nerve neuroma (*arrow*). (a, temporal lobe; b, midbrain; c, pons; d, petrous bone; e, medulla.)

quent and is best seen with CT. The most common sites of a cholesteatoma are the Prussak space between the lateral attic wall and neck of malleus (Figure 37-25). The facial recess is the second most common site for a cholesteatoma. Serious complications of a cholesteatoma include erosion of the lateral semicircular canal resulting in a labyrinthine fistula and facial nerve canal disruption. The hallmark of a cholesteatoma is mass effect with displacement of ossicles and bone destruction.[77]

Granulation tissue, though similar in CT attenuation numbers, does not exert mass effect and only rarely erodes bone. It may result in postinflammatory ossicular fixation resulting from fibrous tissue formation or tympanosclerosis with new bone formation. In contrast to a cholesteatoma, granulation tissue can enhance with gadolinium on MRI. A subtype of granulation tissue is a cholesterol granuloma. It contains a brownish hemorrhagic fluid filled with cholesterol crystals. The cholesterol crystals are the result of hemorrhage and the lesion is therefore bright on T_1W images as well as on T_2 images. The lesion is clinically important, as it has a bluish tint suggesting a paraganglioma. A cholesterol granuloma in the petrous apex is referred to as a cholesterol cyst.[78-81]

In general, CT is the preferred method of evaluating chronic middle ear disease because of its ease in demonstrating bony destruction. If it becomes important to know whether a soft tissue in the middle ear or petrous bone is granulation tissue or a cholesterol cyst vs. a cholesteatoma or paraganglioma, MRI plays a role.

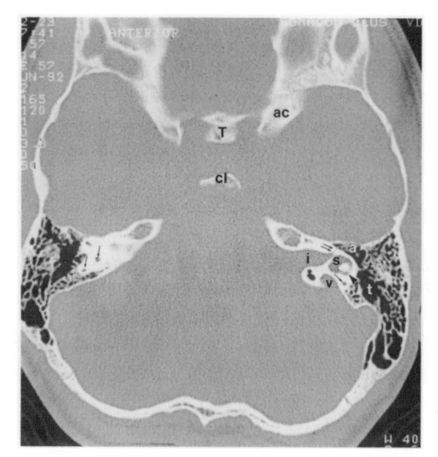

Figure 37-24. Mondini malformation with large vestibular aqueduct. Axial CT scan. (v, dilated vestibular aqueduct; i, internal auditory canal; double arrow, preganglionic facial nerve; a, attic or epitympanic recess; t, antrum; cl, clivus; T, tuberculum sellae; ac, anterior clinoid; arrow, posteior semicircular canal; arrowhead, lateral semicircular canal.)

Cholesteatomas are intermediate intensity on T_1W images and bright on T_2W images. They do not enhance with gadolinium. Granulation tissue enhances intensely with gadolinium, well appreciated on MRI but not on a contrast-enhanced CT. Cholesterol cysts, on the other hand, have a characteristic signal without contrast on MRI.

At present CT is the most accurate method for assessing otosclerosis. The initial change of active otosclerosis is deossification. This can be seen as lucencies along the margins of the oval window or cochlear ducts. A typical sign for cochlear otosclerosis is a double low-attenuation ring paralleling the cochlear turns. In the more mature phase of otosclerosis, foci of denser bone develop. This may lead to total obliteration of the oval window. An MRI may show faint enhancement with gadolinium in the spongiotic areas of the otic capsule. From an imaging standpoint, Paget disease, fibrous dysplasia, and rarefying osteitis of late congenital syphilis are in the differential.[82,83]

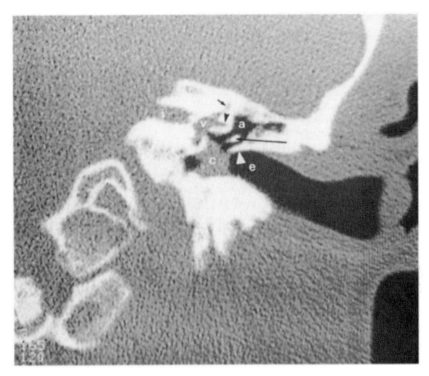

Figure 37-25.   Cholesteatoma. Coronal CT scan. (c, cholesteatoma; a, attic or epitympanic recess; large arrow, incus; black arrowhead, lateral semicircular canal; small arrow, superior semicircular canal; i, internal auditory canal; v, vestibule; e, external auditory canal; white arrowhead, scutum.)

Salivary Glands

Salivary glands can be imaged with both CT and MRI. Cross-sectional imaging has largely replaced sialography for tumor diagnosis. Cross-sectional techniques, with their good visualization of fat planes, allow the determination of whether a tumor is within the gland or outside. Advantages of CT are that calcifications and stones may be better seen. An MRI gives better soft tissue contrast in the parotid and its surrounding structures. The facial nerve can be seen with its main trunk within the parotid gland. This is of great surgical importance, as the intraparotid facial nerve divides the parotid into the superficial and deep lobes. The deep lobe of the parotid is surgically amenable by a submandibular incision; the superficial lobe is amenable to a superficial parotidectomy. If the facial nerve is not well seen, the retromandibular vessels serve as a landmark to differentiate between the deep and superficial lobes on CT as well as MRI. The facial nerve runs lateral to the retromandibular vein. The deep lobe is medial to the vessels, the superficial lobe lateral. This differentiation is less accurate than the direct visualization of the facial nerve. By its three-dimensional display the MRI also demonstrates the relation of the parotid to the stylomastoid foramen better than CT. It can show tumor extending into the facial nerve canal. Gadolinium enhancement shows the extension of the tumor into the canal and also demonstrates perineural spread. Invasion of adjacent structures of the skull base, jugular foramen, hypoglossal foramen, and so forth, is also better demonstrated. Lack of beam artifacts from artificial teeth are in favor of MRI over CT.

Differentiating benign from malignant tumors of the parotid gland is probably not possible. Signal characteristics are unreliable. Invasion of adjacent structures as well as lymphadenopathy are most suggestive of malignancy.

In general, the larger the salivary gland tumor, the greater the chance that the lesion is benign. About 80% of the parotid tumors, 60% of submandibular tumors, and 25 to 40% of sublingual masses are benign.[84] The most common benign tumor of the salivary glands is the pleomorphic adenoma (benign mixed tumor; Figure 37-26). These most commonly occur in the parotid gland. They are lobulated tumors, usually with low signal intensity on T_1W and high signal on T_2W images. They may contain fat. Rarely can a malignancy develop in a benign mixed tumor, the "carcinoma ex pleomorphic adenoma."

Warthin's tumor is the second most common benign parotid tumor. In about 15% of the cases it is bilateral. It may have cystic components. On technetium 99m pertechnetate scans it is "hot," as is the oncocytoma of the parotid, which otherwise has no differentiating features.

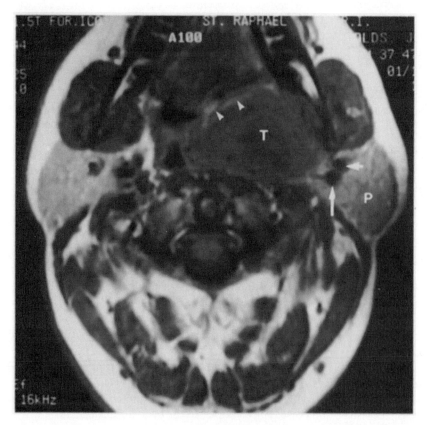

Figure 37-26.   Benign mixed tumor of deep lobe of the parotid. Axial MRI T_1W. (T, tumor; P, superficial lobe of parotid; arrowheads, medially displaced nasoparapharyngeal fat space; small arrow, external carotid; large arrow, retromandibular vein.)

The hemangioma is the most common benign tumor in childhood. It enhances diffusely, is poorly defined, and may contain phleboliths. A hemangioma may coexist with lymphangiomas. Lipoma and intraparotid lymph nodes are rare. The signal intensity of branchial cleft cysts can be variable depending on the protein content. The signal intensity can be that of fluid, but can be very bright on T_1W images and mixed on T_2W images secondary to increased protein. Often one can also see an extension of the cyst through a small canal into the external and middle ear (Figure 37-27).

If intraparotid cysts are bilateral, there is a strong correlation with HIV seropositivity, especially if there is accompanying lymphadenopathy.

Benign inflammatory conditions are often related to a calculus resulting in obstruction and abscess formation. Submandibular duct stones are more common than parotid duct stones. Sjögren's syndrome, often seen in conjunction with connective tissue disease, especially rheumatoid arthritis, is relatively characteristic on CT and MRI. The parotids and possibly also the other salivary glands are diffusely enlarged, appear denser on CT than normal, and contain multiple little cavities secondary to sialectasis. These cavities are filled with small calcifications. Lymphoepithelial masses may be associated.

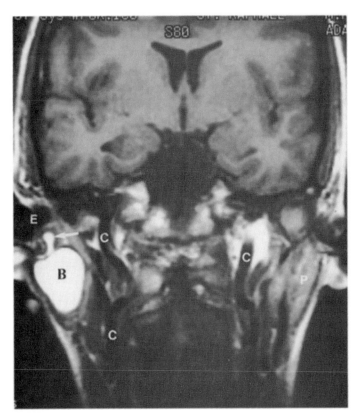

Figure 37-27. Intraparotid branchial cleft cyst type I. Coronal T_1W MRI. (B, branchial cleft cyst; arrow, extension of cyst to external ear canal; E, external ear canal; C, internal carotid artery; P, parotid gland.

Mucoepidermoid carcinomas are the most common parotid malignancies and the second most common submandibular malignancies. The mucoepidermoid carcinoma is the most common salivary gland malignancy in childhood. Adenoid cystic carcinomas (Figure 37-28) are more common in the submandibular gland. They often arise from small salivary glands or gland remnants presenting as primary tumor in the parapharyngeal space remote from glands or mucosa. Acinic cell carcinomas can be bilateral, simulating Warthin's tumors. They also have a tendency to occur in childhood. Adenocarcinomas are very aggressive and metastasize widely. Squamous cell carcinomas arise from ductal epithelial metaplasias and are rare salivary gland tumors.[85–86]

Skull Base, Nasopharynx, and Related Spaces

Both MRI and CT have advantages in imaging of the skull base. The CT scan shows bone very clearly, is superior in demonstrating small calcifications, and demonstrates the bony anatomy including foramina exquisitely. Major disadvantages include decreased soft tissue detail near a bony interface or foramen. Also direct coronal or multiplanar images are difficult to obtain.

An MRI clearly shows the soft tissues near the skull base and allows imaging of the cranial nerves and vascular structures in any plane. It is the preferred method for workup of pituitary tumors, whether macro- or microadenomas. Though bone is not as well seen as on CT, it can be visualized by its bone marrow signal or lack of signal in cortical bone. Soft tissue tumors can easily be demonstrated as they directly invade bone or spread along the foramina or nerves. Contrast enhancement delineates tumors or infection penetrating into bone, as there is high contrast between bone and enhancing tumor, whereas in CT the signal of bone and enhancing tumor may be similar.[87] To determine the operability of skull base lesions, MRI is the preferred method, as it is more accurate in defining the extent of tumor spread and by its multiplanar display allows more accurate surgical planning. The relation of normal soft tissue structures below the skull base is better appreciated than on CT. Fat-suppression techniques allow improved visualization of tumors at the skull base. Fat suppression differentiates the enhancing tumor clearly from fat, which would otherwise have a similar signal to the enhancing tumor. Invasion into fatty bone marrow spaces is also better seen with fat-suppression techniques after gadolinium administration. Gadolinium enhancement with simultaneous fat suppression allows differentiation of edema from enhancing tumor or infection within the bone marrow.[88,89] Spread of tumor into the cavernous sinus is more apparent on MRI than on CT (Figure 37-29). Patency or encasement of major vessels is easily assessed with MRI.[90]

It is important to recognize that the deep facial spaces connect to the skull base and therefore serve as a route of spread to the skull base for tumor or infection. Only a small wedge of the parapharyngeal space reaches the skull base or infratemporal fossa. As the parapharyngeal space contains only fat, it serves as an easy route for infection or tumor.

The masticator space broadly abuts against the skull base and therefore serves as a route for odontogenic infections or oropharyngeal carcinoma. Via the foramen ovale the tumor can spread along the mandibular portion of the trigeminal nerve into the cavernous sinus. Trigeminal neurinomas involving the mandibular portion of cranial nerve V can present as a mass in the masseteric space connecting to the cavernous sinus. Alternatively nasopharyngeal tumors can find a path through the sphenopalatine foramen into the pterygopalatine fossa, and from there via the foramen rotundum along the maxillary portion of the trigeminal nerve into the cavernous sinus or through the infraorbital fissure into the orbit (Figure 37-30). A

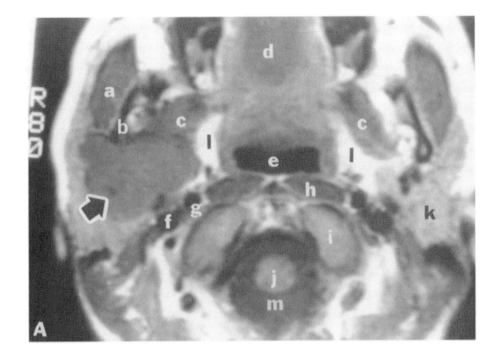

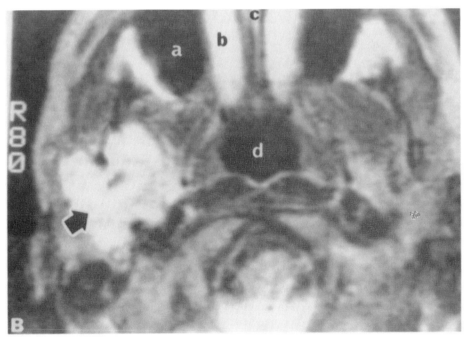

Figure 37-28. Adenocystic carcinoma of the right parotid gland (*arrow*) seen on axial MR scans. A. T₁-weighted image without gadolinium. (a, masseter muscle; b, mandible; c, medial pterygoid muscle; d, palate; e, nasopharynx; f, jugular vein; g, carotid artery; h, longus colli muscle; i, occipital condyle; j, spinal cord; k, normal left parotid gland; l, parapharyngeal space; m, CSF in subarachnoid space.) B. T₂-weighted image clearly showing the tumor. (a, maxillary sinus; b, turbinate; c, septum; d, nasopharynx.)

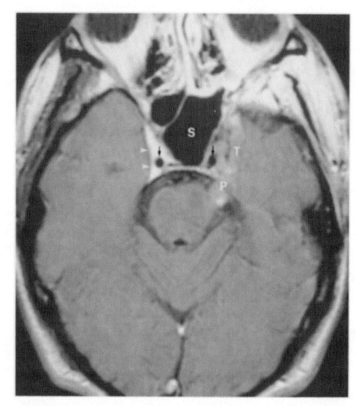

Figure 37-29.   Perineural spread of primary maxillary sinus melanoma along trigeminal nerve into cavernous sinus and preganglionic cisternal portion. Gadolinium-enhanced axial T_1W MRI. (T, tumor in cavernous sinus; P, tumor in preganglionic cisternal portion of trigeminal nerve; arrowheads, normal cavernous sinus; arrow, cavernous sinus portion internal carotid; S, sphenoid sinus.)

common tumor with this kind of spread is a juvenile angiofibroma, which commonly extends laterally into the pterygopalatine fossa. From there it can get access to the middle cranial fossa or cavernous sinus. Further lateral extension is through the pterygomaxillary fissure into the masticator space of the infratemporal fossa.[91] In evaluating nasopharyngeal carcinomas, close attention must be given to these areas. This is best done with MRI, where there is better contrast between normal tissue and tumor tissue. Also its three-dimensional, coronal, and sagittal displays help in visualizing these structures.

Along the carotid space neurogenic tumors such as neuromas, schwannomas, and paragangliomas spread from intracranial into the neck or vice versa. The two foramina involved are the jugular foramen and carotid canal. The carotid space can also serve as a route for infection, especially in perforating injuries. From the carotid space infection can spread via the jugular vein and jugular foramen into the posterior fossa, leading to a brain abscess.

The retropharyngeal spaces connect in a thin portion to the clivus. Deep facial lesions spreading to the retropharyngeal or prevertebral space have access to the clivus and skull

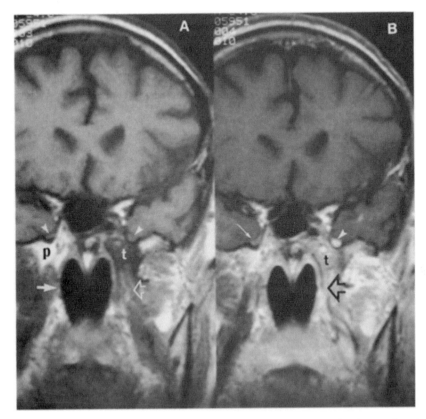

Figure 37-30.   Perineural spread of squamous cell carcinoma of the hard palate to the pterygopalatine fossa and foramen rotundum. A. Nonenhanced T_1W coronal MRI.
(P, normal pterygopalatine fossa filled with fat; t, tumor pterygopalatine fossa; arrow,
fat in normal pterygomaxillary fissure; open arrow, retroantral tumor in pterygomaxillary fissure; arrowhead, second portion of trigeminal nerve in foramen rotundum.)
B. Gadolinium-enhanced coronal T_1W MRI at same location as A. (t, enhanced
tumor in pterygopalatine fossa; open arrow, enhancing tumor in pterygomaxillary
fissure retroantral; arrowhead, enhancing second portion trigeminal nerve in foramen rotundum indicating perineural spread of tumor into cavernous sinus; small
arrow, nonenhancing second portion trigeminal nerve uninvolved side.)

base. Infections originating from pharyngitis or tonsillitis gain access to the retropharyngeal
space, in which they can easily spread upward and downward (Figure 37-31). The prevertebral space is often invaded by infectious processes from vertebral osteomyelitis and discitis.

The constrictor muscle of the mucosal nasopharynx is attached to the skull base by the
pharyngobasilar fascia, a dense aponeurosis. Along the superior posterolateral margin of
this fascia is the sinus of Morgagni. Through this sinus the levator veli palatini muscle and
the eustachian tube enter the nasopharyngeal mucosal space. Nasopharyngeal carcinomas
often arise in the lateral recesses of the nasopharyngeal mucosal space and leave it via the
sinus of Morgagni, thus getting access to the skull base. These tumors block the eustachian

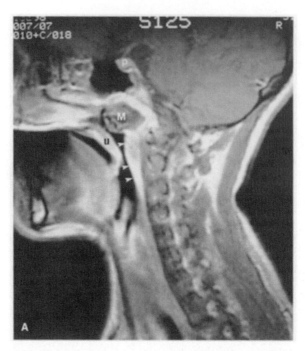

Figure 37-31.   Retropharyngeal fungal abscess (mucormycosis) with clival involvement, carotid invasion, and intracranial epidural extension through jugular foramen. **A.** Sagittal gadolinium-enhanced T_1W MRI. (M, fungal abscess in adenoid region; arrowheads, retropharyngeal extension of abscess; u, uvula; P, pituitary gland.) (*continued*)

tube, which results in retention of fluid in the middle ear and mastoids.[92] Cross-sectional imaging, especially with MRI, allows evaluation of these structures very accurately and is probably the best way to evaluate the submucosal extent of the tumor, which may be more extensive than is appreciated by endoscopy (Figure 37-32).

A typical harmless lesion of the nasopharyngeal mucosal space just below the skull base is the Tornwaldt cyst, which is a notochordal remnant presenting as an epithelial-lined cyst, variable in signal intensity according to its protein content. It is often bright on T_1W images.[93] Chordomas originate from the notochordal remnants and therefore rarely present in the epipharynx.

Oral Cavity and Oropharynx

Evaluation of the mandible, teeth, and alveolar ridges has recently advanced by the introduction of the Dentascan.[94] With this technique, a stack of 1-mm-thick CT slices is acquired and secondary electronic reconstructions in a curved sagittal plane along the mandible or maxillary alveolar ridge are obtained as well as narrowly spaced coronal reconstructions perpendicular to the curve of the mandible. The teeth and their relationship to each other, the mandibular bone, alveolar nerve, and sinuses are displayed in real size. This technique has therefore found widespread acceptance for dental implants, where the relationship of the implant from the alveolar nerve is of paramount importance. This technique is also ideally suited for evaluation of cysts, bone tumors, and bony erosions from tumors adjacent to the mandible.[95-97]

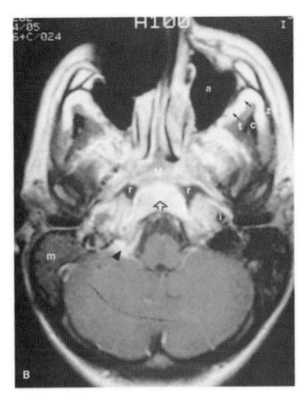

Figure 37-31.   (*Continued*) **B.** Axial gadolinium-enhanced T₁W MRI. (M, fungal abscess adenoid; open arrow, clival enhancement indicating possible osteomyelitis; r, fluid retropharyngeal space; i, internal carotid on left, right internal carotid occluded by fungal invasion; arrowhead, extension of infection through jugular foramen with formation of parameningeal abscess/phlegmon; m, fluid retention mastoid secondary to occlusion of eustachian tube; a, antrum; small arrows, retromaxillary fat space; z, zygomatic arch; c, coronoid process mandible; t, temporalis muscle.)

In the oropharynx, squamous cell carcinoma comprises about 95% of the tumors. Malignant lymphomas account for approximately 5% of tonsillar malignancies and 1 to 2% of the malignancies of the tongue base (Figure 37-33).[98–100]

Squamous cell carcinomas of the tongue and tongue base are usually underestimated on physical examination due to their deep growth (Figure 37-34). Tumors in the tongue base grow to the palatine tonsils when they are lateral in position, whereas tonsillar cancers or cancers of the anterior tonsillar pillar or retromolar trigone often invade the tongue base via the palatoglossal muscles. Lesions of the lateral tongue base grow into the glossotonsillar sulcus and forward into the sublingual space. The extent of the tumor is therefore often not appreciated. Tongue base tumors invade the lateral spaces of the neck all the way to the hyoid via the contiguous sublingual and submandibular spaces, which present no barrier to their growth, whereas the growth of anterior tongue lesions is inhibited by the mylohyoid muscle.

Tumors of the anterior tonsillar pillar spread also to the retromolar trigone, a triangular mucosal region behind the third molar covering the ascending ramus of the mandible. Anterior

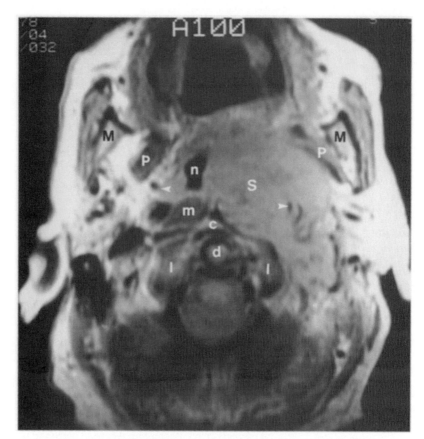

Figure 37-32. Squamous cell carcinoma nasopharynx with large submucosal spread. Axial T_1W MRI. (S, squamous cell carcinoma invading into nasoparapharyngeal space, masseteric space, carotid space, and prevertebral space; arrowheads, internal carotids, note encasement of internal carotid artery on involved side; m, prevertebral muscle on uninvolved side, note infiltration on involved side; c, anterior ring of C1; l, lateral mass C1; d, odontoid; n, displaced nasopharynx; P, medial pterygoid muscle displaced forward on involved side with possible infiltration, nasoparapharyngeal fat space completely obliterated; M, mandible.)

tonsillar pillar tumors grow to the gingival buccal sulcus and buccal mucosa, where they can spread into the infratemporal fossa, the masticator space, and also the parapharyngeal space. Via the palatoglossal muscle they invade the tongue and the soft palate. From the latter location they spread superiorly via the tensor and levator veli palatini into the nasopharynx.

Retromolar trigone lesions behave more like lesions of the gingiva and buccal mucosa. The lesions spread into the mandible either by direct growth or via the inferior alveolar nerve. Perineural spread occurs. Growth along the neurovascular bundle is possible, and tumors can in this way reach the pterygopalatine fossa via the retroantral region. Direct invasion of the pterygomandibular raphe, which serves as attachment for the constrictor muscle and buccinator muscle, occurs. Retroantral spread of tumor into the infratemporal fossa and

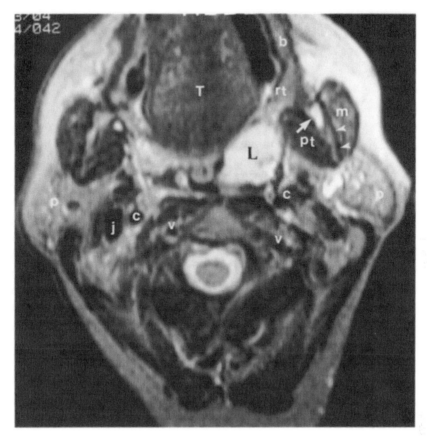

Figure 37-33. Tonsillar lymphoma. Axial T₁W MRI. (L, lymphoma in palatine tonsil; rt, retromolar trigone; arrow, pterygomandibular fat space; m, masseter; arrowheads, mandible; b, buccinator muscle; T, tongue; c, internal carotid; j, jugular vein; p, parotid; v, vertebral artery; pt, medial pterygoid muscle.)

into the retromaxillary fat space results. Once the pterygomaxillary raphe is penetrated, the tumor has access to the masseteric and pterygomandibular space laterally and posteriorly. The latter is a small fat space (see Figure 37-33, arrow) between the mandible and medial pterygoid muscle. The latter space contains the lingual nerve and is continuous with the parapharyngeal space.

Hard palate lesions may invade the nasal cavity by direct growth. Via the greater and lesser palatine foramina the tumors can reach the pterygopalatine fossa and from there spread perineurally into the cavernous sinus (see Figure 37-30).[101]

Lesions of the oral cavity have a very infiltrative growth along muscular planes and neurovascular bundles. The full extent is therefore clinically often not appreciated. Referred pain to the ear is a common presentation for tumors of the tongue base or glossotonsillar sulcus.[102] Trismus is a late sign indicating invasion of the infratemporal fossa and pterygoid muscles.[103] For operative planning, exact imaging with CT or MRI is therefore indispensable. The extent of tumor infiltration often surprises the clinician. As tumor to soft tissue contrast is higher on

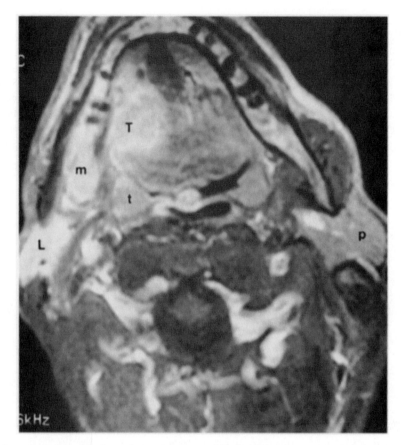

Figure 37-34.   Squamous cell carcinoma of tongue with infiltration of sublingual, submandibular, and parotid space. Axial gadolinium-enhanced T$_1$W MRI. (t, primary tongue carcinoma; m, tumor infiltrating sublingual space and mandible; L, tumor in parotid/submandibular space; t, tonsil; p, parotid gland.)

MRI, and due to its multiplanar capabilities, MRI continues to become the imaging method of choice, though CT is an effective tool in this area if attention is given to avoiding beam-hardening artifacts from artificial teeth by appropriate angulation of the gantry.

Minor salivary gland obstruction in the oral cavity may result in mucoceles, which are referred to as ranulas. If not infected they usually present as pure fluid masses. They can become quite large and present as insinuating masses originating in the sublingual space and extending over the free edge of the mylohyoid muscle into the submandibular space.[104] Epidermoids or dermoids can simulate ranulas. Epidermoids or dermoids occur usually in the midline of the floor of the mouth and less frequently in the soft palate. Presence of fat favors a dermoid cyst; calcifications, a teratoid.

Infrahyoid Neck

A major role in imaging of the neck is to assess the presence and extent of lymphadenopathy. Both CT and MRI are good in visualizing nodes. A CT scan is best done with intravenous contrast. To determine whether a lymph node is abnormal is largely dependent on the size of the node. In general, lymph nodes should not exceed 1 cm in size except for the jugulodigastric node, which can measure up to 1.5 cm. However, size itself does not differentiate between malignant and reactive nodes. The CT scan has an advantage over MRI, as it can possibly show metastatic disease in a normal-sized lymph node. The metastasis appears as a lucent center in a peripherally enhancing node. It is often referred to as a "necrotic" node (Figure 37-35), although necrosis is rarely seen pathologically in small nodes. Probably one sees a less enhancing tumor centrally surrounded by more intensely enhancing normal lymph node tissue.[105–107] Gadolinium-enhanced MRI even with fat suppression does not show this finding consistently. As the amount of enhancement in central tumor and peripheral node are both intense, it may not be appreciated. On noncontrast MRI, tumor within nodes is often intermediate in intensity on both T_1W and T_2W images. Necrotic nodes show a low signal on T_1 and high signal on T_2. Any heterogeneity in signal within a lymph node is suspicious for metastases in MRI. An MRI has an advantage over CT in evaluation of the

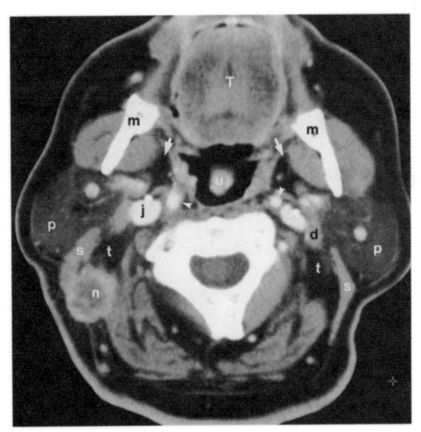

Figure 37-35.   "Necrotic" lymph node metastasis. Axial contrast-enhanced CT. (n, "necrotic" lymph node; s, sternocleidomastoid muscle; t, posterior cervical space; p, parotid gland; j, jugular vein; arrowhead, internal carotid artery; u, uvula; arrow, nasoparapharyngeal space; m, mandible; T, tongue; d, inferior belly digastric muscle.)

retropharyngeal nodes, which do not contrast well from the surrounding musculature on CT. Encasement of vasculature by lymph node masses is also shown more readily by MRI.[108]

Large, homogeneous nodes are suspicious for Hodgkin's or non-Hodgkin's lymphoma and sarcoid or infectious mononucleosis. Densely enhancing lymph nodes on CT are often due to inflammatory processes, especially tuberculosis, metastatic renal or thyroid carcinoma, Kaposi's sarcoma, and angioblastic adenopathies including Castleman disease. Calcified nodes occur especially in old granulomatous disease, metastatic thyroid carcinoma, or mucin-producing tumors such as breast or colon metastases. Following radiation or chemotherapy, calcification can be seen. Partly calcified and at the same time enhancing nodes can be seen in granulomatous diseases or metastatic thyroid carcinoma.[23] If nodes show a variable appearance, ranging from homogeneous to necrotic and calcified, granulomatous disease is likely. It should be remembered that the most common reason for a neck mass in an adult over 40 is metastatic squamous cell carcinoma or thyroid metastasis. Below age 40 a lymphoma is the most common cause for a neck mass. If a primary is unknown, the location of the involved lymph nodes may help in determining a likely site of origin (see Table 37-3).

Reactive lymphadenopathy secondary to an infection is most commonly encountered in the jugulodigastric and the submandibular nodes. Imaging characteristics of an abscess are a ring-enhancing lesion with a central necrotic fluid collection. Differentiation from a necrotic tumor mass may at times be difficult. However, infiltration of adjacent fat, enhancement of fascial planes, and skin thickening are indicators for inflammatory disease. It should be kept in mind that congenital masses can become secondarily infected just as necrotic tumors.

The most common congenital lesion in the infrahyoid neck is a type II branchial cleft cyst. Patients usually present between ages 10 and 40. It is a painless fluctuant mass that often varies in size with respiratory infections. Branchial cleft cysts usually present as well-defined fluid density masses anterior to the sternocleidomastoid muscle in the anterior cervical space displacing the carotid artery and jugular vein medially and posteriorly. The CT appearance is usually that of a nonenhancing low-attenuation mass. On MRI especially, the signal varies depending on the protein content, and can be rather high on T_1W images. It usually is also high in signal on T_2W images. Enhancement can occur peripherally if the cyst is infected.

The second most common congenital lesion is the cystic hygroma or lymphangioma, which is a lymphatic retention cyst due to obstruction or agenesis of afferent lymphatic vessels (Figure 37-36). In contrast to the branchial cleft cyst, cystic hygromas present shortly after birth. Cystic hygromas are most commonly found in the posterior cervical space but can occur in the sublingual or submandibular space. Cystic hygromas usually have fluid density. Fluid-fluid levels are characteristic. Septations are often appreciated. An MRI shows the insinuating nature of the lesion given the great contrast to the surrounding tissues on T_2W images. Loculations of the cyst may have different signal characteristics on T_1W images secondary to the different protein content in the loculations.

Thyroglossal duct cysts are derived of remnants of the incompletely involuted thyroglossal duct, which reaches from the foramen cecum at the tongue base to the thyroid gland. The duct is midline and is intimately related to the hyoid bone. The duct loops around the anterior hyoid bone in midline and may therefore be anterior and/or posterior to the hyoid in the midline. Lower cysts are usually embedded in the strap muscles off midline. If there is solid tissue associated with the cyst, this may represent an ectopic thyroid gland, which also has an increased risk for malignant degeneration.[109,110]

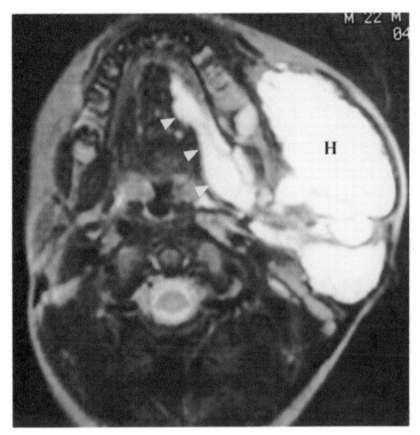

Figure 37-36. Cystic hygroma submandibular and sublingual spaces. Axial T$_2$W MRI. (H, hygroma submandibular space; arrowheads, extension of hygroma into sublingual space.)

Paragangliomas and schwannomas are the most commonly encountered lesions of the carotid space. As the vagus nerve runs between the jugular and carotid, these tumors usually push the carotid anteriorly and medially. The jugular is pushed posteriorly. Only neurogenic tumors separate the carotid artery and jugular vein in this fashion. A special case is the carotid body tumor, which develops in the carotid bifurcation and typically separates the external and internal carotid, resulting in a tulip configuration of the carotid bifurcation. Paragangliomas and carotid body tumors show dense enhancement due to their vascularity. On MRI the paraganglioma may show signal voids due to high-flow vessels in the lesion giving the tumor a salt-and-pepper appearance (Figure 37-37). Neurinomas and schwannomas show variable enhancement characteristics, from densely enhancing to nonenhancing. Lipomatous degeneration is possible.

Carotid aneurysm could potentially mimic neurogenic tumors in the carotid space. Today this problem can usually be solved with MR angiography. Other locations for peripheral neuromas are in the brachial plexus. These lesions may push the anterior scalene muscle anteriorly. Rare locations for other tumors correspond to the location of the nerve they originate from. The phrenic nerve runs anterior to the anterior scalene muscle, the sympa-

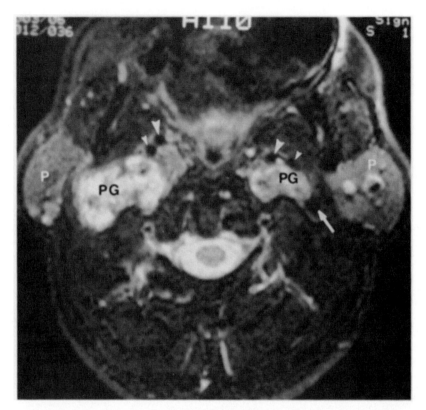

Figure 37-37.   Bilateral paraganglioma. Axial T$_2$W MRI. (PG, paraganglioma; large arrowhead, internal carotid artery; small arrowhead, external carotid artery; arrow, left jugular vein, jugular vein on right is occluded. (Note on left separation of carotid vessel from jugular vein by mass indicating its neurogenic origin in the carotid space; P, parotid.)

thetic trunk anterior to the prevertebral muscle, the accessory nerve in the posterior cervical space, and the recurrent nerve in the tracheoesophageal groove.

For evaluation of masses arising from the thyroid gland, MRI is especially helpful to define the extent of thyroid tumors or substernal goiters. The relationship of the goiter to major vessels is clearly shown without application of contrast. It is therefore preferable to CT, as application of iodine may interfere with the radioisotope workup and potential radioactive iodine therapy. An MRI can show hemorrhagic degeneration. Demonstration of an intact pseudocapsule (low intensity on T$_2$) favors a benign adenoma, whereas penetration of the pseudocapsule favors malignancy.[111]

Evaluation of parathyroid adenomas by MRI compares with nuclear medicine and CT examinations.[112] The signal can be variable depending on the presence or absence of hemorrhagic degeneration of the tumor and depending on the age of the hemorrhage. An MRI is not affected by artifacts from the shoulder girdle at the cervicothoracic junction as is a CT. Mediastinal lesions are easily examined by MRI, in contrast to ultrasound, which is limited in the mediastinum. The great vessels are shown without contrast, facilitating an adenoma detection.[113]

Larynx and Hypopharynx

As endoscopic techniques[114–116] for evaluating the larynx are far advanced, the role of imaging is to demonstrate the pathology not visible by endoscopy. Therefore, imaging has to concentrate on the evaluation of the deep tissues. The two important spaces in the larynx are the pre-epiglottic and paraglottic spaces. The pre-epiglottic space is anterior to the epiglottis. Its most anterior aspect reaches to the thyroid cartilage and superiorly to the thyrohyoid membrane. The pre-epiglottic space is mainly filled with fat. The paraglottic space is more lateral in position. It represents the space deep to the true and false cords. At the level of the false cord the paraglottic space contains mainly fat. At the level of the true cord the space is mainly occupied by the thyroaryepiglottic muscle.

For voice-saving surgery in supraglottic tumors, it is of utmost importance to determine whether the tumor reaches or traverses the true cord, in which case a total laryngectomy has to be performed. It is therefore most important to evaluate whether the tumor invades the paraglottic fat space and reaches to the thyroarytenoid muscle. If the tumor crosses the mucosa of the ventricle, this is usually evident by endoscopy. Tumor may grow submucosally around the ventricle in the paraglottic space and extend into the lateral part of the true cord and below. Tumor may also grow superiorly along the pre-epiglottic space and from there involve the tongue base.

If the tumor arises on the vocal cord, one has to determine whether there is spread along the anterior commissure to the other cord and whether the tumor grows inferiorly. If the tumor reaches the upper margin of the cricoid cartilage, a vertical hemilaryngectomy can no longer be performed. One therefore has to look for tumor within the ring of the cricoid.

It is important to note whether the cartilage is involved. This, however, may be difficult because of the variability of ossification. Subtle infiltration of the cartilage is difficult to detect by either CT or MRI. Nonossified cartilage may have the same attenuation as tumor on CT, whereas on MRI tumor may have a slightly higher signal on T_2W images than bone marrow. Sclerosis of the cartilage, especially if asymmetric, may indicate tumor infiltration on CT, or at least perichondrial spread resulting in adjacent edema and sclerosis.[117]

Hypopharyngeal carcinomas often involve the larynx (Figure 37-38). Therefore the tumor extent has to be determined in relation to the ventricle, vocal cords, and cricoid. Pyriform sinus tumors may extend around the thyroid lamina into the paraglottic space. Laterally, pyriform sinus tumors may involve the carotid.

There is not yet a uniform opinion as to what imaging method is preferred in evaluation of the larynx. An MRI clearly shows better soft tissue contrast, whereas it is handicapped by respiratory motion. Recent improvements in fast imaging may make this less of a problem. A CT scan, on the other hand, is much faster, with imaging times per slice between subseconds and 2 seconds. Using spiral techniques, the larynx can be imaged within a breath hold. Soft tissue contrast, however, does not compare to MRI. The CT scan has an advantage in the evaluation of chondroid lesions, as it depicts the mineralized matrix of the tumors.

Rare lesions in the larynx involve hemangiomas or glomus tumors, which demonstrate dense enhancement after contrast.

Cysts in the larynx are either small retention cysts of minor salivary glands or related to the appendix of the ventricle, which may become obstructed, with resulting development of

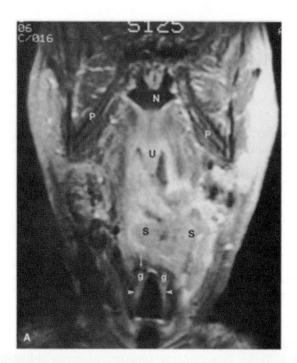

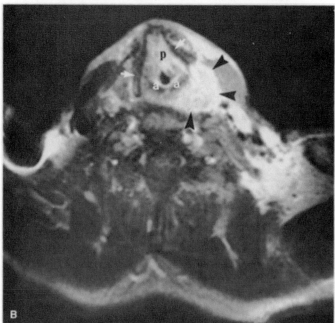

Figure 37-38. Squamous cell carcinoma pyriform sinus. A. Coronal gadolinium-enhanced, fat-suppressed T$_1$W MRI. (S, squamous cell carcinoma pyriform sinus invading into supraglottic larynx with severe compromise of airway; g, glottis; small arrow, compressed laryngeal ventricle; arrowhead, cricoid cartilage; u, uvula; p, medial pterygoid muscle; N, nasopharynx.) B. Axial gadolinium-enhanced, fat-suppressed T$_1$W MRI. (Arrowheads, pyriform sinus tumor; p, invasion into the paraglottic space; a, arytenoid cartilage; arrow, thyroid cartilage.)

either a saccular cyst or an air-filled laryngocele. Large cysts may penetrate through the thyrohyoid membrane into the lateral neck. An obstructing tumor at the ventricle should be looked for. A pharyngocele is continuous with the pyriform sinus and not the laryngeal ventricle.

Recurrent laryngeal nerve palsy results in atrophy of the thyroarytenoid muscle. As a result the ventricle dilates. To determine the etiology of the recurrent nerve palsy, imaging should be performed from the skull base to the aortic arch on the left or subclavian artery on the right. Jugular foramen tumors and carotid sheath tumors affecting the vagus have to be ruled out, as well as mediastinal adenopathy in the aortopulmonic window and tumor in the tracheoesophageal groove compressing the recurrent laryngeal nerve.[40,118]

NEW TECHNOLOGIES

Image-Guided Surgery

Image-guided surgery permits the surgeon to visualize anatomic relationships intraoperatively on a video monitor, which displays the preoperative CT scan.[119,120] This new technology has been most useful in improving the surgeon's confidence during difficult cases of altered anatomy due to severe disease or previous surgery. It requires a special preoperative CT scan with sensors or registration markers to provide positional information. This is a valuable tool in assisting the surgeon in identifying anatomy and disease but does not replace a thorough understanding of the surgical landmarks when performing these operations.

MRA

Significant advances have been made in noninvasive MRI angiograms (MRA). The introduction of stronger gradients in modern MRI machines allows very short acquisition times. With the use of intravenous gadolinium, high-resolution angiography (MRA) can be obtained in about 10 seconds, allowing us to separate the arterial phase from the venous phase of an intravenous gadolinium bolus injection. MRA therefore became a screening tool for evaluation of atherosclerotic carotid and vertebral disease in the neck. It can also be used to demonstrate the vascularity of tumors (Figure 37-39). Secondary reformatting is performed on 3D workstations that allow the cutout of a particular vascular tree and angiotomographic images, avoiding superimposition of vessels. 3D display in multiple projections is easily obtainable.[121–126]

PET

Differentiation of tumor or reactive soft tissue changes after radiation and chemotherapy can be difficult with CT and MRI, as reactive changes or necrosis after radiation can simulate recurrence. The recent introduction of ^{18}F-FDG PET ([18]fluoro-deoxy-D-glucose positron emission tomography) seems to be a promising technique to improve the diagnosis of recurrent tumor and to determine the primary tumor site in head and neck metastatic disease[127,128] (Figure 37-40).

^{18}F-FDG is primarily incorporated into metabolically active tissue, such as brain, myocardium, and tumor. Its uptake increases with time in metabolically active tissue. Though false-positive results are possible due to uptake in inflammatory tissue, serial scanning shows a washout of activity or a constant level in inflammation, as inflammatory tissue is metabolically less active.[128,129]

^{18}F-FDG PET appears to have a higher specificity and sensitivity, especially in cases of prior surgery and radiation therapy, than conventional methods. The ability to screen the whole body makes it an ideal tumor staging tool. Negative results are highly significant. It has been

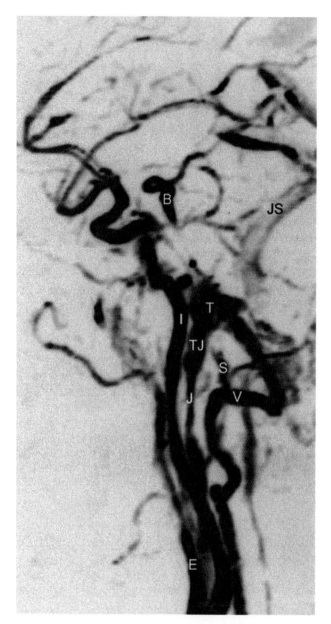

Figure 37-39.   Jugulotympanic glomus tumor: cut out of gadolinium MRA. (T, tumor; TJ, tumor extension into jugular vein; J, AV shunt into jugular vein; S, feeding stylomastoid artery; V, vertebral artery; B, basilar artery; JS, jugular sinus; I, internal carotid; E, external carotid.

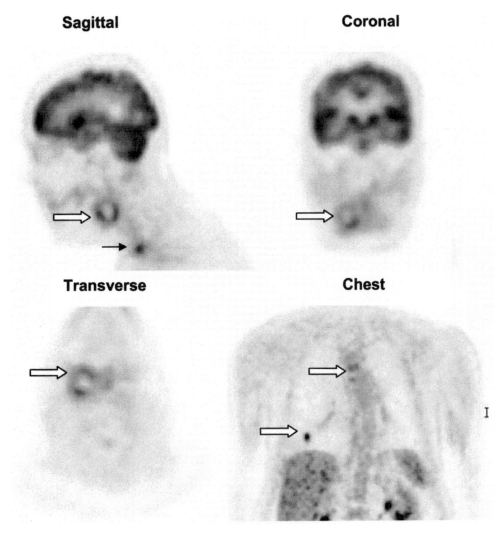

Sagittal

Coronal

Transverse

Chest

Figure 37-40. Metastases from sarcomatoid carcinoma of the larynx after laryngectomy.
Neck: Sagittal, coronal, and transverse images demonstrating a right submandibular lymph node metastasis (block arrow). Site of laryngectomy (small arrow).
Chest: Lung metastases and mediastinal metastases. (*Courtesy Dr. Vincent Caride, Hospital St. Raphael, New Haven.*)

suggested to perform ^{18}F-FDG as primary exam after treatment of head and neck cancers and to follow it with conventional methods such as CT and MRI only when the PET scan is positive, as conventional methods such as MRI and CT show a higher anatomic detail.[129]

Multislice Spiral CT

CT has recently made significant advances by enabling the acquisition of multiple slices within the same rotation of the gantry. This allows us to perform the examination faster, which is advantageous for contrast bolus examinations, as the concentration of contrast can be maintained throughout the exam. Alternatively, one can use the multislice capability to perform thin slices in a short time. Overlapping reconstruction of the spiral multislice data allows production of thin overlapping slices, which can be used for high-resolution reformatted images in planes different from the primary acquisition of the CT slices.[130] High-resolution coronal scans, obtained from the axial data set, approach the resolution of the primary axial slice.[131-133] This is performed after the exam on special 3D workstations. Secondary reformatted high-resolution images of the petrous bones, facial bones, and larynx can thus be obtained from the axial spiral data set, avoiding uncomfortable positioning of the patient and potential streak artifacts from metal implants, especially in teeth. Functional CT imaging during Valsalva maneuvers, breath-hold, and phonation of the larynx are possible, improving tumor detection and staging.[132,133]

References

1. Bergeron RT, Osborn AC, Som PH. *Head and Neck Imaging, Excluding the Brain*. St. Louis: Mosby, 1984.
2. Etter LE. *Roentgenography and Roentgenology of the Middle Ear and Mastoid Process*. Springfield, IL: Charles C Thomas, 1965.
3. Merrill V. *Atlas of Roentgenographic Positions*, 2nd ed. St. Louis: Mosby, 1959, 384–385.
4. Pendergrass EP, Schaeffer JP, Hodes PJ. *The Head and Neck in Roentgen Diagnosis*, 2nd ed. Springfield, IL: Charles C Thomas, 1956.
5. Compere WE. Tympanic cavity and clearance studies. *Trans Am Acad Ophthalmol Otol.* 1958;62:444.
6. Samuel E. *Clinical Radiology of the Ear, Nose, and Throat*. London: Lewis, 1952.
7. Valvassori GE. Radiology of the temporal bone. In Paparella MM, Shumrick DA, eds. *Otolaryngology*. Vol. I. Philadelphia: Saunders, 1973, 1021–1042.
8. Valvassori GE, ed. Symposium on radiology in otolaryngology. *Otolaryngol Clin North Am.* 1973;6.
9. Young BR. *The Skull, Sinuses and Mastoids: A Handbook of Roentgen Diagnosis*. Chicago: Year Book, 1951.
10. Yanagisawa E, Smith HW. Normal radiographic anatomy of the paranasal sinuses. *Otolaryngol Clin North Am.* 1973;6:429–457.
11. Merrell RA Jr, Yanagisawa E. Radiographic anatomy of the paranasal sinuses. I. Waters view. *Arch Otolaryngol.* 1968;87:184–195.
12. Yanagisawa E, Smith HW, Thaler S. Radiographic anatomy of the paranasal sinuses. II.
Lateral view. *Arch Otolaryngol.* 1968;87:196–209.
13. Yanagisawa E, Smith HW, Merrell RA Jr. Radiographic anatomy of the paranasal sinuses. III. Submentovertical view. *Arch Otolaryngol.* 1968;87:299–310.
14. Yanagisawa E, Smith HW, Merrell RA Jr. Radiographic anatomy of the paranasal sinuses. IV. Caldwell view. *Arch Otolaryngol.* 1968;87:311–322.
15. Yanagisawa E, Smith HW. Radiographic anatomy of the paranasal sinuses and related structures. In English GM, ed. *Otolaryngology*. Vol. II. New York: Harper & Row, 1979.
16. Yanagisawa E. Symposium on maxillo-facial trauma III. Pitfalls in the management of zygomatic fractures. *Laryngoscope.* 1973;83:527–546.
17. Dingman RO, Natvig P. *Surgery of Facial Fractures*. Philadelphia: Saunders, 1964.
18. Yanagisawa E, Smith HW, Merrell RA, et al. Radiographic anatomy of the paranasal sinuses. *Arch Otolaryngol.* 1965;82:275.
19. Hudgins PA. The nasopharynx and related spaces. *ASHNR 26th Annual Conference and Postgraduate Course.* Vancouver: ASHNR, 1993, 73–80.
20. Harnsberger HR. Introduction to neck anatomy. *ASHNR 26th Annual Conference and Postgraduate Course.* Vancouver: ASHNR, 1993, 5–11.
21. Harnsberger HR. Head and neck imaging. In Osborne A, Bragg D, eds. *Handbooks in Radiology*. Chicago: Year Book, 1990.

22. Smoker WRK. The infrahyoid neck. *ASHNR 26th Annual Conference and Postgraduate Course.* Vancouver: ASHNR, 1993, 13–19.

23. Holliday RA. Neck nodes and masses. *ASHNR 26th Annual Conference and Postgraduate Course.* Vancouver: ASHNR, 1993, 87–97.

24. Hupke R. The advantages of fast and continuously rotating CT systems. In Fuchs W, ed. *Advances in CT.* New York: Springer-Verlag, 1990.

25. Kalender WA, Vock P, Seissler W. Spiral CT scanning for fast and continuous volume data acquisition. In Fuchs W, ed. *Advances in CT.* New York: Springer-Verlag, 1990.

26. Zwicker C, Astinet F, Langer M, et al. Evaluation of three-dimensional CT in orofacial surgery. In Fuchs W, ed. *Advances in CT.* New York: Springer-Verlag, 1990.

27. Baker HL Jr. The application of magnetic resonance imaging in otolaryngology. *Laryngoscope.* 1986;96:19.

28. Fullerton GD. Physiologic basis of magnetic relaxation. In Stark DD, Bradley WG Jr, eds. *Magnetic Resonance Imaging.* St. Louis: Mosby, 1988, 3–23.

29. Wehrii FW. Principles of magnetic resonance. In Stark DD, Bradley WG Jr, eds. *Magnetic Resonance Imaging.* St. Louis: Mosby, 1988, 36–55.

30. Fullerton GD, Potter JL, Dombluth NC. NMR relaxing of protons in tissues and other macromolecular water solutions. *Magn Reson Imaging.* 1982;1:209.

31. Mitchell DG, Burk DL, Viniitski S, Rifkin MD. The biophysical basis of tissue contrast in extracranial MRI imaging. *AJR.* 1987;149:831–837.

32. Gomori JM, Grossman RI, Hackney DB, et al. Variable appearances of subacute intracranial hematomas on high field spin echo MR. *AJNR.* 1987;8:1019–1026.

33. Thulborn KR, Brady TJ. Iron in magnetic resonance imaging of cerebral hemorrhage. *Magn Reson Q.* 1989;5:23–28.

34. Anderson CM, Lee RE. Time of flight angiography. In Anderson CM, Edelman RR, Turski PA, eds. *Clinical Magnetic Resonance Angiography.* New York: Raven, 1993, 11–42.

35. Gullberg GT, Wehrii FW, Shimakawa A, Simons MA. MR vascular imaging with a fast gradient refocusing pulse sequence and reformatted images from transaxial sections. *Radiology.* 1987;165:241–246.

36. Laub GA, Kaiser WA. MR angiography with gradient motion refocusing. *Comput Assist Tomogr.* 1988;12:377–382.

37. Dumoulin C, Souza S, Walker M, Wagle W. Three-dimensional phase contrast angiography. *Magn Reson Med.* 1989;9:139–149.

38. Turski PA, Korosec FR. Phase contrast angiography. In Anderson CM, Edelman RR, Turski PA, eds. *Clinical Magnetic Resonance Angiography.* New York: Raven, 1993, 43–73.

39. Anderson CM, Turski PA, Edelman RR. Flow quantification. In Anderson CM, Edelman RR, Turski PA, eds. *Clinical Magnetic Resonance Angiography.* New York: Raven, 1993, 127–142.

40. Jabour BA, Lufkin RB, Hanafee WN. Magnetic resonance of the larynx. *Top Magn Reson Imaging.* 1990;2:60–68.

41. Stack JP, Antoun NM, Jenkins JPR, et al. Gadolinium-DTPA as a contrast agent in magnetic resonance imaging of the brain. *Neuroradiology.* 1988;30:145–154.

42. Shellock FG, Morisoli S, Kanal E. MR procedures and biomedical implants, materials, and devices: 1993 update. *Radiology.* 1993;189:587–599.

43. Applebaum EL, Valvassori GE. Effects of magnetic resonance imaging fields on stapedectomy prostheses. *Arch Otolaryngol.* 1985;111:820.

44. Babbel R, Harnsberger HR, Nelson B, et al. Optimization of technique in screening CT of the sinuses. *AJNR.* 1991;12:849–854.

45. Zinreich JS. Imaging for functional endoscopic sinus surgery. *ASHNR 26th Annual Conference and Postgraduate Course.* Vancouver: ASHNR, 1993, 157–160.

46. Zinreich JS, Kennedy DW, Rosenbaum AE, et al. Paranasal sinuses CT imaging requirements for endoscopic surgery. *Radiology.* 1987;163:769–773.

47. Earwaker J. Anatomic variants in sino-nasal CT. *Radiographics.* 1993;13:381–415.

48. Som PM. Neoplasm and inflammation of the sinuses. *ASHNR 26th Annual Conference and Postgraduate Course.* Vancouver: ASHNR, 1993, 139–146.

49. Moore J, Potchen M, Waldenmaier N, et al. High field magnetic resonance imaging of paranasal sinus inflammatory disease. *Laryngoscope.* 1986;96:267–271.

50. Shapiro M, Som PM. MRI of the paranasal sinuses and nasal cavity. *Radiol Clin North Am.* 1989;27:447–475.

51. Weissman JL, Tabor EK, Curtin HD. Magnetic resonance imaging of the paranasal sinuses. *Top Magn Reson Imaging.* 1990;2:27–38.

52. Som PM, Dillon PW, Sze G, et al. Benign and malignant sinonasal lesions with intracranial extension: Differentiation with MRI imaging. *Radiology.* 1989;172:763–766.

53. Lloyd G. Diagnostic imaging of the nose and paranasal sinuses. *J Laryngol Otol.* 1989;103: 453–460.

54. Som PM, Dillon WP, Fullerton GD, et al. Chronically obstructed sinonasal secretions: Observations on T1 and T2 shortening. *Radiology.* 1989;172:515–520.

55. Dillon WP, Som PM, Fullerton GD. Hypointense MR signal in chronically inspissated sinonasal secretions. *Radiology.* 1990;174: 73–78.

56. Som PM. Neoplasm and inflammation of the sinuses. *ASHNR 26th Annual Conference and Postgraduate Course.* Vancouver: ASHNR, 1993, 139–146.

57. Kassel EE, Gruss JS. Imaging of midfacial fractures. *Neuroimaging North Am.* 1991;1: 259–283.

58. Yeates A, Blumenkopf B, Drayer B, et al. Spontaneous CSF rhinorrhea arising from the middle cranial fossa: CT demonstration. *AJNR.* 1984;5:820–821.

59. Johnson DB, Brennan P, Toland J, O'Dwyer AJ. Magnetic resonance imaging in the evaluation of cerebrospinal fluid fistulae. *Clin Radiol* 1996;51(12):837–841.

60. Chakeres DW, Spiegel RK. A systematic technique for comprehensive evaluation of the temporal bone by computed tomography. *Radiology.* 1983;146:97.

61. Valvassori GE. Diagnosis of retrocochlear and central vestibular disease by magnetic resonance imaging. *Ann Otol Rhinol Laryngol.* 1988;97:19–22.

62. Wayman JW, Dutcher PO, Manzione JV, et al. Gadolinium-DTPA-enhanced magnetic reso-

nance scanning in cerebello-pontine angle tumors. *Laryngoscope,* 1989;99:1167–1170.

63. Stack JP, Ramsden RT, Antoun NM, et al. Magnetic resonance imaging of acoustic neuromas: The role of gadolinium-DTPA. *Br J Radiol.* 1988;61:800.

64. Curati WL, Graif M, Kingsley DPE, et al. Acoustic neuromas: Gd-DTPA enhancement in MR imaging. *Radiology.* 1986;158:447–451.

65. Daniels DL, Czervionke LF, Millen SJ, et al. MRI imaging of facial nerve enhancement in Bell's palsy or after temporal bone surgery. *Radiology.* 1989;171:807–809.

66. Seltzer S, Mark AS. Contrast enhancement of the labyrinth on MR scans in patients with sudden hearing loss and vertigo: Evidence of labyrinthine disease. *AJNR.* 1991;12:13–18.

67. Swartz JD, Harnsberger HR. The temporal bone: Magnetic resonance imaging. *Top Magn Reson Imaging.* 1990;2:1–16.

68. Millen SJ, Daniels DL, Meyers GA. Gadolinium-enhanced magnetic resonance imaging in temporal bone lesions. *Laryngoscope.* 1989; 99:257–260.

69. Mikhael M, Wolff AP, Ciric IS. Current concepts in neuroradiological diagnosis of acoustic neuromas. *Laryngoscope.* 1987;97:471–476.

70. Sidman JD, Carrasco VN, Whaley RA, Pillsbury HC. Gadolinium: The new gold standard for diagnosing cerebello-pontine angle tumors. *Arch Otolaryngol Head Neck Surg.* 1989;115: 1244–1247.

71. Tsuruda JS, Hayes C, Dalley R. Phase array coils: Theory and application to the head and neck region. *ASHNR 26th Annual Conference and Postgraduate Course.* Vancouver: ASHNR, 1993, 33–36.

72. Chakeres DW. Temporal bone: Normal anatomy. *ASHNR 26th Annual Conference and Postgraduate Course.* Vancouver: ASHNR, 1993, 21–24.

73. Jackler RK, De La Cruz A. The large vestibular aqueduct syndrome. *Laryngoscope.* 1989; 99:1238–1243.

74. Valvassori GE. The large vestibular aqueduct and associated anomalies of the inner ear. *Otolaryngol Clin North Am.* 1983;16:95–101.

75. Brogan M, Chakeres DW, Schmalbrock P. Comparison of high resolution 3DFT and com-

puted tomography in the evaluation of the otic capsule and vestibular aqueduct. *AJNR.* 1991; 12:1–11.

76. Mafee MF, Charletta D, Kumar A, Belmont H. Large vestibular aqueduct and congenital sensorineural hearing loss. *AJNR.* 1992;13:805–819.

77. Mafee MF, Aimi K, Kahen HL, et al. Chronic otomastoiditis: Conceptual understanding of CT findings. *Radiology.* 1986;160:193–198.

78. Swartz JD. Acute and chronic otomastoiditis. *ASHNR 26th Annual Conference and Postgraduate Course.* Vancouver: ASHNR, 1993, 201–206.

79. Swartz JD, Harnsberger HR. *Imaging of the Temporal Bone,* 2nd ed. New York: Thieme, 1992.

80. Martin N, Sterkers O, Nahum H. Cholesterol granulomas of the middle ear cavities: MR imaging. *Radiology.* 1990;172:521–525.

81. Greenberg JJ, Got RF, Wismer GL, et al. Cholesterol granuloma of the petrous apex. *AJNR.* 1988;9:1205–1214.

82. Valvassori GE. Otosclerosis and otodystrophies. *ASHNR 26th Annual Conference and Postgraduate Course.* Vancouver: ASHNR, 1993, 197–199.

83. Valvassori GE, Dobben GD. CT densitometry of the cochlear capsule in otosclerosis. *AJNR.* 1985;6:661–667.

84. Weissman JL. Salivary gland pathology. *ASHNR 26th Annual Conference and Postgraduate Course.* Vancouver: ASHNR, 1993, 83.

85. Tabor EK, Curtin HD. MR of the salivary glands. *Radiol Clin North Am.* 1989;27:379–392.

86. Holliday RA, Cohen WA, Schinella RA, et al. Benign lymphoepithelial parotid cysts and hyperplastic cervical lymphadenopathy: A new CT appearance. *Radiology.* 1988;168:439–441.

87. Vogl T, Dressel S, Bilaniuk LT, et al. Tumors of the nasopharynx and adjacent areas: MR imaging with Gd-DTPA. *AJNR.* 1990;1:187–194.

88. Tien RD, Hesselink JR, Chu PK, Szumowski J. Improved detection and delineation of head and neck lesions with fat suppression spin echo MR imaging. *AJNR.* 1990;2:69–75.

89. Simon JH, Szumowski J. Chemical shift imaging with paramagnetic contrast material enhancement for improved lesion depiction. *Radiology.* 1989;71:539–543.

90. Teresi LM, Lufkin RB, Vinuela F, et al. MR imaging of nasopharynx and floor of middle cranial fossa, part II. Malignant tumors. *Radiology.* 1987;164:817–821.

91. Curtin HD, Williams R. Computed topographic anatomy of the pterygopalatine fossa. *Radiographics.* 1985;5:429–440.

92. Lanzieri CF, Bangert B. Magnetic resonance imaging of the nasopharynx. *Top Magn Reson Imaging.* 1990;2:49–59.

93. Rao VM. The mid skull base: Anatomy and pathology. *ASHNR 26th Annual Conference and Postgraduate Course.* Vancouver: ASHNR, 1993, 115–121.

94. Yanagisawa K, Friedman CD, Vining EM, Abrahams J. Dentascan imaging of the mandible and maxilla. *Head Neck.* 1993;15:1–7.

95. Abrahams AJ. Mandibular lesions and dental implants. *ASHNR 26th Annual Conference and Postgraduate Course.* Vancouver: ASHNR, 1993, 63–71.

96. Abrahams JJ, Olivierio PJ. Odontogenic cysts: Improved imaging with a dental CT software program. *AJNR.* 1993;14:367–374.

97. Abrahams JJ. CT assessment of dental implant planning. *Oral Maxillofac Surg Clin North Am.* 1992;4:1–18.

98. Mancuso AA. The oropharynx and oral cavity. *ASHNR 26th Annual Conference and Postgraduate Course.* Vancouver: ASHNR, 1993, 51–60.

99. Mancuso AA, Harnsberger HR, Dillon WP. *Workbook for MRI and CT of the Head and Neck,* 2nd ed. Baltimore: Williams & Wilkins, 1989.

100. Som PM, Bergeron RT. *Head and Neck Imaging,* 2nd ed. St. Louis: Mosby, 1991.

101. Parker GD, Harnsberger HR. Clinical-radiologic issues in perineural tumor spread of malignant disease of the extra-cranial head and neck. *Radiographics.* 1991;1:383–399.

102. Yanagisawa K, Kveton JF. Referred otalgia. *Am J Otolaryngol.* 1992;13:323–327.

103. Mancuso AA, Hanafee HN. *Computed Tomography and MRI of the Head and Neck,* 2nd ed. Baltimore: Williams & Wilkins, 1985.

104. McKenna KM, Bradley AJ, Lufkin RB, Hanafee WN. Magnetic resonance imaging of

the tongue and oropharynx. *Top Magn Reson Imaging.* 1990;2:49–59.

105. Yousem DM, Som PM, Hackney DB, et al. Central nodal necrosis and extracapsular neoplastic spread in cervical lymphnodes: MR imaging versus CT. *Radiology.* 1982;182: 753–760.

106. Som PM. Review. Detection of metastasis in cervical lymphnodes: CT and MR criteria and differential diagnosis. Lymph nodes of the neck. *AJR.* 1992;158:961–969.

107. Som PM. Lymph nodes of the neck. *Radiology.* 1983;148:709–723.

108. Jabour BA, Lufkin RB, Layfield LJ, Hanafee WN. Magnetic resonance imaging of metastatic cervical adenopathy. *Top Magn Reson Imaging.* 1990;2:69–75.

109. Johnson JC, Coleman LL. MR imaging of a lingual thyroid gland. *Pediatr Radiol.* 1989; 19:461.

110. Yanagisawa K, Eisen RN, Sasaki CT. Squamous cell carcinoma arising in a thyroglossal duct cyst. *Arch Otolaryngol Head Neck Surg.* 1992;118:538–541.

111. Noma S, Kanaoka M, Minami S, et al. Thyroid masses: MRI imaging and pathologic correlation. *Radiology.* 1988;168:759.

112. Kmbsack AJ, Wilson SD, Lawson TL, et al. Prospective comparison of radio-nuclide, computed tomographic, sonographic, and magnetic resonance localization of parathyroid tumors. *Surgery.* 1989;106:639–646.

113. Aufferman W, Guis M, Taveras NJ, et al. MRI signal intensity of parathyroid adenomas: Correlation with histopathology. *AJR.* 1989;153: 873.

114. Yanagisawa E, Yanagisawa K. Stroboscopic videolaryngography: A comparison of fiberscopic and telescopic documentation. *Ann Otol Rhinol Laryngol.* 1993;102:255–265.

115. Yanagisawa E, Yanagisawa K. Comparison of new telescopic video microlaryngoscopic and standard microlaryngoscopic techniques. *Ann Otol Rhinol Laryngol.* 1992;101:51–60.

116. Yanagisawa E, Yanagisawa R. Laryngeal photography. *Otolaryngol Clin North Am.* 1991; 24:999–1022.

117. Mufioz A, Ranios A, Ferrando J, et al. Laryngeal carcinoma. Sclerotic appearance of the cricoid and arytenoid cartilage: CT-pathologic correlation. *Radiology.* 1993;189:433–437.

118. Curtin HD. The larynx and hypopharynx. *ASHNR 26th Annual Conference and Postgraduate Course.* Vancouver: ASHNR, 1993, 43–49.

119. Roth M, Lanza DC, Zinreich J, et al. Advantages and disadvantages of three-dimensional computed tomography intraoperative localization for functional endoscopic sinus surgery. *Laryngoscope.* 1995;105:1279–1286.

120. Fried MP, Kleefield J, Gopal H, et al. Imageguided endoscopic surgery: Results of accuracy and performance in a multicenter clinical study using an electromagnetic tracking system. *Laryngoscope.* 1997;107:594–601.

121. Modaresi KB, Cox TC, Summers PE, et al. Comparison of intra-arterial digital subtraction angiography, magnetic resonance angiography and duplex ultrasonography for measuring carotid artery stenosis. *Br J Surg* 1999;86(11): 1422–1426.

122. Ho VB, Prince MR, Dong Q. Magnetic resonance imaging of the aorta and branch vessels. *Coron Artery Dis.* 1999;10(3):141–149.

123. Leclerc X, Gauvrit JY, Nicol L, Pruvo JP. Contrast-enhanced MR angiography of the craniocervical vessels: A review. *Neuroradiology* 1999;41(12):867–874.

124. Sardanelli F, Zandrino F, Parodi RC, De Caro G. MR angiography of internal carotid arteries: Breath-hold Gd-enhanced 3D fast imaging with steady-state precession versus unenhanced 2D and 3D time-of-flight techniques. *J Comput Assist Tomogr.* 1999;23(2):208–215.

125. Wetzel S, Bongartz G. MR angiography: Supraaortic vessels. *Eur Radiol.* 1999;9(7): 1277–1284.

126. Scarabino T, Carriero A, Giannatempo GM, Marano R, De Matthaeis P, Bonomo L, Salvolini U. Contrast-enhanced MR angiography (CE MRA) in the study of the carotid stenosis: Comparison with digital subtraction angiography (DSA). *J Neuroradiol.* 1999; 26(2):87–91.

127. Hubner KF, Thie JA, Smith GT, et al. Clinical utility of FDG-PET in detecting head and neck tumors: A comparison of diagnostic methods and modalities. *Clin Positron Imaging.* 2000; 3(1):7–16.

128. Macapinlac HA, Yeung HWD, Larson SM. Defining the role of FDG PET in head and neck cancer. *Clin Positron Imaging.* 1999; 2(6):311–316.

129. Kresnik E, Mikosch P, Gallowitsch HJ, et al. Evaluation of head and neck cancer with $_{18}$F-FDG PET: A comparison with conventional methods. *Eur J Nucl Med.* 2001;28:816–821.

130. Klingenbeck-Regn K, Schaller S, Flohr T, et al. Subsecond multi-slice computed tomography: Basics and applications. *Eur J Radiol.* 1999;31(2):110–124.

131. Baum U, Greess H, Lell M, et al. Imaging of head and neck tumors—methods: CT, spiral-CT, multislice-spiral-CT. *Eur J Radiol* 2000; 33(3):153–160.

132. Lell M, Baum U, Koester M, et al. The morphological and functional diagnosis of the head-neck area with multiplanar spiral CT. *Radiologe.* 1999;39(11):932–938.

133. Bruning R, Sturm C, Hong C, et al. The diagnosis of stages T1 and T2 in laryngeal carcinoma with multislice spiral CT. *Radiologe.* 1999;39(11):939–942.

Pharmacology and Therapeutics

38

HISTAMINE

Histamine is an endogenous amine that is stored in mast cells and basophils. The release of histamine through antigen-antibody reactions or exposure to various chemicals causes a variety of pharmacologic effects of varying intensity throughout the body. These effects range from mild irritation and itching to anaphylaxis and death. Histamine also appears to have a neurotransmitter effect in the central nervous system (CNS). Histamine interacts with specific receptors of the cells in the target tissue, subdivided into H_1, H_2, and H_3. Its effects in this tissue depends on the cell's function and the ratio of H_1:H_2 receptors.

ANTIHISTAMINES

An antihistamine acts as a competitive antagonist by occupying the histamine receptor on effector cells. It does not prevent the release of histamine (as cromolyn does), nor does it destroy histamine. It is now known that histamine acts on at least three distinct receptors. Bronchial and intestinal smooth muscle contraction and increased capillary permeability are mediated by H_1 receptors and antagonized by H_1-receptor blocking agents (conventional "antihistamines"). The action of histamine on gastric secretion and cardiac acceleration is mediated via H_2 receptors. The stimulation of H_2 receptors is antagonized by such agents as famotidine, ranitidine, cimetidine, and nizatidine. The recently described H_3 receptors function as feedback inhibitors in a wide variety of organ systems. H_3 receptor agonists and antagonists are currently available for research purposes only and have no clinical role.

All of the available H_1 receptor antagonists are reversible, competitive inhibitors of the interaction of histamine with H_1 receptors. The first-generation H_1 antagonists can both stimulate and depress CNS function. Depression of the CNS—consisting of decreased alertness, slow reaction times, blurred vision or diplopia, fatigue, and somnolence—are common side effects. The ethanolamines are especially prone to this. Their sedative action is synergistic with that of other CNS depressants such as barbiturates and alcohol. Some antihistamines (diphenhydramine, pyrilamine, and doxylamine) are sold as sleep aids, taking advantage of their CNS-depressant activity. Stimulation of the CNS includes restlessness, nervousness, euphoria, tremor, insomnia, and focal seizures (in patients with pre-existing cerebral lesions) and may be seen in patients taking therapeutic or toxic doses. Phenindamine (Nolahist) is unusual because it stimulates the CNS even at therapeutic doses. The more recently introduced second-generation H_1-receptor antagonists do not cross the blood-brain barrier and therefore are free of the CNS side effects. These include terfenadine, astemizole, loratadine, cetirizine, and fexofenadine, among others. Astemizole has no sedative action or synergistic interaction with alcohol.

986

Azelastine (Astelin) is the first antihistamine to be administered as a topical nasal spray. This agent has been proven to be effective in both seasonal allergic rhinitis and nonallergic vasomotor rhinitis.

Some H_1 receptor antagonists can suppress motion sickness but are less effective against an episode already present. Dimenhydrinate, diphenhydramine, promethazine, and piperazine derivatives are effective in these instances, although they are less effective than the anticholinergic (muscarinic) drug scopolamine. All first-generation antihistamines produce atropine-like activity, giving rise to xerostomia, possible micturition problems, and impotence. It is also possible to experience blurred vision, diplopia, euphoria, elevated blood pressure, anorexia, constipation or diarrhea, and epigastric discomfort. Antihistamines such as diphenhydramine with prominent anticholinergic actions can dry salivary and bronchial secretions, which may adversely affect patients with asthma. The newer "second-generation" antihistamines (loratadine and fexofenadine) have much less anticholinergic activity. Some H_1 antagonists—such as diphenhydramine, promethazine, and pyrilamine—have local anesthetic activity at higher doses (Table 38-1).

H_1-antihistamine therapy is useful to relieve or prevent allergic rhinitis, urticaria, some types of asthma (allergic origin), motion sickness, and the toxic effects of insect bites. Antihistamines alone are of little or no benefit in the treatment of most types of asthma; anaphylactic emergencies; inflammatory disorders of the skin, eyes, and nose; or the common cold and are contraindicated in patients taking monoamine oxidase (MAO) inhibitors.

H_1 antagonists are metabolized by the liver. The duration of action of most antihistamines is about 4 hours. Metabolism may be slower, with a prolonged duration of action, in elderly patients. Symptoms of antihistamine overdose are similar to those of atropine overdose and include CNS excitation and convulsions; treatment is supportive. QT-interval prolongation and torsades de pointes (polymorphic ventricular tachycardia) with possible sudden death is a known complication with increased levels of terfenadine or astemizole, from overdose or due to inhibition of hepatic metabolism. This may be seen with pre-existing hepatic disease and certain cardiovascular conditions or as the result of an interaction with a concurrently administered macrolide antibiotic (erythromycin) or ketoconazole (Nizoral). Because of this, these two agents (terfenadine and astemizole) have been removed from the market.

The H_2 antagonists inhibit gastric secretion caused by histamine, gastrin, and acetylcholine as well as by food. H_2 antihistamines are less lipid-soluble and therefore do not have the sedative, anesthetic, or anticholinergic properties seen in the H_1 antagonists. However, there are H_2 receptors in the brain, and central effects such as agitation, confusion, and depres-

TABLE 38-1. ACTIONS OF STRUCTURAL GROUPS OF TRADITIONAL ANTIHISTAMINES

Class	Antihistaminic Activity	Sedative Effects	Anticholinergic Activity	Antiemetic Effects	GI Side Effects	Duration of Action
Amino alkyl ethers (ethanolamines)	+ to ++	+ to +++	+++	++ to +++	+	4–6 hours
Ethylenediamines	+ to ++	+ to ++	—	—	+++	4–6 hours
Alkylamines (propylamines)	++ to +++	+ to ++	++	—	+	4–25 hours
Phenothiazines	+ to +++	+++	+++	++++	—	4–24 hours

sion can be seen (less so with famotidine than with cimetidine or ranitidine). Cimetidine and ranitidine may inhibit renal clearance of drugs secreted by the renal tubule, and cimetidine can inhibit the cytochrome P450 system.

H_2 antagonists are indicated in hypersecretory states (Zollinger-Ellison syndrome), pancreatic insufficiency, active duodenal ulcer or benign gastric ulcer (short-term treatment), to prevent recurrence of duodenal ulcer (prolonged therapy), to prevent "stress"-induced ulcer in hospitalized patients, to prevent gastric damage induced by nonsteroidal anti-inflammatory drugs, and in the treatment of reflux esophagitis.

Adverse effects seen more with cimetidine than with the other H_2 antagonists include dizziness, confusion (elderly patients), leukopenia, rashes, myalgias, gynecomastia, and impotence. Serious side effects are unusual. Drug interactions can be a problem with cimetidine, which inhibits cytochrome P450 and can decrease the metabolism of many other drugs. Ranitidine, famotidine, and nizatidine normally do not inhibit hepatic drug-metabolizing microsomal enzymes and therefore do not interfere with most other medications.

Receptor subtypes are distributed as follows:

H_1: Smooth muscle, endothelium, brain
H_2: Gastric mucosa, cardiac muscle, mast cells, brain
H_3: Presynaptic—brain, myenteric plexus, other neurons

H_1 Antagonists
First Generation (Table 38-2)
- Rapid oral absorption
- Peak blood concentrations within 1 to 2 hours
- Widely distributed throughout the body (including CNS)
- Metabolized by liver
- Duration of action 4 to 6 hours
- Sedation (excitation at ordinary doses in children and some adults)

Second Generation (Table 38-3)
- Less lipid-soluble.
- Minimal to no CNS penetration.
- Little to no sedation or autonomic blocking effects.
- Longer acting (duration of action 12–24 hours).
- Terfenadine, loratadine, azelastine, and astemizole have active metabolites.

H_2 Antagonists
- Less lipid-soluble.
- Little or no effect on H_1 receptors.
- Inhibit basal (fasting) and nocturnal acid secretions in addition to stimulated secretion (ie, food, chemical, etc.).
- Reduce both the volume and H+ concentration of gastric juice secreted.
- Do not have prominent sedative, anticholinergic, or local anesthetic actions.
- May cause mental confusion (especially in the elderly), agitation, and depression (seen more with cimetidine than with ranitidine or famotidine).
- Ranitidine has a greater potency and less incidence of adverse effects compared to cimetidine.

TABLE 38-2. "FIRST-GENERATION" H_1 ANTIHISTAMINES

	Usual Adult Dose	Comments
Ethanolamines		
Carbinoxamine (Clistin)	4–8 mg	Slight to moderate sedation
Dimenhydrinate (Dramamine)	50 mg	Moderate sedation, antiemetic activity
Diphenhydramine (Benadryl)	25–50 mg	Moderate sedation, antiemetic activity
Doxylamine (Decapryn)	1.25–25 mg	Marked sedation, OTC sleep aids
Clemastine fumarate (Tavist)	1.34–2.68 mg	Minimum sedation
Ethylenediamines		
Antazoline	1–2 drops	Component of ophthalmic solutions
Pyrilamine (Nisavil, Dorantamin, Neo-Antergan)	25–50 mg	Moderate sedation, OTC sleep aids
Tripelennamine (PBZ)	25–50 mg	Moderate sedation
Piperazine derivatives		
Cyclizine (Marezine)	25–50 mg	Slight sedation, anti–motion sickness activity
Meclizine (Antivert, Bonine)	25–50 mg	Slight sedation, anti–motion sickness activity
Hydroxyzine hydrochloride (Atarax)	25 mg	Agent of choice in chronic urticaria and many dermatologic conditions
Hydroxyzine pamoate (Vistaril)	25 mg	
Alkylamines		
Brompheniramine (Dimetane)	4–8 mg	Slight sedation
Chlorpheniramine (Chlor-Trimeton)	4–8 mg	Slight sedation, OTC "cold" aids
Dexchlorpheniramine (Polaramine)	2–4 mg	Slight sedation, active isomer of chlorpheniramine
Dexbrompheniramine (Disomer)	2–4 mg	Minimal sedation
Triprolidine hydrochloride (Actidil, Myidyl)	2.5 mg	Minimal sedation
Phenothiazine derivatives		
Promethazine (Phenergan)	10–25 mg	Marked sedation, antiemetic and antimuscarinic activity
Methdilazine (Tacaryl)	8 mg	Used primarily as antipruritic
Trimeprazine tartrate (Temaril)	2.5 mg	Used primarily as antipruritic
Miscellaneous		
Cyproheptadine (Periactin)	4 mg	Moderate sedation, antiserotonin activity
Azatadine maleate (Optimine)	1–2 mg	Similar to cyproheptadine
Diphenylpyraline hydrochloride (Hispril)	5 mg	Mild sedation
Phenindamine tartrate (Nolahist)	25 mg	May cause drowsiness/excitation can occur

TABLE 38-3. "SECOND-GENERATION" H_1 ANTIHISTAMINES

	Usual Daily Adult Dose	Comments
Piperidines		
Astemizole (Hismanal)	10 mg	Low incidence of sedation
Terfenadine (Seldane)	60 mg	Low incidence of sedation
Loratadine (Claritin)	10 mg	Low incidence of sedation
Levocabastine hydrochloride (Livastin)	1 drop	Ophthalmic preparation
Fexofenadine (Allegra)	180 mg	Low incidence of sedation
Alkylamines		
Acrivastine (Semprex-D)	8 mg	
Piperazines		
Cetrizine hydrochloride (Zyrtec)	5–10 mg	
Phthalazinone		
Azelastine (Astelin)	1096 µg (2 puffs each side of nose BID)	Available as topical nasal spray only

LEUKOTRIENE MODIFIERS

Leukotrienes are biologically active compounds that are derived from the metabolism of arachidonic acid. Phospholipase A_2 releases arachidonic acid from the cell membrane phospholipid bilayer. The arachidonic acid then undergoes oxidative metabolism (via the 5-lipoxygenase pathway) to form the cysteinyl leukotrienes or (via the cyclooxygenase pathway) to generate prostaglandins, prostacyclin, and thromboxanes.

Cysteinyl leukotrienes have been shown to play a significant role in the pathophysiology of asthma. Cysteinyl leukotrienes C_4, D_4, and E_4 induce airway smooth muscle contraction, airway edema via vascular leakage, eosinophil recruitment, and mucous secretion, all contributing to airflow obstruction in asthma.

The action of leukotrienes can be blocked by interfering with their reaction at the receptor or by blocking their synthesis by enzyme inhibition. Zafirlukast (Accolate) and montelukast (Singulair) are leukotriene receptor antagonists, while zileuton (Zyflo) acts by actively inhibiting 5-lipoxygenase.

Zileuton and zafirlukast are two oral leukotriene modifiers that have been approved for prophylaxis and chronic treatment of asthma in adults and children over 12 years of age.

ANTICHOLINERGIC DRUGS

The anticholinergics are considered by many to be the most effective drugs for the prevention and treatment of motion sickness. Their mechanism of action is the competitive inhibition of acetylcholine at muscarinic receptor sites, producing both peripheral and central effects; parasympatholytic, smooth muscle inhibition; and depression of cerebral and medullary centers. Experimental evidence suggests that vestibular receptors are cholinergic, with cortical action contributing to the effect on vestibular function.

Drugs of this class include atropine, scopolamine (hyoscine), and glycopyrrolate (Robinol). Scopolamine is the most effective drug for motion sickness, with fewer side effects than others in its class. All agents used for this purpose should be given prophylactically, as they are much less effective after severe nausea or vomiting has developed. A transdermal preparation, Transderm-Scop, is highly effective when applied about 4 hours prior to exposure, delivering its 0.5-mg dosage over 72 hours. Parenteral glycopyrrolate is commonly given prior to the administration of a general anesthetic to inhibit salivation and respiratory tract secretions, thus facilitating head and neck surgical and diagnostic endoscopic procedures. Atropine is used in the treatment of cardiac bradydysrhythmias. Classic side effects of this class of drugs include xerostomia, tachycardia, drowsiness, headache, gastrointestinal (GI) upset, nightmares, blurred vision, acute glaucoma, and urinary retention.

Ipratropium bromide is the only anticholinergic agent available topically as a nasal spray (Atrovent 0.03 or 0.06%). It has a rapid onset of action and is essentially free of systemic side effects. This agent takes advantage of the fact that rhinorrhea is mainly cholinergic-mediated, and ipratropium competitively binds at the cholinergic sites on the cells. It is equally effective for chronic rhinitis that is allergic, nonallergic, vasomotor, or gustatory-mediated (0.03% strength) in addition to that related to the common cold (0.06% strength). It is less effective for congestion, sneezing, and postnasal drip.

VASOCONSTRICTORS

Epinephrine

1. Very potent stimulatory effects (inotropic and chronotropic) on cardiac muscle (via β_1 receptors) and vasoconstriction (α receptors).
2. Also stimulates β_2 receptors, causing vasodilation of some vessels (skeletal muscle) and bronchodilation.
3. Topical application produces mucous membrane pallor and shrinkage with rapid onset.
4. May be irritating to nasal mucosa (phenylephrine and ephedrine less irritating).
5. Not administered orally.
6. Administered via aerosal (for bronchospasm), topical (nasal), ophthalmic, subcutaneous, or parenteral routes.

Ephedrine

1. Noncatechol sympathomimetic.
2. Causes release of stored catecholamines as well as direct stimulation of receptors.
3. Effects similar to epinephrine (nonselective) in addition to central stimulation, which may produce insomnia, palpations, and nervousness.
4. Prolonged duration of action.
5. Available in oral and topical preparations.
6. May cause urinary retention or extrasystole.
7. Analog pseudoephedrine (Sudafed) is an effective oral decongestant available in time-release form and/or in combination with H_1 antihistamines (Claritin-D, Allegra-D) or mucolytics (Entex).

Phenylephrine

1. Noncatechol sympathomimetic
2. Pure alpha agonist
3. Effective decongestant
4. Available as topical nasal spray (Neo-Synephrine)

Phenylpropanolamine

1. A decongestant that was often combined with antihistamines to counteract their sedative properties and used in many over-the-counter weight-loss preparations.
2. An amphetamine derivative.
3. Recently removed from the market due to a documented increase in incidence of hemorrhagic strokes among patients taking this medication.

Topical

1. Cocaine: a local anesthetic with a peripheral sympathomimetic action by blocking reuptake of catecholamines at sympathetic nerve terminals. Readily enters the CNS and produces a brief but intense amphetamine-like effect. Topical use may result in reactive blood or urine tests for cocaine; therefore the physician needs to inform patients of this and document use in operative reports. Surgeons not wearing latex gloves but handling packs may also test positive.
2. Oxymetazoline (Afrin)
3. Ephedrine
4. Phenylephrine (Neo-Synephrine)
5. Propylhexedrine (Benzedrex)

6. Naphazoline (Privine)
7. Tetrahydrozoline (Tyzine)
8. Xylometazoline (Otrivin)

Chronic use beyond 3 to 5 days may result in tachyphylaxis and rhinitis medicamentosa.

CORTICOSTEROIDS

The adrenal cortex produces many different steroid compounds, all derived from choles-terol. Included among these are androgens, glucocorticoids, and mineralocorticoids.

Mineralocorticoids, which promote Na^+ retention and K^+ secretion, have no anti-inflammatory properties. The main mineralocorticoid is aldosterone, which is responsible for the regulation of salt and water balance. Aldosterone is controlled primarily by the renin-angiotensin system.

Glucocorticoids help regulate protein, lipid, and carbohydrate metabolism. Hydrocor-tisone is the main glucocorticoid; its secretion is controlled by pituitary adrenocorticotropic hormone (ACTH) in a negative feedback system.

The action of glucocorticoids include

1. An increase in gluconeogenesis
2. A decrease in the action of insulin on peripheral tissues
3. An increase in protein catabolism
4. The diuresis of free water
5. Delayed wound healing
6. Stimulation of erythropoiesis
7. An increase in circulating leukocytes
8. Retardation of osseous growth centers and promotion of osteoporesis
9. Inhibition of fibroblast collagen formation and tissue neovascularization
10. Immunosuppression
11. Increase of histamine oxidase
12. Anterior pituitary ACTH suppression

Because of their anti-inflammatory properties, glucocorticoids have been widely used in a number of otolaryngologic disorders and perioperative conditions, including

1. Airway management—croup, supraglottitis, asthma
2. Infectious (short-term, limited use, when covered with appropriate antibiotics)—acute tonsillitis, infectious mononucleosis
3. Perioperatively for microlaryngoscopies, endolaryngeal manipulations, uvulopalato-pharyngoplasties, tonsillectomies, and other oral and oropharyngeal procedures
4. Posttraumatic—facial trauma, laryngeal, facial nerve
5. Sudden idiopathic sensorineural hearing loss (SNHL)
6. Cogan's syndrome
7. Autoimmune SNHL
8. Luetic hearing loss
9. Bell's palsy
10. Nasal polyposis (topical and systemic use)
11. Allergic rhinitis (topical use)
12. Rhinitis medicamentosa (topical and systemic use)

Contraindications to steroid therapy include active tuberculosis, peptic ulcer disease, and psychosis, while relative contraindications include acute viral or bacterial infections, congestive heart failure, severe diabetes, or uremia.

The most commonly used steroids are synthetic derivatives of hydrocortisone and cortisone and include prednisone, Decadron, prednisolone, and methylprednisolone. These compounds have potent anti-inflammatory and other glucocorticoid effects but are relatively low in mineralocorticoid effects—that is, they have low sodium- and water-retention properties. Preparations are available in many different forms, which may be administered via oral, IV, IM, topical, or inhalation routes (Table 38-4).

The normal rate of cortisol secretion by the adrenal cortex is about 20 to 30 mg/day (equivalent to 5 mg of prednisone), and this displays a diurnal variation, with cortisol levels highest in the morning and lowest at night. The suppression of the hypothalmic-pituitary axis that is seen after prolonged therapy with corticosteroids may be slow in returning to normal and may take up to a year or more. Rapid withdrawal of steroid administration after prolonged therapy can result in acute adrenal insufficiency. This may be evident by fevers, myalgia, arthralgia, and malaise. The use of corticosteroids for days or even a few weeks does not lead to suppression of the hypothalmic-pituitary axis. When long-term maintenance therapy is required, every-other-day dosing with a shorter-acting corticosteroid, such as prednisolone, will help limit side effects, including suppression of the hypothalmic-pituitary axis.

Complications associated with the long-term use of corticosteroids include

1. Fluid imbalance
2. Electrolyte disturbances
3. Glycosuria
4. Susceptibility to infections
5. Hypertension
6. Hyperglycemia
7. Peptic ulcers
8. Osteoporosis
9. Cataracts
10. Behavioral disturbances
11. Cushing habitus ("moon face," "buffalo hump")

TABLE 38-4. COMMONLY USED STEROIDS

Generic Name	Trade Name	Relative Dosage	Anti-inflammatory Properties	Cushingoid or Gluconeogenic Properties	Na+ Retention
Hydrocortisone	Solu-Cortef	20	1	1	1
Cortisone		25	0.8	1	1
Prednisone		5	3–5	5	0.8
Prednisolone		5	3–5	5	0.8
Triamcinolone	Kenalog	4	20	20	0
Dexamethasone	Decadron	0.75	20–30	20	0
Methylprednisolone	Medrol Solumedrol Medrol Dose Pak	4	10	10	0

12. Central obesity
13. Acne
14. Hirsuitism

The effects of allergic diseases such as hay fever, bee stings, contact dermatitis, urticaria, and angioneurotic edema may be suppressed by the administration of corticosteroids when given along with the primary therapy. It should be noted, however, that the full effect of the steroids will take some time to develop. Therefore, with severe reactions such as anaphylaxis or airway compromise, therapy should first be initiated with epinephrine 0.3 to 1.0 mg (0.3–1.0 mL of a 1 : 1000 solution) IM or subcutaneously. Dexamethasone (Decadron) 8 to 12 mg may be administered intravenously in life-threatening situations.

Topically administered steroids are available in ointment form. These preparations are usually insoluble and include triamcinolone acetonide or triamcinolone diacetate. Although some systemic absorption can occur from topical administration, the side effects are usually milder and more transient.

Intralesional (Kenalog, 10 mg/mL, 40 mg/mL) and topical corticosteroids are used in the treatment of hypertrophic scars and keloids, to prevent postoperative recurrence after scar revision, and as a prophylaxis in patients with a tendency to form these scars. Injections are performed pre- or intraoperatively and every 4 to 6 weeks for several months postoperatively, with discontinuation of therapy after 8 to 12 months. Dosage should be limited to 120 to 150 mg over 4 to 6 weeks, to avoid suppression of the hypothalamic-pituitary axis. Hypopigmentation and atrophy of subcutaneous and dermal tissues are dose-related side effects.

There is some clinical and experimental evidence that the adverse effects of steroids on wound healing can be counteracted by the administration of vitamin A 20,000 U/day.

Orally inhaled steroids (beclomethasone, triamcinolone, or flunisolide) play an important role in the treatment of bronchial asthma. When inhaled and used as directed, glucocorticoids reduce bronchial hyperactivity and do not cause adrenal suppression.

The intranasal administration of corticosteroids has proven effective for the treatment of seasonal and nonseasonal allergic rhinitis, in addition to certain nonallergic disorders such as rhinitis medicamentosa, rhinitis of pregnancy, and nasal polyposis. Some relief may also be obtained in nonallergic rhinitis with eosinophilia; however, vasomotor rhinitis is less responsive to topical nasal steroids. Through anti-inflammatory and membrane-stabilizing actions, these preparations downregulate the mucosal inflammatory reaction and are believed to facilitate the maintenance of paranasal sinus ostial patency. These actions include vasoconstriction, decreased glandular response to cholinergic stimulation, interference with arachidonic acid metabolism, reduced mediator release, decreased production of cytokines from T lymphocytes, and inhibition of eosinophil influx to the nasal epithelium. Available preparations include beclomethasone (Beconase, Vancinase), budesonide (Rhinocort), dexamethasone (Dexacort), flunisolide (Nasalide), fluticasone (Flonase), triamcinolone (Nasalcort), and mometasone furoate (Nasonex).

When used as directed, systemic side effects and adrenal suppression are not seen. Adverse effects are limited to the nose, with transient irritation, burning, and sneezing being among the most common side effects. The burning sensation is attributed to the carrier vehicles in the sprays, to which the patients often acclimate within days. Use of the aqueous compounds usually avoids this problem. These sprays are safe for children 3 years of age and older. Chronic usage may increase capillary fragility, producing epistaxis. Epistaxis is more commonly due to improper spray application, with the tip of the pump contacting the nasal septum. Several weeks of regular daily use are required to obtain full therapeutic benefit; however, symptomatic relief may be noted within hours of use. Pretreatment with a nasal decongestant spray can increase efficacy, allowing the steroid spray to reach the affected mucosa.

Injecting long-acting corticosteroids into the inferior turbinates is no longer recommended due to the poor long-term results and the severe possible side effects, which include amaurosis due to microembolic vascular occlusion based on particle size.

OTOTOXICITY

Several classes of medications may cause damage to the auditory system; however, antibiotics and diuretics are the most common of these. The first signs of ototoxicity are a high-pitched tinnitus, hearing loss, and vertigo. The hearing loss may be temporary or permanent. With antibiotic therapy, the hearing loss is usually bilateral, but it may be unilateral and usually occurs after 3 to 4 days of therapy. However, the symptoms may be noticeable after the first dose or may even show a delayed onset weeks to months after the completion of therapy. The audiogram pattern of antibiotic-induced ototoxicity is usually a steeply sloping loss in the higher frequencies, while that from diuretic use is usually flat or mildy sloping. Positional nystagmus is an early and sensitive sign of vestibular injury.

Aminoglycosides

Aminoglycosides have a 10% incidence of ototoxicity. The hearing loss is usually a bilateral high-frequency sensorineural loss, which is typically permanent. The amount of hearing loss and the time until onset of symptoms are directly related to renal function and the dose given. Aminoglycosides are excreted mainly by the kidneys; therefore, in patients with impaired renal function, the serum levels will rise, increasing the risk of ototoxicity. Aminoglycosides take longer to clear from the perilymph than they do from the serum. Generally, the ototoxic effects are evident as hair cell loss, which begins in the basilar turn of the cochlea and proceeds toward the apex. The inner row of outer hair cells is affected first, followed by progression to the outer two rows. For reasons that remain unknown, the inner hair cells are protected until frank ototoxicity occurs, with total destruction of the organ of Corti.

Streptomycin and gentamicin are more toxic to the vestibular system; with these agents, vestibular testing may be more useful than audiograms in detecting early signs of ototoxicity. Kanamycin and dihydrostreptomycin tend to be more toxic to the auditory system. The offending agent should be discontinued at the first signs of ototoxicity. One problem, which may delay this, is that the average patient usually does not realize the auditory effects until there is a moderate hearing loss (> 30 dB) that involves the middle (speech) to lower frequencies.

Streptomycin

This drug is primarily vestibulotoxic and therefore causes vertigo before the onset of tinnitus and hearing loss. Because of this, it has been used to treat intractable bilateral Ménière's disease. For this purpose, an average dose of 2 g/day is given until no caloric response is elicited. The vestibulotoxic effect is dose-related. One gram per day for 10 days will give no vestibular symptoms. However, 2 g/day for 14 days has been reported to give vestibular symptoms in 60 to 70% of patients.

Fifty to 60% of the drug is excreted unchanged by the kidneys during the first 24 hours; the larger the dose, the faster the excretion by a normal kidney. This means that any renal insufficiency will result in an elevated serum level. A small fraction is secreted by the liver via the gastrointestinal tract. Peak plasma level is detectable within 1 to 2 hours after IM injection and diminishes by about 50% in 5 hours. The antibiotic can be detected in plasma for at least 8 to 12 hours after administration. Recommended dose for children is 15 to 30 mg/kg/day. Intraoperative semicircular canal perfusion has also been performed for selective vestibular ablation.

The drug continues to be used clinically in multidrug therapy of the most serious forms of tuberculosis.

Histologic findings for streptomycin ototoxicity include

1. Minimal scattered loss of outer hair cells in the upper basal turn of the cochlea. Normal supporting cells.
2. Severe damage to the sensory epithelium of the cristae of all canals. Severe hair cell loss and flattening of the sensory epithelium of the cristae and saccule. The utricular macula is involved, but least so in the vestibular end organs.
3. Stereocilia in the canal's ampullae are swollen and twice their normal diameter.

Dihydrostreptomycin

Dihydrostreptomycin may cause severe and erratic hearing loss even as long as 2 months after discontinuation. The loss is unpredictable and is not dose-related. Due to its excessive ototoxicity and the fact that it offers no advantage over streptomycin, it has been removed from the market in the United States.

Neomycin

Neomycin is not well absorbed when administered topically or orally. Therefore, it is used in bowel preparation and in otic drops, where it carries little risk of ototoxicity. However, repeated use in inflamed tissue has caused irreversible deafness. A parenteral dose of 5 to 8 g over 4 to 6 days has caused tinnitus and irreversible hearing loss. The hearing loss is associated with poor speech discrimination scores. The drug is eliminated by the kidneys. Neomycin, streptomycin, and kanamycin are cleared more slowly from perilymph than from the rest of the body, resulting in delayed ototoxicity occurring as late as 1 to 2 weeks after discontinuation of the drug.

Histologic findings in neomycin ototoxicity include

1. Destruction of inner and outer hair cells, with the outer hair cells slightly less involved. Apical and basal turns are both involved, with the basal turn involvement being more severe.
2. Partial destruction of pillar cells.
3. Partial atrophy of the stria vascularis.
4. Small loss of Deiter's and Hensen's cells.
5. Maculae and cristae remain normal.

Gentamicin

Gentamicin, like streptomycin, preferentially affects the vestibular rather than the auditory system. When used at serum levels of 10 to 12 μg/mL, it usually does not cause ototoxicity. Dosage should be adjusted in patients with renal insufficiency. Idiosyncratic reactions occur and are unrelated to dose/level.

Kanamycin

Kanamycin may not be as ototoxic as neomycin; however, like neomycin, its primary effect is on the cochlea. It produces a characteristic sloping sensorineural hearing loss which is essentially vestibular sparring. Among the aminoglycosides, kanamycin is the most likely to cause unilateral cochlear damage. As with all aminoglycosides, administration must be justified in patients with renal insufficiency, and the minimal effective dose used. In adults with good renal function, 15 mg/kg/day of kanamycin will cause mild to no hearing loss, and repeated administration should not lead to drug accumulation.

Histologic findings in kanamycin ototoxicity include

1. Destruction of inner and outer hair cells. The latter are believed to be destroyed first. More severe degeneration is found in the basal turn, with the apical turn less involved.
2. Usually unaltered supporting cells; hence neural degeneration is insignificant.
3. Normal semicircular canal cristae, and maculae of the utricle and saccule.

Tobramycin

Tobramycin has ototoxic effects similar to those of kanamycin. A high-frequency loss produces a steeply sloping audiogram. Vestibular symptoms are less common.

Amikacin

Amikacin, a derivative of kanamycin, has very little vestibular toxicity and is less ototoxic than gentamicin. Like kanamycin, it may produce a unilateral hearing loss.

Netilmicin and Sisomicin

Netilmicin and sisomicin are much less ototoxic than the other aminoglycosides.

Minocycline

Minocycline may cause reversible vestibular symptoms, which include gait disturbances as well as nausea and vomiting but no nystagmus.

Erythromycin

Symptoms of erythromycin ototoxicity include hearing loss, "blowing" tinnitus, and occasionally vertigo. The mechanism of erythromycin toxicity remains unknown; however, the effects are potentially reversible following the cessation of therapy. The patients particularly at risk include those with hepatic or renal failure, Legionnaire's disease, or advanced age. Doses of greater than 4 g/day pose a higher risk of ototoxicity; symptoms usually appear within 4 days.

High-Ceiling "Loop" Diuretics

Ethacrynic acid, furosemide (Lasix), and bumetanide (Bumex) all have considerable ototoxic potential when given intravenously to patients with renal failure. The ototoxicity appears to stem from the inhibition of cochlear sodium-potassium ATPase, causing changes in the electrolyte composition of the endolymph. The hearing loss from ethacrynic acid and furosemide is usually transient but can be permanent, while bumetanide is less ototoxic than either of these.

Ethacrynic Acid

Ethacrynic acid causes destruction of the intermediate layer of the stria vascularis and outer hair cells of the organ of Corti, most severely in the basal turn. The hearing loss can be transient or permanent. Transient loss may be secondary to the effects on respiratory enzymes (succinate dehydrogenase and adenosine triphosphatase) in the organ of Corti and stria vascularis. Endolymphatic sodium content is decreased. Symptoms include hearing loss, tinnitus, and vertigo.

Furosemide

Lasix in a high dose should be administered over several minutes to minimize its ototoxic effects. Drug-induced changes in the electrolyte composition of the endolymphatic fluid are unique to this class of drugs. Should another potentially ototoxic drug become indicated in a particular case, a diuretic from another class should be substituted.

CHEMOTHERAPEUTIC DRUGS

Cisplatin/carboplatin may produce high-frequency hearing loss with loss of outer hair cells of the basal cochlear turns. Tinnitus, otalgia, and occasionally vestibular symptoms may also occur. Nitrogen mustard produces sensorineural hearing loss through destruction of hair cells. Misonidazole is an agent used to sensitize poorly oxygenated tumor cells to the effects of radiation therapy. The ototoxicity associated with this agent is a sensorineural hearing loss of cochlear origin that may be at least partially reversible upon the completion of therapy. There are reports of hearing returning to pretreatment levels within 1 month of completion of therapy. Bleomycin and 5-fluorouracil may also be ototoxic.

SALICYLATES

Salicylates cause reversible hearing loss and tinnitus. The proposed mechanism of action is the uncoupling of oxidative phosphorylation. These drugs inhibit various transaminase and dehydrogenase enzymes. In humans, discontinuation of high doses of drug will cause the blood level to fall as the drug is excreted, with return to baseline hearing within 24 to 72 hours. No histologic changes have been demonstrated in temporal bone studies. To produce toxicity, 6 to 8 g/day must be taken, resulting in a serum level of 20 mg/dL or greater. However, symptoms have been reported to occur in some individuals taking the minimal recommended dose. Salicylates are rapidly metabolized, with approximately 50% eliminated in 24 hours. Within 48 to 72 hours, all salicylates have been excreted in the urine.

Aspirin is found in the following preparations: Percodan, Fiorinal, Coricidin, Trigesic, Norgesic, Talwin Compound, and Equagesic.

QUININE

Quinine is readily absorbed when taken orally. Ninety-five percent of the drug is metabolized in the liver, so no untoward effects are encountered in renal insufficiency. Most of the drug is excreted in 24 hours. The ototoxic effects of quinine are hearing loss and tinnitus, both of which are reversible. In pregnancy, the ingestion of quinine in therapeutic doses may not give rise to hearing loss in the mother but may affect the fetus, giving rise to bilateral sensorineural hearing loss. Histologically, the outer hair cells and stria vascularis have been noted to be atrophied. The brain stem vestibular and cochlear nuclei have been noted to be normal. Chloroquine taken during pregnancy may be similarly harmful to the fetus.

Other Drugs

Other drugs that are potentially ototoxic include ristocetin, polymixin B, vancomycin, pharmacetin, colistin, the antituberculous drugs viomycin and capreomycin, iodoform alkaloids, tetanus antitoxin, and the beta blocker propranolol.

ANTIEMETICS

Nausea and vomiting may be secondary to motion sickness, pregnancy, GI disorders, the administration of drugs (especially chemotherapeutic agents), or the emergence from general anesthesia. This may cause a delay in the completion of chemotherapy in head and neck cancer patients or may severely affect the postoperative results in otologic, neurosurgical, endoscopic sinus, or aesthetic procedures. Therefore, the postoperative control of nausea and vomiting is critical in head and neck patients. The emetic center of the brain resides in the lateral reticular formation of the medulla. This center, which coordinates the expulsion of gastric contents, receives input from a variety of sources, including visceral afferents, the vestibular system, higher cortical centers, and—most importantly—the chemoreceptor trigger zone in the floor of the fourth ventricle. This zone has dopamine receptors, whereas the emetic center has acetylcholine and histamine receptors, the stimulation of which may induce emesis. Therefore H_1, muscarinic, and dopaminergic antagonists will have varying degrees of antiemetic properties. Dopamine antagonists are the most useful in the treatment of vomiting; these include certain neuroleptic phenothiazines (prochlorperazine, promethazine) and butyrophenones (droperidol). Prochlorperazine (Compazine) is a very effective antiemetic agent but, when given intramuscularly, is associated with a high incidence of dystonias. Chlorpromazine (Thorazine) can prevent vomiting from a number of causes; however, it does not control motion sickness. The butyrophenones (droperidol) have been used intravenously in cancer patients as an alternative to the phenothiazines, since they tend to cause less sedation and hypotension.

Another dopaminergic antagonist with antiemetic properties is metoclopramide (Reglan), a benzamide. Trimethobenzamide (Tigan), another benzamide, has weak antiemetic effects and is not as effective as the phenothiazines or metoclopramide, but it can be given intramuscularly with a low incidence of side effects.

Adverse effects of these agents include extrapyramidal symptoms, drowsiness, dizziness, diarrhea, abdominal discomfort, and anxiety.

H_1 antagonists with prominent anticholinergic properties are used frequently in the prevention of motion sickness. However, these agents (diphenhydramine, scopolamine) are also effective antiemetics and can reduce the incidence of nausea and vomiting in postoperative patients who have been given narcotics such as morphine. When given as part of an antiemetic regimen, these drugs can help reduce the extrapyramidal side effects of the neuroleptics.

Combination regimens may be superior to single-drug therapy, especially in oncology patients. The adjunctive agents may act synergistically with the primary antiemetic; thus, in addition to decreasing the incidence of side effects, they may help to relieve anxiety and anticipatory emesis and provide an amnestic response. Such agents include benzodiazepines (lorazepam), cannabinoids, and corticosteroids. Examples of such regimens include metoclopramide-diphenhydramine-lorazepam; metaclopramide-dexamethasone-lorazepam-benxtropine; or droperidol-diphenhydramine. Selective serotonin 5-HT3 receptor antagonists, ondansetron (Zofran), and granisetron (Krytil) are very effective in the prevention of postoperative and chemotherapy-induced nausea and vomiting. It is not known whether their antiemetic action is on the serotonin 5-HT3 receptors found peripherally in vagal nerve terminals, on those found centrally in the chemoreceptor trigger zone of the fourth ventricle, or both. Due to their selective action, these agents have minimal to no extrapyramidal side effects.

TREATMENT FOR CONTROL OF GASTRIC ACIDITY (GERD, REFLUX ESOPHAGITIS, GASTRIC ULCERS)

Patients with gastroesophageal reflux disease (GERD) commonly present to the otolaryngologist with symptoms of chronic cough or throat clearing, globus sensation, and esophageal, laryngeal, or pulmonary symptoms. They generally are unaware that these problems may be linked to their symptoms. Squamous cell carcinoma of the larynx in some nonsmokers has also been attributed to GERD. This entity may be difficult to diagnose and is often missed. Findings that may or may not be present on endoscopic examination include inflammation and/or erythema to the arytenoids, posterior glottis, and the laryngeal surface of the epiglottis. An increase in vascularization may also be seen.

First-line therapy usually includes dietary changes, elevation of the head at night, and use of antacids, which vary in composition and effectiveness. These may be taken 1 hour after meals, at bedtime, and as needed in between. Overuse of antacids can result in acid-base and other metabolic disturbances. When antacids are ineffective or require too frequent use, H_2 histamine receptor antagonists may be used. These agents inhibit gastric acid secretion by competitively blocking the interaction between histamine and H_2 receptors in gastric mucosa. The degree of inhibition directly parallels the amount of the drug in the blood. When therapy with H_2 antagonists fails or is incomplete, the highly effective H^+,K^+-ATPase inhibitors may be used. These agents (omeprazole, etc.) selectively block the "proton pump" in the apical membrane of the parietal cell, which is responsible for the secretion of the acid. Other drugs used in the treatment of GERD include sucralfate, Gaviscon, metaclopramide, and cisapride.

Muscarinic antagonists are effective in reducing basal gastric acid secretion and to a lesser extent stimulated gastric acid secretion. Pirenzepine and telenzeprine, investigational in the United States, may promote healing of gastric and duodenal ulcers comparable to H_2 antagonists; however, they are less effective than these agents in reducing gastric acid secretion.

Hyoscyamine sulfate (Levsin) is an anticholinergic/antispasmotic that decreases gastric acid secretion and inhibits gastric motility. In addition, it controls secretions in the pharynx, trachea, and bronchi. It acts by specifically inhibiting the action of acetylcholine at the postganglionic nerve endings of the parasympathetic nerves and on smooth muscles that respond to acetylcholine but lack cholinergic innervation. It has no effect on the autonomic ganglia. Levsin may be given sublingually or by mouth; it is rapidly and totally absorbed, and has a short half-life. Potential side effects are similar to those seen with other anticholinergics, including xerostomia, urinary retention, blurred vision, tachycardia, nervousness, and impotence.

Sucralfate (Carafate), which is a complex of sulfated sucrose and aluminum hydroxide, is a cytoprotective agent. It combines topically with exposed proteins of an ulcerated mucosal base to form a protective coating, thus protecting the mucosa from gastric acid and enzymes. Another cytoprotective agent is misoprostol (Cytotec). This prostaglandin analog is effective in treating gastric and duodenal ulcers. Although used as a second-line agent, it is particularly useful in preventing gastric ulcers in patients who require the use of NSAIDs. Its use may be limited by the diarrhea it causes in 30% of patients.

Gaviscon is unique in that it contains alginic acid in addition to the antacids aluminum hydroxide and magnesium trisilicate. This combination allows the formation of a floating "raft foam buffer" on the surface of the gastric contents, which is preferentially refluxed into the esophagus, thus protecting its mucosa. Its action is local; it does not neutralize the entire stomach and has proven effective while the patient is standing or supine.

Metoclopramide has no effect on gastric acid secretion. However, it is effective in the prevention of GERD by increasing the tone of the lower esophageal sphincter, enhancing contractions in the antrum of the stomach, and relaxing the duodenum and pylorus. The result of these actions is increased emptying and decreased reflux of gastric contents. Adverse reactions, although infrequent, may include sedation, altered drug absorption, acute dystonic reactions, and significant extrapyramidal symptoms, including potentially irreversible tardive dyskinesia. Because of these reactions, metoclopramide is reserved for the treatment of severely refractive cases.

Medications Used to Control Gastric Acidity

Antacids: Hydroxides of aluminum and magnesium, sodium bicarbonate, calcium carbonate.

H$_2$ histamine receptor antagonists: Cimetidine (Tagamet), ranitidine (Zantac), famotidine (Pepcid), nizatidine (Axid).

Inhibitors of H$^+$,K$^+$-ATPase: Omeprazole (Prilosec), lansoprazole (Prevacid), rabeprazole (Aciphex), esomeprazole (Nexium), pantoprazole (Protonix).

Cytoprotective agents: Sucralfate, colloidal bismuth, misoprostol (prostaglandin agonist).

Muscarinic antagonists: Hyoscyamine sulfate (Levsin).

Prokinetic agents: Metoclopramide (Reglan) and domperidone (Motilium), which is not available in the United States.

Helicobacter pylori: For eradication in peptic ulcer disease: triple therapy—metronidazole (250 mg t.i.d.), a bismuth compound (Pepto-Bismol, two tablets q.i.d.), and either tetracycline (500 mg q.i.d.), amoxicillin (500 mg t.i.d.), or clarithromycin (500 mg t.i.d.) for 2 weeks, along with an antisecretory agent (H$_2$ antagonist or proton pump inhibitor) for up to 6 months.

MISCELLANEOUS DRUGS

Mucolytics and Expectorants

Mucolytic agents act by depolymerizing mucopolysaccharides, making them smaller and more soluble molecules. Acetylcysteine (Mucomyst, Mucosil) is a mucolytic agent widely used as adjunctive therapy in asthma and is also used as an antidote in acetaminophen toxicity. The mode of action of expectorants is not as well understood, but they probably produce some of their effects through a local or reflex action via vagal pathways. This stimulates secretions by the respiratory tract's secretory glands. Agents in this class include ammonium salts, iodide salts (iodinated glycerol, Organidin), and guaifenesin (available as a single agent or in combination with pseudoephedrine as Duratuss, Entex PSE, or Aquatab D). Decreasing the viscosity and increasing the output of upper respiratory tract secretions aids in the clearance of sinus disease. Dornase alpha (Pulmozyme) is a highly purified recombinant human deoxyribonuclease I, which selectively cleaves DNA. It is administered as an aerosal to patients with cystic fibrosis to reduce sputum viscoelasticity.

Cromolyn Sodium

Cromolyn sodium (disodium cromoglycate) inhibits the release of histamine and other autacoids from sensitized mast cells by preventing mast cell degranulation in response to a variety of stimuli, including the interaction between cell-bound immunoglobulin E (IgE) and specific antigen. Therefore, treatment is most effective when it is initiated before exposure to allergens. Cromolyn sodium has no intrinsic bronchodilator, antihistaminic, or anti-inflammatory activity. The onset of therapeutic effect may take up to 2 to 4 weeks of treatment, and its use should be continued throughout the period of exposure. Transient stinging, burning, irritation, and sneezing are the most common adverse effects noted. Intranasally it is felt to be less effective than nasal steroids, and it must be used 3 to 6 times a day. It is available in various forms, including a nasal solution (Nasalcrom), an ophthalmic solution (Opticrom), capsules for oral use (Gastrocrom), and a dry powder (Intal) or nebulizer for the treatment of asthma.

Hyaluronidase

Hyaluronidase (Wydase) is a protein enzyme that increases the permeability of connective tissue by hydrolyzing the hyaluronic acid in the ground substance. It can be added to local anesthetic agents to increase their dispersion on injection; however, it may also enhance the formation of hematomas.

SMOKING CESSATION THERAPY

Nicorette is a flavored, sugar-free chewing gum containing 2 mg of nicotine bound to an ion-exchange resin in a gum base; it is approved for use in withdrawal from cigarette smoking. On release from the gum, the nicotine is absorbed through the buccal mucosa, with a lower peak concentration and slower onset to peak in comparison to the inhalation of cigarette smoke. Nicotine stimulates central autonomic ganglia, producing the release of catecholamines from the adrenal medulla. Because of its pharmacokinetics, the gum does not produce the same sensation of pleasure that some smokers associate with cigarettes. However, irritability, difficulties in concentration, and other symptoms are relieved. Clinical studies suggest that the drug is effective in maintaining abstinence from smoking. Because of the gum's high viscosity and consequent occlusal stress, fillings and prosthodontic restorations may become displaced with use.

Largely due to this inconvenience, nicotine-releasing transdermal patches have met with much greater popularity. Four products have become available: Habitrol, Nicoderm, and Prostep for 24-hour wear and Nicotrol for 16-hour use. Theoretical advantages of the shorter-term delivery system include mimicking the natural pattern of smoking and avoidance of sleep disturbances, as serum nicotine concentrations wane overnight. A major theoretical disadvantage, however, is failure to prevent early-morning craving. All systems appear to be equally effective and well tolerated. A typical course involves 12 weeks of decreasing-dose therapy at a cost of about $350. All are recommended as part of a more comprehensive behavioral modification program with a maintenance component (relapse prevention) owing to a high short-term but poor long-term abstinence rate. Adverse reactions are largely limited to cutaneous hypersensitivity beneath the patch. Several attempts at suicide by intentional over-dosage have been unsuccessful. A nicotine inhaler is currently under investigation. Bupropion hydrochloride has been used for years as an antidepressant (Wellbutrin, Wellbutrin SR), one "side effect" of which was a decrease in the craving for nicotine. Wellbutrin has been approved for use as an aid to smoking cessation therapy and released under the trade name Zyban. The mechanism by which it enhances smoking cessation is unknown, but its effect may be mediated by noradrenergic or dopaminergic mechanisms. As with other smoking cessation agents, behavioral modification is an important adjunct to therapy.

BOTULINUM-A TOXIN

Botulinum-A toxin (Oculinum, Botox) produces an irreversible blockade of cholinergic synapses at the neuromuscular junction, pharmacologically denervating the muscle. Paresis or paralysis is dose-dependent. The drug is used for the treatment of facial dystonias (blepharospasm, torticollis, hemifacial spasm), effacement of moderate rhytides (eg, glabellar); and spastic dysphonia as a less traumatic alternative to surgical therapy or as an adjunct to surgery.

TREATMENT OF APHTHOUS STOMATITIS

Recurrent minor aphthous ulcers affect 20 to 50% of the population, and mucosal ulcerations play a prominent role in the morbidity associated with chemotherapy, hematologic disease, and recurrent herpetic stomatitis. Regardless of the etiology, the single dominant and consistent feature is severe pain out of proportion to lesion size and clinical appearance. Therapeutic options are very limited and include various topical agents and rinses. Oxidizing mouth rinses [hydrogen peroxide and water, or Cepacol (cetylpyridinium chloride)] are helpful in debriding the region of the lesion and promoting healing. In a recent study comparing the efficacy of various commercially prepared mouth rinses for aphthous stomatitis, Corsodyl mouthwash (chlorhexidine gluconate) and Difflam Oral Rinse (benzydamine hydrochloride) proved to be the most effective.

In cases where pain relief is required, topical steroid preparations may be useful. Examples include oxytetracycline hydrochloride hydrocortisone ointment (Terra-Cortril), triamcinolone (Kenalog in Orabase), or 0.5% fluocinonide (Lidex gel). Aerosolized topical steroids or injectable steroids may also be used. Bioadhesive hydrogel patches made of a cellulose derivative have been shown to effectively control pain and to aid in healing the ulcers.

In cases of diffuse intraoral involvement or generalized mucositis, various "cocktail" rinses may be useful. These may include antibiotics (tetracycline), antifungals (nystatin, clotrimazole), steroids (dexamethasone, hydrocortisone), and various "soothing" agents (viscous xylocaine, diphenhydramine, Maalox).

Zilactin, an over-the-counter agent, is available in liquid or gel form. The liquid form is non-film-forming and relieves the pain, itching, and burning associated with these lesions. It can significantly reduce the size and duration of the outbreak. The gel form produces an occlusive film over the lesion, which provides protection and pain relief that can last up to 6 hours per application.

Topical antiviral agents such as idoxuridine ophthalmic ointment (Stoxil) or acyclovir ointment (Zovirax) may be helpful in recurrent herpes labialis. Occasionally, systemic therapy with antibiotics, antifungals, antivirals, or corticosteroids may be required.

One study has shown benefit from plasmapheresis in patients with chronic relapsing aphthous stomatitis. These patients obtained prolonged remissions and accelerated epithelialization of the mucosa.

TOPICAL ORAL ANTIBIOTIC MOUTH RINSES

Major head and neck surgical and traumatic injuries entering the upper aerodigestive tract through external incisions or lacerations place demands on wound healing unmatched in more conventional injuries. The direct introduction of a large inoculum of polymicrobial aerobic and anaerobic bacteria into the wound may be quantitatively decreased by up to 95% through the use of perioperative topical antibiotic mouth rinses. Studies in colorectal surgery, somewhat analogous to the upper aerodigestive tract, have proven the efficacy of topical antibiotics in reducing septic wound complications. There is also evidence that topical antibiotics may be more effective than systemic antibiotics alone and that combination therapy may be the most effective in the presence of a large inoculum. Clindamycin, neomycin-erythromycin, sanguinaria (Viadent), chlorhexidine (Peridex), and vancomycin have been effective in clinical studies.

TREATMENT OF XEROSTOMIA

Salivary gland hypofunction causing xerostomia is seen frequently in otolaryngology patients as a result of adjuvant radiation therapy, Sjögren's syndrome, or the use of some medications (anticholinergics, antihistamines, antihypertensives, nicotine, and caffeine). Signs and symptoms include cheilitis, mucosal ulceration, dysphagia, masticatory difficulties, dysgeusia, dysphonia, prosthodontic intolerance, oral candidiasis, parotitis, and advanced dental caries. For the medication-induced cases, discontinuation of the agent will usually restore baseline salivary flow. Pilocarpine (Saligan), a cholinergic agonist, may be effective in a select few patients with functioning parenchyma but may be limited by the side effects. However, when delivered topically suspended in a candy-like pastille, it has been shown to produce results similar to those of systemic therapy but with improved tolerance. Another cholinergic agonist, cevimeline (Evoxac), is indicated for the treatment of xerostomia in patients with Sjögren's syndrome. Patients with no salivary reserve will require salivary substitutes.

Frequent sips and ice chips are recommended. As chewing stimulates salivary flow, sugarless or xylitol-based candy or gum may help. Prophylaxis against dental caries should be undertaken with topical fluoride treatments. Commercial nonprescription saliva substitutes containing carboxymethyl or hydroxyethyl cellulose are available in spray, aerosol, swab, and liquid preparations and are more effective than water- or glycerin-based solutions. Mucopolysaccharide (Mouth-Kote) and mucin-containing products may provide even better lubrication.

HEMOSTATICS

Desmopressin acetate (DDAVP) has been found to temporarily increase the concentration of antihemophilic factor VIII:C and von Willebrand factor in blood. It may improve bleeding times enough to effect hemostasis in minor surgical procedures (eg, tonsillectomy/adenoidectomy) in patients with hemophilia A, type 1 von Willibrand disease, or prolonged bleeding times secondary to renal failure. As the oral cavity contains a high concentration of plasminogen activators, oral procedures are particularly severe tests of hemostasis. The use of DDAVP may cause the release of tissue-type plasminogen activators. To counteract these factors, antifibrinolytic agents (Amicar/EACA, tranexamic acid) are also used in the perioperative treatment of these patients. Desmopressin is mainly given intravenously at a dose of 0.3 μg/kg body weight, and its effects are seen in about 30 minutes. It is also administered as a nasal spray for treatment of primary nocturnal enuresis and central cranial diabetes insipidus. Bismuth subgallate is an insoluble, poorly absorbed heavy metal supplied in powder form (Mallinckrodt) that can be mixed into a paste-like solution with saline, with or without epinephrine, and applied directly as a topical hemostatic agent in adenotonsillectomy procedures. Although its use began empirically, it is now known to be an astringent as well as an activator of factor XII (Hageman), greatly accelerating the intrinsic clotting cascade. The agent is without known side effect in over 20 years of use.

Topical bovine thrombin (Thrombinar) may be used as an aid in hemostasis for oozing and minor capillary bleeding. It clots the fibrinogen of blood directly. Topical gelatin (Gelfoam) and collagen foam (Helistat) or microfibrillar collagen (Avitene, Instat) are available adjuncts to hemostatic technique.

VACCINATION/ANTIVIRAL THERAPY
Hepatitis B

Recombinant hepatitis B vaccine (Recombivax HB, Energix-B) has replaced pooled plasma-derived vaccines and is much safer, eliminating the worry of blood-transmitted pathogens. Infants who are born to HBsAg-negative mothers should receive 2.5 μg of Recombivax HB vaccine or 10 μg of Energix-B vaccine. The second dose of vaccine should be given between 1 and 4 months of age provided that at least 1 month has elapsed since the first dose. A third dose is recommended between 6 and 18 months of age.

Infants who are born to HBsAg-positive mothers should receive 0.5 mL hepatitis B immunoglobulin (HBIG) within 12 hours of birth and either 5 mg of Recombivax HB or 10 mg of Energix-B at a separate site. The second dose of vaccine should be given at 1 month of age and the third at 6 months of age.

Haemophilus influenzae Type B

Haemophilus influenzae type b is a common pathogen implicated in sinusitis, otitis media, and epiglottitis. Despite effective antibiotic therapy, significant morbidity and mortality persist. Three conjugated vaccines are available for use in infants: HbOC (HbTITER), PRP-T (ActHIB; OmniHIB), and PRP-OMP (Pedvax HIB). Three doses are recommended, at 2, 4, and 6 months of age. Children receiving PRP-OMP at 2 and 4 months of age do not require a dose at 6 months of age. After the primary infant *H. influenzae* type b vaccine series is completed, a booster dose at 12 to 15 months of age is recommended. A significant reduction in the incidence of childhood epiglottitis has been seen since the introduction of the vaccine.

Diphtheria, Tetanus, and Pertussis

Vaccine for these three entities is given together (DTP) at 2, 4, and 6 months of age. A fourth dose may be given between 12 and 18 months of age provided that at least 6 months have elapsed since the third dose. Diphtheria and tetanus toxoids and acellular pertussis vaccine (DTaP) may be used for the fourth and/or fifth dose of DTP vaccine in children 15 months of age or older and may be preferred for children in these age groups. Combined DTP–*H. influenzae* type b vaccines may be used when these two vaccines are to be given simultaneously.

Polio Vaccine

The polio vaccine (OPV) is normally administered at 2 and 4 months of age, with a third dose between 6 and 18 months of age and a fourth dose between 4 and 6 years of age.

Measles, Mumps, and Rubella

The first dose of the measles, mumps, and rubella (MMR) vaccine is administered between 12 and 15 months of age, with a second dose given at either 4 to 6 years of age or 11 to 12 years of age.

Polyvalent-inactivated influenza vaccines are prepared for each season and are recommended for medical personnel to protect themselves and their patients. They can be effective in anyone who cannot afford to be incapacitated by illness. Rimantidine (Flumadine) is indicated for the prophylaxis and treatment of illness caused by various strains of influenza A virus. It is an oral preparation reported to significantly improve flu-like symptoms and to decrease viral shedding of the influenza A virus. Another agent, oseltamivir (Tamiflu) is indicated for the treatment of uncomplicated acute illness due to influenza infection in adults who have been symptomatic for no more than 2 days.

AESTHETIC DRUGS

Minoxidil 2% (Rogaine) is available as a topical preparation for the treatment of male-pattern baldness. The drug is a potent peripheral vasodilating antihypertensive agent that increases scalp blood flow and may stimulate epidermal DNA synthesis. Good to excellent results may be found in one-third of patients, with best response in smaller areas of balding, shorter duration of baldness, and the most indeterminate type hairs at onset. Tachyphylaxis, or decreased beneficial effect with prolonged usage, may occur. Adverse effects are unusual and long-term effectiveness and toxicity are unknown. Topical tretinoin (Retin-A) is being used without FDA approval to improve the appearance of aging skin. Increased dermal blood flow, hyperplasia of atrophic epidermis, promotion of normal dermal and epidermal differentiation, thickening of the epidermal stratum granulosum, decreased melanin content, and enhanced density of collagen in the papillary dermis with modest clinical reversal of signs of epidermal damage result from the topical application of this drug. Retinoid dermatitis (erythema, photosensitivity, dryness, and scaling) is seen in almost all patients, requiring the addition of topical steroid creams in some and at least an aggressive moisturizer regimen. The effectiveness of this drug is, at present, unimpressive. A more established application of Retin-A is in the preparation of the skin for chemical exfoliation procedures. The drug is typically applied for a 4- to 8-week prepeel period, often with the addition of a hydroquinone preparation (eg, Melanex) to minimize potential pigmentary changes.

Actinic exposure of the skin results in acute (sunburn) and chronic injury (eg, degenerative changes, decreased immune reactivity, and malignant lesions). Ultraviolet-B radiation is the most damaging, with most rays reaching the earth between 10 A.M. and 3 P.M. in most U.S. latitudes. Most sunscreens exhibit peak absorption in this range and are applied in a cream, oil, lotion, or gel vehicle. Physical sunscreens (eg, zinc oxide) are radiopaque formulations that scatter light and are cosmetically unacceptable to many. Effective sunscreens may prevent skin cancer, but chronic changes may occur despite their use. *Substantivity* refers to the tendency of the product to remain on the skin during prolonged activity. PABA and its derivatives are the most effective; however, some patients will be sensitive to these compounds. Mineral oils lubricate the skin and alter its optical properties but do not protect against actinic injury or promote tanning. Altitude, reflectivity, clothing, and atmospheric conditions also affect the results of exposure. Patients with exposed cervicofacial incisions and lacerations are advised to protect these areas specifically for at least 1 year postinjury to avoid relative hyperpigmentation.

PERIOPERATIVE DRUGS

With the increase in same-day surgery and office surgical suites, ultra-short-acting benzodiazepines, narcotics, and nondepolarizing neuromuscular blocking agents have come into prominent use, largely replacing the longer-acting agents diazepam, morphine, Demerol, and pancuronium in these settings.

Midazolam (Versed) is a parenteral benzodiazepine indicated for short surgical, diagnostic, or endoscopic procedures; induction of general anesthesia; and as a hypnotic drug in balanced anesthesia regimens. It is ideal because of its lack of tissue irritation, faster onset of action, and rapid hepatic elimination (the half-life is 1 to 4 hours); moreover, the level of sedation is easily and smoothly titrated. Midazolam is also commonly used to avoid adverse effects during the use of ketamine (Ketalar), which remains in widespread use. Flumazenil (Mazecon) is a parenteral benzodiazepine receptor antagonist that may be used for the reversal of conscious sedation in surgical procedures or in overdose situations. Although reversal of sedation, prevention of further amnesia, and improved psychomotor performance are observed, the extent to which respiratory depression can be reversed is variable and is only partly effective at best. Recurrence of sedation may require redosing within several hours.

Similarly, triazolam (Halcion) has been developed as an oral benzodiazepine for use in the treatment of insomnia. In this regard, it is as effective as longer-acting benzodiazepines in decreasing time to onset of sleep and frequency of awakening, and in increasing total sleep time, although, because of its short 2- to 3-hour half-life, it is less likely to produce residual hypnotic effects on the morning following administration.

Fentanyl (Sublimaze) is the prototype short-acting synthetic opioid, which is used in local-standby and balanced general anesthetic techniques as above. This class of narcotic analgesics produces fewer cardiovascular side effects than morphine and more effectively suppresses undesirable hemodynamic reflex and hormonal responses to surgical stimulation. These characteristics, and a brief 30- to 60-minute duration of action, make this drug a more appropriate choice for use in outpatient, emergency, and intensive care settings. As expected, narcotic antagonists such as naloxone (Narcan) effectively reverse typical adverse/overdosage effects of these opioid analgesics. The fentanyl patch (Duragesic) may be used in the treatment of chronic cancer pain syndromes.

Vecuronium (Norcuron) and atracurium (Tracrium) are short-acting (1 hour) nondepolarizing neuromuscular blockers whose duration of action is about half that of pancuronium (Pavulon), making their pharmacokinetic profile more desirable for short procedures under general anesthesia or assisted ventilation.

Propofol (Diprivan) is an intravenous sedative-hypnotic agent used widely in monitored anesthesia care, sedation procedures in conjunction with local/regional anesthetic techniques, and brief diagnostic (eg, endoscopy) procedures. Assets include rapid, smooth onset of action, easy titration of a continuous infusion to a desired anesthetic endpoint, and smooth and rapid emergence from anesthesia without adverse after effects.

Ketorolac (Toradol) is the first injectable (IM) nonsteroidal anti-inflammatory drug (NSAID) released for short-term (5-day) analgesic use in the United States. It is comparable to 12 mg IM morphine or 100 mg IM meperidine (Demerol) and is also available in oral form. There is no respiratory depression, no physiologic addictive potential, and less nausea, vomiting, and sedation than with the latter drugs. Inasmuch as NSAIDs affect platelet aggregation (reversible inhibition) and may prolong bleeding time, this drug is not recommended as a premedication or for anesthesia support. Unlike the irreversible inhibition of acetylsalicylic acid (ASA), the hemostatic effects of ketorolac disappear as the drug is eliminated. Although several clinical studies have not found excessive bleeding, many anecdotal case reports exist that implicate this drug in postoperative hematoma. Careful consideration should be given, therefore, to its use in certain types of procedures (eg, rhytidectomy, blepharoplasty).

MEDICATIONS ASSOCIATED WITH A HIGHER INCIDENCE OF TINNITUS

(As reported on product labeling listed in PDR)
Alprazolam (Xanax tablets) 6.6%
Bepridil hydrochloride (Vascor tablets 200 and 300 mg), up to 6.52%
Butorphanol tartrate (Stadol injectable and Stadol NS nasal spray), 3 to 9%
Choline magnesium trisalicylate (Trilisate liquid and tablets), less than 20%
Clomipramine hydrochloride (Anafranil capsules), 4 to 6%
Fenoprofen calcium (Nalfon 200 pulvules and tablets), 4.5%
Fosphenytoin sodium (Cerebyx injection), 8.9%
Mefloquine hydrochloride (Lariam tablets), among most frequent
Nabumetone (Relafen tablets), 3 to 9%
Naproxen sodium (Anaprox, EC-Naprosyn Delayed Release, Naprelan, Naprosyn suspension and tablets), 3 to 9%
Salsalate (Disalcid capsules and tablets), among most common
Tacrolimus (Prograf), greater than 3%
Xylocaine with and without epinephrine injections, among most common

MEDICATIONS ASSOCIATED WITH ANOSMIA

(As reported on product labeling listed in PDR)
Beclomethasone dipropionate (Beclovent and Beconase Inhalation Aerosol, Beconase AQ Nasal Spray), rare
Ciprofloxacin (Cipro IV and Tablets), less than 1%
Dexamethasone (Dexacort Phosphate in Turbinaire)
Enalaprilat (Vasotec IV)
Enalapril maleate (Vasotec Tablets), 0.5 to 1.0%
Enalapril maleate/hydrochlorothiazide (Vaseretic Tablets)
Flunisolide (Aerobid and Aerobid-M Inhaler Systems), 3 to 9%
Flunisolide (Nasalide Nasal Solution 0.025%)
Ganciclovir sodium (Cytovene-IV), one report

MEDICATIONS ASSOCIATED WITH A HIGHER INCIDENCE OF VERTIGO

(As reported on product labeling listed in PDR)
Anistreplase (Eminase), less than 10%
Buprenorphine (Buprenex Injectable), 5 to 10%

Clozapine (Clozaril Tablets), more than 5 to 19%
Dexfenfluramine hydrochloride (Redux Capsules), 3.1%
Doxazosin mesylate (Cardura Tablets), 2 to 23%
Enoxacin (Penetrex Tablets), 3%
Flumazenil (Romazicon), 10%
Interferon alfa-2B (Intron A for Injection), less than 5% to 23%
Leuprolide acetate (Lupron Depot-3 month 22.5 mg), 6.4%
Metoprolol tartrate/hydrochlorothiazide (Lopressor HCT Tablets), 10%
Mitotane (Lysodren Tablets), 15%
Nalbuphine hydrochloride (Nubain Injection), 5%
Primidone (Mysoline Suspension and Tablets), among most frequent
Riluzole (Rilutek Tablets), 2.5 to 4.5%
Salsalate (Disalcid Capsules and Tablets), among most common
Sumatriptan succinate (Imitrex Injection), 11.9%
Terazosin hydrochloride (Hytrin Capsules), 0.5 to 21%
Tocanide hydrochloride (Tonocard Tablets), 8.0 to 25.3%
Tramadol hydrochloride (Ultram Tablets 50 mg), 26 to 33%

MEDICATIONS ASSOCIATED WITH OTOTOXICITY

(As reported on product labeling listed in PDR)
Amikacin sulfate (Amikin Injectable)
Carboplatin (Paraplatin for Injection), 1 to 13%
Cetirizine hydrochloride (Zyrtec Tablets), less than 2%
Cisplatin (Platinol and Platinol-AQ for Injection) up to 31%
Furosemide (Lasix Injection, Oral Solution, and Tablets)
Gentamicin (Garamycin Injectable)
Neomycin sulfate/dexamethasone sodium phosphate (Neodecadron Topical Cream)
Neomycin sulfate/polymyxin B (Neosporin G.U. Irrigant)
Netilmicin (Netromycin Injection 100 mg/mL)
Polymyxin B sulfate/neomycin sulfate/hydrocortisone acetate (Cortisporin Cream, Otic
    Solution and Suspension, Pediotic Suspension)
Polymyxin B sulfate/bacitracin zinc/neomycin sulfate/hydrocortisone acetate (Cortisporin
    Ointment)
Streptomycin sulfate
Tobramycin sulfate (Nebcin Vials, Hyporets, and ADD-Vantage)
Torsemide (Demadex Tablets and Injectable)
Vancomycin hydrochloride (Vancocin HCL, Oral Solution and Pulvules, Vials and ADD-
    Vantage)

MEDICATIONS ASSOCIATED WITH A HIGHER INCIDENCE OF RHINITIS

(As reported on product labeling listed in PDR)
Atovaquone (Mepron Suspension), 5%
Bisoprolol fumarate (Zebeta Tablets), 2.9 to 4.0%
Butorphanol tartrate (Stadol Injectable and NS Nasal Spray), 3 to 9%

Calcitonin (synthetic) (Miacalcin Nasal Spray), 12%

Clomipramine hydrochloride (Anafranil Capsules), 7 to 12%

Daunorubicin estrate (DaunoXome), up to 12%

Desmopressin acetate (DDAVP Nasal Spray and Rhinal Tube), 3 to 8%

Didanosine (Videx Tablets, Powder for Oral Solution, & Pediatric Oral Solution), 48%

Diltiazem hydrochloride (Dilacor XR Extended-release Capsules), 2.9 to 9.6%

Diphtheria and Tetanus Toxoids and Acellular Pertussis Vaccine Adsorbed, 6%

Doxazosin mesylate (Cardura Tablets), 3%

Felbamate (Felbatol), 6.9%

Flunisolide (Aerobid and Aerobid-M Inhaler Systems), 3 to 9%

Fluvastatin sodium (Lescol Capsules), 4.7%

Gabapentin (Neurontin Capsules), 4.1%

Ipratropium bromide (Atrovent Nasal Spray 0.03%), 2.0 to 5.1%

Lamotrigine (Lamictal Tablets), 13.6%

Loracarbef (Lorabid Suspension and Pulvules), 1.6 to 6.3%

Mesalamine (Asacol Delayed-Release Tablets), 5%

Mupirocin calcium (Bactroban Nasal), 1.0 to 6.0%

Mycophenolate mofetil (CellCept Capsules), more than or equal to 3%

Nafarelin acetate (Synarel Nasal Solution for Central Precocious Puberty), 5%

Naproxen sodium (Naprelan Tablets), 3 to 9%

Nedocromil sodium (Tilade Inhaler), 4.6%

Nizatidine (Axid Pulvules), 9.8%

Pentostatin (Nipent for Injection), 10 to 11%

Pergolide mesylate (Permax Tablets), 12.2%

Pilocarpine hydrochloride (Salagen Tablets), 5 to 14%

Riluzole (Rilutek Tablets), 7.8 to 8.9%

Risperidone (Risperdal Tablets), 8 to 10%

Sargramostim (Leukine), 11%

Tacrine hydrochloride (Cognex Capsules), 8%

Tacrolimus (Prograf), greater than 3%

Ursodiol (Actigall Capsules), 5.2%

MEDICATIONS ASSOCIATED WITH ANGIOEDEMA

(As reported on product labeling listed in PDR)

Albuterol (Ventolin Syrup, Tablets, Inhalation Aerosol & Solution, Proventil Inhaler Aerosol), rare

Amlodipine besylate/benazepril hydrochloride (Lotrel Capsules), about 0.5%

Aspirin (Easprin)

Auranofin (Ridaura Capsules)

Azithromycin (Zithromax Capsules, Tablets, Oral Suspension), 1% or less

Beclomethasone dipropionate (Vanceril Inhaler, Vancenase PocketHaler, Beconase Inhalation Aerosol, AQ Nasal Spray, Beclovent Inhalation Aerosol), rare

Butabarbital sodium (Butisol Sodium Elixir and Tablets), less than 1%

Captopril (Capoten Tablets), approximately 1 in 1000 patients

Captopril/hydrochlorothiazide (Capozide Tablets), approximately 1 in 1000 patients

Carisoprodol/aspirin (Soma Compound Tablets with and without codeine), less common

Ceftazidime (Ceptaz, Fortaz), very rare

Cephalexin hydrochloride (Keftab Tablets, Keflex Pulvules and Oral Suspension)

Ciprofloxacin (Cipro IV, Tablets), 1% or less

Clonidine hydrochloride (Catapres Tablets), about 5 in 1000 patients

Chloramphenicol sodium succinate (Chloromycetin Sodium Succinate)

Cromolyn sodium (Intal Inhaler, Nasalcrom Nasal Solution), infrequent

Diclofenac potassium (Voltaren Tablets and XR-Tablets, Cataflam Tablets), less than 1%

Enalaprilat (Vasotec IV), 0.5 to 1%

Enalapril maleate (Vasotec Tablets)

Enalapril maleate/hydrochlorothiazide (Vaseretic Tablets), 0.6%

Etidronate disodium (diphosphate) (Didronel Tablets)

Fenoprofen calcium (Nalfon 200 Puvules and Nalfon Tablets)

Hepatitis B immune globulin (Human) (Hep-B-Gammagee)

Hepatitis B vaccine (Recombivax HB), less than 1%

Indomethacin (Indocin Capsules, SR Capsules, Oral Suspension, Suppositories), less than 1%

Lisinopril (Zestril Tablets), 0.1%

Lisinopril (Prinivil Tablets), 0.3 to 1.0%

Lithium carbonate (Eskalith Capsules and CR Controlled Release Tablets)

Mephobarbital (Mebaral Tablets)

Metoclopramide hydrochloride (Reglan Injectable, Syrup, Tablets), rare

Methocarbamol/aspirin (Robaxisal Tablets)

Nalidixic acid (NegGram Caplets and Suspension)

Nitrofurantoin (Macrodantin Capsules)

Nitrofurantoin monohydrate (Macrobid Capsules)

Norfloxacin (Noroxin Tablets)

Pentobarbital sodium (Nembutal Sodium Capsules, Solution, and Suppositories), less than 1%

Pentoxifylline (Trental Tablets), less than 1%

Phenobarbital (Phenobarbital Elixir and Tablets), less than 1%

Piroxicam (Feldane Capsules), less than 1%

Quinidine gluconate (Quinaglute Dura-Tabs Tablets)

Quinidine polygalacturonate (Cardioquin Tablets)

Quinidine sulfate (Quinidex Extentabs)

Secobarbital sodium (Seconal Sodium Pulvules), less than 1%

Thiabendazole (Mintezol Chewable Tablets & Suspension)

Trimethoprim/sulfamethoxazole (Septra Tablets, DS Tablets, Suspension, IV Infusion, Bactrim Tablets, DS Tablets, Pediatric Suspension, IV Infusion)

MEDICATIONS ASSOCIATED WITH A HIGHER INCIDENCE OF XEROSTOMIA

(As reported on product labeling listed in PDR)

Acrivastine/pseudoephedrine hydrochloride (Semprex-D Capsules), 7%

Alprazolam (Xanax Tablets), 14.7%

Amoxapine (Asendin Tablets), 14%

Anastrozole (Arimidex Tablets), 4.5 to 5.7%

Apraclonidine hydrochloride (Iopidine 0.5%), 10%

Astemizole (Hismanal Tablets), 5.2%

Bromocriptine mesylate (Parlodel Capsules and SnapTabs), 4%

Brompheniramine maleate/phenylpropanolamine hydrochloride/codeine phosphate (Dimetane-DC Cough Syrup), most frequent

Brompheniramine maleate/pseudoephedrine hydrochloride/dextromorphan hydro-bromide (Bromofed-DM Cough Syrup), among most frequent

Bupropion hydrochloride (Wellbutrin Tablets), 27.6%

Buspirone hydrochloride (BuSpar Tablets), 3%

Butorphenol tartrate (Stadol Injection and Stadol NS Nasal Spray), 3 to 9%

Cetirizine hydrochloride (Zyrtec Tablets), 5%

Chlordiazepoxide/amitriptyline hydrochloride (Limbitrol DS Tablets), among most frequent

Chlorpheniramine maleate/pseudophedrine hydrochloride (Atrohist Pediatric Suspension), among most common

Clomipramine hydrochloride (Anafranil Capsules), 63 to 84%

Clonidine hydrochloride (Catapres Tablets), 40%

Clonidine hydrochloride (Catapres-TTS), 25%

Clonidine hydrochloride/chlorthalidone (Combipres Tablets), 40%

Clozapine (Clozaril Tablets), more than 5 to 6%

Cyclobenzaprine hydrochloride (Flexeril Tablets), 7 to 27%

Dexfenfluramine hydrochloride (Redux Capsules), 12.5%

Dicyclomine hydrochloride (Bentyl 10 and 20 mg Tablets, Injection, and Syrup), 33%

Disopyramide phosphate (Norpace and Norpace CR Capsules), 32%

Doxepin hydrochloride (Zonalon Cream), 1 to 10%

Etretinate (Tegison Capsules), 1 to 10%

Fenfluramine hydrochloride (Pondimin Tablets), among most common

Fentanyl (Duragesic Transdermal System), 10% or more

Flumazenil (Romazicon), 3 to 9%

Fluvoxamine maleate (Luvox Tablets), 14%

Fluoxetine hydrochloride (Prozac Pulvules and Liquid, Oral Solution), 5 to 12%

Fosphenytoin sodium (Cerebyx Injection), 4.4%

Guanfacine hydrochloride (Tenex Tablets), 5 to 54%

Interferon alfa 2B (Intron A for Injection), up to 28%

Ipratropium bromide (Atrovent Inhalation Solution), 3.2%

Isotretinoin (Accutane Capsules), up to 80%

Leuprolide acetate (Lepron Depot 3.75 mg), less than 5%

Loratadine (Claritin Tablets), 3%, (Claritin-D Tablets), 14%

Maprotiline hydrochloride (Ludiomil Tablets), 22%

Mazindol (Sanorex Tablets), among most common

Mirtazapine (Remeron Tablets), 25%

Moricizine hydrochloride (Ethmozine Tablets), 2 to 5%

Nalbuphine hydrochloride (Nubain Injection), 4%

Nefazodone hydrochloride (Serzone Tablets), 25%

Oxycodone hydrochloride (OxyContin Tablets), 6%

Paroxetine hydrochloride (Paxil Tablets), 1.0 to 20.6%

Pergolide mesylate (Permax Tablets), 3.7% frequent

Pimozide (Orap Tablets), 5 of 20 patients

Propafenone hydrochloride (Rythmol Tablets 150 mg, 225 mg, 300 mg), 0.9 to 5.7%

Scopolamine (Transderm Scopolamine), 66%

Selegiline hydrochloride (Eldepryl Capsules), 6%

Sertraline hydrochloride (Zoloft Tablets), 16.3%

Terfenadine (Seldane Tablets), 2.3 to 4.8% (Seldane-D Extended Release Tablets), 21.7%

Tramadol hydrochloride (Ultram Tablets), 5 to 10%

Trazodone hydrochloride (Desyrel and Desyrel Dividose), 14.8 to 33.8%

Trihexyphenidyl hydrochloride (Artane Elixir and Tablets), 30 to 50%

Tripelennamine hydrochloride (PBZ and PBZ-SR Tablets), among most frequent

Venlafaxine hydrochloride (Effexor), 2 to 22%

Zolpidem tartrate (Ambien Tablets), 3%

Bibliography

Aledort LM. Treatment of von Willebrand's disease. *Mayo Clin Proc* 1991;66:841–846.

Borisova OV, El'kova NL, Shcherbachenko OI, et al. The use of plasmaphoresis in treating recurrent aphthous stomatitis. *Stomatologiia (Mosk)* 1997;76(3):23–25.

Clark WG, Brater DC, Johnson AR. *Goth's Medical Pharmacology,* 13th ed. St. Louis: Mosby, 1992.

Craig CR, Stitzel RE. *Modern Pharmacology,* 2nd ed. Boston: Little, Brown, 1986.

Drouin M, Yang WH, Bertrand B, et al. Once daily mometasone furoate aqueous nasal spray is as effective as twice daily beclomethasone dipropionate for treating perennial allergic rhinitis. *Ann Allergy Asthma Immunol* 1996;77(2):153–160.

Edres MA, Scully C, Gelbier M. Use of proprietary agents to relieve recurrent aphthous stomatitis. *Br Dent J* 1997;182(4):144–146.

Fee WE, Aminoglycoside ototoxicity in the human. *Laryngoscope* 1980;90(suppl 24).

Graft D, Aaronson D, Chervinsky P. A placebo and active controlled randomized trial of prophylactic treatment of seasonal allergic rhinitis with mometasone furoate aqueous nasal spray. *J Allergy Clin Immunol* 1996;98(4):724–731.

Hamlar DD, Schuller DE, Gahbauer RA, et al. Determination of the efficacy of topical oral pilocarpine for postradiation xerostomia in patients with head and neck carcinoma. *Laryngoscope* 1996;106(8):972–976.

Hardman JG, Limbird LE, Molinoff PB, et al, eds. *Goodman and Gilman's The Pharmacologic Basis of Therapeutics,* 9th ed. New York: McGraw-Hill, 1996.

Hebert JR, Nolop K, Lutsky BN. Once daily mometasone furoate aqueous nasal spray (Nasonex) in seasonal allergic rhinitis: an active and placebo controlled study. *Allergy* 1996;51(8):569–576.

Horwitz RJ, Mcgill KA, Busse WW. The role of leukotriene modifiers in the treatment of asthma. *Am J Respir Crit Care Med* 1998; 157(5):1363–1371.

Judkins JH, Dray TG, Hubbell RN. Intraoperative ketorolac and posttonsillectomy bleeding. *Arch Otolaryngol Head Neck Surg* 1996;122:937–940.

Katzung BG. *Basic and Clinical Pharmacology,* 6th ed. Norwalk, CT: Appleton & Lange, 1995.

Lee KJ. *Essential Otolaryngology,* 6th ed. Norwalk, CT: Appleton & Lange, 1995.

Madore DV. Impact of immunization on *Haemophilus influenzae* type b disease. *Infect Agents Dis* 1996;5(1):8–20.

Mahdi AB, Coulter WA, Woolfson AD, Lamey PJ. Efficacy of bioadhesive patches in the treatment of recurrent aphthous stomatitis. *J Oral Pathol Med* 1996;25(8):416–419.

Marlowe FI. Ototoxic agents. *Otolaryngol Clin North Am* 1978;11(3):791–800.

Paparella MM, Shumrick DA, Gluckman JL, Meyerhoff WL. *Otolaryngology,* 3rd ed. Philadelphia: Saunders, 1991.

Physician's Desk Reference (PDR), 55th ed. Montvale, NJ: Medical Economics, 2001.

Physician's Desk Reference for Nonprescription Drugs, 22nd ed. Montvale, NJ: Medical Economics, 2001.

Physicians GenRx, The Complete Drug Reference. St. Louis: Mosby, 1996.

Rosenwasser LJ. Leukotriene modifiers: new drugs, old and new reactions. *J Allergy Clin Immunol* 1999;103:374–375.

Senior BA, Radkowski D, MacArthur C, et al. Changing patterns in pediatric supraglottitis: a multi-institutional review, 1980 to 1992. *Otolaryngol Head Neck Surg* 1994;110(2):203–210.

Waltzman SB, Cooper JS. Nature and incidence of misonidazole-produced ototoxicity. *Arch Otolaryngol* 1981;107:52–54.

Highlights and Pearls 39

HIGHLIGHTS AND PEARLS

1. Chronic tympanic membrane perforation may allow epithelial migration into the middle ear.
2. Chronic eustachian tube dysfunction can generate negative pressures to 600 cm H_2O with resultant retraction pocket formation.
3. Epithelial migration or retraction pocket formation with internal desquamation, enzymatic erosion, and osteitis allow formation and progression of cholesteatoma.
4. Cholesteatoma in Prussak's space most commonly spreads between the lateral mallear ligament and lateral incudal fold to involve the incus before entering the antrum.
5. Cholesteatoma/keratoma
   A. Mesotympanic keratoma
      (1) Originates from a marginal or central retraction or perforation.
      (2) Passes underneath the lateral incudal fold.
      (3) Usually involves the posterior tympanum (facial recess, sinus tympani, etc).
      (4) May enter the epitympanum by passing medial to the body of the incus.
      (5) Once in the epitympanum, spread continues posteromedially to the aditus between the superior mallear and superior incudal folds.
   B. Epitympanic keratoma
      (1) Originates in the epitympanum from a pars flaccida retraction or perforation.
      (2) Enters Prussak's space.
      (3) Three routes of egress from Prussak's space
         (a) Posterior route
            (i) Most common.
            (ii) Spread lateral to the body of the incus between the lateral mallear fold and the lateral incudal fold, around the superior incudal fold, and into the aditus.
         (b) Inferior route. Spread between the lateral and posterior mallear folds into the posterior pouch of von Troltsch and into the mesotympanum.
         (c) Anterior route. Spread anterior to the neck of the malleus via a dehiscence in the anterior mallear fold into the anterior pouch of von Troltsch and into the protympanum.
6. Complications of cholesteatoma in order of frequency
   A. Semicircular canal erosion/fistula and dizziness
   B. Extradural or perisinus abscess
   C. Serous or suppurative labyrinthitis
   D. Facial nerve paralysis
   E. Meningitis secondary to tegmental erosion
   F. Epidural, subdural, or parenchymal brain abscess
   G. Sigmoid sinus thrombosis/phlebitis

H. Subperiosteal abscess/Bezold's abscess due to erosion of the mastoid cortex

I. Recurrence of cholesteatoma (attic is most common)

7. The anterior and posterior tympanic isthmuses communicate the epitympanum with the mesotympanum.

A. The anterior tympanic isthmus is bounded by the tensor tympani tendon, body of the incus, stapes suprastructure, and bony labyrinth.

B. The posterior tympanic isthmus is bounded by the posterior incudal ligament, posterior canal wall, pyramidal process, and medial incudal fold.

8. The tympanic ring continues to expand and thicken into adult life.

9. The vestibular aqueduct (also called the aqueduct/canal of Cotugno) transmits the endolymphatic duct and is parallel to the cochlear aqueduct. It also carries a plexus of veins known as the veins of the vestibular aqueduct.

10. The cochlear aqueduct is filled only with periotic tissues and contains no other structures.

11. Hyrtle's fissure is an embryologic remnant that normally obliterates but may persist as a hypotympanic connection to the subarachnoid space; this may allow transmission of middle ear or mastoid infections to the cerebrospinal fluid (CSF).

12. Foramen of Huschke is an embryologic remnant that may persist as a communication from the anteroinferior aspect of the medial external auditory canal. Allows the spread of tumors and infection to or from the preauricular area/glenoid fossa/parotid.

13. Fissures of Santorini are lymphatic channels that connect the anteroinferior aspect of the cartilaginous ear canal with the preauricular area/glenoid fossa/parotid and allow the spread of infection or tumor.

14. The dilator tubae portion of the tensor veli palatini muscle is primarily responsible for eustachian tube opening; tubal closure is passive.

15. The natural resonance of the external auditory canal is 3000 Hz; of the middle ear, 800 Hz; of the tympanic membrane, between 800 and 1600 Hz.

16. The phase difference between the oval and round windows is 4 dB when the tympanic membrane is intact.

17. Both myelinated and unmyelinated neurons attach to the base of the cochlear hair cells. Afferent and efferent neurons attach to both types of hair cells and regulate the specificity of Reissner's membrane.

18. The primary auditory cortex corresponds to Brodmann's area 41, which is located in the superior portion of the temporal lobe along the floor of the lateral cerebral fissure.

19. One in 200 children is born with some degree of congenital hearing loss. One-third to three-fourths of these losses have a genetic component. Of those with a genetic component, one-third are part of an identifiable syndrome, whereas others have hearing loss as their only finding.

20. More than 70 syndromes have been identified with a genetic basis involving hearing loss.

A. Usher syndrome—caused by one of five possible mutations at 1q, 3q, 11p, 11q, and 14q, all autosomal-recessive

B. Waardenburg syndrome—caused by one of two possible mutations, 2q (codes for PAX3) and 3p (codes for MITF), both autosomal-dominant

C. Alport syndrome—most due to mutation at Xq (codes for COL4A5), with X-linked recessive transmission; few cases of mutation at 2q (codes for COL4A3 and COL4A4) with autosomal-dominant

D. Stickler syndrome (hearing loss, detached retina, myopia, and micrognathia)—mutation at 6p (COL11A2) or 12q (COL2A1), autosomal-dominant

E. Osteogenesis imperfecta—mutation at 5p (COL1A2) or 17q (COL1A1), autosomal-dominant

F. Norries syndrome (exudative retinopathy, hearing loss)—mutation at Xp11 (codes for NDP), X-linked recessive

G. X-linked hearing impairment—rare syndrome with stapes fixation and perilymph gusher from mutation on Xq (codes for BRN1)

21. Nonsyndromic hearing loss occurs in association with no other physical findings. Locations of several genes found. Three recessive genes at 11q, 13q, and 17p. Two dominant genes at 1p and 5q.

22. Symphalangia, ankylosis of the proximal interphalangeal joints of the hands and feet, associated with conductive hearing loss secondary to stapes fixation.

23. Waardenburg syndrome causes 2% of all deafness and affects 1:42,000 new births. Affects at least 18 different human characteristics; these effects can be classified as major or minor or may be nonpenetrant. WS1, the most common variant, must express two major effects or one major effect and two minor effects. Patients with WS that do *not* have dystopia canthorum have WS2.

   Patients with WS1 have gene mutations of PAX3; PAX3 is located on chromosome 2. Patients with WS2 have gene mutations at MITF, EDNRB (endothelin receptor B) or EDN3 (endothelin 3). PAX3 and MITF encode proteins called transcription factors which regulate the activities of other genes.

   WS major effects:
   A. Hearing loss
   B. Heterochromia irides or isochromia irides (sapphire blue)
   C. White hair as forelock (poliosis), eyebrows, or eyelashes on other parts of the body
   D. Dystopia canthorum (widely spaced inner canthi)
   E. First-degree relative with diagnosis of WS

   WS minor effects:
   A. Skin without pigmentation
   B. Fusion of the eyebrows (synophrys)
   C. Broad nasal bridge
   D. Thin nasal alae
   E. Premature gray hair

24. Diagnosis of congenital hearing loss is usually delayed until approximately 2.5 years of age.

25. Infant hearing loss is associated with certain high-risk groups who should have early auditory brain response or otoacoustic emission testing.

   A. Bacterial meningitis, especially type b *Haemophilus influenzae*. (Although streptococci are the most common cause of childhood meningitis, a greater percentage of those children with *H. influenzae* develop hearing loss.)

  B. Congenital perinatal infections (TORCH).
   (1) Toxoplasmosis
   (2) Other/(eg, syphilis)
   (3) Rubella
   (4) Cytomegalovirus
   (5) Herpes
  C. Positive family history of congenital hearing loss.
  D. Concomitant head and neck anomalies.
  E. Birth weight less than 1500 g.
  F. Hyperbilirubinemia.
  G. Initial Apgar score < 4 at birth, no spontaneous respirations at birth, or prolonged hypotonia persisting to 2 hours of age.
  H. Prolonged NICU stay (5 to 10% of post-NICU infants have some degree of measurable hearing loss).

26. Sudden sensorineural hearing loss occurs in 10.7 per 100,000 population and has many causes; it may be the presenting symptom in as many as 10% of acoustic neuromas.

27. Sudden hearing loss prognostic factors
  A. Good
   (1) Minimal hearing loss
   (2) Low-frequency loss
   (3) Absence of vestibular symptoms
   (4) Early treatment (within 3 days)
   (5) No changes in N_1 latency in electrocochleography (ECoG)
  B. Poor
   (1) Advanced age
   (2) Total deafness
   (3) Objective vestibular symptoms
   (4) Other vascular risk factors
   (5) Delay of treatment

28. Between 40 and 70% of patients with sudden hearing loss recover some hearing without treatment.

29. Low-dose aminoglycoside ototoxicity is associated with a mutation of the 12S mitochondrial rRNA gene. Vestibular studies in low-dose aminoglycoside ototoxicity are usually normal, whereas vestibular abnormalities are common in normal aminoglycoside toxicity.

30. Differential diagnosis of dizziness
  A. Organic
   (1) Vascular
   (2) Vestibular
   (3) Neurologic, nonvestibular
    (a) Central
    (b) Peripheral
  B. Psychogenic
  C. True vertigo alone
   (1) Vestibular neuronitis
   (2) Recurrent vestibulopathy

          (3)   Benign positioning vertigo
          (4)   Dysequilibrium of aging
          (5)   Multiple sclerosis
          (6)   Epilepsy
          (7)   Migraine
          (8)   Vertebrobasilar insufficiency
      D.   Vertigo, tinnitus, and deafness
          (1)   Hydrops
          (2)   Labyrinthitis
          (3)   Ototoxic medications
          (4)   Trauma
          (5)   Acoustic neuroma
          (6)   Fistula
          (7)   Central nervous system (CNS) tumor
          (8)   CNS infection
          (9)   Inflammatory disorder

31.   Differential diagnosis of hydrops
      A.   Allergy
      B.   Ménière's disease
      C.   Mumps
      D.   Syphilis
      E.   Hypothyroidism
      F.   Mondini deformity
      G.   Elevated anti-HSV (herpes simplex virus) IgG in perilymph suggests role of HSV; does not correlate with serum anti-HSV IgG, but does correlate with serum anti-HSV IgE.

32.   Hearing aid components
      A.   Power supply
      B.   Microphone (transducer)
      C.   Amplifier
      D.   Receiver
      E.   Earmold

33.   Gain measurement of a hearing aid is the difference between the level of the input signal and the level of the output signal at a given frequency.

34.   To decrease the amount of gain in the low frequencies in patients with high-frequency neural loss, consider:
      A.   Open venting of the earmold.
      B.   Shorten the canal of the earmold.
      C.   Enlarge the sound bore.

35.   In the use of hearing aids, a vented aid allows low-frequency sounds to escape (low-frequency attenuation), thus selectively amplifying high-frequency sounds. A closed mold provides a more uniform amplification. In general, a patient with a dynamic range of more than 45 dB is a good hearing aid candidate, whereas a patient with a dynamic range of 25 to 45 dB is a fair candidate.

36.   Saccades of any origin are mediated by the cerebellum for accurate precision of their amplitudes and latencies.

37. Saccades are dependent on the integrity of the maculae and degree of consciousness.

38. Deflection of the stereocilia toward the kinocilium causes an decrease in the resting discharge of the hair cells.

39. Polarization of hair cells in the horizontal canal is opposite that of the posterior and superior canals. Ampullopetal flow increases the resting discharge rate in the horizontal superior semicircular canal (SCC), whereas ampullofugal flow increases this rate in the posterior and SCC.

40. The narrowest portion of the membranous labyrinth is the ductus reuniens between the cochlea and saccule.

41. Diagnostic criteria for acute labyrinthitis
    A. Acute unilateral peripheral dysfunction without hearing loss.
    B. Occurrence predominantly in middle age.
    C. One single episode of prolonged vertigo (hours to days).
    D. Decreased electronystagmography (ENG) caloric response in one ear.
    E. Spontaneous and complete resolution of symptoms within 6 months.

42. Lesions of the peripheral vestibular apparatus usually produce a horizontal-torsional nystagmus. Positioning nystagmus is predominantly vertical-torsional. Nystagmus of central origin is usually purely torsional or purely vertical, but can have horizontal components (especially cerebral cortical lesions). Smooth pursuit is also affected in central lesions. Purely torsional is usually brain stem/vestibular nuclei. Down-beating vertical is usually craniocervical junction. Up-beating vertical is usually pontomedullary or fourth ventricle. Periodic alternating nystagmus usually arises in dorsal medulla/cerebellum.

    Gaze-evoked nystagmus is seen as a side effect of some medications as well as brain stem lesions. If this changes to the opposite direction, it is termed centripetal nystagmus. If it then returns to the initial side, it is rebound nystagmus. Gaze-evoked nystagmus that increases with prolonged eccentric gaze is associated with myasthenia gravis. Latent nystagmus is associated with strabismus. Pendular nystagmus shows sinusoidal oscillation of the slow phase and can be congenital or acquired; if acquired, it is often associated with multiple sclerosis or brain stem infarct. This can be associated with palatal myoclonus. Convergence–retraction nystagmus occurs with midbrain lesions and is often associated with upward gaze paralysis (Parinaud syndrome).

43. Acute peripheral vestibular lesions have nystagmus that beats away initially, and with time converts to beat toward the lesion.

44. The facial nerve has a natural dehiscence along its inferior margin superior to the oval window in nearly 50% of normal specimens.

45. The iter chordae posterior is the small canal through which the chorda tympani passes as it branches from the facial nerve in the fallopian canal and enters the middle ear.

46. The iter chordae anterior is the small canal in the anterior petrotympanic fissure where the chorda tympani exits the middle ear (also called the canal of Huguier).

47. Cerumen has an acidic pH and is bacteriostatic, especially for gram-positive organisms, and fungistatic.

48. Cholesterol granuloma is a nonspecific response but is seen most often in atelectatic ears. Cholesteatoma must have a keratinizing epithelium with keratin debris but need

not have an intact matrix, cholesterol crystals, tympanic membrane perforation, or a sac-like structure.

49. In cases of suspected SCC fistula from cholesteatoma, a positive fistula test (positive Hennebert's sign) results when positive external auditory canal pressure causes ampullopetal stimulation of the horizontal SCC with horizontal nystagmus to the ipsilateral side; with negative pressure, the nystagmus reverses.

50. Severe or total sensorineural hearing loss (SNHL) develops in 8% of lateral canal fistulae and in over 50% of more extensive fistulae; limited losses are the result of the membranous labyrinth sealing the fistula. Less SNHL with SCC fistulae than with cochlear fistulae. Safe to remove matrix if fistula less than 2 mm.

51. In 10% of the population, the anterior petrous cell tract is pneumatized, whereas 30% have pneumatization of the posterior tract. Cholesterol granulomata of the petrous apex occur within these pneumatized cell tracts.

52. Dorello's canal is formed between the petrous portion of the temporal bone laterally and the petroclinoid ligament superomedially; this canal conveys cranial nerve VI and the inferior petrosal sinus.

53. Petrous apicitis may result in Gradenigo syndrome: retro-orbital headache, otorrhea, and diplopia secondary to irritation of cranial nerve VI within Dorello's canal.

54. Meckel's cave is a depression in the anteromedial aspect of the petrous portion of the temporal bone in which rests the gasserian ganglion of cranial nerve V.

55. Approximately 150 to 200 mL of cerebrospinal fluid (CSF) is present in the normal adult; it is replenished four times daily.

56. Referred otalgia
    CN V: Oral cavity, mandible, temporomandibular joint (TMJ), palate, preauricular region
    CN VII: External auditory canal, postauricular region
    CN IX: Tonsil, tongue base, nasopharynx, eustachian tube, pharynx (transmitted via Jacobsen's nerve)
    CN X: Hypopharynx, larynx, trachea (transmitted via Arnold's nerve)

57. Hitzelberger's sign is numbness of the postauricular area associated with compression of the facial nerve by an acoustic neuroma.

58. Jacobsen's nerve is a branch of the glossopharyngeal nerve that arises from the inferior (petrous) ganglion of cranial nerve IX and enters the middle ear by ascending through the tympanic canaliculus between the internal jugular vein and internal carotid artery to join the tympanic plexus.

59. Arnold's nerve arises from branches of the superior (jugular) ganglion of the vagus nerve in the neck, which unite to form the ramus auricularis of cranial nerve X, which passes through the jugular fossa and through the substance of the lateral temporal bone to innervate the external auditory canal and postauricular area.

60. The acoustic reflex arc consists of the cochlea, cranial nerve VIII, cochlear nuclei, and contralateral olivary complex via the trapezoid body to the motor nucleus of cranial nerve VII and then via the nerve to the stapedius. A unilateral stimulus results in bilateral contraction.

61. By convention, the ear in which the probe is placed is called the probe ear. The ear to which the acoustic reflex soliciting tone is presented can be either the probe ear (ipsilateral) or the opposite ear (contralateral reflex).

62. Reflex decay is measured at 500 Hz, 10 dB above threshold, for 10 seconds. Abnormal decay is decay to less than 50% of the original amplitude in 10 seconds. That finding is indicative of a probable eighth nerve or brain stem lesion.

63. Factors that can affect the acoustic reflex:
    A. Conductive losses of 40 dB for the ear receiving the reflex-eliciting tone or as little as 10 dB for the probe ear
    B. Cochlear hearing losses of greater than 70 dB
    C. Eighth nerve lesions
    D. Multiple sclerosis
    E. Brain stem lesions

64. Eighth nerve or central nervous system (CNS) lesions may have the following acoustic reflex responses:
    A. Normal reflexes
    B. Elevated reflex thresholds without decay
    C. Normal or elevated reflex thresholds with decay
    D. Absent reflexes

65. Basic rules of masking
    A. Masking is always presented by air conduction, whether the testing is of air or bone conduction.
    B. Air conduction signals cross over at 50 dB.
    C. Bone conduction signals cross over at 0 dB.
    D. Crossover will occur to the cochlear threshold of the opposite ear.
    E. The purpose of masking is to eliminate the nontest ear from participating in the test and should be used under these circumstances:
        (1) Testing air conduction whenever there is a difference between the level of the signal and the bone conduction of the nontest ear exceeding 50 dB.
        (2) Testing bone conduction any time the unmasked audiogram shows an air–bone gap.
    F. Bilateral 50-dB air–bone gaps create a masking dilemma that requires special audiometric techniques.

66. Behavioral audiometric tests can be grouped into categories based on an attempt to determine whether a patient has an auditory recruitment or auditory fatigue.
    A. Recruitment is an abnormal growth in loudness. It indicates a cochlear lesion. When an acoustic neuroma is present, the finding of recruitment probably overrides the finding of auditory fatigue.
    B. Fatigue, known as tone decay or adaptation, is a change of auditory threshold resulting from continued acoustic stimulation. It is the classic sign of eighth nerve or low brain stem site of lesion.

67. Tests of recruitment include the following:
    A. Speech test of dynamic range between speech reception threshold and discomfort level. The normal range is 95 dB. The more narrow the range, the greater the recruitment.
    B. Alternate binaural loudness balance (ABLB) test compares the loudness of a constant tone as perceived by the two ears separately; if the points of equal loudness on the laddergram are parallel, recruitment is absent. If the points tend to converge, recruitment is on the side of the convergence.

C. The short increment sensitivity index (SISI) test is an indirect test of loudness recruitment, requiring perception of 1-dB increments of the same signal intensity presented at approximately 20 dB above the subject's pure tone threshold.

D. The narrow threshold crossings of 2 to 3 dB on continuous tone presentation of the Békésy test are an indication of auditory recruitment near threshold.

E. Acoustic reflex thresholds compared to pure tone thresholds is called the Metz recruitment test. In the normal ear, the range between pure tone threshold and acoustic reflex threshold is 85 dB. When that range is reduced below 60 dB, auditory recruitment is undoubtedly present.

68. Tests of auditory fatigue include several tone decay tests.

A. The Carhart tone decay test and the modified tone decay test of Rosenberg are both presented at threshold.

B. The Olson–Noffziger tone decay test is presented 20 dB above threshold.

C. The Jerger suprathreshold adaptation test is presented at 90 to 100 dB hearing level. In all cases, the examiner seeks to determine if threshold changes occur with ongoing tonal presentations.

D. The adaptation shown on type III Békésy tracings, where continuous tone thresholds fall markedly below pulsed-tone threshold tracings, is also suggestive of a retrocochlear lesion.

E. A gradual relaxation of the stapedial reflex, known as reflex decay, in the presence of a continuous tonal presentation is also suggestive of a retrocochlear lesion.

F. A decrease of speech discrimination at high intensities, known as rollover, is a result of cochlear distortion of eighth nerve adaptation. Normal hearing and conductive loss are not associated with rollover. In cochlear distortion, there is mild rollover. With retrocochlear lesions, there is often significant rollover; a decrease of more than 20% is suspicious.

69. As a battery, behavioral audiometric tests have a sensitivity of 70% and a specificity of 90%. Patient cooperation is the limiting factor.

70. The most common cause of conductive hearing loss between the ages of 15 and 50 is otosclerosis. Elevated anti-measles virus IgG in perilymph in otosclerosis; does not correlate with serum anti-measles IgG.

71. Even with otosclerotic lesions completely obliterating the oval window, it is unusual to find air–bone gaps greater than 50 dB.

72. An air–bone gap of greater than 50 dB suggests ossicular discontinuity.

73. The most common and earliest lesion in otosclerosis is firm, bony ankylosis located at the anterior edge of the oval window.

74. Clinical features of otosclerosis

A. Caucasian

B. Women twice as often as men

C. Pregnancy often coincides with the onset of otosclerosis or with an increase in activity of the lesions

D. About 50% of patients have a family history

E. Middle age

75. Temporal bone studies have shown histologic evidence of otosclerosis in 9.7% of adult Caucasian men, 18.5% of adult Caucasian women, and less than 1% of African-

American adults. However, it is estimated that only 12% of histologic lesions become clinically significant.

76. Severe thiamine (vitamin B_1) deficiency may lead to sensorineural hearing loss or tinnitus.

77. Severe niacin deficiency may cause nystagmus.

78. Perilymph fistulae (PLFs) in adults and children can cause sudden hearing loss, dysequilibrium, or both. Congenital anomalies may render children more susceptible than adults. Widely patent cochlear aqueducts increase susceptibility. Exploratory tympanotomy is the ultimate diagnostic aid. PLFs are the most common cause of cochlear hearing loss after stapedectomy.

79. Closure of PLFs usually results in a clearing of vestibular symptoms with little or no recovery in hearing. Most leaks are from the margins of the round or oval windows.

80. Tinnitus may be the first presenting symptom of an acoustic neuroma.

81. The region of the cochlea closest to the middle ear promontory serves the frequency range between 3 and 5 kHz.

82. Damage to the ossicular chain with an eardrum perforation usually causes a conductive hearing loss between 30 and 50 dB.

83. Ossicular discontinuity behind an intact eardrum causes a conductive loss of 55 to 65 dB.

84. Ninety-eight percent of patients with palatal cleft develop velar muscle dysfunction with resultant eustachian tube dysfunction, persistent serous otitis, and recurrent acute otitis media.

85. The most likely sites for the production of endolymph are the secretory cells of the stria vascularis of the cochlea and the dark cells of the vestibular labyrinth.

86. Synkinesis is defined as a single axon innervating widely separated facial muscles; it is not seen as a result of neuropraxia or axonotmesis.

87. "Crocodile tears" can be sequelae of facial nerve paralysis. These result from cross-innervation from the lesser superficial petrosal nerve, a branch of cranial nerve IX, carrying parasympathetic axons from the inferior salivatory nucleus to the parotid gland, to the greater superficial petrosal nerve, a branch of cranial nerve VII, carrying parasympathetic axons from the superior salivatory nucleus to the lacrimal gland.

88. Frey syndrome, also known as gustatory sweating, is seen in as many as 60% of postparotidectomy patients and can be diagnosed by Minor's starch-iodide test. Cross-innervation of parasympathetic nerves from the lesser superficial petrosal nerve (a branch of cranial nerve IX) from the inferior salivatory nucleus to the sweat glands of the skin flap. Treat with topical antiperspirant roll-on, topical glycopyrrolate, or topical atropine.

89. Homograft tympanoplasty is often recommended for slag burns of the tympanic membrane.

90. In the evaluation of hearing loss following administration of ototoxic medications, supra-audiometric testing often reveals subtle sensorineural losses before routine audiometric testing becomes positive.

91. During auditory brain response (ABR) testing, demyelination prolongs latency, and recruitment affects thresholds.

92. Brain stem function can be identified on ABR testing at approximately 28 weeks' gestational age with the appearance of waves I, III, and V. "Maturity" is not reached until approximately 18 months after birth.

93. Approximately 30% of patients with Ménière's disease develop bilateral symptoms during their lifetime.

94. In the evaluation of a patient for a retrocochlear lesion, an audiogram and ABR should be the first screening tests obtained. Then, based on the clinical history and other findings, the patient should undergo gadolinium-DTPA enhanced magnetic resonance imaging (MRI). Any patient with an abnormal ABR and also patients who are being screened for neurofibromatosis should also undergo MRI because of the high incidence of acoustic neuromata in type II von Recklinghausen disease.

95. Retrocochlear lesions should be suspected if ABR results show the following:
    A. Significant absolute wave V latency greater than 4.6 msec.
    B. Prolonged I–V latencies.
    C. Internal wave V latency difference greater than 0.3 msec.

96. Enhanced computed tomography (CT) scanning is the procedure of choice in the diagnosis of temporal bone fractures.

97. Temporal bone fractures

Longitudinal	**Transverse**
70 to 90%	10 to 20%
Lateral skull trauma	Frontal/occipital

Paralysis of cranial nerve VII seen in 10 to 20% and often delayed due to edema
Seventh nerve paralysis seen in 40 to 50% and immediate due to crush or laceration in the labyrinthine portion
Often associated with a conductive hearing loss secondary to ossicular injury
Often associated with a sensorineural loss due to direct cochlear injury
Vestibular symptoms rare, as is SNHL, both due to inner ear concussion
Sudden onset vestibular symptoms due to direct SCC injury

98. Pseudotumor cerebri may cause pulsatile tinnitus.

99. Malignant tumors metastatic to the temporal bone are found from breast, kidney, lung, stomach, larynx, prostate, and thyroid; route of spread via valveless Batson's plexus.

100. Viruses associated with SNHL
     A. Rubella
     B. Herpes simplex 1 and 2
     C. Varicella (chickenpox or zoster oticus)
     D. Variola (smallpox)
     E. Epstein–Barr virus
     F. Polio
     G. Influenza
     H. Adenovirus
     I. Cytomegalovirus
     J. Measles
     K. Mumps (most common cause of acquired unilateral SNHL)
     L. Hepatitis

101. *Aspergillus niger* is the most commonly identified organism in otomycosis. Small numbers of yeast species are often isolated from chronic otitis externa.

102. The most common complication of pressure equalizing (PE) tube insertion is persistent otorrhea. This is thought to be due to persistent transudate formation or a result of chronic mucositis rather than a foreign-body reaction to the tube.

103. Large-bore PE tubes are associated with a higher rate of perforation, especially after prolonged intubation, tube retention, or multiple episodes of intubation.

104. Necrotizing external otitis/malignant otitis externa is a rapidly progressive infection of the external canal and skull base that is caused by *Pseudomonas.* The diagnosis is made with a combination of technetium-99 and gallium-67 scanning. Repeat gallium-67 scanning is used to follow the resolution of the disease. Appropriate antibiotics are essential; intravenous ticarcillin plus tobramycin or oral ciprofloxacin. CT may be used for confirmation of osteomyelitis, although 30 to 50% of the trabecular bone of the mastoid must be destroyed before the CT becomes obviously positive. Surgery may be required when scan results are nonconfirmatory, for nerve decompression, for tissue debridement, or for continued disease despite appropriate treatment. Use of hyperbaric oxygen may be of some help.

105. Agents for otomycosis
    A. Merthiolate 1:1000
    B. 1.5% acetic acid
    C. 79 to 95% isopropyl alcohol
    D. Methyl cresyl-acetate
    E. Nystatin suspension, cream, ointment, or powder
    F. Clotrimazole cream, lotion, or solution

106. Agents for external otitis
    A. Neomycin—an aminoglycoside with a spectrum covering *Escherichia coli,* Enterobacteriaceae, *Klebsiella, Proteus, Haemophilus influenzae, Staphylococcus aureus,* and *Streptococcus faecalis.* Of note is that 6 to 8% of patients develop a hypersensitivity reaction to the topical application of this antibiotic.
    B. Polymyxin B—a combination of polymyxin B_1 and B_2 with a spectrum covering Enterobacteriaceae, *E. coli, Klebsiella,* and *Pseudomonas. Serratia, Proteus, Neisseriae,* and *Providencia* are resistant.
    C. Colistin—also known as polymyxin E, with a spectrum covering the same organisms as polymyxin B and with the same resistances. Certain *Pseudomonas* species may become resistant to polymyxin B but retain their sensitivity to colistin.
    D. Combinations.

107. The most commonly cultured organisms in chronic otomastoiditis are *Pseudomonas, Proteus, Klebsiella,* and *Staphylococcus.* Chronic otitis without cholesteatoma is prevalent in Native Americans.

108. The organisms most commonly found in septic lateral sinus thrombosis are hemolytic streptococci and type III pneumococci. The onset of sinus thrombosis is characterized by a high spiking temperature, severe toxic symptoms, rapid pulse, chills, and sweating. The following signs indicate possible impending complications in chronic ear disease: headache (especially parietal or occipital), drowsiness, nausea, and vomiting. A positive Queckenstedt test is also often associated.

109. Otoscopy—tympanic membrane redness correlates poorly with actual active disease due to the flare reaction elicited by insertion of the speculum into the external auditory canal.

110. Tympanocentesis—20 to 30% sterile despite apparently active disease.

111. Effusions—antibiotics have no proven effectiveness in eradication of effusions without acute bacterial otitis media or other bacterial upper airway infection.

112. Acute otitis media organisms
    A. *Streptococcus pneumoniae*, 30%
    B. *Haemophilus influenzae*, 20% (30% beta-lactamase positive)
    C. *Moraxella catarrhalis*, 15% (75% beta-lactamase positive)
113. Griesinger's sign is edema and tenderness over the mastoid cortex and is associated with thrombosis of the mastoid emissary vein as a result of lateral sinus thrombosis. This can also be associated with cavernous sinus thrombosis.
114. Approximately 70% of patients have a residual middle ear effusion 2 weeks after the treatment of an episode of acute otitis media, 40% after 1 month, 20% after 2 months, and 10% after 3 months (ie, 90% of middle ear effusions persistent after an episode of treated acute otitis media resolve within 90 days).
115. In children with middle ear effusion, air conduction thresholds average 20 to 27 dB; the bone conduction threshold is not affected. The otoscopic examination of an air–fluid level or bubbles in the middle ear is associated with less hearing loss and impairment. A predicted relationship between hearing levels and tympanogram characteristics cannot be shown. Twenty-five to 50% of children with chronic otitis media with effusion have positive cultures. Impedance audiometry is less sensitive in the group from newborn to 7 months of age due to external canal collapse.
116. Cerebellar abscesses secondary to otitis media usually form through preformed pathways, whereas temporal lobe abscesses result from seeding through bone erosion.
117. Keratitis obturans vs. external canal cholesteatoma
    A. Keratitis
        (1) Otalgia
        (2) Hearing loss
        (3) Otorrhea (rare)
        (4) Bilateral involvement
        (5) Erosion of the external canal
        (6) Associated with bronchiectasis, sinusitis, and chronic obstructive pulmonary disease
        (7) Younger patients
        (8) Periodic debridement is essential
        (9) Topical steroids may be helpful
        (10) No association with ciliary dysmotility
    B. Canal cholesteatoma
        (1) No hearing loss
        (2) Otorrhea (common)
        (3) Older patients
        (4) Medical/surgical treatment
118. Familial periodic cerebellar ataxia—discrete episodes of cerebellar disturbance with dysarthria, ataxia, and dysequilibrium often precipitated by stress or exercise. Results from abnormal intracellular pH homeostasis. Treated with acetazolamide.
119. Auditory brain stem response wave associations (mnemonic: *E. coli*).
    I: Eighth nerve
    II: Cochlear nucleus
    III: Superior olivary nucleus
    IV: Lateral lemniscus

      V: Inferior colliculus

      VI: Medial geniculate

      VII: Auditory radiation (Brodmann's area 41)

120. Most basal cell carcinomas and epidermoid carcinomas of the auricle involve the helix.

121. External auditory canal osteomas are usually single and occur in the suture lines. Exostoses are usually multiple and are frequently associated with cold H_2O exposure. Although cerumen impaction and external otitis are frequent, conductive hearing loss is generally not seen until greater than 90% obstruction of the external auditory canal occurs.

122. Fifty percent of patients with myxedema have reversible SNHL.

123. Achondroplasia is the most common skeletal dysplasia, is autosomally dominant, and occurs in 1 in 26,000 live births. It is a disorder of endochondral bone formation. Associated abnormalities include a narrow foramen magnum with potential for brain stem compression, hydrocephalus, spinal canal stenosis, respiratory infections, apnea, otitis, and hearing loss. Abnormal skull base cephalometrics, temporal bone malformation, maxillary hypoplasia, nasal bone and septal hypoplasia, and abnormal orientation of the eustachian tube, internal auditory canal, external auditory canal, labyrinth, and jugular bulb have all been reported. Approximately 60% have some type of hearing loss, with the conductive type being the most common. Greater than 50% of these children require insertion of middle ear ventilation tubes. It has been suggested that the insertion of these tubes results in a higher rate of tympanic membrane perforation. It has also been reported that serum IgG deficiency, cell-mediated immune deficiencies, and combined immune deficiencies are associated with short-limbed dwarfism.

124. Branchio-oto-renal (Melnick–Fraser) syndrome occurs in 1 in 40,000 live births. It is seen in 2% of profoundly deaf children. Inheritance is autosomal-dominant with variable penetrance; gene localized to 8q. Associated findings include the following (incidences of F through J are unknown):

    A. Hearing loss, 89%

    B. Preauricular pits, 77%

    C. Renal dysplasia, 66%

    D. Branchial anomalies, 63%

    E. Pinna abnormalities, 41%

    F. Middle ear malformations

    G. Inner ear malformations

    H. Lacrimal duct stenosis

    I.   Bifid uvula

    J. Facial paresis/paralysis

125. Newborn infants have a subglottic lumen that averages 6 mm in diameter; 5 mm is regarded as borderline normal, and 4 mm is definitely stenotic.

126. During rigid bronchoscopy in the pediatric age group, one must always be aware that the actual internal and external diameters of the bronchoscope are consistently larger than designated; this will prevent inadvertent mucosal and submucosal trauma during instrumentation.

127. Most common cause of tracheal collapse in infant is tracheomalacia. Most common cause of tracheal compression is an aberrant subclavian artery.

128. During the neonatal period, prolonged intubation by the oral route is advocated by some because of the relative ease of intubation and pulmonary toilet, lack of bacterial contamination from the nose, avoidance of soft tissue injury in the nasal cavities and nasopharynx, and decreased tube movement. Others advocate nasal intubation as tube stabilization is better; therefore endolaryngeal trauma from tube telescoping is minimized.

129. Neonates are obligate nasal breathers until approximately 6 weeks of age; should distress occur, patency of the nasal airways must be confirmed with the transnasal insertion of a catheter; choanal atresia occurs in one of every 5000 to 7000 live births and is twice as common in females. It is unilateral more often than bilateral; when unilateral, it is twice as often on the right as on the left. About 90% are bony and 10% are membranous.

130. Venturi jet ventilation is used in pediatric endoscopic procedures, excision of laryngeal papillomata, and endolaryngeal laser procedures. Possible complications of this technique include hypoventilation, pneumothorax, pneumomediastinum, subcutaneous emphysema, abdominal distention, mucosal dehydration, and distal seeding of malignant cells or papillomavirus particles.

    These hazards can be minimized by recognizing those patient factors likely to predispose to complications. Obesity decreases chest, lung, and abdominal compliance, necessitating higher ventilation pressures. Short, stiff, or arthritic cervical spines make laryngoscope placement difficult with possible hypoventilation or air leak. Aerophagia can be minimized with adequate premedication. Relaxation will increase chest wall compliance and prevent vocal fold adduction. Appropriate jets and pressure settings must be determined for each patient; smaller-diameter tracheal lumens also increase intra-airway pressures with an increased risk of complications. In patients with large obstructive lesions, outlet obstruction may occur; ventilation should periodically be terminated to allow adequate exhalation.

    A nasogastric tube can be inserted to decrease gastric distention. During laryngeal instrumentation, ventilation must be suspended to prevent distal seeding. Moisture is essential to prevent cast formation and mucosal dehydration. In many instances, a small endotracheal tube can be inserted beyond the obstructing lesion that allows adequate ventilation and yet provides access to the lesion, thus eliminating the need and risk of this modality.

131. Cystic fibrosis
    A. Hereditary disease of children and young adults.
    B. Generalized dysfunction of exocrine glands.
    C. Features
        (1) Pancreatic insufficiency
        (2) Chronic obstructive pulmonary disease/bronchiectasis/pneumonia
        (3) Malabsorption
        (4) Cirrhosis of the liver
        (5) Nasal polyps/chronic sinusitis
        (6) High sweat chloride/salt wasting
        (7) Dehydration
    D. Diagnosis: sweat chloride values greater than 60 mEq/L.

E. Aggressive management of polyps and sinusitis with steroids, regular sinus irrigations with tobramycin, and endoscopic sinus surgery.

132. Ciliary dysmotility. Numerous forms. Clinical tests of ciliary function using methylene blue and saccharin. Electron microscope study of cilia biopsy in glutaraldehyde. Kartagener syndrome—a triad of recurrent sinusitis, bronchiectasis, and situs inversus—lacks dynein side arms on A-tubules.

133. In children, the blood volume (mL) is approximately 7.5% of body weight (g).

134. Laryngomalacia is often seen in association with other findings resulting from delay of development of neuromuscular control; these may include gastroesophageal reflux, central or obstructive apneae, hypotonia, failure to thrive, and pneumonia.

135. Cri-du-chat syndrome is associated with a deletion of the short arm of chromosome 5. The endolarynx is narrowed, diamond-shaped, and has a persistent interarytenoid cleft.

136. VATER association involves congenital malformations of vertebral, anal, tracheoesophageal, radial, and renal structures; three of these malformations are required to make this diagnosis.

137. VACTERL association is similar to the above but also involves congenital anomalies of cardiac and limb structures.

138. Crouzon syndrome—mutation at 10q for fibroblast growth factor (FGF) gene; autosomal-dominant transmission.

139. Treacher Collins syndrome—mutation on 5q with autosomal-dominant transmission.

140. Infantile lobar emphysema often requires lobectomy and is often associated with congenital cardiac defects.

141. Malignant hyperthermia occurs in 1 in 15,000 children and 1 in 50,000 to 100,000 adults. Autosomal-transmission with reduced penetrance and variable expressivity. No associated physical stigmata, no specific laboratory tests, no historical facts related to susceptibility. If history is suspicious, a full neuromuscular evaluation is required, including a muscle biopsy and serum creatine phosphokinase (CPK), lactic dehydrogenase (LDH), alkaline phosphatase, and urinary myoglobin. This occurs due to a sudden increase in the calcium concentration in the muscle sarcoplasm due to either decreased uptake or excessive release of calcium from the sarcoplasmic reticulum. It is usually associated with halogenated inhalational anesthetic agents and depolarizing muscle relaxants. Approximately 40% of cases of malignant hyperthermia have been found to occur during ear, nose, and throat cases. There is a slight increase in males and a slight decrease among African Americans. Approximately 70% have positive caffeine/halothane muscle stimulation test. Dantrolene 1 mg/kg slow IV push until symptoms abate, or to a maximum dose of 10 mg/kg, plus cooling, 100% oxygen.

142. Choanal atresia occurs in 1 of 8000 births with female predominance. Ten percent of atresia plates are mucosal only, while 90% have a bony and/or cartilaginous component. Two-thirds are unilateral, more commonly on the right side. Fifty percent are associated with congenital anomaly: CHARGE association (*C*oloboma, *H*eart defects, choanal *A*tresia, *R*etarded growth, *G*enital hypoplasia, *E*ar abnormality), Apert syndrome, Crouzon disease, Treacher Collins syndrome, trisomy 18 syndrome, and velo-cardiofacial syndrome. Bilateral atresia presents at birth with cyclical apnea and crying, and urgently requires an oral airway and surgical correction before hospital discharge. Unilateral atresia presents later in childhood. Initial treatment is usually transnasally although transpalatal approaches have less recurrence.

143. Cervical adenopathy in the pediatric population is more frequently infectious rather than neoplastic in origin. The most common etiologic bacteria are *Staphylococcus aureus* and group A streptococci. Adenopathy usually responds to penicillinase-resistant antibiotics. Tuberculous and fungal and granulomatous diseases must be considered.

144. Cat-scratch disease, most common cause of chronic cervical adenopathy in children and adolescents. Causative agent, *Rochalimaea henselae,* is intracellular pleomorphic bacterium in the Rickettsiaeae family. Other *Rochalimaea* species responsible for bacillary angiomatosis in immunosuppressed or immunocompromised patients, trench fever, and Q fever. Questionable cat–flea vector.

145. Down syndrome is associated with
     A. Frequent upper respiratory infections
     B. Frequent otitis media secondary to eustachian tube dysfunction (ETD)
     C. Abnormal nasopharynx shape
     D. Poor tone of tensor veli palatini
     E. Congenital ossicular deformities

146. Unilateral exophthalmos in children is most often a result of orbital cellulitis; bilateral disease can be due to leukemia or metastatic neuroblastoma. Rhabdomyosarcoma is the most common unilateral orbital malignancy in the pediatric age group; dermoids and hemangiomas are the most common benign masses. Rule out orbital apex syndrome.

147. Histiocystosis X is a family of granulomatous diseases of unknown etiology, manifest by a proliferation of mature histiocytes and with multiple presentations.
     A. Eosinophilic granuloma. Chronic course in adults and children with osteolytic bone lesions (often frontal or temporal). Proptosis is seen with frontal or sphenoid involvement. Acute mastoiditis, middle ear granulations, and tympanic membrane perforations are common. Facial paralysis is possible. Surgical excision/debridement is the recommended treatment for single lesions; chemotherapy and radiotherapy have been used for recurrences and inaccessible lesions.
     B. Hand-Schüller-Christian disease. Subacute course in children and younger adults; lytic skull lesions are often associated with proptosis and diabetes insipidus or pituitary insufficiency secondary to erosion of the sphenoid roof into the sella (this constellation occurs in about 10%). Mastoid and middle ear lesions are common and can cause ossicular erosion and acute mastoiditis; facial paralysis is seen in 2%. External auditory canal polyps are also seen. Mandibular involvement with loss of teeth, hepatosplenomegaly, and adenopathy may also be associated. There can be a 30% mortality (especially with heart, lung, brain, or pituitary involvement); chemotherapy and/or radiotherapy are recommended.
     C. Letterer-Siwe disease. Acute, rare, rapidly progressive form seen in infants less than 2 years of age, characterized by fever, proptosis, splenomegaly, hepatomegaly, adenopathy, multiple bony lesions, anemia, thrombocytopenia, and exfoliative dermatitis. Chemotherapy is the treatment of choice, but the response is poor. Radiotherapy can be used for localized or unresponsive lesions.

148. Cystic hygroma (lymphangiomatous ectasia) frequently produces airway or feeding problems that require intervention. Spontaneous remission is uncommon; early surgical intervention is recommended, and multiple procedures are often required.

149. The most commonly encountered malignancy in the pediatric age group is lymphoma. A thorough evaluation should include a fine needle aspiration biopsy (under sedation if necessary) with appropriate staining techniques to determine the cell of origin, posterior-anterior and lateral chest films, intravenous pyelogram (IVP), bone marrow aspirate, and scans as indicated. The overall mortality is about 30%. Stages: 1, localized; 2, limited above diaphragm with systemic symptoms; 3, diffuse disease.

150. Stridor in children
    A. Laryngeal, 60%
        (1) Laryngomalacia, 60%
        (2) Subglottic stenosis, 20%
        (3) Vocal cord palsy, 13%
        (4) Others, 7%
    B. Tracheal, 15%
        (1) Tracheomalacia, 45%
        (2) Vascular compression, 45%
        (3) Stenosis, 5%
    C. Bronchial, 5%
    D. Infection, 5%
    E. Miscellaneous, 15%

151. Nasal dermal sinus
    A. Foramen cecum: Anterior neuropore at anterior floor of cranial vault.
    B. Prenasal space: Potential space beneath nasal bone running from frontal bone/foramen cecum area to anterior aspect of nasal bone.
    C. Fonticulus frontalis: Embryologic gap between nasal and frontal bones.
    D. Dura and nasal skin lie in close proximity and become separated with foramen cecum closure. Persistent dural–dermal connection via foramen cecum and prenasal space (or less frequently via fonticulus frontalis) produces gliomas, meningoceles, or encephaloceles projecting from above. Projecting from below may be dermal sinuses or dermoids.
    E. Incidence: 1 in 20,000 to 40,000 births.

152. Differential diagnosis of nasal masses
    A. Congenital: Glioma, encephalocele, dermoid, teratoma
    B. Infectious: Tuberculosis, rhinoscleroma, rhinosporidiosis
    C. Inflammatory/Granulomatous: Allergic polyp, sarcoid
    D. Benign tumors: Squamous and Schneiderian papilloma, juvenile angiofibroma, paraganglioma, leiomyoma, schwannoma, adenoma
    E. Malignant tumors: Squamous cell carcinoma, salivary gland carcinoma, esthesioneuroblastoma, chordoma, melanoma, lymphoma, plasmacytoma, histiocytosis X, rhabdomyosarcoma

153. Subglottic hemangiomas of infancy usually present by 3 months of age and occur more commonly in the left posterolateral quadrant. Fifty percent of laryngeal lesions are associated with cutaneous manifestations. Treatment is reserved only for symptomatic infants; steroids are controversial, and laser excision and debulking is currently favored.

154. Signs and symptoms of adult obstructive sleep apnea include daytime hypersomnolence, snoring, morning headaches, decreased productivity, lethargy, and depression.

Over extended periods, intellectual deterioration, impotence, cardiac arrhythmias, and pulmonary hypertension may result.

The diagnosis of the site of obstruction is essential. Fiberoptic endoscopy in the supine position with Müller maneuver is helpful in determining the site of lesion. Cephalometric measurements are required in many cases. Medical evaluation and treatment must include nasal congestion and obstruction, allergies, and sinusitis. Weight loss is often important. Soporific medications and narcotics should be avoided, as these tend to increase the apnea index.

Several devices are available and have found some use in selected patients, including nasal airways, nasal valve supports, tongue-advancement devices, and bite prostheses to maintain an open bite. Nasal continuous positive airway pressure (CPAP) is available, but patient tolerance is often a limiting factor. Surgical treatment must address any significant nasal obstruction that may be present in addition to adenoidectomy, tonsillectomy, partial midline or posterior glossectomy, uvulo-palato-pharyngoplasty, hyoid suspension, mandibular advancement, maxillary advancement, and/or tracheotomy. A thorough workup is essential to determine the site of obstruction prior to attempting surgical repair.

155. Airway lengthening techniques
   A. Mobilization after blunt dissection of the larynx and trachea (3 cm)
   B. Incision of the annular ligaments on one side of the trachea proximal to the anastomosis and on the opposite side distally (1.5 cm)
   C. Laryngeal release
      (1) Suprahyoid (5 cm)
      (2) Infrahyoid (often results in dysphagia)

156. The true vocal fold is 1.7 mm in thickness. The most important laryngeal muscle of respiration and airway protection is the posterior cricoarytenoid; it is the only muscle of vocal fold abduction and is innervated by the external branch of the superior laryngeal nerve (SLN). The internal branch of the SLN is sensory to the supraglottic larynx.

157. Vocal cord medialization requires injection lateral to vocalis muscle. Teflon is most often used for permanent paralysis, but collagen (especially autologous) is gaining favor. Gelfoam may be used for temporary paralysis. Laryngoplasty is another option.

158. TMJ syndrome often is associated with the following:
   A. Bruxism
   B. Dental trauma or dental surgery
   C. Mandibular trauma/abnormalities/asymmetry
   D. Myofacial or cervical tension
      Treatment begins with soft diet, warm compresses, and nonsteroidal anti-inflammatory drugs (NSAIDs). A thorough dental/maxillofacial evaluation is advised.

159. Paragangliomas including carotid body tumors, chemodectomas, and glomus tumors—about 10% multiple, about 10% malignant, and about 10% hormonally active. If symptoms are consistent with hormonal activity (flushing, sweating, headache), urinary vanillylmandelic acid (VMA) and metanephrines and serum catecholamines should be measured.

160. Some patients require cricopharyngeal (CP) myotomy for successful speech utilizing a tracheoesophageal fistula (TEF); insufflation testing is helpful in determining

which patients will develop successful TEF speech; pharyngeal plexus block can assist in determining the result of the CP myotomy.

161. Laryngoceles are more commonly external than internal, and they exit through the thyrohyoid membrane.

162. Approximately 90% of congenital facial paralysis resolves spontaneously. Possible causes include difficult delivery, cephalopelvic disproportion, dystocia, high forceps delivery, or intrauterine trauma. If no resolution after a period of observation, ENoG can be used to determine excitability. CT and MRI may be required for adequate evaluation.

163. The orbicularis oris requires two-point fixation and symmetry for adequate function.

164. Flaps
    A. Regional skin
        (1) Deltopectoral, first to fourth perforators from internal mammary artery
        (2) Forehead, superficial temporal artery plus possible occipital branch
        (3) Nape of neck, occipital artery
    B. Myocutaneous
        (1) Pectoralis majoris (PM), thoracoacromial artery and internal mammary artery perforators
        (2) Trapezius, occipital, suprascapular, and transverse cervical arteries
        (3) Sternocleidomastoid
            (a) Occipital artery (loops around twelfth cranial nerve)
            (b) Superior thyroid artery
            (c) Transverse cervical artery (good for use in buccal defects, but use is contraindicated after radial neck dissection)
        (4) Platysma, occipital, postauricular, facial, superior thyroid, and transverse cervical
        (5) Latissimus dorsi, thoracodorsal artery (long, bulky, reliable with longest pedicle)
    C. Osteomyocutaneous
        (1) Trapezius with scapular spine
        (2) Sternocleidomastoid with clavicle
        (3) PM with rib
    D. Free flaps

165. Extracapsular spread in lymph node involved with metastatic spread portends a poor prognosis. Gadolinium (Gd)- DTPA enhanced MRI with fat suppression appears useful in determining this preoperatively.

166. The treatment of choice for carcinoma in situ of the glottis has been serial microlaryngoscopy and stripping until eradication of the malignancy. Current trends include laser excision after biopsy documentation.

167. The most common site of verrucous carcinoma formation is the buccal mucosa. Surgery has been recommended for this variant because of the suggestion that radiation therapy may cause a transformation of this histologic type into a more aggressive squamous cell variant; despite this, radiation may be used in selected cases.

168. Squamous carcinoma of the paranasal sinuses requires aggressive treatment including surgery and radiation therapy, and in some cases chemotherapy. Again Gd-DTPA MRI with fat suppression assists in determining invasion of the orbit and anterior cranial fossa to assist in surgical planning.

169. Inactivation of tumor suppressor genes (TSGs) is important in the development of head and neck cancers. Cytogenetic analyses and loss of heterozygosity (LOH) are used to identify key regions in the human genome that encode TSGs. High incidence of LOH in squamous cell carcinoma of the head and neck (SCCHN) on the short arm of chromosome 3 in the region of 3p24-p25.

170. Genetic amplification of proto-oncogenes is seen in some SCCHN. MYC proto-oncogene has been identified in SCCHN. MYC amplification seen in 10 to 15% of SCCHN. Seems to correlate closely with T stage but *not* with lymph node metastases, local recurrence rate, distant metastases, or long-term survival.

171. Interleukin 2 plus interleukin 12, in combination, produce the greatest activation of nature killer cell cytolysis of tumor cells in SCCHN than either cytokine alone.

172. Apoptosis is programmed cell death and is a process with characteristic and specific morphologic changes at the nuclear level. Tumor necrosis factor–alpha receptor binding results in apoptosis of SCCHN cells with oligonucleosomal fragmentation of DNA and typical morphologic changes. This dsDNA lysis is thought to be the result of the activation of an endogenous endonuclease which cuts the DNA at specific linker regions.

173. Warthin's tumor (papillary cystadenoma lymphomatosum) now comprises up to 20% of all parotid tumors, second only to the benign mixed variant. Its peak incidence is in the 5th decade, and there is an increasing appearance in females. It most often occurs in the right parotid. A Tc-99 scan is usually positive in Warthin's tumor.

174. Cystic hygroma (lymphangiomatous ectasia) frequently produces airway or feeding problems that require intervention. Spontaneous remission is uncommon, early surgical intervention is recommended, and multiple procedures are often required.

175. Esthesioneuroblastoma. Rare tumor of neuroepithelium presenting as nasal roof mass with epistaxis, obstruction, anosmia, pain, and mass effect. Neck metastases develop in 10 to 20% and distant metastases in 12 to 18%. Treated with craniofacial resection plus radiotherapy. Recurrence occurs in 50% and is usually local. Salvage with surgery, radiotherapy, and/or chemotherapy. Ten-year survival, 53 to 71%.

176. Flap failure rates
    A. Free, 16 to 30%
    B. Deltopectoral, 11 to 20%
    C. PM, < 5%

177. Relapsing polychondritis. This rare inflammatory disorder of cartilage and connective tissue is presumed to be of autoimmune etiology. Manifestations include chondritis of the auricle, nose, and respiratory tract; nonerosive polyarthritis; ocular inflammation; and potentially cochleovestibular involvement. 50% of patients experience auricular inflammation and arthritis; fewer patients have the other symptoms. Chondritis develops rapidly and resolves in 1 to 2 weeks; recurrent episodes produce cartilaginous deformity. The sedimentation rate is elevated. Steroids are used in severe cases.

178. *Rhinoscleroma.* Slowly progressive granulomatous infection of *Klebsiella rhinoscleromatis* endemic to hot, dry climates which involves primarily the nose but also larynx and trachea. Catarrhal, granulomatous, and sclerotic-cicatricial stages occur. Histology shows granulation, pseudoepitheliomatous hyperplasia, Russell bodies, and Mikulicz cells. Treatment is difficult and involves debridement with various antibiotics for months to years.

179. Rhinophyma. Nasal enlargement due to sebaceous hypertrophy with nodular, telangiectatic, and hypervascular changes. There is no association with alcohol use, though chronic *Demodex follicularum* infection has been suggested as a cause. Treatment involves decortication and recontouring of the nose with dermabrasion, cold technique, or laser.

180. *Frontal sinus ablation and obliteration.*
    A. Ablation: Removal of either the frontal sinus wall (Reidel procedure) or posterior wall (cranialization), removal of any mucosa, and plugging of duct.
    B. Obliteration: Performed via osteoplastic flap approach and removing all sinus mucosa, occluding the nasofrontal ostium, and filling the sinus space with fat harvested from the lower *left* abdominal wall. These procedures are performed due to the high incidence of nasofrontal ostium stenosis after sinusotomy and resulting long-term potential for frontal sinus mucocele.

181. Anosmia may be associated with chronic rhinitis, chronic sinusitis, nasal polyps, nasal allergy, head trauma with or without cribriform fracture, postviral congenital malignancy of the nasal cavity/nasopharynx/ethmoid sinus/frontal sinus, psychiatric disorders, medications, nasal surgery, and hypogonadism (Kallmann syndrome).

182. Nasal obstruction
    A. Septal deviation, turbinate hypertrophy, nasal narrowing, trauma, nasal valve collapse, tip ptosis, choanal atresia, nasopharyngeal obstruction/mass, septal hematoma
    B. Nasal tumor, foreign body
    C. Inflammation due to nasal/sinus infection, allergy, granulomatous process, atrophic rhinitis, septal abscess
    D. Medication, hypothyroidism, pregnancy
    E. Psychogenic, hyperpatency

183. "M," "n," and "ng" are normal nasal consonants, and their production is associated with an open velopharyngeal port. Velopharyngeal incompetence (VPI) is associated with nasal escape during the production of other consonants. Repair of VPI with a pharyngeal flap attempts to reduce this abnormal escape; caution must be taken to create ports less than 20 mm^2 to prevent continued nasal escape. Ports that are of insufficient size may result in chronic nasopharyngitis, anterior rhinorrhea, and otitis.

184. Optic chiasm lesions may result in bitemporal hemianopsia, whereas optic tract lesions result in a contralateral hemianopsia.

185. Complications after mandibular fracture increase approximately 300% when repair is delayed 7 to 10 days.

186. Mandibular osteomyelitis after fracture is associated with a fracture through a tooth root.

187. Medial orbital blowout fractures are unusual. Signs and symptoms include swelling, ecchymosis, and diplopia during medial or lateral gaze due to medial rectus muscle entrapment.

188. Serious cosmetic deformity or airway obstruction following nasal trauma in children should be dealt with using open as opposed to closed methods. Produces good results with minimal risk to growth centers.

189. Repair of mandibular fractures using biphasic devices or open reduction with internal fixation utilizing compression plates is often recommended for the following [in place of intermaxillary fixation (IMF)]:

    A. Multiple comminuted fractures
    B. Elderly patients
    C. Severe pulmonary disease
    D. Children
    E. Mentally handicapped/seizures
    F. Alcoholic
    G. Pregnant

190. Tuberculosis of the larynx is most common in the interarytenoid area and the laryngeal surface of the epiglottis.

191. Gutman's sign is associated with SLN paralysis. In the normal individual, lateral pressure over the thyroid cartilage causes an increased voice pitch, whereas anterior pressure causes a decrease. In SLN paralysis, the reverse is true.

192. Pseudotumor of the orbit is an idiopathic condition that involves inflammatory edema of the medial rectus muscle. Treatment includes steroids and possible immunotherapy.

193. Brissaud phenomenon (facial tonic or clonic spasms) may be the result of nerve irritation due to compression by a mass lesion or a vascular loop; it may also be due to a lesion or infarct of the pons involving the facial nuclei or efferent pathways. Brissaud syndrome is hysterical glossolabial spasm.

194. Turbinectomy. The utility and safety of inferior turbinectomy for nasal obstruction are debated. Various techniques exist, including submucous resection, cautery, laser, cryosurgery, and simple resection. Removal of the anteroinferior portion is probably as effective as total resection unless large posterior "mulberry" hypertrophy exists. Some individuals believe there is a long-term risk of causing atrophic rhinitis with turbinectomy, particularly in hot, dry climates.

195. *Internal maxillary artery (IMA) ligation.* Performed for posterior-inferior epistaxis resistant to packing or other conservative measures. Failure occurs due to inadequate ligation, contralateral collateral blood flow, or bleeding due to anterior or posterior ethmoid artery source. Angiographic embolization is an alternative option but often cannot be done after IMA ligation since the surgery often occludes access vessels necessary for arteriography. Complications include facial edema, cellulitis, sinusitis, oroantral fistula, and injury to orbital contents, infraorbital nerve, teeth, and vidian nerve.

196. Pupillary reflex—direct and consensual components. Optic nerve, optic tract, superior colliculus to pretectal area; pretectal neurons ipsilateral and contralateral via posterior commissure to visceral nuclei of oculomotor complex; preganglionic fibers via cranial nerve III to ciliary ganglion; postganglionic fibers from ciliary ganglion to sphincter of the iris.

197. Corneal reflex—ophthalmic branch of the trigeminal nerve, with body in trigeminal ganglion, ipsilateral and contralateral innervation to motor nuclei of cranial nerve VII with innervation of orbicularis oculi.

198. DISH syndrome (diffuse idiopathic skeletal hyperostosis), previously known as Forestier disease, results in paraspinous ligament calcification; it can be associated with similar disease of other joints. It can be a cause of dysphagia due to cervical osteophytes compressing the esophageal lumen or from inflammation of the periesophageal soft tissues. Lateral neck radiographs and barium esophagography are helpful. Rigid and flexible endoscopy must be performed with extreme caution to

prevent perforation. NSAIDs may decrease soft tissue inflammation, and resection may be indicated.

199. Immunosuppression (acquired/iatrogenic) results in an increase in lymphoproliferative disorders and should be kept in mind when evaluating lesions of Waldeyer's ring, salivary glands, or cervical nodes.

200. Osler-Weber-Rendu disease (hereditary hemorrhagic telangiectasia) has autosomal-dominant transmission. Several genes implicated in pathogenesis. 9q33-34 endoglin and transforming growth factor beta-2 receptor, 3p22, are involved; 9q33-34 locus associated with pulmonary and CNS manifestations. Another site has been identified at 12q, but the gene at that site has not been identified; 12q associated with telangiectases and epistaxis.

201. Arteriovenous malformations (AVMs), hemangiomata, and epistaxis may be amenable to embolization as an adjunctive or definitive therapy.

202. Complications of laser use include burns beyond the operative site, endotracheal tube ignition, cottonoid ignition, pneumothorax, and subcutaneous emphysema. Secondary complications include endotracheal tube (ETT) obstruction, burns resulting from reflection of laser energy from surgical instruments, hemorrhage, and perichondritis. Delayed complications include glottic webbing, cicatrix, and stenosis.

203. Meleney ulcer is associated with *S. aureus* and nonhemolytic streptococci.

204. Marjolin ulcer is a skin ulceration at the site of an old scar, often from burns, with propensity for malignant degeneration.

205. Temporal arteritis is characterized by giant cells within the tunica media.

206. Trigeminal neuralgia (tic douloureux) most often affects the second and third divisions of the fifth cranial nerve (V_2 and V_3).

207. Passavant's ridge is a constriction of the superior margin of the superior constrictor muscle seen in many patients during velopharyngeal closure.

208. Chordoma. Rare skull base/nasopharyngeal malignancy of notochord remnant. Histology demonstrates characteristic physaliferous cells with "soap bubble" appearance and compressed nucleus. Treatment is surgical with radiotherapy for incomplete excision; chemotherapy is not useful. Twenty percent 5-year survival.

209. Granular cell myoblastoma may cause pseudoepitheliomatous hyperplasia of the larynx; it is seen in the tongue, skin, breast, subcutaneous tissues, and respiratory tract. Three percent become malignant.

210. Schneiderian papilloma. These arise from respiratory (Schneiderian) epithelium and are associated with human papillomaviruses 6 and 11. These are usually unilateral, and there are three types: (1) septal papilloma (50%) presents as a verrucoid, pedunculated, or sessile nasal septal lesion; (2) inverting papilloma (47%) is usually a polypoid mass growing from the lateral nasal wall; and (3) cylindrical papilloma (3%) is a red-brown papillary lesion of the lateral wall. Treatment requires complete excision, which may be difficult. Malignant degeneration occurs in 10 to 15% and is usually squamous cell carcinoma. The individual cells are rich in glycogen and are filled with cristae-laden senescent mitochondria.

211. Nasal resistance. Blacks have lower resistance than whites, 24% less by anterior rhinomanometry and 17% less by posterior rhinomanometry. Mean total airway resistance by anterior method was 0.136 Pa/cm³/s in blacks and 0.179 Pa/cm³/s in whites. By posterior method, 0.134 Pa/cm³/s in blacks and 0.161 Pa/cm³/s in whites.

212. Hutchinson's rule. Herpes zoster involvement of the nasal tip is associated with a high incidence of herpes zoster ophthalmicus due to retrograde spread via the nasociliary nerve; early ophthalmology consultation advised. (*Am J Ophthalmol* 1972;74:142.)

213. Reed–Sternberg cells are seen in Hodgkin disease, but not in lymphosarcoma or reticulum cell sarcoma.

214. Noma (cancrum oris) is an aggressive destructive infection of the soft tissues of the face. It usually begins at the mucous membrane and infiltrates locally at the oral commissure or buccal space. It is a mixed infection of both aerobic and anaerobic bacteria, especially *Borrelia,* staphylococci, and anaerobic streptococci. It is often seen in debilitated, malnourished, or immunosuppressed patients.

215. Pemphigus is associated with suprabasal intraepidermal bullae; it affects the oral cavity in approximately two-thirds. In those with oral cavity involvement, about half subsequently develop skin lesions. Autoantibodies are present to the epithelial intercellular substance; acantholysis is seen on biopsy, and there is a positive Nikolsky sign. All areas of the GI tract can become involved and are the usual source of sepsis and death. Steroids are the method of treatment. Vulgaris is the rapid acute form, and vegetans is a more indolent chronic form.

216. Pemphigoid occurs in two forms: bullous and benign mucous membrane. In the latter, lesions are usually limited to the oral cavity and conjunctiva. Oral lesions are seen in only one-third of those with the bullous form. Subepidermal bullae are present and tend to be smaller and more tense. These rupture less easily, and the Nikolsky sign is negative. No acantholysis is present on biopsy. Autoantibodies are present to the basement membrane. Both forms are more successfully treated with intermittent systemic steroids. Penicillamine may allow healing in resistant cases.

217. Cherubism presents with painless, symmetric enlargement of the body and ramus of the mandible. It may rarely involve the maxillae. It is autosomally dominant in transmission. Radiographs reveal multiloculated lucencies. Biopsy reveals giant cells with hemosiderin deposits. No bone formation occurs, and no evidence of fibrous dysplasia is present. Self-limited and ceases at puberty. Bony remodeling may cause some mild cosmetic deformity.

218. Hyperostosis frontalis interna is a form of localized dysplasia limited to the inner table of the frontal bone and occurs mainly in elderly females. Headaches may be associated with it. Obesity, dizziness, psychologic disturbances, and inverted sleep rhythms may be seen. This constellation of symptoms is known as the Morgagni-Stewart-Morel syndrome.

219. Hyperostosis of the calvarial bones may also be associated with the following:
    A. Chronic osteomyelitis
    B. Meningioma
    C. Osteoblastic metastases
    D. Fibrous dysplasia
    E. Paget disease
    F. Infantile cortical hyperostosis
    G. Albers-Schönberg disease (osteopetrosis)

220. Caseating necrosis is associated with the following:
    A. Tularemia
    B. Brucellosis

     C. Tuberculosis

     D. Fungus

221. Septal perforation. Most common etiologies are iatrogenic, cocaine use, septal abscess, and nose picking, but also due to infections such as syphilis, tuberculosis, leprosy, and rhinoscleroma. Inflammatory etiologies include Wegener's granulomatosis, sarcoid, lupus, and other collagen vascular disease, while neoplasms include nasal lymphoma and other malignancy. Symptoms include epistaxis, crusting, obstruction, and whistling. Clean, smooth perforations are more likely due to trauma, surgery, or cocaine. Suspicious lesions should be evaluated with fluorescent treponemal antibody-absorption test (FTA-ABS), complete blood count (CBC), erythrocyte sedimentation rate (ESR), urinalysis, blood urea nitrogen (BUN), creatinine, and other tests as indicated. Treatment includes nasal irrigation, septal buttons, or closure with mucosal flaps. Perforations larger than 2 cm are difficult to close.

222. Eagle syndrome is dysphagia associated with a calcified stylohyoid ligament or an elongated styloid process; a calcified stylohyoid ligament is an incidental finding in about 4% of the normal population.

223. Leukoplakia has the microscopic characteristics of the following:

     A. Hyperkeratosis

     B. Parakeratosis

     C. Dyskeratosis

     D. No pleomorphism

     E. No anaplasia

     F. No desmoplasia

224. Nevi

     A. Intraepithelial—benign

     B. Junctional—premalignant

     C. Intradermal—benign

     D. Blue (Spitz)—benign

     E. Mixed—benign

225. CSF otorrhea

     A. Associated with 6% of basilar skull fractures.

     B. Ninety percent seal spontaneously.

     C. Middle fossa leaks heal rapidly due to the extensive fibrosis promoted by the rich arachnoid mesh in this area.

     D. Posterior fossa leaks close more slowly, as little arachnoid is present in this area.

226. Indications for repair of CSF leak

     A. Persistent leak for longer than 2 weeks despite bed rest with head elevation.

     B. Recurrent meningitis.

     C. Brain or meningeal herniation.

     D. Penetration of brain by bony spicule.

227. Lymph node metastasis rates (at presentation)

     A. Laryngeal cancer

         (1) Glottic

            (a) Mobile mid-true vocal cord (TVC), 1 to 4%

            (b) Fixed TVC, 7%

      (c) Anterior commissure, 15%

      (d) $T_3 > 3$ cm, 25%

      (e) T_4 (> 5 mm subglottic or across ventricle), 45%

  (2) Supraglottic

      (a) T_1, 13 to 40%

      (b) T_2, 38 to 45%

      (c) T_3, 40 to 55%

      (d) T_4, 50 to 65%

      [Suprahyoid epiglottis, aryepiglottic fold (AEF), and arytenoid lesions tend to metastasize earlier than infrahyoid epiglottis and false vocal fold lesions; also of note is that supraglottic lesions tend to produce not only ipsilateral, but contralateral, bilateral, occult, and fixed lesions. CT and MRI help identify these metastases.]

  (3) Subglottic

      (a) Primary (often with cricoid erosion)

      (b) Secondary (greater than 5 mm extension from glottis, often with cartilage invasion), 23%

  (4) Transglottic

      (a) All lesions, 25 to 50%

      (b) T_3, 25 to 35%

      (c) T_4, 40 to 50%

      (Many lesions have clinically occult metastases, which may be contralateral or bilateral; transglottic lesions originating in the epiglottis and false and true vocal folds tend to have more occult metastases.)

  (5) Hypopharynx

      (a) Pyriform, 50 to 70%

      (b) Marginal (AEF), 35 to 45%

      (c) Postcricoid/posthypopharynx, 50 to 60%

      (Many lesions have occult metastases, and contralateral and bilateral disease is not uncommon; also, when ipsilateral disease is present, there is about 33% probability that occult contralateral disease is present in lesions of the tongue base, supraglottis, and subglottis.)

B. Lip carcinoma

  (1) T_2, 52%

  (2) T_3, 73%

C. Floor of mouth

  (1) T_2, 65%

  (2) T_3, 71%

  (3) Frequent occurrence of contralateral, bilateral, and occult adenopathy

D. Buccal mucosa

  (1) Half have adenopathy at presentation

E. Tongue

  (1) Anterior

      (a) T_2, 43%

      (b) T_3, 72%

      (c) Occult-positive nodes present in 65%

    F.   Retromolar trigone
- (1) 60+% with adenopathy at presentation
- (2) 25% with contralateral nodes

228. Carcinoma of the lip
- A. Basal cell carcinoma (often upper lip)
- B. Squamous carcinoma
  - (1) Often lower lip
  - (2) Infrequent metastases (6–8%) from lower lip lesions
  - (3) Upper lip lesions metastasize early

229. Cervical metastases from occult primary tumors
- A. Five percent of cases present with adenopathy.
- B. Squamous is predominant histologic type.
- C. Ninety percent of primaries eventually found with repeated examination, biopsies, and scanning.
- D. Frequent sites of primary
  - (1) Base of tongue
  - (2) Nasopharynx
  - (3) Tonsil
  - (4) Larynx/hypopharynx
  - (5) Lung
  - (6) GI tract
  - (7) Thyroid
- E. Treatment
  - (1) Panendoscopy and directed biopsies
  - (2) Neck dissection alone
  - (3) Neck dissection with radiation to probable sites
  - (4) Radiation to neck and probable sites
- F. Prognosis
  - (1) Five-year survival 30% despite type of treatment
  - (2) If primary lesion discovered, prognosis worse

230. Rhabdomyosarcoma
- A. Most common soft tissue malignancy of the head and neck in children.
- B. Sites of involvement
  - (1) Orbit
  - (2) Neck
  - (3) Face
  - (4) Temporal bone
  - (5) Tongue
  - (6) Palate
  - (7) Larynx
- C. Often presents before age 10.
- D. Rapid growth.
- E. Orbital tumors are unique in that they tend toward locally aggressive behavior, but metastasize rarely; the converse is true of other sites.
- F. Chemotherapy and radiation are the main modalities of treatment after biopsy-proven diagnosis; surgery is reserved for unresponsive lesions.
- G. Three-year survivals up to 80%.

231. Paraganglioma
    A. Sites of occurrence (in order of frequency)
        (1) Carotid body
        (2) Jugulotympanic
        (3) Intravagal
        (4) Laryngeal
        (5) Nasal
        (6) Nasopharyngeal
        (7) Orbital
    B. Ten percent multicentric (of which 8% are associated with another malignancy).
    C. Familial tendency.
    D. Two to 6% metastasize.
    E. Ten percent hormonally active; if symptoms suggest activity, serum catecholamines and urinary VMA and metanephrines should be checked.
    F. Angiography indicated in most cases.
    G. CT and MRI both supply valuable information.
    H. Embolization is a treatment modality in some cases; often surgical excision is required.
    I. Morbidity related to location and size at presentation. Order of morbidity is as follows:
        (1) Jugulare
        (2) Tympanum
        (3) Vagale
        (4) Carotid body
232. Craniopharyngioma
    A. Arises from a nest of squamous cells in the area of Rathke's pouch
    B. Clinical presentation
        (1) Headaches
        (2) Visual loss (possible bitemporal hemianopsia)
        (3) Optic atrophy
        (4) Hypopituitarism
        (5) Enlargement of sella turcica
        (6) Parasellar calcifications
    C. Differential diagnosis
        (1) Optic glioma
        (2) Primary pituitary tumors
        (3) Parasellar metastases
233. Osteomas
    A. Benign, slow-growing, osteogenic
    B. Usually affect the bones of the face and skull
    C. Usually painless, but may cause pain, headache, or facial pressure
    D. Sites of predilection
        (1) Mandible
        (2) Temporal bone
        (3) Frontal sinus
        (4) Ethmoid sinus

      (5)   Maxillary sinus
      (6)   Sphenoid sinus
- E.   Treat with surgical excision
- F.   Associated with Gardner syndrome
      (1)   Autosomal dominant
      (2)   Osteomata, soft tissue tumors, and colon polyps
      (3)   Polyps have 40% rate of malignant degeneration

234. Localized compact osteomata are more common in the frontal sinus, and localized cancellous osteomata are more common in the maxillary antrum and ethmoid sinuses.

235. Teratomas
- A.   Tumors of pluripotent embryonal cells
- B.   Occur in 1 in 4000 births
- C.   Females more often afflicted
- D.   Majority recognized by age of 1 year
- E.   Polyhydramnios is present in 18%
- F.   Often occur near thyroid gland
- G.   Rarely become malignant, but when this happens, early aggressive, combined treatment is required
- H.   Usual sites of origin
      (1)   Sacrococcygeal
      (2)   Mediastinal
      (3)   Retroperitoneum
      (4)   Gonadal
- I.   Ten percent occur in the head and neck
      (1)   Orbital
      (2)   Nasal
      (3)   Nasopharynx
      (4)   Oral cavity
      (5)   Neck
- J.   Four types
      (1)   Dermoid cyst
      (2)   Teratoid cyst
      (3)   Teratomoma
      (4)   Epignathi

236. Dermoid cyst
- A.   Most common.
- B.   Contain epidermal and mesodermal remnants.
- C.   Polypoid masses covered with skin and epidermal appendages.
- D.   In neck, occur in submental region deep to or superficial to mylohyoid membrane; those superficial may appear in the floor of mouth and may be confused with ranulae.
- E.   May cause obstruction of breathing or deglutition.
- F.   Excision is the treatment of choice.

237. Teratoid cyst
- A.   Composed of all three germ layers.
- B.   Often cystic with an epithelial lining.
- C.   Differentiation of tissues is minimal.

238. Teratomoma
    A. Composed of all three germ layers.
    B. Usually solid.
    C. Cellular differentiation allows recognition of organ structure.
    D. Often fatal.
239. Epignathi
    A. Composed of all three germ layers.
    B. Most differentiated of all forms; complete organs and body parts identifiable.
    C. Often arise from midline or lateral basisphenoid and protrude through mouth.
    D. Often fatal.
240. Amyloid gives a positive metachromatic crystal violet stain and green birefringence with Congo-red stain.
241. The parotid duct is found along a line from the tragus to the midportion of the upper lip.
242. Adenocystic carcinoma constitutes 6% of all salivary gland tumors.
243. The histologic derivation of parotid tumors is as follows: acini—acinous cell tumor, intercalated duct cell—mixed tumor, and epithelial—myoepithelial carcinoma; excretory duct—mucoepidermoid carcinoma and squamous cell carcinoma.
244. All components of all salivary glands are ectodermal derivatives.
245. A scan with technetium 99m reveals Warthin's tumor or oncocytoma as a "hot" nodule.
246. The accuracy of fine needle aspiration biopsies and frozen section specimens in salivary gland lesions varies with the experience of the pathologist.
247. Well-differentiated thyroid carcinoma is associated with Gardner syndrome (familial colonic polyposis) and with Cowden disease (familial goiter and skin hamartomata).
248. Twenty-five to 35% of medullary thyroid carcinomata associated with multiple endocrine neoplasia 2 (MEN2). Ninety percent of individuals with MEN2 will develop thyroid carcinoma. Autosomal-dominant inheritance.
249. RET proto-oncogene not normally expressed in normal thyroid follicular cells; codes for a tyrosine kinase enzyme. Chromosome 10 rearrangement results in RET being inserted near one of three promoter regions in nucleus of follicular cell and then expressed, with the development of a follicular cell carcinoma.
250. RET proto-oncogene is normally expressed in parafollicular C cells of the thyroid. Five point mutations of this gene have been found in 95% of hereditary medullary thyroid carcinoma; 80% of these point mutations occur at codon 634. Other codons include 609, 611, 618, 620, 768, 804, and 918; 95% of individuals with MEN2B have codon 918 mutation.
251. Lifetime penetrance of medullary thyroid carcinoma in MEN2A is 90% and in MEN2B is nearly 100%. Recommend thyroidectomy at age 6 years in MEN2A and at birth in MEN2B due to observed distant metastases as early as age 6 in MEN2A and soon after birth in MEN2B.
252. Hürthle cell tumors. Mean age of occurrence 45 to 50 years of age with a 2 to 1 female predominance. Cell with abundant granular cytoplasm filled with mitochondria (similar to oncocytoma). Benign are encapsulated without capsular or vascular invasion. Malignant if capsular, vascular, or thyroid parenchyma invasion. Usually negative on iodine-123, iodine-131, and technetium-99m scans.
253. Papillomas of the oral cavity are most frequently seen on the tonsillar pillars and soft palate. May be premalignant.

254. The incidence of carcinoma of the esophagus is increased in patients with the following:
    A. Achalasia
    B. Oculopharyngeal syndrome
    C. Caustic burns
    D. Plummer-Vinson syndrome
    E. Pernicious anemia
255. Herpangina: Minute vesicles on the anterior tonsillar pillars and soft palate, coxsackie A; hand, foot, and mouth disease includes involvement of hands and feet.
256. Leiomyoma is the most common benign tumor of the esophagus.
257. Scleroderma: Unknown etiology, likely autoimmune reaction to connective tissues. Most common sites in GI tract are esophagus and small bowel. Upper esophagus is not usually involved. More prevalent in women than in men. Physiologic abnormalities include decreased motility of the esophagus and esophagitis. Pathologically the mucosa and the submucosa are involved; however, the longitudinal muscles are seldom involved. Typical barium swallow reveals a flaccid, dilated esophagus that is similar to that of achalasia. Dysphagia in 39%, decreased mouth opening in 28%, and sicca syndrome in 80%.

258.

Parameter	Dermatomyositis	Scleroderma
Dysphagia	Pharyngeal	Esophageal
Nasal regurgitation	Frequent	Absent
Stage of disease	Severe muscle involvement	Extensive skin disease
Remissions	With steroids	None
Complications	Rare	Esophagitis, herniation
Findings at esophagoscopy	Normal	Esophageal ulceration
X-ray findings	Loss of peristalsis	Loss of peristalsis
Motility	Decreased	Decreased
Site of maximum involvement in the esophagus	Upper one-third	Lower two-thirds

259. Esophagus: Esophageal pressures
    A. 5 to 10 mmHg normal resting pressure of lower esophageal sphincter.
    B. 40 to 60 mmHg characteristic of achalasia.
    C. 10 mmHg compatible with scleroderma or gastroesophageal reflux.
260. The protean manifestations of Marfan syndrome result from an absence of the microfibrillar-fiber system in the various connective tissues of the body.
261. Chemical face peeling
    A. Multiple agents: Glycolic acid, trichloroacetic acid, phenol, Croton oil
    B. Indications: Fine rhytids, erasure of dermabrasion demarcation
    C. Precautions
        (1) Pigmented areas may lose pigmentation temporarily or permanently.
        (2) Peel regions rich in adnexal structures.
        (3) Peels for pigmentation must be superficial.
        (4) Phenol toxicity can cause headache, nausea, hypotension, CNS depression, and arrhythmias.

    D. Complications
- (1) Hypopigmentation.
- (2) Irregular hyperpigmentation.
- (3) Perioral scarring: Avoid facelift at same sitting.
- (4) Prominent skin pores: Avoid deep peel in young patients for pigmentation.

    E. Healing timetable
- (1) 5 days, epidermis regenerates
- (2) 7 days, epidermis loosely attached to dermis
- (3) 2 weeks, new collagen deposited, fills out dermis, giving youthful appearance
- (4) 1 month, pigmentation returns, milia possible and require opening
- (5) 6 months, epidermis normal thickness
- (6) 10 months, dermis normalizes

262. Facelift

    A. Sun exposure is the most significant factor in premature aging.

    B. Diseases of premature aging (all autosomal-recessive) include the following:
- (1) Cutis laxa, associated with hernias, emphysema, aneurysms—repeated lifting may help.
- (2) Progeria, associated with growth retardation and early atherosclerosis—lifting is not recommended.
- (3) Werner syndrome, associated with high-pitched voice, diabetes, osteoporosis—lifting not recommended.

    C. Most authorities recommend dissection superficial to platysma, but beneath galea temporally to avoid hair follicles.

    D. Complications: hematoma 1 to 8%, usually within 24 hours, presents with pain—more common in men; hair loss, skin slough, nerve injury, salivary cysts (which usually respond to aspiration and pressure).

263. Scar revision in adults at 9 to 12 months; in children, 18 months.

264. Nylon suture retains 75% of its tensile strength for 2 years. Polyglycolic acid loses approximately 40% of its strength in 7 days and 80% in 14 days. A wound does not obtain normal tensile strength until 6 weeks after repair. It has approximately 10% of its normal tensile strength from day 14 and 25% of its normal tensile strength on day 21 following.

265. Skin elasticity is greatest during infancy. Children are more likely to form hypertrophic scars.

266. The most difficult to treat delayed complication of orbital blowout fracture is enopthalmos.

267. The most common cause of lagophthalmos after blepharoplasty is the excision of too much lid skin.

268. Due to the relative size of the face to the skull, maxillofacial trauma in children is less common. Skull fractures and intracranial injuries are more common.

269. Hypertrophic scars contain more type III collagen.

270. Tar should be cleaned from a wound with ether; anecdotal reports have suggested mayonnaise is also effective.

271. When performing a W-plasty, the base should be no longer than 6.0 mm and the sides no longer than 6.5 mm.

272. The pectoralis major myocutaneous flap in women should have its incision placed in the inframammary crease.
273. Tip dynamics:
   A. Tip-narrowing procedures
      (1) Thinning resection
      (2) Morselization
      (3) Triangular wedge excisions
      (4) Removal of subcutaneous fat and tissue
      (5) Vertical dome division (Goldman rhinoplasty)
   B. Superior tip rotation
      (1) Lateral crural flap
      (2) Rim strip
      (3) Lateral crural detachment
      (4) Complete strip and excision of caudal septum
      (5) Vertical dome division
   C. Tip retrodisplacement
      (1) Rim strip
      (2) Lateral crural flap
      (3) Lateral crural detachment
      (4) Medial crural detachment
      (5) Lateral crural excisions
      (6) Medial crural excisions
   D. Increasing tip projection
      (1) Plumping
      (2) Suturing medial crura together
      (3) Septocolumellar sutures
      (4) Struts
      (5) Battens
      (6) Vertical dome division
274. Most common nerve injury during facelift: Auriculotemporal branch of cranial nerve V.
275. Most common branches of facial nerve injury
   A. Marginal mandibular
   B. Temporal
   C. Buccal
276. Most commonly injured cranial nerves
   A. I (viral, surgery, trauma)
   B. VIII (viral, ototoxin, barotrauma, acoustic trauma, surgery, fracture, concussion)
   C. X
   D. VII
277. Fibro-osseous lesions. Definition: An unrelated group of lesions sharing the same histologic features as their common denominator (benign cellular fibrous tissue containing variable amounts of mineralized material). Diagnosis is often impossible by microscopy alone and requires clinical and radiographic information.
   There are three types of fibro-osseous lesions, all differing in treatment.
   A. Osseous dysplasia cementoma
      (1) Character: A reactive lesion
      (2) Clinical findings

           (a) Occurs predominantly in African-American women over age 20.

           (b) Most common location is periapical alveolar bone of mandibular anteriors.

           (c) Asymptomatic.

      (3) X-ray findings

           (a) Early lesion periapical lucency or multiple lucencies resembling periapical granuloma or cyst, but tooth is always vital.

      (4) Subtype

           (a) Florid osseous dysplasia.

           (b) Extensive lesion in multiple quadrants associated with expansion, dull pain, and traumatic (simple) bone cysts.

  B. Fibrous dysplasia

      (1) Character: A developmental lesion

      (2) Clinical findings

           (a) Young age group (first to second decade).

           (b) Diffuse, painless bony swelling with facial deformity.

           (c) Does not cross midline.

      (3) X-ray findings

           (a) Ground glass, multilocular, radiolucent, or irregularly mottled opaque and lucent.

           (b) Fusiform tapered expansion.

           (c) Diffuse margins.

           (d) Involves and incorporates lamina dura and cortical bone.

      (4) Types

           (a) Monostotic: Only one bone affected (75%).

           (b) Polyostotic: More than one bone affected (20%); associated with Albright syndrome (5%) (precocious puberty and café au lait spots).

           (c) Juvenile aggressive: Rapidly growing, markedly deforming lesion of maxilla that destroys tooth buds and is refractory to treatment.

  C. Ossifying fibroma (cementifying fibroma)

      (1) Character: A benign neoplasm

      (2) Clinical findings

           (a) Causes painless bulge in cortex.

           (b) Teeth displaced.

           (c) Any age or location but more common in mandible in female young adults.

      (3) X-ray finding

           (a) Well-demarcated lucency with no scant or dense opacity.

           (b) Causes divergence of tooth roots.

      (4) Subtype

           (a) Juvenile active ossifying fibroma.

           (b) Can grow to enormous proportions and cause death by encroachment of vital structures; found in children and adolescents and appears as a huge expansile cannonball lesion on x-ray film.

278. Cervical metastases of occult infraclavicular primaries comprise 1 to 2% of all neck metastases.

    A. Subclavicular metastases to the neck
        (1) Lung
        (2) Pancreas
        (3) Kidney
        (4) Esophagus
        (5) Ovary
    B. Pathology of subclavicular metastases to the neck
        (1) Squamous cell carcinoma, 60%
        (2) Adenocarcinoma, 20%
        (3) Undifferentiated, 10%
        (4) Melanoma, 10%
    C. Five-year survival after treatment for subclavicular metastases to the neck
        (1) Squamous cell carcinoma, 50%
        (2) Adenocarcinoma, 0%
        (3) Undifferentiated, 50%
        (4) Melanoma, 0 to 10%

279. Differential diagnosis of neck mass
    A. Midline
        (1) Thyroglossal duct cyst
        (2) Dermoid
        (3) Sebaceous cyst
        (4) Delphian node
        (5) Aberrant thyroid tissue
        (6) Thyroid isthmus tumor
    B. Lateral
        (1) Lymph node
        (2) Submandibular gland tumor
        (3) Branchial cleft cyst
        (4) Carotid body tumor
        (5) Lipoma
        (6) Neurofibroma
        (7) Sebaceous cyst
        (8) Parathyroid cyst
        (9) Primary soft tissue tumor
        (10) Infection (tuberculosis, syphilis)
        (11) Cystic hygroma
    C. Multiple
        (1) Nonspecific
        (2) Specific adenitis
             (a) HIV
             (b) Epstein–Barr virus, cytomegalovirus
             (c) Toxoplasmosis
             (d) Bacterial
             (e) Fungal
             (f) Tuberculosis
             (g) Lymphoma
             (h) Metastatic disease

280. Differential diagnosis of cerebellopontine angle tumors
    A. Acoustic neuroma
    B. Neurofibroma
    C. Meningioma
    D. Cholesteatoma
    E. Aneurysm
    F. Glioma
    G. Metastases
    H. Glomus tumors
    I. Osteoma, lipoma
281. Melanoma
    A. Incidence
        (1) 7 per 100,000
        (2) 20% in head and neck area
        (3) 1% of all cancer in the United States
        (4) 3% of all cutaneous neoplasms
    B. Etiology
        (1) Congenital moles, 15 mm
        (2) Dysplastic nevi: Junctional nevus
        (3) Solar cofactor
    C. Classification
        (1) Lentigo maligna
        (2) Superficial spreading
        (3) Nodular
        (4) Subungual
    D. Clinical features
        (1) Variegated color
        (2) Irregular border
        (3) Increase in size
        (4) Irregular surface
    E. Treatment
        (1) Wide surgical excision with or without regional lymphadenectomy as
            indicated
        (2) Radiation therapy
        (3) Chemotherapy
        (4) Regional hyperthermia
        (5) Immunotherapy
    F. Five-year survival
        (1) Clark I, 100%
        (2) Clark II, 93%
        (3) Clark III, 74%
        (4) Clark IV, 39%
    G. Prognosis poor if
        (1) Large size
        (2) Ulceration
        (3) Satellites
        (4) BANS (back, upper arm, posterolateral neck, posterior scalp), nail beds,
            mucosal

282. Wegener's granulomatosis. Idiopathic, probably autoimmune disease, classically with triad of upper/lower airway necrotizing granulomas, systemic vasculitis, and focal glomerulonephritis. Ninety percent have head and neck symptoms at presentation, typically nasal obstruction, discharge, sinusitis, epistaxis, deformity, and pain. Otologic disease is common, usually with serous otitis media. Pulmonary involvement reported in >95% and renal in >80%. Other symptoms include arthralgia/myalgia, auricular chondritis, polyarticular arthritis, ocular inflammation, and purpura. Laboratory findings include elevated ESR and C-reactive protein. Classic antineutrophil cytoplasmic antibody (c-ANCA) is reported, 78 to 100% sensitive in disseminated disease and 60 to 70% in isolated upper airway disease. Treatment is begun with steroids until control is obtained, and then changed to methotrexate, which is continued for about 1 year.

283. Lethal midline granuloma syndrome. Confusing, obsolete terminology previously described to include Wegener's granulomatosis, polymorphic reticulosis, idiopathic midline destructive disease, and non-Hodgkin lymphoma. Now separated into Wegener's granulomatosis and angiocentric T cell lymphoma.

284. Angiocentric nasal T cell lymphoma. Rare disease in western countries but common in Asia and China. Associated with Epstein–Barr virus. Presents as midline destructive lesion with obstruction, epistaxis, crusting, ulceration, midfacial destruction, and systemic symptoms. May be confused with other nasal granulomatous processes, particularly Wegener's granulomatosis. Radiotherapy is used for treatment and should be done before dissemination.

285. Sjögren syndrome
    A. Described as xerostomia and xerophthalmia; all types show positive antinuclear antibodies (ANA), positive radio frequency (RF), and elevated ESR.
    B. Primary disease is not associated with connective tissue disorder; it is characterized by positive SS-A, positive SS-b, HLA B8, and Dw3.
    C. Secondary disease is associated with connective tissue disorders with rheumatoid arthritis–lupus erythematosus (RA–LE) characterized by positive SS-A and HLA Dw4.
    D. Peak incidence 40 to 60 years of age.
    E. Females to males, 9 : 1.
    F. Second most common connective tissue disease after RA.
    G. Biopsy reveals lymphocytic and histiocytic infiltrate with glandular atrophy.
    H. Extraglandular symptoms may be seen in addition to primary exocrine gland pathology (eg, bronchiectasis).
    I. Increased risk of lymphocytic malignancy with:
        (1) Parotid enlargement
        (2) Primary Sjögren syndrome
        (3) Lymphadenopathy
        (4) Splenomegaly
        (5) Decreased total IgM on serum protein electrophoresis (SPEP)
    J. Myoepithelial cells are present in biopsy specimens of Sjögren syndrome but not in lymphoma (may be done of lip, sputum, palate).
    K. Must be distinguished from sicca-like syndromes, which have xerostomia and/or xerophthalmia, but with negative tests and biopsy. Associated with the following:

      (1) Aging

      (2) Medications (diuretics, anticholinergics, antihistamines, antidepressants)

      (3) Other diseases (hepatitis, autoimmune disorders)

      (4) Chronic dehydration

286. Actinomycosis

    A. Etiology: *Actinomyces israelii.*

    B. Culture: Branching, anaerobic, or microaerophilic gram-positive rods (must be grown on blood agar in anaerobic conditions).

    C. Associations

      (1) Mucous membrane trauma

      (2) Poor oral hygiene

      (3) Dental abscess

      (4) Aspiration

      (5) Diabetes

      (6) Immunosuppression

    D. Treatment

      (1) Penicillin, 4 to 6 weeks by mouth.

      (2) Sulfonamides, 4 to 6 weeks by mouth.

      (3) Failures may require intravenous therapy.

      (4) Incision and drainage required in some cases.

287. Nocardiosis

    A. Subtype of actinomycosis caused by another species of the actinomycetes, *Nocardia.*

    B. Soil saprophyte, inhaled and causes primary lung disease with secondary hematogenous spread.

    C. Usually associated with diabetes or immunosuppression.

    D. Cultures reveal aerobic, weakly acid-fast organism, which on Sabouraud's agar reveals branching, beaded, refractile hyphae.

    E. Usually presents as pneumonia, but tissue trauma may be associated with primary skin lesion.

    F. Treatment may require incision and drainage, and/or prolonged treatment with sulfonamides.

288. Rhinocerebral mucormycosis. Rapidly progressive disease caused by fungi of family Mucoraceae: *Rhizopus, Mucor,* and *Absidia,* less commonly by *Aspergillus* species. This occurs almost exclusively in diabetic ketoacidosis, other immunocompromised states, and renal disease, but is surprisingly rare in HIV. These fungi invade blood vessel walls, producing thrombosis, ischemic infarction, and necrosis and allowing spread of disease. Patients are acutely ill, with fever, lethargy, facial pain, and visual impairment. Examination demonstrates dark, necrotic turbinates and nasal septum and granular serosanguinous rhinorrhea. Black facial necrosis and septal or palatal perforation may occur. Gomorri silver methenamine (GMS) and KOH preparations demonstrate hyphae. CT demonstrates sinus disease, although bony destruction appears late. MRI delineates major vessel and intracranial involvement. Treatment involves control of predisposing metabolic disorder, radical debridement, and amphotericin B. Survival approaches 80% and is best in diabetics, because their underlying disorder (ketoacidosis) is usually controllable.

289. Histoplasmosis
    A. Etiology
       (1) *Histoplasma capsulatum*
       (2) Endemic in Missouri and Ohio River valleys
    B. Clinical features
       (1) Lung involvement
       (2) Rhinitis, pharyngitis, epiglottitis
       (3) Nodular lesions of tongue, lip, and oral mucosa (oral lesions much more common than in *Blastomyces* and *Coccidioides*)
       (4) Dirty white mucosa or true cords
    C. Pathology: Epithelioid granulomas
    D. Diagnosis
       (1) Skin test
       (2) Complement fixation
       (3) Latex agglutination
       (4) Laryngeal lesions require direct laryngoscopy (DL) and biopsy with fungal stains
    E. Treatment: Amphotericin B
290. Coccidioidomycosis
    A. Etiology
       (1) *Coccidioides immitis*
       (2) San Joaquin Valley fever
    B. Clinical features: Involvement of skin, mucous membranes, thyroid, eyes, trachea, salivary glands; severe erosions of epiglottis
    C. Diagnosis
       (1) Skin test
       (2) Complement fixation
       (3) Chest x-ray—coin lesions
    D. Treatment: Amphotericin B
291. Blastomycosis
    A. Etiology: Soil saprophyte, *Blastomyces dermatitides*
    B. Regional: Midwest, Mississippi and Ohio River valleys
    C. Clinical features
       (1) Red laryngeal ulcers
       (2) Vocal cord involvement
       (3) Glottic or subglottic stenosis
       (4) May involve tongue, palate, buccal mucosa
       (5) Hoarseness may be first ENT manifestation
       (6) Primary site is usually lung, with secondary hematogenous spread
       (7) Most frequent extrapulmonary sites: skin, bone, genitourinary (GU), adrenal, larynx mucosa
    D. Diagnosis
       (1) Biopsy reveals pseudoepitheliomatous hyperplasia, intraepithelial micro-abscesses, multinucleated giant cells (has been confused with squamous carcinoma).

        (2)   Culture reveals thermal dimorphic fungus, with birefringent broad-based buds (must be grown on Sabouraud's agar and stained with methenamine-silver or silver-chromate).

   E.   Treatment: Amphotericin B

292. Cryptococcosis
   A.   Etiology: *Cryptococcus neoformans*
   B.   Predisposing factors: Immunosuppression, lymphoma
   C.   Clinical features: Membranous nasopharyngitis, meningitis, hearing loss
   D.   Diagnosis: Fluorescent antibody test
   E.   Treatment: Amphotericin B

293. Rhinosporidiosis
   A.   Etiology: *Rhinosporidium seeberi,* never cultured; may be nanocyte stage of cyanobacterium, *Microcystis aeruginosa*
   B.   Southern India, Sri Lanka, Pakistan
   C.   Clinical features: Friable, red polypoid lesions in nasal cavity and pharynx; nasal obstruction, rhinorrhea, epistaxis, sneezing, hyponasal speech
   D.   Treatment: Surgery and cauterization; 10% recur. Dapsone/amphotericin for recalcitrant cases

294. Aspergillosis
   A.   Etiology: *Aspergillus fumigatus*
   B.   Clinical features
      (1)   Unilateral painless proptosis
      (2)   Laryngeal involvement
      (3)   Bone erosion
      (4)   Associated with immunosuppression or malignancy in many
   C.   Biopsy: Acute, branching, septate hyphae when grown on Sabouraud's agar
   D.   Treatment: Surgery

295. Candidiasis
   A.   Predisposing factors
      (1)   Antibiotics, steroids
      (2)   Infants, elderly
      (3)   Diabetes, malnutrition, immunosuppression
   B.   Diagnosis: Sabouraud's medium
   C.   Clinical features: Patches of creamy white pseudomembrane, odynophagia, dysphagia, angular cheilitis, laryngitis
   D.   Treatment: Nystatin, amphotericin B

296. Neurogenic tumors
   A.   Von Recklinghausen disease
      (1)   Definition: Hamartomatous disorder
      (2)   Epidemiology
         (a)   Autosomal dominant, type 2 localized to 22q mutation
         (b)   1 in 2500 to 3300 births
         (c)   50% apparent at birth
      (3)   Pathology: Multiple, plexiform neurofibromas, sarcomatous changes

      (4)   Clinical features:
          (a)   Skin: Café au lait spots, tumors, vitiligo
          (b)   Bone: Osteolysis, abnormalities of bone growth
          (c)   CNS: Glioma, acoustic neuroma (may be bilateral in type 2), meningioma, and/or spina bifida
      (5)   Treatment: Conservative surgery and close observation due to increased incidence of sarcoma formation

  B. Neuroblastoma
      (1)   Definition: Malignant tumor that arises from ganglion cells
      (2)   Epidemiology: Most common soft tissue neoplasm in children; rarely primary in head and neck, although commonly metastasizes to head and neck
      (3)   Clinical features: Mass
      (4)   Treatment: Surgery plus chemotherapy plus radiotherapy

  C. Neurofibrosarcoma
      (1)   Definition: Malignant tumor that arises from neurofibromas
      (2)   Epidemiology: All ages; 5% of all sarcomas
      (3)   Treatment: Surgery plus chemotherapy plus radiotherapy
      (4)   Prognosis: 40% 5-year survival

297. Osteogenic sarcoma
  A. Definition: Malignant tumor of bone that characteristically produces osteoid
  B. Epidemiology
      (1)   0.07 per 100,000 population
      (2)   20% of all bone malignancies
      (3)   7% occur in jaws, mandible, maxilla
      (4)   Equal among sexes
  C. Etiology
      (1)   Paget disease
      (2)   Fibrous dysplasia
      (3)   Radiotherapy
      (4)   Trauma
      (5)   Osteochondroma
  D. Pathology: Osteoblastic, chondroblastic, fibroblastic
  E. Clinical features
      (1)   Mass (body of mandible, alveolar ridge of maxilla)
      (2)   Paresthesias
      (3)   Pain
      (4)   Loose dentition
  F. Investigations: X-ray films—"sunburst" appearance (found in 25% of cases), osteolysis and osteoblastosis
  G. Differential diagnosis
      (1)   Benign
          (a)   Odontogenic cyst
          (b)   Ossifying fibroma, fibrous dysplasia
          (c)   Central giant cell granuloma

        (d) Histiocytosis X

        (e) Arteriovenous malformation

        (f) Hemangioma

    (2) Malignant

        (a) Multiple myeloma

        (b) Metastatic neoplasm

        (c) Ameloblastoma

        (d) Fibrosarcoma

        (e) Reticulum cell sarcoma

        (f) Squamous cell carcinoma

  H. Treatment: Surgery plus radiotherapy plus chemotherapy; prognosis: 40% 5-year survival

298. Tumors of maxilla and mandible

  A. Developmental

    (1) Dental origin

        (a) Periodontal, from epithelial rests within periodontal ligament

            (i)   Periapical

            (ii)   Lateral

            (iii)   Residual (affect extraction)

        (b) Dentigerous

            (i)   Cystic odontoma, from enamel

            (ii)   Eruption cyst, from enamel of third molar

        (c) Odontogenic keratocyst, usually involves mandibular ramus, lined by keratinizing epithelium; malignant potential?

        (d) Calcifying odontogenic cyst, same as c, above, but with deposition of calcium

    (2) Nondental origin

        (a) Fissural, epithelium trapped between fusion planes

            (i)   Nasoalveolar

            (ii)   Median

            (iii)   Incisive (nasopalatine duct)

            (iv)   Globulomaxillary

  B. Extravasational cysts, secondary to trauma

  C. Metabolic—osteolytic lesions associated with lipid dystrophy, cherubism, osteitis fibrosa cystica, other conditions

  D. Inflammatory—fungal, syphilis, other infections

  E. Neoplastic

    (1) Noninvasive benign

        (a) Gingival hyperplasia

        (b) Fibroma

        (c) Lipoma

        (d) Osteoma

        (e) Chondroma

        (f) Odontoma (most common tumor of maxilla and mandible, hamartomatous—all tooth tissues)

        (g) Papilloma

    (2) Invasive benign
- (a) Giant cell tumor of bone
- (b) Central giant cell granuloma of bone
- (c) Myxoma
- (d) Hemangioma
- (e) Lymphangioma
- (f) Endothelioma
- (g) Neurogenic
- (h) Adenoma
- (i) Mixed cell tumor
- (j) Fibro-osteoma
- (k) Ameloblastoma—usually mandibular tumor, appears in males in their 30s; loculated cystic cavity with displacement of tooth roots, vessels, and nerves

    (3) Malignant
- (a) Epithelial
  - (i) Squamous
  - (ii) Adenocarcinoma
  - (iii) Malignant ameloblastoma
  - (iv) Transitional cell (lymphoepithelioma)
  - (v) Basal cell
- (b) Mesothelial
  - (i) Fibrosarcoma
  - (ii) Myosarcoma
  - (iii) Angiosarcoma
  - (iv) Osteogenic sarcoma
  - (v) Chondrosarcoma
- (c) Lymphoma
- (d) Melanoma
- (e) Myeloma (Ewing sarcoma)
- (f) Multiple myeloma

299. Screening test

	True	**Results**
Screening test (+)	+	−
Results (−)	A	B
B = false-positive	C	D
C = false-negative		

$$\text{Sensitivity} = \frac{A \times 100}{A + C}$$

$$\text{Specificity} = \frac{D \times 100}{B + D}$$

$$\text{Predictive value of a positive test} = \frac{A \times 100}{A + B}$$

300. Fluids
    A. Daily fluid requirement is 2200 mL/24 hours (for adults).
    B. Daily output of fluid
        (1) 700 mL via respiration
        (2) 200 mL in the feces
        (3) 100 mL via perspiration (without fever)
        (4) 1200 mL in the urine
301. Contrast studies of the aortic arch are necessary following cervicomediastinal injuries that result in the following:
    A. Widened mediastinum
    B. Pulse rate deficit
    C. Supraclavicular hematoma
    D. Brachial plexus injury
    E. Cervical bruit
302. Vancomycin is the antibiotic of choice in the treatment of pseudomembranous colitis associated with *Clostridium difficile* overgrowth; administered orally, nonabsorbed and nonototoxic.
303. Acute lead poisoning may cause colic, constipation or diarrhea, anorexia, weakness, paralysis, convulsions, and coma. Red blood cell (RBC) basophilic stippling is present. Whole blood lead level is greater than 0.08 mg/dL, and urinary levels are greater than 0.15 mg/L. Glycosuria is present, and urinary levels of delta aminolevulinic acid and coproporphyrin III are increased. Radiographs show linear opacifications along the length of the long bones or circular opacifications around ossification centers. Treatment includes avoidance of further exposure and the use of chelating agents.
304. Cervical injuries are generally divided into zone 1 (below the top of the sternal notch), zone 2 (between the sternal notch and the mandibular angle), and zone 3 (above the mandibular angle). There has been a trend away from mandatory exploration of all penetrating neck wounds. Factors such as subcutaneous emphysema, hemoptysis, hematemesis, hematoma, significant bleeding, dysphagia, dysphonia, or neurologic injury infer that important structures may have been injured. Angiography and esophagography are often used to obtain further information. If any of the above factors or studies are positive, immediate surgical exploration is also indicated for zone 2. For injuries to zones 1 and 3, angiography is indicated in almost all cases. Exploration is also done more frequently for injuries in these areas.
305. Autacoids
    A. Histamine
        (1) Histamine is found in mast cells, platelets, leukocytes, and the parietal cell region of the stomach.
        (2) Physiology
            (a) Contracts smooth muscles.
            (b) Increases dilation and permeability of capillaries and venules.
            (c) Dilates arterioles and venules via a direct action on the musculature.
            (d) Contracts larger vessels.
            (e) Stimulates exocrine glands.
            (f) Increases gastric secretion.

B. Serotonin
   (1) Serotonin is found in platelets, cerebral tissues, and the mucosa of the GI tract. It is not found in mast cells in humans.
   (2) Increases capillary permeability.
   (3) Contracts smooth muscle.
C. Kinins
   (1) Kallidin I (bradykinin) is found in plasma and increases capillary permeability, smooth muscle contraction, and vasodilation. It is formed by the action of enzymes on plasma globulin.
   (2) Kallidin II is a decapeptide. It has properties similar to those of kallidin I but is formed by different enzymes. One of these enzymes may be kallikrein.
D. Prostaglandins (PGs)
   (1) Produced by nearly all body tissues.
   (2) Thousands of analogs (eg, PGE, PGF, PGG, PGH).
   (3) Actions
      (a) Potent vasodilators.
      (b) Increased cardiac output.
      (c) Regulate platelet aggregation.
      (d) PGFs contract bronchial and tracheal muscles; PGEs cause relaxation of these muscles.
      (e) Promote diuresis.
      (f) May stimulate or depress the CNS.
      (g) Cause the release of ACTH, luteinizing hormone (LH), and thyrotropin (may abort early pregnancies).
      (h) Appear to amplify pain by sensitizing the nerve endings.
   (4) Mechanism of action is by stimulating cyclic adenosine monophosphate (cAMP) or cyclic guanosine monophosphate (cGMP) production.

306. Visual acuity and the condition of the globe should always be examined first in any ocular injury prior to palpation.

307. Cardiac tamponade symptoms include the following:
   A. Low cardiac output manifests as low blood pressure and increased heart rate.
   B. Muffled cardiac sounds.
   C. Increased central venous pressure.
   D. Decreased amplitude on ECG.
   E. Diagnosis by pericardiocentesis.

308. Air embolism can be associated with head and neck trauma or with venous perforation during routine head and neck procedures.
   A. It manifests as "to-and-fro" murmur and decreased cardiac output as described for cardiac tamponade, above.
   B. Treatment with elevation of head of bed and patient placement in the left lateral decubitus position.
   C. Cardiac puncture may be required for aspiration of air (also possible with a Swan–Ganz catheter).

309. Patients suffering from long-term airway obstruction may develop apnea after tracheotomy. This occurs because respiration is driven by hypoxia in these patients; resolution of this hypoxia results in CO_2 narcosis. Postobstructive pulmonary edema may also result due to the sudden elimination of high intralumenal pressures. This is

the same phenomenon that occurs after excision in some children suffering from obstruction as a result of adenoid or tonsillar hypertrophy. Positive end expiratory pressure (PEEP) can prevent and treat this accumulation.

310. CSF leaks may be documented and localized by intrathecal metrizamide followed by scanning. Fluorescein is also used with visual documentation of leak absorbed by intranasal pledgets. Intrathecal radionuclides can also be used with scanning of the patient and of intranasal pledgets to localize the site(s).

311. False-positive serology (VDRL) may be associated with the following:
    A. Malaria
    B. Leprosy
    C. Lupus
    D. Collagen-vascular diseases
    E. Rheumatoid arthritis
    F. Measles
    G. Smallpox
    H. Hepatitis
    I. Infectious mononucleosis

312. False-positive heterophile antibody may be associated with the following:
    A. Serum sickness
    B. Rheumatoid arthritis
    C. Hodgkin disease
    D. Brucellosis
    E. Hepatitis

313. Malignant hyperthermia is caused by the release of calcium in large amounts from the sarcoplasmic reticulum, usually associated with the use of depolarizing anesthetic agents. Prophylactic treatment in known patients and acute treatment in newly diagnosed patients with dantrolene sodium at a dose of 1 mg/kg is required. Anesthetic agents should be discontinued, 100% oxygen initiated, acidosis corrected, and cooling blankets and ice bags applied; treatment of arrhythmias may be necessary. Steroids and procainamide have been recommended as needed. The use of an unused anesthetic machine is also recommended for known malignant hyperthermia patients.

314. The most common organisms in postoperative wound infections after head and neck surgery are *Staphylococcus aureus* and beta-hemolytic streptococci in early cases and mixed oral flora in late infection. Necrotizing fasciitis is a rapid and dangerous anaerobic infection requiring aggressive debridement, blood sugar control, and antibiotics; in some cases, hyperbaric oxygen has been useful.

315. Chyle fistula can result from dissection in the supraclavicular fossa. Volumes of less than 150 mL/day can be treated with direct pressure and a low-fat diet; if using hyperalimentation, medium-chain triglyceride (MCT) oil can be used as a caloric source, as it provides only medium-chain triglycerides, which do not increase chyle production. For volumes greater than 150 mL/day, exploration and ligation are recommended.

316. The head and neck constitute 9% of the total body surface area, with the head comprising 7% and the neck 2%.

317. Hypercalcemia associated with parathyroid pathology results from adenoma in 80% and diffuse hyperplasia in 20%. Normal variation reveals that 90% have 5 parathyroids, 5% have 3, and 3% have only a single gland.

318. Stress or injury causes an increase in adrenal steroid production, epinephrine release, gluconeogenesis, growth hormone release, and white blood cell (WBC) count. It does not cause increased thyroid hormone release or production.

319. Chronic obstructive lung disease results in a decreased forced expiratory volume (FEV_1)/forced vital capacity (FVC) ratio, whereas restrictive lung disease results in preservation of this ratio.

320. Differential diagnosis of headache
    A. Extracranial etiology
        (1) Muscle contraction/tension
        (2) Vascular: Distention of scalp arteries, throbbing—triggered by menses, alcohol, stress
            (a) Classic migraine: Vasoconstriction followed by vasodilation
                (i) Aura (sensory, motor, behavioral)
                (ii) Family history
                (iii) Childhood onset
                (iv) Hemicranial
                (v) Epiphenomena (photophobia, diarrhea)
                (vi) Treatment: Ergotamine
            (b) Complicated migraine
                (i) Intracranial (brain stem)
                (ii) Ophthalmic
                (iii) Nausea, vomiting, photophobia
                (iv) Women greatly outnumber men
            (c) Common migraine
                (i) Late onset, no prodrome
                (ii) Warning: Change in mood, appetite
                (iii) Treatment: Ergotamine
            (d) Cluster
                (i) Older age
                (ii) Bouts of episodes
                (iii) Hyperlacrimation, rhinorrhea
                (iv) Hemicranial
                (v) Treatment: Ergotamine
            (e) Mixed (migraine and tension)
        (3) Others
            (a) Inflammatory infections (sinusitis, dental)
            (b) Intracranial etiology
                (i) Traction headache: Space-occupying lesion; papilledema; early morning headache, nausea, vomiting
                (ii) Vascular: Widespread vasodilation of cerebral vessels; aneurysm and subarachnoid hemorrhage: worst headache associated with depressed sensorium, central signs
                (iii) Inflammatory: Meningitis, cerebritis/encephalitis
            (c) Ocular
                (i) Oculomotor imbalance
                (ii) Increased intraocular pressure

        (d)   Tic douloureux
            (i)   Excruciating paroxysms of lancinating pain lasting seconds
           (ii) Usually V_2, V_3
          (iii) Treatment: Tegretol, Dilantin, percutaneous radio frequency destruction, or alcohol injection
        (e)   Temporomandibular joint dysfunction

321. Differential diagnosis of hemoptysis
    A. Recent
       (1) Pneumonia
          (a) Primary
          (b) Secondary
             (i)   Tumor
            (ii) Foreign body
           (iii) Aspiration
       (2) Pulmonary infarct
       (3) Acute bronchitis
       (4) Infection: Bronchitis, abscess, tuberculosis
       (5) Iatrogenic: Tracheotomy, intubation, bronchoscopy, needle biopsy
       (6) Cancer
    B. Chronic
       (1) Tuberculosis
       (2) Bronchial carcinoma
    C. Recurrent
       (1) Chronic bronchitis
       (2) Neoplasm
       (3) Bronchiectasis
       (4) Cystic fibrosis
       (5) Pulmonary hypertension
       (6) Osler-Weber-Rendu syndrome
       (7) Arteriovenous fistula
       (8) Cardiovascular disease
          (a) Mitral valve disease
          (b) Left ventricular failure
          (c) Pulmonary embolus
    D. Investigations
       (1) Chest x-ray film
       (2) Endoscopy with or without laser coagulation
       (3) Cytology
       (4) Culture and sensitivity tests
       (5) Occasional bronchogram, angiogram, lung scan

322. Daily caloric need for an average adult ranges from 1800 to 3000 calories depending on the metabolic rate.

323. During surgery, when the skin incision is made, there is a sudden increase in serum catecholamines, growth hormones, cortisol, and antidiuretic hormone (ADH) levels, leading to an increase in serum glucose and glucagon, gluconeogenesis, a decrease in insulin receptor sites, and decreased urinary output.

324. Water intoxication symptoms are lethargy, seizures, and coma. (Serum sodium in the range of 115–120 mEq/L.) Can lead to congestive heart failure, decreased glomerular flow rate, and renal failure.

325. SIADH (syndrome of inappropriate ADH) can be caused by chlorpropamide (Diabinese), clofibrate (Atromid), vincristine, cyclophosphamide (Cytoxan), meperidine (Demerol), and morphine sulfate. The findings are low serum sodium, increased urinary sodium, and increased urine osmolality (> 300 mOsm).

326. Metabolic acidosis can be caused by lactic acidosis, which can be secondary to excessive ethanol intake, obstructive pulmonary disease, sepsis, DBI, and acetazolamide (Diamox). Sepsis is a common cause of lactic acidosis in postoperative patients.

327. Metabolic alkalosis can be caused by vomiting, nasogastric tube suction, decreased extracellular fluid volume, decreased chloride and potassium, increased aldosterone levels, and diuretics. One of the treatments is replacement of chloride.

328. Hyperosmolar coma (ie, >340 mOsm/L, where the normal value is 285 to 290 mOsm/L) is a condition that can be caused by phenytoin (Dilantin), steroids, thiazide diuretics, myocardial infarction, and stroke. Serum sodium, BUN, and glucose are elevated. Despite elevated serum glucose, there is no ketoacidosis.

329. Normal serum values (mEq/L)
   - Na = 140
   - K = 4
   - Cl = 95 to 105
   - HCO_3 = 28

330. Normal arterial blood gases
   - Po_2 = 95 to 100
   - pH = 7.4
   - Pco_2 = 40
   - Oxygen saturation = 97 to 100%

331. Weight loss, decreased serum albumin, and decreased total iron-binding capacity are indications of malnutrition in a postoperative patient. A decrease in caloric intake leads to ketosis, which in turn leads to decreased urinary excretion of uric acid, which can cause gout symptoms.

OTOLOGY

1. Cochlear emissions are generated by outer hair cells.
2. Evoked otoacoustic emissions are not detectable in patients with hearing loss greater than 55 dB.
3. Evoked emissions are not helpful in tracking acoustic neuromas because there is no outer hair cell involvement.
4. Why does microtia work precede atresia work? To preserve soft tissue and provide a thin epithelial envelope free of scar to receive cartilage framework.
5. When do you treat unilateral atresia? Usually in the teenage years, unlike microtia, which is usually at 7 years of age.
6. The most common audiometric finding in congenital aural atresia is a 50- to 60-dB hearing loss with normal nerve function.
7. Unilateral atresia occurs six times greater than bilateral atresia.

8. Regarding auditory amplification, it is important to provide stimulation to the infant at 4 to 6 months with bone conduction aids.

9. Implantable bone conduction aids must be held off until $2\frac{1}{2}$ to 3 years to guarantee adequate skull thickness.

10. Overall, only 50% of aural atresia patients are surgical candidates. Success is increased if the middle ear and mastoid space are at least two-thirds normal size and if all three ossicles, although deformed, are identified.

11. There is a 20% association of facial nerve abnormalities in congenital atresia.

12. When evaluating a patient for necrotizing otitis externa, technetium-99m scan evaluates the bone involvement. A gallium-67 scan evaluates the efficacy of therapy by measuring the presence of WBCs.

13. According to Bluestone, chemoprophylaxis in chronic otitis media is indicated in patients with a history of
    a. Three infections in 6 months
    b. Four to five infections in 12 months

14. There is no indication for the prophylactic use of Bactrim or Septra in any age group.

15. When considering the use of exogenous corticosteroids, remember that the body produces 20 mc of cortisol per day, which is equivalent to 5 mg of prednisone per day. This is equivalent to 4 mg of methylprednisolone or 0.75 mg of Decadron.

16. Effectiveness of adenoidectomy of chronic otitis media with effusion is unrelated to size.

17. The hallmark sign of fungal infection of the ear is granulation tissue at the short process of the malleus.

18. Tympanosclerosis of the tympanic membrane is secondary to poor vascularity with subsequent hyalin formation.

19. Reasons for a persistently draining mastoid cavity are inadequate meatoplasty, dependent tip cell, high facial ridge, exposed eustachian tube.

20. Regarding cholesteatoma, the number one ossicle eroded is the long process of the incus.

21. The cholesteatoma matrix is completely removed except for the following situations: (a) the matrix is adherent to the dura, (b) the matrix is adherent to the superior semicircular canal, (c) the matrix is firmly adherent to the facial nerve, (d) extends into the mesotympanum covering the footplate.

22. In the patient with a greater than 45-dB conductive hearing loss and a high-frequency sensorineural hearing loss (HFSNHL), you should think of cochlear otosclerosis and recommend amplification rather than surgery.

23. In general, therapy for sudden sensorineural hearing loss is limited to patients seen within 3 weeks of symptom onset because of extremely poor prognosis for hearing recovery beyond that time.

24. Recurrent meningitis in infants and children may be secondary to the presence of Hyrtyl's fissure, which is a communication between the middle ear space and the subarachnoid space.

25. Beta$_2$-transferrin is a protein marker specific to CSF and perilymph.

26. The goal of diuretic therapy in Ménière's disease is not diuresis but to drive the kidney to maintain relatively constant urine output, minimizing rapid shifts in systemic fluid and electrolyte balance.

27.   There is only a 24% true-positive result using the fistula test to diagnose a perilymphatic fistula.

FACIAL PLASTICS

1.   There is no significant difference in the melanocyte density between African Americans (AA) and Caucasians. The melanocytes are more reactive in AA.
2.   Following laser resurfacing, bio-occlusive dressings provide a pathway of proper moisture and humidity, decreasing epithelial closure time by up to 50%.
3.   Accutane causes sebaceous gland atrophy and must be discontinued 6 months prior to dermabrasion or laser resurfacing.
4.   When constructing a bilobe transposition flap, the most common mistake is creating the base of flap A too narrow.
5.   Basic rules for Z-plasty flaps.
   a.   No Z-plasty with angles greater than 90 degrees
   b.   No Z-plasty with arms greater than
      (1)   1 cm on the face
      (2)   1.5 cm in the neck
   c.   No angles less than 30 degrees to avoid tip necrosis
6.   The line of maximum extensibility (LME) represents the perpendicular to the resting skin tension lines (RSTL), resulting in a closure that produces the least amount of tension. Increase of tension greater than 250 g results in decreased blood flow in the flap.
7.   The endpoint of dermabrasion or laser resurfacing is determined by punctate bleeding, signifying the papillary dermis.
8.   Regarding tissue expanders, the number one complication is dehiscence at the incision site. The highest complication rate occurs in the cheek and neck: 69%.
9.   The number one error in upper lid blepharoplasty is underestimating the amount of medial fat to excise.
10.   The thickness of the eyelid skin is on average 10/1000 inch.
11.   The musculi orbicularis oculi is composed of
   a.   Orbital portion
   b.   Palpebral portion
      (1)   Pretarsal-superior position
      (2)   Preseptal-inferior position
12.   The number one fat pad missed during lower blepharoplasty is the lateral fat pad. Removal of fat from the medial and central compartments first will make it difficult to assess the amount of fat to be removed from the lateral compartment.
13.   The number one complication associated with lower lid blepharoplasty is ectropion. The number one etiology of ectropion is decreased lid laxity. Therefore, always perform lid SNAP and distraction tests.
14.   Basic fibroblast growth factor (BFGF) has shown to enhance growth (budding) of the fat graft.
15.   When using bovine collagen (Zyderm/Zyplast) 3% of patients will experience an allergic reaction. Of those negative tests, 0.6% will test positive upon a second skin test. This is due to a delayed hypersensitivity reaction, where the first test dose elicits the production of antibodies and the second test dose results in the positive test.

16. Zyderm possesses a higher amount of water; therefore, you must overcorrect by 150 to 200%. Zyplast contains less water; thus no overcorrection is required.
17. Etiology of the polly-beak deformity: Scar formation at the anterior septal angle, inadequate soft tissue removed initially, and excessive bony dorsum reduction.

TRAUMA

1. The most common error in orbital wall reconstruction is failure to repair the posterior orbital floor.
2. The only indication for immediate exploration of the orbit in blowout fractures is rapid onset of serious intraorbital bleeding with visual acuity compromise. Other indications are entrapment and enophthalmos.
3. Facial nerve injury occurs more often with transverse fractures, but since longitudinal fractures occur more often, facial nerve injury is more often associated with longitudinal fractures.
4. Cerebrospinal fluid leaks are associated after temporal bone fracture 11 to 27% of the time.
5. The most common cause of posttraumatic vertigo is concussive injury to the membranous labyrinth.
6. The most common cause of a persistent conductive hearing loss associated with temporal bone fractures is ossicular disruption at the incudostapedial joint dislocation.

PEDIATRICS

1. A foreign body should be ruled out if a child has unilateral wheezing.
2. Tube obstruction is the most common complication in infant tracheotomy.
3. Hypoactive neuromuscular control has been the most current theory for laryngomalacia.
4. Cytomegalovirus infection is a possibility in newborn sensorineural hearing loss (SNHL).
5. Meningitis will commonly cause high-frequency hearing loss.
6. Consider immunologic deficiency in children with chronic sinusitis.
7. Reflux may cause endolaryngeal granulation tissue.
8. Radical surgery for rhabdomyosarcoma is reserved for residual disease following chemotherapy and radiation.
9. Patients with choanal atresia have a high association with other congenital anomalies.
10. Purulent rhinorrhea is the most common presenting sign for sinusitis in children.
11. Oral steroids should be used initially in children with symptomatic airway hemangiomas to stimulate involution.
12. Hemangioma is the most common benign pediatric parotid tumor.
13. Facial trauma in children most commonly results in dental injuries.
14. There is a high association of subglottic stenosis in Down syndrome patients.
15. The best treatment for unilateral pediatric vocal cord paralysis is speech therapy.
16. Amoxicillin is the drug of choice in treating pediatric Lyme disease.
17. Otorrhea is the most common complication following ventilation tube placement.
18. Studies suggest that adenoidectomy, regardless of adenoidal size, is helpful in children with chronic otitis media with effusion requiring multiple sets of tubes.
19. Cystic fibrosis is autosomal recessive.
20. Children with cystic fibrosis who undergo polypectomy alone will experience a 90% recurrence.

21. Children with cystic fibrosis who undergo endoscopic removal along with a sinus procedure experience a 35% recurrence.

GENERAL OTOLARYNGOLOGY

1. Bitter sensation is better appreciated through the glossopharyngeal nerve.
2. Sensation for ammonia and hot chili peppers is mediated by the trigeminal nerve. It is considered a function of common chemical sense.
3. Only 3% of patients with olfactory loss following head trauma recover their sense of smell.
4. Voice fundamental frequency increases in aging men but decreases in aging women.
5. Diabetes insipidus is commonly seen in histiocytosis X.
6. Persistent adenoid tissue in a young adult with recurrent serous otitis media should be tested for HIV.
7. Bactrim and erythromycin may elevate cyclosporin levels in transplant patients.
8. Cervical adenopathy is the most common head and neck manifestation in sarcoidosis.
9. Airway obstruction in sarcoidosis involves the supraglottis.
10. Proximal myalgia is the most common presenting symptom of giant cell arteritis.
11. A biopsy which shows cysts and trophozoites is suggestive of *Pneumocystis carinii*.
12. A biopsy which shows Zimmerman cells is suggestive of a hemangiopericytoma.
13. Patients with primary Sjögren disease have a risk for non-Hodgkin lymphoma.
14. If there is a high suspicion for temporal arteritis but the arterial biopsy is negative, try the contralateral side.
15. Mild cases of Wegener's granulomatosis can be treated with sulfamethoxazole-trimethoprim instead of cyclophosphamide.
16. Cystitis limits the use of cyclophosphamide.
17. Serous otitis media is the most common otologic manifestation in Wegener's.
18. Multiple pulmonary nodules are the most common chest x-ray finding in Wegener's.
19. Rising antineutrophil cytoplasmic antibody (ANCA) levels in Wegener's suggest relapsing disease.
20. Malignant hyperthermia crisis should be treated in the following manner:
    a. Turn off all potent inhalation agents and hyperventilate with 100% O_2.
    b. Call for help.
    c. Check arterial blood gas.
    d. Administer dandrolene sodium.
    e. Cool patient off (ie, cooling blanket, gastric lavage).
    f. Treat for arrhythmia if necessary.
    g. Close urine monitoring.
    h. Treat hyperkalemia with glucose and insulin if necessary.
    i. Observe in ICU.
    j. Monitor temperature, blood gases, electrolytes, urine output, urine myoglobin, and serum creatine phosphokinase (CPK).
21. Angiotensin-converting enzyme (ACE) inhibitors elevate the cough threshold by increasing bradykinin levels.
22. Airway collapse is the cause for mortality in patients with relapsing polychondritis.
23. Scleroderma is associated with a decreased lower esophageal sphincter (LES) pressure.
24. Achalasia is associated with an increased LES pressure.

25. Dandy's syndrome (oscillopsia) is an inability to fixate eyes while moving.
26. Polymorphic reticulosis should be considered a T cell lymphoma.
27. Some 25% of all patients presenting with a skin malignancy have more than one lesion at the time of diagnosis.
28. Systemic diseases associated with skin cancers include albinism, xeroderma pigmentosum (SCCA), Gorlin's syndrome (basal cell carcinoma), dysplastic nevus syndrome (melanoma), Bowen's disease (SCCA).
29. Basal cell carcinoma is the number one nonmelanoma skin cancer. The second most common is squamous cell carcinoma, with a 30% rate of metastasis.
30. Indications for Mohs surgery:
    a. Recurrent disease
    b. Morpheaform carcinoma
    c. Lesion approaches embryonic fusion planes
    d. Long-standing lesion
    e. Poorly differentiated squamous cell carcinoma (SCCA)
    f. Need to preserve soft tissue—ie, eyelid
31. Lymphoscintigraphy (technetium 99m) identifies anatomil lymph nodes at risk but not whether tumor is within those nodal groups. This allows planning of selective lymph node dissection.
32. Mucosal melanoma is very rare (2%) and carries a 5-year survival rate of 10% and recurrence rate of 50%. The major failure is local recurrence, not regional lymph node metastases. ELND is *not* beneficial.
33. The corneal apex is 15 to 18 mm anterior to the lateral orbital rim. Anything greater than 21 mm or a 2-mm difference between each eye is significant.
34. Causes of adult and pediatric unilateral proptosis in decreasing order of occurrence
    a. Adult: Graves' orbitopathy>> infection> pseudotumors> paranasal tumor> hemangioma> lacrimal gland tumor> lymphoma/leukemia> metastasis> neurofibroma/meningioma> dermoid/epidermoid.
    b. Pediatric: Infection>> pseudomotor> dermoid> hemangioma/lymphangioma> rhabdomyosarcoma> leukemia> neurofibroma> optic nerve glioma> metastasis> paranasal tumor
35. Rhabdomyosarcoma is the most common orbital malignancy in children.
36. Metastatic disease is most likely from lung>> breast> systemic lymphoma> kidney
37. *Pattern of orbitopathy*
    a. Mild cases
       (1) First 6 to 12 months—congestion and inflammation
       (2) Next 1 to 2 years—resolution
    b. Moderate to severe
    c. Chronic stage—mucopolysaccharide deposition and fibrosis.
38. *Indications for surgical decompression*
    a. Compression-induced optic neuropathy or glaucoma
    b. Exposure keratitis unresponsive to ophthalmic lubricants
    c. Cosmesis
39. *Treatment of orbitopathy*
    a. Prednisone 80 to 100 mg every day for 3 to 4 weeks followed by a slow taper until signs regress.
    b. External beam therapy: 20 Gy over 2 weeks (if failed prednisone)

40. There is a 5 to 10% chance of malignant transformation (SCCA) in inverting papilloma.
41. Approaches for surgical resection of inverting papilloma
    a. Transnasal/transantral: Only 5% can be approached this way and no involvement of ethmoid.
       (1) Cells should be present
    b. Degloving approach: Inferior turbinate or maxillary sinus with minimal involvement of the inferior ethmoid cells.
       (1) Cannot be performed if within the ethmoid labyrinth.
    c. Lateral rhinotomy and medial maxillectomy: "gold standard."
42. Wegener's granulomatosis histology composed of angiocentric, epithelial-type *necrotizing granulomas* with the presence of giant cells and histiocytes.
43. Head and neck involvement occurs in 45%.
    a. 10% subglottic and upper tracheal involvement
    b. 20% conductive/sensorineural hearing loss or both
44. The stain of choice in fungal sinusitis is Gomori-methanamine.
45. Significant points regarding choanal atresia:
    a. 1/8000 live births
    b. Females>males
    c. 50% of patients have associated anomalies
    d. 90% membranous/10% bony
    e. Two-thirds unilateral and one-third bilateral
    f. Failure of the nasobuccal membrane to rupture
    g. Failure to pass a #5 or #6 Fr catheter at least 3 cm into the nasal cavity
    h. CT scan to verify
46. *Velopharyngeal dysfunction*
    a. Intelligibility of speech is affected more by articulation rather than resonance.
    b. The hypernasal child nasalizes nonnasal phonemes/d/,/b/,t/.
    c. Diagnosis:
       (1) Endoscopic evaluation of Passavant's ridge
       (2) Videofluoroscopy
    d. Treatment:
       (1) Speech therapy directed toward articulation and increasing resonance
       (2) Maximize before any surgery attempted
    e. Prosthetics:
       (1) Indicated in children whose gap is large because of little to no motion of the velopharyngeal sphincter
    f. Obturator
    g. Palatal lift: Not indicated in a child with a short palate
    h. Surgery:
       (1) Pharyngeal flap
           Success depends on lateral wall motion, since the lateral walls must approximate flap for proper speech.
       (2) Posterior wall augmentation
           Increase anteroposterior (AP) projection of the posterior pharyngeal wall to contact velum. Injectables—ie, Gelfoam, Teflon, collagen.
       (3) Sphincter pharyngoplasty

Web created to build up both the lateral and posterior walls; therefore, closure can be obtained without lateral wall motion. *Must possess velar motion.*

47. Cleft lip (CL) and cleft palate (CP)
   a. Syndromic versus nonsyndromic—multifactorial inheritance etiology
   b. Consider syndromic until proven otherwise
   c. *Risk factors for CL/CP*
      (1) Single gene transmission
      (2) Chromosome aberrations (trisomy D+E)
      (3) Teratogens: alcohol, thalidomide, vitamin A
      (4) Environmental: Amniotic band syndrome, maternal diabetes
   d. *Sequelae from unrepaired CL/CP*
      (1) Collapse of alveolar ridge
      (2) Midface retrusion
      (3) Malocclusion
   e. When to repair CL (rule of 10s): 10 to 14 weeks, 10 lb, hemoglobin 10
   f. When to repair CP: At 10 to 18 months of age
   g. Cleft palate flaps are based on the descending palatine, which is located in the greater palatine foramen.
48. Surgery for obstructive sleep apnea (OSA) versus snoring
   a. 50% of patients have associated hypertension
   b. Prognosis: 50% success for OSA, 80% success for snoring
   c. Risk factors for potential airway problems:
      (1) Apnea index of >70
      (2) Oxygen saturation of <80%
      (3) Difficult airway—thick neck, mesomorph habitus, retrognathic/microgenic
      (4) *Important pearl:* When excising any portion of the soft palate, one must remember that the middle one-third of the palate is the most important from a functional standpoint. Therefore, remove more laterally rather than centrally.
49. *Recurrent respiratory papillomatous pearls (RRPs):*
   a. Always avoid tracheotomy in the face of RRP because of the risk of stomal involvement
   b. The papilloma virus resides in the superficial epithelial layer
   c. Associated with human papillomavirus 6 and 11
   d. Viral capsid antigen resides in the outer layer of diseased epithelium, therefore, must remove *all* exophytic lesions
   e. Two occult sites for RRP to reside:
      (1) Nasopharynx-nasopharyngeal surface of the soft palate
      (2) Undersurface of the true vocal folds
   f. Treatments:
      (1) Direct laryngoscopy with stripping and/or CO_2 laser ablation
      (2) Alpha interferon
      (3) *Pearl:* Avoid jet ventilation, since this can potentially seed lower respiratory airways
50. Contact ulcer versus granuloma of the larynx (1 : 5)

    a. Acute ulcer
- (1) Dysphonia/aphonia
- (2) Pain
- (3) Odynophagia/dysphagia
- (4) Large, inflamed, raggy lesion

    b. Chronic ulcer
- (1) Vocal fatigue
- (2) Referred otalgia/odynophonia
- (3) Odynophagia/dysphagia
- (4) Single with uniform appearance

    c. Granuloma
- (1) Dysphonia/vocal fatigue
- (2) No pain
- (3) Globus larynges
- (4) Smooth, shiny, white/gray lesion

HEAD AND NECK

1. Hyperfractionated radiation techniques permit a higher cumulative dose per treatment.
2. Skin malignancies in the areas surrounding the tragus and pretragus can often spread to the stylomastoid foramen.
3. Postoperative compared to preoperative radiation in head and neck squamous carcinoma improves locoregional control, although overall survival is unchanged.
4. Postlaryngectomy patients have a high likelihood of recurrence when a Delphian node is involved.
5. The preauricular area has the highest rate of recurrence following Mohs surgery for basal cell carcinoma of the face.
6. Rigid fixation is preferred over wire fixation for mandibular osteotomies because the former is associated with a lower rate of nonunion with infection.
7. Retinoids appear to reduce the likelihood of developing second primaries in patients with head and neck squamous carcinomas.
8. Human papillomavirus 16 is associated with head and neck squamous carcinoma.

FOREIGN BODY OF THE AERODIGESTIVE TRACT

1. Children <6 years of age do not possess molars to grind nuts and raw vegetables.
2. Clinical signs and symptoms

    a. Tracheal/bronchial
- (1) Stridor/wheezing
- (2) Cough without associated illness
- (3) Recurrent or migratory pneumonia
- (4) Acute aphonia

    b. Esophageal
- (1) Odynophagia
- (2) Drooling
- (3) Vomiting/spitting
- (4) Airway compromise due to impingement of posterior trachea

3. Radiograph
   a. Chest x-ray
      (1) Visualize foreign body
      (2) Evaluate for atelectasis on side affected
      (3) Overinflation due to air trapping
   b. Lateral decubitus
      (1) Evaluates for mediastinal shift
      (2) Uninvolved side down results in shift of mediastinum down secondary to gravity
      (3) Involved side down results in no shift due to air trapping
4. Anesthesia
   a. Deep inhalational
      (1) Allows patient to spontaneously ventilate
   b. Neuromuscular paralysis
      (1) Must determine whether patient can ventilate if paralyzed
      (2) This will prevent laryngospasm (also consider topical lidocaine on vocal cords)
      (3) Prevents patient movement during retrieval
5. Five levels at which a foreign body is likely to lodge in the esophagus:
   a. Cricopharyngeus muscle
   b. Thoracic inlet
   c. Level of aortic arch
   d. Tracheal bifurcation
   e. Gastroesophageal junction
6. Ingestion of disc battery
   a. Contains lithium, NaOH, KOH, +/− mercury.
   b. 1 hour—mucosal damage.
   c. 2 to 4 hours—damage to muscular layer.
   d. 8 to 12 hours—potential perforation.
   e. If battery passed into stomach, demonstrated by x-ray.
   f. Send home and monitor stool for battery.
   g. Repeat x-ray if not passed in 4 to 7 days.
   h. With larger batteries (23 mm), repeat x-ray in 48 hours following observation of battery in stomach.
   i. If still in stomach, remove endoscopically.

LASERS

1. Visible
   a. Argon (514 nm)—vascular and pigmented lesions
   b. KTP (532 nm)
   c. Tunable yellow (577 nm)—cutaneous vascular lesions
   d. Tunable red (633 nm)—photodynamic therapy
   e. Nd:YAG (1060 nm)
2. Invisible
   a. CO_2 (10,600 nm)—numerous surgical applications including skin, ear, larynx, tracheobronchial

ANTIBIOTICS

1. Penicillins (beta-lactam family)
   a. Penicillin G and V: Effective against *Streptococcus pyogenes* (beta-hemolytic group A), *S. pneumoniae,* and actinomycosis; inactivated by penicillinase.
   b. Penicillinase resistant: Methicillin, oxacillin, cloxacillin, dicloxacillin, and nafcillin.
   c. Aminopenicillins: Ampicillin and amoxacillin; spectrum includes gram-negatives—*Escherichia coli, Proteus,* and *Haemophilus influenzae.*
   d. Augmented penicillins: Augmentin and Unasyn; spectrum includes *Staphylococcus, H. influenzae, M. catarrhalis,* and anaerobes. Ticarcillin with clavulanate (Timentin) effective against *Pseudomonas.*

2. Cephalosporins
   a. First generation: Cephalexin, cephradine, and cefadroxil; good against gram-positive organisms.
   b. Second generation: Cefuroxime; good gram-positive coverage and ampicillin-resistant *H. influenzae* and *M. catarrhalis.* Cefaclor, cefprozil, cefpodoxime, and loracarbef are others.
   c. Third generation: Cefixime, ceftriaxone, ceftazidime, cefotaxime, and cefoperazone; less gram-positive and anaerobe coverage; good CNS penetration.

3. Macrolides
   a. Erythromycin: Effective against streptococci, pneumococci, *Mycoplasma, Chlamydia, Legionella,* diphtheria, and pertussis; in combination with sulfa (Pediazole), effective against *H. influenzae.*
   b. Azithromycin and clarithromycin longer acting and effective for *H. influenzae.*
   c. Clindamycin: Highly effective against gram-positive organisms and anaerobes; high bone concentrations.

4. Tetracyclines: Effective against *Mycoplasma* and *Legionella.* Stains tooth-forming enamel; should not be used under age 10 years or in pregnancy. Photosensitivity.

5. Chloramphenicol: Broad spectrum against most gram-positive and negative organisms but not against *Pseudomonas.* Good CSF penetration. Bone marrow suppression 1:24,000.

6. Vancomycin: Good gram-positive coverage including methicillin-resistant *Staphylococcus.* Ototoxic intravenously; not ototoxic orally.

7. Metronidazole: Highly effective for anaerobes; second line for pseudomembranous colitis.

8. Aminoglycosides: Gentamicin, tobramycin, amikacin, and netilmicin; highly effective against *Pseudomonas.* Very ototoxic when given intravenously; questionable when used topically.

9. Quinolones: Ciprofloxacin and ofloxacin; active against *Pseudomonas, H. influenzae,* and *M. catarrhalis.*

DEFINITIONS

Acanthosis: Increased thickness of prickle cell layer.
Anaplasia: Change in a cell or tissue to a less highly differentiated form.

Atrophy: Diminution in the size of cells, organ, or tissue after a stage of full development.

Carcinoma in situ: Growth disturbance in which there is sufficient atypicality of the epithelial cells and their arrangement to warrant the diagnosis of cancer in the absence of invasion.

Choristoma: Similar to hamartoma except the component tissues are not normally present in that part of the body.

Desmoplasia: Connective tissue reaction to tumor.

Dyskeratosis: Production of keratin at lower layers.

Dysplasia: Change affecting the size, shape, and orientational relationship.

Ectopic: Normal-appearing tissue in abnormal location.

Hamartoma: Circumscribed overgrowth of tissues normally present in that part of the body.

Hyperkeratosis: Increased thickness of keratinized layers.

Hyperplasia: Increase in the number of cells per unit of tissue or organ of origin.

Hypertrophy: Increase in individual cell size.

Keratoacanthosis: Large acanthoma, surface keratosis.

Metaplasia: Change of one type of adult cell or tissue to another.

Metastasis: Secondary discontinuous cancerous growths.

Neoplasm: Proliferation of cells and formation of a mass.

Parakeratosis: Migration of nucleated cells to the surface.

Pleomorphism: More than one form of a single cell type.

Repair: Cell proliferation to repair and restore toward normal structure and function.

Tumor: Any swelling from whatever cause.

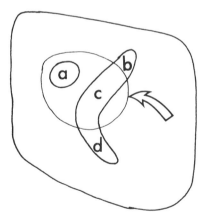

Figure 39–1. Left orbit. Arrow points to tendon of Zinn, which divides the orbital fissures into three compartments. Structures passing through (a) are the optic nerve and the ophthalmic artery. Structures passing through (b) are the trochlear nerve and the lacrimal and frontal divisions of V_1 as well as the supraorbital vein. Structures passing through (c) are the oculomotor and abducens nerves and the nasociliary division of V_1. Structures passing through (d) are the zygomaticofacial and zygomaticotemporal divisions of V_2 and the inferior ophthalmic vein.

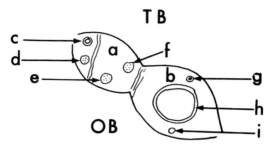

Figure 39–2. Right jugular foramen. (TB, temporal bone; OB, occipital bone; a, pars nervosa; b, pars vasculara; c, inferior petrosal sinus; d, glossopharyngeal nerve; e, vagus nerve; f, accessory nerve; g, posterior meningeal artery; h, internal jugular vein; i, nodes of Krause.)

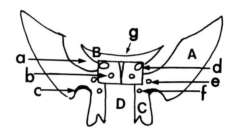

Figure 39–3. Sphenoid bone. [A, greater wing; B, lesser wing; C, pterygoid process; D, nasal cavity; a, foramen rotundum; b, pterygoid canal; c, jugum. *Note:* Pterygoid processes have medial and lateral plates (the lateral plate is the origin for both pterygoid muscles) and the hamulus (for tensor palati).]

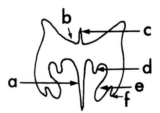

Figure 39–4. Ethmoid bone. (a, perpendicular plate; b, cribriform plate; c, crista galli, d, superior turbinate; e, middle turbinate; f, uncinate process.)

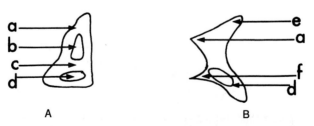

Figure 39–5. Right arytenoid. A. Anterior view. B. Lateral view. (a, colliculus; b, triangular pit; c, arcurate crest; d, oblong pit; e, corniculate; f, vocal process.)

1076

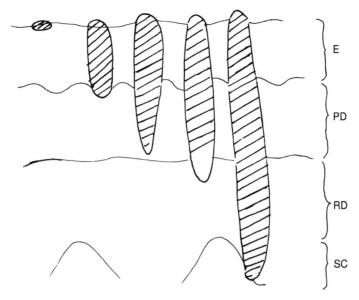

Figure 39–6. Clinicopathologic staging of melanoma. (E, epidermis; PD, papillary dermis; RD, reticular dermis; SC, subcutaneous tissue; BANS, back, upper arm, posterolateral neck, posterior scalp.)

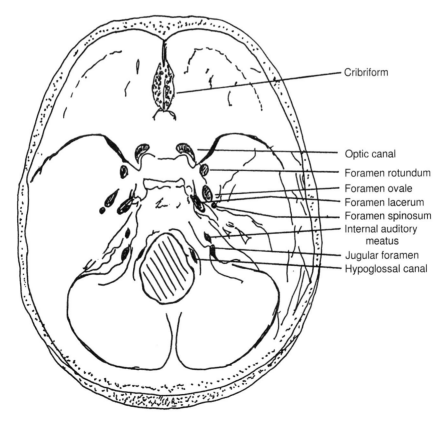

Figure 39–7. Base of skull, internal aspect.

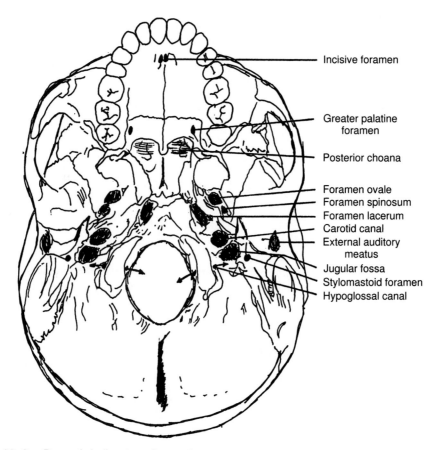

Figure 39–8. Base of skull, external aspect.

TABLE 39-1. AIRWAY OBSTRUCTION IN CHILDREN

Site	Voice	Stridor	Retractions	Mouth	Feeding	Cough
Nasal nasopharynx	Hyponasal	Sonorous inspiratory	Entire chest, especially when asleep	Open	Poor, choking and aspiration	Normal
Oropharynx	Muffled	Inspiratory coarse, snore	Entire chest	Open	Difficult, saliva pooling, aspiration	Normal
Supraglottis	Muffled	Inspiratory sonorous	None until late	Open, tripod	Impossible	Wet
Subglottis	Hoarse	Inspirations early, expirations late	Early; xiphoid and intercostal. Late; whole	Closed, alar flaring	Normal or dysphagia	Barking
Tracheobronchial	Normal	Expiratory wheezing to and from	Xiphoid and sternal prolonged, expiratory hyperinflation	Closed, alar flaring	Normal	Brassy

TABLE 39-2. LABORATORY VALUES IN COAGULATION DEFECTS

Factor Defect	Platelets	Bleeding Time	Partial Thromboplastin Time	Prothrombin Time	Thrombin Time
I	N	I or N	I	I	I
II	N	N	I	I	N
V	N	N	I	I	N
VII	N	N	N	I	N
VIII	N	N	I	N	N
IX	N	N	I	N	N
X	N	N	I	I	N
XI	N	N	I	N	N
XII	N	N	I	N	N
XIII	N	N	I	N	N
Von Willebrand	N[a]	I	I	N	N

[a]Poor platelet adhesiveness.

N, normal; I, increased.

TABLE 39-3. CONGENITAL NASAL MASSES

Parameter	Dermoid	Glioma	Encephalocele
Contents	Ecto/mesoderm: hair follicles, sweat + sebaceous glands	Neural tissue	Neural tissue/CSF
Location	Anywhere nasal dorsum to cribriform. Usually lower one-third of nose going beneath nasal bones	60% external; 30% internal; 10% combined. At or lateral to nasal root if external. Internal at lateral nasal wall	Nasofrontal, nasoethmoid, naso-orbital, or skull base
Morphology	Cyst, dermal sinus, or dural connection	15–20% with dural stalk	Soft, bluish, compressible
Diagnosis (+)	CT ± MR. Furstenburg (−)	CT ± MR. Furstenburg (−)	CT and MRI. Furstenburg
Treatment	External excision; neuro-surgical assistance	External excision unless dural connection	Intracranial then extracra-nial excision

TABLE 39-4. SYNDROMES OR DISEASES WITH ORAL LESIONS

Syndrome, Lesion, or Disease	Etiology
Koplik spots	Measles virus
Herpangina	Enteroviruses
Herpetic stomatitis	Herpes simplex virus
Aphthous stomatitis	Unknown
Pharyngoconjunctival fever	Adenoviruses
Vincent's stomatitis (trench mouth)	Anaerobic mouth bacteria
Thrush	*Candida* species

TABLE 39-5. ETIOLOGIC AGENTS IN THE COMMON COLD[a]

Agent	Prevalence[b]
Viruses	
Rhinoviruses	++++
Coronaviruses	++
Parainfluenza viruses	++
Respiratory syncytial virus	++
Adenoviruses	+
Enteroviruses	+
Influenza viruses	+
Reovirus	+
Other	
M. pneumoniae	+

[a] An acute, communicable, usually viral disease characterized by nasal stuffiness, sneezing, coryza, throat irritation (without pharyngitis), and no or minimal fever.
[b] ++++, most common; ++, common; +, rare as causative agent.

TABLE 39-6. ETIOLOGIC AGENTS IN ACUTE OTITIS MEDIA

Agent[a]	Prevalence[b]
Bacteria	
S. pneumoniae	++++
H. influenzae[c]	+++
B. catarrhalis[d]	+
Group A streptococci	+
Other: enteric bacteria, *S. aureus,*	
S. epidermidis, P. aeruginosa,	+
M. pneumoniae	+

[a] Otitis media is common in respiratory viral infections (adenoviruses, influenza viruses, parainfluenza viruses, rhinoviruses, coronaviruses, and respiratory syncytial virus), but in most instances middle ear disease is caused by secondary or concomitant bacterial infection.
[b] ++++, most common; +++, very common; +, rare as causative agent.
[c] Less common cause in children more than 10 years old.
[d] Predominantly noted in young children.

TABLE 39-7. ETIOLOGIC AGENTS IN SINUSITIS[a]

Infection	Aerobes		Anaerobes
Acute sinusitis	*S. pneumoniae*	*S. pyogenes*	*Peptostreptococcus*
	H. influenzae		*Fusobacterium*
	M. catarrhalis		*Bacteroides*
Chronic sinusitis	*S. aureus*		*Prevotella*
	S. pneumoniae		*Porphyromonas*
	H. influenzae		*Fusobacterium*
Nosocomial	Standard acute pathogens		
	K. pneumoniae	*P. mirabilis*	
	P. aeruginosa	*E. coli*	
	Enterobacter		

[a] Pediatric bacteriology is as above. Fifty to 88% of chronic sinusitis cultures grow anaerobes. Middle meatal cultures are useful, while nasal cultures are inaccurate.

TABLE 39-8. ETIOLOGIC AGENTS IN ORBITAL AND PERIORBITAL CELLULITIS

Agent	Prevalence[a]
H. influenzae	++++
S. aureus	+++
Group A streptococci	++
S. pneumoniae	++
Bacteroides species	+
Peptostreptococci	+
Veillonella	+

[a]++++, most common; +++, very common; ++, common; +, rare as causative agent.

TABLE 39-9. ETIOLOGIC AGENTS IN CHILDREN WITH CERVICAL ADENITIS AS THE PRIMARY FINDING

Agent	Prevalence[a]
Bacteria	
S. aureus	++++
Group A streptococci	++++
S. epidermidis	++
Atypical mycobacteria	++
M. tuberculosis	+
Gram-negative enterics	+
A. israelii	+
H. influenzae	+
Anaerobes of mouth flora	+
C. diphtheriae	+
F. tularensis	+
Other	
Cat-scratch disease agent	+
Herpes simplex virus	+
Fungi	+
T. gondii	+

[a]++++, most common; ++, common; +, rare as causative agent.

TABLE 39-10. ETIOLOGIC AGENTS IN LARYNGOTRACHEITIS

Agent	Prevalence[a]
Viruses	
Parainfluenza virus type 1[b]	++++
Parainfluenza virus type 2[b]	++
Parainfluenza virus type 3	++
Influenza virus A[b]	+++
Influenza virus B[b]	+
Other: respiratory syncytial virus, adenoviruses, rhinoviruses, enteroviruses, herpes simplex	+
M. pneumoniae	+
C. diphtheriae	+

[a]++++, most common; +++, very common; ++, common; +, rare as causative agent.
[b]Associated with outbreaks of croup.

TABLE 39-11. JUGULAR FORAMEN SYNDROMES

Syndrome	Nerve IX Taste	Nerve X Vocal Cord	Nerve X Palate	Nerve XI Shoulder	Nerve XII Tongue
Collect–Sicard	+	+	+	+	+
Hughlings–Jackson		+	+	+	+
Vernet	+	+	+	+	
Schmidt		+	+	+	
Avellis		+	+		
Tapia		+			+
Villaret	+	+	+		+

ANATOMY

1. Branches of the external carotid artery
    A. Superior thyroid artery (*Note:* 85% of superior thyroid arteries arise from the external carotid and 15% arise directly from the common carotid)
        (1) Infrahyoid artery
        (2) Superior laryngeal artery
        (3) Sternomastoid artery
        (4) Cricothyroid artery
    B. Lingual artery
        (1) Suprahyoid artery
        (2) Dorsalis linguae artery
        (3) Sublingual artery
    C. Facial artery
        (1) Cervical branches
            (a) Ascending palatine artery
            (b) Tonsillar artery
            (c) Submaxillary artery
            (d) Submental artery
            (e) Muscular branches
        (2) Facial branches
            (a) Muscular branches
            (b) Inferior labial artery
            (c) Inferior coronary artey
            (d) Superior coronary artery
            (e) Lateral nasal artery
            (f) Angular artery
    D. Occipital artery
        (1) Muscular branches
        (2) Sternomastoid artery
        (3) Auricular artery
        (4) Meningeal branches

E.   Posterior auricular artery
    (1)   Stylomastoid branch posterior tympanic artery
    (2)   Auricular branch
    (3)   Mastoid branch
F.   Ascending pharyngeal artery
    (1)   Prevertebral branches
    (2)   Pharyngeal branches
    (3)   Inferior tympanic branch
G.   Superficial temporal artery
    (1)   Transverse facial artery
    (2)   Middle temporal artery
    (3)   Anterior auricular branches
H.   Internal maxillary artery
    (1)   Maxillary portion
        (a)   Anterior tympanic branch
        (b)   Deep auricular branch
        (c)   Middle meningeal artery
        (d)   Accessory meningeal artery
        (e)   Inferior dental artery
    (2)   Pterygoid portion
        (a)   Deep temporal branch
        (b)   Pterygoid branch
        (c)   Masseteric artery
        (d)   Buccal artery
    (3)   Sphenomaxillary portion
        (a)   Posterior superior alveolar artery
        (b)   Infraorbital artery
        (c)   Descending palatine artery
        (d)   Vidian artery
        (e)   Pterygopalatine artery
        (f)   Sphenopalatine artery
        (g)   Posterior nasal artery

2.   Blood supply to the tonsil
  A.   Facial artery
    (1)   Tonsillar artery
    (2)   Ascending palatine artery
  B.   Dorsal lingual branch of the lingual artery
  C.   Internal maxillary artery
    (1)   Descending palatine artery
    (2)   Greater palatine artery
  D.   Ascending pharyngeal artery

3.   Blood supply to the adenoids
  A.   Ascending palatine branch of facial artery
  B.   Ascending pharyngeal artery
  C.   Pharyngeal branch of internal maxillary artery
  D.   Ascending cervical branch of thyrocervical trunk

4. Ethmoid arteries
   A. Ethmoid arteries are branches of the ophthalmic artery and are found in the fron-toethmoid suture line. This suture line delineates level of the anterior cranial fossa floor.
   B. Anterior ethmoid artery is usually 24 mm behind the anterior lacrimal crest, the posterior is about 12 mm behind that, and the optic nerve about 6 mm behind that (24-12-6 rule).
5. Contents of skull foramina, fissures, canals, and sinuses
   A. Cavernous sinus
      (1) Internal carotid artery
      (2) Cranial nerve III
      (3) CN IV
      (4) CN V_1 and V_2
      (5) CN VI
   B. Superior orbital fissure
      (1) CN III
      (2) CN IV
      (3) CN V_1 branch
         (a) Frontal nerve
         (b) Lacrimal nerve
         (c) Nasociliary nerve
      (4) CN VI
      (5) Superior ophthalmic vein
      (6) Inferior ophthalmic vein branch
      (7) Middle meningeal artery (orbital branch)
   C. Inferior orbital fissure
      (1) CN V_2 branch
         (a) Zygomatic nerves
         (b) Sphenopalatine branch
   D. Optic canal
      (1) Optic nerve
      (2) Ophthalmic artery
      (3) Central retinal artery
   E. Carotid canal
      (1) Internal carotid artery
      (2) Carotid plexus of sympathetic nerves
      (3) Lymphatics
      (4) Emissary vein
   F. Jugular foramen (three compartments)
      (1) Anterior
         (a) Inferior petrosal sinus
      (2) Middle
         (a) CN IX
         (b) CN X
         (c) CN XI
      (3) Posterior

    (a) Internal jugular vein
    (b) Meningeal branches from the occipital and ascending pharyngeal arteries
    (c) Nodes of Krause
G. Foramen lacerum
    (1) Cartilage
    (2) Fibrous tissue
    (3) Internal carotid artery
    (4) Sympathetic nerve
H. Foramen ovale
    (1) CN V_3
    (2) Small meningeal artery
    (3) Small petrosal nerve
    (4) Emissary vein
I. Foramen rotundum
    (1) Maxillary division of V
J. Foramen spinosum
    (1) Middle meningeal artery and vein
    (2) Lymphatics
K. Hypoglossal canal
    (1) CN XII
    (2) Emissary vein
    (3) Lymphatics
L. Innominate canal
    (1) Lesser superficial petrosal nerve
M. Foramen magnum
    (1) Medulla
    (2) CN XI
    (3) Vertebral arteries
    (4) Anterior and posterior spinal arteries
6. Cranial nerve central connections
A. First nerve
    (1) Subcallosal portion of hippocampal gyrus, area of the uncus.
    (2) Each optic tract carries crossed and uncrossed fibers.
B. Second nerve. Afferent fibers only via the optic nerve chiasm tract, then via the lateral geniculate body, superior colliculus, and pretectal area. Secondary fibers from the lateral geniculate radiate to the visual cortex (area striata) in the occipital cortex, which corresponds with Brodmann's area 17. Secondary fibers from the pretectal area terminate in the nucleus of Edinger-Westphal.
C. Third nerve
    (1) Motor (somatic) nucleus—cell bodies for contralateral innervation of levator palpebrae and all extraocular muscles except superior oblique and lateral rectus.
    (2) Autonomic nucleus (2 parts)
        (a) Lateral nucleus of Edinger-Westphal contains preganglionic parasympathetic fibers to the ciliary muscles (96%) and the sphincter pupillae (4%).

        (b)   Medial nucleus—small motor cells for fine-tuning motor movements (variable third central nucleus of Perlia supplying additional neurons to the superior rectus muscle).

D.   Fourth nerve. Trochlear arises from the motor (somatic) nucleus and carries ipsilateral fibers to the superior oblique muscle.

E.   Fifth nerve. Largest cranial nerve.
    (1)   General somatic sensory for pain, thermal, and tactile sense from skin of face and forehead, mucous membranes of nose and mouth, the teeth, and large portions of the dura; all three peripheral branches (ophthalmic, maxillary, and mandibular) contribute fibers to the dura. Proprioceptive inputs from teeth, periodontal ligaments, hard palate, and temporomandibular joint. Stretch receptors of muscles of mastication.
    (2)   Special visceral efferents to muscles of mastication (temporalis, masseter, lateral, and medial pterygoid), mylohyoid, anterior digastric, tensor tympani, and tensor veli palatini.

F.   Sixth nerve: Abducens carries only somatic motor fibers for the lateral rectus muscle and has the longest intracranial course of the cranial nerves.

G.   Seventh nerve.
    (1)   Nervus intermedius
        (a)   Somatic sensory to the external auditory canal.
        (b)   Visceral afferent—sensation in the nose, palate, and pharynx.
        (c)   Special visceral afferent—taste from the anterior two-thirds of the tongue with cell bodies located in the geniculate ganglion; afferent fibers ascend via the tractus solitarius to synapse in the ganglion of the solitary tract.
        (d)   General visceral efferent—autonomic fibers that arise from the superior salivatory nucleus and travel via the nervus intermedius and chorda tympani to the submandibular and sublingual glands, and also via the greater superficial petrosal nerve to the pterygopalatine ganglion and then to the lacrimal gland and the minor salivary glands of the nasal cavity and palate.
    (2)   Motor fibers
        (a)   Special visceral efferent fibers from the motor nucleus of VII to the stapedius, posterior belly of digastric, and muscles of facial expression; the lower face receives only crossed fibers, whereas the upper face receives both crossed and uncrossed fibers.

H.   Eighth nerve
    (1)   Spiral ganglion fibers ascend to the dorsal and ventral cochlear nuclei then via the inferior cerebellar peduncle to the ipsilateral superior olivary nucleus, or may cross via the reticular formation and the trapezoid body to the opposite olivary nucleus. Both crossed and uncrossed fibers ascend via the lateral lemniscus to the nucleus of the same name, the inferior colliculus or the medial geniculate body. All fibers ascend to terminate in the cortex of the superior temporal gyrus.
    (2)   Vestibular afferent fibers may ascend to the vestibular nuclei or descend via the medial longitudinal fasciculus to the vestibulospinal tract. The

medial vestibular nucleus has multiple connections to the reticular formation, motor nuclei of the cranial nerves, and autonomic nuclei. The superior nucleus sends ascending fibers to the cerebellum and the medial longitudinal fasciculus. The lateral nucleus forms the direct vestibulospinal tract, which is the chief antigravity mechanism in the CNS.

- I. Ninth nerve
  - (1) Special visceral afferents convey taste from the posterior one-third of the tongue to the inferior (petrosal) ganglion and then via the tractus solitarius to its nucleus.
  - (2) General visceral afferents convey sensation from the oral cavity, oropharynx, and hypopharynx, again via the tractus solitarius.
  - (3) Special visceral efferents from the inferior salivatory nucleus via Jacobson's nerve to the otic ganglion and thence to the parotid.

- J. Tenth nerve
  - (1) Somatic afferents via Arnold's nerve and meningeal branches to the superior (jugular) ganglion convey sensation from the external auditory canal and posterior auricle.
  - (2) Visceral afferents via the tractus solitarius to its nucleus for receptors of respiration, cardiac activity, gastric secretion, biliary function, and so forth.
  - (3) Special visceral afferents convey taste from the epiglottis and larynx via the inferior (nodose) ganglion and via the tractus solitarius to its nucleus.
  - (4) Special visceral efferents from the nucleus ambiguus to the striated muscles of the velum, pharynx, and larynx.
  - (5) General visceral efferents from the dorsal nucleus to the smooth muscle of the esophagus, stomach, small intestine, upper colon, gallbladder, pancreas, lungs, and inhibitory fibers to the heart.

- K. Eleventh nerve
  - (1) Cranial part—arises in the nucleus ambiguus and contains special and general visceral efferent fibers that join with the vagus and are distributed with it.
  - (2) Spinal part—arises from motor cells in the first five segments of the cervical spinal cord and travels upward via the foramen magnum, across the occipital bone to the jugular fossa, where it pierces the dura and turns caudad via the jugular foramen into the neck, to innervate the sternocleidomastoid and trapezius.

- L. Twelfth nerve. The hypoglossal nerve carries only somatic efferent motor fibers for the muscles of the tongue.

7. Ganglia
  - A. The ciliary ganglion is a parasympathetic ganglion and receives preganglionic fibers from the Edinger-Westphal nucleus. The synapses are within the ganglion. The postganglionic fibers go to the ciliary muscles and the sphincter pupillae muscle. It also receives the postganglionic sympathetic fibers en route to the vasculature of the globe. There is no sympathetic synapse within this ganglion. The nasociliary branch of cranial nerve V_1 carries sensation back to the CNS via the ganglion. There is no synapse for this sensory innervation within this ganglion.

    B.   The sphenopalatine ganglion is a parasympathetic ganglion. It receives its preganglionic parasympathetic fibers via the greater superficial petrosal nerve from the superior salivatory nucleus. The postganglionic fibers innervate the lacrimal gland via the zygomatic nerve. Sensory nerves of V_2 pass through it without synapses. The sympathetic postganglionic nerve also passes through it without synapse.

    C.   The submandibular ganglion has synapses for parasympathetic innervation. The preganglionic fibers are from the superior salivatory nucleus via the chorda tympani. The postganglionic parasympathetic fibers go to the submandibular gland. The sensory fibers are from nerve V_3, and the postganglionic sympathetic fibers from the facial artery pass through it without synapses. This ganglion also receives preganglionic parasympathetic fibers from the inferior salivatory nucleus via Jacobsen's nerve (branch of CN IX) and a small contribution from the superior salivatory nucleus via the lesser superficial petrosal nerve (branch of CN VII). The sensory branch of V_3 and the postganglionic sympathetics from the middle meningeal artery pass through this ganglion without synapses.

8.   Skull bones. The bones of the skull are of two types: those derived from endochondral ossification of cartilage and those that form from ossification of tissues without the intervening cartilaginous phase.

    A.   Endochondral bones (mnemonic: POEMS)

       (1) Petrous

       (2) Occipital

       (3) Ethmoid

       (4) Mastoid

       (5) Sphenoid

    B.   Membranous bones

       (1) Sphenoid

       (2) Parietal

       (3) Frontal

       (4) Lacrimal

       (5) Nasal

       (6) Maxillae

       (7) Mandible

       (8) Palate

       (9) Zygoma

      (10) Premaxilla

      (11) Tympanic ring

      (12) Squamosa

      (13) Vomer

      (14) Bony modiolus

9.   Orbit. Includes components of the maxillary, frontal, ethmoid, zygomatic, sphenoid, palatal, and lacrimal bones. The lacrimal gland rests in the zygomatic process of the frontal bone. The lacrimal sac in the fossa bounded by the lacrimal bone and the frontal process of the maxilla.

10.   Zygoma. Four processes: frontal, maxillary, temporal, and sphenoid.

11.   Maxilla. Four processes: frontal, zygomatic, palatine, and alveolar.

12.   Mandible. May be partly endochondral formation of Meckel's cartilage. It is the only facial bone capable of pathologic fracture.

13. Pharyngeal constrictors
    A. Superior—spans from the median raphe and the pharyngeal tubercle of the occipital bone to the pterygomandibular ligament, mandible, and medial pterygoid plate.
    B. Middle—spans from the median raphe to the hyoid bone and the stylohyoid ligament.
    C. Inferior—spans from the median raphe to the oblique line of the thyroid cartilage, cricoid cartilage, and cricothyroid muscle.
14. Esophageal dehiscences
    A. Killian—between the cricopharyngeus and thyropharyngeus muscles (site of Zenker's diverticulum).
    B. Killian-Jamieson—between the cricopharyngeus and the circular fibers of the esophagus.
    C. Lamier-Hackman—between the circular and longitudinal fibers of the esophagus.
15. Soft palate
    A. Five muscular components
        (1) Palatopharyngeus from the pharynx to the soft palate.
        (2) Palatoglossus from the base of tongue to the soft palate.
        (3) Musculus uvulae from the posterior nasal spine to the soft palate.
        (4) Levator veli palatini originates from the petrous portion of the temporal bone, from the superior constrictor and the eustachian tube, to insert on the soft palate.
        (5) Tensor veli palatini arises from the sphenoid bone, medial pterygoid plate, and eustachian tube and inserts in the soft palate. It is the only muscle of the group innervated by the pharyngeal plexus.
16. Pterygomandibular raphe is between the buccinator muscle and the superior constrictor muscle.
17. Parapharyngeal space
    A. Boundaries
        (1) Superiorly—base of skull
        (2) Laterally—ramus of mandible, medial pterygoid muscle
        (3) Posterolaterally—parotid fascia
        (4) Medial—superior constrictor muscle, buccopharyngeal fascia
        (5) Anteriorly—pterygoid fascia, pterygomandibular raphe
        (6) Posteriorly—carotid sheath, vertebral fascia
        (7) Inferiorly—lesser cornu of the hyoid
    B. Three compartments
        (1) Prestyloid compartment
            (a) Internal maxillary artery
            (b) Inferior alveolar nerve
            (c) Lingual nerve
            (d) Auriculotemporal nerve
        (2) Retrostyloid compartment
            (a) Internal carotid artery
            (b) Internal jugular vein
            (c) Cranial nerves IX to XII
            (d) Cervical sympathetic chain

          (3) Retropharyngeal compartment
             (a) Lymphatics
             (b) Node of Rouvière

18. Soft tissue spaces of the head and neck
    A. Canine
    B. Buccal
    C. Submental
    D. Sublingual
    E. Submandibular
    F. Pterygomandibular
    G. Masseteric
    H. Temporal (F to H combined form the masticator space)
    I. Carotid
    J. Parotid
    K. Lateral pharyngeal
    L. Retropharyngeal (skull base to C_7–T_1)
    M. Prevertebral (skull base to diaphragm: also known as danger space 4)

(Note: Upper limits of normal prevertebral soft tissues on lateral neck film are 7 mm at C_2 and 20 mm at C_6.)

HISTOLOGY

    A. Ear
        (1) Middle ear—nonciliated cuboidal epithelium in general, although in the area near the eustachian tube orifice there is a transition to ciliated cuboidal.
        (2) Eustachian tube—pseudostratified, ciliated columnar epithelium with goblet cells.
        (3) Mastoid and epitympanum—pavement epithelium without cilia.
        (4) Endolymphatic duct and proximal portion of endolymphatic sac—columnar epithelium with villi.
        (5) Distal endolymphatic sac—smooth cuboidal epithelium.
    B. Nose
        (1) Lower two-thirds of septum and lateral wall inferior to superior turbinate is respiratory epithelium, which is pseudostratified ciliated columnar epithelium with irregular basal cells and goblet cell (also called Schneiderian epithelium).
        (2) Upper one-third of septum and lateral wall superior to superior turbinate and roof of nose is pseudostratified nonciliated, columnar epithelium with serous glands of Bowman.
        (3) Olfactory membrane is composed of bipolar cells of olfaction as well as supporting and basal cells.
        (4) Vestibule is lined with stratified squamous epithelium with some sebaceous glands.
    C. Nasopharynx
        (1) Upper one-half ciliated columnar epithelium.
        (2) Lower one-half nonkeratinizing squamous epithelium.
    D. Paranasal sinuses and nasolacrimal duct has pseudostratified ciliated columnar epithelium.

E. Junction between nasopharynx and oropharynx transitional zone.
F. Oropharynx and hypopharynx stratified squamous epithelium.
G. Palatine tonsils—stratified squamous epithelium.
H. Adenoid—ciliated columnar epithelium.
I. Lingual tonsil—stratified squamous epithelium.
J. Larynx
    (1) True cord, false cord, and upper two-thirds of epiglottis, aryepiglottic folds: pseudostratified nonkeratinizing stratified squamous epithelium.
    (2) All other structures are pseudostratified ciliated columnar epithelium.
    (3) Mucous glands are present in the ventricle, saccule, laryngeal surface of the epiglottis, and margin of the aryepiglottic fold.
K. Trachea and bronchi—pseudostratified ciliated columnar epithelium with goblet cells.
L. Esophagus
    (1) Upper two-thirds—stratified squamous epithelium with inner circular muscular layer and outer longitudinal muscular layer.
    (2) Lower one-third—villous columnar epithelium with same muscular layers.

MISCELLANEOUS HISTOLOGIC TERMS

Charcot-Leyden crystals: Crystal-like material seen in eosinophilic infitrate of allergic fungal sinusitis.

Homber-Wright rosettes: Pseudorosette pattern seen in grade I esthesioneuroblastoma.

Flexner-Wintersteiner rosettes: True neural rosettes of grade III and IV esthesioneuroblastoma.

Warthin-Starry stain: Used to identify cat-scratch bacillus.

Paraganglioma tumors: Composed of cell nests, or "zellballen," surrounded by sustentacular cells.

Psyalliferous cells: "Soap bubble" cells of chordomas.

Congo-red stain: Used for amyloid to show apple-green birefringence.

Church-spire keratosis: Peaked surface keratinization of verrucous carcinoma. Also shows broad rete pegs with pushing margins.

Bibliography

Anderson GJ, Tom LWC, Womer RB, et al. Rhabdomyosarcoma of the head and neck in children. *Arch Otolaryngol Head Neck Surg.* 1990;116: 428–431.

Black FO, Presznecker S, Norton T, et al. Surgical management of perilymph fistulas. *Arch Otolaryngol Head Neck Surg.* 1991;117:641–648.

Brookhouser PE, Auslander MC. Aided auditory thresholds in children with postmeningitic deafness. *Laryngoscope.* 1989;99:800–808.

Campbell SM, Montanaro A, Bardana EJ. Head and neck manifestations of autoimmune disease. *Am J Otolaryngol.* 1983;4(3):187–215.

Cramer HB, Kartush JM. Testing facial nerve function. *Otolaryngol Clin North Am.* 1991;24(3): 555–571.

DiNardo LJ, Wetmore RF. Head and neck manifestations of histiocytosis-X in children. *Laryngoscope.* 1989;99:721–724.

Donowitz GR, Mandell GL. Beta-lactim antibiotics (Pt. 2). *N Engl J Med.* 1988;318(8):490.

Enjolis O, Riche MC, Merland JJ, et al. Management of alarming hemangiomas in infancy: A review of 25 cases. *Pediatrics.* 1990;85:491–498.

Ferguson BJ, Allen NB, Farmer JC Jr. Giant cell arteritis and polymyalgia rheumatica: Review for the otolaryngologist. *Ann Otol Rhinol Laryngol.* 1987;96:373–379.

Fulp SR, Castell DO. Scleroderma esophagus. *Dysphagia.* 1990;5:204–210.

Furuta Y, Shinohara T, Sano K, et al. Molecular pathologic study of human papillomavirus infection in inverted papilloma and squamous cell carcinoma of the nasal cavities and paranasal sinuses. *Laryngoscope.* 1991;101:79–85.

Gates GA, Avery CA, Prihoda TJ. Effect of adenoidectomy upon children with chronic otitis media with effusion. *Laryngoscope.* 1988;98: 58–63.

Gaulard P, Henni T, Marolleau JP, et al. Lethal midline granuloma (polymorphic reticulosis) and lymphomatoid granulomatosis. *Cancer.* 1988;62: 705–710.

Gianoli GJ, Miller RH, Guarisco JL. Tracheotomy in the first year of life. *Ann Otol Rhinol Laryngol.* 1990;99:896.

Grundfast K, Harley E. Vocal cord paralysis. *Otolaryngol Clin North Am.* 1989;22(3):569–597.

Healy GB. Management of tracheobronchial foreign bodies in children: An update. *Ann Otol Rhinol Laryngol.* 1990;99:889–891.

Hellman D, Laing T, Petri M, et al. Wegener's granulomatosis: Isolated involvement of the trachea and larynx. *Ann Rheum Dis.* 1987;46:628–631.

Hong WK, Lippman SM, Itri LM, et al. Prevention of second primary tumors with isoretinoin in squamous-cell carcinoma of the head and neck. *N Engl J Med.* 1990;9:795–801.

Horak FB, Jones-Rycewicz C, Black FO, et al. Effects of vestibular rehabilitation on dizziness and imbalance. *Otolaryngol Head Neck Surg.* 1992;106:175–180.

Horiot JC, Le Fur R, N'Guyen T, et al. Hyperfractionated compared with conventional radiotherapy in oropharyngeal carcinoma: An EORTC randomized trial. *Eur J Cancer.* 1990;26(7): 779–780.

Hughes GB, Barna BP, Kinney SE, et al. Clinical diagnosis of immune inner-ear disease. *Laryngoscope.* 1988;98:251–253.

Jahrsdoerfer RA, Thompson EG, Johns ME, et al. Sarcoidosis and fluctuating hearing loss. *Ann Otol.* 1981;90:161–163.

Kemink JL, Telian SA, El-Kashlan H, et al. Retrolabyrinthine vestibular nerve section: Efficacy in disorders other than Meniere's disease. *Laryngoscope.* 1991;101:523–528.

Krespi YP, Mitrani M, Husain S, et al. Treatment of laryngeal sarcoidosis with intralesional steroid injection. *Ann Otol Rhinol Laryngol.* 1987;96: 713–715.

Lonsbury-Martin BL, Whitehead ML, Martin GK. Clinical applications of otoacoustic emissions. *J Speech Hear Res.* 1991;34:964–981.

Lusk R. Endoscopic sinus surgery in children with chronic sinusitis: A pilot study. *Laryngoscope.* 1990;100:654.

Mandel EM, Rockette HE, Bluestone CD, et al. Myringotomy with and without tympanostomy tubes for chronic otitis media with effusion. *Arch Otolaryngol Head Neck Surg.* 1989;115: 1217–1224.

Maniglia AJ, Kline SN. Maxillofacial trauma in the pediatric age group. *Otolaryngol Clin North Am.* 1983;16(3):717–730.

Mattox DE, Lyles CA. Idiopathic sudden sensorineural hearing loss. *Am J Otol.* 1989;10:242–247.

Morgan D. Current management of choanal atresia. *Int J Pediatr Otorhinolaryngol.* 1990;19:1–4.

Mott AE, Leopold DA. Disorders in taste and smell. *Med Clin North Am.* 1991;75(6):1321–1353.

Muntz H. Nasal antral windows in children: A retrospective study. *Laryngoscope.* 1990;100:643.

Murty GE. Wegener's granulomatosis: Otorhinolaryngological manifestations. *Clin Otolaryngol.* 1990;15:385–393.

Narcy P, Contencin P, Fligny I, et al. Surgical treatment for laryngotracheal stenosis in the pediatric patient. *Arch Otolaryngol Head Neck Surg.* 1990; 116:1047–1050.

Niparko JK, Swanson NA, Baker SR, et al. Local control of auricular, periauricular, and external canal cutaneous malignancies with Mohs surgery. *Laryngoscope.* 1990;100:1047–1051.

Peckham CS, Stark O, Dudgeon JA, et al. Congenital cytomegalovirus infection: A cause of sensorineural hearing loss. *Arch Dis Child.* 1987;62: 1233–1237.

Poole MD, Postma DS. Characterization of cough associated with angiotensin-converting enzyme inhibitors. *Otolaryngol Head Neck Surg.* 1991; 105(5):714–715.

Quiney RE, Mitchell DB, Djazeri B, et al. Recurrent meningitis in children due to inner ear anomalies. *J Laryngol Otol.* 1989;103:473–480.

Schwaber MK, Larson TC, Zealear DL, et al. Gadolinium-enhanced magnetic resonance imaging in Bell's palsy. *Laryngoscope.* 1990;100: 1264–1269.

Shindo ML, Hanson DG. Geriatric voice and laryngeal dysfunction. *Otolaryngol Clin North Am.* 1990;23(6):1035–1044.

Singer PA. Thyroiditis: Acute, subacute, and chronic. *Med Clin North Am.* 1991;75(1):61–77.

Specks U, DeRemee RA. Granulomatous vasculitis: Wegener's granulomatosis and Churg–Strauss syndrome. *Rheum Dis Clin North Am.* 1990;16:377–396.

Steere AC. Lyme disease. *N Engl J Med.* 1989; 321:586–596.

Sullivan PK, Fabian RF, Driscoll D. Mandibular osteotomies for tumor extirpation: The advantage of rigid fixation. *Laryngoscope.* 1992;102:73–80.

Teixido M, Kron TK, Plains EM. Head and neck sequelae of cardiac transplantation. *Laryngoscope.* 1990;100:231–236.

Thedinger BA, Nadol JB, Montgomery WW, et al. Radiographic diagnosis, surgical treatment, and long-term follow-up of cholesterol granuloma of the petrous apex. *Laryngoscope.* 1989;99:896–907.

Tupchong L, Scott CB, Blitzer PH, et al. Randomized study of preoperative versus postoperative radiation therapy in advanced head and neck carcinoma: Long-term follow-up of RTOG study 73-03. *Int J Radiat Oncol Biol Phys.* 1991;20:21–28.

Wackym PA, Abdul-Rasool IH. Prospective management of malignant hyperthermia in the otolaryngological patient. *J Laryngol Otol.* 1988;102:513–516.

Zalzal GH, Anon JB, Cotton RT. Epiglottoplasty for the treatment of laryngomalacia. *Ann Otol Rhinol Laryngol.* 1987;96:72.

Index

Note: Page numbers followed by f indicate figures; those followed by t indicate tables.